Handbook of Devel Psychopathology

Third Edition

MW00991525

Michael Lewis • Karen D. Rudolph

Editors

Handbook of Developmental Psychopathology

Third Edition

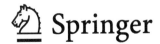 Springer

Editors
Michael Lewis
Institute for the Study
  of Child Development
Rutgers University
New Brunswick, NJ, USA

Karen D. Rudolph
Department of Psychology
University of Illinois
Urbana-Champaign
Champaign, IL, USA

ISBN 978-1-4614-9607-6 (hardcover)   ISBN 978-1-4614-9608-3 (eBook)
ISBN 978-1-4899-7672-7 (softcover)
DOI 10.1007/978-1-4614-9608-3
Springer New York Heidelberg Dordrecht London

Library of Congress Control Number: 2014931987

Printed on acid-free paper

Springer is part of Springer Science+Business Media (www.springer.com)

Preface

The *Handbook of Developmental Psychopathology* presents cutting-edge theory and research in the field of developmental psychopathology; as such, it is one of the primary resources for the field. It has been 10 years since the publication of the second edition of the *Handbook*. During this time, there has been a burgeoning of work in the field of developmental psychopathology. The dynamic nature of the field necessitates an updated volume that considers advancements in theory, research methodology, and empirical findings. The first edition of the *Handbook* sought to combine the fields of developmental science and psychopathology, arguing that the origins of psychopathology in adulthood could be found in childhood. A primary focus was placed on traditional psychiatric diagnostic schemes, drawn primarily from adult psychiatry, to parse the field of psychopathology into particular disorders. As the field grew, emphasis changed from a primary focus on diagnostic categories to a focus on developmental perspectives on the emergence and growth of psychopathology. This shift in emphasis required a more comprehensive volume that considered multiple perspectives on psychopathology as reflected in biological, psychological, and contextual frameworks. The second edition met this challenge by supplementing descriptions of the presentation, course, and etiology of particular disorders with chapters devoted to varying conceptual paradigms, such as biological, cognitive, social, and ecological perspectives. This edition underscored the idea that psychopathology cannot merely be viewed in terms of developing individual characteristics but also must be considered within the dynamic framework of shifts in children's developmental contexts across the life span.

Since the publication of the second edition, the field has continued to mature such that theory and research emphasize not only the importance of understanding varying levels of development but also the need for integrative multilevel models reflecting interactions and transactions among multiple vulnerabilities, risks, and protective factors that shape development trajectories of health and psychopathology. Perhaps one of the fastest growing areas of the field in recent years is the intersection of neuroscience and psychopathology. This rapid growth is reflected in recent research on molecular genetics and epigenetics, brain imaging, and the role of early experience in the development of biological systems. Cutting-edge developments in this area are reflected in two new chapters, with an eye toward considering how developing biological systems are influenced by, and influence, psychological and social processes underlying risk for psychopathology. Also reflecting this interface between biology and context, new chapters include a focus on the effect of early deprivation on cognitive, emotional, and biological systems and on the role of pubertal development in psychopathology. Another growing area in the field is a greater integration of theory and research on early temperament, personality, and psychopathology, as well as new work exploring early indicators of personality pathology during childhood and adolescence. A third area of rapid growth is the development of sophisticated statistical procedures for tracking change, allowing for a more nuanced understanding of continuity and change in psychopathology over time; these advances are reflected in a chapter on research methodology. Providing a balanced view of the field, this edition considers processes underlying resilience from psychopathology in high-risk youth, with an integration of contemporary theory and research on positive psychology. The sections on specific disorders are updated and expanded to include chapters on substance use and suicide. In sum, the third edition strives to retain the strengths of the earlier editions while integrating state-of-the-art theory and empirical research that reflect contemporary multidisciplinary perspectives on developmental psychopathology.

This edition is divided into nine Parts. The first concerns general issues and theories. The second focuses on environmental contexts, including family, schooling, peers, life stress, and culture. The third Part brings together cutting-edge work on individual-level processes involved in psychopathology, including genetics and neuroscience, the interactive role of early experience and biology, as well as temperament and pubertal development. The next three Parts focus on specific disorders, including early childhood disorders, disruptive behavior disorders (ADHD, aggression, conduct problems), and emotional disorders (depression, suicide, anxiety, and obsessions and compulsions). Control disorders are presented in the seventh Part. Part 8, Chronic Developmental Disorders, includes chapters on autism spectrum disorders, intellectual disability, gender dysphoria, and personality pathologies. Last, Part 9 covers Trauma Disorders, including maltreatment, posttraumatic stress, and dissociative disorders.

Finally, a word in regard to the new DSM manual. Although the first edition of the *Handbook* utilized the DSM classification system, the second edition of the *Handbook* moved more toward a developmental perspective. This emphasis has continued in this third edition. When necessary, the new and revised chapters have taken the new DSM manual into account. The commitment of the NIMH to move the field of psychopathology from symptom-based toward a more dynamic classification system mirrors our belief that a more research-oriented system of psychopathology is especially relevant to studying the development of psychopathology.

New Brunswick, NJ, USA   Michael Lewis
Champaign, IL, USA   Karen D. Rudolph

Contents

Part I   Issues and Theories

1   **Toward the Development of the Science
    of Developmental Psychopathology** 3
    Michael Lewis

2   **A Dialectic Integration of Development
    for the Study of Psychopathology** 25
    Arnold J. Sameroff

3   **Nature–Nurture Integration** 45
    Michael Rutter

4   **Developmental, Quantitative, and Multicultural
    Assessment of Psychopathology** 67
    Thomas M. Achenbach

5   **Developmental Epidemiology** 87
    Katie A. McLaughlin

6   **Modeling Strategies in Developmental Psychopathology
    Research: Prediction of Individual Change** 109
    Sonya K. Sterba

7   **Resilience and Positive Psychology** 125
    Suniya S. Luthar, Emily L. Lyman,
    and Elizabeth J. Crossman

Part II   Context and Psychopathology

8   **Family Context in the Development of Psychopathology** 143
    Patrick T. Davies and Melissa L. Sturge-Apple

9   **Schooling and the Mental Health of Children
    and Adolescents in the United States** 163
    Robert W. Roeser and Jacquelynne S. Eccles

10 **Peer Relationships and the Development
    of Psychopathology** 185
    Sophia Choukas-Bradley and Mitchell J. Prinstein

11   The Influence of Stressors on the Development
     of Psychopathology 205
     Kathryn E. Grant, Susan Dvorak McMahon,
     Jocelyn Smith Carter, Russell A. Carleton,
     Emma K. Adam, and Edith Chen

12   Culture and Developmental Psychopathology............................ 225
     Xinyin Chen, Rui Fu, and Lingli Leng

Part III   Neuroscience and Psychopathology

13   Developmental Behavioral Genetics.. 245
     Thomas G. O'Connor

14   Functional Magnetic Resonance Imaging in Developmental
     Psychopathology: The Brain as a Window into the
     Development and Treatment of Psychopathology...................... 265
     Johnna R. Swartz and Christopher S. Monk

15   The Contributions of Early Experience
     to Biological Development and Sensitivity to Context.............. 287
     Nicole R. Bush and W. Thomas Boyce

16   Temperament Concepts in Developmental Psychopathology.... 311
     John E. Bates, Alice C. Schermerhorn, and Isaac T. Petersen

17   Puberty as a Developmental Context
     of Risk for Psychopathology.. 331
     Karen D. Rudolph

Part IV   Early Childhood Disorders

18   Attachment Disorders: Theory, Research,
     and Treatment Considerations 357
     Howard Steele and Miriam Steele

19   Early Deprivation and Developmental Psychopathology.......... 371
     Elisa A. Esposito and Megan R. Gunnar

20   Prematurity and Failure to Thrive: The Interplay
     of Medical Conditions and Development................................... 389
     Stephanie Blenner, L. Kari Hironaka,
     Douglas L. Vanderbilt, and Deborah A. Frank

21   Sleep Interventions: A Developmental Perspective................... 409
     Eleanor L. McGlinchey and Allison G. Harvey

Part V   Disruptive Behavior Disorders

22   A Developmental Perspective
     on Attention-Deficit/Hyperactivity Disorder (ADHD) 427
     Susan B. Campbell, Jeffrey M. Halperin,
     and Edmund J.S. Sonuga-Barke

23   A Developmental Model of Aggression and Violence: Microsocial and Macrosocial Dynamics Within an Ecological Framework... 449
Thomas J. Dishion

24   Conduct Disorder.. 467
Karen L. Bierman and Tyler R. Sasser

Part VI   Emotional Disorders

25   Depression in Children and Adolescents 489
Judy Garber and Uma Rao

26   A Developmental Model of Self-Inflicted Injury, Borderline Personality, and Suicide Risk.................................. 521
Christina M. Derbidge and Theodore P. Beauchaine

27   The Developmental Psychopathology of Anxiety...................... 543
Michael W. Vasey, Guy Bosmans, and Thomas H. Ollendick

28   Obsessions and Compulsions: The Developmental and Familial Context................................. 561
Catherine K. Kraper, Timothy W. Soto, and Alice S. Carter

Part VII   Control Disorders

29   Alcoholism: A Life Span Perspective on Etiology and Course... 583
Brian M. Hicks and Robert A. Zucker

30   The Epidemiology and Etiology of Adolescent Substance Use in Developmental Perspective.. 601
John Schulenberg, Megan E. Patrick, Julie Maslowsky, and Jennifer L. Maggs

31   Developmental Trajectories of Disordered Eating: Genetic and Biological Risk During Puberty............................ 621
Kelly L. Klump

32   Enuresis and Encopresis: The Elimination Disorders.............. 631
Janet E. Fischel and Kate E. Wallis

Part VIII   Chronic Developmental Disorders

33   Autism Spectrum Disorder: Developmental Approaches from Infancy through Early Childhood..................................... 651
Helen Tager-Flusberg

34   Intellectual Disability... 665
Barbara Tylenda, Rowland P. Barrett, and Henry T. Sachs, III

35   Gender Dysphoria.. 683
Kenneth J. Zucker

36   Personality Pathology.. 703
Daniel N. Klein, Sara J. Bufferd, Margaret W. Dyson,
and Allison P. Danzig

Part IX   Trauma Disorders

**37   A Developmental Psychopathology Perspective
on Child Maltreatment**.. 723
Dante Cicchetti and Adrienne Banny

38   Posttraumatic Stress Disorder in Children and Adolescents.... 743
Stephanie M. Keller and Norah C. Feeny

39   Dissociative Disorders in Children and Adolescents 761
Joyanna L. Silberg

About the Editors... 777

Author Index 779

Subject Index... 829

Contributors

Thomas M. Achenbach, Ph.D. Departments of Psychiatry and Psychology, University of Vermont, Burlington, VT, USA

Emma K. Adam, Ph.D. School of Education and Social Policy, and Faculty Fellow, Cells to Society Center and The Institute for Policy Research, Northwestern University, Evanston, IL, USA

Adrienne Banny, M.A. Institute of Child Development, University of Minnesota, Minneapolis, MN, USA

Rowland P. Barrett, Ph.D. Alpert Medical School of Brown University, Providence, RI, USA

John E. Bates, Ph.D. Department of Psychological and Brain Sciences, Indiana University, Bloomington, IN, USA

Theodore P. Beauchaine, Ph.D. Department of Psychology, The Ohio State University, Columbus, OH, USA

Karen L. Bierman, Ph.D. Department of Psychology, The Pennsylvania State University, University Park, PA, USA

Stephanie Blenner, M.D. Boston University School of Medicine, Boston, MA, USA

Guy Bosmans, Ph.D. Parenting and Special Education Research Group, University of Leuven, Leuven, Belgium

W. Thomas Boyce, M.D. School of Population and Public Health, University of British Columbia, Vancouver, BC, Canada

Sara J. Bufferd, Ph.D. Department of Psychology, California State University San Marcos, San Marcos, CA, USA

Nicole R. Bush, Ph.D. Department of Psychiatry, University of California – San Francisco, San Francisco, CA, USA

Susan B. Campbell, Ph.D. Department of Psychology, University of Pittsburgh, Pittsburgh, PA, USA

Russell A. Carleton, Ph.D. Department of Psychology, DePaul University, Chicago, IL, USA

Alice S. Carter, Ph.D. Psychology Department, University of Massachusetts Boston, Boston, MA, USA

Jocelyn Smith Carter, Ph.D. Department of Psychology, DePaul University, Chicago, IL, USA

Edith Chen, Ph.D. Department of Psychology, and Faculty Fellow, Institute for Policy Research, Northwestern University, Evanston, IL, USA

Xinyin Chen, Ph.D. Graduate School of Education, University of Pennsylvania, Philadelphia, PA, USA

Sophia Choukas-Bradley, M.A. Department of Psychology, University of North Carolina at Chapel Hill, Chapel Hill, NC, USA

Dante Cicchetti, Ph.D. Institute of Child Development, University of Minnesota, Minneapolis, MN, USA
Mt. Hope Family Center, University of Rochester, Rochester, NY, USA

Elizabeth J. Crossman, M.A. Department of Human Development, Teachers College, Columbia University, New York, NY, USA

Allison P. Danzig, M.A. Department of Psychology, Stony Brook University, Stony Brook, NY, USA

Patrick T. Davies, Ph.D. Department of Clinical and Social Sciences in Psychology, University of Rochester, Rochester, NY, USA

Christina M. Derbidge, Ph.D. George E. Wahlen, Department of Veterans Affairs Medical Center, 500 Foothill Drive, Salt Lake City, UT, USA

Thomas J. Dishion, Ph.D. Department of Psychology and Prevention Research Center, Arizona State University, Tempe, AZ, USA

Margaret W. Dyson, Ph.D. Child and Adolescent Services Research Center, University of California – San Diego, La Jolla, CA, USA

Jacquelynne S. Eccles, Ph.D. School of Education, University of California, Irvine, CA, USA

Elisa A. Esposito, M.A. Institute of Child Development, University of Minnesota, Minneapolis, MN, USA

Norah C. Feeny, Ph.D. Department of Psychological Sciences, Case Western Reserve University, Cleveland, OH, USA

Janet E. Fischel, Ph.D. Department of Pediatrics, Stony Brook University and Stony Brook Long Island Children's Hospital, Stony Brook, NY, USA

Deborah A. Frank, M.D. Grow Clinic for Children, Boston Medical Center, Boston University School of Medicine, Boston, MA, USA

Rui Fu, M.S. Graduate School of Education, University of Pennsylvania, Philadelphia, PA, USA

Judy Garber, Ph.D. Department of Psychology and Human Development, Vanderbilt University, Nashville, TN, USA

Kathryn E. Grant, Ph.D. Department of Psychology, DePaul University, Chicago, IL, USA

Megan R. Gunnar, Ph.D. Institute of Child Development, University of Minnesota, Minneapolis, MN, USA

Jeffrey M. Halperin, Ph.D. Department of Psychology, Queens College and the Graduate Center, City University of New York, Flushing, NY, USA

Allison G. Harvey, Ph.D. Department of Psychology, The Golden Bear Sleep and Mood Research Clinic, Clinical Science Program and Psychology Clinic, University of California, Berkeley, CA, USA

Brian M. Hicks, Ph.D. Department of Psychiatry, University of Michigan, Ann Arbor, MI, USA

L. Kari Hironaka, M.D., M.P.H. Boston University School of Medicine/ Boston Medical Center, Boston, MA, USA

Stephanie M. Keller, M.A. Department of Psychological Sciences, Case Western Reserve University, Cleveland, OH, USA

Daniel N. Klein, Ph.D. Department of Psychology, Stony Brook University, Stony Brook, NY, USA

Kelly L. Klump, Ph.D. Department of Psychology, Michigan State University, East Lansing, MI, USA

Catherine K. Kraper, M.A. Psychology Department, University of Massachusetts Boston, Boston, MA, USA

Lingli Leng, M.Ed. Department of Social Work and Social Administration, Hong Kong University, Hong Kong, China

Michael Lewis, Ph.D. University Distinguished Professor and Director, Institute for the Study of Child Development, Rutgers Robert Wood Johnson Medical School, New Brunswick, NJ, USA

Suniya S. Luthar, Ph.D. Department of Psychology, Arizona State University, Tempe, AZ, USA

Emily L. Lyman, M.A. Department of Counseling and Clinical Psychology, Teachers College, Columbia University, New York, NY, USA

Jennifer L. Maggs, Ph.D. Human Development and Family Studies, The Pennsylvania State University, University Park, PA, USA

Julie Maslowsky, Ph.D. Health Behavior and Health Education, Department of Kinesiology and Health Education, The University of Texas at Austin, Austin, TX, USA

Eleanor L. McGlinchey, Ph.D. Division of Child and Adolescent Psychiatry, Columbia University Medical Center, New York State Psychiatric Institute, New York, NY, USA

Katie A. McLaughlin, Ph.D. Department of Psychology, University of Washington, Seattle, WA, USA

Susan Dvorak McMahon, Ph.D. Department of Psychology, DePaul University, Chicago, IL, USA

Christopher S. Monk, Ph.D. Department of Psychology, University of Michigan, Ann Arbor, MI, USA

Thomas G. O'Connor, Ph.D. Wynne Center for Family Research, Department of Psychiatry, University of Rochester Medical Center, Rochester, NY, USA

Thomas H. Ollendick, Ph.D. Child Study Center, Department of Psychology, Virginia Polytechnic Institute and State University, Blacksburg, VI, USA

Megan E. Patrick, Ph.D. Institute for Social Research, University of Michigan, Ann Arbor, MI, USA

Isaac T. Petersen Department of Psychological and Brain Sciences, Indiana University, Bloomington, IN, USA

Mitchell J. Prinstein, Ph.D., A.B.P.P. Department of Psychology, University of North Carolina at Chapel Hill, Chapel Hill, NC, USA

Uma Rao, M.D. Department of Psychiatry, Vanderbilt University, Nashville, TN, USA

Robert W. Roeser, Ph.D. Department of Psychology, Portland State University, Portland, OR, USA

Karen D. Rudolph, Ph.D. Department of Psychology, University of Illinois, Champaign, IL, USA

Michael Rutter, M.D. MRC Social, Genetic and Developmental Psychiatry Centre, Institute of Psychiatry, King's College London, London, UK

Henry T. Sachs, III, M.D. Alpert Medical School of Brown University, Providence, RI, USA

Arnold J. Sameroff, Ph.D. University of Michigan, Ann Arbor, MI, USA

Tyler R. Sasser, M.S. Training Interdisciplinary Education Scientists Program, The Pennsylvania State University, University Park, PA, USA

Alice C. Schermerhorn, Ph.D. Department of Psychology, University of Vermont, Burlington, VT, USA

John Schulenberg, Ph.D. Institute for Social Research, University of Michigan, Ann Arbor, MI, USA

Joyanna L. Silberg, Ph.D. The Sheppard Pratt Health System, Baltimore, MD, USA

Edmund J.S. Sonuga-Barke, Ph.D. Department of Psychology, University of Southampton, Southampton, SO, UK
and
Ghent University, Ghent, Belgium

Timothy W. Soto, M.A. Psychology Department, University of Massachusetts Boston, Boston, MA, USA

Howard Steele, Ph.D. Department of Psychology, New School for Social Research, New York, NY, USA

Miriam Steele, Ph.D. Department of Psychology, New School for Social Research, New York, NY, USA

Sonya K. Sterba, Ph.D. Psychology and Human Development Department, Vanderbilt University, Nashville, TN, USA

Melissa L. Sturge-Apple, Ph.D. Department of Clinical and Social Sciences in Psychology, University of Rochester, Rochester, NY, USA

Johnna R. Swartz, M.S. Department of Psychology, University of Michigan, Ann Arbor, MI, USA

Helen Tager-Flusberg, Ph.D. Department of Psychology, Boston University, Boston, MA, USA

Departments of Anatomy & Neurobiology and Pediatrics, Boston University School of Medicine, Boston, MA, USA

Barbara Tylenda, Ph.D., A.B.P.P. ABPP, Clinical Associate Professor of Psychiatry and Human Behavior, Alpert Medical School of Brown University, Providence, RI, USA

Douglas L. Vanderbilt, M.D. Keck School of Medicine, University of Southern California, Los Angeles, CA, USA

Michael W. Vasey, Ph.D. Department of Psychology, The Ohio State University, Columbus, OH, USA

Kate E. Wallis, M.D., M.P.H. Department of Pediatrics, New York University School of Medicine, New York, NY, USA

Kenneth J. Zucker, Ph.D. Gender Identity Service, Child, Youth, and Family Services, Centre for Addiction and Mental Health, Intergenerational Wellness Centre, Beamish Family Wing, Toronto, ON, Canada

Gender Identity Service, Child, Youth, and Family Services, Centre for Addiction and Mental Health, Toronto, ON, Canada

Robert A. Zucker, Ph.D. Departments of Psychiatry and Psychology, Addiction Research Center, University of Michigan Medical School, Ann Arbor, MI, USA

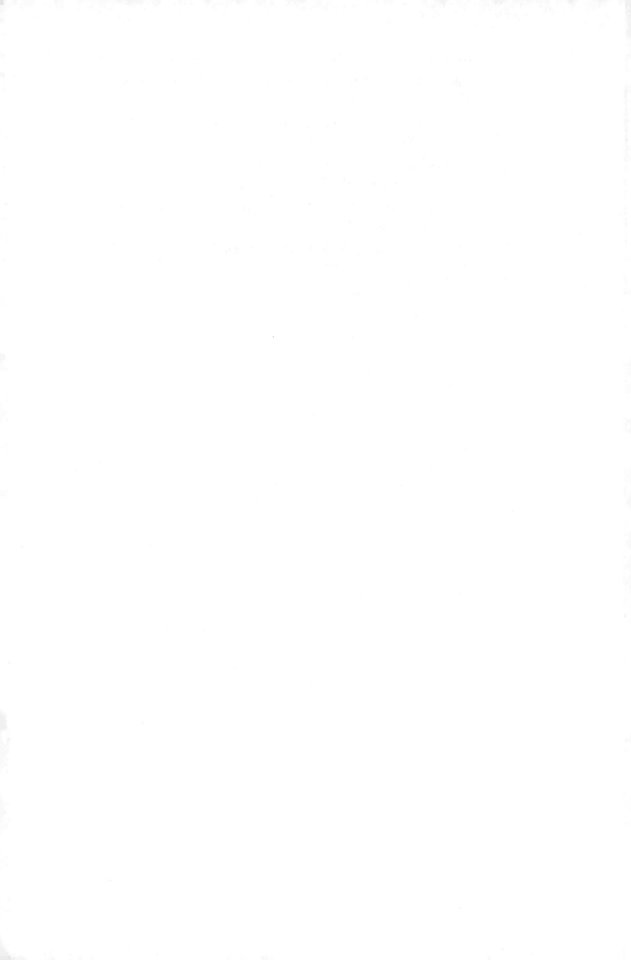

Part I

Issues and Theories

Toward the Development of the Science of Developmental Psychopathology

Michael Lewis

It is almost 30 years since the seminal paper by Sroufe and Rutter (1984) and nearly 25 years since the first edition of the *Handbook of Developmental Psychopathology* (Lewis & Miller, 1990). Much has changed in the study of pathology since then, including our models of development, the definitions of psychopathology—with some newer types added and others removed—and in particular new measurements and new statistical techniques. Nevertheless I think it is still appropriate to define our field as "the study of the prediction of development of maladaptive behaviors and the processes that underlie them." As we have said, the thrust of the definition of developmental psychopathology requires something more than a simple combination of two sets of interests. Besides the study of change and development of maladaptive behaviors, the combination of issues of development with that of psychopathology informs both areas of interest. But perhaps of equal importance is that our study of the development of pathology forces us to look at individual differences.

In a recent book on attachment and psychoanalysis, Morris Eagle (2013) tried to reconcile the different points of view of attachment theory and psychoanalysis. He tried to understand the differences and similarities around the problem of how actual events versus the construction of a child's reality or fantasy affect the child's development. For him, attachment theory is more concerned with the actual events, that is, what really happened in the opening year of life, rather than what psychoanalysis has been concerned with, the concern for fantasy or the construction of reality.

This dichotomy is of special interest for the study of psychopathology, even though the work of Mary Main has tried to bridge the gap though her emphasis on attachment models as the mechanism connecting what happened to the idea of what happened (Main, Kaplan, & Cassidy, 1985). For her, these models are dependent on what actually happened vis-a-vis the earlier mother–child interaction. This is consistent with much of the interest in articulating the nature of the development of psychopathology since it is predicated on finding the relation between what really happened as it affects the child's development. While longitudinal studies gives us some clues as to what really happened, our emphasis on discovering the past as a reality is bound to give us only weak associations. This is likely always to be the case given what we know about the human condition, namely, that our experiences and our memories are constructions even as they occur, let alone when we recall them, and these constructions bear only a weak association to what really happened (Lewis, 1997). Given these facts in regard to human behavior, we must remember that the notion of what really happened cannot be the bases of a predictive science. An example of this dilemma can readily be seen in a longitudinal

M. Lewis, Ph.D. (✉)
Institute for the Study of Child Development,
Rutgers Robert Wood Johnson Medical School,
New Brunswick, NJ 08901, USA
e-mail: lewis@rwjms.rutgers.edu

M. Lewis and K.D. Rudolph (eds.), *Handbook of Developmental Psychopathology*,
DOI 10.1007/978-1-4614-9608-3_1, © Springer Science+Business Media New York 2014

study of attachment. For this study we obtained attachment ratings of a large number of one-year-olds in a slightly modified standard attachment paradigm and followed them until they were 18 years old (Lewis, Feiring, & Rosenthal, 2000). We found that their attachment rating did not predict their AAI scores nor their psychopathology scores at 18 years. What did predict these scores at 18 was the nature of their family structure, namely, whether or not their parents were divorced. Of particular interest was the finding that their memory of their childhood, which was unrelated to their earlier attachment, was related to their AAI scores at 18 but only if we took the family structure into account.

I mention these findings to remind us of how children construct their experiences and memories; how they respond to events in their worlds rather than what really has happened is an important addition to the study of the development of psychopathology. Thus, when we talk about the various models that we use to study these problems, we need keep in mind that individual difference in the construction of reality need be taken into account. The question that still needs to be addressed is how individual children construct their reality. This has to include how earlier experiences influence later ones and how individual differences in temperament may affect these constructions. Thus individual differences in temperament not only affect how a child may respond to an event but in addition affect the nature of the construction of the event and memories of it.

Models of Developmental Psychopathology

Models of development always represent world views about human nature and environments that create a human life course. Models of abnormal development also reflect these different world views. So, for example, the trait notion of personality (Block & Block, 1980) and the invulnerable child (Anthony, 1970; Garmezy, 1974; Rutter, 1981) both share the view that some fixed pattern of behavior may be unaffected by environmental factors. Likewise, information in regard to the

regression of a child's behavior to old behavioral patterns under stress requires that we reconsider the idea that all developmental processes are transformational, that is, that all old behavioral patterns are changed or transformed into new ones.

Two views of human nature have predominated in our theories of development. In the first, the human psyche is acted on by its surrounding environment—both its biological and its external physical and social environments. In the second view, the human organism acts on and in a bidirectional fashion interacts with the biological, physical, and social environments (Overton, 2006). The reactive view has generated a dichotomy of two major theoretical paradigms: biological determinism and social determinism. The active view, in contrast, has generated what has recently come to be known as the *relational developmental systems perspective* (Lerner, 2006). Let us consider the views in their more extreme forms to show how their respective theories might treat the issues of development.

In both the biological-motivational and social-determinism paradigms, the causes of behavior or action are forces that act on the organism, causing it to behave. These may be internal biological features of the species, including species-specific action patterns. In all cases, within this world view, the organism is acted on and the causes of its action (including its development) are external to it. Thus, for example, the major determinant of sex-role behavior is thought to be biological, that is, determined by sex and in this case by the effects of hormones. Alternatively, sex-role behavior can be determined externally by the shaping of effect of the social environment, either the differential rewards of conspecifics (Fagot, 1973). Examples of the former are already well known (e.g., parental praising or punishing of specific sex-role-appropriate actions, such as playing with particular toys; see Goldberg & Lewis, 1969; Rheingold & Cook, 1975). Examples of determinism by the social world include giving the child a male or female name or specific toys to play with. This view does not have to imply reinforcement control but structural control. In all such external control paradigms, we need not infer a self or consciousness and with it a will, intention, or plans.

In contrast with this passive or reactive view is the relational developmental systems perspective based on the world view that the organism is inherently active, acting on, and being acted on the biological, physical, and social environment in a bidirectional fashion (Lewis, 2010; Lewis & Rosenblum, 1974). Within this perspective the organism has a self and consciousness and as such has desires and plans (Lewis, 1979). These desires and goals are constructed, as are most of the actions enabling the organism to behave adaptively. This view does not necessitate discarding either biological imperatives or social control as potential determinants of behavior, because from this relational perspective, humans are both biological and social creatures, and both must impact on behavior. I prefer to think of these biological and social features as nothing more than the raw materials or resources for the construction of cognitive structures subsumed under a self and consciousness, which include goals and desires, plans, and action. Taking the example of sex-role behavior, I have argued that hormones and social control become material for the construction of self-cognitive structures. These structures might take the form "I am male or female," "Males or females behave this way or that way," or "To receive the praise of others (a desired goal) I should act either this way or that" (Lewis, 1985). Cognitions of this sort and their accompanying goals and desires, together with cognitions concerning information about the world, enable the child to *intentionally act,* that is, to consciously construct a plan as described.

These two world views are present in all psychological inquiry. The reactive organism mechanistic model receives support in the case of the biological study of action (e.g., T cells tracing foreign proteins that have entered the body). Relational developmental systems views are supported by theories of the mind. It should not go unnoticed that with the growth of cognitive science, the idea of constructing mental representations, in particular of the self (that do not correspond in any one-to-one fashion with the "real" world) and with it plans and intentions, had become more acceptable to psychology proper by the 1980s but is still somewhat lacking

in the study of developmental psychopathology (Gardner, 1985).

Models of development have been considered by many writers, and the interested reader is referred to Overton (2006) and as well as Sameroff (2014). I particularly like Riegel's (1978) scheme for considering models that involve the child and the environment. In this scheme, each of these elements can be active or passive agents. The passive child-passive environment model is of relatively less interest because it arose from John Locke and David Hume and now receives little attention. In such a model, the environment does not try to affect behavior, and the child is a passive "blank tablet" upon which is received information from the world around it. Such models originally had some use, for example, in our understanding of short-term memory where memories were likened to a small box that was sequentially filled. When a new memory was entered and there was no more room, the first (or oldest) memory dropped out. Although such a view of memory is no longer held, other views, especially in perception, share many of the features of this model. Gibson's (1969) notion of affordance, for example, suggests such a model because innate features of the child extract the given features of the environment. Such models are by their nature mechanistic although the infant has to have locomotion in its world in order for it to occur.

The passive child-active environment model is an environmental control view because here the environment actively controls, by reward and punishment, the child's behavior. The characteristics of this environment may differ, as may the nature of the different reinforcers, but the child's behavior is determined by its environment. We are most familiar with this model in operant conditioning. It is a model much favored by many therapists and is used in diverse areas, such as behavior modification treatment to alter maladaptive behavior or in the treatment of autism, as well as in theories that explain normal sex-role learning by parental or peer reinforcement (Bem, 1987).

The third model is that of an active person and a passive environment. These models have in common an active child extracting and constructing its world from the material of the environment. Piaget's theory fits well within this framework (Piaget, 1952), although some have argued that Piaget may be a preformationalist—passive child-passive environment—in that all the structures children create are identical (Bellin, 1971). Given the active organismic view of Piaget, it is easy to see that although the child needs the environment to construct knowledge, the environment itself plays little role in the knowledge itself (Lewis, 1983). Linguistic theories, such as those held by Chomsky (1957, 1965), suggest that biological linguistic structures are available for children to use in their construction of language in particular environments. More recently, we have suggested that innate early action patterns in interaction with the environment produce the different feeling states which we call emotions, such as fear and happiness (Lewis, 2014). Whether such views are better placed in the passive child-passive environment model can be questioned, although the critical feature of this model should not be lost. In psychopathology and therapy, we often employ such a model when we attempt to help patients alter their behavior—active person—but discount the role of the environment outside the therapeutic environment.

The last model is most familiar to those studying development because of its interactive nature. An active person and an active environment are postulated as creating, modifying, and changing behavior. These interactive models take many forms, varying from the interactional approach of Lewis (Lewis, 1972; Lewis & Feiring, 1991), to the transactional models of Sameroff and Chandler (1975), to the epigenetic models of Zhang and Meaney (2010). They also include Chess and Thomas (1984) and Lerner's (1984) goodness-of-fit model and, from a developmental psychopathology point of view, the notion of vulnerability and risk status (Garmezy, Masten, & Tellegen, 1984; Rutter, 1979).

Even though Riegel's (1978) approach is useful, other systems of classification are available. For example, both passive child and passive and active environment models are mechanistic in that either biological givens within the organism or environmental structures outside the organism

act on the child. On the other hand, both active child models must be interactive because organisms almost always interact in some way with their environment, which, given its structure (whether active or passive), affects the ongoing interaction. In the models of development as they are related to maladaptive and abnormal behavior, we use a combination of approaches.

With this in mind, three models of development psychopathology have been suggested: these include a *trait model,* a *contextual or environmental model,* and an *interactional model.* Although each of these models has variations, the interactional model is the most variable. Because attachment theory remains central to normal and maladaptive development, it is used often as an example in our discussion. These three models, which are prototypes of the various views of development and developmental psychopathology, make clear how such models diverge and how they can be used to understand the etiology of pathology. Unfortunately, by describing sharp distinctions, we may draw too tight an image and, as such, may make them caricatures. Nevertheless, it is important to consider them in this fashion in order to observe their strengths and weaknesses.

Trait or Status Model

The trait or status model is characterized by its simplicity and holds to the view that a trait, or the status of the child at one point in time, is likely to predict a trait or status at a later point in time. A trait model is not interactive and does not provide for the effects of the environment. In fact in the most extreme form, the environment is thought to play no role either in affecting its display or in transforming its characteristics. A particular trait may interact with the environment but the trait is not changed by that interaction.

Traits are not easily open to transformation and can be processes, coping skills, attributes, or tendencies to respond in certain ways. Traits can be innate features, such as temperament or particular genetic codes. More important from our point of view is that traits can also be acquired through learning or through more interactive processes.

However, once a trait is acquired, it remains relatively unaffected by subsequent interactions. The trait model is most useful in many instances, for example, when considering potential genetic or biological causes of subsequent psychopathology. A child who is born with a certain gene or a set of genes is likely to display psychopathology at some later time. This model characterizes some of the research in the genetics of mental illness. Here, the environment, or its interaction with the genes, plays little role in the potential outcome. The early work of Kallman (1946), for example, on heritability of schizophrenia supports the use of such a model, as does the lack or presence of certain chemicals on the development depression (see Puig-Antich's early work, 1982). In each of these cases, the presence of particular features is hypothesized as likely to affect a particular type of pathology. Although a trait model is appealing in its simplicity, there are any number of problems with it; for example, not all people who possess a trait or have a particular status at one point in time are *all* likely to show subsequent psychopathology or the same type of psychopathology (Saudino, 1997). Another example is the genetic traits related to breast cancer (BRCA). While some with such a trait develop cancer, most will not do so.

That all children of schizophrenic parents do not themselves become schizophrenic or that not all monozygotic twins show concordance vis-a-vis schizophrenia suggests that other variables need to be considered (Gottesman & Shields, 1982; Kringlon, 1968). We return to this point again; however, it is important to note that the failure to find a high incidence of schizophrenic children of schizophrenic parents leads to the need to postulate such concepts as resistance to stress, coping styles, and resilience. Each of these terms has a trait-like feature to them.

This model is also useful when considering traits that are not genetically or biologically based. For example, the attachment model as proposed by Bowlby (1969) and Ainsworth (1973) holds that the child's early relationship with his/her mother in the first year of life will determine the child's adjustment throughout life. The security of attachment that the child shows at the end

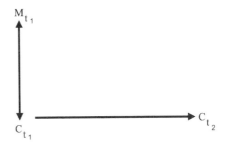

Fig. 1.1 Trait model using the attachement construct

of the first year of life is the result of the early interaction between the mother and the child. Once the attachment is established, it acts as a trait affecting the child's subsequent behavior. Attachment as a trait is established through the interaction of the child with his/her mother but, once established, acts like any other trait: that is, it may interact with the environment at any time but is not altered by it (see Ainsworth, 1989).

Figure 1.1 presents the trait model using the traditional attachment construct. Notice that the interaction of the mother and child at T_1 produces the intraorganism trait, C_{t1} in this case, a secure or an insecure attachment. Although attachment is the consequence of an interaction, once established, it is the trait (C_{t1}) residing in the child that leads to C_{t2}. There is no need to posit a role of the environment except as it initially produces the attachment. The problems with a trait view of the attachment model have been addressed by many (Lamb, Thompson, Gardner, & Charnov, 1985; Lewis et al., 2000) nevertheless; it is a widely held view that the mother–child relationship in the first year of life can affect the child's subsequent socio-emotional life as well as impact on its mental health. Interestingly, more recently Sroufe, Coffino, and Carlson (2010) in their longitudinal study of early attachment also have found that attachment at 1 year of life does not predict later psychopathology without taking the subsequent environment into account (see Lewis et al., 2000, for a similar view).

Moreover, there is the belief that this attachment trait can act as a protective factor in the face of environmental stress. Secure attachment is often seen as a resiliency factor. The concept of

Fig. 1.2 Invulnerability
model from point of view
of an acquired trait

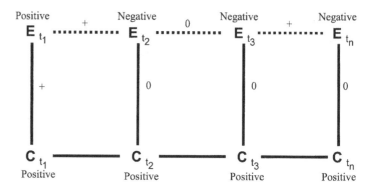

resilience is similar to a trait model, since there are aspects of children that appear to protect them from subsequent environmental stress. These resiliency traits serve to make the child stress resistant. Such a mechanism is used to explain why not all at-risk children develop psychopathology. Garmezy (1989) and Rutter (1979) have mentioned factors that can protect the child against stress and, therefore, psychopathology. The problem here is that besides intellectual ability and an easy temperament, it is not clear what other factors on an a priori basis we can say are protective factors unless we wish to consider that early positive social experiences are themselves protective factors. In that case, the protective factors reside in the environment rather than in the person, which now starts to resemble an environmental model.

Figure 1.2 presents the invulnerability or resilience model from the point of view of an acquired trait. Notice that at t_1 the environment is positive, so the child acquires a protective attribute. At t_2, the environment becomes negative (stress appears); however, the attribute acquired at t_1 protects the child (the child remains positive). At each additional point in time (t_3, t_4,..., t_n), the environment may change; however, it has little effect on the child because the intraorganism trait is maintained.

Of some question is the prolonged impact of a stress given the protective factor. It is possible to consider such a factor in several ways. In the first place, a protective factor can act to increase the threshold before a stress can affect the child. Stress will have an effect, but it will do so only after a certain level is past. A threshold concept

applies not only for intensity but also for duration; that is, invulnerability may represent the ability to sustain one or two stress events but not prolonged stress, or, alternatively, it may protect the child against long-term stress. Specific to secure attachment, it is increasingly clear that it is not a protective factor in terms of the child's reaction to subsequent stress (Lewis et al., 2000; Sroufe et al., 2010). There are, however, newer findings on Romanian children in orphanages which suggests a critical period effect such that attachment failures after a year or so lead to permanent psychopathology including such biological differences as in cortisol regulation (see Rutter, 2013). While these data are impressive and support a trait-like model, only continued study of these children will reveal how these failures interact with environmental differences. To date across many areas of inquiry, the idea of critical periods in development, unaltered by subsequent environmental forces, has received only mixed findings (Lewis, 1997). Even psychoanalytic theory, while postulating critical periods on the one hand, also suggests that environmental forces such as psychoanalytic treatment can alter the past's effect on the future.

Trait models in personality theory are not new (Allport & Allport, 1921), and the problems identified in personality research apply here as well. The major problem related to trait models is the recognition that individual traits are likely to be situation specific (Mischel, 1965). As such, they can only partially characterize the organism. For example, a child may be securely attached to his/her mother but insecurely attached to his/her father or his/her older sibling. It would therefore be hard to characterize the child as insecurely attached simply because he/she was insecurely attached to one family member but not to the others (Fox, Kimmerly, & Schafer, 1991). Accurate prediction from an insecure attachment trait to subsequent psychopathology would be difficult without knowing the child's complete attachment pattern. Such data might dilute attachment from a trait located within the individual to a set of specific relationships. Thus, to characterize the child in a simple way, such as secure or insecure, may miss the complex nature of traits, especially those likely to be related to subsequent psychopathology.

Equally problematic with the trait notion is the fact that such models leave little room for the impact of environment on subsequent developmental growth or dysfunction. Environments play a role in children's development in the opening year of life and continue to do so throughout the life span (Lewis, 1997). The idea of a secure attachment trait as a protection from environmental stress or of an insecure attachment trait as vulnerability factor, while undergoing modification within attachment theory, is still widely held (see Steele & Steele, 2014).

The Environmental Model

The prototypic environmental model holds that exogenous factors mostly influence development. There are several problems in using this model. To begin with there is considerable problems in defining what environments are. They might be the physical properties of the world around the child. So, for example, the HOME Scale to characterize the physical characteristics, including the number of books or toys in the home, has been used and meets this definition. Environments may be defined as the parental behaviors or the emotional tone in which the child lives. These problems of defining environments have recently been considered by Mayes and Lewis (2013), in whose book the wide range of possible environmental factors likely to influence the child are presented.

A more serious problem for testing this model is the failure to consider the impact of environ-ments throughout the life span. In fact, the strongest form of the environmental or contextual model argues that adaptation to current environment, throughout the life course, is a major influence in our socioemotional life. As environments change, so too does the individual (Lewis, 1997; Sroufe, Egeland, Carlson, & Collins, 2005). This dynamic and changing view of environments and adaptation is in strong contrast to the earlier models of environments as forces acting on the individual and acting on the individual *only* in the early years of life. Let us consider them in detail, recognizing that the nature or the classification of types of environments lags far behind our measurement of individual characteristics.

In the simplest environmental model, the child's behavior, normal or maladaptive, is primarily a function of the environmental forces acting on it at any point in time. In such a model, a child shows behavior x but not behavior y because behavior x is positively rewarded by his/her parents while y is punished. Notice that in this model, the environmental forces act on the organism, who is passive to them, and the behavior emitted is a direct function of this action. Although this model may apply for some behavior, it is more likely the case that environmental forces act on the child directly at one point in time and indirectly at later points in time. Our hypothetical child may later do behavior x, not because of the immediate reward value but because the child remembers that x is a rewarded behavior. Clearly, much of our behavior is controlled by this indirect form of environmental pressure acting on our constructed models of how the world works. Many other forms of indirect reward and punishment have been observed. For example, consider the situation in which a child is present when the mother scolds the older sibling for writing on the walls of the house. The younger child, although not directly punished, does learn that writing on walls is not an action to be performed (Lewis & Feiring, 1981). Unfortunately, these indirect forms of reward and punishment have received little attention, although there is some current interest in triadic interaction where indirect effects can be considered (Feiring, Lewis, & Starr, 1984; Repacholi, Meltzoff, & Olsen, 2008).

There are many different types of environmental forces. For example, we see an advertisement for a product "that will make other people love us." We purchase such a product in the hopes that others will indeed love us. We can be rewarded or punished in many direct and indirect ways; however, it is important to note that the more the organism has to construct the nature or purpose of the environmental forces, the more we move from the passive child-active environment to the active child-active environment model. The social-cognitive theories of personality are examples of this active-active model (Bandura, 1986; Mischel, 1965). In all cases, the environment supplies the information that the child uses. Thus, in some sense the environment is passive, while the child is active in constructing meaning. Here we can see again that it is the children's construction of meaning which influences their behavior and that their construction and the reality as seen by another may be quite different.

Because other people make up one important aspect of our environment, the work on the structures of the *social* environment is particularly relevant, and attempts have been made to expand the numbers of potentially important people in the child's environment (Lewis, 2013), as well as to create an analysis of the structure of the social environment itself (Lewis, 2014). Although considerable effort has been focused on the importance of the mother on the child, other persons, including fathers, siblings, grandparents, and peers, clearly have importance in shaping the child's life (Bronfenbrenner & Crouter, 1983). Given these diverse features of environments and the important roles attributed to them, it is surprising that so little systematic work has gone into their study. For the most part, mothers and, to some extent, families have received the most attention, and we therefore use them in our examples; however, without a more complete theory about the role of the social nexus, our work on the development of psychopathology will be incomplete.

The role of environments in the developmental process has been underplayed because most investigators seek to find the structure and change within the organism itself. Likewise, in the study of psychopathology, even though we recognize that environments can cause disturbance and abnormal behavior, we prefer to treat the person—to increase coping skills or to alter specific behaviors—rather than change the environment (Lewis, 1997). Yet we can imagine the difficulties that are raised when we attempt to alter specific maladaptive behaviors in environments in which such behaviors are adaptive—a point well taken years ago by Szasz (1961).

Our belief that the thrust of development resides in the organism rather than in the environment, in large part, raises many problems. At cultural levels, we assume that violence (and its cure) must be met in the individual—a trait model—rather than in the structure of the environment. The murder rate using handguns in the USA is many times higher than in most other Western societies. We seek responsibility in the nature of the individual (e.g., XYY males, or the genetics of antisocial behavior), when the nature of the environment is also likely to be involved. In this case, murders in the USA may be more due to the nonrestriction of automatic guns than to people characteristics. Thus, we can either conclude that Americans are by nature more violent than Europeans or that because other Western societies do not allow handguns or automatic weapons, they therefore have lower murder rates (Cairns & Cairns, 2000).

A general environmental model suggests that children's behavior is a function of the environment in which the behavior occurs, because the task of the individual is to adapt to its current environment. As long as the environment appears consistent, the child's behavior will be consistent: if the environment *changes,* so too will the child's behavior. If a more active organism model is used, it is still the case that maladaptive environments produce abnormal behavior; however, the abnormal behavior is produced by the child's perception and construction of his/her reality. From a developmental psychopathology point of view, maladaptive behavior is caused by maladaptive environment; if we change those environments, we alter the behavior.

Figure 1.3 presents this model. The environment (E) at t_1, t_2, and t_3 all impact on the child's behavior at each point in time. The child's behavior at

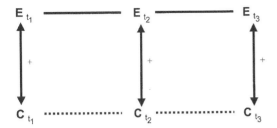

Fig. 1.3 Model of change as a function of the environment

C_{t1}, C_{t2}, and C_{t3} appears consistent, and it is, as long as E remains consistent. In other words, the continuity in C is an epiphenomenon of the continuity of E across time. Likewise, the lack of consistency in C reflects the lack of consistency in the environment. The child's behavior changes over t_1 to t_3 as the environment produces change. Even though it appears that C is consistent, it is so because E *is* consistent. Consistency and change in C are supposed by exogenous rather than by endogenous factors.

Such a model of change as a function of the environment can be readily tested but rarely is it done. This failure reflects the bias of the trait model. Again, consider the case of the attachment model. Although it is recognized that the environment affects the attachment at t_1, the child's status or trait at t_1 (C_{t1}) is hypothesized to determine the child's other outcomes, C_{t2}, C_{t3}, and so forth. Rarely is the environment and the consistency of the environment factored into the model as a possible cause of subsequent child behavior. Consider that poor parenting produces an insecure child at C_{t1} and this parenting remains poor at t_2 and t_3. Without considering the continued effects of poor parenting, it is not possible to make such a conclusion. That most research in this area fails in this regard constitutes evidence for the lack of interest in the environmental model. It should be pointed out that the recent longitudinal study of Sroufe and colleagues has begun to alter this model in light of their findings (Sroufe et al., 2005).

Other forms of maladaptive behavior development have a similar problem. Depressed women are assumed to cause concurrent as well as subsequent depression in children (Zahn-Waxler, Cummings, McKnew, & Radke-Yarrow, 1984). What is not considered is the fact that depressed mothers at t_1 are also likely to be depressed at t_2 or t_3. What role does the mother's depression at these points play in the child's subsequent condition? We can only infer the answer given the limited data available. The question that needs to be asked is what would happen to the child if the mother was depressed at t_1 but was not depressed at t_2 or t_3? This type of question suggests that one way to observe the effect of the environment on the child's subsequent behavior is to observe those situations in which the environment changes.

The environmental change can occur in two ways: a positive environment can become negative or a negative environment can become positive. In each case, the change in the child's behavior should inform us as to the role of the environment in affecting behavior. In the former case, we would expect an increase in the child's maladaptive behavior, whereas in the latter, we would expect to see a decrease. There are several studies that can be of help in answering this question. Thompson, Lamb, and Estes (1982), for example, examined children's attachment between 1 year and 18 months. They found that the change in the child was related to the mother's going back to work. When the child's environment changed by going from less to more stress, there was an increase in the negative behavior of the child. When there was no change in the stress environment, there was little change in the child's behavior. The Romanian study, in particular the Bucharest Early Intervention Program, shows what may happen when the environment changes from high to low stress. Children who were placed in foster care rather than being in the orphanage showed that the positive environment resulted in increased cortical white matter as well as cognitive capacity relative to the children who remained in the orphanage (see Nelson et al., 2007; Sheridan, Fox, Zeanah, McLaughlin, & Nelson, 2012; Sheridan, Sarsour, Jutte, D'Esposito, & Boyce, 2012).

Abused children are found not to be securely attached and also have poor peer relationships (Schneider-Rosen & Cicchetti, 1984). The trait model holds that the insecure attachment produces subsequent poor peer relationships. Alternatively, an environmental model would state that abusive parents also are likely not to encourage or promote good peer relationships; thus, both insecure attachment and poor peer relationships are due to poor parenting at both points in time. Moreover, if peer relationships could be encouraged by placing these children in supervised day care, then peer relationships should improve even though the attachment characteristic did not change. Such findings would support an environmental model and at the same time suggest that social behavior, especially to peers, is not a function of the mother–infant attachment (see also Harlow & Harlow, 1965, for a similar view about the independence of the peer and parent relationships). In an earlier study we reported that although initial peer behavior in abused children was different than that in a nonabused group, after 1 month in a day care setting the behavior of the two groups could not be distinguished even though the child–mother relationship remained poor (Lewis & Schaeffer, 1981). Findings such as these suggest that not only past but also concurrent environmental influences need to be given more attention.

Although the environmental model can be made more complex, this general model suggests, in all cases, that the child's concurrent mental health status is determined by the current environment as well as past ones (Lewis, 1997). Should the environment change, then the child's status is likely to change. The degree to which the environment remains consistent, and in our case psychopathogenic, is the degree to which psychopathology will be consistently found within the subject. Therefore, the environmental model can be characterized by the view that the constraints, changes, and consistencies in children's psychopathology rest not so much with intrinsic structures located in the child as in the nature and structure of the environment of the child. The caveat is that the construction of children's belief about the nature of the current environment and memories of the past should also be taken into account.

Prior Experience

The environmental model also raises again the issue of the nature and degree of prior experience, that is, the notion of a critical period. Certain environmental influences may have a greater effect at some points in time but not others. For example, a responsive environment in the first year and a less-responsive environment in the second year should lead to better consequences than a nonresponsive environment in the first year and a responsive environment in the second year. Although critical periods suggest some organismic characteristics, the effects of the environment as a function of past experience remain relevant here. In its simplest form, when a series of positive events is followed by a negative event, it is important to know whether the impact of the negative event depends on the number or the timing of the preceding positive ones. In similar fashion, the same question applies for a series of negative events.

For example, Child A has four positive environmental events prior to the negative one, whereas Child B has only two. Is the negative event more negative for Child B than for Child A? The simplest environmental model would suggest no difference because such models argue for a passive child and, given such, past experiences have little effect. On the other hand, memory systems are likely to be ones in which past experiences are registered and processed. Given this fact, the four positive past experiences for Child A might dilute the effects of the negative event. A more complex model provides for a more active child, and here the child's memory and construction of all the past positive events allow for a reconstruction of the negative one. The effect of the past events might serve to buffer the effect of the next event.

Besides the effects of past experiences on the behavior of the child, particular time periods may be critical for some environmental events something which the Romanian orphanages data suggests. For example, a limited number of negative events in early life may have a greater impact than the same number of events later in life.

Attachment theory suggests that the failure of the child to securely attach in the first year may predispose him/her to serious maladaptive behavior, even though the environment thereafter is altered in the positive direction. The data for this position are mixed and suggest that, at least for socioemotional development, ongoing poor environments may be more critical than just the early ones. Nevertheless, the models of the effect of past experience, critical periods, and current environments are in need of continued testing over a long period of years if we are to understand the importance of an environmental model of developmental psychopathology. We need long-term observation since we do not have any developmental theory which informs us of when in development the effects of early negative experiences can be altered by new positive ones.

Whatever model we choose, it is clear that the study and treatment of maladaptive behavior require that the environment across the life span be considered. Although some maladaptive behavior of the child may be altered within the therapeutic situation, the child usually returns to the same environment in which these maladaptive behaviors were formed. If such behavior is to be modified, we have to modify the environment. A strong environmental model suggests that, in many cases, this may be sufficient.

The Child by Environment Models

Interactional Model

While both the trait and the environmental models continue to receive support from research, it is the interactional models—which incorporate characteristics of the child, be they attachment status, genetic factors, or temperament as they interact with the environment—which have for the most part captured our attention in the study of development in general and developmental psychopathology in particular. The number and diversity of these models and the ways of measuring these are considerable (see, for example, Sterba, 2014).

These models have some general features and while Sameroff (2014) has called them transactional we have called them interactional (Lewis, 1972). Both transactional and interactional models have in common the belief that we need to consider both child and environment in determining the course of development. Such models usually require an active child and an active environment; however, they need not be so. What they do require is the notion that behavior is shaped by its adaptive ability and that this ability is related to environments. Maladaptive behavior may be misnamed because the behavior may be adaptive to a maladaptive environment. The stability and change in the child need to be viewed as a function of both factors, and as such, the task of any interactive model is to draw us to the study of both features. In our attachment example, the infant who is securely attached, as a function of the responsive environment in the first year, will show competence at a later age as a function of the earlier events as well as the nature of the environment at later ages (see Lewis, 1997; Sroufe et al., 2005).

One of the central issues of the developmental theories that are interactive in nature is the question of transformation. Two models of concurrent behavior as a function of traits and environment can be drawn. In the first, both trait and environment interact and produce a new set of behaviors. However, neither the traits nor the environment are altered by the interaction.

From a developmental perspective, this is an additive model because new behaviors are derived from old behaviors and their interaction with the environment, but these new behaviors are added to the repertoire of the set of old behaviors (Lewis, 1997). For example, an insecurely attached child (−ATT) can interact with a positive environment (+E) so that a positive outcome (+O) occurs:

$$(-ATT) \times (+E) \rightarrow +O$$

In this case, the trait of (−ATT) remains unaffected by the interaction and (+O) is added to the set of behaviors including (−ATT). Likewise, (+E) is not altered by the interaction. This model is very useful for explaining such diverse phenomena as regression, vulnerability, and goodness of fit.

Transformational Model

A transformational model can be contrasted to the interactional model, but having already discussed one we can be more brief here. This type of model requires that all features that make up an interaction are themselves comprised of all features and are transformed by their interaction. These are called *transactional models* (see Sameroff, 2014). For example, if we believe in Fig. 1.3 that the child's characteristics at C_{t1} interact with the environment E_{t1} to produce a transformed C_{t2} and E_{t2}, then it is likely that C_{t1} and E_{t1} also were transformed from some earlier time $t_{(n-1)}$ and that, therefore, each feature is never independent of the other. The general expression of this then is

$$\left(C_{t1} \times E_{t1} \right) \rightarrow C_{t2}, E_{t2}, \text{where}$$

$$C_{t1} = \int \left(C_{tn-1} \times E_{tn-1} \right) \text{ and}$$

$$E_{t1} = \int \left(E_{tn-1} \times C_{tn-1} \right).$$

Such models reject the idea that child or environmental characteristics are ever independent or exist as pure forms; there is here an ultimate regression effect. Moreover, these features interact and transform themselves at each point in development. The linear functions that characterize the other models are inadequate for the transformational view. The parent's behavior affects the child's behavior; however, the parent's behavior was affected by the child's earlier behavior.

An example of this is a study where we found that intrusive mothers of 3-month-olds are likely to have insecurely attached children at 1 year. However, their overstimulation appears to be related to their children's earlier behavior. Children who do not appear socially oriented at 3 months, preferring to play with and look at toys rather than people, become insecurely attached. These children have mothers who are over stimulating. Thus, earlier child characteristics—non-sociability—lead

to maternal overstimulation which in turn leads to insecure attachments (Lewis & Feiring, 1989). However, this analysis still gives us two relatively separate measures of C and E and thus is interactional rather than transformational.

On the other hand, an insecure attachment at 1 year can be transformed given the proper environment, and an insecure attachment can transform a positive environment into a negative one. Consider the irritable child who interacts with a positive environment and produces a negative environment that subsequently produces a negative, irritable child. The causal chain does not simply pass in a continuous fashion either through the environment or through the irritable child as a trait or environmental model would have it. In fact, it is a circular pattern of child causes affecting the environment and the environmental causes affecting the child. Such models have intrinsic appeal but are by their nature difficult to test. However, as Sterba (2014) shows, the new statistical procedures may be able to address this type of problem. Nevertheless, the problems of colinearity and high correlations found in environmental and child measures continue to make the testing of such models difficult. Most of the models employ regression-like analyses which in general require linear functions. The use of linear function themselves may be open to question given that linearity may be a limit function in human behavior. Even so, it is difficult not to treat a child or an environmental characteristic as a "pure" quantity, though we might know better. As such, we tend to test the interactive models that require less transformation.

Goodness-of-Fit Model

According to the goodness-of-fit model, pathology arises when the child's characteristics do not match the environmental demand, or, stated another way, the environmental demand does not match the child's characteristic (Lerner, 1984; Thomas & Chess, 1977). Notice that maladjustment is the consequence of the *mismatch*. It is not located in either the nature of the child's characteristic or in the environmental demand. Some might argue that certain environmental demands, by their nature, will cause pathology in the same way that certain child characteristics, by their nature, will cause them. Although this may be the case in extremes, the goodness-of-fit model suggests that psychopathology is the consequence of the mismatch between trait and environment, and, as such, it is an interactive model.

Consider the case of the temperamentally active child. If such a child is raised in a household where activity and noise are valued and where there is a match between the active child and the environment, no maladaptive behavior results. However, if this same child is raised in a household where quiet behavior and inhibition are valued, we would expect to see more adjustment problems. Similarly, for the quiet, lethargic child, again, dependent on the match between the behavior and the environment, different degrees of maladjustment would occur.

In terms of transformation, such a model is relatively silent. Even so, it would seem reasonable to imagine that new behaviors arise due either to the match or mismatch, but these new behaviors do not require the old behaviors to be transformed. The active child may learn to move more slowly, but the trait of activity is not lost or transformed. The environment, too, may change, because less is required of the child, but the values or goals underlying the requirement remain and are not changed.

An example of this goodness-of-fit model can be seen in one of our studies of sex-role behavior. We obtained early sex-role behavior in children as well as maternal attributes about sex role and asked how these two factors might affect subsequent adjustment. A goodness-of-fit model appeared to best explain the data. The sex-role behavior of 2-year-olds in terms of how much the children played with male and female sex-role toys were observed. There were large individual differences: some boys played more with boy toys than girl toys, and some boys played more with girl toys than boy toys. The same was true for the girls. Mothers were given the Bem Scales, and we were able to determine their sex-role orientation. Some mothers showed traditional sex-role beliefs, whereas others were more androgynous in their beliefs. We found that

school adjustment, as rated by the teacher, was dependent on neither the mother's belief nor the child's sex-role play. Rather, adjustment was dependent upon the goodness of fit between the child's play and the mother's belief. For example, boys showed subsequently better adjustment if their mothers were androgynous in belief, and they played equally with boy and girl toys, as well as if mothers were traditional and the boys played more with boy than girl toys. Adjustment at 6 years was worse if there was no fit, for example, if the mothers were traditional and the boys were androgynous, or if the mothers were androgynous and the boys were more male-toy oriented. The same was true for girls. The goodness of fit between the individual and its environment rather than the nature of the child's behavior itself may be more important for the development of maladaptive behavior (Lewis, 1987). One therapeutic solution, then, is to alter the maladaptive behavior of the individual: the other is to alter the nature of the fit. Matching children by their characteristics to teachers' traits reduces educational mismatch and may increase academic achievement.

The non-transformational feature of the goodness-of-fit model is particularly relevant for the development of psychopathology in two areas: the phenomenon of regression and the vulnerable child. Regression is a problem for any transactional model in which old behaviors are transformed and become new behaviors (Piaget, 1952). If old behaviors are transformed, they should disappear from the child's repertoire and should be unavailable for use once the new behaviors appear. This should be the case for the growth of intellectual or social behaviors. Nevertheless, it is clear that regression is a common occurrence in all domains and, as such, challenges the transformational model. It is not possible to use old behaviors if they were transformed. The appearance of regression requires that old behaviors do not disappear but are retained when new behaviors develop. New behaviors may have a greater likelihood of being elicited; however, old behaviors will occur, especially under stress.

The vulnerable or resilient child is another example of the usefulness of a non-transformational or interactive model. A vulnerable child possesses some characteristics that place him/her at risk. If the environment is positive, the at-risk features are not expressed and the child appears to be adjusted. Over repeated exposures to the positive environment, the child appears adjusted; however if given an instant or two of a negative environment, the child will appear maladjusted, showing abnormal behavior. For example, Sroufe (1983) once wrote that "even when children change rather markedly, the shadows of the earlier adaptation remain, and in times of stress, the prototype itself may be clear" (p. 74). It is obvious from this example that the positive environmental experiences were unable to transform the at-risk features that remained independent of their interaction with the environment. Likewise, if the child is resilient, then nonnegative experiences are likely to change this. This may be likely, however in the extreme may not be so (Rutter, 2012). If the at-risk features remain independent of the environment and are displaced as positive or negative adjustment only as the environment changes, then a goodness-of-fit model, rather than a transformational model, best explains the data. It is possible that at-risk features are influenced by the environment such that repeated positive exposures make the response to a negative event less severe—a type of threshold view. Under such conditions, we approach a transformational model.

Epigenetic Model

Of particular interest and one receiving considerable recent attention are the epigenetic models. While they are interactional they are not necessarily transactional; since the child characteristics may change, the environment usually remains consistent as does the child's DNA. The epigenetic model explores the effect of experience on gene expression and then gene expression and both brain and behavior. For the most part, the work has focused on how environmental stress impacts on the HPA axis which in turn modifies gene transcription. These models and data that support them can be seen in the recent work by Meany and associates (see Bush & Boyce, 2014, for more details).

Although not often discussed, there seems to be some indication that when the environmental perturbation stops, the gene expression may change back to a more normal state (Masterpasqua, 2009). The finding that placing pups of low-licking/-grooming mothers in a high-licking/-grooming situation suggests that environment change can change the gene expression in both a negative and positive way. These findings are also relevant for a discussion of critical periods since they indicate that pathological behaviors (even at the gene level) can right themselves when environments change.

Defining Maladaptive

In this section I will raise a number of issues having to do with defining maladaptive behavior and include the issues of (1) discrete versus continuous behavior, (2) who defines maladaptive behavior, (3) changes in maladaptive behavior with development, (4) predictions and the notion of sudden change, and finally (5) the construction of reality and maladaptive behavior.

Discrete Versus Continuous Behavior

We have little trouble in defining psychopathology when we observe psychoses, since behaviors such as hallucinations or deeply disturbed thinking patterns indicate a clear pattern.

On the other hand, there are behaviors we label as maladaptive. In deciding whether we wish to call the behaviors psychotic or disturbed, our classification system becomes more of a problem (see Achenbach, 2000). The issue here is whether all classes of psychopathology should be thought of as a yes-no, has or has not the disorder, or considered as a continuum. Psychotic disorders are usually thought of as yes-no: one cannot be a little psychotic. How about depression? It can be considered a yes-no disturbance, especially if we use a DSM-like classification system. On the other hand, it can be considered as a continuum, with the pathology classification representing one end of the continuum. Such problems continue to cause difficulties in the study of developmental psychopathology because of these sampling and classification issues. The classification issues have to do with many problems, including what should be considered an outcome measure.

Sampling issues arise when we use a yes-no classification system given the relatively low base rate of most clinical disorders. In order to study the development of these disorders, very large samples need to be collected. Select subjects, who are at high risk for a disorder, can be used, but the likelihood of obtaining a high rate of disorder, though increased, does not give us a very large number of subjects. Moreover, the selection of unique samples of high-risk children has its own problem. For example, the selection of a large schizophrenia sample for a study of its development requires the examination of schizophrenic mothers (Garmezy & Rutter, 1983; Sameroff & Seifer, 1981). We know that the number of children showing early disorders, but not schizophrenia, is relatively lower than would be expected (Garmezy et al., 1984). Parenthetically, this finding is related to our interest in resilience and the issue of invulnerability (Garmezy, 1981, 1989).

Perhaps of greatest concern is the use of ratings such as the CBCL (Achenbach, 1991). While the validity of the scales were established by a cutoff value which differentiated a clinical from a nonclinical sample, there have been no validations of pathology in values below the cutoff levels. Nevertheless, a large number of studies do not use the cutoff values but instead use the scales as a continuum. The reasons for this are, as we have pointed out, the low level of pathology in a sample as defined by the cutoff values. Even in large samples there are few subjects who qualify as having a maladaptive behavior. To solve this sampling problem, the maladaptive scales are used in a continuous fashion. In one highly reported study of the effects of day care, it was reported that while those in all day infant care had subsequently higher scores on the aggression subscale of the CBCL than those either not in infant day care or those with fewer hours of day care, none of the day-care groups had levels above the cutoff for this scale. The low level of psychopathology in the population leads to these types of difficulty, and one wonders how many findings reported which use the continuous measure to study the development of psychopathology can be replicated.

Who Defines Maladaptive or Psychopathology?

Still another problem related to the outcome measures is the issue of not only what the classification of children should be but also who classifies them. Typically, children themselves do not determine that they are disordered. Rather, a parent or teacher usually identifies signs of disorders and refers a child to a clinician. An examination of childhood disorder must include parents' and teachers' perceptions of the child as well as the child's own perceptions. However, studies of child disorder, for example, depression, show that different people's assessments of the same child do not agree (Jensen, Salzberg, Richters, & Watanabe, 1993; Stavrakaki, Vargo, Roberts, & Boodoosingh, 1987). Patterns of agreement are no more consistent when outside raters such as clinicians, teachers, or peers are employed. Kazdin, French, Unis, and Esveldt-Dawson (1983), for example, found that parents and clinicians were in stronger agreement than children and clinicians, but Moretti, Fine, Haley, and Marriage (1985), Poznanski, Mokros, Grossman, and Freeman (1985), and Stavrakaki et al. (1987) reported the opposite. Research examining agreement between teachers and children also shows low levels of agreement (Achenbach, 1991; Jacobsen, Lahey, & Strauss, 1983; McConaughy, Stanger, & Achenbach, 1992; Saylor, Finch, Baskin, Furey, & Kelly, 1984). Peer ratings sometimes correlate with children's self-reported depression (Jacobsen et al., 1983; Lefkowitz & Testiny, 1980; Saylor et al., 1984) but only in normal samples. This raises the general issue of whether the assessment of the child's characteristics is consistent across raters or different measures. If this is not so, then factors that impact on individual differences may vary depending on who measures the outcome.

Raters may disagree about the same child for a number of reasons. First, different instruments are usually used to obtain ratings from different people, and the instruments might not be compatible (Achenbach, 1991; McConaughy et al., 1992; Stanger, McConaughy, & Achenbach, 1992). Second, low rates of agreement about child disorder also may be due to the fact that some raters might not know the child well enough to draw clinical conclusions. This is particularly important for syndromes such as depression, which may reflect a child's "inner state." A third reason for low rates of agreement may be due to the rater's own problems. For example, mothers who are more depressed perceive their children as more depressed (Richters, 1992).

Finally, it is likely that people's perceptions are based on the child's behavior in different situations. Teachers and parents experience the child in different circumstances that require different coping skills. That children are seen in different situations that elicit different behaviors is likely to be an important factor. Situationally determined behavior has been well documented. There is evidence that different observers base their judgments on different characteristics of the child (Routh, 1990). For example, as long ago as 1985, Kazdin, Moser, Colbus, and Bell showed that parents and children emphasize different facets of the child's functioning. Children focused on internal feelings and expectancies for the future, while parents focused on the child's overt social behavior and outward manifestations of affect. Mischel (1990) has suggested that while behavior differs across situations, it may be consistent within situations. While parents, teachers, and children may disagree about the child, they may provide accurate assessments *within particular contexts.*

These problems support two ideas that need attention in any study of psychopathology. The first idea is that of an individual having characteristics that are enduring across situations and time. In general, while there may be some consistency across raters or scales and situations, the variance accounted for remains rather low considering the power of the idea of personality transcending

situation, context, and other people. The second idea is that from a developmental point of view, the idea of predicting individual differences in psychopathology over time may be difficult if there is low agreement in terms of the classification of children and adults in terms of their psychopathology.

Prediction and the Notion of Sudden Change

Predictability in the study of developmental psychopathology constitutes an important aspect of our definition (Sroufe & Rutter, 1984). Such a focus on prediction as a central feature is understandable because the origins of maladaptive behavior require an understanding of continuity and change. Even so, it is surprising that such a focus is required. Freud (1920/1955) doubted the ability of prediction. In truth, he appeared to be cognizant of the fact that retrospective prediction was much easier than prospective predication (see also Freeman, 1984). His belief about the complexity involved in the development of maladaptive as well as normal behavior made him skeptical about the ability to predict outcome. Even more important for our discussion is the recognitions that elaborate debate exists within the domain of normal development to question the issue of continuity and therefore of prediction. It would be a mistake to assume that prediction is always possible or even a desired goal. The relationship between continuity and prediction allows us to view this problem from a developmental perspective. Much has been written on this topic over the last 50 years (Lewis, 1997; Reese & Overton, 1970).

The idea of continuity also involves the idea of gradualism. As espoused by Darwin (1871), gradualism assumes that a series of small changes can account for the development of complex outcomes. Gradualism in evolution has been questioned by Eldredge and Gould (1972), who propose a theory of gradual change punctuated by sudden change. When applied to individual development, notions of continuity and gradualism take several forms, the most common form assuming that a person's development is an intraindividual process. Such theories assume that what the person is like now will determine what the person will be like in the future, the "trait" notion of development which predominates, especially in theories of social development.

Of course, general interactive models assume that an individual's development is the result of the continuing interactive process in which people adapt to their changing environments, which in turn affect the environments themselves. Such models by their nature make prediction difficult, since if the environment changes by some processes, they are in many cases random. Consider the effect of wars and military service on men's lives. Wars are exogenous (and presumably random) and yet profoundly affect lives, altering them in ways not readily predicted even if we were to have an accurate historical record of lives before the war (Elder, 1986). We could consider less dramatic events, such as death, illness, floods, and fires, all of which are random to lives and may profoundly alter them.

Any model that depicts development of psychopathology as a trajectory undisturbed by surrounding events, although created from the events earlier in time, needs reconsideration. As we have suggested, individuals develop in the presence of random events and their development may be more characterized by zigs and zags than by some predetermined connected and linear pattern. It is only when we understand how organisms are influenced by their environments now and how people's ideas for their future can affect their desires and behaviors that we can understand the nature of pathology.

The Construction of Reality

Any discussion of the interaction of the child's characteristics with the environment raises an important issue in the study of developmental psychopathology which has to do with the question raised about the difference between attachment and psychoanalytic theories which we characterized at the beginning of this chapter, that is, the question of the importance of the environment itself or the child's construction of it.

This is an interesting question since in attachment theory both of these views are measured. Consider that in infancy we measure the child's behavior toward the mother once she returns. In the AAI we measure the grown child's construction of the attachment model. While we assume these are the same, the first causing the second, this has not proven always to be the case (Lewis et al., 2000).

J.J. Gibson, in a wonderful article on the nature of the stimulus, raised this issue over 50 years ago (Gibson, 1960). Clearly, what we measure in the environment may not be what the child perceives or even constructs about the environment. In some sense, then, our measurement of the environment reflects a perspective which may not be reflected by the child we study. So, for example, we measure the level of depression that the child's mother reports about herself; however we do not measure the children's perception or even their construction of their mother's depression. Children may differ in their perceptions or constructions of reality for many reasons, including the mixed messages of the environment, such as the mother's saying "I am tired," rather than that she is depressed. We know, for example, that Chinese and American cultures differ in the degree of somatization versus psychological explanations used and this is likely to exist on an individual family basis. Child characteristics may also affect the child's perception and construction of its environment. The same parental punishment for a temperamentally fearful child may be expressed as quite different from a child who is not temperamentally fearful.

A particular case of some interest is related to how the child comes to experience one parent from the comments of the other. For example, a father who is absent, that is, has few interactions with his child, can be perceived in two different ways depending on how the child's mother explains his absence; in one case, "He is working hard to earn extra money for your education" versus "He is doing what he wants to do." In both cases the measurement of the time spent in interaction with his daughter is the same; however, the child's construction of her model of the father–child relationship is likely to be different.

While our measures of the environment become more complex, without considering the child's perspective of the nature of their environment, we assume that the nature of the structure (or environment) is what we measure rather than what the child perceives or constructs. However, before we even start our study of the child's perceptions and constructs, we need to recognize that children, certainly by the end of the second year of life, have an active self-referential system, a self system, which is active in creating plans and has intentionality and that their perceptions and constructs of their social and emotional worlds involve the interaction of this active self with their environment and that psychopathology may center in this constructed self-system.

References

Achenbach, T. M. (1991). *Manual for the child behavior checklist and 1991 child behavior profile*. Burlington, VT: University of Vermont, Department of Psychiatry.

Achenbach, T. M. (2000). Assessment of psychopathology. In A. J. Sameroff, M. Lewis, & S. M. Miller (Eds.), *Handbook of developmental psychopathology* (2nd ed., pp. 41–56). New York: Plenum.

Ainsworth, M. D. S. (1973). The development of infant-mother attachment. In B. M. Caldwell & H. N. Rissiuti (Eds.), *Review of child development research* (Vol. 3, pp. 1–95). Chicago: University of Chicago Press.

Ainsworth, M. D. S. (1989). Attachment beyond infancy. *American Psychologist, 44*, 709–716.

Allport, F. H., & Allport, G. W. (1921). Personality traits: Their classification and measurement. *Journal of Abnormal Psychology and Social Psychology, 16*, 6–40.

Anthony, E. J. (1970). The behavior disorders of children. In P. H. Mussen (Ed.), *Carmichael's manual of child psychology* (pp. 667–764). New York: Wiley.

Bandura, A. (1986). *Social foundations of thought and action: A social cognitive theory*. Englewood Cliffs, NJ: Prentice-Hall.

Bellin, H. (1971). The development of physical concepts. In T. Michel (Ed.), *Cognitive development and epistemology* (pp. 85–119). New York: Academic Press.

Bem, S. L. (1987). Masculinity and femininity exist only in the mind of the perceiver. In J. M. Reinisch, L. A. Rosenblum, & S. A. Sanders (Eds.), *Masculinity/femininity: Basic perspectives* (pp. 304–314). New York: Oxford University Press.

Block, J., & Block, T. H. (1980). The role of ego control and ego resiliency in the organization of behavior. In W. Collins (Ed.), *Minnesota Symposium on Child Psychology* (Vol. 13, pp. 325–377). Hillsdale, NJ: Erlbaum.

Bowlby, J. (1969). *Attachment and loss: Vol. 1. Attachment*. New York: Basic Books.

Bronfenbrenner, U., & Crouter, A. C. (1983). The evolution of environmental models in developmental research. In W. Kessen & P. H. Mussen (Eds.), *History, theory, and methods: Handbook of child psychology* (Vol. 1, pp. 357–414). New York: Wiley.

Bush, N. R., & Boyce, W. T. (2014). The contributions of early experience to biological development and sensitivity to context. In M. Lewis & K. Rudolph (Eds.), *Handbook of developmental psychopathology* (3rd ed.). New York: Springer.

Cairns, R. B., & Cairns, B. D. (2000). The natural history and developmental functions of aggression. In A. J. Sameroff, M. Lewis, & S. M. Miller (Eds.), *Handbook of developmental psychopathology* (2nd ed., pp. 403–429). New York: Plenum.

Chess, S., & Thomas, A. (1984). *Origins and evolution of behavior disorders*. New York: Brunnser/Mazel.

Chomsky, N. (Ed.). (1957). *Syntactic structures*. The Hague: Mouton.

Chomsky, N. (Ed.). (1965). *Aspects of the theory of syntax*. Cambridge, MA: MIT Press.

Darwin, C. (1871). *On the origin of species*. London: John Murray.

Eagle, M. N. (2013). *Attachment and psychoanalysis: Theory, research, and clinical implications*. New York: Guilford Press.

Elder, G. H., Jr. (1986). Military times and turning points in men's lives. *Developmental Psychology, 22*, 233–245.

Eldredge, N., & Gould, S. J. (1972). Punctuated equilibria: An alternative to phyletic gradualism. In T. J. Schopf (Ed.), *Models in paleobiology* (pp. 83–115). San Francisco, CA: Truman Cooper.

Fagot, B. I. (1973). Sex-related stereotyping of toddlers' behaviors. *Developmental Psychology, 9*, 429.

Feiring, C., Lewis, M., & Starr, M. D. (1984). Indirect effects and infants' reaction to strangers. *Developmental Psychology, 20*, 485–491.

Fox, N. A., Kimmerly, N. L., & Schafer, W. D. (1991). Attachment to mother/attachment to father: A meta-analysis. *Child Development, 62*(1), 210–225.

Freeman, M. (1984). History, narrative, and life-span development knowledge. *Human Development, 27*, 1–19.

Freud, S. (1955). The psychogenesis of a case of homosexuality in a woman. In J. Strachey (Ed. and Trans.), *The standard edition of the complete psychological works of Sigmund Freud* (Vol. 18, pp. 118–139). London: Hogarth. (Original work published 1920).

Gardner, H. (1985). *The mind's new science*. New York: Basic Books.

Garmezy, N. (1974). The study of competence in children at risk for severe psychopathology. In E. Anthony & C. Koupernik (Eds.), *The child in his family* (Vol. 3, pp. 77–98). New York: Wiley.

Garmezy, N. (1981). Children under stress: Perspectives on antecedents and correlates of vulnerability and resistance to psychopathology. In A. I. Rabin, J. Arnoff, A. M. Barclay, & R. A. Zucker (Eds.), *Further explorations in personality* (pp. 126–145). New York: Wiley.

Garmezy, N. (1989). Stress-resistant children: The search for protective factors. In J.E. Stevenson (Ed.), *Aspects of current child psychiatry research (Journal of Child Psychology and Psychiatry Book Supplement, No. 4*, pp. 213–233). Oxford: Pergamon Press.

Garmezy, N., Masten, A. S., & Tellegen, A. (1984). The study of stress and competence in children: A building block for developmental psychopathology. *Child Development, 55*, 987–1111.

Garmezy, N., & Rutter, M. (1983). *Stress, coping, and development in children*. New York: McGraw-Hill.

Gibson, J. J. (1960). The concept of the stimulus in psychology. *American Psychologist, 15*, 694–703.

Gibson, J. J. (1969). *Principles of perceptual learning and development*. New York: Appleton.

Goldberg, S., & Lewis, M. (1969). Play behavior in the year-old infant: Early sex differences. *Child Development, 40*, 21–31.

Gottesman, I., & Shields, J. (1982). *Schizophrenia: The epigenetic puzzle*. New York: Cambridge University Press.

Harlow, H. F., & Harlow, M. K. (1965). The affectional systems. In A. M. Schrier, H. F. Harlow, & F. Stollnitz (Eds.), *Behavior of nonhuman primates* (Vol. 2). New York: Academic Press.

Jacobsen, R. H., Lahey, B. B., & Strauss, C. C. (1983). Correlates of depressed mood in children. *Journal of Abnormal Child Psychology, 11*, 29–40.

Jensen, P. S., Salzberg, A. D., Richters, J. E., & Watanabe, H. K. (1993). Scales, diagnoses, and child psychopathology: I. CBCL and DISC relationships. *Journal of the American Academy of Child and Adolescent Psychiatry, 32*, 397–406.

Kallman, F. J. (1946). The genetic theory of schizophrenia: An analysis of 691 schizophrenic twin index families. *American Journal of Psychiatry, 103*, 309–322.

Kazdin, A. E., French, N. H., Unis, A. S., & Esveldt-Dawson, I. (1983). Assessment of childhood depression: Correspondence of child and parent ratings. *Journal of the American Academy of Child Psychiatry, 22*, 157–164.

Kazdin, A. E., Moser, J., Colbus, D., & Bell, R. (1985). Depressive symptoms among physically abused and psychiatrically disturbed children. *Journal of Abnormal Psychology, 94*, 298–307.

Kringlon, E. (1968). An epidemiological twin study of schizophrenia. In D. Rosenthal & S. Kety (Eds.), *The transmission of schizophrenia* (pp. 49–63). New York: Pergamon Press.

Lamb, M. E., Thompson, R., Gardner, W., & Charnov, E. (1985). *Infant-mother attachment: The origins and developmental significance of individual differences in strange situation behavior*. Hillsdale, NJ: Erlbaum.

Lefkowitz, M. M., & Testiny, E. P. (1980). Assessment of childhood depression. *Journal of Consulting and Clinical Psychology, 48*, 43–50.

Lerner, R. M. (1984). *On the nature of human plasticity*. New York: Cambridge University Press.

Lerner, R. M. (2006). Developmental science, developmental systems, and contemporary theories of human development. In R. M. Lerner (Ed.), W. Damon & R. M. Lerner (Editors-in-chief), *Handbook of child psychology: Vol. 1. Theoretical models of human development* (6th ed., pp. 1–17). Hoboken, NJ: Wiley.

Lewis, M. (1972). State as an infant-environment interaction: An analysis of mother-infant interaction as a function of sex. *Merrill-Palmer Quarterly, 18*, 95–121.

Lewis, M. (1979). The self as a developmental concept. *Human Development, 22*, 416–419.

Lewis, M. (1983). Newton, Einstein, Piaget, and the concept of the self. In L. S. Liben (Ed.), *Piaget and the foundations of knowledge* (pp. 141–177). Hillsdale, NJ: Erlbaum.

Lewis, M. (1985). Age as a social dimension. In T. Field & N. Fox (Eds.), *Social perception in infants* (pp. 299–319). New York: Academic Press.

Lewis, M. (1987). Early sex role behavior and school age adjustment. In J. M. Reinisch, L. A. Rosenblum, & S. A. Sanders (Eds.), *Masculinity/Femininity: Basic perspectives* (pp. 202–226). New York: Oxford University Press.

Lewis, M. (1997). *Altering fate: Why the past does not predict the future*. New York: Guilford Press.

Lewis, M. (2010). The emergence of consciousness and its role in human development. In R. Lerner & W. Overton (Eds.), *The handbook of lifespan development* (Cognition, biology, and methods, Vol. 1, pp. 628–670). Hoboken, NJ: Wiley.

Lewis, M. (2013). Beyond the dyad. In L. Mayes & M. Lewis (Eds.), *The Cambridge handbook of environment in human development* (pp. 103–116). New York: Cambridge University Press.

Lewis, M. (2014). *The rise of consciousness and the development of emotional life*. New York: Guilford Press.

Lewis, M., & Feiring, C. (1981). Direct and indirect interactions in social relationships. In L. Lipsitt (Ed.), *Advances in infancy research, 1* (pp. 129–161). New York: Ablex.

Lewis, M., & Feiring, C. (1989). Infant, mother and mother-infant interaction behavior and subsequent attachment. *Child Development, 60*, 831–837.

Lewis, M., & Feiring, C. (1991). Attachment as personal characteristic or a measure of the environment. In J. L. Gewirtz & W. M. Kurtines (Eds.), *Intersections with attachment* (pp. 1–21). Hillsdale, NJ: Erlbaum.

Lewis, M., Feiring, C., & Rosenthal, S. (2000). Attachment over time. *Child Development, 71*(3), 707–720.

Lewis, M., & Miller, S. (1990). *Handbook of developmental psychopathology*. New York: Plenum.

Lewis, M., & Rosenblum, L. (Eds.). (1974). *The effect of the infant on its caregiver: The origins of behavior, 1*. New York: Wiley.

Lewis, M., & Schaeffer, S. (1981). Peer behavior and mother-infant interaction in maltreated children. In M. Lewis & L. Rosenblum (Eds.), *The uncommon child: The genesis of behavior, 3* (pp. 193–223). New York: Plenum.

Main, M., Kaplan, N., & Cassidy, J. (1985). Security in infancy, childhood, and adulthood: A move to the level or representation. In I. Bretherton & W. Waters (Eds.), *Growing points of attachment theory and research. Monographs of the Society for Research in Child*

Development (Vol. 50(1–2, Serial No. 209), pp. 66–104).

Masterpasqua, F. (2009). Psychology and epigenetics. *Review of General Psychology, 13*(3), 194–201.

Mayes, L., & Lewis, M. (Eds.). (2013). *The Cambridge handbook of environment in human development*. New York: Cambridge University Press.

McConaughy, S. H., Stanger, C., & Achenbach, T. M. (1992). Three-year course of behavioral/emotional problems in a national sample of 4- to 16-year-olds: I. Agreement among informants. *Journal of the American Academy of Child and Adolescent Psychiatry, 31*, 932–940.

Mischel, W. (1965). *Personality assessment*. New York: Wiley.

Mischel, W. (1990). Personality dispositions revisited and revised: A view after three decades. In L. Pervin (Ed.), *Handbook of personality: Theory and research* (pp. 111–134). New York: Guilford Press.

Moretti, M. M., Fine, S., Haley, G., & Marriage, K. (1985). Childhood and adolescent depression: Child-report vs. parent-report information. *Journal of the American Academy of Child Psychiatry, 24*, 298–302.

Nelson, C. A., Zeanah, C. H., Fox, N. A., Marshall, P. J., Smyke, A. T., & Guthrie, D. (2007). Cognitive recovery in socially deprived young children: The Bucharest early intervention project. *Science, 318*(5858), 1937–1940.

Overton, W. F. (2006). Developmental psychology: Philosophy, concepts, methodology. In R. M. Lerner & W. Damon (Eds.), *Handbook of child psychology. Theoretical models of human development* (6th ed., Vol. 1, pp. 18–88). Hoboken, NJ: Wiley.

Piaget, J. (1952). *The origins of intelligence in children* (M. Cook, Trans.) New York: International Universities Press. (Original work published 1936).

Poznanski, E., Mokros, H. B., Grossman, J., & Freeman, L. N. (1985). Diagnostic criteria in childhood depression. *American Journal of Psychiatry, 142*, 1168–1173.

Puig-Antich, J. (1982). Psychobiological correlates of major depressive disorder in children and adolescents. In L. Greenspan (Ed.), *Psychiatry 1982: Annual Review* (pp. 41–64). Washington, DC: American Psychological Association.

Reese, H. W., & Overton, W. F. (1970). Models of development and theories of development. In L. R. Goulet & P. B. Baltes (Eds.), *Life-span developmental psychology: Research and theory* (pp. 115–145). New York: Academic Press.

Repacholi, B. M., Meltzoff, A. N., & Olsen, B. (2008). Infants' understanding of the link between visual perception and emotion: "If she can't see me doing it, she won't get angry.". *Developmental Psychology, 44*(2), 561–574.

Rheingold, H. L., & Cook, K. V. (1975). The content of boys' and girls' rooms as an index of parents' behavior. *Child Development, 46*, 459–563.

Richters, J. E. (1992). Depressed mothers as informants about their children: A critical review of the evidence for distortion. *Psychological Bulletin, 112*, 485–499.

Riegel, K. F. (1978). *Psychology, mon amour: A countertext*. Boston, MA: Houghton Mifflin.

Routh, D. K. (1990). Taxonomy in developmental psychopathology: Consider the source. In M. Lewis & S. M. Miller (Eds.), *Handbook of developmental psychopathology* (pp. 53–62). New York: Plenum Press.

Rutter, M. (1979). Protective factors in children's responses to stress and disadvantage. In M. W. Kent & J. G. Rolf (Eds.), *Primary prevention of psychopathology* (Social competence in children, Vol. 3, pp. 150–162). Hanover, NH: University Press of New England.

Rutter, M. (1981). Stress, coping and development: Some issues and some questions. *Journal of Child Psychology and Psychiatry, 22*, 323–356.

Rutter, M. (2012). 'Natural experiments' as a means of testing causal inferences. In C. Barzini, P. Dawid, & L. Bernardinelli (Eds.), *Causality: Statistical Perspectives and Applications* (pp. 253–272). Chichester: Wiley.

Rutter, M. (2013). Nature-nurture integration. In M. Lewis & K. Rudolph (Eds.), *Handbook of developmental psychopathology* (3rd ed.). New York: Springer.

Sameroff, A. J. (2014). A dialectic integration of development for the study of psychopathology. In M. Lewis & K. Rudolph (Eds.), *Handbook of developmental psychopathology* (3rd ed.). New York: Springer.

Sameroff, A. J., & Chandler, M. J. (1975). Reproductive risk and the continuum of caretaking causality. In F. D. Horowitz (Ed.), *Review of child development research* (Vol. 4, pp. 187–244). Chicago, IL: University of Chicago Press.

Sameroff, A. J., & Seifer, B. (1981). The transmission of incompetence: The offspring of mentally ill women. In M. Lewis & L. Rosenblum (Eds.), *The uncommon child: The genesis of behavior, 3* (pp. 63–90). New York: Plenum.

Saudino, K. J. (1997). Moving beyond the heritability question: New directions in behavioral genetic studies of personality. *Current Directions in Psychological Science, 6*(4), 86–90.

Saylor, C. F., Finch, A. J., Baskin, C. H., Furey, W., & Kelly, M. (1984). Construct validity for measures of childhood depression: Application of a multitrait-multimethod methodology. *Journal of Consulting and Clinical Psychology, 52*, 977–985.

Schneider-Rosen, K., & Cicchetti, D. (1984). The relationship between affect and cognition in maltreated infants: Quality of attachment and the development of visual self-recognition. *Child Development, 55*, 648–658.

Sheridan, M. A., Fox, N. A., Zeanah, C. H., McLaughlin, K. A., & Nelson, C. A. (2012). Variation in neural development as a result of exposure to institutionalization early in childhood. *Proceedings of the National Academy of Sciences, 109*(32), 12927–12932.

Sheridan, M. A., Sarsour, K., Jutte, D., D'Esposito, M., & Boyce, W. T. (2012). The impact of social disparity on prefrontal function in childhood. *PLoS ONE, 7*(4). doi:10.1371/journal.pone.0035744.

Sroufe, L. A. (1983). Infant-caregiver attachment and patterns of adaptation in preschool: The roots of maladaptation and competence. In M. Perlmutter (Ed.),

Minnesota Symposium in Child Psychology (Vol. 16, pp. 41–83). Hillsdale, NJ: Erlbaum.

Sroufe, L. A., Coffino, B., & Carlson, E. A. (2010). Conceptualizing the role of early experience: Lessons from the Minnesota longitudinal study. *Developmental Review, 30*(1), 36–51.

Sroufe, L. A., Egeland, B., Carlson, E. A., & Collins, W. A. (2005). *The development of the person: The Minnesota study of risk and adaptation from birth to adulthood*. New York: Guilford.

Sroufe, L. A., & Rutter, M. (1984). The domain of developmental psychopathology. *Child Development, 55*, 17–29.

Stanger, C., McConaughy, S. H., & Achenbach, T. M. (1992). Three-year course of behavioral/emotional problems in a national sample of 4–16 year olds: II. Predictors of syndromes. *Journal of the American Academy of Child and Adolescent Psychiatry, 31*, 941–950.

Stavrakaki, C., Vargo, B., Roberts, N., & Boodoosingh, L. (1987). Concordance among sources of information for ratings of anxiety and depression in children. *Journal of the American Academy of Child and Adolescent Psychiatry, 26*, 733–737.

Steele, H., & Steele, M. (2014). Attachment disorders: Theory, research, and treatment considerations. In M. Lewis & K. Rudolph (Eds.), *Handbook of developmental psychopathology* (3rd ed.). New York: Springer.

Sterba, S. (2014). Modeling strategies in developmental psychopathology research: Prediction of individual change. In M. Lewis & K. Rudolph (Eds.), *Handbook of developmental psychopathology* (3rd ed.). New York: Springer.

Szasz, T. S. (1961). *The myth of mental illness*. New York: Harper & Row.

Thomas, A., & Chess, S. (1977). *Temperament and development*. New York: Brunner/Mazel.

Thompson, R. A., Lamb, M. E., & Estes, D. (1982). Stability of infant-mother attachment and its relationship to changing life circumstances in an unselected middle class sample. *Child Development, 53*, 144–148.

Zahn-Waxler, C., Cummings, E. M., McKnew, D. H., & Radke-Yarrow, N. (1984). Altruism, aggression, and social interactions in young children with a manic-depressive parent. *Child Development, 55*, 112–122.

Zhang, T.-Y., & Meaney, M. J. (2010). Epigenetics and the environmental regulation of the genome and its function. *Annual Review of Psychology, 61*, 439–466.

A Dialectic Integration of Development for the Study of Psychopathology

Arnold J. Sameroff

The field of developmental psychopathology was initially focused on efforts to understand the etiology of adult mental disorders by studying children and their disorders. However, this effort produced unanticipated changes in our understanding of pathology, individual development, and the role of social context. Among these modifications were the blurring of the division between mental illness and mental health, the need to attend to patterns of adaptation rather than personality traits, and the powerful influences of the social world on individual development. Current developmental views place deviancy in the dynamic relation between individuals and their contexts. From another perspective, the history of developmental psychopathology is an example of universal dialectical processes where action in the world, that is, research on mental illness, produces results that contradict the models that inspired that action, that is, linear models of individual psychopathology. Dialectical developmental processes are evident as we trace how patterns of adaptation by researchers, expressed in theoretical models and empirical paradigms, increasingly have come to match the complexities of human mental health and illness.

The attention of philosophers and then scientists to human development has always begun with a concern that children should grow up to be good citizens who would contribute to society through diligent labor, moral family life, and civil obedience, and, more recently, to be happy while making these contributions. The motivation for these concerns was that there were many adults who were not. Although attention was paid to the socialization and education of children, it was ultimately in the service of improving adult performance. The societal concern has always had a lifespan perspective. Without healthy, productive adults no culture could continue to be successful.

With these civic motivations and supports, there have been major advances in our understanding of the intellectual, emotional, and social behavior of children, adolescents, and adults. Moreover these understandings have increasingly involved multilevel processes cutting across disciplinary boundaries in the social and natural sciences. This progress has forced conceptual reorientations as earlier unidirectional views that biological or social circumstance controlled individual behavior have become multidirectional perspectives where individual behavior reciprocally changes both biological and social circumstance.

Understanding continuity was the basis of traditional developmental science. Understanding discontinuity is the basis of contemporary developmental science. Why is it that a biological gene or human trait does not always lead to the same outcome? More complexly, why is it that some children who are doing well end up as adults with many problems, and more hopefully, why is it that some children with many problems end up doing very well as adults? The answer lies in the

A.J. Sameroff, Ph.D. (✉)
University of Michigan, Ann Arbor, MI 48109, USA
e-mail: sameroff@umich.edu; sameroff@gmail.com

series of development steps where context amplifies or reduces the effects of prior steps. Multidisciplinary efforts in the biological and social sciences continue to demonstrate that successful developmental predictions from prior genetic or psychological measures are highly contingent on the child's environment. For those concerned with improving developmental outcomes, explaining discontinuities has a high priority because they offer opportunities to change the course of development through therapeutic interventions. Understanding such discontinuities requires integrating analyses of individual behavior with constructs from the full range of life and social sciences.

The theoretical history of developmental psychopathology has been characterized by swings between beliefs that determinants of an individual's behavior could be found either in their irreducible fundamental units or in their irreducible fundamental experiences. The growth process between babyhood and adulthood could be explained by appeals either to *intrinsic* properties of the child or to *extrinsic* properties of experience—the nature-nurture dilemma. Current research continues to document how deterministic conceptualizations of either emphasize the limitations of both approaches. In a collaborative study of the genetic determinants of height, one of the most heritable human traits, with a combined sample of 63,000 individuals and assessing 500,000 genetic variations, three genes were found to be related to the outcome (Visscher, 2008). Combined they explained only 3 % of the variance. If 97 % of the variance is left unexplained in this classic quantitative trait, what can we expect for much more complex psychological characteristics? On the environmental side one of the most universal transmitted traits is culture. However, when culture is examined as a predictor, more variation for psychological traits is found within cultures than between them. Similarly more psychological variation is found within neighborhoods than between, within schools than between and within families than between (Furstenburg, Cook, Eccles, Elder, & Sameroff, 1999).

Practically, the nature-nurture question comes into play when a child has a problem, and the question arises, "Who is responsible?" Most parents' first response is to blame the child, and most professionals' first response is to blame the parents. However, most scientists know that it is both. It is both child and parent, but it is also neurons and neighborhoods, synapses and schools, proteins and peers, and genes and governments. But that conclusion does not explain how it is both. Explicating the probabilistic transactions between individual and context will be the topic of this chapter. In what follows I will present a contemporary summary of what developmental models should contain and offer a suggestion for an integrated view of psychopathology that captures much of the variance that needs explaining.

Roots of Developmental Psychopathology

There is a set of unresolvable dialectical contradictions inherent in any discipline, and it is within these contradictions that the sources of progress can be found. Some of these contradictions are inherent in the study of psychology, some in the study of development, and some unique to the study of developmental psychopathology. One of the basic contradictions in each of these domains is between the labels used to divide and categorize the phenomena of concern and the dynamic reality which comprises the phenomena themselves. Unique to the study of pathology is the contradiction between the abstracted diagnostic schemes used for categorizing individuals and the complex dynamic processes of the individuals themselves.

Another contradiction is the contrast between the study of serious mental disorders and mental health. Whereas clinicians have needed to center their attention on children who are in the greatest therapeutic need, most developmentalists who have entered the field have viewed the study of pathology in the few as a means for understanding the roots of mental health in the many. The study of mental disorder may be inseparable from the study of mental health, and it may be that the study of each is required for the understanding of the other (Sroufe, 1990).

The field is labeled with a concern for pathology, that is, disease. Here we find another important dialectical contradiction in the name developmental psychopathology. By using a developmental approach in the study of pathology, we may find that the disease disappears when understood as one of many adaptational processes between an individual and life experiences. The final contradiction lies in the nature-nurture dichotomy where we find that by studying the environment we obtain a better understanding of the individual and by studying the individual we obtain a better understanding of the environment. The better we understand the sources of these contradictions, the better will we be at understanding and changing the mental health of children. The theoretical issues in developmental psychopathology can be captured in three major areas, the conceptualizations of pathology, individual development, and the role of the environment.

How Do We Define Pathology?

Is it a qualitative or quantitative judgment? Can individuals be placed on universal dimensions, or are there qualitative distinctions to be made that place people in one category or another? This is one aspect of the continuity vs. discontinuity issue, here between one kind of individual and another.

The discipline of developmental psychopathology has been promoted as the foundation for major advances in our ability to understand, treat, and prevent mental disorders (Cicchetti, 1989). One assumption underlying this expectation is that the perspectives of developmentalists and psychopathologists offer different conceptualizations of the same phenomena and that their unification would produce a clarification of the appearance and etiology of psychological disturbances. In this vein Rutter and Garmezy (1983) characterized this difference as the developmentalist's concern with *continuity* in functioning such that severe symptoms are placed on the same

dimension as more normal behaviors in contrast to the pathologist's concern with *discontinuity* where the abnormal is differentiated from the normal. The division of the field into those who approach the problem from a developmental perspective and those that approach from a clinical perspective has served to mask the fact that there are many different kinds of developmentalists and many different kinds of psychopathologists. These differences arise in contrasting interpretations of behavioral development and ultimately in contrasting views of the sources of behavioral deviation as either deterministic or probabilistic.

There are two basic questions that need to be addressed for understanding childhood psychopathology. One is *what does it mean to be disordered,* and the other is *are disordered children different in kind or in degree.* These issues have been best described by Zigler and Hodapp (1986) in their interpretation of mental retardation. In their view there are two kinds of children with low intelligence scores. One group is dimensional and identified by the diagnostic test. They are part of the normal distribution of any attribute and represent, in the case of mental retardation, the less than 3 % of individuals who are two standard deviations below the mean. Labeling them as retarded is an artifact of the normal distribution and not of the individuals themselves. It also produced the artifact of the 6-hour retarded child, who only manifests the difficulty when assessed through the lens of scholastic standards, yet shows adequate social competence in the worlds of work and social relationships. This categorical view of retardation is further undermined by the major reduction in the percentage of mentally retarded individuals after 18 years of age when they leave the academic environment and are no longer subject to normed tests of development (Berkson, 1978).

There is a second group of individuals who score in the retarded range who are indeed different in kind from the first. They are organically impaired, and the correlates of their low scores on the IQ test will be different than those who are only at the low end of the normal distribution. Because their biology is different, the processes by which they develop may be different, and the therapeutic treatments required to improve their status may be different from the first group of children who are at the low end of the normal distribution. Behavioral genetic research has provided some confirmation for this dichotomy in that siblings of severely retarded children with IQs less than 50 tend to have normal average IQs of around 100, whereas siblings of mildly retarded children with IQs in the 60s had a lower average IQ of 85 and 20 % were themselves retarded (Nichols, 1984).

When we move from mental retardation to mental illness, we are struck with the same question. Do the children with whom we are concerned represent the lowest part of a normal distribution, or are they different in kind from the rest of the population? The answer to this question will have powerful implications for our understanding and treatment of their mental health problems. Community surveys of mental health routinely diagnose many more individuals as having psychopathology than make their way to clinical facilities. Are these results because of the lack of adequate services or because their aberrant behavior is compensated by their life circumstances? Are there mental health criteria that distinguish those who are "really" deviant from those who are not? Moreover will these criteria apply to individuals regardless of their context or only reflect deviance between individuals and their specific contexts?

How Do We Understand Individuals and Their Development?

Is it through a search for stable characteristics of the individual independent of context, or is it the search for patterns of functioning in context? Moreover, when these characteristics change over time, is it the unfolding of some maturational pattern or a reaction to new contextual demands as each individual interacts with an expanding social domain? Again the continuity-discontinuity issue is of central concern.

Progress in the technology of molecular genetics has led to hopes that the etiology of mental disorders will soon be revealed and that their treatment and prevention will follow. Although we may view this as a technological statement of fact, it can alternatively be interpreted as the expression of a particular belief system about the nature of the child and especially the nature of pathology. The basis for such linear hopes is a view of humans as determined by their biology and a view of development as an unfolding of predetermined lines of growth. Among these hypothesized lines of development are those that produce the emotionally disturbed, such as schizophrenics and depressives; the cognitively disturbed, such as the learning disabled and the retarded; and the undisturbed, that is, normal individuals.

But does this model fit those individuals who do not stay on their predicted trajectories? There have been many full-term healthy infants who were predicted to have a happy course but instead ended up with a variety of mental disorders later in life. In these cases one could argue that we have not yet developed the sophisticated diagnostic tools to identify their inherent deviancy at birth. However, how would one explain those infants who had already shown major disabilities and yet somehow did not progress to adult forms of disturbance (Sameroff & Chandler, 1975)? The biographies of many individuals that were certain candidates for a life of institutionalization but whose fate was altered to a happier end have been well documented (cf. Garmezy, 1985).

The Rochester Longitudinal Study (RLS) that my colleagues, Melvin Zax, Ronald Seifer, Ralph Barocas, and Alfred and Clara Baldwin, have been involved in for 40 years (Sameroff, Seifer, Baldwin, & Baldwin, 1993; Sameroff, Seifer, & Zax, 1982; Sameroff & Zax, 1973) was an example of an old research model that centered on a linear analysis of the effects of parental psychopathology on child behavior. During the course of the study, however, adaptive changes were forced upon the investigators because of the lack of congruence between hypotheses and data. This dialectical process produced changes in the analytic strategy as well as the investigators' understanding of development—from a study of genetic influences on behavior to an investigation of the interaction of complex dynamic processes between individual and context. Bridging the gap between the unlimited complexity of dynamic developmental conceptualizations and the limited complexity of possible empirical investigations characterizes the scientific problem for the discipline of developmental psychopathology.

In 1968, we (Sameroff & Zax, 1973) initiated a study using the high-risk approach to examine the early development of children of parents who had a variety of psychiatric diagnoses with special attention to schizophrenia. At the outset we considered three major hypotheses: (1) that deviant behavior in the child would be attributed to variables associated with a specific maternal diagnosis, e.g., schizophrenia; (2) that deviant behavior would be attributable to variables associated with characteristics of mental illness in general, like the severity and chronicity of the disorder, but no diagnostic group in particular; and (3) that deviant behavior would be associated with social circumstances, exclusive of parental psychopathology.

The first hypothesis found little support. Most of the significant differences found for the schizophrenic group occurred during the prenatal period, and these differences were in the mothers, not in the children. The schizophrenic mothers were the most anxious and least socially competent. They also had the worst prenatal obstetric status. The second hypothesis, that mental illness in general would produce substantial effects, was supported more strongly. In almost every instance where there was a difference between diagnostic groups, it could be explained by a corresponding difference in the severity and/or chronicity of the illness. In addition, there were a large number of developmental effects produced by severity and/or chronicity differences that did not have corresponding diagnostic differences. When the number of significant outcomes was compared for differences in the diagnostic, mental illness, and social status dimensions, the highest density was found in the social class contrasts, the third hypothesis. One of the more interesting results was that the differences found between offspring of women with psychiatric diagnoses and those without were almost the same as those between offspring of lower and higher social status women.

From these analyses a relatively clear picture could be seen. Among the mental illness measures, severity and chronicity of maternal disturbances were better predictors of risk than their specific diagnoses, but even stronger effects on development were found from social status variables. At Rochester we were struck by how our attempts to study the child out of context were defeated by the profound effects of social variables on the lives of the children in our investigation. The contradiction here was that research devoted to understanding the nature of the child at risk for schizophrenia brought to the fore information that it may be the nature of the environment that was as important as any biological heritage for their future mental health.

How Do We Conceptualize the Environment?

Is it a passive set of additive experiences that maximizes or minimizes innate individual potential as in the concept of genetic ranges of reaction, or does experience have nonlinear transformative effects as it interacts and transacts with dynamic individual developmental processes? This issue will be fully explored in the following description of a unified theory of development.

A Unified Theory of Development

In tune with the advanced understanding of molecular genetics, there is a contemporary zeitgeist emphasizing dynamic conceptualizations within most scientific disciplines. In his spirit, I recently proposed that contemporary theories of development require at least four models for understanding human psychological change: a *personal* one, a *contextual* one, a *regulation* one, and a *representational* one (Sameroff, 2010). However, a fifth model for *evolutionary* change has become essential. The *personal model* is necessary for understanding the progression of competencies from infancy on. It requires unpacking the changing complexity of the individual as he or she moves from the sensorimotor functioning of infancy to increasingly intricate levels of cognition, from early attachments with a few caregivers to relationships with many peers, teachers, and others in the world beyond home and school, and from the early differentiation of self and other to the multifaceted personal and cultural identities of adolescence and adulthood. The *contextual model* is necessary to delineate the multiple sources of experience that augment or constrain individual development. The growing child is increasingly involved with a variety of social settings and institutions that have direct or indirect impact as exemplified in Bronfenbrenner's (1977) view of the social ecology. The *regulation model* adds a dynamic systems perspective to the relation between person and context. During early development, human regulation moves from the primarily biological to the psychological and social. What begins as the regulation of temperature, hunger, and arousal soon turns to regulation of attention, behavior, and social interactions. The *representational model* is where an individual's here and now experiences in the world are given a longer term existence in thought. These representations are the cognitive structures where experience is encoded at abstracted levels that provide an interpretive structure for new experiences, as well as a sense of self and other. Finally the *evolutionary* model is necessary to explain the codevelopment of genetic polymorphisms, psychological, and social functioning. Combining these five models offers a comprehensive view of the multiple parts, wholes, and interconnecting processes that comprise human development, especially as they are related to psychopathology. Moreover, within each model there is evidence of discontinuities that can expand or contract the developmental success of children.

Personal Model

Because psychology's central focus is on individuals, developmental psychopathology's main concerns have been on how children change over time, especially how early characteristics lead to mental health problems. How one thinks about change will have a clear influence on research objectives. Three ways of conceptualizing change are notions about trait, growth, and development. If one believes that an individual consists of a set of unchanging traits, then there is no need for developmental research. Thinking about change as a growth process allows for change but only on quantitative dimensions, more words, more numbers, more ideas. Viewing personal change as development implies qualitative changes where there is a period of stability of functioning followed by a transition to a structurally different period of stability presumed to reflect more encompassing cognitive and social functioning. The classic examples of stages are in the writings of Freud and Piaget. Although there have been major revisions or rejections of their specific formulations, there are some generally accepted notions that within many domains individuals move in steps from novices, to experts, to masters where they do not just do things better, they do things differently (Ericsson & Charness, 1994). Qualitative or structural reorganizations of the individual are the points of discontinuity where children can enter different trajectories for better or worse. The study of depression and conduct disorder in children are examples of empirical complexities in attempts to use specific diagnoses as continuing individual characteristics.

Depression

The criteria for identifying children with depression vary from high scores on a parent checklist to careful diagnostic interviews. Compas and Hammen (1994) did an extensive analysis of the meaning of such scores, and they raised three questions overlapping with our present concerns. The questions were whether a depressive disorder in childhood takes the same form as a depressive disorder in adulthood, whether high depression scores are different in quality or merely quantity from low depression scores, and whether depression is a unitary construct that can be separated from the symptoms of other disorders—the comorbidity question.

Their conclusions increase the complexity of the diagnostic problem because there appear to be three levels of depressive phenomena with similar degrees of sadness—depressed mood, depressive syndromes, and depressive disorders. It is only the latter with criteria for an extended duration and accompanying functional impairment that qualifies for the categorical diagnosis. But the bigger difficulty is that it is rare for children who have depression problems to only have depression problems. There is a tendency for emotional and behavioral problems to cluster or co-occur in the same individual. This co-occurrence can be variously thought of as covariation, interrelatedness, or comorbidity.

Comorbidity is a fascinating issue. It should be rare for an individual to have one serious disorder much less two. Because one has diabetes should not make it more likely to have cancer. But for psychiatric disorders this seems to be the case. For depression comorbidity is the rule not the exception. A review of community epidemiological studies found the range of comorbidity to be between 33 and 100 % (Flemming & Offord, 1990). Anxiety conditions are most frequently comorbid with depression, so one might think that this could be easily explained because they are both internalizing disorders. But the co-occurrence with externalizing disorders is equally as high, ranging from 17 to 79 %, including conduct disorders, oppositional-defiant disorders, attention-deficit disorder, and alcohol and drug abuse. Moreover, the worse the course of the child's depression the more likely that she or he would have a concurrent non-affective comorbid condition (Keller et al., 1988).

For a while when depression was first being discovered in children, it was believed that everything was a symptom of depression. The concept of masked depression was posited as an explanation for all these other symptoms (Cytryn & McKnew, 1974). Now we understand that these other conditions are not simple expressions of underlying depression. They are symptoms and disorders in their own right.

Compas and Hammen end their review with a provocative idea that high rates of covariation and comorbidity of depressive phenomena are the result of the exposure of high-risk children to multiple sources of risk that contribute independently to negative outcomes. We will return to this idea when we consider the whole issue of risk and resilience.

Conduct Disorder

Externalizing problems are much more intrusive than internalizing problems into the lives of those around affected children. Crime is mostly committed by teenagers and young adults, but it does not easily fit in with mental illness categories because for most individuals it is self-limiting. For one reason or another, children start and then stop, most within a one-year period of time (Elliott, Huizinga, & Ageton, 1985). Although adult antisocial behavior is generally preceded by childhood antisocial behavior, most antisocial children do not become antisocial adults because most adults are not antisocial (Robins, 1978). There does appear to be a group of early offenders who are persistent through early adulthood. Stattin and Magnusson (1991) found that this group accounted for only 5 % of their sample but 62 % of the crimes. If there was going to be a valid diagnosis of conduct disorder, this would appear to be the group that would have it. Yet this group also has the highest levels of comorbidity. Boys who were only aggressive were less likely to become persistent offenders than boys who were aggressive and hyperactive, for example. They are also more likely to have a variety of nondiagnostic problems including academic deficiencies, poor interpersonal relationships, and deficiencies in social problem solving skills.

Developmental pathways associated with conduct disorder have been increasingly studied (cf. NICHD Early Child Care Research Network, 2004). An interesting example is a developmental analysis of boys from childhood to adolescence by Rolf Loeber and his colleagues (Loeber et al., 1993). They were able to distinguish three pathways: (a) an early authority conflict pathway characterized by stubborn behavior, defiance, and authority avoidance; (b) a covert pathway characterized by minor covert behaviors, property damage, and moderate to serious forms of delinquency; and (c) an overt pathway characterized by aggression, fighting, and violence. This information is very important for appreciating the developmental trajectories that children follow through these behavior patterns, but does it throw light on any trait for conduct disorder in these youth? Not as much as we would hope. The worse the disorder, in this case delinquency, the more likely the boys were to be in more than one pathway, with the highest rates for youth who were in all three pathways. As in other such studies, comorbidity is rampant in this sample with attention-deficit hyperactivity and substance abuse especially associated with the overt pathway. The result is that not only the more serious the disturbance the more comorbidity between disorders but also the more deviant pathways within a disorder.

What we have learned from this discussion of individual behavior is that children are integrated wholes rather than collections of diagnostic traits. When they show evidence of serious dysfunction, it is not restricted to single domains unless the study only measures single domains of dysfunction. The worse the problems, the more likely it is that more than one behavioral area is involved. This conclusion is in keeping with one of the more articulate redefinitions of psychopathology in developmental terms provided by Sroufe and Rutter (1984) who saw the discipline as the study of patterns of adaptation rather than individual traits.

Contextual Model

Although developmental psychopathology is focused on individuals, it has become clear that understanding change requires an analysis of an individual's experience. Behavior, in general, and development, in particular, cannot be separated from the social context. Our understanding of experience has moved from a focus on primary caregivers to multiple other sources of socialization. There were many predecessors who felt that families, schools, neighborhoods, and culture had influences on development, but Bronfenbrenner (1977) turned these ideas into a comprehensive framework with predictions of how these settings affect the child but also how they affect each other. Although his terminology of microsystems, mesosystems, macrosystems, exosystems, and chronosystems may not be universally accepted, his principle that the family,

school, and community are all intertwined in explaining any particular child's progress is now universally acknowledged.

The analysis of social ecologies proposed by Bronfenbrenner described a range of social influences from the parent practices that have direct influence on the child to community and economic factors that can only impinge on the child through the action of others. Depending on disciplinary background different sets of these social variables have been proposed to explain the sources of mental health problems. Economists have focused on poverty and deprivation, sociologists have implicated problems in the community and family structure, educators blame the school system, and psychologists have focused on processes within the family and its members as the environmental influences that most profoundly affect successful development. Rather than viewing these as competing hypotheses, each can be interpreted as a contributor to a positive or negative mental health trajectory. The ecological model emphasizes the contributions of multiple environmental variables at multiple levels of social organization to multiple domains of child development.

Traditionally, social contacts were considered to expand from participation wholly in the family microsystem into later contact with the peer group and school system. Today, however, many infants are placed in out-of-home group childcare in the first months of life. Each of these settings has its own system properties such that their contributions to the development of the child are only one of many institutional functions. For example, the administration of a school setting needs attention to financing, hiring, training of staff, and building maintenance before it can perform its putative function of caring for or educating children (Maxwell, 2009). Thus, a sociological analysis of such settings provides information about its ability to impact children.

Attention to the effects on children of changing settings over time must be augmented by attention to changing characteristics of individuals within a setting. Contemporary social models take a life course perspective that includes the interlinked life trajectories of not only the child but other family members (Elder, Johnson & Crosnoe, 2003). For example, experience for the child may be quite different if the mother is in her teens with limited education or in her 30s after completing professional training and entry into the job force.

For the purposes of this discussion of issues in developmental psychopathology, I will restrict this review to two environmental issues, the multiple risk model and the contrast among risk, protective, and promotive factors. Although a central role of epidemiology is the identification of the causes of poor health, Costello and Angold (1996) point out that in the study of complex physical disorders, the preponderance of studies have identified risk factors rather than causes. Moreover, such comprehensive efforts as the Framingham Study of heart disease have discovered that no single influence is either sufficient or necessary to produce the disorder. In the domain of mental illness, a variety of studies beginning with Rutter (1979) have noted that it may be the quantity rather than the quality of risk factors that is most predictive when data from multiple environmental influences are combined.

Capturing the complex effects of multiple environmental situations has been a daunting enterprise requiring vast sample sizes to capture the unique contributions of each setting. An alternative methodology to dimensionalize the negative or positive quality of a child's experience has been the use of multiple or cumulative risk or promotive factor scores. In the Rochester Longitudinal Study, we combined ten environmental risk variables to calculate a multiple risk score for each child when they were 4 years old. These included (1) a history of maternal mental illness; (2) high maternal anxiety; (3) parental perspectives that reflected rigidity in the attitudes, beliefs, and values that mothers had in regard to their child's development; (4) few positive maternal interactions with the child observed during infancy; (5) head of household in unskilled occupations; (6) minimal maternal education; (7) disadvantaged minority status; (8) single parenthood; (9) stressful life events; and (10) large family size. The resulting score was highly correlated with child mental health; there was a significant

linear function. The more risk factors the greater the prevalence of clinical symptoms in the preschoolers (Sameroff, Seifer, Zax, & Barocas, 1987). These effects were also found when multiple environmental risk scores were correlated to child's mental health at 13 and 18 years of age (Sameroff, Bartko, Baldwin, Baldwin, & Seifer, 1998).

Another opportunity to examine the effects of multiple environmental risks on child development was provided by data emerging from a study of adolescents in a large sample of Philadelphia families (Furstenberg et al., 1999). We took a more conceptual approach in designing the project so that there were 20 environmental measures spread among six ecological levels. These were *family processes* that included support for autonomy, behavior control, parental involvement, and family climate; *parent characteristics* that included mental health, sense of efficacy, resourcefulness, and level of education; *family structure* that included the parents' marital status and socioeconomic indicators of household crowding and welfare status; *family management* comprised of variables of institutional involvement, informal networks, social resources, and adjustments to economic pressure; *peers* that included indicators of association with prosocial and antisocial peers; and *community* that included census tract information on average income and educational level of the neighborhood, a parent report of neighborhood problems, and measures of the adolescent's school climate. In addition to the large number of ecological variables, we used a wide array of youth developmental outcomes in five domains: *psychological adjustment, self-competence, conduct problems, extracurricular involvement,* and *academic performance.*

For the environmental risk analyses, each of the 20 variables was dichotomized with approximately a quarter of the families in the high-risk group and then the number of high-risk conditions summed. When we examined the relation between the multiple risk factor score and the five adolescent outcomes, there were large declines in outcome with increasing risk and a substantial overlap in slope for each (Sameroff, 2006). Although this kind of epidemiological research does not unpack the processes by which each individual is impacted by contextual experience, it does document the multiple factors in the environment that are candidates for more specific analyses.

The concern with preventing developmental failures has often clouded the fact that the majority of children in every social class and ethnic group are not failures. They get jobs, have successful social relationships, and raise a new generation of children. The concern with the source of such success has fostered an increasing concern with the development of competence and the identification of protective factors as in the work of Masten and Garmezy (1985). However, the differentiation between risk and protective factors is far from clear, and there continue to be many theoretical and methodological limitations in their identification (Luthar & Zigler, 1991).

Some have argued that protective factors can only have meaning in the face of adversity (Rutter, 1987), that is, much reduced effects for advantaged children. But in most cases protective factors appear to be simply the positive pole of risk factors (Stouthamer-Loeber et al., 1993), that is, they help everybody (Guttman, Sameroff, & Eccles, 2002). In this sense a better term for the positive end of the risk dimension would be *promotive* rather than protective factors. To test this simplification we created a set of promotive factors by identifying families at the positive pole of each of our risk factors (Sameroff, Seifer, & Bartko, 1997). For example, where a negative family climate had been a risk factor, a positive family climate now became a promotive factor, or where a parent's poor mental health was a risk factor, her good mental health became promotive. We then summed these promotive factors and examined their relation to adolescent outcomes. The results mirrored the effects of multiple risks. Families with many promotive factors did substantially better than families from contexts with few promotive factors. For the youth in this study, there did not seem to be much difference between the influence of risk and promotive variables. The more risk factors the worse the outcomes; the more promotive factors the better the outcomes. In short, when taken as part of a constellation of environmental influences on child development, most contextual variables in the parents, the family, the neighborhood, and the culture at large seem to be dimensional, aiding in general child development at one end and inhibiting it at the other.

Of interest here is how the ecological model affects our understanding of continuity and discontinuity. What one would expect is that good families, good schools, and good neighborhoods go together, and conversely bad families, bad schools, and bad neighborhoods are highly correlated. But it turns out this is only true at the aggregate level from one community to another. When one uses individual children as the level of analysis, then the correlations between the quality of the family, peer group, school, and neighborhood become quite modest. Each child can have a quite different experience with a different set of positive or negative contextual features influencing his or her development, but the conclusion does not change in that the more good things in a children's lives, the better their outcomes.

Of great significance for the life course, these effects play out over time as a manifestation of the Matthew effect, "To the man who has, more will be given until he grows rich; the man who has not will lose what little he has" (Matthew 13:12). In a study of high- and low-IQ 4-year-olds, we tracked their academic achievement through high school (Gutman, Sameroff, & Cole, 2003). The low-IQ group living in low contextual risk conditions consistently did better than the high-IQ group living in high-risk conditions. Over time promotive or risky contextual effects either fostered or wiped out prior individual competence.

Regulation Model

The third component of the unified theory is the *regulation model* reflecting the dynamic systems orientation of modern science (Sameroff, 1995). The developmental approach expands upon traditional views of mental disease by incorporating biological and behavioral functioning into a general systems model of developmental regulation. Within this approach underlying entities do not exist independent of developmental organization.

The expression of biological vulnerabilities can occur only in relation to the imbalance between coping skills and stresses in each individual's life history. Continuities in competence or incompetence from childhood into adulthood cannot be simply related to continuities in underlying pathology or health.

The relations between earlier and later behavior have to be understood in terms of the continuity of ordered or disordered experience across time interacting with an individual's unique biobehavioral characteristics. To the extent that experience becomes more organized, problems in adaptation will diminish. To the extent that experience becomes more chaotic, problems in adaptation will increase. What the developmental approach contributes is the identification of factors that influence the child's ability to organize and regulate experience and, consequently, the child's level of adaptive functioning.

Growing attention is being given to the biological regulators of development not only at the somatic level but also at the genetic. New advances in biological research are forcing more attention to be paid to analyzing environmental influences. At the molecular level we have learned that despite the fact that every cell in an organism has the same genotype, each will have different characteristics and a different history. This differentiation is a function of the differing experiences of each cell; these are environmental effects.

The idea that the child is in a dynamic rather than passive relationship with experience has become a basic tenet of contemporary developmental psychology. However, most of the rhetoric is about "self"-regulation. Whether it is Piaget's assimilation-accommodation model in cognition or Rothbart's (1981) reactivity and self-regulatory view of temperament, equilibration is primarily a characteristic native to the child. The context is necessary as a source of passive experiences that stimulate individual adaptation, but has no active role in shaping that adaptation. These views promote a belief that regulation is a property of the person. However, self-regulation mainly occurs in a social surround that is actively engaged in "other"-regulation. At the biological level the self-regulatory activity of

genes is intimately connected to the other-regulatory activity of the epigenome and the surrounding cell cytoplasm.

This issue of the developmental expansion of self-regulation to include other-regulation is captured by the *ice-cream-cone-in-a-can* model of development (Sameroff & Fiese, 2000), depicted in Fig. 2.1. The developmental changes in the relationship between individual and context are represented as an expanding cone within a cylinder. The balance between other-regulation and self-regulation shifts as the child is able to take on more and more responsibility for his or her own well-being. The infant, who at birth could not survive without the caregiving environment, eventually reaches adulthood and can become part of the other-regulation of a new infant, beginning the next generation.

It is parents who keep children warm, feed them, and cuddle them when they cry; peers who provide children with knowledge about the range and limits of their social behavior; and teachers who socialize children into group behavior as well as regulate cognition into socially constructed domains of knowledge. Although these other-regulators can be considered background to the emergence of inherent individual differences in regulatory capacities, there has been much evidence from longitudinal research among humans and cross-fostering studies in other animals that "self"-regulatory capacities are heavily influenced by the experience of regulation provided by caregivers. The capacity for self-regulation arises through the actions of others. This regulation by others provides the increasingly complex social, emotional, and cognitive experiences to which the child must self-regulate and the safety net when self-regulation fails. Moreover, these regulations are embedded not only in the relation between child and context but also in the additional relations between family and their cultural and economic situations (Raver, 2004). These regulatory systems range from the here-and-now experiences of parent–child interactions to governmental concern with the burden of national debt that will be passed on the next generation and to conservationists' concerns with the fate of the planet as a viable environment for future generations of humans.

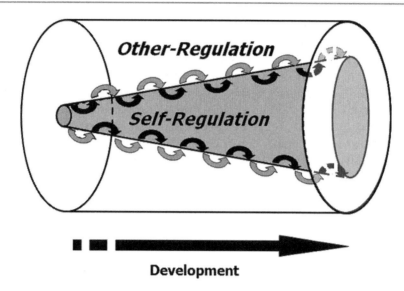

Fig. 2.1 Transactional relations between self-regulation and other-regulation

Early functional physiological self-regulation of sleep, crying, and attention is augmented by caregiving that provides children with regulatory experiences to help them quiet down on the one hand and become more attentive on the other. Sleep is an interesting example where biological regulation becomes psychological regulation through social regulation. As wakefulness begins to emerge as a distinct state, it is expanded and contracted by interactions with caregivers who stimulate alertness and facilitate sleepiness. Although it remains an essential biological process, eventually it takes on a large degree of self-regulation as the child increasingly makes active decisions about waking time and sleeping time. But this agentic decision-making remains intimately connected with other-regulation in terms of the demands of school and work for specific periods of wakefulness.

The relation between self- and other-regulation has implications for diagnostic systems for the psychopathology of children. In an attempt to define mental health diagnoses for infants, Sameroff and Emde (1989) argued for a position that infant diagnoses could not be separated from relationship diagnoses. Our point was that in early development life is a "we-ness" rather than an "I-ness." The developmental and clinical question in this case is when does a diagnosis become indi-vidualized, at what stage does a child have a self-regulation problem instead of an other-regulation problem? One answer is to identify the point in development when areas of self-regulation become independent of initial regulatory contexts and are carried into new relationships.

The previous discussion of the need for a construct of other-regulation to complete an understanding of self-regulation leads now to how the relation between self and other operates developmentally, and for this we turn to the transactional model (Sameroff & Chandler, 1975). Transactions are omnipresent. Everything in the universe is affecting something else or is being affected by something else. In the transactional model the development of the child is a product of the continuous dynamic interactions of the child and the experience provided by his or her social settings. What is core to the transactional model is the analytic emphasis placed on the interdependent effects of the child and environment and is depicted in the bidirectional arrows between self and other in Fig. 2.1. The transactional model helps to explain many of the continuities and discontinuities in development. Interactions are typified by continuity where there may be a mutual dependence between one's behavior and another's, but there is not restructuring—there is a stable pattern of correlations. Transactions occur when one partner changes their behavior such that there is a new pattern of interaction—a discontinuity—that can move in a positive or negative direction. Transactions are opportunities for interventionists to aim for the more positive outcome.

In a recent book on the topic (Sameroff, 2009), a number of researchers documented transactional processes in cognitive and social-emotional domains where agents in the family, school, and cultural contexts altered the course of children's development in both positive and negative directions. Transactional examples have been typically in the behavioral domain with an emphasis on parent–child mutual exacerbations producing problem behavior in both partners (Patterson, 1986). More recently, transactions have been recognized in teacher–student relationships where the effects of the teacher on the child in one grade will change the reaction of the teacher in the next moving the student to higher or lower levels of competence (Morrison & Connor, 2009). Multilevel transactions have also been documented where not only the parent and child are transacting with each other but both are also transacting with cultural practices (Bornstein, 2009).

Representational Model

Since the beginnings of psychodynamic thinking, representations have been used to explain psychopathology and as targets for psychotherapeutic interventions. Representations are encodings of experience that are more or less elaborated internal summaries of the external world. They include the cognitive representations where the external world is internalized, the social representations where relationships become working models, the cultural representations of different ethnicities or social classes, and even the developmental theories discussed here. Representations are obviously not the same as what they represent. They have the function of bringing order to a variable world, producing a set of expectations of how things should fit together that are generally adaptive but in the case of psychopathology tend more toward the maladaptive.

We have long been familiar with such representations as perceptual constancy in which objects are perceived as being a certain size even when the sensory size is manipulated. In such a summation certain aspects are selected and others ignored. In the representation of a square, for example, the size, color, and texture of the square object may be ignored. Analogously, when representations are made of a social object such as a parent, certain features are included in the representation and others are ignored. Research using the adult attachment interview (Main & Goldwyn, 1984) has emphasized that representations of parents are often idealized, where only positive aspects are included in the mental model. Although the links between the quality of representations of child–parent relationships during infancy and those during adulthood are far from direct, early working models of attachment do seem to have long-term consequences for adult development (Sroufe, Egeland, Carlson, & Collins, 2005).

Similarly, parents create representations of their children that emphasize certain aspects, deemphasize others, and have stability over time independent of the child's actual characteristics. We had parents rate their infants' temperament during the first year of life following a structured interaction sequence (Seifer, Sameroff, Barrett, & Krafchuk, 1994). We also had them rate the temperament of six unfamiliar infants engaged in the same interaction sequence. The average correlation in temperament ratings of the unfamiliar infants between mothers and trained observers was 0.84 with none below 0.60. The average correlation in temperament ratings between mothers and trained observers for their own children was 0.35 with a range down to −0.40. Mothers were very good raters of other people's children, but very poor raters of their own due to the personal representations that they imposed on their observations. Documenting such differences in parent representations would be of no more than intellectual interest, if there were not consequences for the later development of the child. For example, infants whose mothers perceived them as problematic criers during infancy increased their crying during toddlerhood and had higher problem behavior scores when they were preschoolers

(McKenzie & McDonough, 2009). Representations are further examples of the ubiquity of discontinuities in development. Individuals, parents in this case, interpret the same reality in quite different ways leading to quite different outcomes from the same initial child conditions.

Individual well-being is also a result of meaningful cultural engagement with desirable everyday routines that have a script, goals, and values (Weisner, 2002). Meaningfulness, a key component of cultural analyses, is primarily found in coherent representations. Meaning systems can have a positive influence as where family routines provide a narrative representation for the family members that allows the whole to continue adaptive functioning despite the variability in the behavior of the parts (Fiese and Winter, 2009), for example, an alcoholic parent or an ill child. The negative effect of a lack of meaningfulness was found in a study of native Canadian youth who showed much higher levels of suicide and other problem behavior when there were large inconsistencies in cultural continuity from one generation to another (Chandler, Lalonde, Sokol, & Hallett, 2003). The order or disorder in a family or society's representation of itself affects the adaptive functioning of its members.

Evolutionary Model

Historically, evolutionary psychologists have tended toward reductionism, explaining current psychological and social organization as the result of Darwinian selective processes on the genome during the history of the species. More recent formulations have added more dynamic conceptualizations to our understanding of both historic evolutionary forces and contemporary gene expression. In each case there is an intimate relationship between the evolving or developing organism and its experiential surround. Of empirical interest are the reformulations of gene–environment interactions in terms of differential susceptibility theory and epigenetics.

The original descriptions of gene–environment interactions (cf. Caspi et al., 2003) found that certain gene alleles produced a greater mental health

vulnerability to abusive environments and described these polymorphisms categorically as vulnerability genes. Further research has enlarged the concept of gene–environment interaction into a U-shaped function labeled as differential susceptibility (Ellis, Boyce, Belsky, Bakermans-Kranenburg, & van IJzendoorn, 2011), such that the same allele can produce worse mental health in stressful contexts but better mental health in more supportive social contexts. These opposite effects where the same polymorphism can express itself as either a risk factor or a promotive factor depending on social experience emphasize the lack of determinism in even the most basic individual biological characteristics.

Advances in epigenetics have reframed what we consider to be the basic biological units, from the unchanging genome to the epigenome where experiences are dynamically coded (Meaney, 2010). A fundamental premise of the transmission of genes from one generation to another was that the genotype is not influenced by the experience of the phenotype. This is no longer the case when the more inclusive epigenome is taken into consideration. Not only is the activation of the genome influenced by the experience of the individual, but such changes are transmitted from one generation to another. Researches in both differential susceptibility and epigenetics are further demonstrations of how discontinuities can be found at every level of functioning. Initial conditions alone are not predictive of future development.

From the systems perspective evolutionary theory has provided a fruitful analog for understanding the transitions that lead from one developmental stage to another in the personal model described above. As opposed to the gradualist understanding of evolutionary changes originally proposed by Darwin that would look like the growth model of individual change, Eldredge and Gould (1972) argued that evolution was characterized by continuity evidenced in long periods of stasis where there were only modest changes, alternating with discontinuity, where there were short periods of rapid change, which they labeled *punctuated equilibrium*. The implication was that there was a balance between species and their ecosystems until it was interrupted by either large changes in the species or large changes in the environment that required a new equilibration. In terms of understanding developmental disconti- nuities in the individual, we would need to search for such changes in the child or the context that create pressures for a new equilibration leading to future mental order or disorder.

Unifying the Theory of Development

Now that the five models necessary for a theory of development have been described, we can attempt to integrate them into a comprehensive view that contains most known influences on developmental psychopathology using both a structural model that describes all the pieces and then a functional model that shows how their interactions and transactions unfold over time.

The self has often been described as a set of interacting psychological and biological pro- cesses as depicted in Fig. 2.2. The psychological domains overlap in cognitive and emotional realms of intelligence, mental health, social com- petence, and identity, among others. Here they are depicted as the set of grey, overlapping circles comprising the psychological part of the self. Each of these psychological domains is subserved by and interacts with a set of biological processes,

including neurophysiology, neuroendocrinology, proteomics, epigenomics, and genomics that are depicted as a set of black, overlapping circles. Together the grey and black circles comprise the *biopsychological* self-system. This self-regula- tion system transacts with the other-regulation system, depicted by the surrounding white cir- cles, representing the many settings of the social ecology, including family, school, neighborhood, community, and overarching geopolitical influ- ences. Taken together the three sets of overlap- ping circles comprise the *biopsychosocial* aspects of an individual in context.

Next, the developmental model of personal change is added to the biopsychosocial model, where there are qualitative shifts in organization reflecting changing relationships among the bio- psychosocial aspects as seen in Fig. 2.3. These periods of changing organization are analogous to the evolutionary shifts described in the theory of punctuated equilibria. The leading edge for these changes can originate in the individual, repre- sented by the arrows pushing outward in the figure, or from the context, as represented by the arrows pushing inward, resulting in points of inflection, that is, developmental change. It is the relation between shifts in the child and shifts in the context that mark new stages. Such individual shifts can be tied to personal changes as mundane as beginning to walk or as complicated as adolescence.

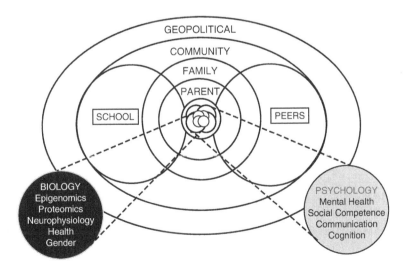

Fig. 2.2 Biopsychosocial ecological system

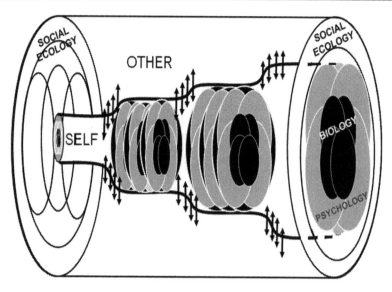

Fig. 2.3 Unified theory of development including the personal change, context, and regulation models

Puberty is a biological achievement of the child, but adolescence is a socially designated phase between childhood and adulthood (Worthman, 1993). Puberty is universal but adolescence is not, in either historical or cross-cultural perspective. In many cultures adolescence is directly tied to biological changes, but in modernizing cultures it is more closely tied to age-based transitions into middle and high schools. Depending on the culture sexual participation can be encouraged at an early age before biological maturity or discouraged until individuals are well into adulthood. These pressures from changes in the child and the context are represented by the up and down arrows around the adolescent transition in Fig. 2.3. In western societies, adolescence is generally recognized, but the quality of the adolescent experience is quite variable and may be heavily dependent on stage-environment fit. Depending on the particular family or school system, desires for autonomy and intimacy can be fostered or thwarted moving the adolescent into better or worse future functioning. Negative psychological changes associated with adolescent development often result from a mismatch between the needs of developing adolescents and the opportunities afforded them by their social environments (Eccles et al., 1993).

The recent emphasis on identifying developmental cascades in psychopathology offers many empirical examples of the interplay between individual and contextual shifts over time (cf. Masten & Cicchetti, 2010). An informative example is the work of Dodge et al. (2009) explaining the predictive cascade between child, parents, and peer group leading from a difficult temperament in infancy to substance abuse in adolescence. The direct correlation between infant and adolescent characteristics is negligible, but becomes amplified as infant problems lead to parent problems that lead to peer problems and back again to later parenting and peer problems and finally to the adverse adolescent outcome.

The unified theory depicted in Fig. 2.3 combines the personal change, contextual, and regulation model, but it would become overly complex to add the representational model to the figure as well. Suffice it to say that representation suffuses every aspect of the model in the interacting identities, attitudes, beliefs, and attributions of the child, the family, the culture, and the organizational structure of social institutions. Moreover, the way developmental science conceptualizes the child may be only one of a number of possible cultural inventions (Kessen, 1979). The most important representation for current purposes is captured in the depiction of a unified theory of development. Like most theories the unified view does not make specific predictions, but does specify what will be necessary for explaining the developmental phenomena in psychopathology. It is a reversal of the usual bottom-up empirical stance where the researcher maintains as narrow focus as possible unless forced to enlarge the scope by some contradictory findings. The top-down theoretical stance is that researchers need to be aware that they are examining only a part of a larger whole consisting of multiple interacting dynamic systems where each influences the outcome of interest. Over time the body changes, the brain changes, the mind changes, and the environment changes along courses that may be somewhat independent of each other and somewhat a consequence of experience with each other. It should be a very exciting enterprise to fill in the details of how biological, psychological, and social experiences foster and transform each other to explain both adaptive and maladaptive functioning across the life course.

I have summarized a universal theory of development that can be used to explain both ordered and disordered adaptive processes using the same models. Within this framework are answers to the questions of defining pathology, understanding individuals and their development, and conceptualizing the environment. All children are constantly adapting to and requiring adaptations from their caregiving environment. Individual differences from the genome on have the potential to lead to more positive mental health outcomes. Which path will be taken is the result of a continuous dynamic with the ability of the context to support or subvert developmental achievements. The extent of our understanding of the elements of this dynamic will limit or increase our ability to plan intervention efforts to move children toward adaptive solutions.

Development and Psychopathology

The field of developmental psychopathology has introduced an important reorientation to the study of mental health and disorder. The principles of development that apply to the achievement of healthy growth are now seen as the same ones that apply to the achievement of illness (Sroufe & Rutter, 1984). In this view most illnesses are indeed achievements that result from the active strivings of each individual to reach an adaptive relation to his or her environment. The nutrients or poisons that experience provides will flavor that adaptation. No complex human accomplishment has been demonstrated to arise without being influenced by experience. The study of linkages across time is perhaps the most defining of developmental psychopathology in that it contains the basis for continuities and discontinuities. The perspective taken by developmental psychopathology offers a powerful alternative to nondevelopmental approaches because principles of process are integrated into an understanding of behavioral deviancy. Where traditional views have seen deviancy as inherent in the individual, developmental views place deviancy in the dynamic relation between the individual and the internal and external context.

References

Berkson, G. (1978). Social ecology and ethology of mental retardation. In G. P. Sackett (Ed.), *Observing behavior, Vol. I: Theory and applications in mental retardation* (pp. 403–409). Baltimore, MD: University Park Press.

Bornstein, M. H. (2009). Toward a model of culture-parent–child transactions. In A. Sameroff (Ed.), *The transactional model of development: How children and contexts shape each other* (pp. 139–161). Washington, DC: American Psychological Association.

Bronfenbrenner, U. (1977). Toward an experimental ecology of human development. *American Psychologist, 32,* 513–531.

Caspi, A., Sugden, K., Moffitt, T. E., Taylor, A., Craig, I., Harrington, H., et al. (2003). Influence of life stress on depression: Moderation by a polymorphism in the 5-HTT gene. *Science, 301,* 386–389.

Chandler, M. J., Lalonde, C. E., Sokol, B. W., & Hallett, D. (2003). Personal persistence, identity development, and suicide: A study of native and non-native North American adolescents. *Monographs of the Society for Research in Child Development, 68*(2, Series No. 273)

Cicchetti, D. (1989). Developmental psychopathology: Some thought on its evolution. *Development & Psychopathology, 1,* 1–4.

Compas, B. E., & Hammen, C. L. (1994). Child and adolescent depression: Covariation and comorbidity in development. In R. J. Haggerty, L. R. Sherrod, N. Garmezy, & M. Rutter (Eds.), *Stress, risk, and resilience in children and adolescents: Processes, mechanisms, and interventions* (pp. 225–267). New York: Cambridge University Press.

Costello, E. J., & Angold, A. (1996). Developmental psychopathology. In R. B. Cairns, G. H. Elder Jr., & E. J. Costello (Eds.), *Developmental science* (pp. 168–189). New York: Cambridge University Press.

Cytryn, L., & McKnew, D. H. (1974). Factors influencing the changing clinical expression of the depressive process in children. *American Journal of Psychiatry, 131*, 879–881.

Dodge, K. A., Malone, P. S., Lansford, J. E., Miller, S., Pettit, G. S., & Bates, J. E. (2009). A dynamic cascade model of the development of substance-use onset. *Monographs of the Society for Research in Child Development, 74*(3), 1–134.

Eccles, J. S., Midgley, C., Wigfield, A., Buchanan, C. M., Reuman, D., Flanagan, C., et al. (1993). Development during adolescence: The impact of stage-environment fit on young adolescents' experiences in schools and in families. *American Psychologist, 48*, 90–101.

Elder, G. H., Jr., Johnson, M. K., & Crosnoe, R. (2003). The emergence and development of life course theory. In J. T. Mortimer & M. J. Shanahan (Eds.), *Handbook of the life course* (pp. 3–19). New York: Kluwer Academic/Plenum.

Eldredge, N., & Gould, S. J. (1972). Punctuated equilibria: An alternative to phyletic gradualism. In T. J. M. Schopf (Ed.), *Models in paleobiology*. San Francisco, CA: Freeman Cooper.

Elliott, D. S., Huizinga, D., & Ageton, S. S. (1985). *Explaining delinquency and drug use*. Beverly Hills, CA: Sage.

Ellis, J. E., Boyce, W. T., Belsky, J., Bakermans-Kranenburg, M. J., & van IJzendoorn, M. H. (2011). Differential susceptibility to the environment: An evolutionary–neurodevelopmental theory. *Development and Psychopathology, 23*, 7–28.

Ericsson, K. A., & Charness, N. (1994). Expert performance: Its structure and acquisition. *American Psychologist, 49*(8), 725–747.

Fiese, B. H., & Winter, M. A. (2009). The dynamics of family chaos and its relation to children's socioemotional well being. In G. W. Evans & T. D. Wachs (Eds.), *Chaos and its influence on children's development: An ecological perspective* (pp. 55–76). Washington, DC: APA Books.

Flemming, J. E., & Offord, D. R. (1990). Epidemiology of childhood depressive disorders: A critical review. *Journal of American Academy of Child and Adolescent Psychiatry, 29*, 571–580.

Furstenberg, F. F., Jr., Cook, T. D., Eccles, J., Elder, G. H., Jr., & Sameroff, A. (1999). *Managing to make it: Urban families and adolescent success*. Chicago: University of Chicago Press.

Garmezy, N. (1985). Stress-resistant children: The search for protective factors. In J. E. Stevenson (Ed.), *Recent research in developmental psychopathology* (pp. 213–233). Oxfort: Pergamon Press.

Gutman, L. M., Sameroff, A. J., & Cole, R. (2003). Academic growth curve trajectories from first to twelfth grades: Effects of multiple social risk and preschool child factors. *Developmental Psychology, 39*, 777–790.

Gutman, L. M., Sameroff, A. J., & Eccles, J. S. (2002). The academic achievement of African American students during early adolescence: An examination of multiple risk, promotive, and protective factors. *American Journal of Community Psychology, 30*(3), 367–399.

Keller, M. B., Beardslee, W., Lavori, P. W., Wunder, J., Dils, D. L., & Samuelson, H. (1988). Course of major depression in non-referred adolescents: A retrospective study. *Journal of Affective Disorders, 15*, 235–243.

Kessen, W. (1979). The American child and other cultural inventions. *American Psychologist, 34*, 815–820.

Loeber, R., Wung, P., Keenan, K., Giroux, B., Stouthamer-Loeber, M., Van Kammen, W. B., et al. (1993). Developmental pathways in disruptive child behavior. *Development and Psychopathology, 5*, 103–133.

Luthar, S. S., & Zigler, E. (1991). Vulnerability and competence: A review of research on resilience in childhood. *American Journal of Orthopsychiatry, 61*, 6–22.

Main, M., & Goldwyn, R. (1984). Predicting rejection of their infant from mother's representation of her own experience: Implications for the abused and abusing intergenerational cycle. *Child Abuse and Neglect, 8*, 203–217.

Masten, A. S., & Cicchetti, D. (2010). Developmental cascades. *Development and Psychopathology, 22*, 491–495.

Masten, A. S., & Garmezy, N. (1985). Risk, vulnerability, and protective factors in developmental psychopathology. In B. B. Lahey & A. E. Kazdin (Eds.), *Advances in clinical child psychology* (Vol. 8, pp. 1–52). New York: Plenum.

Maxwell, L. E. (2009). Chaos outside the home: The school environment. In G. W. Evans & T. D. Wachs (Eds.), *Chaos and its influence on children's development: An ecological perspective* (pp. 117–136). Washington, DC: APA Books.

McKenzie, M. J., & McDonough, S. C. (2009). Transactions between perception and reality: Maternal beliefs and infant regulatory behavior. In A. Sameroff (Ed.), *The transactional model of development: How children and contexts shape each other* (pp. 35–54). Washington, DC: American Psychological Association.

Meaney, M. J. (2010). Epigenetics and the biological definition of gene X environment interactions. *Child Development, 81*(1), 41–79.

Morrison, F. J., & Connor, C. M. (2009). The transition to school: Child instruction transactions in learning to read. In A. Sameroff (Ed.), *The transactional model of development: How children and contexts shape each other* (pp. 183–201). Washington, DC: American Psychological Association.

NICHD Early Child Care Research Network. (2004). Trajectories of physical aggression from toddlerhood to middle childhood. *Monographs of the Society for Research in Child Development, 69*(4), Whole No. 278.

Nichols, P. (1984). Familial mental retardation. *Behavior Genetics, 14*, 161–170.

Patterson, G. R. (1986). Performance models for antisocial boys. *American Psychologist, 41*, 432–444.

Raver, C. C. (2004). Placing emotional self-regulation in sociocultural and socioeconomic contexts. *Child Development, 75*, 346–353.

Robins, L. (1978). Sturdy childhood predictors of adult antisocial behaviour: Replications from longitudinal studies. *Psychological Medicine, 8*, 611–622.

Rothbart, M. K. (1981). Measurement of temperament in infancy. *Child Development, 52*, 569–578.

Rutter, M. (1987). Continuities and discontinuities from infancy. In J. Osofsky (Ed.), *Handbook of infant development* (2nd ed., pp. 1256–1296). New York: Wiley.

Rutter, M., & Garmezy, N. (1983). Development psychopathology. In E. M. Hetherington (Ed.), *Carmichael's manual of child psychology: Vol. 4. Social and personality development* (pp. 775–911). New York: Wiley.

Rutter's, M. (1979). Protective factors in children's responses to stress and disadvantage. In M. W. Kent & J. E. Rolf (Eds.), *Primary prevention of psychopathology Vol. 3: Social competence in children* (pp. 49–74). Hanover, NH: University of New England Press.

Sameroff, A. J. (1995). General systems theories and developmental psychopathology. In D. Cicchetti & D. Cohen (Eds.), *Manual of developmental psychopathology* (Vol. 1, pp. 659–695). New York: Wiley.

Sameroff, A. J. (2006). Identifying risk and protective factors for healthy youth development. In A. Clarke-Stewart & J. Dunn, J. *Families count: Effects on child and adolescent development* (pps. 53–76). Cambridge, UK: Cambridge University Press.

Sameroff, A. J. (Ed.). (2009). *The transactional model of development: How children and contexts shape each other.* Washington, DC: American Psychological Association.

Sameroff, A. J. (2010). A unified theory of development: A dialectic integration of nature and nurture. *Child Development, 81*, 6–22.

Sameroff, A. J., Bartko, W. T., Baldwin, A., Baldwin, C., & Seifer, R. (1998). Family and social influences on the development of child competence. In M. Lewis & C. Feiring (Eds.), *Families, risk, and competence* (pp. 1161–1183). Mahwah, NJ: Lawrence Erlbaum Associates.

Sameroff, A. J., & Chandler, M. J. (1975). Reproductive risk and the continuum of caretaking casualty. In F. D. Horowitz, M. Hetherington, S. Scarr-Salapatek, & G. Siegel (Eds.), *Review of child development research* (Vol. 4, pp. 187–244). Chicago: University of Chicago.

Sameroff, A. J., & Emde, R. N. (Eds.). (1989). *Relationship disturbances in early childhood: A developmental approach.* New York: Basic Books.

Sameroff, A. J., & Fiese, B. H. (2000). Transactional regulation: The developmental ecology of early intervention. In J. P. Shonkoff & S. J. Meisels (Eds.), *Early intervention: A handbook of theory, practice, and analysis* (2nd ed., pp. 135–159). New York: Cambridge University Press.

Sameroff, A. J., Seifer, R., Baldwin, A. L., & Baldwin, C. A. (1993). Stability of intelligence from preschool to adolescence: The influence of social and family risk factors. *Child Development, 64*, 80–97.

Sameroff, A. J., Seifer, R., & Bartko, W. T. (1997). Environmental perspectives on adaptation during childhood and adolescence. In S. S. Luthar, J. A. Barack, D. Cicchetti, & J. Weisz (Eds.), *Developmental psychopathology: Perspectives on risk and disorder.* Cambridge, MA: Cambridge University Press.

Sameroff, A. J., Seifer, R., & Zax, M. (1982). Early development of children at risk for emotional disorder. *Monographs of the Society for Research in Child Development, 47*(7, Serial No. 199).

Sameroff, A. J., Seifer, R., Zax, M., & Barocas, R. (1987). Early indicators of developmental risk: The Rochester longitudinal study. *Schizophrenia Bulletin, 13*, 383–393.

Sameroff, A. J., & Zax, M. (1973). Neonatal characteristics of offspring of schizophrenic and neurotically-depressed mothers. *Journal of Nervous and Mental Diseases, 157*, 191–199.

Seifer, R., Sameroff, A. J., Barrett, L. C., & Krafchuk, E. (1994). Infant temperament measured by multiple observations and mother report. *Child Development, 65*, 1478–1490.

Sroufe, L. A. (1990). Considering the normal and abnormal together: Te essence of developmental psychopathology. *Development and Psychopathology, 2*, 335–347.

Sroufe, L. A., Egeland, B., Carlson, E. A., & Collins, W. A. (2005). *The development of the person: The Minnesota study of risk and adaptation from birth to adulthood.* New York: Guilford.

Sroufe, L. A., & Rutter, M. (1984). The domain of developmental psychopathology. *Child Development, 55*, 17–29.

Stattin, H., & Magnusson, D. (1991). Stability and change in criminal behaviour up to age 30. *British Journal of Criminology, 31*(4), 327–346.

Stouthamer-Loeber, M., Loeber, R., Farrington, D. P., Zhang, Q., van Kammen, W., & Maguin, E. (1993). The double edge of protective and risk factors for delinquency: Interrelations and developmental patterns. *Development and Psychopathology, 5*, 683–701.

Visscher, P. M. (2008). Sizing up human height variation. *Nature Genetics, 40*(5), 489–490.

Weisner, T. S. (2002). Ecocultural understanding of children's developmental pathways. *Human Development, 45*, 275–281.

Worthman, C. M. (1993). Biocultural interactions in human development. In M. E. Pereira & L. A. Banks (Eds.), *Juvenile primates: Life history, development, and behavior* (pp. 339–358). New York: Oxford University Press.

Zigler, E., & Hodapp, R. M. (1986). *Understanding mental retardation.* New York: Cambridge University Press.

Nature–Nurture Integration

3

Michael Rutter

The two key features of developmental psychopathology (DP) concern the importance of continuities and discontinuities across the span of development and the span between normality and disorder (Rutter, 1988; Rutter & Sroufe, 2000; Sroufe & Rutter, 1984). Both, however, required a shift from what has been traditional in developmental psychology and in child psychiatry (Rutter, 2013). Thus, developmental psychology has tended to focus particularly on developmental universals and on trait continuities over time, whereas DP demands a focus on individual differences and on the growing psychological cohesion that may extend across traits and on the modifications and changes that derive from altered circumstances. Child psychiatry, on the other hand, has tended to concentrate on the causes and course of individual diagnostic conditions. Of course, these are important, but what is different about a DP perspective is that it is necessary to go on to pose questions such as those involving age-related variations in susceptibility to stress, the extent to which development of disorder is dependent on prior circumstances at an earlier age, the query as to whether there are points in development when psychological qualities become relatively stabilized, and the question as to why some psychopathological patterns

become so much more common during adolescence than they had been in childhood. DP concepts emphasize that *both* continuities and discontinuities have to be considered and that a central concern has to involve determination of the mediating mechanisms involved in both change and stability.

DP, therefore, is not a theory and it is not a discipline. Rather, it is a perspective that has important implications for both research and clinical practice (Rutter, 2008). DP perspectives have also required an appreciation that there is often a two-way interplay between individuals and their environment; that there may be heterotypic, as well as homotypic, continuity in psychopathological progressions; and that in some circumstances risk effects may actually be protective, with resulting resilience. In addition, it has become clear that most disorders involve multifactorial causation—meaning not only that a mixture of genetic and nongenetic causal influences but also that the particular mix varies from individual to individual and that in most cases there is not one causal process but several. As will be discussed in more detail, gene–environment interplay is crucially important in relation to these multiple DP issues. Finally, psychiatrists have had to accept that the notion of utterly distinct diagnostic categories that differ from all others and which involve "clear water" between them does not hold up (Rutter, 2013). Although, of course, there are important meaningful differences between diagnostic categories, there is much more overlap than used to be appreciated,

3

M. Rutter, M.D. (✉)
MRC Social, Genetic and Developmental
Psychiatry Centre, Institute of Psychiatry,
King's College London, London SE5 8AF, UK
e-mail: Camilla.azis@kcl.ac.uk

M. Lewis and K.D. Rudolph (eds.), *Handbook of Developmental Psychopathology*,
DOI 10.1007/978-1-4614-9608-3_3, © Springer Science+Business Media New York 2014

as is evident in the case of autism, ADHD, and schizophrenia as well as that between schizophrenia and bipolar disorders.

Genetic Influences

Other chapters in this volume deal in detail with various aspects of genetics and epigenetics, but it is not possible to discuss nature–nurture interplay without first emphasizing a few of the key genetic concepts and findings (Rutter, 2012a). First, it used to be assumed that genes operated (via messenger RNA) only through their effects on proteins which then indirectly led on to the behavioral or phenotypic effects, through a process that remains ill-understood in almost all cases. It created a puzzle, in that it was found that these accounted for so little of the effects of genes. Attention then turned to what had previously been regarded as "junk DNA," and it became clear that, far from being junk, it was crucially important; multiple DNA elements were involved in gene actions (Rutter, 2006, 2012a). Many genes with important phenotypic effects do not have effects on proteins (e.g., the serotonin transporter promoter (5-HTTLPR) that has been much studied in relation to gene–environment interactions (GxE) brings about its effects through promoting the action of other genes and not through a direct action itself on proteins).

Second, it has been necessary to abandon the concepts of genes "for" any individual disorder (Kendler, 2005). The effects of the individual genes that have been identified so far are tiny with respect to each gene, with an odds ratio rarely exceeding 1.3 and mostly far below that. In addition, as will be discussed in relation to GxE, some genes operate on biological pathways that occur in individuals without psychopathology (Hyde, Bogdan, & Hariri, 2011; Meyer-Lindenberg & Weinberger, 2006) and not just in those with some specified disorder. It has also become apparent that genetic influences may operate on features within a diagnostic category, rather than on the disorder as a whole—as exemplified by the catechol-*O*-methyltransferase (COMT) effect on antisocial behavior in individuals with attention-deficit/hyperactivity disorder

(ADHD) but not on antisocial behavior otherwise and not on ADHD in the absence of antisocial behavior (Caspi et al., 2008; Thapar et al., 2005). Moreover, it has been shown that most forms of psychopathology operate dimensionally rather than categorically and that genes may exert their effects through quantitative trait loci having an effect on continuously distributed dimensions (Rutter, 2003).

Third, it has been found that some genetic influences on psychopathology do not follow the usual patterns. For example, some conditions (such as the fragile X syndrome) operate through the transgenerational expansion of trinucleotide repeats. Others involve genomic imprinting with the result that the phenotypic effects differ according to whether the mutant gene comes through the mother or the father. Thus, this is the case with the Prader–Willi syndrome and the Angelman syndrome, both of which are due to a deletion on chromosome 15 but with the difference that paternal inheritance leads to Prader–Willi and maternal inheritance to Angelman syndrome.

A further anomaly is that most genes have multiple (pleiotropic) effects and not just effects on one particular outcome (Flint, Greenspan, & Kendler, 2010). A different issue is posed by the observation that although both autism and schizophrenia have a high heritability but low fecundity (rate of having children), they have not died out (Uher, 2009). It is not obvious quite why that is the case, but part of the answer might lie in the role of rare, highly penetrant, pathogenic mutations—although these would not account for the high familiality of these disorders.

Finally, although most of the writings on genes in the psychopathological arena concern genes that provide a susceptibility or liability, cancer genetics makes clear that effects of genes need to be considered in relation to protection as well as liability. Note that this is not simply the other end of a risk effect. The genes involved in oncogenesis (i.e., the liability to cancer) are not the same as the tumor-suppressant genes, and the mechanisms involved are not the same.

As will be discussed more fully in relation to nature–nurture integration, it is clear that genes may have their main effect through influences on environmental risk exposure (through gene–environment correlations—rGE) or through environmental susceptibility (through gene–environment interactions—GxE). In both cases, there is a gene–environment coaction and not independent effects of each. For a long time, it had been assumed that environments cannot influence genetic effects, but it is known now that they can, by virtue of epigenetic mechanisms (Meaney, 2010). Environments cannot alter gene sequences; they are present from the outset and do not change throughout life. Nevertheless, genes can only bring about effects if they are expressed, and this comes about through processes that can and do change over time as a result of the coming together of genetic, environmental, and chance (stochastic) effects. It is through such mechanisms that genes become, in effect, "switched on" and "switched off." The most obvious example of this is the genetic influence on the timing of the menarche, but there are many others.

Nongenetic Influences

The conceptualization of nongenetic influences has had to change a good deal over the years (Academy of Medical Sciences, 2007). First, there has come to be an appreciation that these need to include prenatal as well as postnatal influences. This was obvious with respect to the evidence that prenatal exposure to alcohol (as derived through the mother's alcohol consumption) led to a distinctive clinical picture that came to be called the fetal alcohol syndrome and then, later, fetal alcohol spectrum. The effects of thalidomide in leading to gross limb defects were an even more dramatic example. The findings on the effects of maternal smoking in leading to an increased likelihood of low birth weight were less dramatic but were very important in terms of the much higher rate of prenatal exposure. Most recently, it has become clear that the prenatal effects can include high maternal anxiety and not just toxins (Mueller & Bale, 2008; Sillaber, Holsboer, & Wotjak, 2009).

The second major change was the appreciation that nongenetic effects needed to include

random, or stochastic, effects and not just the effects of differences in environmental exposure. This was first demonstrated in terms of the increased risk for Down syndrome associated with being born to an older mother, but, in recent years, it has become clear that there are also, albeit different, risks associated with high paternal age. Both maternal and paternal age effects have been demonstrated in relation to autism, but it probably applies more widely (Reichenberg, Gross, Kolevzon, & Susser, 2011; Sandin et al., 2012). The mechanisms associated with maternal age effects and paternal age effects are likely to be different. The mother's eggs have been in her ovaries since before birth, so the risk probably derives from the eggs being "old" and, as it were, past their "sell-by" date. No cell divisions are involved. By contrast, male's sperms are produced de novo throughout life, involving multiple cell divisions. The evidence indicates that the likelihood of mutations rises with the number of cell divisions (Kong et al., 2012), thereby increasing risk. The finding serves as a reminder that biological development is probabilistic and not deterministic. Thus, so far as the brain is concerned, initial neuronal overproduction is followed by neuronal pruning to correct initial errors and to enhance neuronal connections that support brain activity that seems to be useful. The probabilistic nature of development means that minor congenital anomalies are very common. It has been found that these anomalies are more common in disorders such as autism, ADHD, and schizophrenia, but they occur at quite a high frequency in individuals without disorder.

What is currently under discussion is whether the concept of these developmental perturbations needs to include chromosome anomalies and copy-number variations. Again, they are substantially more common in individuals with mental disorders such as autism, schizophrenia, and ADHD, but they also occur in many people without disorder. It seems unlikely that most of these developmental perturbations have direct effects on psychological or psychopathological development, but, equally, it does seem that they may have causal effects of a less specific kind.

The third change in concept concerns the appreciation that environmental influences do not just impinge on a passive organism. Rather, from infancy onwards, individuals interpret and process their experiences. This means that it has become necessary to distinguish between the "objective" and "effective" (or subjectively experienced) environment. It might seem obvious that the objective environment is more important, but recent evidence indicates that the reverse may actually be the case (Rutter, 2012d). Thus, it seems that people's self-rating of their own social status is more influential than social class as measured by education and occupation.

Fourth, individuals both select and shape their environments—something that is associated with "active" and "evocative" gene–environment correlations. A somewhat related issue concerns the distinction between "shared" and "non-shared" environmental effects (Rutter, 2006). Despite the terminology, this does not actually mean sharing or non-sharing of the environment but rather whether the environmental effects tend to make siblings more alike or less alike. That has no direct connection with the objective environment as such. Fifth, although much of the research and clinical literature is concerned with family influences, it is obvious that psychosocial influences extend to include the peer group, the school, and the community, often with a complicated network of interactions among them.

Sixth, there has been a shift of focus from the possible effects of some environments in provoking the onset of some mental disorder to effects that endure long after the particular experience has come to an end (Uher et al., 2011). This was most dramatically shown in the follow-up into late adolescence of individuals who experienced profound deprivation in Romanian institutions and who were then, subsequently, adopted into UK families (Rutter, Kumsta, Schlotz, & Sonuga-Barke, 2012; Rutter & Sonuga-Barke, 2010). The markedly beneficial change in environment was certainly associated with substantial improvement in developmental functioning, but the effects of institutional deprivation were still strong more than a dozen years after the children left the institutions. Other studies have shown the same, and the findings have necessarily led to the question of the biological embedding of experiences (Rutter, 2012d) or, put more colloquially, how environments "get under the skin." Possible mediating mechanisms (intervening processes) are many and various, but attention has come to be particularly focused on epigenetic mechanisms and on the effects of stress and adversity on hypothalamic–pituitary–adrenal (HPA) axis. In addition, the mediating mechanisms might also include changes in the mental models (the meanings that are attached to experiences) that individuals acquire with respect to the experiences that they have gone through.

Finally, there has been a growing awareness of the need to test hypotheses about environmentally mediated effects, rather than assume them. Quantitative genetic research has long shown the importance of environmental influences on phenotypic variation (Plomin, DeFries, & Loehlin, 1977), but it has been much less successful in identifying the specific environments that have such effects. Eaves, Prom, and Silberg's (2010) development of the longitudinal twin and parent design (LTAP) has provided one good way forward. The findings showed a strong effect of antisocial parents on antisocial behavior in the children—an effect that was substantially environmentally mediated via the effect of parental neglect.

However, the development of more than a dozen variations of "natural experiment" that serve to "pull apart" variables that ordinarily go together has provided a substantial range of tests for environmental mediation (Rutter, 2007, 2012b). These have shown the reality of major environmental effects for certain key environmental features (such as discord, disharmony, and neglect). The analysis of nature–nurture integration has to begin with a clear testing of the separate effects of each. Van IJzendoorn et al. (2011) have argued for the value of using a randomized controlled trial to test for the environmental effect of the E in GxE studies—citing three relatively small studies that used this approach (Bakermans-Kranenburg, Van IJzendoorn, Pijlman, Mesman, & Juffer, 2008; Beach, Brody, Lei, & Philibert, 2010; Kegel, Bus, & van IJzendoorn, 2011). Overbeek,

Weeland, and Chhangur (2012) put forward the same argument—adding a further example (Cicchetti, Rogosch, & Toth, 2011) and a further paper on the Brody/Beach study (Brody, Beach, Philibert, Chen, & Murry, 2009). However, as Rutter (2012c) pointed out, although an RCT is indeed the best way of testing the effect of an intervention, the findings cannot be extrapolated backwards to an E effect years earlier—a serious limitation in the light of Karg, Burmeister, Shedden, and Sen (2011) finding that GxE with respect to the serotonin transporter polymorphism mainly applied to maltreatment in childhood as the E but with depression in adult life as the resulting phenotype.

With respect to both epigenetics and HPA effects, there is abundant evidence that there are environmental effects, but what is not clear at the moment is the extent to which such effects account for individual differences (e.g., in whether the stress effects are sensitizing (i.e., increasing vulnerability) or steeling (i.e., strengthening stress resistance); whether they are, or are not, associated with psychopathology; and whether or not they persist over time). One of the problems in investigating epigenetic effects in humans is the fact that the effects tend to be tissue specific. Because epigenetic changes cannot be examined in the brain during life, there has had to be reliance on either postmortem studies or studies of other tissues in the hope that these may adequately reflect what is going on in the brain. So far as HPA effects are concerned, it is clear that the effects of acute stress are rather different from those of chronic adversity, and it is also apparent that we do not know how far HPA effects are associated with the individual differences in psychopathology following adverse experiences (Gunnar & Vazquez, 2001, 2006; Loman & Gunnar, 2010).

Gene–Environment Correlations (rGE)

Gene–environment correlations (rGE) concern genetic influences on individual variations in people's exposure to particular sorts of environments. Plomin et al. (1977) differentiated among "passive," "active," and "evocative" rGE. Passive means that the rGE derives from parental genes influencing the rearing provided. The child's genes and the child's behavior are not implicated. Passive rGE needs to be studied through twin studies of parents (Neiderhiser et al., 2004), with a focus on the phenotype of the rearing environment. Note that this is not synonymous with a shared environmental effect because it cannot be assumed that passive rGE will affect all children in the same way or to the same degree (Rutter, Moffitt, & Caspi, 2006).

"Active" and "evocative" rGE are different because they concern the child's genes. "Active" rGE concerns the genetic effects on the child's behavior that serves to select or shape the environments experienced. Thus, this will be influenced by the child's genetically influenced behaviors, attitudes, and interests. Some children, for example, spend their free time reading on their own, others will be out with peers on the football field, yet others will be practicing some musical instrument, and many will be out playing and chatting with friends or hanging around street corners up to some mischief with other members of a gang. These experiences will, in turn, play a role in the child's development. "Evocative" rGE is different because it is solely concerned with the interpersonal aspects of the social environment. Thus, children's tendency to annoy others, or have fun with them, or to exercise leadership will play a role in shaping the environment experienced by means of an effect on other people's treatment of them.

Child-based designs are needed to assess "active" and "evocative" rGE. For example, adoption designs may be used to determine if genetically influenced features of the biological parents who did *not* rear them are associated with effects on the rearing provided by the adoptive parents who do not share the children's genes (Ge et al., 1996; O'Connor, Deater-Deckard, Fulker, Rutter, & Plomin, 1998).

There are strong reasons for expecting to find substantial rGE. It is well demonstrated by animal models that there is significant niche construction by animals such as beavers, weaver birds, and termites who modify their physical environment through building dams or constructing nursery environments for their offspring (Kendler & Gardner, 2010). In addition to effects on their physical environment, in social animals, there will be shaping and selecting through parent–offspring, mate, and adult–peer relationships. In humans, too, there is ample evidence that individuals do shape and select their environments. Because this will come about through the behavior of either the parents or the children, genetic influences on those behaviors will result in a genotype–environment correlation. Kendler and Baker (2007) undertook a systematic review of 55 independent studies in humans, using genetically sensitive designs in order to estimate the heritability of the environmental measures. Thirty-five environmental measures were examined by means of at least two studies, and the weighted heritability estimates mainly fell in the 15–35 % range with a weighted heritability mean of 27 %. Heritability was 29 % for self-report measures, 26 % for informant report measures, and 14 % for direct rater or videotape observations. The last finding that observation measures had a much lower heritability might suggest that the heritability reflected perceptions of the environment and not the actual environment. However, most of the observational measures were based on very short observations (typically about 10 min), whereas self-reports and informant reports were based on a much greater time period. If it was the time period, rather than the method of rating, that was responsible for the lower heritability, it should follow that the heritability ought to be much higher when it was examined across time periods. This was indeed what was found by Foley, Neale, and Kendler (1996) measured over a 12-month period and by Kendler (1997) over a 5-year period. In both studies, the heritability of the temporally stable aspects of the environment was about twice as great as those obtained by measurements on one occasion. Kendler and Baker (2007) appropriately concluded that heritability was not solely the result of subjective perceptions but rather reflected "real" environmental experiences. There was also some evidence that the heritability of the environment might increase during adolescence as individuals became more able to control and influence their environment.

Kendler and Baker (2007) found that experiences that are largely dependent on an individual's own behavior (as would be the case with family discord or conflict) are more heritable than "fateful" events independent of the person's own actions (such as bereavement). Secondly, whether reported by the parent or the child, parenting behavior reflecting the emotional quality of the parent–child relationship was more heritable than parenting behavior related to disciplinary styles. They suggested that the latter might be more like a social attitude in which parenting learned through their own experience was applied equally to all of their children, whereas emotional quality was impacted by the genetically influenced temperament of both parent and child. Evidence also indicated that genes from each person involved in a relationship appeared to contribute to its quality. Obviously, genetic factors cannot in any direct way "code" for specific environments. Rather, the rGE derives out of genetic influences on some form of behavior. Adoption studies provide a way of studying mediation effects with a design that separates the influences from biological parentage from the influences associated with rearing. Studies by Ge et al. (1996) and by O'Connor et al. (1998) showed that children born to (but not reared by) mothers with drug or alcohol problems had adoptive mothers who showed more negativity towards them. More detailed analyses showed that this effect was mediated by the evocative effect of the children's disruptive behavior on their adoptive mothers and, moreover, that this was found to a broadly similar degree in children not at genetic risk. This certainly means that research attention needs to be focused on the behaviors rather than on the genetics as such. The first implication, nevertheless, is that, because of rGE, it follows that part of the mediation of a risk factor that is descriptively environmental in nature (such as marital conflict and breakup, sexual abuse, or lack of social support) is likely to be genetic, and that is indeed what has been found. The clear implication is that it is essential to test for, not just assume, environmental mediation, and that is where natural experiments come into their own (Rutter, 2007, 2012a).

Although the focus of research needs to be on the behaviors involved in shaping or selecting the environments, multivariate genetic analyses can be highly useful in identifying the behaviors that mediate the genetic effect. This is done by treating the E as a phenotype. Sometimes the answers have been surprising. For example, Braungart, Plomin, DeFries, and Fulker (1992) found that only 23 % of the genetic variance on the HOME measure was accounted for by the child's score on the Bayley test of mental development. A further study showed that task orientation seemed to be the key mediator. Similarly, Kendler, Jacobson, Myers, and Eaves (2008) examined the mediating elements in the association between peer deviance (PD) and conduct disorder (CD). The study involved adult male twins and used a life history calendar to assess CD and PD. There were strong genetic influences on CD, with consequent environmental effects on PD through the peer network. In turn, PD had consequent effects on CD. In other words, the findings suggested a bidirectional process. rGE was found for peer deviance, which had an environmentally mediated effect on CD. The rGE for peer deviance was largely mediated through the social selection of like-minded deviant peers.

Sometimes, geneticists write and talk as if the correlation is truly between genes and environment, which implies that DNA could be in the environment. The same applies to niche construction (as with the beaver example given above). The implication is that the niche is genetically driven to create an environment that is maximally suited to the individual. The key point, however, is that the rGE has to operate through some behavior. This could bring about an adaptive, or a maladaptive, environment. In humans, the mediating behavior most studied has concerned the child's disruptive behavior, but the range of possibilities is much wider than that.

Gene–Environment Interactions (GxE)

Until the 1990s, most behavioral geneticists tended to dismiss GxE as sufficiently unimportant and sufficiently rare that it was safe to ignore it in partitioning the variance between G and E (Plomin, DeFries, & Fulker, 1988). This dismissal was based on the infrequency with which interactions have been found between anonymous genes and anonymous environments, both considered as a whole. That was not the appropriate focus because a universally operative GxE was most unlikely and because known examples of GxE applied only to specifics (Rutter & Pickles, 1991).

There are four positive reasons why GxE was expected to be quite common (Rutter et al, 2006). First, genetically influenced differential responses to the environment constitute the mechanism that has been thought to give rise to evolutionary change. To reject GxE would mean rejection of the cornerstone of evolutionary thinking. Second, to suppose that there is no GxE would require the assumption that responsivity to the environment is the one biological feature that is uniquely outside of genetic influence. That seems implausible in the extreme. Third, a wide range of human and other animal, naturalistic, and experimental studies have shown huge heterogeneity in response to all manner of environmental features—both physical and psychosocial. It is implausible that this variation involves no genetic influence. Fourth, behavioral genetic studies have provided many pointers to likely GxE—particularly in relation to depression and antisocial behavior (Rutter & Silberg, 2002). However, this evidence is rather circumstantial, and the situation became transformed by the molecular genetic advances that allowed individual susceptibility genes to be identified and by the increasing range of "natural experiment" strategies that allowed a better testing for environmental mediation of effects.

Before turning to the substantive findings on GxE, it is important to note five key methodological issues. Thus, first, it is important to check whether scaling variations have resulted in artifactual GxE. That is because it has long been known that changes in scale can either introduce artifactual GxE or alternatively artifactually eliminate true GxE. That is, changes in scale can either eliminate true GxE or create a false impression of GxE when, in reality, there is no biological GxE. Second, synergistic GxG interactions could account for apparent GxE, and it is necessary to use strategies that can separate the two. In other words, what seems on the surface to be GxE is in fact representing two or more genes reinforcing the actions of each other. Third, both additive and multiplicative synergistic interactions must be examined. Geneticists have tended to favor multiplicative GxE that uses a log scale, whereas most biologists consider that additive synergistic interactions appear more plausible (Kendler & Gardner, 2010). The conventional terminology is unfortunate because the term "additive" suggests a lack of interaction, whereas here it means there is an interaction, but it is one that does not require a logarithmic scale. Fourth, it is known that rGE can sometimes give rise to a misleading impression of apparent GxE and, again, that possibility must be tested in a rigorous fashion. Finally, as always, proper attention must be paid to multiple tests, and findings should be corrected appropriately.

Risch et al. (2009) have argued that it is improper to test for interactions if there is no statistical main effect, but statisticians are divided on this. Both forward and backward modeling have a mixture of plusses and minuses, and dogmatic assertions that there is only one acceptable approach have to be rejected (Rutter, Thapar, & Pickles, 2009). Human epidemiological studies of GxE were first put on the map through the Dunedin studies using identified candidate genes (selected on the basis of biological findings) and measured environments. The pattern of findings was similar in all their studies. That is, there was no genetic main effect; there were a weak environmental main effect and a much stronger GxE effect. Risch et al. (2009) are correct that if there is GxE, there must be some genetic main effect, but the main conclusion from the Dunedin studies is that, with a sample size of about 1,000, the genetic main effect was too small to be identified (Caspi, Hariri, Holmes, Uher, & Moffitt, 2010).

Risch et al.'s (2009) meta-analytic review dismissed the Dunedin findings as likely to be artifactual. However, the Risch et al. (2009) study was based on an unrepresentative, and biased, selection of studies, an exclusively statistical concept of GxE, and a failure to consider either the specific steps taken in the Dunedin studies to

test for possible scaling effects, possible GxG, possible effects of rGE, etc., as well as completely ignoring basic science, human experiments, and animal models (Caspi et al., 2010; Uher & McGuffin, 2009). Thus, Caspi and his colleagues tested GxE using several different measures of outcome that varied in their scaling properties. They tested for GxE using a different gene that was similar in scaling, but differed in its biology, and, again, found no GxE. This indicated that the GxE was a function of the biology and not of the scaling. Similarly, they tested the possible effects of GxG by examining the timing of the interaction. If the interaction reflected GxG, it should not show a timing effect, whereas if it was a true GxE, the interaction should apply only to E that preceded the interaction. The latter was found to be the case. In addition to all of that, Risch et al. (2009) focused exclusively on the use of life events as the measure of E—despite the fact that GxE had been found with maltreatment as well as with life events.

The topic of GxE needs to be considered from two different perspectives. First, the epidemiological findings need to be complemented by the experimental findings—both human and those using animal models. Secondly, attention needs to be focused on whether the findings apply in the same way to life events and to maltreatment and other adversities.

With respect to the latter, it is relevant that a much more extensive meta-analysis was undertaken by Karg et al. (2011). They dealt with 54 studies of interaction between 5-HTTLPR and various forms of stress in relation to the development of depression. The most important finding from this study was that there was only a weak, marginally significant, GxE in relation to life events but a highly significant, much stronger, GxE using maltreatment as the E. That means that the GxE applied to an E operating in early childhood in relation to an outcome that only became manifest in adolescence or early adult life. The clear implication is that the biological causal pathway was likely to operate over a long time span. That means that it is probably a mistake to focus on the effects of stress in provoking the onset of a disorder, and, instead, attention needs to be focused on the effects of adverse experiences in increasing the liability to a disorder (not just its timing). In that connection, too, Uher et al. (2011) found that the interaction between childhood maltreatment and the serotonin transporter promoter genotype in the Dunedin cohort applied only to persistent (i.e., chronic or recurrent) depression as the outcome variable.

Human experimental studies of GxE with respect to the 5-HTTLPR used an intermediate phenotype. The intermediate phenotype, to be useful, must be on the same biological pathway that leads to disorder, must involve a stress challenge that is open to manipulation, and must give rise to an immediate or non-delayed response that can be objectively measured; Hariri et al. (Hariri et al., 2002; Hyde et al., 2011) examined the amygdala activation response to fearful stimuli with the key comparison being the short- and long-allele versions of the 5-HTTLPR genotype. They found a significantly greater activation in those with a short allele—in other words, the same as found in the epidemiological studies (Hariri et al., 2005; Heinz et al., 2004). The findings, and others using similar techniques, confirmed the reality and meaningfulness of the GxE, but it was a crucially important methodological feature that the samples used were all screened to be free of psychopathology. This means that the GxE is not confined to individuals with the outcome variable in question—whether that be depression or antisocial behavior. Rather, it applies to a biological pathway that applies to everyone. However, studies using clinical samples (Caspi et al., 2010) showed the same, so that clearly it is relevant for psychopathologies.

The same broad conclusions derived from animal models. Thus, the short allele of the 5-HTTLPR was associated with serotonin metabolites in the cerebrospinal fluid (Bennett et al., 2002), visual response to stimuli (Champoux et al., 2002), increased adrenocorticotropic hormone (ACTH) levels (Barr et al., 2004), coping responses (Spinelli et al., 2007), and brain morphology (Jedema et al., 2009). Suomi's research group used rhesus monkeys to examine the effects of the interaction between the 5-HTTLPR genotype and the pattern of rearing (Nelson et al., 2009).

They used a chronic experience and not an acute stress. The chronic experience concerned rearing by peers, which their own research, as well as that by others, had shown to carry substantial risk effects. Other studies using infant rhesus macaques have focused on the acute response to a human intruder (Kinnally et al., 2010). The fact that the findings were less clear-cut may well be a consequence of using a single social separation–relocation procedure, rather than a different maladaptive form of rearing.

Rodent Studies

Rodents show functional variation in the 5-HTT gene, but there is no equivalent of the repeat length polymorphisms (i.e., short or long) seen in humans. Nevertheless, there are other polymorphisms at other regions of the 5-HTT gene (Caspi et al., 2010). These have been investigated in two rather different ways. First, knockout rat mutants (and those with transgenic overexpression of 5-HTTLPR) have been studied. The findings have shown that the neural consequences extend well beyond those stemming from 5-HTTLPR and its role in 5-HTTLPR availability. Caspi et al. (2010) argued that the 5-HTT modulates stress reactivity through its effects on neurolimbic circuitry (Hariri, Drabant, & Weinberger, 2006). The second approach has been to study directly the only known single-nucleotide polymorphism (SNP) in the coding region of the rat's 5-HTTLPR homologue (Belay et al., 2011). The findings showed a GxE with respect to the effects of the prenatal environment on the HPA axis and with the postnatal environment on behavior. Once more, the findings suggested a developmental, as well as stress reactivity, effect. The fact that the prenatal and postnatal effects differ is also in keeping with the hypothesis that the genetic effect is on a general environmental susceptibility (see below). The findings also showed a prenatal stress interaction for glucocorticoid mRNA levels, emphasizing the biological impact.

Most of the discussion of GxE focuses on it as representing a genetic moderation of a response to adverse environments. However, both Belsky and Boyce and their coworkers have pointed out that evolutionary considerations mean that it is more likely that susceptibility applies to most environments and not just adverse ones (Ellis, Boyce, Belsky, Bakermans-Kranenburg, & Van IJzendoorn, 2011). They put forward some evidence that the same polymorphic variance associated with vulnerability in adverse environments is also associated with a better response to positive ones. It is much too early to accept or reject the hypothesis about the so-called plasticity genes, but the evidence in support is growing. Nevertheless, there has yet to be direct testing of the hypothesis that the polymorphism associated with vulnerability in the context of adversity is also associated with a greater beneficial response to positive environments such as therapeutic interventions in the same individuals. Until that has been done, there has to be caution over the claims. However, the study by Simons et al. (2012) provides findings that come closest to what is needed (see discussion below on the monoamine oxidase A (MAOA) genotype).

GxE with Respect to the MAOA Genotype and Antisocial Behavior

The most space has been given to the 5-HTTLPR findings because they have given rise to the most research. However, it is necessary to note the parallel findings on the MAOA gene and the interaction with maltreatment in relation to antisocial behavior in the children (Caspi et al., 2002). Maltreatment was selected as the E variable because of the evidence that it has lasting neurochemical correlates in both humans and other animals. The gene concerned a functional polymorphism in the promoter region of MAOA gene. The findings showed that maltreated children whose genotype gave rise to low levels of MAOA were more likely to develop antisocial behavior as measured in several different ways. Similar methodological checks were undertaken to those employed with the 5-HTTLPR. The result held up, (Foley et al. 2004; Fergusson, Boden, Horwood, Miller, and Kennedy 2012) as did the findings of a meta-analysis (Kim-Cohen et al., 2006; Taylor & Kim-Cohen, 2007).

The Fergusson et al. (2012) report, based on the Christchurch longitudinal study, brought out several other important findings. The findings confirmed the Caspi et al. (2002) finding of GxE with the low-activity variant of the MAOA gene in males. This is in keeping with most other published reports (but not all) (Huizinga et al., 2006; Prichard, Mackinnon, Jorm, & Easteal, 2008), but the findings suggested that the GxE also applied to other environmental factors (such as smoking and maternal deprivation) and personal factors (such as IQ). Queries need to be raised about the assumption that these represented causal influences. Thus, three different types of actual experiment (D'Onofrio et al., 2008; Obel et al., 2011; Thapar et al., 2009) have shown that the risks associated with prenatal smoking exposure probably reflect genetic, and not environmental, mediation of risk (Thapar & Rutter, 2009).

A key study is that by Nikulina, Widom, and Brzustowicz (2012) using a prospective cohort design involving court-substantiated cases of child abuse and a comparable control group—both followed up into adult life and interviewed. The study was innovative in looking for possible sex and ethnicity differences and in examining depressive and alcohol abuse phenotypes, as well as antisocial behavior. The findings were complicated by the number of 3-way interactions but were important in showing that the high-activity variant predisposed to depressive phenotypes in females (but not males). No sex differences were found with respect to alcoholism. With respect to depressive phenotypes, the low-activity variant was protective in whites, but the high-activity variant was protective in nonwhites. There are too few studies to draw firm conclusions on ethnic differences.

Findings from the Iowa Adoption Studies confirmed the GxE with respect to the MAOA genotype and antisocial behavior (Beach et al., 2010) but also showed that a new variable nucleotide repeat (VNTR) added to the variance explained in predicting antisocial personality disorder in females.

Recent research has sought to investigate further the possible moderating role of variations in the social context. For example, Mertins, Schote, Hoffeld, Griessmair, and Meyer (2011) used an experimental design to vary information about other people's behavior in relation to private and public investment. In the first round (in which there was no information on other people's behavior), male participants contributed approximately half of their point endowment. Further rounds showed that low-MAOA-activity males contributed less to the public good than high-activity males. The reverse, however, applied in females. In keeping with other research (Meyer-Lindenberg & Weinberger, 2006), it is clear that MAOA associations usually show a sex by genotype interaction—meaning that the effects in males and females differ and may even work in opposite directions. Lee (2011) studied the association between deviant peer affiliation and antisocial behavior as possibly moderated by the MAOA genotype. The sample studied prospectively was a large group of male Caucasian adolescents and young adults from the Add Health study. Low-activity MAOA was associated overall with significantly more overt antisocial behavior (ASB), but deviant peer affiliation predicted ASB more strongly in individuals with the high-activity MAOA genotype. Thus, there was an apparently main effect of low-activity MAOA on ASB but (perhaps because of neural effects) (Buckholtz & Meyer-Lindenberg, 2008) a significant GxE with respect to high-activity MAOA. Note that although this is the opposite of what Caspi et al. (2002) found, Caspi's GxE referred to maltreatment, whereas this concerned a deviant peer group, which is likely to operate rather differently.

Simons et al. (2012) using longitudinal data from a sample of several hundred African American males focused on adherence to a street code of violent identity as the social context variable in relation to a hostile demoralized community. Possible genetic differential susceptibility combined three genes 5-HTTLPR, the dopamine receptor gene DRD-4, and the MAOA gene. A hostile environment had significant effects on street code and on aggression, whereas the plasticity genes did not. Respondents with several plasticity alleles were *more* likely to engage in aggression when exposed to a hostile environment but *less* likely in its absence—a crossover effect indicating GxE. Further analyses showed

that adopting the street code served as a mediator of the effects of a hostile environment on aggression. The findings provide probably the best support so far for Belsky's differential susceptibility hypothesis (Belsky & Beaver, 2011; Belsky & Pluess, 2009).

Animal models, using rhesus macaques, have given rise to findings that are difficult to interpret. Newman et al. (2005) found that mother-reared monkeys with the low-activity MAOA genotype were more aggressive than low-activity nursery-reared animals or any animals with a high-activity genotype. The authors raised queries about the compatibility with abusive human environments. Karere et al. (2009) somewhat similarly examined social context variations—contrasting infants reared with mothers and up to 150 other animals in large cages, reared with mothers in a smaller group, reared with mother and access at most to one other mother–infant pair, and reared with same-aged peers in a nursery. All groups were exposed to a brief social challenge at 3–4 months. Low-activity genotype animals reared under adverse conditions were at the greatest risk of adverse outcomes. However, adverse rearing that involved exposure to more aggression facilitated the impact of genotype on anxiety, but adverse conditions that did not involve such exposure did not. As the title of the article noted, the findings raise questions on what is meant by an adverse environment and on human parallels. The primate studies note the role of GxE, but they neither support nor reject the specifics of the human studies.

Schizophrenia and Other Outcomes

Although this chapter has provided a broad coverage of the research literature, there are other genotypes and other outcomes that have not been considered—such as physical assault in suicide attempts (Ben-Efraim, Wasserman, Wasserman, & Sokolowski, 2011), unusual deprivation-specific patterns (Kumsta, Rutter, Stevens, & Sonuga-Barke, 2010), and response to interventions on "externalizing behavior" (Bakermans-Kranenburg et al., 2008) and mother–infant separation (D'Amato et al., 2011). These and numerous other reports underline the fact that, so far, gene–environment interdependence has been examined in relation to rather a narrow range of genotypes and of environments. Nevertheless, the principles appear broadly similar across the range although, of course, the specifics vary.

Meyer-Lindenberg (2011) has argued that GxE research in schizophrenia needs to start with evidence on neural system findings in the disorder—noting the role of dopaminergic mechanisms, which suggested the likely importance of COMT. He also noted that the GxE focus might be better placed on neural effects than on a behavioral phenotype. He noted the evidence showing the role of 5-HTTLPR in amygdala activation (Munafò, Brown, & Hariri, 2008). Regarding E, he pointed to the evidence implicating migration, urbanicity, and social status (van Os & Poulton, 2008). Meyer-Lindenberg argued that the neural evidence suggested attention to social status, and Zink et al. (2008) designed an experimental strategy that could manipulate perceived social status. The findings showed that the brain responses to superiority and inferiority were dissociable.

In keeping with the need to start with the evidence on neural features and on cannabis effects, various prospective population studies found that cannabis greatly increased the risk for schizophrenia (Arseneault et al., 2002; Fergusson, Horwood, & Swain-Campbell, 2003; Henquet et al., 2005; van Os et al., 2002; Zammit, Allebeck, Andreasson, Lundberg, & Lewis, 2002). However, the same research showed that despite odds ratios of 2 to 3, many individuals used cannabis without developing schizophrenia and many people with schizophrenia had not taken cannabis. The research findings showed that the risk was greatest in the case of those first using cannabis in adolescence rather than adult life and in those with heavy cumulative exposure to cannabis. Using the biological findings of COMT effects on the dopamine system (Harrison & Weinberger, 2004), Caspi et al. (2005) used the Dunedin longitudinal study to investigate the hypothesis that COMT genotype might moderate the cannabis risk effect on schizophrenia. They found that the greatest increase in schizophrenia was in those with the

Val/Val genotype, a lesser increase in those with the Val/Met, and no increase in the Met/Met individuals. The finding that the schizophrenia risk stemmed only from cannabis use and not heroin or cocaine suggested that the mediation was through biochemical pathways rather than social stressors (Rutter et al., 2006).

Research since the Caspi et al. (2005) paper was sought to take understanding of the postulated GxE forward in several different ways. First, it appears that it is important to consider the role of dosage. Di Forti et al. (2009) found that people with a first episode of psychosis, as compared with controls, had used cannabis for longer and with a greater frequency. In addition, they were much more likely to have used high-potency cannabis (sinsemilla or "skunk"). The implication is that the psychosis risk is a function of heavy, prolonged exposure to Δ9-THC.

Estrada et al. (2011) in a study of young psychiatric patients (mean age 17 years)—80 with schizophrenia spectrum disorders and 77 with other nonpsychotic disorders—showed that age at first cannabis use correlated with age at onset of psychiatric disorder (so that earlier cannabis use was associated with earlier onset). The Val158Met genotype was not associated with either diagnosis or cannabis use, but the Val/Val genotype was associated with an earlier age of onset than with Met carriers. Pelayo-Terán et al. (2010) also examined the age of onset in a cross-sectional study of 174 patients with a first episode of psychosis. Among nonusers of cannabis, the age of onset was later, and duration of psychosis was longer in met homozygotes—suggesting that the GxE reflected a moderator effect of cannabis in suppressing the delay effect of the met allele.

Zammit, Owen, Evans, Heron, and Lewis (2011) by contrast, in a study of a subsample (2,630) of the Avon Longitudinal Study of Parents and Children (ALSPAC) at ages 14 and 16 years, found that the 168 individuals who had used cannabis at age 14 had an odds ratio of 2.5 for psychotic-like symptoms at age 16 years. GxE was examined only using a multiplicative model (despite Kendler and Gardner (2010) putting forward reasons for preferring an additive synergistic model). No GxE was found—thus not confirming the Caspi et al. (2005) findings. Despite the message of the paper, limited weight should be attached to the negative findings—because of the misleading reliance on psychotic-like symptoms in adolescence rather than a schizophrenia spectrum disorder, because of an equally misleading reliance on a multiplicative model, and because of the small subsample studied.

Henquet and colleagues (Henquet et al., 2009; Henquet, Rosa, Krabbendam, & Sergi Papiol, 2006) used an experimental approach to test the causal inference of the Val158Met polymorphism GxE effect. In the first study, they used a sample of patients, relatives and controls, to give a single dose of THC—the psychoactive ingredient of cannabis (or placebos). Those with the homozygous Val genotype were more likely to develop THC-induced psychotic symptoms, but this was contingent on previous evidence of psychosis liability. The later study used a structured diary technique to investigate if exposure to cannabis increased the level of psychotic symptoms and if this was moderated by the COMT Val158Met genotype. The findings were broadly in line with the first study but with the additional indication that hallucinations were a more sensitive phenotype than delusions. The implication is that there is a GxG synergism as well as a GxE.

There is no acceptable animal model of schizophrenia, but studies of both rats (Pistis et al., 2004; Schneider & Koch, 2004) and mice (O'Tuathaigh et al., 2010) have examined neurocognitive phenotypes on the grounds that schizophrenia involves cognitive features that are likely to be effected by cannabis (Ayhan, Sawa, Ross, & Pletnikov, 2009). The findings are not entirely consistent, but there is evidence of greater THC effects on cognition during adolescence and that there is suggestive COMT modulation of adolescent THC effects.

Human studies of the effects of cannabis use in adolescence on brain structure and function are limited, but there is growing evidence of lasting effects on neurodevelopment and cognitive performance (Casadio, Fernandes, Murray, & Di Forti, 2011; Meier et al., 2012).

Putting together all sources, there is strong evidence that cannabis has a contributory causal role in the etiology of some psychotic illnesses and that this risk is strongest in the case of heavy early use in individuals with a preexisting vulnerability to psychosis. The evidence of a GxE effect in which individuals with the Val158Met polymorphism are most vulnerable is also strong, although not completely overwhelming. However, it is most unlikely that cannabis use constitutes the only environmental risk. Thus, Harley et al. (2010) showed that both cannabis use and childhood trauma were independently associated with psychotic symptoms but the risk was greatest when they were both present. As already noted, it is also clear that many individuals develop schizophrenia in the absence of cannabis use and many people use cannabis without developing schizophrenia.

Methodological Matters

Because of the unavoidable complexity of trying to analyze gene–gene and gene–environment interactions, there have been several attempts at developing rule-based algorithms using both additive and multiplicative interactions as well as a range of different types of genetic models (Amato et al., 2010; Ding, Källberg, Klareskog, Padyukov, & Alfredsson, 2011; Lehr, Yuan, Zeumer, Jayadev, & Ritchie, 2011; Peng, 2010; Wakefield, De Vocht, & Hung, 2010). They have mainly been recommended as tools for the preselection of attributes to be used in more complex computationally intensive approaches. However, doubt needs to be expressed regarding the focus on purely statistical approaches to GxE, without concern for the biology (Caspi et al., 2010).

There have been increasing concerns in recent years over the problem of publication bias (Duncan & Keller, 2011; Ioannidis, 2005). There can be no doubt that the problem of publication bias is a real one, but valid concerns are sometimes used unfairly to damn good work. Critics of GxE research have usually argued for exact replications with a narrowly defined environmental feature. That does not seem a sensible way forward because none of the research suggests that GxE applied only to very specific stressors and the pooling of such stressors as advocated by Karg et al. (2011) and by Fergusson et al. (2012) appears a valuable way of moving forward. Sugden et al.'s (2010) study, showing that serotonin transporter gene moderated emotional problems following bullying victimization, uses the same way of proceeding. Robins (1978), years ago, argued that sturdy replication means that similar results should be found despite variations in sample characteristics, phenotype measurement, and environmental exposure. That needs to be the requirement with respect to the biology, and it is foolish to demand an exact copying of the details. A valid finding should be robust to variations in the details.

Clinical, Conceptual, and Research Implications of Gene–Environment Interdependence

First, the findings on developmental perturbations, such as congenital anomalies, chromosome anomalies, and copy-number variations (CNVs), highlight the need to consider both their causes and their effects. High maternal age and high paternal age increase the likelihood of such anomalies occurring, but the anomalies do not account for individual variations in psychopathological consequences. By what mechanisms do raised maternal and paternal age have their effects? Why are all of these developmental perturbations more common in certain mental disorders but not in others? Insofar as any of these have causal effects on psychopathology, as seems very likely to be the case with CNVs—how do the causal effects arise and why are they so diagnostically nonspecific? All of us need to be more aware of the probable importance of these developmental perturbations, as well as appreciate the uncertainty as to whether it is valid to group them all together and accept the uncertainty.

The epigenetic findings have shown that experiences can alter the biology by influencing gene expression. This constitutes one possible mediating mechanism for the biological embedding of environmental experiences. Its conceptual importance is that it serves as a reminder that the effects of experiences are part of biology and are not

separate from it. The finding that the epigenetic effects of gene expression are neurochemically mediated means that it could turn out to be appropriate to consider using medication to treat the effects of psychosocial adversities, although that remains highly speculative at the moment. As discussed, although it is well demonstrated through research that spans several different species that experiences do bring about epigenetic effects, two major questions remain unanswered. First, do these explain the individual differences in response to experiences, and, second, do the epigenetic effects account for effects on the mental disorder outcome when that occurs? This query needs to be addressed at several different levels. Thus, epigenetic effects are likely to bring about the changes in HPA functioning, but is it the epigenetic effects or is it the HPA axis effects that actually account for the phenotypic variations in the development of mental disorder (Rutter, 2012d)?

The findings on rGE have two important implications. First, the existence of rGE means that part of the mediation of the risk effects of adverse experiences may be genetic rather than environmental, making treatment strategies focusing on reducing the environmental risk possibly less efficacious than hoped for. But it is probably even more important that the main mediating effect of the supposed genetic influence on the environment lies in the evocative role of disruptive child behaviors rather than any direct genetic effect. The clinical implication is that there should be interventions focused on the negative evocative effects on parents (and others) of certain child behaviors. Children can, and do, select and shape their environments, and part of the risk effects may involve these effects. But is the main mediator the child's disruptive behavior, or are other behaviors also influential?

The implications of GxE are even more important, but, in some respects, they are less self-evident. First, the human experimental data showing that the neural effects of GxE are found in individuals without psychopathology, as well as in those with it, means that there must be a dimensional perspective in relation to risk effects. This is, of course, one of the two central features of developmental psychopathology. The second essential feature is the importance of considering continuities and discontinuities over the span of development. The finding that GxE is mainly concerned with effects that are initiated in childhood but persist into adult life underlines the importance of this point.

There has been a temptation by some people to suppose that the GxE findings mean that seriously adverse experiences such as abuse or neglect may not matter if someone does not have the allele associated with environmental susceptibility. That would be a wrong interpretation of the evidence because the findings show that GxE effects are to a considerable extent outcome specific. Thus, the 5-HTTLPR GxE is relevant for depression but not for antisocial behavior. The converse applies to the MAOA gene. Doubtless in time, other genes will be found to have effects on other outcomes. What that clearly means is that it cannot be assumed that the GxE as studied so far means that abuse and neglect are harmless for some individuals because there may be ill effects on outcomes other than depression and antisocial behavior. Yet a different reason for it being wrong to assume that abuse or neglect may not matter if someone does not have the allele associated with environmental vulnerability concerns the evidence (which is so far suggestive rather than conclusive) that the same polymorphic variance associated with vulnerability to adverse environments is also associated with better response to positive ones. The implication is that GxE should be an encouragement for the likely value of therapeutic or preventive interventions, rather than the reverse (which many have wrongly assumed).

Despite a few destructive critiques based on looking at only a small portion of the relevant evidence, it may be expected that future research findings will confirm the basic principles of gene–environment interdependence. On the other hand, as is evident from the modifications on details that have come about through research during the last few years, it is certainly likely that details will need to be altered. The future of research into gene–environment interplay is bright, and the findings are already altering our understanding of both normal and abnormal psychological developments.

Conclusion

Concepts of genes (nature) and environment (nurture) have changed dramatically over recent decades. Genes were previously thought of as single features that had, via messenger RNA, a unitary effect on particular proteins which in turn led, through ill-understood pathways, to some phenotypic outcome. No one now thinks of genes in that fashion. In the first place, each gene actually involves multiple DNA elements and not just one. Gene effects are entirely dependent on gene expression—a process that involves multiple DNA elements, chance, and the environment—thus, in a stroke, destroying the qualitative difference between nature and nurture. The notion that the only genes that matter being those with effects on proteins, the rest being "junk" DNA, has also gone. Many of the most important gene actions operate through the promotion of other genes, there being no effect as such on proteins. The idea that each gene has just one effect has also had to be abandoned in view of the evidence that most genes have pleiotropic actions. Finally, it is now realized that some genes have their effects, at least in part, through influences on environmental exposure (through rGE) and on environmental susceptibility (through GxE). In this way, genes, as it were, get "outside the skin." In addition, the actions of some genes depend on synergistic interaction with other genes.

Our understanding of the environment has undergone a similarly great transformation. First, there has come a realization that because a feature describes an environment, that does not mean that the risks are environmentally mediated. A wide range of "natural experiments" have been devised to test environmental mediation hypotheses. Second, environments do not just involve socialization experiences, as implied by the word "nurture." Environments involve prenatal, as well as postnatal, effects (as illustrated, e.g., by fetal alcohol influences); and they involve physical, as well as psychosocial, features (as shown by the importance of cannabis effects). During the late 1960s, there was a debate on the extent to which apparent socialization effects reflected children's influences on their parents, rather than the other way round. It is now clear that the effects can work in either direction, with bidirectional effects common. Finally, it has come to be appreciated that environmental effects get biologically embedded—i.e., get "inside the skin." In the past, too, much attention was paid to the effects of acute events, whereas now (at least with respect to GxE) it has been shown that serious chronic or recurrent adversities (such as physical abuse or sexual abuse) are more influential.

With respect to gene–environment interplay, it appears that the processes are not fixed and unchanging. Rather, there are ill-understood variations according to social context, sex, and ethnicity. This is particularly apparent in the findings on both the COMT and MAOA effects. It is clear that the same gene (or the same environment) may have, in different circumstances, both a "direct" or "main" effect and one depending on gene–environment interplay. The notion of the so-called plasticity genes is an attractive one, and although the "crossover" effect according to the presence or absence of adversity is plausible, it remains to be rigorously tested. rGE effects are important, not because they have much useful to say about genes, but because they highlight the need to study which behaviors account for both shaping/selecting of environments and evocative effects influencing other people's responses. There is a particular interest in studying environments, such as the peer group, which may have either deviance-enhancing or protective effects.

In my opinion, there is nothing to suggest that there is any value in screening the genome for G–E interplay when it is defined as a statistical phenomenon. Rather, the need is for research to identify the biological pathways involved. So far, the range of both genes and environments that have been studied has been quite narrow. Moreover, all too often the focus has been on a particular disease or disorder outcome, ignoring the fact that genes do not code for psychiatric diagnoses or psychological traits. The future of research into nature–nurture integration is bright, and the likely payoff in terms of clinical gains is also substantial, but the challenges to be dealt with and the hazards to be overcome remain substantial.

References

Academy of Medical Sciences. (2007). *Identifying the environmental causes of disease: How should we decide what to believe and when to take action?* London: Academy of Medical Sciences.

Amato, R., Pinelli, M., D'Andrea, D., Miele, G., Nicodemi, M., Raiconi, G., et al. (2010). A novel approach to simulate gene-environment interactions in complex diseases. *BMC Bioinformatics, 11*(8).

Arseneault, L., Cannon, M., Poulton, R., Murray, R., Caspi, A., & Moffitt, T. E. (2002). Cannabis use in adolescence and risk for adult psychosis: Longitudinal prospective study. *British Journal of Psychiatry, 325,* 1212–1213.

Ayhan, Y., Sawa, A., Ross, C. A., & Pletnikov, M. V. (2009). Animal models of gene-environment interactions in schizophrenia. *Behavioural Brain Research, 204,* 274–281.

Bakermans-Kranenburg, M. J., Van IJzendoorn, M. H., Pijlman, F. T. A., Mesman, J., & Juffer, F. (2008). Experimental evidence for differential susceptibility: Dopamine D4 receptor polymorphism (DRD4 VNTR) moderates intervention effects on toddlers' externalizing behavior in a randomized controlled trial. *Developmental Psychology, 44,* 293–300.

Barr, C. S., Newman, T. K., Shannon, C., Parker, C., Dvoskin, R. L., Becker, M. L., et al. (2004). Rearing condition and rh5-HTTLPR interact to influence limbic-hypothalamic-pituitary-adrenal axis response to stress in infant macaques. *Biological Psychiatry, 55,* 733–738.

Beach, S. R. H., Brody, G. H., Lei, M. K., & Philibert, R. A. (2010). Differential susceptibility to parenting among African American youths: Testing the DRD4 hypothesis. *Journal of Family Psychology, 24,* 513–521.

Belay, H., Burton, C. L., Lovic, V., Meaney, M. J., Sokolowski, M., & Fleming, A. S. (2011). Early adversity and serotonin transporter genotype interact with hippocampal glucocorticoid receptor mRNA expression, corticosterone, and behavior in adult male rats. *Behavioral Neuroscience, 125,* 150–160.

Belsky, J., & Beaver, K. M. (2011). Cumulative-genetic plasticity, parenting and adolescent self-regulation. *Journal of Child Psychology and Psychiatry, 52,* 619–626.

Belsky, J., & Pluess, M. (2009). Beyond diathesis stress: Differential susceptibility to environmental influences. *Psychological Bulletin, 135,* 885–908.

Ben-Efraim, Y. J., Wasserman, D., Wasserman, J., & Sokolowski, M. (2011). Gene–environment interactions between CRHR1 variants and physical assault in suicide attempts. *Genes, Brain, and Behavior, 10,* 663–672.

Bennett, A. J., Lesch, K. P., Heils, A., Long, J. C., Lorenz, J. G., Shoaf, S. E., et al. (2002). Early experience and serotonin transporter gene variation interact to influence primate CNS function. *Molecular Psychiatry, 7,* 118–122.

Braungart, J. M., Plomin, R., DeFries, J. C., & Fulker, D. W. (1992). Genetic influence on tester-rated infant temperament as assessed by Bayley's infant behavior record: Nonadoptive and adoptive siblings and twins. *Developmental Psychology, 28*, 40–47.

Brody, G. H., Beach, S. R. H., Philibert, R. A., Chen, Y., & Murry, V. M. B. (2009). Prevention effects moderate the association of 5-HTTLPR and youth risk behavior initiation: Gene × Environment hypotheses tested via a randomized prevention design. *Child Development, 80*, 645–661.

Buckholtz, J. W., & Meyer-Lindenberg, A. (2008). MAOA and the neurogenetic architecture of human aggression. *Trends in Neurosciences, 31*, 120–129.

Casadio, P., Fernandes, C., Murray, R. M., & Di Forti, M. (2011). Cannabis use in young people: The risk for schizophrenia. *Neuroscience and Biobehavioral Reviews, 35*, 1779–1787.

Caspi, A., Hariri, A. R., Holmes, A., Uher, R., & Moffitt, T. E. (2010). Genetic sensitivity to the environment: The case of the serotonin transporter gene and its implications for studying complex diseases and traits. *American Journal of Psychiatry, 167*, 509–527.

Caspi, A., Langley, K., Milne, B., Moffitt, T. E., O'Donovan, M., Owen, M. J., et al. (2008). A replicated molecular genetic basis for subtyping antisocial behavior in children with attention-deficit/hyperactivity disorder. *Archives of General Psychiatry, 65*, 203–210. doi:10.1001/archgenpsychiatry.2007.24.

Caspi, A., McClay, J., Moffitt, T. E., Mill, J., Martin, J., Craig, I. W., et al. (2002). Role of genotype in the cycle of violence in maltreated children. *Science, 297*, 851–854.

Caspi, A., Moffitt, T. E., Cannon, M., McClay, J., Murray, R., Harrington, H. L., et al. (2005). Moderation of the effect of adolescent-onset cannabis use on adult psychosis by a functional polymorphism in the catechol-O-methyltransferase gene: Longitudinal evidence of a gene X environment interaction. *Biological Psychiatry, 57*, 1117–1127.

Champoux, M., Bennett, A., Shannon, C., Higley, J. D., Lesch, K. P., & Suomi, S. J. (2002). Serotonin transporter gene polymorphism, differential early rearing, and behavior in rhesus monkey neonates. *Molecular Psychiatry, 7*, 1058–1063.

Cicchetti, D., Rogosch, F. A., & Toth, S. L. (2011). The effects of child maltreatment and polymorphisms of the serotonin transporter and dopamine D4 receptor genes on infant attachment and intervention efficacy. *Development and Psychopathology, 23*, 357–372.

D'Amato, F. R., Zanettini, C., Lampis, V., Coccurello, R., Pascucci, T., Ventura, R., et al. (2011). Unstable maternal environment, separation anxiety, and heightened CO2 sensitivity induced by gene-by-environment interplay. *PLoS One, 6*, e18637.

D'Onofrio, B. M., Hulle, C. A., Waldman, I. D., Rodgers, J. L., Harden, K. P., Rathouz, P. J., et al. (2008). Smoking during pregnancy and offspring externalizing problems: An exploration of genetic and environmental confounds. *Development and Psychopathology, 20*, 139–164.

Di Forti, M., Morgan, C., Dazzan, P., Pariante, C., Mondelli, V., Marques, T. R., et al. (2009). High-potency cannabis and the risk of psychosis. *British Journal of Psychiatry, 195*, 488–491.

Ding, B., Källberg, H., Klareskog, L., Padyukov, L., & Alfredsson, L. (2011). GEIRA: Gene-environment and gene–gene interaction research application. *European Journal of Epidemiology, 26*, 557–561.

Duncan, L. E., & Keller, M. C. (2011). A critical review of the first 10 years of candidate gene-by-environment interaction research in psychiatry. *American Journal of Psychiatry, 168*, 1041–1049.

Eaves, L. J., Prom, E. C., & Silberg, J. L. (2010). The mediating effect of parental neglect on adolescent and young adult anti-sociality: A longitudinal study of twins and their parents. *Behavior Genetics, 40*, 425–437.

Ellis, B. J., Boyce, W. T., Belsky, J., Bakermans-Kranenburg, M. J., & Van IJzendoorn, M. H. (2011). Differential susceptibility to the environment: An evolutionary-neurodevelopmental theory. *Development and Psychopathology, 23*, 7–28.

Estrada, G., Fatjó-Vilas, M., Munoz, M. J., Pulido, G., Minano, M. J., Toledo, E., et al. (2011). Cannabis use and age at onset of psychosis: Further evidence of interaction with COMT Val158Met polymorphism. *Acta Psychiatrica Scandinavica, 123*, 485–492.

Fergusson, D. M., Boden, J. M., Horwood, L. J., Miller, A., & Kennedy, M. A. (2012). Moderating role of the MAOA genotype in antisocial behaviour. *British Journal of Psychiatry, 200*, 116–123.

Fergusson, D. M., Horwood, L. J., & Swain-Campbell, N. R. (2003). Cannabis dependence and psychotic symptoms in young people. *Psychological Medicine, 33*, 15–21.

Flint, J., Greenspan, R. J., & Kendler, K. S. (2010). *How genes influence behavior*. Oxford & New York: Oxford University Press.

Foley, D. L., Eaves, L. J., Wormley, B., Silberg, J. L., Maes, H. H., Kuhn, J., et al. (2004). Childhood adversity, monoamine oxidase A genotype, and risk for conduct disorder. *Archives of General Psychiatry, 61*, 738.

Foley, D. L., Neale, M. C., & Kendler, K. S. (1996). A longitudinal study of stressful life events assessed at interview with an epidemiological sample of adult twins: The basis of individual variation in event exposure. *Psychological Medicine, 26*, 1239–1252.

Ge, X., Conger, R. D., Cadoret, R. J., Neiderhiser, J. M., Yates, W., Troughton, E., et al. (1996). The developmental interface between nature and nurture: A mutual influence model of child antisocial behavior and parent behaviors. *Developmental Psychology, 32*, 574–589.

Gunnar, M. R., & Vazquez, D. M. (2001). Low cortisol and a flattening of expected daytime rhythm: Potential indices of risk in human development. *Development and Psychopathology, 13*, 515–538.

Gunnar, M. R., & Vazquez, D. M. (2006). Stress, neurobiology and developmental psychopathology. In D. Cicchetti & D. Cohen (Eds.), *Developmental psychopathology* (Vol. 2, pp. 533–577). New York: Wiley.

Hariri, A. R., Drabant, E. M., Munoz, K. E., Kolachana, B. S., Mattay, V. S., Egan, M. F., et al. (2005). A susceptibility gene for affective disorders and the response of the human amygdala. *Archives of General Psychiatry, 62*, 146–152.

Hariri, A. R., Drabant, E. M., & Weinberger, D. R. (2006). Imaging genetics: Perspectives from studies of genetically driven variation in serotonin function and corticolimbic affective processing. *Biological Psychiatry, 59*, 888–897.

Hariri, A. R., Mattay, V. S., Tessitore, A., Kolachana, B., Fera, F., Goldman, D., et al. (2002). Serotonin transporter genetic variation and the response of the human amygdala. *Science, 297*, 400–403.

Harley, M., Kelleher, I., Clarke, M., Lynch, F., Arseneault, L., Connor, D., et al. (2010). Cannabis use and childhood trauma interact additively to increase the risk of psychotic symptoms in adolescence. *Psychological Medicine, 40*, 1627–1634.

Harrison, P. J., & Weinberger, D. R. (2004). Schizophrenia genes, gene expression, and neuropathology: On the matter of their convergence. *Molecular Psychiatry, 10*, 40–68.

Heinz, A., Braus, D. F., Smolka, M. N., Wrase, J., Puls, I., Hermann, D., et al. (2004). Amygdala-prefrontal coupling depends on a genetic variation of the serotonin transporter. *Nature Neuroscience, 8*, 20–21.

Henquet, C., Krabbendam, L., Spauwen, J., Kaplan, C., Lieb, R., Wittchen, H. U., et al. (2005). Prospective cohort study of cannabis use, predisposition for psychosis, and psychotic symptoms in young people. *British Medical Journal, 330*, 11.

Henquet, C., Rosa, A., Delespaul, P., Papiol, S., Faňanás, L., Van Os, J., et al. (2009). COMT Val158Met moderation of cannabis-induced psychosis: A momentary assessment study of 'switching on' hallucinations in the flow of daily life. *Acta Psychiatrica Scandinavica, 119*, 156–160.

Henquet, C., Rosa, A., Krabbendam, L., & Sergi Papiol, L. F. (2006). An experimental study of catechol-O-methyltransferase Val158Met moderation of Δ-9-tetrahydrocannabinol-induced effects on psychosis and cognition. *Neuropsychopharmacology, 31*, 2748–2757.

Huizinga, D., Haberstick, B. C., Smolen, A., Menard, S., Young, S. E., Corley, R. P., et al. (2006). Childhood maltreatment, subsequent antisocial behavior, and the role of monoamine oxidase A genotype. *Biological Psychiatry, 60*, 677–683.

Hyde, L. W., Bogdan, R., & Hariri, A. R. (2011). Understanding risk for psychopathology through imaging gene-environment interactions. *Trends in Cognitive Sciences, 15*, 417–427.

Ioannidis, J. P. (2005). Differentiating biases from genuine heterogeneity: Distinguishing artefactual from substantive effects. In H. R. Rothstein, A. J. Sutton, & M. Borenstein (Eds.), *Publication bias in meta-analysis: Prevention, assessment and adjustments* (pp. 287–302). Sussex: Wiley.

Jedema, H. P., Gianaros, P. J., Greer, P. J., Kerr, D. D., Liu, S., Higley, J. D., et al. (2009). Cognitive impact of genetic variation of the serotonin transporter in primates is associated with differences in brain morphology rather than serotonin neurotransmission. *Molecular Psychiatry, 15*, 512–522.

Karere, G. M., Kinnally, E. L., Sanchez, J. N., Famula, T. R., Lyons, L. A., & Capitanio, J. P. (2009). What is an "adverse" environment? Interactions of rearing experiences and MAOA genotype in rhesus monkeys. *Biological Psychiatry, 65*, 770–777.

Karg, K., Burmeister, M., Shedden, K., & Sen, S. (2011). The serotonin transporter promoter variant (5-HTTLPR), stress, and depression meta-analysis revisited: Evidence of genetic moderation. *Archives of General Psychiatry, 68*, 444–454.

Kegel, C. A. T., Bus, A. G., & van IJzendoorn, M. H. (2011). Differential susceptibility in early literacy instruction through computer games: The role of the dopamine D4 receptor gene (DRD4). *Mind, Brain, and Education, 5*, 71–78.

Kendler, K. S. (1997). Social support: A genetic-epidemiologic analysis. *American Journal of Psychiatry, 154*, 1398–1404.

Kendler, K. S. (2005). "A gene for…". The nature of gene action in psychiatric disorders. *American Journal of Psychiatry, 162*, 1243–1252.

Kendler, K. S., & Baker, J. H. (2007). Genetic influences on measures of the environment: A systematic review. *Psychological Medicine, 37*, 615–626.

Kendler, K. S., & Gardner, C. O. (2010). Dependent stressful life events and prior depressive episodes in the prediction of major depression: The problem of causal inference in psychiatric epidemiology. *Archives of General Psychiatry, 67*, 1120–1127.

Kendler, K. S., Jacobson, K., Myers, J. M., & Eaves, L. J. (2008). A genetically informative developmental study of the relationship between conduct disorder and peer deviance in males. *Psychological Medicine, 38*, 1001–1011.

Kim-Cohen, J., Caspi, A., Taylor, A., Williams, B., Newcombe, R., Craig, I. W., et al. (2006). MAOA, maltreatment, and gene–environment interaction predicting children's mental health: New evidence and a meta-analysis. *Molecular Psychiatry, 11*, 903–913.

Kinnally, E. L., Karere, G. M., Lyons, L. A., Mendoza, S. P., Mason, W. A., & Capitanio, J. P. (2010). Serotonin pathway gene–gene and gene–environment interactions influence behavioral stress response in infant rhesus macaques. *Development and Psychopathology, 22*, 35–44.

Kong, A., Frigge, M. L., Masson, G., Besenbacher, S., Sulem, P., Magnusson, G., et al. (2012). Rate of de novo mutations and the importance of father's age to disease risk. *Nature, 488*, 471–475.

Kumsta, R., Rutter, M., Stevens, S., & Sonuga-Barke, E. J. (2010). IX. Risk, causation, mediation, and moderation. *Monographs of the Society for Research in Child Development, 75*(1), 187–211. doi:10.1111/j.1540-5834.2010.00556.x.

Lee, S. S. (2011). Deviant peer affiliation and antisocial behavior: Interaction with monoamine oxidase A

(MAOA) genotype. *Journal of Abnormal Child Psychology, 39*, 321–332.

Lehr, T., Yuan, J., Zeumer, D., Jayadev, S., & Ritchie, M. D. (2011). Rule based classifier for the analysis of gene-gene and gene-environment interactions in genetic association studies. *BioData Mining, 4*(4).

Loman, M. M., & Gunnar, M. R. (2010). Early experience and the development of stress reactivity and regulation in children. *Neuroscience and Biobehavioral Reviews, 34*, 867–876.

Meaney, M. J. (2010). Epigenetics and the biological definition of gene × environment interactions. *Child Development, 81*, 41–79.

Meier, M. H., Caspi, A., Ambler, A., Harrington, H. L., Houts, R., Keefe, R. S. E., et al. (2012). Persistent cannabis users show neuropsychological decline from childhood to midlife. *Proceedings of the National Academy of Sciences, 109*(40), E2657–E2664.

Mertins, V., Schote, A. B., Hoffeld, W., Griessmair, M., & Meyer, J. (2011). Genetic susceptibility for individual cooperation preferences: The role of monoamine oxidase A gene (MAOA) in the voluntary provision of public goods. *PLoS One, 6*(6), e20959.

Meyer-Lindenberg, A. (2011). Neurogenetic mechanisms of gene-environment interactions. In K. A. Dodge & M. Rutter (Eds.), *Gene-environment interactions in developmental psychopathology* (pp. 71–86). New York: Guilford Press.

Meyer-Lindenberg, A., & Weinberger, D. R. (2006). Intermediate phenotypes and genetic mechanisms of psychiatric disorders. *Nature Reviews. Neuroscience, 7*, 818–827.

Mueller, B. R., & Bale, T. L. (2008). Sex-specific programming of offspring emotionality after stress early in pregnancy. *The Journal of Neuroscience, 28*, 9055–9065.

Munafò, M. R., Brown, S. M., & Hariri, A. R. (2008). Serotonin transporter (5-HTTLPR) genotype and amygdala activation: A meta-analysis. *Biological Psychiatry, 63*, 852–857.

Neiderhiser, J. M., Reiss, D., Pedersen, N. L., Lichtenstein, P., Spotts, E. L., Hansson, K., et al. (2004). Genetic and environmental influences on mothering of adolescents: A comparison of two samples. *Developmental Psychology, 40*, 335–351.

Nelson, E. E., Herman, K. N., Barrett, C. E., Noble, P. L., Wojteczko, K., Chisholm, K., et al. (2009). Adverse rearing experiences enhance responding to both aversive and rewarding stimuli in juvenile rhesus monkeys. *Biological Psychiatry, 66*, 702–704.

Newman, T. K., Syagailo, Y. V., Barr, C. S., Wendland, J. R., Champoux, M., Graessle, M., et al. (2005). Monoamine oxidase A gene promoter variation and rearing experience influences aggressive behavior in rhesus monkeys. *Biological Psychiatry, 57*, 167–172.

Nikulina, V., Widom, C. S., & Brzustowicz, L. M. (2012). Child abuse and neglect, MAOA, and mental health outcomes: A prospective examination. *Biological Psychiatry, 71*, 350–357.

O'Connor, T. G., Deater-Deckard, K., Fulker, D., Rutter, M., & Plomin, R. (1998). Genotype–environment correlations in late childhood and early adolescence: Antisocial behavioral problems and coercive parenting. *Developmental Psychology, 34*, 970–981.

O'Tuathaigh, C. M. P., Hryniewiecka, M., Behan, A., Tighe, O., Coughlan, C., Desbonnet, L., et al. (2010). Chronic adolescent exposure to Δ-9-tetrahydrocannabinol in COMT mutant mice: Impact on psychosis-related and other phenotypes. *Neuropsychopharmacology, 35*, 2262–2273.

Obel, C., Olsen, J., Henriksen, T. B., Rodriguez, A., Järvelin, M. R., Moilanen, I., et al. (2011). Is maternal smoking during pregnancy a risk factor for hyperkinetic disorder? Findings from a sibling design. *International Journal of Epidemiology, 40*, 338–345.

Overbeek, G., Weeland, J., & Chhangur, R. (2012). Research on gene-environment interdependence: Honing the tools and examining the angles. *European Journal of Developmental Psychology, 9*, 413–418.

Pelayo-Terán, J. M., Pérez-Iglesias, R., Mata, I., Carrasco-Marín, E., Vázquez-Barquero, J. L., & Crespo-Facorro, B. (2010). Catechol-O-Methyltransferase (COMT) Val158Met variations and cannabis use in first-episode non-affective psychosis: Clinical-onset implications. *Psychiatry Research, 179*, 291–296.

Peng, B. (2010). Simulating gene-environment interactions in complex human diseases. *Genome Medicine, 2*, 21.

Pistis, M., Perra, S., Pillolla, G., Melis, M., Muntoni, A. L., & Gessa, G. L. (2004). Adolescent exposure to cannabinoids induces long-lasting changes in the response to drugs of abuse of rat midbrain dopamine neurons. *Biological Psychiatry, 56*, 86–94.

Plomin, R., DeFries, J. C., & Fulker, D. W. (1988). *Nature and nurture during infancy and early childhood.* Cambridge: Cambridge University Press.

Plomin, R., DeFries, J. C., & Loehlin, J. C. (1977). Genotype-environment interaction and correlation in the analysis of human behavior. *Psychological Bulletin, 84*, 309–322.

Prichard, Z., Mackinnon, A., Jorm, A. F., & Easteal, S. (2008). No evidence for interaction between MAOA and childhood adversity for antisocial behavior. *American Journal of Medical Genetics. Part B, Neuropsychiatric Genetics, 147*, 228–232.

Reichenberg, A., Gross, R., Kolevzon, A., & Susser, E. (2011). Parental and perinatal risk factors for autism. In E. Hollander, A. Kolevzon, & J. Coyle (Eds.), *Textbook of autism spectrum disorders* (pp. 239–246). Washington, DC: American Psychiatric Publishing Inc.

Risch, N., Herrell, R., Lehner, T., Liang, K. Y., Eaves, L., Hoh, J., et al. (2009). Interaction between the serotonin transporter gene (5-HTTLPR), stressful life events, and risk of depression. *Journal of the American Medical Association, 301*, 2462–2471.

Robins, L. (1978). Sturdy childhood predictors of adult antisocial behaviour: Replications from longitudinal studies. *Psychological Medicine, 8*, 611–622.

Rutter, M. (1988). Epidemiological approaches to developmental psychopathology. *Archives of General Psychiatry, 45*, 486–495.

Rutter, M. (2003). Categories, dimensions, and the mental health of children and adolescents. *Annals of New York Academy of Sciences, 1008*, 11–21.

Rutter, M. (2006). *Genes and behavior: Nature-nurture interplay explained.* Oxford: Blackwell Scientific.

Rutter, M. (2007). Proceeding from observed correlation to causal inference: The use of natural experiments. *Perspectives on Psychological Science, 2*, 377–395.

Rutter, M. (2008). Developing concepts in developmental psychopathology. In J. J. Hudziak (Ed.), *Developmental psychopathology and wellness: Genetic and environmental influences* (pp. 3–22). Arlington: American Psychiatric Publishing Inc.

Rutter, M. (2012a). Gene-environment interdependence. *European Journal of Developmental Psychology, 9*, 391–412.

Rutter, M. (2012b). 'Natural experiments' as a means of testing causal inferences. In C. Barzini, P. Dawid, & L. Bernardinelli (Eds.), *Causality: Statistical perspectives and applications* (pp. 253–272). Chichester: Wiley.

Rutter, M. (2012c). Response to commentaries on discussion paper "gene-environment interdependence". *European Journal of Developmental Psychology, 9*, 426–431.

Rutter, M. (2012d). Achievements and challenges in the biology of environmental effects. *Proceedings of the National Academy of Sciences, 109*, 17149–17153.

Rutter, M. (2013). Developmental psychopathology: A paradigm shift or just a relabeling? *Development and Psychopathology* (25th Edn.), *25*, 1201–1213.

Rutter, M., Kumsta, R., Schlotz, W., & Sonuga-Barke, E. (2012). Longitudinal studies using a "natural experiment" design: The case of adoptees from Romanian institutions. *Journal of the American Academy of Child & Adolescent Psychiatry, 51*, 762–770.

Rutter, M., Moffitt, T. E., & Caspi, A. (2006). Gene-environment interplay and psychopathology: Multiple varieties but real effects. *Journal of Child Psychology and Psychiatry, 47*, 226–261.

Rutter, M., & Pickles, A. (1991). Person-environment interactions: Concepts, mechanisms, and implications for data analysis. In T. D. Wachs & R. Plomin (Eds.), *Conceptualization and measurement of organism-environment interaction* (pp. 105–141). Washington, DC: American Psychological Association.

Rutter, M., & Silberg, J. (2002). Gene-environment interplay in relation to emotional and behavioral disturbance. *Annual Review of Psychology, 53*, 463–490.

Rutter, M., & Sonuga-Barke, E. J. (2010). Deprivation-specific psychological patterns: Effects of institutional deprivation. *Monographs of the Society for Research in Child Development, 75*(1).

Rutter, M., & Sroufe, L. A. (2000). Developmental psychopathology: Concepts and challenges. *Development and Psychopathology, 12*(3), 265–296.

Rutter, M., Thapar, A., & Pickles, A. (2009). Gene-environment interactions: Biologically valid pathway or artifact? *Archives of General Psychiatry, 66*, 1287–1289. doi:10.1001/archgenpsychiatry.2009.167.

Sandin, S., Hultman, C. M., Kolevzon, A., Gross, R., MacCabe, J. H., & Reichenberg, A. (2012). Advancing maternal age is associated with increasing risk for autism: A review and meta-analysis. *Journal of the American Academy of Child & Adolescent Psychiatry, 51*, 477–486.

Schneider, M., & Koch, M. (2004). Deficient social and play behavior in juvenile and adult rats after neonatal cortical lesion: Effects of chronic pubertal cannabinoid treatment. *Neuropsychopharmacology, 30*, 944–957.

Sillaber, I., Holsboer, F., & Wotjak, C. T. (2009). Animal models of mood disorders. In D. S. Charney & E. J. Nestler (Eds.), *Neurobiology of mental illness* (3rd ed., pp. 378–391). New York: Oxford University Press.

Simons, R. L., Lei, M. K., Stewart, E. A., Beach, S. R. H., Brody, G. H., Philibert, R. A., et al. (2012). Social adversity, genetic variation, street code, and aggression. *Youth Violence and Juvenile Justice, 10*, 3–24.

Spinelli, S., Schwandt, M. L., Lindell, S. G., Newman, T. K., Heilig, M., Suomi, S. J., et al. (2007). Association between the recombinant human serotonin transporter linked promoter region polymorphism and behavior in rhesus macaques during a separation paradigm. *Development and Psychopathology, 19*, 977–987.

Sroufe, L. A., & Rutter, M. (1984). The domain of developmental psychopathology. *Child Development, 55*, 17–29.

Sugden, K., Arseneault, L., Harrington, H. L., Moffitt, T. E., Williams, B., & Caspi, A. (2010). Serotonin transporter gene moderates the development of emotional problems among children following bullying victimization. *Journal of the American Academy of Child & Adolescent Psychiatry, 49*, 830–840.

Taylor, A., & Kim-Cohen, J. (2007). Meta-analysis of gene-environment interactions in developmental psychopathology. *Development and Psychopathology, 19*, 1029–1037.

Thapar, A., Langley, K., Fowler, T., Rice, F., Turic, D., Whittinger, N., et al. (2005). Catechol O-methyltransferase gene variant and birth weight predict early-onset antisocial behavior in children with attention-deficit/hyperactivity disorder. *Archives of General Psychiatry, 62*, 1275–1278.

Thapar, A., Rice, F., Hay, D., Boivin, J., Langley, K., van den Bree, M., et al. (2009). Prenatal smoking might not cause attention-deficit/hyperactivity disorder: Evidence from a novel design. *Biological Psychiatry, 66*, 722–727. doi:10.1016/j.biopsych.2009.05.032.

Thapar, A., & Rutter, M. (2009). Do prenatal risk factors cause psychiatric disorder? Be wary of causal claims. *British Journal of Psychiatry, 195*, 100–101. doi:10.1192/bjp.bp.109.062828.

Uher, R. (2009). The role of genetic variation in the causation of mental illness: An evolution-informed framework. *Molecular Psychiatry, 14*, 1072–1082.

Uher, R., Caspi, A., Houts, R., Sugden, K., Williams, B., Poulton, R., et al. (2011). Serotonin transporter gene moderates childhood maltreatment's effects on persistent but not single-episode depression: Replications and implications for resolving inconsistent results. *Journal of Affective Disorders, 135,* 56–65.

Uher, R., & McGuffin, P. (2009). The moderation by the serotonin transporter gene of environmental adversity in the etiology of depression: 2009 update. *Molecular Psychiatry, 15,* 18–22.

van IJzendoorn, M. H., Bakermans-Kranenburg, M. J., Belsky, J., Beach, S., Brody, G., Dodge, K. A., et al. (2011). Gene-by-environment experiments: A new approach to finding the missing heritability. *Nature Reviews Genetics, 12*(12), 881.

van Os, J., Bak, M., Hanssen, M., Bijl, R. V., De Graaf, R., & Verdoux, H. (2002). Cannabis use and psychosis: A longitudinal population-based study. *American Journal of Epidemiology, 156,* 319–327.

van Os, J., & Poulton, R. (2008). Environmental vulnerability and genetic-environmental interactions.

In H. J. Jackson & P. D. McGorry (Eds.), *The recognition and management of early psychosis: A preventive approach* (2nd ed., pp. 47–60). Cambridge: Cambridge University Press.

Wakefield, J., De Vocht, F., & Hung, R. J. (2010). Bayesian mixture modeling of gene-environment and gene-gene interactions. *Genetic Epidemiology, 34,* 16–25.

Zammit, S., Allebeck, P., Andreasson, S., Lundberg, I., & Lewis, G. (2002). Self reported cannabis use as a risk factor for schizophrenia in Swedish conscripts of 1969: Historical cohort study. *British Medical Journal, 325,* 1199.

Zammit, S., Owen, M. J., Evans, J., Heron, J., & Lewis, G. (2011). Cannabis, COMT and psychotic experiences. *British Journal of Psychiatry, 199,* 380–385.

Zink, C. F., Tong, Y., Chen, Q., Bassett, D. S., Stein, J. L., & Meyer-Lindenberg, A. (2008). Know your place: Neural processing of social hierarchy in humans. *Neuron, 58,* 273–283.

Developmental, Quantitative, and Multicultural Assessment of Psychopathology

4

Thomas M. Achenbach

In the chapter that I wrote for the first edition of this *Handbook* (Achenbach, 1990), I focused mainly on how to conceptualize developmental psychopathology. In the second edition of the *Handbook* (Achenbach, 2000), my chapter focused on assessment of psychopathology within the conceptual framework of developmental psychopathology. In light of growing awareness of quantitative and cultural variations in people's needs for help, the time has come to integrate developmental, quantitative, and multicultural concepts, methods, and findings in order to advance both our understanding of behavioral, emotional, and social problems and our efforts to ameliorate them.

In this chapter, I focus on assessment as a central nexus where concepts and research related to developmental aspects of psychopathology interface with the practical challenges of validly identifying each individual's characteristics and needs for help. Developmental research on psychopathology has mainly concerned the period of rapid development from infancy through adolescence. (For brevity, I use "children" and "childhood" in reference to this entire period.) However, because developmental, quantitative, and multicultural findings are relevant across the life span, I also address their growing applications to adults.

Until recently, most publications, theory, and research related to psychopathology have been based on a few rather similar societies. Yet, to advance knowledge and its potential benefits beyond those few societies, research and practical applications must involve more diverse populations. Quantitative data on individuals in multiple populations are essential both for advancing the science of developmental psychopathology and for taking account of the many similarities and differences within and between populations.

It is important to highlight some theoretical differences between traditional cross-cultural research and the quantitative multicultural approach illustrated in this chapter. Traditional cross-cultural research conceptualizes findings from different populations (often designated as "cultures") as if they uniformly characterize most members of each population. As an example, when cross-cultural researchers compare Populations A and B that adhere to different religions, the religious beliefs endorsed by samples of Population A versus Population B may indeed reflect categorical differences between beliefs held by most members of Population A versus most members of Population B. However, as argued by the Dutch cross-cultural psychologists Hubert Hermans and Harry Kempen (1998), the use of categorical labels such as "individualism versus collectivism" for other kinds of differences between populations may falsely represent "cultures as internally homogeneous and externally distinctive" (p. 1119). In other words, comparisons between populations in terms of categorical

T.M. Achenbach, Ph.D. (✉)
Departments of Psychiatry and Psychology,
University of Vermont, Burlington, VT 05401, USA
e-mail: thomas.achenbach@uvm.edu

M. Lewis and K.D. Rudolph (eds.), *Handbook of Developmental Psychopathology*,
DOI 10.1007/978-1-4614-9608-3_4, © Springer Science+Business Media New York 2014

labels may incorrectly imply that all members of a population are the same (i.e., that the population is internally homogeneous) and that all members of each population are different (i.e., externally distinct) from all members of other populations.

In contrast to categorical comparisons of populations, this chapter illustrates measurement of quantitative variations in problems reported for large representative samples of individuals in many populations. The data thus obtained can then be used to empirically determine whether populations are "internally homogeneous and externally distinctive," i.e., whether members of one population all have a similar level of problems and whether that level differs from the levels found for members of other populations.

Developmental Framework

It is now widely recognized that psychopathology needs to be understood in relation to developmental processes and to differences in levels of biological, cognitive, social, emotional, and educational development. Even if there is continuity from particular kinds of developmental perturbations at early periods to similar or different kinds of perturbations at later periods, so many characteristics change over the course of development that most perturbations are unlikely to have the same consequences or to be assessable in the same way in different developmental periods.

Diagnostic Categories

Diagnostic categories of the American Psychiatric Association's (2000; 2013) *Diagnostic and Statistical Manual* (*DSM*) and the World Health Organization's (1992) *International Classification of Diseases* (*ICD*) lack evidence-based models for relations between development and psychopathology. As an example, the criteria for one of the most frequently used *DSM* diagnostic categories, Attention Deficit Hyperactivity Disorder (ADHD), require that "Some hyperactive-impulsive or inattentive symptoms that caused impairment were present before age 7 years" (American Psychiatric Association,

2000, p. 92); changed to 12 years in DSM-5. Yet, research on ADHD has not supported this criterion (Barkley & Biederman, 1997). Furthermore, for children who are assessed well after the age of 7, it is not realistic to expect most parents or children to accurately report whether ADHD symptoms that caused impairment were present before age 7. Because a diagnosis of ADHD requires that at least 6 out of 9 (DSM-5 requires 5 out of 9 for ages >16 years) particular symptoms of either inattention or hyperactivity-impulsivity have "persisted for at least 6 months to a degree that is maladaptive and inconsistent with developmental level" (p. 92), it is also unclear how this 6-month criterion should be applied retrospectively to parent and/or child reports of problems occurring before age 7. Consequently, it appears that, for children older than 7, retrospective parent and/or child reports cannot be assumed to validly rule in or rule out ADHD. Even for symptoms that are present at the time of a diagnostic assessment, the *DSM*'s failure to specify assessment operations for determining whether the symptoms are "maladaptive and inconsistent with developmental level" makes it hard to determine which symptoms should count toward the diagnostic threshold.

Another kind of developmentally important issue is raised by diagnostic criteria that are similar for all ages. To continue with ADHD as an example, the same symptom lists and diagnostic thresholds are applied to children of all ages, even though the base rates and the relevance of the criterial behaviors change greatly from preschool through adolescence. The criteria are also the same for males and females, despite possible gender differences in the prevalence, effects, and developmental course of the criterial behaviors. Equally important, changes in criteria from one edition of a nosology to another and differences between the *DSM* and *ICD* cause differences in who qualifies for particular diagnoses, which in turn affects associations between the diagnoses and developmental parameters. After release of the *DSM-5* and *ICD-11*, years of research may be needed to test associations between the new versions of diagnoses and developmental parameters, gender, clinical status, cultural factors, treatment effects, other diagnoses, etc.

"Bottom-Up" Approach to Psychopathology

Rather than relying on *DSM* and *ICD* categories, a more empirical, "bottom-up," approach to the developmental study of psychopathology assesses broad spectra of characteristics relevant to successful and unsuccessful adaptation within each developmental period. Not only the characteristics but also the assessment methods, the sources of data, and the taxonomic organization of the data need to suit the developmental levels of the individuals being assessed. For example, before about 18 months of age, verbal communication and peer relationships are less relevant than at later periods, and parents and other caregivers are typically the main sources of assessment data. The taxonomic organization of assessment data is also apt to be less differentiated than at later periods.

After about 18 months of age, more diverse aspects of functioning become important, additional assessment methods become feasible, and relevant sources of assessment data expand to include teachers, self-reports, and eventually intimate partners. Taxonomic possibilities also become more differentiated to include problems with attention, learning, self-regulation, reality testing, social relationships, rule-breaking behavior, substance use, aggression, personal responsibility, etc.

Standardized Assessment of Psychopathology

Standardized, developmentally appropriate assessment methods need to be applied to large representative samples of individuals in order to identify characteristics that distinguish between individuals who are apt to need professional help and those who are developing well. As an example, cognitive tests have been used for over a century (Binet & Simon, 1905) to assess individuals' performance on standardized, developmentally appropriate tasks for comparison with the performance of normative samples of age-mates.

Standardized assessment of behavioral, emotional, and social problems has a much shorter history than standardized cognitive assessment. Moreover, unlike cognitive tests, assessment of behavioral, emotional, and social problems requires data on individuals' functioning in various everyday contexts rather than in standardized test situations. An additional difference is that—unlike assessment of cognitive abilities in terms of correct versus incorrect responses to specific standardized tasks—the assessment of psychopathology involves people's judgments of behavioral, emotional, and social problems occurring in response to diverse unstandardized situations.

People differ in what aspects of functioning they observe, how they judge and remember what they observe, and their candor in reporting their knowledge of the individual who is being assessed. Reflecting these differences, meta-analyses of many studies have yielded only low to moderate correlations between reports of psychopathology by various informants and also between self-reports and reports by various informants for both child and adult psychopathology (Achenbach, Krukowski, Dumenci, & Ivanova, 2005; Achenbach, McConaughy, & Howell, 1987; Duhig, Renk, Epstein, & Phares, 2000). Because no single informant can provide a complete and accurate picture, data from multiple informants are needed to provide comprehensive assessment of behavioral, emotional, and social problems for which professional help may be needed. The kinds of informants who are potentially relevant depend on the developmental level of the individuals who are being assessed.

Although assessment of psychopathology differs in multiple respects from assessment of cognitive abilities, it is nevertheless similar in requiring comparisons of standardized data with developmentally appropriate norms in order to determine the degree to which results for individuals resemble or differ from results for representative samples of age-mates. As argued in the following section, quantitative approaches to assessment are needed to take account of variations in functioning related to development, gender, clinical status, informants, and normative populations.

Quantitative (Including Dimensional) Assessment

Quantification can be applied to assessment procedures and data in various ways. For ADHD diagnoses, the *DSM-5* requires at least six out of nine inattention or hyperactivity-impulsivity symptoms to be judged present for ages <17 years. This implies a rudimentary kind of quantification, because the diagnostic threshold is defined in terms of the number of symptoms. Diagnostic thresholds for other diagnoses are also defined in terms of particular numbers of symptoms. Examples include 4 out of 8 symptoms for Oppositional Defiant Disorder (ODD), 3 out of 15 symptoms for Conduct Disorder (CD), and 5 out of 9 symptoms for Major Depressive Disorder (American Psychiatric Association, 2013). However, other than defining the diagnostic threshold, variations in the numbers of symptoms judged to be present are not intended to affect the overall conclusion about whether an individual has a particular disorder.

To consider possibilities for what it calls "dimensional" diagnostic criteria, the American Psychiatric Association appointed a task force to consider dimensional approaches to *DSM-5*. Based on reports by experts in many forms of child and adult psychopathology, the task force recommended that *DSM-5* include dimensional criteria (Helzer et al., 2008). Dimensional criteria might involve simply counting the number of symptoms judged present in order to provide a score rather than merely specifying the number of symptoms for a yes/no diagnostic threshold. Thus, for example, when being assessed for ADHD, individuals would receive scores of 0 to 9 for the number of symptoms of inattention judged to be present. Dimensional criteria could also involve quantifying the judgments of each symptom by rating the symptom. For example, if each of the 9 criterial symptoms of inattention were rated as 0, 1, or 2 to reflect the severity and/or frequency of each symptom, the symptom ratings could be summed to yield scores for inattention ranging from 0 to 18.

If criteria are dimensionalized by tabulating the number of symptoms judged to be present or by summing ratings of symptoms, how should the resulting numbers be used? It is easy to see that a score of 0 would argue against a diagnosis, whereas a very high score (e.g., 9 on a 0–9 scale or 18 on a 0–18 scale) would argue for a diagnosis. But how would the many individuals who score between the extremes be diagnosed? If the architects of *DSM-5* followed past practices, committees of experts would select the number needed to define a yes/no diagnostic threshold. Field trials might be used to see whether the number selected to define the diagnostic threshold seems to make sense. However, more effort would be needed to make full use of the dimensional scores to take account of important variations related to developmental level, gender, clinical status, informant, and differences in relevant populations. Although use of dimensional scores to take account of these important variations might sound utopian, researchers from some 50 societies have collaborated in taking these additional steps, as detailed later. The value of dimensional assessment of psychopathology has been supported by meta-analytic findings of 15% better reliability and 37% better validity than found for categorical assessment of psychopathology (Markon, Chmielewski, & Miller, 2011).

Actualizing Quantitative Assessment

The increasing availability of electronic computers in the 1960s facilitated the use of quantitative methods to model patterns of associations among children's behavioral, emotional, and social problems (e.g., Achenbach, 1966; Conners, 1969; Dreger et al., 1964; Miller, 1967; Quay, 1964; Rutter, 1967). Various factor analytic and cluster analytic methods were used to identify sets of problems that tended to co-occur. Despite differences in the rating instruments, the samples that were rated, and the analytic methods, reviews of findings from these instruments revealed convergence on two broadband groupings of problems (Achenbach & Edelbrock, 1978; Quay, 1979). One broadband grouping comprised problems of anxiety, depression, social withdrawal, and somatic complaints without known physical causes. The second broadband grouping comprised problems of aggressive and rule-breaking behavior. The broadband groupings were given various names, including Internalizing versus Externalizing, Personality Problems versus Conduct Problems, and Overcontrolled versus Undercontrolled (Achenbach & Edelbrock, 1978; Quay, 1979).

The reviews of the findings also revealed convergence on several narrowband syndromes of problems. For example, separate syndromes were found for overtly aggressive behaviors such as fighting and physically attacking people versus covertly delinquent ("rule-breaking") behaviors such as lying, stealing, and truancy. Several of the narrowband syndromes were found to be hierarchically related to the broadband Internalizing and Externalizing groupings. For example, children whose problems corresponded to either the aggressive behavior or rule-breaking behavior syndrome were classified together according to the problems comprising the broadband Externalizing grouping (Achenbach, 1966).

The quantitative findings on patterns of children's problems fostered the use of standardized instruments for obtaining ratings of children's problems by parents, teachers, and children themselves. The ratings of problem items that were associated with a syndrome or with a broadband grouping could be summed to provide a child's score for the syndrome and/or broadband grouping. These scores could be analyzed in relation to other variables for research purposes. Very high and very low scores could also be clinically useful for distinguishing between children who were most likely and those who were least likely to need help. However, in order to make the full range of scores on syndromes and broadband groupings more meaningful for clinical assessment of individual children and to provide standard metrics for comparing and combining data across samples, additional steps were needed, as outlined in the following sections.

Psychometric Advances

Test–retest correlations in the .80s and .90s were reported for scale scores obtained from parent and teacher ratings over periods of 1 week to 1 month for several of the early instruments [reviewed by Achenbach and Edelbrock (1978)]. These findings indicated high levels of consistency in the rank ordering of scale scores obtained from parents and teachers over periods when children's behavior was presumably not changing much.

To test various forms of validity and to provide valid normative metrics for clinical assessment and for generalizing the findings, representative general population samples need to be assessed. Although scores were reported for some nonclinical samples assessed with several of the early instruments, most of these samples were not randomly selected to be representative of the general population of children residing in diverse localities. An exception was a randomly selected sample of 1,300 parents in Washington, D.C., Maryland, and Virginia. In a home interview survey, parents completed the Child Behavior Checklist (CBCL) for 4- to 16-year-olds (Achenbach & Edelbrock, 1981). The data were then used to test the validity with which scores on every CBCL problem and competence item and scale discriminated between children from the general population sample who had not received mental health services in the preceding 12 months and demographically matched children who were receiving mental health or special education services. US national samples were subsequently assessed with slightly revised versions of the CBCL, plus the parallel Teacher's Report Form (TRF) and the Youth Self-Report (YSR) completed by 11- to 18-year-olds (Achenbach, 1991; Achenbach & Rescorla, 2001).

Similar methodology was used to develop, norm, and validate the Child Behavior Checklist for Ages 1½–5 (CBCL/1½–5) and the Caregiver-Teacher Report Form for Ages 1½–5 (C-TRF; Achenbach, 1992, 1997, Achenbach & Rescorla, 2000), as well as the Adult Self-Report (ASR) and Adult Behavior Checklist (ABCL) for ages 18–59 (Achenbach & Rescorla, 2003) and the Older Adult Self-Report (OASR) and Older Adult Behavior Checklist (OABCL) for ages 60–90+ (Achenbach, Newhouse, & Rescorla, 2004). The CBCL/1½–5 and 6–18, C-TRF, TRF, YSR, ASR, ABCL, OASR, OABCL, and related instruments are collectively known as the Achenbach System of Empirically Based Assessment (ASEBA).

Many kinds of validity data have been published for successive editions of the CBCL, TRF, and YSR and their scoring scales (Achenbach & Rescorla, 2001 provide details). These have included tests of the ability of every problem and competence item and scale to discriminate between demographically matched general population samples and samples of children referred for mental health or special education services; confirmatory factor analytic (CFA) tests of syndromes that were initially derived by exploratory factor analytic (EFA) methods; and significant correlations with psychiatric diagnoses and with other instruments for assessing psychopathology, such as the Conners (1997) Rating Scales (CRS) and the Behavior Assessment System for Children (BASC; Reynolds & Kamphaus, 1992). Additional validity findings have included significant prediction of psychiatric diagnoses and referral for mental health services, as well as signs of disturbance including suicidal behavior, substance abuse, and trouble with the law over periods of as much as 24 years (Reef, Diamantopoulou, van Meurs, Verhulst, & van der Ende, 2009). Extensive validity data have also been published for the ASEBA preschool and adult instruments (Achenbach & Rescorla, 2000, 2003, 2010, 2014).

Multi-informant Assessment

As pointed out previously, various informants tend to provide different information about children's functioning. As standardized ratings of children's problems by their parents, teachers, and the children themselves have been found to be reliable and valid, each kind of informant can potentially provide useful information. Furthermore, genetic research has shown that discrepancies between mothers' and fathers' ratings reflect different genetic and environmental influences on children's functioning (Bartels, Boomsma, Hudziak, van Beijsterveldt, & van den Oord, 2007; Van der Valk, van den Oord, Verhulst, & Boomsma, 2003). In other words, the discrepancies between mothers' and fathers' ratings of their children reflect real differences in aspects of

children's functioning elicited, noticed, and reported by each parent, rather than parental "biases" or errors. Genetic research has also shown that discrepancies between ratings by mothers and teachers reflect different genetic and environmental influences on children's functioning at home versus school (Derks, Hudziak, Dolan, Ferdinand, & Boomsma, 2006).

Most professionals who work with troubled children now recognize the need to obtain assessment data from mothers, fathers, multiple teachers, and the children themselves whenever possible. To facilitate both clinical and research applications of multi-informant data, scales scored from each ASEBA form are displayed on profiles in relation to norms for ratings by the kind of informant who completed the form (e.g., parent, caregiver, teacher, youth). After children have been rated by multiple informants, users can visually compare the parallel profiles scored from each informant's ratings to identify similarities and differences between patterns of scale scores. The ASEBA computer software also provides more precise comparisons between up to eight sets of parent, teacher, and self-ratings. The comparisons include side-by-side displays of ratings of each problem item by up to eight informants, plus bar graphs where each bar reflects a scale score obtained from ratings by a particular informant standardized in relation to norms for the child's age and gender, the type of informant (parent, teacher, self), and the relevant society (explained later). The software also displays correlations between problem item ratings from each pair of informants, with comparisons to correlations between similar pairs of informants in large reference samples.

Multicultural Assessment

Most mental health literature, diagnostic categories, and clinical practices originated in a handful of rather similar societies. (I use "societies" to include distinctive regions within countries, such as Flanders, the Flemish-speaking region of Belgium, and commonwealths, such as Puerto Rico, as well as countries.) The growing interconnectedness of societies around the world and the many immigrants to host societies very different from the immigrants' home societies argue for mental health assessment instruments and research designed to identify similarities and differences in psychopathology between members of different societies and cultural groups.

A standardized diagnostic interview (SDI), the Composite International Diagnostic Interview (CIDI), has been used to obtain prevalence estimates for diagnoses in epidemiological samples of adults assessed in 14 societies (World Health Organization, 2004). The prevalence of ≥1 CIDI diagnosis ranged from 4.3 % in Shanghai, China, to 26.4 % in the USA.

Considering the cost and logistical challenges of administering SDIs to epidemiological samples of children and their parents, it is not surprising that no studies like the WHO study of adults have been done for diagnoses of children. In fact, as of this writing, there appears to be only one published study that directly compared the prevalence of child diagnoses in as many as two societies. This study compared diagnoses made with the Development and Well-Being Assessment (DAWBA) in a UK national sample versus a sample from the city of Taubaté, Brazil (Fleitlich-Bilyk & Goodman, 2004). Children aged 7–14 and their parents were administered structured interviews, and teachers completed questionnaires about the children. The data were fed into a computer program which generated *DSM* diagnoses. Clinicians then reviewed the computer output and decided whether to accept or change the computer-generated diagnoses. Based on a comparison of 14 diagnostic categories, significantly more Taubaté children (12.7 %) than UK children (9.7 %) received ≥1 diagnosis.

Single-society studies have used the DAWBA or the Diagnostic Interview Schedule for Children (DISC) to assess epidemiological samples of ≥300 children (the minimum required to obtain adequate statistical power for population samples; Nunnally & Bernstein, 1994) in several societies. Although none of these studies reported statistical comparisons of prevalence estimates from different societies, a review of the published studies found that the prevalence of ≥1 diagnosis ranged from 1.8 % in Goa, India, to 50.6 % in a study of three US areas and Puerto Rico (Achenbach, Rescorla, & Ivanova, 2012; Pillai et al., 2008; Shaffer et al., 1996).

The methodology of the studies differed in many ways, such as 1-stage versus 2-stage epidemiological designs; use of the DAWBA versus the DISC; different editions of the DISC and *DSM* criteria; ages of the children; interviews with parent, child, or both; methods for combining multi-informant data; sampling; recruitment procedures; and completion rates. The many methodological differences preclude conclusions about whether the differences in estimated prevalence reflect true differences in prevalence. Although the difference between the 1.8 % prevalence in Goa, India, and the 50.6 % prevalence in three areas of the USA and Puerto Rico suggests that Indian children have far fewer disorders than American children, another study in India obtained a prevalence of 12.0 % (Srinath et al., 2005), while a US national study obtained a prevalence of 13.1 % (Merikangas et al., 2010). The very small difference between prevalence estimates from the latter two studies thus contradicts the impression of a much lower prevalence in India versus the USA, which was implied by the studies in Goa, India, versus three US areas and Puerto Rico. Furthermore, a local psychiatrist in Goa observed "that Indian informants were understating child mental health symptoms" (Goodman et al., 2012). Consequently, much needs to be done before conclusions can be drawn about true differences in the prevalence of diagnosed disorders for children in different societies. Because diagnostic criteria have changed in *DSM-5* and will change in *ICD-11* (scheduled for release in 2015), SDIs will need to be changed to apply the new diagnostic criteria.

Standardized Multicultural Assessment

To advance knowledge about variations in child psychopathology across different societies, better standardization of assessment in more societies is needed than has heretofore been afforded by

SDIs. Certain standardized rating instruments for obtaining dimensional scale scores have been used in multiple societies, as summarized in the following sections.

Strengths and Difficulties Questionnaire

The Strengths and Difficulties Questionnaire (SDQ) has been used in numerous societies. Describing it as "a brief behavioural screening questionnaire" (p. 581), Robert Goodman (1997) constructed the SDQ to assess dimensions designated as Conduct Problems, Emotional Symptoms, Hyperactivity, Peer Problems, and Prosocial. Each dimension is assessed with five items that are rated *0 = not true, 1 = somewhat true,* and *2 = certainly true.* The 0-1-2 ratings are summed to yield a score for each dimension, and the scores for the first four dimensions are summed to yield a Total Difficulties score.

Confirmatory factor analyses (CFAs) have supported Goodman's five dimensions in samples from some societies, but CFAs of other samples have supported broadband internalizing and externalizing problem dimensions, plus a dimension that includes the prosocial items and favorably worded items that are reverse scored to count on the problem dimensions (Achenbach et al. (2012) provide a review of the SDQ findings.) An example of a reverse-scored item is *Has at least one good friend,* which is reverse scored to count on the Peer Problems dimension. In analyses of British parent, teacher, and self-ratings, the SDQ internalizing and externalizing dimensions were concluded to be more valid than the Conduct Problems, Emotional Symptoms, Hyperactivity, and Peer Problems dimensions for low-scoring epidemiological samples, although the narrowband dimensions were acknowledged to be potentially useful in higher scoring clinical samples (Goodman, Lamping, & Ploubidis, 2010).

Comparisons of mean SDQ dimensional scores from six societies (Lai et al., 2010) and comparisons of the percentage of total difficulties scores above a clinical cutpoint in 12 societies (Ravens-Sieberer, Erhart, Gosch, Wille, & European KIDSCREEN Group, 2008) have yielded significant differences among societies.

Table 4.1 Societies included in ASEBA multicultural norm group 1, 2, or 3

Albania	Greece	Poland
Argentina	Hong Kong	Portugal
Australia	Iceland	Puerto Rico
Austria	India (Telugu)	Romania
Bangladesh	Iran	Russia
Belgium (Flanders)	Israel	Serbia
Brazil	Italy	Singapore
Chile	Jamaica	Spain
China	Japan	Sweden
Colombia	Korea (South)	Switzerland (German)
Croatia	Kosovo	Taiwan
Czech Republic	Lebanon	Thailand
Denmark	Lithuania	Tunisia
Ethiopia	Netherlands	Turkey
Finland	Norway	United Arab Emirates
France	Pakistan	United States
Germany	Peru	Uruguay

Note. Societies included in multicultural norm group 1, 2, or 3 for ≥1 ASEBA instrument for ages 1½–59 (Achenbach & Rescorla, 2007, 2010, 2014 provide details)

Societal differences in scores have suggested that "population-specific SDQ norms may be necessary for valid international comparisons" (Goodman et al., 2012), but such norms have not been published to date.

ASEBA Instruments

There are published reports of the use of ASEBA instruments from 104 societies and cultural groups (Bérubé & Achenbach, 2014). Uniform CFA procedures have been used to test statistically derived ASEBA syndrome models in the 52 societies listed in Table 4.1 (Achenbach & Rescorla, 2014, Ivanova, Achenbach, Dumenci, et al., 2007, Ivanova, Achenbach, Rescorla, Dumenci, Almqvist, Bathiche, et al., 2007; Ivanova, Achenbach, Rescorla, Dumenci, Almqvist, Bilenberg, et al., 2007; Ivanova et al., 2010, 2011; Rescorla et al., 2012). According to the root mean square error of approximation (RMSEA)—the fit index found to perform best for the type of data and CFAs that were used (Yu & Muthén, 2002)—the ASEBA syndrome models achieved acceptable or good fit in all samples that were tested. The Comparative Fit

Index (CFI) and Tucker-Lewis Index (TLI) also indicated acceptable or good fit in most samples, although these indices have not performed as well as the RMSEA for the types of data and CFAs that were used (Yu & Muthén, 2002).

Cross-society correlations between mean item scores obtained in different societies averaged in the .70s for every instrument (Achenbach & Rescorla, 2014; Rescorla et al., 2011, 2012). These findings indicate considerable consistency in the items that received low, medium, or high ratings by particular kinds of informants in different societies.

Analyses of variance (ANOVAs) have been used to test age, gender, and societal differences in scores on syndromes, internalizing, externalizing, Total Problems, and *DSM*-oriented scales scored from each instrument (Rescorla, Achenbach, Ginzburg, et al., 2007; Rescorla et al., 2007a, 2007b; 2011, 2012). (The *DSM-oriented* scales were constructed by having experts from many societies identify ASEBA items that they judged to be very consistent with *DSM* diagnostic categories.) The ANOVAs revealed age and gender effects that were very consistent across societies, with negligible interactions of society with age and gender. However, differences between societies were statistically significant on most scales, with effect sizes (ESs) ranging from small to medium according to Cohen's (1988) criteria.

Multicultural Norms

The CFAs supporting the statistically derived ASEBA syndrome models in 52 societies indicate that those syndrome models can be used to represent patterns of co-occurring problems in the societies where they were supported. The cross-society similarities in ratings of particular problem items as low, medium, or high indicated by correlations between societies averaging in the .70s also indicate considerable consistency in how informants in different societies tend to interpret the items.

Despite the support for the syndrome models and the cross-society similarity in items rated low, medium, or high, the significant societal differences in scale scores mean that a particular scale score in Society A may signify a different degree of deviance from most scores in that society than the same scale score in Society B. Because assessment of behavioral, emotional, and social problems depends on informants' awareness, judgments, and reports of specific problems, there is no objective gold standard for assessing such problems. As is now widely recognized for reports of children's problems, no single informant's judgments are sufficient for comprehensive assessment, because children's functioning may differ from one context to another and because different informants may perceive, remember, and report different problems. Although the need for multi-informant assessment of adults may be less widely recognized, meta-analyses have shown that correlations between ratings of psychopathology by different informants are not materially better for adults than for children (Achenbach et al., 2005).

The differences found between reports by different informants as well as the differences between scale scores in different societies argue for norms that take account of both differences between kinds of informants and differences between societies. Does this mean that separate norms are needed for each kind of informant in every single society?

The bars in Fig. 4.1 depict CBCL/6–18 Total Problems scores ranging from the 5th to the 95th percentile in 31 societies. The star in the middle of each bar represents the mean Total Problems score for the society. Although there are statistically significant differences between the mean Total Problems scores in the different societies, there is also a great deal of overlap between the distributions of Total Problems scores obtained in each society and every other society. If you look at the leftmost bar, which represents Japanese parents' CBCL ratings, and then look at the rightmost bar, which represents Puerto Rican parents' CBCL ratings, you can see that most Japanese children's CBCL scores overlap with most Puerto Rican children's CBCL scores. Thus, even though Japan had the lowest mean Total Problems score and Puerto Rico had the highest, the distributions

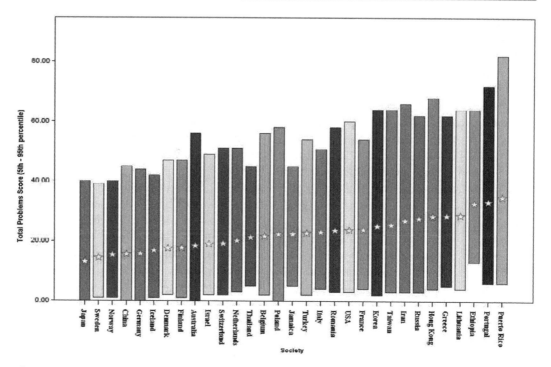

Fig. 4.1 Distributions of CBCL Total Problems scores: 5th to 95th percentiles. *Stars* indicate the mean Total Problems score for each society (From Achenbach, 2009, p. 54. Reproduced by permission)

of their scores reveal considerable overlap. Similar overlaps were found among all societies on all instruments for ages 1½ to 59 years, the ages for which ASEBA data have been compared for many societies. In other words, no society has yet been found where the ASEBA Total Problems scores fail to overlap with all the other societies for which normative data have been obtained on the same instrument.

Another important point to note is that societal differences may differ for different informants. As an example, even though Japanese parents rated their children's problems lower than parents in all the other societies in Fig. 4.1, Japanese youths' self-ratings of problems on the YSR placed then at the middle of the distribution of mean YSR Total Problems scores. A similar pattern was found for Mainland China, where parents' mean CBCL Total Problems scores were at the low end of the societies that were compared, but Chinese youths' self-ratings on the YSR were in the middle of the societies whose mean YSR Total Problems scores were compared.

The evidence from the many societies in which ASEBA instruments have been used to assess population samples thus indicates that (a) no society is categorically different from any other society with respect to distributions of problem scores obtained from a particular kind of informant, and (b) no one kind of informant should be used as the gold standard for the level of problems characterizing individuals in a society.

Constructing Multicultural Norms

Findings of significant differences between mean Total Problems scores from different societies but also substantial overlaps between distributions of scores indicate that: (a) Different sets of norms are needed to take account of differences between societies, but (b) the differences between many of the societal mean scores and distributions of scores are too small to warrant different sets of norms for every society. Furthermore, findings of important differences between the Total Problems scores from different informants, as well as differences between a particular society's rank among societies according to different informants, indicate that informant-specific norms are needed. Similar findings for the narrowband and broadband problem scales likewise argue that informant-specific norms are needed for those scales as well.

To enable clinicians, trainees, and researchers to evaluate individuals in relation to norms for relevant societies, norms based on societies having similarly low, medium, or high Total Problems scores have been constructed for the ASEBA problem scales. The norms are called "multicultural" because of the cultural variations across the societies included in the norms.

For ASEBA instruments that have been used to assess general population samples from multiple societies, the mean Total Problems scores have been found to form normal distributions. An *omnicultural mean* (Ellis & Kimmel, 1992) has been computed for the mean Total Problems scores obtained for each instrument by averaging the mean Total Problems scores from all the societies having general population samples for that instrument. Consistent with the common practice of using ± 1 standard deviation (*SD*) from the mean to demarcate the medium range of scores, societies having Total Problems scores within ± 1 *SD* of the omnicultural mean have been used to form a medium-score group, designated as Group 2. Societies having mean Total Problems scores >1 *SD below* the omnicultural mean have been used to form a low-score group, designated as Group 1. And societies having mean Total Problems scores >1 *SD above* the omnicultural mean have been used to form a high-score group, designated as Group 3. Group 1, 2, and 3 norms are constructed for each gender, age range, and scale on each instrument as detailed by Achenbach and Rescorla (2007, 2010, 2014).

To display an individual's scale scores in relation to norms appropriate for a particular society, the user chooses the society from the list of societies for which norms are available. If data needed to determine a society's norm group have not been obtained, users can choose to have an individual's scale scores displayed in relation to Group 1, 2, or 3 norms based on the group for which a similar society qualified. As another alternative, users can have an individual's scale scores displayed in relation to Group 1 and/or Group 2 and/or Group 3 norms to see whether the individual's scale scores are in the clinical range according to any set of norms. As illustrated in the following section, there are also additional reasons for displaying the same individual's scale scores in relation to more than one set of norms.

Practical Applications of Developmental, Quantitative, and Multicultural Assessment

The use of developmentally calibrated standardized instruments to assess many general population and clinical samples in dozens of societies provides the research basis for assessment of children and adults for many purposes in diverse contexts. Two cases will be used to illustrate practical applications of the research-based assessment procedures. The names and other personal details are fictional.

The Case of Kristin, Age 5

Kristin and her parents were natives of a Scandinavian country designated here as Society A. Kristin's parents both worked for a multinational firm, which transferred them to a Western European country, designated here as Society C, when Kristin was 3. After the family moved to Society C, Kristin attended a half-day nursery school for 2 years and learned the language of society C. At age 5, she entered an all-day kindergarten in Society C. After the first 2 months of kindergarten, Kristin's teacher met with Kristin's parents to discuss her concerns about unevenness in Kristin's development and her lack of developmental progress. Although Kristin's language and reading readiness skills were within the normal range, her motor skills were less developed and she tended to daydream and become distracted. Kristin's parents had not been aware of these problems, but because they had noticed that she seemed unhappy and discouraged about school, they consented to have the school psychologist evaluate Kristin.

As part of the evaluation, the psychologist sought to document how Kristin's functioning appeared at school and home in terms of ratings of specific problems, quantitative scale scores, and comparisons with relevant norms. To document how Kristin's functioning in school appeared to her teachers, the psychologist asked the kindergarten teacher and assistant teacher to complete C-TRF forms. Kristin's mother and father were asked to complete CBCL/1½–5 forms, which have many of the same items as the C-TRF but differ with respect to some items specific to home versus group settings such as school and day care. Although the psychologist offered Kristin's parents the opportunity to complete the CBCL/1½–5 translation for their native language, they were sufficiently fluent in the language of Society C to complete the CBCL/1½–5 in its language.

The C-TRF and CBCL/1½–5 are both scored on six syndromes that were derived from EFAs and CFAs of ratings of thousands of 1½–5-year-olds (Achenbach & Rescorla, 2000) and that have been supported by CFAs in many societies (Ivanova et al., 2010, 2011). The syndromes scored from both forms are designated as *Emotionally Reactive, Anxious/Depressed, Somatic Complaints, Withdrawn, Attention Problems*, and *Aggressive Behavior*. An additional syndrome, designated as *Sleep Problems*, comprises sleep-related items that are rated only on the CBCL/1½–5. In addition to the syndromes, each form is scored on broadband Internalizing and Externalizing scales comprising the first four and last two syndrome scales, respectively. Each form is also scored on a Total Problems scale comprising all the problem items on the form, plus a Stress Problems scale derived from clinical research on posttraumatic stress disorder (Achenbach & Rescorla, 2010) and on five *DSM-oriented* scales designated as *Affective Problems, Anxiety Problems, Pervasive Developmental Problems, Attention Deficit Hyperactivity Problems*, and *Oppositional Defiant Problems*.

CBCL/1½–5 Profiles

To see whether conclusions about the parents' ratings would differ in relation to norms for their home Society A (a Group 1 Society) versus norms for Society C (a Group 2 society), the psychologist displayed Kristin's CBCL scores on profiles in relation to Group 1 norms and then in relation to Group 2 norms. Figure 4.2 shows the profile of syndrome scales scored from the CBCL/1½–5 completed by Kristin's mother. The scores are displayed in relation to the Group 1 norms appropriate for the family's home society.

As can be seen in Fig. 4.2, scores for the Anxious/Depressed and Attention Problems syndromes were both in the clinical range (above the top broken line on the profile, i.e., T score >69, >97th percentile) according to Group 1 norms. Kristin's mother endorsed all five Attention Problem items with ratings of 1 or 2. Scores for all the other syndrome scales were in the normal range. When displayed in relation to the Group 2 norms appropriate for Society C where the family now resided, the Attention Problem syndrome score remained in the clinical range, but the Anxious-Depressed syndrome score was now in borderline clinical range, between the two broken lines on the profile (i.e., $T = 65–69$, 93rd–97th percentile). Thus, whether scored in relation to Group 1 or Group 2 norms, Kristin's mother reported enough problems of the Anxious-Depressed and Attention Problems syndromes to be of clinical concern.

Cross-Informant Comparisons

In order to directly compare scale scores for ratings by both parents and both teachers, the psychologist had the scoring software display the bar graphs shown in Fig. 4.3 for the syndrome and Stress Problems scales and in Fig. 4.4 for the *DSM-oriented* scales. In the box for each scale, the leftmost bar indicates the scale score from the mother's ratings, standardized in relation to the Group 1 norms. The next bar to the right indicates the same scale scored from the father's ratings, standardized in relation to the Group 1 norms. The next two bars indicate the same scales scored from the mother's and father's ratings, respectively, but standardized in relation to the Group 2 norms. The rightmost bars indicate the scores obtained from ratings by Kristin's teacher and assistant teacher, standardized in relation to the Group 2 norms appropriate for their society.

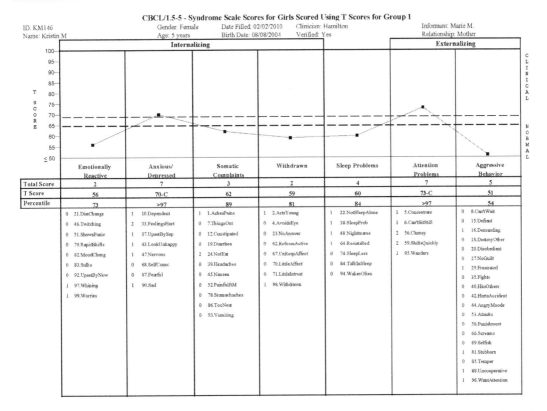

Fig. 4.2 Kristin's profile of syndrome scales scored from the CBCL completed by her mother in relation to Group 1 norms (From Achenbach & Rescorla, 2010, p. 13. Reproduced by permission)

As can be seen in Fig. 4.3, five of the six bars for the Attention Problems syndrome (the middlemost box) are in the borderline or clinical range, indicating high enough levels of attention problems to be of clinical concern. The only exception is for the father's score standardized in relation to the Group 2 norms, although the T score of 62 indicates more attention problems than were reported for 88% of the Group 2 normative sample. For the other syndromes, three of the six bars were in the borderline or clinical range for the Anxious/Depressed syndrome, indicating that this is another area in which Kristin is apt to need help. Other areas of possible concern include Sleep Problems, for which the father's ratings reached the borderline range in relation to Group 1 norms, and Stress Problems, for which both parents' ratings reached the borderline range in relation to Group 1 norms. The very low scores for the Aggressive Behavior syndrome in ratings

by all informants indicate that aggressive behavior is definitely not a problem area.

As shown in Fig. 4.4 for the *DSM*-oriented scales, there was less consistency among scores for the *DSM*-oriented Attention Deficit Hyperactivity Problems scale than for the statistically derived Attention Problems syndrome. Although the bars from ratings by both teachers are in the borderline clinical range, scores represented by the four bars for ratings by Kristin's parents ranged from $T=52–59$ (51st–81st percentiles). This suggests that although all informants agreed in reporting relatively high levels of problems on the empirically based Attention Problems syndrome, there was less consistent evidence for the combination of attentional and behavioral problems that characterize *DSM*-defined ADHD, which may have been evident only in school. The fact that four out of the six bars were in the borderline or clinical range for

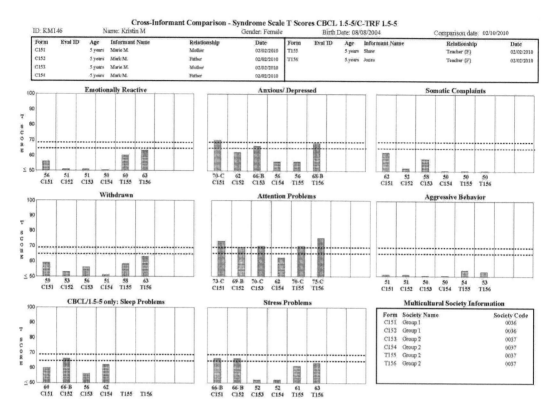

Fig. 4.3 Cross-informant comparisons of Kristin's scores on the syndrome and Stress Problems scales. As explained in the text, the C151 and 152 bars show mother's and father's ratings in relation to Society A (Group 1) norms. The C153 and 154 bars show mother's and father's ratings in relation to Society C (Group 2) norms. The T155 and T156 bars show the teacher's and assistant teacher's ratings in relation to Society C (Group 2) norms (From Achenbach & Rescorla, 2010, p. 18. Reproduced by permission)

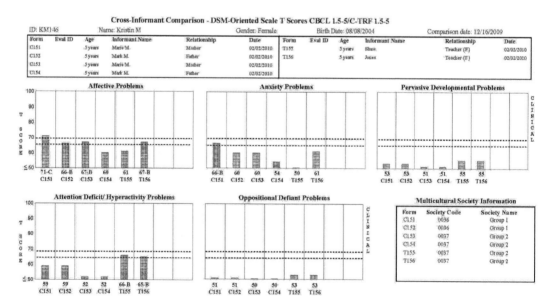

Fig. 4.4 Cross-informant comparisons of Kristin's scores on the DSM-oriented scales. The C151 and C152 bars show mother's and father's ratings in relation to Society A (Group 1) norms. The C153 and C154 bars show mother's and father's ratings in relation to Society C (Group 2) norms. The T155 and T156 bars show the teacher's and assistant teacher's ratings in relation to Society C (Group 2) norms (From Achenbach & Rescorla, 2010, p. 28. Reproduced by permission)

Affective Problems indicates a need for help in this area, as did the elevated levels of three out of the six bars for the Anxious/Depressed syndrome shown in Fig. 4.3. The unanimously low scores for the Pervasive Developmental Problems and Oppositional Defiant Problems scales are evidence for a lack of problems in these areas.

In addition to obtaining ratings from Kristin's parents and teachers, the psychologist tested Kristin's cognitive abilities, pre-academic skills, and visual-motor development. Based on observations of Kristin's behavior during the tests, the psychologist completed the Test Observation Form (TOF; McConaughy & Achenbach, 2004) and scored it in relation to norms for girls' ages 2–5 in Society C. Kristin's score was in the borderline clinical range on the TOF Attention Problems syndrome, but in the normal range on the other TOF scales. The test results indicated good verbal comprehension and working memory, reading readiness, and number skills, but developmental delays in processing speed and visual-motor integration skills. Based on discussions of the findings with Kristin's parents and teachers, it was decided to implement a behavioral plan to reward Kristin with stickers for staying on task and completing her work during each school day. At the end of each school week, Kristin could choose a reward based on the number of stickers she had earned. To address Kristin's delays in processing speed and visual-motor integration, an occupational therapist worked with Kristin's parents and teachers on ways to help Kristin improve her skills.

The Case of Robert, Age 11

Robert's family lived in an Asian country, designated here as Society D. Robert and his mother were natives of Society D, but Robert's father had grown up in a different Asian country, designated here as Society E. When Robert was in 6th grade, his teacher became concerned about his aggressive and bullying behavior toward classmates. Robert's mother was also concerned about Robert's getting into trouble in the neighborhood. At the urging of Robert's teacher, his mother took

him to the local community mental health service. As part of the intake evaluation, each parent was asked to complete the CBCL/6–18, Robert was asked to complete the YSR, and the parents were asked to permit Robert's teacher to complete the TRF. Because Society D was in Group 1 for CBCL/6–18 and TRF norms, the mother's CBCL and the TRFs were scored in relation to Group 1 norms. Although there were some differences between the mother's CBCL and the teacher's TRF standardized scale scores, both forms yielded scores in the borderline or clinical range on the Aggressive Behavior and Rule-Breaking Behavior syndromes, as well as on the *DSM*-oriented Conduct Problems scale.

Because Society D was in Group 2 for YSR norms, Robert's YSR was scored in relation to Group 2 norms. Although Robert endorsed some of the same items as his mother and teacher on the Aggressive Behavior and Rule-Breaking syndrome scales, his scores on these scales were below the borderline clinical range for Group 2 norms.

Society E, where Robert's father grew up and still had strong family, cultural, and linguistic ties, was in Group 3 for the CBCL/6–18 norms. Although Robert's father also endorsed several aggressive and rule-breaking items, all the scale scores from his CBCL were in the normal range. These findings were consistent with his view that Robert's behavior was not troublesome enough to warrant mental health services, although he did consent to accompany Robert's mother to a meeting with the mental health clinician.

The clinician obtained the teacher's consent to show the TRF profile to Robert's parents and obtained each parent's consent to show the other parent the profile from their respective CBCLs. The clinician then encouraged the parents to discuss their views of Robert and whether they saw any need for changing his behavior. Thereafter, the clinician showed the parents the TRF and CBCL syndrome profiles, explained how the profiles compared Robert's scores with scores of typical peers, and encouraged the parents to comment on any similarities and differences that they saw between the profiles. Both parents mentioned that the scores on the Aggressive Behavior and Rule-Breaking Behavior scales were higher on the TRF profile and on the mother's CBCL profile than on the father's CBCL profile. They also mentioned that the father had endorsed several of the same aggressive and rule-breaking items as the teacher and mother. The clinician explained why the father's scale score was nevertheless lower because it was compared to CBCL ratings typical of Society E, the father's home society.

After the parents fully understood the reasons for the differences between the elevations of the scales on the father's CBCL profile versus the other profiles, the clinician encouraged discussion of how some behaviors might be more common and acceptable in Society E than in Society D, where the behaviors were apt to get a child in trouble at school and in the neighborhood. This led to a discussion of how to help Robert develop more acceptable behavior in his school and neighborhood and to a treatment plan that would include helping Robert's father model and reinforce behaviors more appropriate for Society D than Society E.

Summary and Conclusions

This chapter focused on assessment as a central nexus where concepts and research related to the development of psychopathology interface with practical challenges of identifying each individual's characteristics and needs for help. Existing "top-down" diagnostic categories for psychopathology lack evidence-based models for relating development to psychopathology.

A more "bottom-up" approach to psychopathology quantitatively assesses broad spectra of characteristics relevant to adaptation within each developmental period, using developmentally appropriate methods and sources of data. Standardized assessment data for large representative samples of individuals have been statistically analyzed to identify syndromes of co-occurring problems and to construct norms for syndrome scales, broadband Internalizing and Externalizing scales, and *DSM*-oriented scales comprising items judged to be very consistent with *DSM* diagnostic categories.

Comparisons of developmentally calibrated scale scores from many societies show that the distributions of scale scores from every society overlap with the distributions of scores from every other society studied to date. Despite differences in mean scale scores, these findings indicate that none of the studied societies is categorically different from any other society in terms of problems reported for representative samples of members of those societies. Instead, for standardized assessment of behavioral, emotional, and social problems, the findings indicate that quantitative multicultural assessment reflects similarly broad ranges of problems that characterize individuals within each society as well as providing models for comparing and coordinating findings across diverse societies.

Normed, quantitative (dimensional) scales make it possible to take account of differences in problems related to developmental level, gender, type of informant, and society. Multicultural norms have been constructed on the basis of ratings by different kinds of informants in many societies. Ratings of individuals are entered into software that can display scale scores in relation to user-selected multicultural norms appropriate for the individuals being assessed and for the informants who rate them. Whether or not official diagnostic systems eventually incorporate dimensional criteria that take account of developmental, gender, informant, and societal differences, there will be continuing needs to tailor assessment of psychopathology to empirically identified patterns and distributions of problems in diverse populations.

References

Achenbach, T. M. (1966). The classification of children's psychiatric symptoms: A factor-analytic study. *Psychological Monographs, 80*(7), 1–37.

Achenbach, T. M. (1990). Conceptualization of developmental psychopathology. In M. Lewis & S. M. Miller (Eds.), *Handbook of developmental psychopathology*. New York: Plenum Press.

Achenbach, T. M. (1991). *Integrative guide for the 1991 CBCL/4-18, YSR, and TRF profiles*. Burlington, VT: University of Vermont, Department of Psychiatry.

Achenbach, T. M. (1992). *Manual for the Child Behavior Checklist/2-3 and 1992 Profile*. Burlington, VT: University of Vermont, Department of Psychiatry.

Achenbach, T. M. (1997). *Guide for the Caregiver-Teacher Report Form for Ages 2–5*. Burlington, VT: University of Vermont, Department of Psychiatry.

Achenbach, T. M. (2000). Assessment of psychopathology. In A. J. Sameroff, M. Lewis, & S. M. Miller (Eds.), *Handbook of developmental psychopathology* (2nd ed.). New York: Plenum Press.

Achenbach, T. M. (2009). *The Achenbach System of Empirically Based Assessment (ASEBA): Development, findings, theory, and applications*. Burlington, VT: University of Vermont, Research Center for Children, Youth, and Families.

Achenbach, T. M., & Edelbrock, C. (1978). The classification of child psychopathology: A review and analysis of empirical efforts. *Psychological Bulletin, 85*, 1275–1301. doi:10.1037/0033-2909.85.6.1275.

Achenbach, T. M., & Edelbrock, C. (1981). Behavioral problems and competencies reported by parents of normal and disturbed children aged four to sixteen. *Monographs of the Society for Research in Child Development, 46* (1, Serial No. 188). doi:10.2307/1165983

Achenbach, T. M., Krukowski, R. A., Dumenci, L., & Ivanova, M. Y. (2005). Assessment of adult psychopathology: Meta-analyses and implications of cross-informant correlations. *Psychological Bulletin, 131*, 361–382. doi:10.1037/0033-2909.131.3.361.

Achenbach, T. M., McConaughy, S. H., & Howell, C. T. (1987). Child/adolescent behavioral and emotional problems: Implications of cross-informant correlations for situational specificity. *Psychological Bulletin, 101*, 213–232. doi:10.1037/0033-2909.101.2.213.

Achenbach, T. M., Newhouse, P. A., & Rescorla, L. A. (2004). *Manual for the ASEBA older adult forms & profiles*. Burlington, VT: University of Vermont, Research Center for Children, Youth, and Families.

Achenbach, T. M., & Rescorla, L. A. (2000). *Manual for the ASEBA preschool forms & profiles*. Burlington, VT: University of Vermont, Research Center for Children, Youth, and Families.

Achenbach, T. M., & Rescorla, L. A. (2001). *Manual for the ASEBA school-age forms & profiles*. Burlington, VT: University of Vermont, Research Center for Children, Youth, and Families.

Achenbach, T. M., & Rescorla, L. A. (2003). *Manual for the ASEBA adult forms & profiles*. Burlington, VT: University of Vermont, Research Center for Children, Youth, and Families.

Achenbach, T. M., & Rescorla, L. A. (2007). *Multicultural supplement to the Manual for the ASEBA School-Age Forms & Profiles*. Burlington, VT: University of Vermont Research Center for Children, Youth, and Families.

Achenbach, T. M., & Rescorla, L. A. (2010). *Multicultural supplement to the Manual for the ASEBA Preschool Forms & Profiles*. Burlington, VT: University of Vermont Research Center for Children, Youth, and Families.

Achenbach, T. M., & Rescorla, L. A. (2014). *Multicultural supplement to the Manual for the ASEBA Adult Forms & Profiles*. Burlington, VT: University of Vermont, Research Center for Children, Youth, and Families.

Achenbach, T. M., Rescorla, L. A., & Ivanova, M. Y. (2012). International epidemiology of child and adolescent psychopathology: 1. Diagnoses, dimensions, and conceptual issues. *Journal of the American Academy of Child and Adolescent Psychiatry, 51*, 1261–1272.

American Psychiatric Association. (2000; 2013). *Diagnostic and statistical manual of mental disorders* (4th ed. text rev.; 5th ed.). Washington, DC: Author.

Barkley, R. A., & Biederman, J. (1997). Toward a broader definition of the age-of-onset criterion for attention-deficit hyperactivity disorder. *Journal of the American Academy of Child and Adolescent Psychiatry, 36*, 1204–2110.

Bartels, M., Boomsma, D. I., Hudziak, J. J., van Beijsterveldt, T. C. E. M., & van den Oord, E. J. C. G. (2007). Twins and the study of rater (dis)agreement. *Psychological Methods, 12*, 451–466. doi:10.1037/1082-989X.12.4.451.

Bérubé, R. L., & Achenbach, T. M. (2014). *Bibliography of published studies using the Achenbach system of Empirically Based Assessment (ASEBA)*. Burlington, VT: University of Vermont, Research Center for Children, Youth, and Families.

Binet, A., & Simon, T. (1905). New methods for the diagnosis of the intellectual level of subnormals. L'Année Psychologique, 1916. Translated in A. Binet, & T. Simon, *The development of intelligence in children*. Baltimore: Williams & Wilkins.

Cohen, J. (1988). *Statistical power analysis for the behavioral sciences* (2nd ed.). New York: Academic Press.

Conners, C. K. (1969). A teacher rating scale for use in drug studies with children. *American Journal of Psychiatry, 126*, 884–888.

Conners, C. K. (1997). *Conners' Rating Scales-Revised technical manual*. North Tonawanda, NY: Multi-Health Systems.

Derks, E. M., Hudziak, J. J., van Beijsterveldt, T. C. E. M., Dolan, C. V., & Boomsma, D. I. (2006). Genetic analyses of maternal and teacher ratings on attention problems in 7-year-old Dutch twins. *Behavior Genetics, 36*, 833–844. doi:10.1007/s10519-006-9084-5.

Dreger, R. M., Lewis, P. M., Rich, T. A., Miller, K. S., Reid, M. P., Overlade, D. C., et al. (1964). Behavioral classification project. *Journal of Consulting Psychology, 28*, 1–13. doi:10.1037/h0046180.

Duhig, A. M., Renk, K., Epstein, M. K., & Phares, V. (2000). Interparental agreement on internalizing, externalizing, and total behavior problems: A meta-analysis. *Clinical Psychology: Science and Practice, 7*, 435–453.

Ellis, B. B., & Kimmel, H. D. (1992). Identification of unique cultural response patterns by means of item response theory. *Journal of Applied Psychology, 77*, 177–184. doi:10.1037/0021-9010.77.2.177.

Fleitlich-Bilyk, B., & Goodman, R. (2004). The prevalence of child psychiatric disorders in Southeast Brazil. *Journal of the American Academy of Child and Adolescent Psychiatry, 43*, 727–734.

Goodman, A., Heiervang, E., Fleitlich-Bilyk, B., Alyahri, A., Patel, V., Mullick, M. S., et al. (2012). Cross-national differences in questionnaires do not necessarily reflect comparable differences in disorder prevalence. *Social Psychiatry and Psychiatric Epidemiology, 47*, 1321–1331. doi:10.1007/s00127-011-0440-2.

Goodman, A., Lamping, D. L., & Ploubidis, G. B. (2010). When to use broader internalising and externalising subscales instead of the hypothesized five subscales on the Strengths and Difficulties Questionnaire (SDQ): Data from British parents, teachers and children. *Journal of Abnormal Child Psychology, 38*, 1179–1191.

Goodman, R. (1997). The Strengths and Difficulties Questionnaire: A research note. *Journal of Child Psychology and Psychiatry, 38*, 581–586. doi:10.1111/j.1469-7610.1997.tb01545.x.

Helzer, J. E., Kraemer, H. C., Krueger, R. F., Wittchen, H.-U., Sirovatka, P. J., & Regier, D. A. (Eds.). (2008). *Dimensional approaches in diagnostic classification: Refining the research agenda for DSM-V.* Washington, DC: American Psychiatric Association.

Hermans, H. J. M., & Kempen, H. J. G. (1998). Moving cultures: The perilous problems of cultural dichotomies in a globalizing society. *American Psychologist, 53*, 1111–1120. doi:10.1037//0003-006X.53.10.1111.

Ivanova, M. Y., Achenbach, T. M., Dumenci, L., Rescorla, L. A., Almqvist, F., Weintraub, S., et al. (2007). Testing the 8-syndrome structure of the CBCL in 30 societies. *Journal of Clinical Child and Adolescent Psychology, 36*, 405–417. doi:10.1080/15374410701444363.

Ivanova, M. Y., Achenbach, T. M., Rescorla, L. A., Bilenberg, N., Bjarnadottir, G., Denner, S., et al. (2011). Syndromes of preschool psychopathology reported by teachers and caregivers in 14 societies using the Caregiver Teacher Report Form (C-TRF). *Journal of Early Childhood and Infant Psychology, 7*, 87–103.

Ivanova, M. Y., Achenbach, T. M., Rescorla, L. A., Dumenci, L., Almqvist, F., Bathiche, M., et al. (2007). Testing the Teacher's Report Form syndromes in 20 societies. *School Psychology Review, 36*, 468–483.

Ivanova, M. Y., Achenbach, T. M., Rescorla, L. A., Dumenci, L., Almqvist, F., Bilenberg, N., et al. (2007). The generalizability of the Youth Self-Report syndrome structure in 23 societies. *Journal of Consulting and Clinical Psychology, 75*, 729–738. doi:10.1037/0022-006X.75.5.729.

Ivanova, M. Y., Achenbach, T. M., Rescorla, L. A., Harder, V. S., Ang, R. P., Bilenberg, N., et al. (2010). Preschool psychopathology reported by parents in 23 societies. Testing the seven-syndrome model of the Child Behavior Checklist for Ages 1.5-5. *Journal of the American Academy of Child and Adolescent Psychiatry, 49*, 1215–1224. doi:10.1016/j.jaac.2010.08.019.

Lai, K. Y. C., Luk, E. S. L., Leung, P. W. L., Wong, A. S. Y., Law, L., & Ho, K. (2010). Validation of the Chinese version of the Strengths and Difficulties Questionnaire in Hong Kong. *Social Psychiatry and Psychiatric Epidemiology, 45*, 1179–1186.

Markon, K. E., Chmielewski, M., & Miller, C. J. (2011). The reliability and validity of discrete and continuous measures of psychopathology: A quantitative review. *Psychological Bulletin, 137*, 856–879.

McConaughy, S. H., & Achenbach, T. M. (2004). *Manual for the Test Observation Form for Ages 2–18.* Burlington, VT: University of Vermont, Research Center for Children, Youth, and Families.

Merikangas, K. R., He, J. P., Brody, D., Fisher, P. W., Bourdon, K., & Koretz, D. S. (2010). Prevalence and treatment of mental disorders among US children in the 2001–2004 NHANES. *Pediatrics, 125*, 75–81.

Miller, L. C. (1967). Louisville Behavior Checklist for males, 6–12 years of age. *Psychological Reports, 21*, 885–896.

Nunnally, J. C., & Bernstein, I. H. (1994). *Psychometric theory* (3rd ed.). New York: McGraw-Hill.

Pillai, A., Patel, V., Cardozo, P., Goodman, R., Weiss, H. A., & Andrew, G. (2008). Non-traditional lifestyles and prevalence of mental disorders in adolescents in Goa, India. *British Journal of Psychiatry, 192*, 45–51.

Quay, H. C. (1964). Personality dimensions in delinquent males as inferred from the factor analysis of behavior ratings. *Journal of Research in Crime and Delinquency, 1*, 33–37.

Quay, H. C. (1979). Classification. In H. C. Quay & J. S. Werry (Eds.), *Psychopathological disorders of childhood* (2nd ed., pp. 1–42). New York: Wiley.

Ravens-Sieberer, U., Erhart, M., Gosch, A., Wille, N., & European KIDSCREEN Group. (2008). Mental health of children and adolescents in 12 European countries – Results from the European KIDSCREEN study. *Clinical Psychology and Psychotherapy, 15*, 154–163.

Reef, J., Diamantopoulou, S., van Meurs, I., Verhulst, F., & van der Ende, J. (2009). Child to adult continuities of psychopathology: A 24-year follow-up. *Acta Psychiatrica Scandinavica, 120*, 230–238.

Rescorla, L. A., Achenbach, T. M., Ginzburg, S., Ivanova, M. Y., Dumenci, L., Almqvist, F., et al. (2007). Consistency of teacher-reported problems for students in 21 countries. *School Psychology Review, 36*, 91–110.

Rescorla, L. A., Achenbach, T. M., Ivanova, M. Y., Bilenberg, N., Bjarnadottir, G., Denner, S., et al. (2012). Behavioral/emotional problems of preschoolers: Caregiver/teacher reports from 15 societies. *Journal of Emotional and Behavioral Disorders 20*, 68–81.

Rescorla, L. A., Achenbach, T. M., Ivanova, M. Y., Dumenci, L., Almqvist, F., Bilenberg, N., et al. (2007a). Behavioral and emotional problems reported by parents of children ages 6 to 16 in 31 societies. *Journal of Emotional and Behavioral Disorders, 15*, 130–142. doi:10.1177/10634266070150030101.

Rescorla, L. A., Achenbach, T. M., Ivanova, M. Y., Dumenci, L., Almqvist, F., Bilenberg, N., et al. (2007b). Epidemiological comparisons of problems and positive qualities reported by adolescents in 24 countries. *Journal of Consulting and Clinical Psychology, 75*, 351–358. doi:10.1037/0022-006X.75.2.351.

Rescorla, L. A., Achenbach, T. M., Ivanova, M. Y., Harder, V. S., Otten, L., Bilenberg, N., et al. (2011). International comparisons of behavioral and emotional problems in preschool children: Parents' reports from 24 societies. *Journal of Clinical Child and Adolescent Psychology, 40*, 456–467.

Rescorla, L. A., Ivanova, M. Y., Achenbach, T. M., Begovac, I., Chahed, M., Drugli, M. B., et al. (2012). International epidemiology of child and adolescent psychopathology: 2. Integration and applications of dimensional findings from 44 societies. *Journal of the American Academy of Child and Adolescent Psychiatry* 51, 1273–1283.

Reynolds, C. R., & Kamphaus, R. W. (1992). *Behavior assessment system for children*. Circle Pines, MN: American Guidance Service.

Rutter, M. (1967). A children's behaviour questionnaire for completion by teachers: Preliminary findings. *Journal of Child Psychology and Psychiatry, 8*, 1–11.

Shaffer, D., Fisher, P., Dulcan, M. K., Davies, M., Piacentini, J., Schwab-Stone, M. E., et al. (1996). The NIMH Diagnostic Interview Schedule for Children version 2.3. (DISC-2.3): Description, acceptability,

prevalence rates, and performance in the MECA study. *Journal of the American Academy of Child and Adolescent Psychiatry, 35*, 865–877.

Srinath, S., Girimaji, S. C., Gururaj, G., Seshadri, S., Subbakrishna, D. K., Bhola, P., et al. (2005). Epidemiological study of child & adolescent psychiatric disorders in urban & rural areas of Bangalore, India. *Indian Journal of Medical Research, 122*, 67–79.

Van der Valk, J. C., van den Oord, E. J. C. G., Verhulst, F. C., & Boomsma, D. I. (2003). Using shared and unique parental views to study the etiology of 7-year-old twins' internalizing and externalizing problems. *Behavior Genetics, 33*, 409–420.

World Health Organization. (1992). *Mental disorders: Glossary and guide to their classification in accordance with the tenth revision of the International Classification of Diseases* (10th ed.). Geneva: World Health Organization.

World Health Organization World Mental Health Survey Consortium. (2004). Prevalence, severity, and unmet need for treatment of mental disorders in the World Health Organization world mental health surveys. *Journal of the American Medical Association, 291*, 2581–2590. doi:10.1001/jama.291.21.2581.

Yu, C. Y., & Muthén, B. O. (2002). *Evaluation of model fit indices for latent variable models with categorical and continuous outcomes* (Technical Report). Los Angeles: University of California at Los Angeles, Graduate School of Education and Information Studies.

Developmental Epidemiology

5

Katie A. McLaughlin

This chapter examines the contribution of epidemiological research to our understanding of developmental psychopathology. I first review some basic information about the field of epidemiology: the goals and scope of epidemiological research, a brief history of the discipline, and how epidemiological approaches differ from other study designs in developmental psychopathology. The bulk of the chapter is devoted to consideration of the types of research questions in developmental psychopathology that can be uniquely addressed using epidemiological research designs and a review of hallmark findings produced by developmental epidemiology. The chapter ends with a discussion of how epidemiological approaches can be incorporated into one's own research program, with an eye towards encouraging researchers to capitalize on the increasing armamentarium of publicly available epidemiological datasets that can be used to advance our understanding of developmental psychopathology. This chapter builds on seminal reviews of this topic by Jane Costello and Adrian Angold (Angold & Costello, 1995; Costello & Angold, 1995; Costello, Egger, & Angold, 2005; Costello, Foley, & Angold, 2006) that describe

K.A. McLaughlin, Ph.D. (✉)
Department of Psychology, University
of Washington, Box 351525, Seattle, WA 98195, USA
e-mail: mclaughk@uw.edu

the central methods of developmental epidemiology and their application to questions in developmental psychopathology.

What Is Developmental Epidemiology?

Epidemiology is the study of the distribution and determinants of health and disease in populations (Susser, 1973). Central to this approach is the notion that an individual's risk for disease is based not only upon risk and protective factors at the individual level but also is a function of disease risk in the society in which they are embedded (Rose, 1992). Epidemiology thus seeks to understand not only why a particular individual develops an illness but also why a particular population experiences a specific distribution of risk for that illness. The history of epidemiology has witnessed several major shifts in the predominant paradigms used to study the distribution of disease in populations. The discipline of epidemiology began during the Industrial Revolution as massive societal change related to urbanization produced overcrowding, poor sanitation, and marked disparities in health across social classes. At this time, epidemiologists focused on social and economic factors driving risk for disease and implemented structural solutions such as closed sewage and draining systems and regular garbage collection. As advances in microbiology

M. Lewis and K.D. Rudolph (eds.), *Handbook of Developmental Psychopathology*,
DOI 10.1007/978-1-4614-9608-3_5, © Springer Science+Business Media New York 2014

improved understanding of how specific agents (i.e., germs) were involved in the etiology of specific diseases, epidemiology became more narrowly focused on mechanistically identifying microbial causes of infectious diseases and controlling them with vaccines or medication. During the period of infectious disease epidemiology, consideration of social and economic factors as determinants of disease faded. Following World War II, however, the focus of epidemiology shifted again to a risk factor approach based on the notion that combinations of factors acted in concert to shape the probability of illness, particularly of chronic diseases including mental disorders. With the advent of modern epidemiological study designs—particularly cohort and case–control studies—individual-level factors associated with increased probability of disease were identified (e.g., cigarette smoking and lung cancer), and attempts to control risk factors through lifestyle (e.g., smoking cessation) and environmental change (e.g., reduce passive smoke exposure) were implemented (Susser & Susser, 1996). Over the past two decades, a modern era of epidemiology has emerged that considers risk factors operating at multiple levels, including macrosocial, individual, and biological, and seeks to identify the mechanisms through which risk factors ultimately increase the probability of disease (Krieger, 1994; Susser, 1998). Although the field previously involved a predominant focus on factors operating at only one of these levels, current approaches to epidemiology are explicitly multilevel and concerned with identifying *causes* of health states (Krieger, 1994; Susser, 1998), with the ultimate goal of preventing disease onset.

Modern epidemiology thus shares the fundamental multilevel and mechanistic perspectives of developmental psychopathology. So what is unique about an epidemiological approach? At the most basic level, epidemiology is concerned with identifying exposure–disease relationships. This does not differ fundamentally from the goals of developmental psychopathology, but the methods employed in epidemiology differ in important ways from those used in other study designs. I focus here on several key aspects of

epidemiology that are distinct from other methods used to study child and adolescent mental health, as a thorough review of study designs and measures of association in epidemiology is beyond the scope of this chapter. Readers are referred elsewhere for greater detail about epidemiological methods and their application to the study of psychopathology (Rothman, Greenland, & Lash, 2008; Susser, Schwartz, Morabia, & Bromet, 2006).

First, epidemiology is explicitly interested in characterizing the *distribution* of diseases in populations. This task typically involves the counting of cases to determine the proportion of individuals in the population that meet criteria for a particular disorder (i.e., prevalence) and, in longitudinal studies, the number of new cases that develop over a period of time (i.e., incidence rate). Major advances in the surveillance of child and adolescent mental disorders have occurred over the past four decades, following the advent of diagnostic interviews that combine information from multiple informants to generate youth psychiatric diagnoses (Angold & Costello, 1995). Efforts to count cases of youth mental disorders occurred first in regional studies (Cohen et al., 1993; Costello, Mustillo, Erkanli, Keeler, & Angold, 2003) and more recently national studies (Kessler, Avenevoli, Costello, Georgiades, et al., 2012). Epidemiology is also focused on identifying *disparities* in health outcomes. The distribution of youth mental disorders varies by sex, age, race/ethnicity, nativity, socioeconomic status, and sexual orientation. Epidemiology is explicitly concerned with identifying socially disadvantaged subgroups of the population that experience disproportionate risk for particular adverse health outcomes in order to better target preventive interventions.

Second, epidemiologic studies seek to identify factors that *explain* nonrandom distribution of disease across population subgroups, across space, and across time with the goal of preventing the onset of ill health. Whereas psychology and clinical medicine focus predominantly on the treatment of health problems, the goal of identifying risk factors in epidemiology is to inform efforts to *prevent* disease onset by altering the

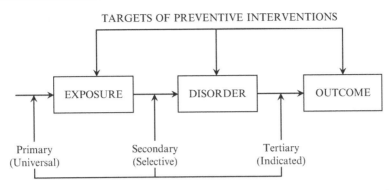

Fig. 5.1 Epidemiology explicitly includes disease *prevention* as a goal. Figure 5.1 depicts the targets of the three major classes of preventive interventions in epidemiology: primary, secondary, and tertiary. Adapted from Costello and Angold (1995)

distribution of risk factors in the population (Rose, 1992). Primary, or universal, prevention is the mainstay of epidemiology and involves efforts to lower the incidence of a disease by shifting the distribution of risk factors in the population in a way that reduces risk exposure and thus the number of new cases (see Fig. 5.1). Secondary, or indicated, prevention aims to reduce disease onset among individuals who have already been exposed to causal risk factors or are already showing signs or symptoms of disease. Finally, tertiary prevention is concerned with reducing the amount of disability associated with a disease among already diagnosed cases. A combined primary and secondary prevention approach is being used in the Durham Family Initiative (DFI) to prevent the occurrence of child maltreatment in Durham County, North Carolina. Based on evidence that risk factors for child maltreatment operate at the level of children, parents, families, neighborhood, and community levels, the DFI has created a preventive system of care that seeks to reduce risk factors at each of these levels through universal screening, early intervention for high-risk families, neighborhood- and community-level interventions, and collaboration among government agencies to provide these services (Dodge et al., 2004).

Finally, epidemiology is concerned with *populations*. A first step in any epidemiologic research study is to identify the source population or the population of individuals that will be the focus of study (e.g., children born in New York City in the year 2000). Because it is rarely feasible to recruit every person from the source population into a study, participants are sampled from the source population to create a study population. Epidemiologic studies frequently rely on probability sampling, which means that every person in the source population has a known probability of being included in the study (Lohr, 1999). Sampling weights are typically constructed that correct for nonresponse and differential selection probabilities, allowing accurate inferences to be made about the source population based on observations in the study population. For example, Patricia Cohen's study of child mental health first enumerated all households in two counties in upstate New York (Cohen et al., 1993). A multistage random sample was created by first randomly selecting households and, second, randomly selecting one child aged 1–10 years within households for families with more than one child in the eligible age range. Epidemiology is also concerned with exposure–disease associations that can be measured *only* at the level of the population, such as the population attributable risk proportion, described in more detail below.

Developmental epidemiology applies these principles to examine variation in the distribution and determinants of health, particularly mental health outcomes, across development. Developmental epidemiology shares fundamental assumptions with developmental psychopathology. Both perspectives emphasize the reciprocal and integrated nature of our understanding of normal and abnormal development;

normal developmental patterns must be characterized to identify developmental deviations, and abnormal developmental outcomes shed light on the normal developmental processes that lead to maladaptation when disrupted (Cicchetti, 1993; Sroufe, 1990). Both approaches conceptualize development as cumulative and hierarchical, meaning that it is influenced not only by genetics and the environment but also by previous development (Lewis, 1997; Sroufe, 2009; Sroufe, Egeland, & Kreutzer, 1990). Acquisition of competencies at one point in development provides the scaffolding upon which subsequent skills and competencies are built, such that capabilities from previous periods are consolidated and reorganized in a dynamic, unfolding process across time. Developmental deviations from earlier periods are carried forward and have consequences for the successful accomplishment of developmental tasks in a later period (Cicchetti & Toth, 1998). Finally, both perspectives consider the dynamic interplay between risk and resilience factors operating at multiple levels (Cicchetti & Toth, 2009). This includes a focus on neurobiological, psychological, and social development and the importance of social context in shaping each of these aspects of development (Cicchetti, 1996; Lynch & Cicchetti, 1998).

Incorporating a developmental perspective into epidemiological approaches is critical for understanding how developmental processes influence psychopathology at the population level for several reasons. First, the prevalence and distribution of mental disorders varies across development. For example, the prevalence of major depression is only 2.8 % in children under the age of 13 and increases to 5.6 % in adolescents aged 13–18 (Costello, Erkanli, & Angold, 2006). By adulthood, the lifetime prevalence of depression is 16.2 % (Kessler et al., 2003). The incidence of depression remains relatively low prior to puberty and rises most dramatically between ages 15 and 18 (Hankin et al., 1998; Kessler et al., 2003). Although the prevalence of childhood depression is similar for boys and girls, females are more likely than males to develop depression beginning at age 13 and continuing through adolescence and adulthood

(Hankin et al., 1998; Kessler et al., 2003; Nolen-Hoeksema & Twenge, 2002). Second, the developmental timing and persistence of symptom expression has implications for what we classify as a mental disorder. Drawing on epidemiologic data from numerous sources, Moffitt (1993) proposed a widely accepted developmental taxonomy of antisocial behavior in which antisocial behavior that is evident in early childhood and persistent across the life course is pathological, whereas antisocial behavior that is limited to adolescence is considered developmentally normative and, potentially, adaptive. Third, risk factors for specific mental disorders change with development. For example, a wide range of early childhood risk factors, including perinatal insults, motor deficits, and caretaker instability, are associated with onset of major depression during childhood and adolescence but are not associated with depression onset in adulthood (Jaffee et al., 2002). Finally, the manifestation of disorders and expression of symptoms also change with development. For example, children with separation anxiety disorder are more likely to experience nightmares about separation and excessive distress upon separation from caregivers than adolescents, whereas adolescents are more likely than children to experience physical complaints related to school attendance (Francis, Last, & Strauss, 1987).

What Can We Learn from Developmental Epidemiology?

For the most part, the types of research questions that are investigated using developmental epidemiology methods are similar to the questions examined with other developmental psychopathology methods. However, through the use of population-based sampling, developmental epidemiology studies can provide unique information about developmental psychopathology that is not available through other means. This section focuses specifically on the types of information we can glean from developmental epidemiology studies that are difficult to obtain using other study designs.

Prevalence, Comorbidity, and Distribution of Psychopathology

The most basic type of information provided by developmental epidemiology studies relates to the prevalence of mental disorders and other conditions in the population. Until very recently, information about the prevalence of mental disorders in children was based on findings from regional studies, such as the Great Smoky Mountain Study (Costello et al., 1996) and the Methods for the Epidemiology of Child and Adolescent Mental Disorders (MECA) Study (Shaffer et al., 1996). The US National Comorbidity Survey Replication Adolescent Supplement (NCS-A), conducted by Ronald Kessler, Kathleen Merikangas, and colleagues, is the first nationally representative survey of youth mental disorders among 13–17-year-olds. The results of this survey are just becoming available. They suggest that the prevalence of mental disorders in US adolescents is high, with 40.3 % of adolescents meeting criteria for a past-year disorder, a prevalence estimate that closely resembles lifetime prevalence in adults (Kessler, Avenevoli, Costello, Georgiades, et al., 2012). The prevalence of mental disorders decreases sharply, however, when a threshold of functional impairment must be crossed to meet the diagnostic criteria for a disorder. Indeed, NCS-A data indicate that 8.0 % of adolescents meet the Substance Abuse and Mental Health Services Administration definition of serious emotional disturbance (SED) in the past year and that the majority of adolescent disorders (58.2 %) are mild in severity (Kessler, Avenevoli, Costello, Green, et al., 2012).

Patterns of disorder comorbidity can also be investigated using epidemiological data. Although comorbidity has frequently been studied in clinical samples, representative estimates of disorder co-occurrence and the temporal sequencing of comorbid disorders in the population must be obtained using epidemiological samples. Understanding the temporal progression of disorder onset can aid in identification of causal pathways of risk among disorders over the life course and provides valuable information for targeting intervention efforts to prevent the subsequent development of comorbid disorders. The Great Smoky Mountain Study has been used to identify patterns of both concurrent and sequential comorbidity in children and adolescents (Costello, Mustillo, et al., 2003). Findings from this study suggest that youths who met criteria for a mental disorder at one point in time were more than three times as likely to meet criteria for a disorder at a subsequent time as compared to children with no previous diagnosis. Controlling for concurrent comorbidity, prior diagnosis of anxiety disorder was associated with the later onset of depression and substance abuse, previous major depression predicted subsequent anxiety disorders, attention-deficit/hyperactivity disorder was associated with onset of oppositional defiant disorder, and conduct disorder predicted the later onset of substance abuse (Costello, Compton, Keeler, & Angold, 2003). Both concurrent and sequential comorbidity were more prominent among girls, particularly for internalizing disorders. This pattern is consistent with findings from other epidemiological studies of disorder comorbidity in children and adolescents (McGee, Feehan, Williams, & Anderson, 1992).

Epidemiological studies also provide important information regarding the distribution of psychopathology in the population or the degree to which disorder prevalence varies across sociodemographic groups. Identifying such differences is critical for understanding health disparities, identifying high-risk groups to target with preventive interventions, and as a first step in determining the mechanisms through which vulnerability to psychopathology is conferred differentially across groups. Although prevalence differences are frequently inferred using data from convenience, clinical, or school samples, limitations in sample selection and population representativeness of such designs preclude firm conclusions regarding the distribution of psychopathology in the population. Epidemiological data can be particularly useful in resolving discrepancies observed in such studies. For example, despite mixed findings from convenience and clinical samples (Meyer, 2003), epidemiological studies from the past decade consistently suggest that the prevalence of mental disorders is elevated among sexual minorities in the USA and other developed countries. The prevalence of mood, anxiety, and substance use disorders as well as suicide attempts is higher among individuals who identify as lesbian, gay, or bisexual (LGB) as compared to heterosexuals (Cochran & Mays, 2000a, 2000b). These disparities emerge early in the life course. Population-based studies of adolescents reveal markedly higher rates of psychiatric disorders and suicide attempts among LGB youths relative to their heterosexual peers (Fergusson, Horwood, & Beautrais, 1999; Russell & Joyner, 2001). Identification of these disparities has sparked theoretical advances in the conceptualization of minority stress as it applies to LGB populations (Meyer, 2003) and in the identification of mechanisms underlying the relationship between sexual orientation and psychopathology across development (Hatzenbuehler, 2009), as well as innovations in the development of preventive interventions for LGB youths (Ryan, Russell, Huebner, Diaz, & Sanchez, 2010).

Identifying Risk and Protective Factors

Epidemiological studies are frequently used to identify risk and protective factors for psychopathology. Although many study designs in developmental psychopathology can be used to identify relationships between specific exposures and mental health outcomes, epidemiological studies can be particularly useful in examining the influence of timing, duration, and magnitude of exposure on psychopathology. To accurately quantify such relationships, it is necessary to have a sufficient number of respondents within different levels of exposure. For example, to examine the influence of timing of child maltreatment on risk of major depression it is necessary to have a dataset that includes an adequate number of respondents who experienced maltreatment at specific age periods of interest as well as a sufficient number of non-maltreated children. This type of data structure is typically available only in large population-based studies.

Timing of Exposure

A central tenet in the study of development is that timing of exposure matters. The primary developmental tasks occurring at the time of exposure to a risk factor are thought to be the most likely to interrupted or disrupted by the experience. In a set of pioneering studies in psychiatric epidemiology, Susser (Susser et al., 1996) identified prenatal maternal malnutrition as a risk factor for offspring schizophrenia using data on pregnancies that occurred during the Dutch Hunger Winter during World War II. The risk of schizophrenia was found to be elevated only among offspring whose mothers experienced extreme malnutrition during the first trimester of pregnancy (Susser & Lin, 1992). The relationship between childhood poverty and educational attainment also varies according to timing of exposure, such that poverty experienced in the first 5 years of life has a more marked influence on the probability of finishing high school than poverty experienced in later developmental periods (Duncan, Yeung, Brooks-Gunn, & Smith, 1998). The degree to which timing of exposure to adverse childhood experiences influences subsequent risk for psychopathology is currently a topic of considerable interest that epidemiologic studies are well suited to investigating.

Duration of Exposure

Certain risk and protective factors may influence psychopathology only if they are experienced for a sufficient duration of time. Research consistently suggests that childhood poverty has a particularly detrimental influence on developmental outcomes when it is experienced chronically over time. Children raised in persistent poverty are more than twice as likely to experience detriments in cognitive ability, poor school achievement, and elevations in behavior problems as compared to children who experience transient poverty (Duncan, Brooks-Gunn, & Kato Klebanov, 1994; Korenman, Miller, & Sjaastad, 1995).

Magnitude of Exposure

Epidemiological studies can also be utilized to study the impact of magnitude or severity of exposure on mental health outcomes. For example, Jaffee, Caspi, Moffit, Polo-Tomás, and Taylor (2007) used data from the Environmental Risk (E-Risk) Longitudinal Twin Study to examine predictors of resilience (defined as low levels of antisocial behavior) in maltreated children and to evaluate whether these factors were associated with resilience at all levels of exposure to stress. High IQ and positive temperament were associated with resilience, but only for children with relatively low stress exposure; no association between high IQ and positive temperament with resilience was observed for children who experienced five or more cumulative stressors (Jaffee et al., 2007). These findings are consistent with other studies suggesting that once the number of stressors crosses a threshold, very few children exhibit resilient functioning (Forehand, Biggar, & Kotchick, 1998). In another study of resilience, numerous putative protective factors were examined as predictors of resilience (defined as low levels of externalizing behaviors) among respondents with exposure to early childhood adversity in the Christchurch Study. High IQ, low affiliation with delinquent peers, and low novelty seeking predicted resiliency in adolescents exposed to childhood adversity, and these resiliency factors had accumulating effects such that resilience was most commonly observed among adolescents who possessed all three of these factors (Fergusson & Lynskey, 1996).

Population-Level Inferences

Certain types of relationships are observable only at the population level, and epidemiological studies are uniquely positioned to elucidate these relationships. One example of an effect measure used in epidemiology to characterize a population-level phenomenon is the population attributable risk proportion (PARP). PARP represents the proportion of cases of a particular disease or disorder

in the population that are statistically explained by a particular exposure. In epidemiology, a PARP is interpreted as the proportion of cases of disease in the population that could be eliminated or prevented if a particular exposure were eradicated, assuming stable distributions of other risk factors in the population (Rockhill, Newman, & Weinberg, 1998). The PARP is a joint function of the strength of association between an exposure and outcome and the prevalence of the exposure in the population. The PARP is therefore a valuable effect measure for estimating population burden. Traditional measures of exposure–outcome relationships are inadequate for characterizing population burden. For example, even if the relationship between a particular exposure and outcome is quite strong, that exposure will not play a substantial role in explaining cases in the population if it is rare. In contrast, an exposure that has a weak association with an outcome but has high prevalence may explain a high proportion of cases in the population. The relationship between trauma types and post-traumatic stress disorder (PTSD) provides an illustrative case. Although rape is an event associated with an extremely high conditional risk of PTSD and sudden unexpected death of a loved one is associated with a low conditional risk of PTSD, data from the NCS-A suggest that unexpected death of a loved one explains a substantially greater proportion of adolescent PTSD cases in the population than rape because it is more than three times as common (McLaughlin, Koenen, Hill, Petukhova, & Kessler, 2013).

PARPs and other population-based effect measures can also provide useful information for targeting preventive interventions. For example, data from the National Comorbidity Survey Replication (NCS-R) and the NCS-A were recently used to examine the relationships between type and number of adverse childhood experiences (e.g., maltreatment, parental psychopathology, domestic violence) and subsequent first onset of mental disorders in adolescents and adults. PARPs were calculated in each of these studies, and the results were consistent across the adolescent and adult data in suggesting that slightly less than one-third of mental disorder onsets in the US population

(28.2 % and 32.0 %, respectively) are associated with exposure to childhood adversities (Green et al., 2010; McLaughlin et al., 2012). The large PARPs associated with these exposures suggest that adverse childhood experiences are very important either as determinants of mental disorder onsets (causal risk factors) or as markers of other determinants (risk markers) and as such represent promising targets for preventive interventions. Another example comes from the Dunedin Multidisciplinary Health and Development Study, a population-based birth cohort. Kim-Cohen and colleagues (2003) estimated PARPs of adult mental disorders associated with child and adolescent disorders. Approximately three-quarters (73.9 %) of adult mental disorder cases had met the criteria for a mental disorder before age 18 and, one-half (50.0 %) had met the criteria for a disorder prior to age 15 (Kim-Cohen et al., 2003). PARPs ranged from 23.0 to 46.0 % across adult diagnoses, indicating that more than one-quarter of adult mental disorders are attributable to prior child–adolescent disorders. These findings suggest that early effective treatment of juvenile diagnoses may have meaningful preventive effects on disorder progression and subsequent disorder onsets.

Age–Period–Cohort Effects

Time is a central construct in all studies of development. Yet, understanding the influence of time on disorder risk is a complicated undertaking. In epidemiology, attempts are frequently made to deconstruct the effects of time into age effects, period effects, and cohort effects. Age effects reflect the influence of aging and development on risk for a disorder; this is the typical way in which time is conceptualized in developmental psychopathology. As described earlier, the process of development has numerous implications for psychopathology propensity and manifestation. The prevalence of various disorders varies with age, as do risk factors and characteristic symptom expressions of psychopathology. But time can influence psychopathology in other ways. Period and cohort effects are used to examine how the time period in which one is born and lives influences health

(Holford, 1991). A period effect is the result of a widespread change in exposure at the population level that influences all individuals alive at that time, regardless of age. Examples of period effects are the occurrence of a natural or man-made disaster, introduction of an environmental pollutant, or widespread changes in social norms. Period effects are not typically studied in relation to psychopathology, because it is difficult to imagine that there are exposures that have similar mental health effects on individuals of all ages. As a result, cohort effects are more frequently used in developmental epidemiology to examine the influence of historical changes in risk and protective factors on mental health outcomes according to one's year of birth. Although different definitions of cohort effects have been proposed, recent conceptualizations describe cohort effects as the result of changes in the distribution of exposures at the population level that differentially influence people according to age; in other words, cohort effects represent an interaction between age and period of birth in shaping disease susceptibility (Keyes, Utz, Robinson, & Li, 2010).

The use of age–period–cohort effect analysis methods has proven to be particularly useful in understanding variation over time in substance use and substance disorders. For example, using data from 1979 to 2005, Kerr and colleagues (Kerr, Greenfield, Bond, Ye, & Rehm, 2009) document a divergence in historical trends of alcohol use according to age. Although the average alcohol volume consumed and frequency of binge drinking has declined over time for individuals aged 26 and older, average alcohol volume consumed and frequency of binge drinking has increased over time for individuals aged 18–25 (Kerr et al., 2009). Increased alcohol consumption and binge drinking among adolescents and young adults was specifically observed among those born after 1975. Social factors that contribute to substance use have also been studied using age–period–cohort methods. A recent study documented substantial variation across time in adolescent social norms regarding approval of marijuana use and a strong association between such norms and adolescent marijuana use (Keyes et al., 2011). The odds of adolescent marijuana use were more than 3.5

times higher in cohorts where fewer than half of adolescents disapproved of marijuana use compared to cohorts where most adolescents disapprove of its use, controlling for one's own attitudes towards marijuana use. Although cohort-specific approval of marijuana use was strongly related to adolescent patterns of use, period-specific approval was not. These findings suggest that adolescent substance use behavior is influenced mostly by social norms of similar-aged peers rather than broader societal norms regarding substance use (Keyes et al., 2011).

Importantly, interpretation of age–period–cohort effects remains challenging. Strong collinearity among age, period, and cohort creates difficulty in estimating standard statistical models to quantify effects, although new methods have been developed that mitigate the influence of collinearity on age, period, and cohort estimates (Keyes & Li, 2010; Yang & Land, 2008). Caution is especially warranted in interpreting age–period–cohort effects that are based on retrospective reporting in cross-sectional surveys. For example, findings from several epidemiological surveys of adults suggested that the lifetime prevalence of major depression was higher in younger birth cohorts than in older birth cohorts (i.e., increasing over time) and that the average age of depression onset was becoming increasingly younger (Burke, Burke, Rae, & Regier, 1991; Kessler et al., 2003). The existence of this "epidemic" of depression was, in turn, widely publicized in the media. However, recall bias is a concern when adults are asked to report retrospectively about child and adolescent episodes of depression, and recall failure of episodes among older individuals might contribute to the appearance of higher prevalence in younger cohorts in the absence of a real cohort effect. To address this issue, Costello and colleagues (Costello, Erkanli, & Angold 2006) conducted a meta-analysis of epidemiologic studies of children and adolescents from successive birth cohorts with observations of over 60,000 youths. Their analysis revealed no changes in the prevalence of depression across birth cohorts, suggesting that previously reported findings of such a cohort effect were likely due to recall bias in older adults (Costello, Erkanli, et al., 2006).

Geographic, Social, and Contextual Influences

Health and developmental outcomes exhibit marked geographical variation, and epidemiology has long acknowledged the importance of place as a determinant of risk exposure and health status. Research examining the influence of neighborhoods on health has increased dramatically in the past two decades. The upsurge in research on this topic is attributable to advances in multilevel modeling and statistical approaches that allow for simultaneous estimation of individual- and neighborhood-level effects and account for nonindependence of observations from multiple individuals living in the same neighborhood, as well as renewed interest in the social determinants of health (Diez Roux, 2001). At the most basic level, the physical characteristics and location of one's neighborhood may influence health and development through exposure to hazards such as lead and other toxins, pollutants, graffiti, and ambient noise, as well as by determining access to healthy food and social services and the availability of alcohol and illicit drugs (Aneshensel & Sucoff, 1996). The place in which one lives also determines numerous aspects of social context including education and employment opportunities, formal and informal institutions, presence of stable adult role models, social norms, and exposure to crime, violence, and delinquent behavior (Sampson, Morenoff, & Gannon-Rowley, 2002). Research on neighborhoods and individual outcomes naturally lends itself to an epidemiological approach, because respondents must be drawn from a sufficiently large number of areas to obtain adequate variability in neighborhood characteristics; at the same time, measurement of individual-level characteristics must be performed to simultaneously estimate the effects of both neighborhood and individual-level factors on the outcome of interest. Epidemiological study designs that examine neighborhood effects on child health and development include national or regional studies that sample respondents from a large number of areas, as well as neighborhood-based designs that identify neighborhood characteristics of interest and sample individuals living in neighborhoods with those particular characteristics (e.g., proportion of residents living in poverty) (Leventhal & Brooks-Gunn, 2000). Neighborhoods are almost always defined using geographic boundaries defined by the Census Bureau. Ecological designs that link aspects of place to aggregate population-based measures of health, such as rates of mortality or premature birth, can also be used to examine geographic variation in health. These have less commonly been used to study questions in developmental psychopathology.

Existing evidence suggests that neighborhood characteristics are, indeed, important determinants of child mental health and developmental outcomes. Even after controls for individual- and family-level factors are considered, youths residing in low SES neighborhoods (based on average income, educational attainment, and/or employment status of adults in the neighborhood) exhibit lower achievement scores and cognitive ability (Chase-Lansdale & Gordon, 1996; Sampson, Sharkey, & Raudenbush, 2008), higher levels of externalizing behavior problems in early childhood (Duncan et al., 1994), and greater engagement in delinquent and criminal behavior in adolescence (Peeples & Loeber, 1994) than youths from more affluent neighborhoods. Rates of exposure to child maltreatment, a potent risk factor for child and adolescent psychopathology, are also elevated in socioeconomically disadvantaged neighborhoods as well as in neighborhoods characterized by residential instability, overcrowding, and greater access to alcohol and illicit drugs (Coulton, Crampton, Irwin, Spilsbury, & Korbin, 2007; Freisthler, Needell, & Gruenewald, 2004). Other neighborhood characteristics that have been linked to psychopathology and substance use include residential instability, ambient hazards and dangers, physical disorder (e.g., broken windows, graffiti), and density of alcohol outlets (Aneshensel & Sucoff, 1996; Keyes et al., 2012; Kuntsche, Keundig, & Gmel, 2008). Recent research has identified specific social processes through which neighborhoods influence child developmental outcomes. The degree of social cohesion among neighborhood members and their willingness to intervene for the common good—a construct known as collective efficacy—has been

shown to mediate the effects of concentrated poverty and neighborhood disadvantage on crime, violence, children's antisocial behavior, and composite measures of child mental health (Sampson, Raudenbush, & Earls, 1997; Xue, Leventhal, Brooks-Gunn, & Earls, 2005).

A primary methodological question raised in research on neighborhoods and health involves the role of selection; it is difficult to disentangle whether associations between neighborhood characteristics and developmental outcomes reflect actual neighborhood effects or whether differential selection of individuals into neighborhoods explains these associations (Sampson et al., 2002). Advanced statistical methods have been developed to try to model selection effects (Sampson, Sharkey, & Raudenbush, 2007), but they remain a persistent challenge in neighborhood research. The Moving to Opportunity (MTO) Study, an experimental study that randomized families living in public housing in high-poverty neighborhoods to receive relocation and rent assistance in order to move to a low-poverty area, provides more rigorous evidence for the importance of neighborhoods on child development and health outcomes. Longitudinal follow-up of these families found that parents who moved to low-poverty neighborhoods reported less distress than those who stayed in high-poverty neighborhoods, and boys who moved to low-poverty neighborhoods exhibited lower symptoms of anxiety and depression than those who did not move (Leventhal & Brooks-Gunn, 2003).

Policy-Level Influences

One of the more exciting recent developments in developmental epidemiology involves the use of epidemiological data to investigate the influence of public policies on child health and developmental outcomes. National tracking surveys (i.e., cross-sectional surveys that are repeated at regular intervals such as the National Health Interview Survey [NHIS] and the Youth Risk Behavior Surveillance System [YRBSS]) provide an excellent opportunity to examine the associations of public policies with mental health and health behaviors at the population level. An important consideration in this type of research is to ensure that the dataset selected to examine health outcomes can be aggregated at the appropriate level for the policy being examined. If a state-level policy is of interest, a dataset must be used that classifies respondents based on state of residence; if county-level policy is the focus, aggregation of respondents at the county level must be possible. Policies at the school, county, and state levels have been shown to have important influences on child mental health and development. For example, a recent study suggests that school-level policies and other aspects of the social environment are associated with suicide attempts among LGB adolescents. Hatzenbuehler (2011) determined the proportion of schools in each county in Oregon that had implemented antidiscrimination and anti-bullying policies that specifically protected sexual minority youths and had gay-straight alliances on campus; this measure of school policy was combined with several other markers of the social environment (e.g., proportion of same-sex couples in each county) and linked to individual-level mental health data from the Oregon YRBSS, aggregated at the county level. The findings indicated that LGB adolescents are at elevated risk for suicide attempts in counties with a smaller proportion of schools that have protective policies and gay-straight alliances (Hatzenbuehler, 2011). Epidemiological research has also documented relationships between the amount of state excise taxes on cigarettes and child exposure to smoke within the home (Hawkins, Chandra, & Berkman, 2012), between state-level alcohol taxes and the prevalence of alcohol dependence (Henderson, Liu, Diez Roux, Link, & Hasin, 2004), and between state-level school nutrition and physical education policies and the prevalence of child/adolescent obesity (Riis, Grason, Strobino, Ahmed, & Minkovitz, 2012). Studies that directly examine public policies in this way have the advantage of providing clear guidance regarding policy interventions that might ameliorate developmental outcomes at the population level.

Epidemiological data that is collected over multiple time points can also be used to monitor changes in population-level health following changes in public policy. An innovative example of this type of research is a study conducted by Costello and colleagues (Costello, Compton, Keeler, & Angold, 2003) using data from the Great Smoky Mountain Study, which began annual data collection in 1993. During this ongoing data collection, a change in public policy resulted in the opening of a casino on an American Indian reservation that included children in the Great Smoky Mountain Study (Costello, Compton, et al., 2003). The casino opening resulted in an income supplement for all families living on the reservation, as well as increased employment opportunities. A meaningful proportion of families living in poverty at the beginning of the study were no longer poor 8 years later. Before the casino opened, children living in families that would be moved out of poverty had similar levels of psychopathology as children living in families that would remain persistently poor; both of these groups had higher psychopathology than children living in nonpoor families. Following the casino opening, children living in families that were no longer poor experienced a decrease in externalizing symptoms such that they had lower levels of symptoms than children whose families remained poor and similar levels of symptoms to children in families that were never poor (Costello, Compton, et al., 2003). No changes in internalizing symptoms were observed as a result of the intervention. These findings provided strong evidence for social causation theories of the relationship between poverty and mental illness, particularly for child externalizing behavior.

National tracking data can be used in a similar fashion to monitor changes in mental health at the population level following major events, such as natural or man-made disasters. If survey data are not collected in close enough proximity to an event to determine changes in psychopathology following that event, study designs can draw on the measures used in national tracking surveys to use in original data collection. For example, the NHIS has administered the Strengths and Difficulties Questionnaire (Goodman, 1999) to parents in every year since 2001 to estimate the prevalence of serious emotional disturbance

(SED) among US children. This same measure was administered to a population-based sample of adults following Hurricane Katrina. This study estimated that 15.1 % of youths aged 4–17 in hurricane-affected areas had SED following the storm compared to 4.7 % in hurricane-affected areas prior to the storm based on NHIS data from the previous year using the same measure (McLaughlin et al., 2009). Information of this sort can be useful to policy makers for mental health service planning purposes.

Service Utilization

Epidemiological data can also be utilized to examine the use of mental health services among children and youths in order to generate estimates of unmet need for treatment and identify factors that influence service utilization. Data from the Great Smoky Mountain Study indicate that service use is strongly associated with need; children and adolescents with SED are nearly 10 times as likely to receive mental health services than youths without a disorder (Burns et al., 1997). However, only 40 % of youths who meet criteria for a mental disorder and experience significant functional impairment (thus qualifying as having SED) received mental health services in the 3 months preceding the survey, and only 20 % received services in the specialty mental health sector (Burns et al., 1995). Among children and adolescents who receive mental health treatment, the vast majority obtain it in the education sector, typically from guidance counselors and school psychologists (Burns et al., 1995, 1997). Youths who have public insurance (i.e., Medicaid) are more than four times as likely to receive mental health services than those without insurance coverage, although children and adolescents with private insurance are no more likely that youths without coverage to receive services (Burns et al., 1997). Together, these findings suggest substantial unmet need for mental health services among youths with functionally impairing mental disorders, the substitution of school-based services for services in the specialty mental health sector, and potential problems with access to treatment for uninsured youths and those with private insurance.

Using Epidemiological Data

This section focuses on how researchers in developmental psychopathology can use epidemiological data in their own research. An increasing number of developmental epidemiology datasets are publicly available and can be either downloaded or requested for use by researchers for little or no cost. These datasets provide researchers the opportunity to utilize population-based data and to incorporate epidemiological research methods into an existing program of research. Table 5.1 provides a description of publicly available epidemiological datasets that are well suited to addressing research questions in developmental psychopathology. Although this list is far from exhaustive, the highlighted datasets include a selection of different study designs (e.g., cross-sectional, longitudinal), different sampling strategies (e.g., nationally representative, birth cohort), and a focus on diverse sets of risk and protective factors for psychopathology. Many of these datasets—and others not included in this review—are available from the Inter-University Consortium for Political and Social Research (ICPSR) at the University of Michigan: http://www.icpsr.umich.edu/icpsrweb/ICPSR.

There are several advantages to incorporating publicly available epidemiological datasets into one's research program. The most obvious benefit is the savings in terms of time and expense associated with collecting data. Of course, not all research questions can be investigated using epidemiological data. But many can, and using existing data is typically more efficient than obtaining funding and collecting data on one's own. Moreover, most publicly available epidemiological datasets include large numbers of participants (typically 10,000+), providing greater power to examine risk and protective factors and other exposure–outcome relationships than is often possible when collecting one's own data. Another advantage of using epidemiological data is that the sampling frame and sampling strategies are articulated (typically in the study documentation), allowing you to make more accurate inferences about the study population than is possible when using convenience or clinical samples or other study designs that do not involve

Table 5.1 Characteristics of a sampling of publicly available developmental epidemiology datasets

Study name	Study design	N	# of waves	Age range	Sampling strategy	Mental health outcomes	Notable exposures
National Longitudinal Study of Adolescent Health (Add Health)[a]	Cohort	Wave 1: 90,118 (in school), 20,745 (in home) Waves 2–4: 14,000+	4	Wave 1: Grades 7–12 Wave 2: Grades 8–12 Wave 3: 18–26 Wave 4: 24–32	Stratified, random sample of all high schools in the United States at wave 1; Stratified random sample of respondents for in-home interviews for waves 1–4	Depressive symptoms, alcohol and drug use, symptoms of alcohol and drug abuse, suicidal ideation, suicide attempts, and healthcare utilization	Sexual behaviors, social networks, romantic relationships, sexual attraction, sexual orientation, timing and frequency of exposure to physical and sexual abuse, numerous aspects of social context, biomarkers including BMI, C-reactive protein, glycosylated hemoglobin, blood pressure, and DNA
Avon Longitudinal Study of Parents and Children (ALSPAC)[b]	Birth cohort	14,000+	10+ and ongoing	Data available beginning at birth and through age 15	Attempted to enroll all pregnant women in Avon County, UK with expected delivery dates between 4/1/1991 and 12/31/1992 using numerous sampling methods	Depressive symptoms and MDD, anxiety symptoms disorders, attention and hyperactivity, oppositional and antisocial behavior, psychosis, borderline personality disorder symptoms, eating disorders, and self harm	Parenting, temperament, personality, social cognition and communication, diet and lifestyle, daycare, schooling, achievement, cognitive ability, physical health, housing, pollutants, parent-reported stressors, bullying, peer and romantic relationships, serum collection of C-reactive protein and interleukin-6, and DNA
Project on Human Development in Chicago Neighborhoods[c]	Cohort	6,000+ at wave 1	3	Wave 1: age 6 months, 3, 6, 9, 12, 15, or 18 years	Multistage clustered area probability survey	Antisocial behavior, substance use, depressive symptoms, generalized anxiety disorder, conduct disorder and oppositional defiant disorder, and suicidal behavior	In-depth information on structural conditions and organization of neighborhoods, including organizational and political structure, cultural values, informal social control, formal social control, social cohesion, relationships among neighbors, crime, violence, graffiti, social norms, alcohol and drug use, and use of police force. Good information on family and developmental factors
National Health Interview Survey (NHIS)[d]	Repeated cross sectional	75,000+ annually (10,000+ children of adult respondents)	11 since expanded child mental health questions added	18+ (with numerous questions about children of adult participants)	Multistage area probability survey	ADHD, mental retardation, developmental delay, autism, and emotional and behavioral problems (measured using the Strengths and Difficulties Questionnaire[e] beginning in 1991; items from the Child Behavior Checklist[f] are used for children aged 2–3)	Parent and child physical health status, parent and child injuries, parent mental health, child mental health service utilization, family SES, health insurance coverage, and healthcare access and utilization
Monitoring the Future[c]	Repeated cross sectional	50,000+ annually	37 and ongoing	8th, 10th, and 12th graders	Multistage clustered area probability survey	Use of illicit drugs, alcohol, and tobacco	Sexual risk behaviors, parental monitoring, beliefs about substance use, exposure to drug education, engagement in school activities, exposure to crime and violence, and religious beliefs.

(continued)

Table 5.1 (continued)

Study name	Study design	N	# of waves	Age range	Sampling strategy	Mental health outcomes	Notable exposures
National Survey on Drug Use and Health	Repeated cross sectional	70,000+ annually	24 and ongoing	12+ years	Multistage area probability survey	Use of illicit drugs, alcohol, and tobacco, past-month distress, and suicidal ideation	Neighborhood environment, illegal activities, drug use by friends, social support, extracurricular activities, exposure to substance abuse prevention and education programs, and perceived adult attitudes towards drug use
Youth Risk Behavior Surveillance Survey (YRBSS)	Repeated cross sectional; conducted biannually since 1991	10,000+ at each wave	23 and ongoing	Grades 9–12	Three-stage cluster sample design	Alcohol and other drug use, tobacco use, and suicidal behavior	Risk behaviors that contribute to unintentional injuries and violence, sexual behaviors, sexual orientation, unhealthy dietary behaviors, inadequate physical activity, and bullying
National Comorbidity Survey Replication Adolescent Supplement (NCS-A)[c]	Cross sectional	10,484	1	13–17 years	Dual-frame household and school samples: (1) adolescent residents of households participating in the NCS-R selected using a multistage clustered area probability sample; (2) probability sample of schools in NCS-R primary sampling units, probability samples of students within schools	DSM-IV diagnoses assessed using the Composite International Diagnostic Interview Schedule for DSM-IV (CIDI) including mood (major depression/ dysthymia, bipolar disorder), anxiety (panic disorder, GAD, social phobia, specific phobia, PTSD, separation anxiety disorder), behavior (conduct disorder, ODD, ADHD, IED), substance disorders (alcohol and drug abuse and dependence), and suicidal behavior	Childhood adversities (maltreatment, domestic violence, parental separation), traumatic events, family socioeconomic status, peer and family relationships, romantic relationships and sexual behavior, physical health, cognitive function, academic achievement, and parent mental health
Collaborative Psychiatric Epidemiology Surveys (CPES)[c]	Cross sectional	20,013	1	18+ years	Multistage clustered area probability	DSM-IV diagnoses assessed using the Composite International Diagnostic Interview Schedule for DSM-IV (CIDI)	Oversample of Black, Hispanic, and Asian Americans; discrimination experiences, acculturation, and ethnic identity
National Epidemiological Survey of Alcohol and Related Conditions (NESARC)[g]	Longitudinal	Wave 1: 43,093 Wave 2: 34,653	2	18+ years	Multistage clustered area probability	DSM-IV diagnoses assessed using the Alcohol Use Disorder and Associated Disability Interview Schedule—DSM-IV Version (AUDADIS); extensive assessment of alcohol and drug use disorders	Sexual orientation, discrimination, childhood adversity (wave 2), trauma exposure (wave 2), and social support

[a]More details available at http://www.cpc.unc.edu/projects/addhealth

[b]More details available at http://www.bristol.ac.uk/alspac/

[c]Data available at the Inter-University Consortium for Political and Social Research: http://www.icpsr.umich.edu/icpsrweb/ICPSR/

[d]More details available at http://www.cdc.gov/nchs/nhis.htm

[e]Goodman (1999)

[f]Achenbach and Edelbrock (1979)

[g]More details available at http://niaaa.census.gov/data.html

probability sampling. Finally, as reviewed in the previous sections, epidemiological studies are well suited to addressing a variety of research questions that are difficult to investigate using other study designs, especially research questions that require data collected at multiple levels of analysis (e.g., biological, psychological, and social/contextual). Leveraging publicly available data provides an opportunity to incorporate these types of research questions into one's own research program.

Using publicly available data is not without disadvantages, however. Using a dataset that was not designed or collected specifically to answer your research question of interest presents several challenges. Most notably, the measures used to assess a given construct of interest are likely to be shorter or more cursory than what would be included in a study designed specifically to address your research question. In general, epidemiological datasets are not constructed to answer one specific research question; rather, they are collected to provide a general population-based resource for addressing numerous questions about a particular outcome or set of outcomes (e.g., mental disorders). As a result, many studies focus on breadth rather than depth when assessing risk and protective factors. This requires adaptability on the part of the researcher in terms of determining how available measures can be used to address one's research question. It is also important to acknowledge that beginning to use an existing dataset involves a significant time commitment. Although the investment of time is often less than what would be required to collect a new dataset of one's own, ample time is needed to familiarize oneself with the data structure, variables, and idiosyncrasies of a new dataset. This investment of time is most useful when a dataset can be used to address multiple questions of interest in one's research program.

Selecting a Study

In addition to the general advantages and disadvantages of using publicly available epidemiological data, each of the primary epidemiological study design types involve specific methodological benefits and costs that are important to consider before selecting a dataset. This section reviews the advantages and disadvantages of using cohort, cross-sectional, and case–control studies to investigate questions in developmental psychopathology.

Cohort studies are typically the design type of choice in developmental epidemiology because they are prospective and can directly examine developmental changes in psychopathology and in exposure–outcome relationships. A classic cohort study enrolls individuals with and without a particular exposure (e.g., maternal smoking during pregnancy) and follows them over time to ascertain disease outcomes as a function of exposure. Most cohort studies in developmental epidemiology use a more general approach of recruiting a large sample and following respondents over time, rather than selecting on the basis of a specific exposure. An example of this type of cohort study is the National Longitudinal Study of Adolescent Health (Add Health). More specifically, many developmental epidemiology cohort studies are birth cohorts. Birth cohorts recruit as many respondents as possible who were born in a particular place at a particular time and follow them longitudinally. Examples of birth cohort studies include the Dunedin Multidisciplinary Study of Health and Development, the Avon Longitudinal Study of Parents and Children, and the Christchurch Study.

Cohort studies involve numerous methodological advantages. These include the ability to estimate the risk ratio, which is the risk of disease among individuals exposed to particular risk factor divided by the risk of disease among the unexposed. The risk ratio is the gold standard measure of effect in developmental epidemiology (Tu, 2003). Critically, cohort studies also allow the temporal ordering of risk and protective factors relative to disorder outcomes to be established. They also provide the opportunity to model developmental trajectories to estimate how symptoms and disorders vary over time within individuals and how risk and protective factors influence these developmental trajectories. Cohort studies are thus particularly well suited to studying the course of mental disorders, identifying risk factors for disorder persistence, and examining the temporal sequencing of comorbid disorders. Together, these advantages make cohort studies the mainstay of developmental epidemiology.

Cohort studies are not without disadvantages, however. First, cohort studies are not well suited to studying rare outcomes (e.g., body dysmorphic disorder), because there are typically not enough cases available in a given sample to provide reliable estimates of association. Attrition is a major challenge in cohort studies. Participant loss to follow-up threatens the careful probability sampling involved in epidemiological studies and influences the types of inferences that can be made about the study population. Attrition is a particular problem when it occurs differentially (i.e., when it is not random). If participants with a specific mental disorder (i.e., depression) or with a specific risk factor (i.e., child maltreatment) are more likely to drop out of the study, this introduces bias in estimating prevalence and the associations between risk factors and outcomes. For example, the association between child maltreatment and substance disorders will be underestimated if participants who have a history of maltreatment and a substance disorder are more likely to drop out of the study than participants with maltreatment exposure who do not have a substance disorder. An additional challenge in cohort studies involves measurement of constructs across development. Often, different measures are used to assess the same construct in childhood as compared to adolescence or adulthood. For example, depressive symptoms are typically assessed using different instruments at different developmental periods. This introduces challenges in modeling change over time and may require the use of latent variable approaches. Finally, some prominent birth cohort studies (e.g., the Dunedin Multidisciplinary Study of Health and Development) were started before reliable and valid measures had been created to assess many constructs of interest in developmental psychopathology. As such, assessment of childhood characteristics in these studies is frequently based on measures that might be outdated as compared to current gold standards.

One additional limitation of cohort studies, from the perspective of the investigators collecting the data, is that they are costly and time consuming. Many years of follow-up are typically needed to track participants through risk periods of interest, requiring substantial investments of time and money. Accelerated cohort designs, also called cross-sequential cohorts, present a solution to this issue. Accelerated cohorts enroll separate cohorts of participants (i.e., groups of participants born in the same year) into the study at baseline. Participants are then followed across time and complete additional assessments at regular intervals. Comparison of developmental changes across cohorts provides the ability to determine whether these effects are similar across birth cohorts or whether they differ according to year of birth or time of measurement. This type of study design also allows greater efficiency in studying developmental change than in a typical cohort design, because developmental changes can be examined over a longer time period than the actual follow-up period of the study. The Great Smoky Mountain Study (Costello et al., 1996) is an example of an accelerated cohort design. Three cohorts of children were recruited at baseline, aged 9, 11, and 13 years. Children were reassessed annually, and data from this study have produced numerous important findings regarding incidence, prevalence, comorbidity, and developmental changes in psychopathology from middle childhood through adolescence (Costello, Mustillo, et al., 2003). An additional advantage of this study design is the ability to examine age–period–cohort effects, described earlier in the chapter. A disadvantage with this study design is that there are fewer participants at the tails of the age distribution (i.e., the oldest and youngest age groups) at any given time point.

Cross-sectional studies are also frequently used to answer developmental epidemiology research questions. In a cross-sectional study, participants complete study assessments at a single point in time and are not followed longitudinally. Cross-sectional studies are often used for estimating disorder prevalence, distribution, and comorbidity. An example of a cross-sectional epidemiological study designed to study these constructs is the NCS-A (Kessler et al., 2009). Cross-sectional studies can also be used to study relationships of risk and protective factors with mental disorders and are particularly well suited to studying exposures that do not change with time (e.g., sex, race/ethnicity). If data are carefully collected regarding disorder age of onset and timing of exposure, it may also be possible to estimate associations between temporally prior risk and protective factors and subsequent disorder onset using survival analysis or other regression-based techniques. This approach has frequently been used in cross-sectional epidemiological datasets by Ronald Kessler and colleagues to study exposure–disorder relationships, for example, the relationship between temporally prior mental disorders and subsequent onset of secondary comorbid disorders (Kessler, Avenevoli, McLaughlin, et al., 2012). From a data collection perspective, cross-sectional studies are less time consuming and costly than cohort studies. As a result, cross-sectional epidemiological studies often include much larger samples than cohort studies. Another primary advantage of cross-sectional studies is that attrition is not a concern. Probability sampling techniques and weighting can be applied to ensure that inferences based on the study sample are generalizable to the source population of interest. Some cross-sectional epidemiological surveys are repeated at regular intervals, typically annually, resulting in numerous unique samples of the population across time. Examples of repeated cross-sectional surveys include the Monitoring the Future Study (http://www.monitoringthefuture.org), the NHIS (http://www.cdc.gov/nchs/nhis.htm), and the YRBSS (http://www.cdc.gov/HealthyYouth/yrbs/index.htm).

The primary disadvantage in using cross-sectional studies is that the temporal ordering of exposures and disorder onset cannot be firmly established. Retrospective recall is required to estimate the developmental timing of events, and numerous recall biases may influence the validity of these estimates. Although procedures have

been developed to improve the accuracy of these reports (Knauper, Cannell, Schwarz, Bruce, & Kessler, 1999), recall bias is difficult to eliminate completely. It is important to note, however, that retrospective recall is required even in prospective studies. In the absence of daily monitoring of participants, which is not a method typically employed in epidemiological studies, respondent reports of events occurring over some previous time period must be used to assess most constructs of interest. Cohort studies provide the advantage of reducing the period of time for which participant recall is required. An additional disadvantage of cross-sectional studies is incidence-prevalence bias. Cross-sectional studies typically focus on prevalent cases (e.g., current cases of major depression). Because prevalent cases often differ in important ways from incident cases, identification of risk factors among prevalent cases may confound factors associated with disorder onset with factors associated with disorder persistence.

Case–control studies are also frequently used in epidemiological studies. Case–control studies involve selecting participants with and without a specific disease or disorder (cases and controls, respectively) and collecting an exposure history to determine exposure–outcome relationships. Case–control studies are less frequently used in developmental epidemiology and are typically conducted to answer a focused research question. For example, this type of study design has been used to investigate risk factors for autism, including maternal autoimmune disorders (Croen, Grether, Yoshida, Odouli, & Van de Water, 2005; Smeeth et al., 2004). Case–control studies are advantageous for studying rare outcomes more cheaply and efficiently than cohort studies but have numerous methodological disadvantages. Recall bias is a prominent concern, particularly if recall bias differs among cases and controls. This is a likely possibility in many cases, particularly if parents of children with and without a disorder are being interviewed about past exposures. Parents of children with a mental disorder may be more invested in accurately recalling past exposures or may have better memory for events that could be related to their child's condition. Case–control studies that use existing medical record or archival data that were collected prior to the ascertainment of cases and controls can overcome this methodological weakness. A second primary concern is that cases and controls are often selected using different methods and therefore represent different source populations. Finally, the measure of effect used in case–control studies, the odds ratio, often overestimates the risk ratio—the gold standard association between an exposure and outcome (Tu, 2003). Nested case–control studies eliminate most of these disadvantages. Nested case–control studies involve selecting cases and controls from an ongoing cohort study and using exposure data collected at a previous time point as part of the cohort study. In this type of study, the odds ratio is a valid estimate of the risk ratio because cases are included in the sampling frame for selection of controls, and recall bias is not a concern. For example, data from longitudinal population registers in Denmark were used to examine risk factors for suicide in youth aged 10–21. A nested case–control study was conducted by examining all completed suicides over a 16-year period (cases) and a sample of controls matched on age and sex. Using previously collected data in the registry, investigators identified parental and respondent mental illness as the factors most strongly associated with youth suicide (Agerbo, Nordentoft, & Mortensen, 2002). Because case–control studies are typically initiated to study a fairly specific research question, no such studies are included in Table 5.1.

Conclusion

Developmental psychopathology is centrally concerned with the dynamic interplay between risk and protective factors operating at multiple levels to influence developmental outcomes. This includes a focus on neurobiological, psychological, and social development and, in particular, the importance of social context and social ecology in shaping each of these aspects of development. Developmental epidemiology methods are uniquely suited to addressing these types of complex multilevel questions. Indeed, epidemiological approaches offer the ability to simultaneously explore risk and protective factors operating within individuals, families, schools, neighborhoods, and society. Developmental epidemiology methods can also be leveraged to identify the forces driving population-level patterns of youth mental disorder prevalence and comorbidity, service use, and mental health disparities across population subgroups, space, and time. An increasing number of epidemiological studies of child and adolescent mental illness have been conducted that are freely available to researchers in developmental psychopathology, providing unique opportunities to investigate the multitude of interacting determinants of child mental health and development in the population.

References

Achenbach, T. M., & Edelbrock, C. S. (1979). The child behavior profile: II. Boys aged 12–16 and girls aged 6–11 and 12–16. *Journal of Consulting and Clinical Psychology, 47*, 223–233.

Agerbo, E., Nordentoft, M., & Mortensen, P. B. (2002). Familial, psychiatric, and socioeconomic risk factors for suicide in young people: Nested-case control study. *British Medical Journal, 325*, 74–79.

Aneshensel, C. S., & Sucoff, C. A. (1996). The neighborhood context of adolescent mental health. *Journal of Health and Social Behavior, 37*, 293–310.

Angold, A., & Costello, E. J. (1995). Developmental epidemiology. *Epidemiologic Reviews, 17*, 74–81.

Burke, K. C., Burke, J. D., Rae, D. S., & Regier, D. A. (1991). Comparing age at onset of major depression and other psychiatric disorders by birth cohorts in five US community populations. *Archives of General Psychiatry, 48*, 789–795.

Burns, B. J., Costello, E. J., Angold, A., Tweed, D. L., Stangl, D. K., Farmer, M. E., et al. (1995). Children's mental health service use across service sectors. *Health Affairs, 14*(3), 147–159.

Burns, B. J., Costello, E. J., Erkanli, A., Tweed, D. L., Farmer, E. M. Z., & Angold, A. (1997). Insurance coverage and mental health service use by adolescents with serious emotional disturbance. *Journal of Child and Family Studies, 6*, 89–111.

Chase-Lansdale, P. L., & Gordon, R. (1996). Economic hardship and the development of five- and six-year-olds: Neighborhood and regional perspectives. *Child Development, 67*, 3338–3367.

Cicchetti, D. (1993). Developmental psychopathology: Reactions, reflections, projections. *Developmental Review, 13*, 471–502.

Cicchetti, D. (1996). Contextualism and developmental psychopathology. *Development and Psychopathology, 10*, 137–141.

Cicchetti, D., & Toth, S. L. (1998). The development of depression in children and adolescents. *American Psychologist, 53*, 221–241.

Cicchetti, D., & Toth, S. L. (2009). The past achievements and future promises of developmental psychopathology: The coming of age of a discipline. *Journal of Child Psychology and Psychiatry, 50*, 16–25.

Cochran, S. D., & Mays, V. M. (2000a). Lifetime prevalence of suicide symptoms and affective disorders among men reporting same-sex sexual partners: Results from NHANES III. *American Journal of Public Health, 90*, 573–578.

Cochran, S. D., & Mays, V. M. (2000b). Relation between psychiatric syndromes and behaviorally defined sexual orientation in a sample of the US population. *American Journal of Epidemiology, 151*, 516–523.

Cohen, P., Cohen, J., Kasen, S., Velez, C. M., Hartmark, C., Johnson, J., et al. (1993). An epidemiological study of disorders in late childhood and adolescence-I. Age- and gender-specific prevalence. *Journal of Child Psychology and Psychiatry, 34*, 851–867.

Costello, E. J., & Angold, A. (1995). Developmental epidemiology. In D. Cicchetti & D. Cohen (Eds.), *Developmental psychopathology, Vol. 1: Theory and methods*. New York: Wiley & Sons.

Costello, E. J., Angold, A., Burns, B. J., Stangl, D. K., Tweed, D. L., Erkanli, A., et al. (1996). The great smoky mountains study of youth: Goals, design, methods, and the prevalence of DSM-III-R disorders. *Archives of General Psychiatry, 56*, 1129–1136.

Costello, E. J., Compton, S. N., Keeler, G., & Angold, A. (2003). Relationships between poverty and psychopathology: A natural experiment. *JAMA: Journal of the American Medical Association, 290*, 2023–2029.

Costello, E. J., Egger, H., & Angold, A. (2005). 10-year research update review: The epidemiology of child and adolescent psychiatric disorders: I. Methods and public health burden. *Journal of the American Academy of Child and Adolescent Psychiatry, 44*(10), 972–986.

Costello, E. J., Erkanli, A., & Angold, A. (2006). Is there an epidemic of child or adolescent depression? *Journal of Child Psychology and Psychiatry, 47*(12), 1263–1271.

Costello, E. J., Foley, D. L., & Angold, A. (2006). 10-year research update review: The epidemiology of child and adolescent psychiatric disorders: II. Developmental epidemiology. *Journal of the American Academy of Child and Adolescent Psychiatry, 45*, 8–25.

Costello, E. J., Mustillo, S., Erkanli, A., Keeler, G., & Angold, A. (2003). Prevalence and development of psychiatric disorders in childhood and adolescence. *Archives of General Psychiatry, 60*, 837–844.

Coulton, C. J., Crampton, D. S., Irwin, M., Spilsbury, J. C., & Korbin, J. E. (2007). How neighborhoods influence child maltreatment: A review of the literature and alternative pathways. *Child Abuse and Neglect, 31*, 1117–1142.

Croen, L. A., Grether, J. K., Yoshida, C. K., Odouli, R., & Van de Water, J. (2005). Maternal autoimmune diseases, asthma and allergies, and childhood autism spectrum disorders. *Archives of Pediatrics and Adolescent Medicine, 159*.

Diez Roux, A. V. (2001). Investigating neighborhood and area effects on health. *American Journal of Public Health, 91*, 1783–1789.

Dodge, K. A., Berlin, L., Epstein, M., Spitz-Roth, A., O'Donnell, K., Kaufman, M., et al. (2004). The Durham family initiative: A preventive system of care. *Child Welfare, 83*, 109–128.

Duncan, G. J., Brooks-Gunn, J., & Kato Klebanov, P. (1994). Economic deprivation and early childhood development. *Child Development, 65*, 296–318.

Duncan, G. J., Yeung, W. J., Brooks-Gunn, J., & Smith, J. R. (1998). How much does childhood poverty affect the life chances of children? *American Sociological Review, 63*, 406–423.

Fergusson, D. M., Horwood, L. J., & Beautrais, A. (1999). Is sexual orientation related to mental health problems and suicidality in young people? *Archives of General Psychiatry, 56*, 876–880.

Fergusson, D. M., & Lynskey, M. T. (1996). Adolescent resiliency to family adversity. *Journal of Child Psychology and Psychiatry, 37*, 281–292.

Forehand, R., Biggar, H., & Kotchick, B. A. (1998). Cumulative risk across family stressors: Short- and long-term effects for adolescents. *Journal of Abnormal Child Psychology, 26*, 119–128.

Francis, G., Last, C. G., & Strauss, C. C. (1987). Expression of separation anxiety disorder: The roles of age and gender. *Child Psychiatry and Human Development, 18*, 82–89.

Freisthler, B., Needell, B., & Gruenewald, P. J. (2004). Is the physical availability of alcohol and illicit drugs related to neighborhood rates of child maltreatment. *Child Abuse and Neglect, 29*, 1049–1060.

Goodman, R. (1999). The extended version of the strengths and difficulties questionnaire as a guide to child psychiatric caseness and consequent burden. *Journal of Child Psychology and Psychiatry, 40*, 791–799.

Green, J. G., McLaughlin, K. A., Berglund, P., Gruber, M. J., Sampson, N. A., Zaslavsky, A. M., et al. (2010). Childhood adversities and adult psychopathology in the National Comorbidity Survey Replication (NCS-R) I: Associations with first onset of DSM-IV disorders. *Archives of General Psychiatry, 62*, 113–123.

Hankin, B. L., Abramson, L. Y., Moffitt, T. E., Silva, P. A., McGee, R., & Angell, K. E. (1998). Development of depression from preadolescence to young adulthood: Emerging gender differences in a 10-year longitudinal study. *Journal of Abnormal Psychology, 107*, 128–140.

Hatzenbuehler, M. L. (2009). How does sexual minority stigma "get under the skin?" A psychological mediation framework. *Psychological Bulletin, 135*, 707–730.

Hatzenbuehler, M. L. (2011). The social environment and suicide attempts in lesbian, gay, and bisexual youth. *Pediatrics, 127*, 896–903.

Hawkins, S. S., Chandra, A., & Berkman, L. F. (2012). The impact of tobacco control policies on disparities in children's secondhand smoke exposure: A comparison of methods. *Maternal and Child Health Journal, 16*, S70–S77.

Henderson, C., Liu, X., Diez Roux, A. V., Link, B. G., & Hasin, D. S. (2004). The effects of US state income inequality and alcohol policies on symptoms of depression and alcohol dependence. *Social Science and Medicine, 58*, 565–575.

Holford, T. R. (1991). Understanding the effects of age, period, and cohort on incidence and mortality rates. *Annual Review of Public Health, 12*, 425–457.

Jaffee, S. R., Caspi, A., Moffit, T. E., Polo-Tomás, M., & Taylor, A. (2007). Individual, family, and neighborhood factors distinguish resilient from non-resilient maltreated children: A cumulative stressors model. *Child Abuse and Neglect, 31*, 231–253.

Jaffee, S. R., Moffit, T. E., Caspi, A., Fombonne, E., Poulton, R., & Martin, J. (2002). Differences in early childhood risk factors for juvenile-onset and adult-onset depression. *Archives of General Psychiatry, 58*, 215–222.

Kerr, W. C., Greenfield, T. K., Bond, J., Ye, Y., & Rehm, J. (2009). Age-period-cohort modelling of alcohol volume and heavy drinking days in the US National Alcohol Surveys: Divergence in younger and older adult trends. *Addiction, 104*, 27–37.

Kessler, R. C., Avenevoli, S., Costello, E. J., Georgiades, K., Green, J. G., Gruber, M. J., et al. (2012). Prevalence, persistence, and socio-demographic correlates of DSM-IV disorders in the U.S. National Comorbidity Survey Replication Adolescent (NCS-A) supplement. *Archives of General Psychiatry, 69*, 372–380.

Kessler, R. C., Avenevoli, S., Costello, E. J., Green, J. G., Gruber, M. J., McLaughlin, K. A., et al. (2012). Severity of 12-month DSM-IV disorders in the National Comorbidity Survey Replication Adolescent Supplement. *Archives of General Psychiatry, 69*, 381–389.

Kessler, R. C., Avenevoli, S., McLaughlin, K. A., Green, J. G., Lakoma, M. D., et al. (2012). Lifetime prevalence and comorbidity of DSM-IV disorders in the National Comorbidity Survey Replication Adolescent Supplement (NCS-A). *Psychological Medicine, 42*, 1997–2010.

Kessler, R. C., Avenevoli, S., Costello, E. J., Green, J. G., Gruber, M. J., Heeringa, S., et al. (2009). National comorbidity survey replication adolescent supplement (NCS-A): II. Overview and design. *Journal of the American Academy of Child & Adolescent Psychiatry, 48*, 380–385.

Kessler, R. C., Berglund, P., Demler, O., Jin, R., Koretz, D., Merikangas, K. R., et al. (2003). The epidemiology of major depressive disorder: Results from the National Comorbidity Survey Replication (NCS-R). *Journal of the American Medical Association, 289*, 3095–3105.

Keyes, K. M., & Li, G. (2010). A multi-phase method for estimating cohort effects in age-period contingency table data. *Annals of Epidemiology, 20*, 779–785.

Keyes, K. M., McLaughlin, K. A., Koenen, K. C., Goldmann, E., Uddin, M., & Galea, S. (2012). Child maltreatment increases sensitivity to adverse social contexts: Neighborhood physical disorder and incident drinking in Detroit. *Drug and Alcohol Dependence, 122*, 77–85.

Keyes, K. M., Schulenberg, J. E., O'Malley, P. M., Johnston, L. D., Bachman, J. G., Li, G., et al. (2011). The social norms of birth cohorts and adolescent marijuana use in the United States, 1976–2007. *Addiction, 106*, 1790–1800.

Keyes, K. M., Utz, R. L., Robinson, W., & Li, G. (2010). What is a cohort effect? Comparison of three statistical methods for modeling cohort effects in obesity prevalence in the United States, 1971–2006. *Social Science and Medicine, 70*, 1100–1108.

Kim-Cohen, J., Caspi, A., Moffitt, T. E., Harrington, H., Milne, B. J., & Poulton, R. (2003). Prior juvenile diagnoses in adults with mental disorder: developmental follow-back of a prospective-longitudinal cohort. *Archives of General Psychiatry, 60*(7), 709–717.

Knauper, B., Cannell, C. F., Schwarz, N., Bruce, M. L., & Kessler, R. C. (1999). Improving the accuracy of major depression age of onset reports in the US National Comorbidity Survey. *International Journal of Methods in Psychiatric Research, 8*, 39–48.

Korenman, S., Miller, J., & Sjaastad, J. (1995). Long-term poverty and child development in the United States: Results from the NLSY. *Children and Youth Services Review, 17*, 127–155.

Krieger, N. (1994). Epidemiology and the web of causation: Has anyone seen the spider? *Social Science and Medicine, 39*, 887–903.

Kuntsche, E., Keundig, H., & Gmel, G. (2008). Alcohol outlet density, perceived availability and adolescent alcohol use: A multilevel structural equation model. *Journal of Epidemiology and Community Health, 62*, 811–816.

Leventhal, T., & Brooks-Gunn, J. (2000). The neighborhoods they live in: The effects of neighborhood residence on child and adolescent outcomes. *Psychological Bulletin, 126*, 309–337.

Leventhal, T., & Brooks-Gunn, J. (2003). Moving to opportunity: An experimental study of neighborhood effects on mental health. *American Journal of Public Health, 93*, 1576–1582.

Lewis, M. (1997). *Altering fate: Why the past does not predict the future*. New York: Guilford Press.

Lohr, S. L. (1999). *Sampling: Design and analysis*. Pacific Grove, CA: Brooks/Cole Publishing.

Lynch, M., & Cicchetti, D. (1998). An ecological-transactional analysis of children and contexts: The longitudinal interplay among child maltreatment, community violence, and children's symptomatology. *Development and Psychopathology, 10*, 235–257.

McGee, R., Feehan, M., Williams, S., & Anderson, J. (1992). DSM-III disorders from age 11 to age 15 years. *Journal of the American Academy of Child and Adolescent Psychiatry, 31*(1), 50–59.

McLaughlin, K. A., Fairbank, J. A., Gruber, M. J., Jones, R. T., Lakoma, M. D., Pfefferbaum, B., et al. (2009). Serious emotional disturbance among youths exposed to Hurricane Katrina 2 years postdisaster. *Journal of the American Academy of Child and Adolescent Psychiatry, 48*, 1069–1078.

McLaughlin, K. A., Green, J. G., Gruber, M. J., Sampson, N. A., Zaslavsky, A., & Kessler, R. C. (2012). Childhood adversities and first onset of psychiatric disorders in a national sample of adolescents. *Archives of General Psychiatry, 69*(11), 1151–1160.

McLaughlin, K. A., Koenen, K. C., Hill, E., Petukhova, M., & Kessler, R. C. (2013). Trauma exposure and posttraumatic stress disorder in a US national sample of adolescents. *Journal of the American Academy of Child and Adolescent Psychiatry, 52*(8), 815–830.e14.

Meyer, I. H. (2003). Prejudice, social stress, and mental health in lesbian, gay, and bisexual populations: Conceptual issues and research evidence. *Psychological Bulletin, 129*, 674–697.

Moffitt, T. E. (1993). Adolescence-limited and life-course persistent antisocial behavior: A developmental taxonomy. *Psychological Review, 100*, 674–701.

Nolen-Hoeksema, S., & Twenge, J. M. (2002). Age, gender, race, socioeconomic status, and birth cohort difference on the children's depression inventory: A meta-analysis. *Journal of Abnormal Psychology, 111*, 578–588.

Peeples, F., & Loeber, R. (1994). Do individual factors and neighborhood context explain ethnic differences in juvenile delinquency? *Journal of Quantitative Criminology, 10*, 141–157.

Riis, J., Grason, H., Strobino, D., Ahmed, S., & Minkovitz, C. (2012). State school policies and youth obesity. *Maternal and Child Health Journal, 16*, S111–S118.

Rockhill, B., Newman, B., & Weinberg, C. (1998). Use and misuse of population attributable fractions. *American Journal of Public Health, 88*, 15–19.

Rose, G. (1992). *The strategy of preventive medicine* (Vol. 1). Oxford: Oxford University Press.

Rothman, K. J., Greenland, S., & Lash, T. L. (2008). *Modern epidemiology* (3rd ed.). Philadelphia, PA: Lippincott Williams & Wilkins.

Russell, S. T., & Joyner, K. (2001). Adolescent sexual orientation and suicide risk: Evidence from a national study. *American Journal of Public Health, 91*, 1276–1281.

Ryan, C. E., Russell, S. T., Huebner, D., Diaz, R. M., & Sanchez, J. (2010). Family acceptance in adolescence and the health of LGBT young adults. *Journal of Child and Adolescent Psychiatric Nursing, 23*, 205–213.

Sampson, R. J., Morenoff, J. D., & Gannon-Rowley, T. (2002). Assessing "neighborhood effects": Social processes and new directions. *Annual Review of Sociology, 28*, 443–478.

Sampson, R. J., Raudenbush, S., & Earls, F. (1997). *Neighborhoods and violent crime: A multilevel study of collective efficacy Science, 277*, 918–924.

Sampson, R. J., Sharkey, P., & Raudenbush, S. (2007). Durable effects of concentrated disadvantage on verbal ability among African-American children. *Proceedings of the National Academy of Sciences, 105*, 845–852.

Sampson, R. J., Sharkey, P., & Raudenbush, S. (2008). Durable effects of concentrated disadvantage on verbal ability among African-American children. *Proceedings of the National Academy of Sciences, 105*, 845–852.

Shaffer, D., Fisher, P., Dulcan, M. K., Davies, M., Piacentini, J., Schwab-Stone, M. E., et al. (1996). The NIMH Diagnostic Interview Schedule for Children Version 2.3 (DISC-2.3): Description, acceptability, prevalence rates, and performance in the MECA study. *Journal of the American Academy of Child and Adolescent Psychiatry, 35*, 865–877.

Smeeth, L., Cook, C., Fombonne, E., Heavey, L., Rodrigues, L. C., Smith, P. G., et al. (2004). MMR vaccination and pervasive developmental disorders: A case–control study. *Lancet, 364*, 963–969.

Sroufe, L. A. (1990). Considering normal and abnormal together: The essence of developmental psychopathology. *Development and Psychopathology, 2*, 335–347.

Sroufe, L. A. (2009). The concept of development in developmental psychopathology. *Child Development Perspectives, 3*, 178–183.

Sroufe, L. A., Egeland, B., & Kreutzer, T. (1990). The fate of early experience following developmental change: Longitudinal approaches to individual adaptation in childhood. *Child Development, 61*, 1363–1373.

Susser, E. S. (1973). *Causal thinking in the health sciences: Concepts and strategies in epidemiology.* New York: Oxford Press.

Susser, M. (1998). Does risk factor epidemiology put epidemiology at risk? Peering into the future. *Journal of Epidemiology and Community Health, 52*, 608–611.

Susser, E. S., & Lin, S. (1992). Schizophrenia after prenatal exposure to the Dutch Hunger Winter of 1944–1945. *Archives of General Psychiatry, 49*, 983–988.

Susser, E. S., Neugebauer, R., Hoek, H. W., Brown, A. S., Lin, S., Labovitz, D., et al. (1996). Schizophrenia after prenatal famine. *Archives of General Psychiatry, 53*, 25–31.

Susser, E. S., Schwartz, S., Morabia, A., & Bromet, E. J. (2006). *Psychiatric epidemiology.* New York: Oxford Press.

Susser, M., & Susser, E. S. (1996). Choosing a future for epidemiology: I. Eras and paradigms. *American Journal of Public Health, 86*, 668–673.

Tu, S. (2003). Developmental epidemiology: A review of three key measures of effect. *Journal of Clinical Child and Adolescent Psychology, 32*, 187–192.

Xue, Y., Leventhal, T., Brooks-Gunn, J., & Earls, F. (2005). Neighborhood residence and mental health problems in 5- to 11-year-olds. *Archives of General Psychiatry, 62*, 554–563.

Yang, Y., & Land, K. C. (2008). Age-period-cohort analysis of repeated cross-section surveys: Fixed or random effects? *American Sociological Review, 36*, 297–326.

Modeling Strategies in Developmental Psychopathology Research: Prediction of Individual Change

6

Sonya K. Sterba

Developmental psychopathologists often seek to explain change over time in psychiatric syndromes and behavioral constructs. Because the rate and form of change may be unique to particular children, complex interactions among person-level characteristics, environmental characteristics, genetic/biological characteristics, and time are often hypothesized and investigated (e.g., Petersen et al., 2012). However, before we can assess change over time in such constructs and before we can investigate how change differs across children, we must consider how to conceptualize the psychiatric constructs themselves, and we must consider what assumptions are required for quantifying change. In order to address these issues, we first briefly discuss preliminary statistical and conceptual issues involving the categorical versus continuous representation of psychopathological constructs at a given time point. Second, we discuss some preconditions for quantifying change in such constructs across development. The third and fourth sections of this chapter focus on methods for describing and predicting longitudinal change in psychopathological constructs; these methods allow recovery of interactions between

person characteristics and time. We conclude with extension topics relevant to the longitudinal modeling of psychopathology and some design and data considerations for such studies.

Conceptualizing Psychiatric Syndromes as Categorical or Continuous

Symptoms such as anhedonia, weight change, and depressed mood covary or co-occur in the population at large. At certain severities, frequencies, and durations, the joint presence of these symptoms, along with several others, is conventionally considered to define an (unobserved) depression syndrome in the Diagnostic and Statistical Manual of Mental Disorders V (American Psychiatric Association, 2013). More generally, a psychiatric syndrome may be conceptualized as a dimensional or a categorical underlying construct. Dimensional models of psychopathology posit that associations among such depression symptoms occur because they mutually depend on the same underlying dimensional syndrome (i.e., a depressogenic liability distribution). Categorical models of psychopathology posit that there are homogeneous groups with unique symptom profiles and furthermore that observed associations among such depression symptoms arise due to the mixing together of groups with different mean profiles. For instance, one group might have a mean profile with high anhedonia and insomnia and moderate levels of

6

6

S.K. Sterba, Ph.D. (✉)
Psychology and Human Development Department, Quantitative Methods Program, Vanderbilt University, Peabody #552; 230 Appleton Place, Nashville, TN 37203, USA
e-mail: Sonya.Sterba@Vanderbilt.edu

other symptoms, whereas another group might have a mean profile with high depressed mood and concentration problems but moderate levels of other symptoms.

There have been attempts to discriminate statistically between categorical and continuous representations of psychiatric constructs (for reviews, see Helzer, van den Brink, & Guth, 2006; Kraemer, Shrout, & Rubio-Stipec, 2007; Krueger, Markon, Patrick, & Iacono, 2005; Widiger & Samuel, 2005). Recent approaches (e.g., Brown & Barlow, 2005; Conway, Hammen, & Brennan, 2012; Gillespie, Neale, Legrand, et al., 2011; Hallquist & Pilkonis, 2012; Lubke, Muthén, & Moilanen, et al., 2007; Muthén, 2006; Trull & Durrett, 2005; Walton, Ormel, & Krueger, 2011; Witkiewitz et al., 2013) involving analyses of symptom-level data have often involved comparing the fit of alternative statistical models that explain associations among symptoms using either latent dimensions—factor analysis models—or categories—mixture models such as latent class or latent profile models. Representations that combine both categories and continua have also been considered and have received attention in DSM-V (Regier, Kuhl, & Kupfer, 2013). Although there is no guarantee that the better fitting model corresponds to the true nature of psychiatric syndromes in the population (Bollen, 1989; Lubke et al., 2007), this assumption often seems to be employed. The ability to accurately discriminate between these categorical and continuous representations of psychopathology has been shown to depend on, for instance, sample size and the separation among classes, if classes exist (Lubke, 2012; Lubke & Neale, 2006, 2008). Historically, taxometric methods have also been used for discriminating classes from continua for psychiatric constructs (see Haslam, Holland, & Kuppens, 2012; Waller & Meehl, 1998), though these approaches have recently been shown to have key limitations compared to mixture models for this purpose (see Lubke & Tueller, 2010).

Ongoing interest in representing psychiatric constructs categorically often stems from the fact that ultimately categorical decisions will need to be made regarding who will get treatment (cases) and who will not (Costello & Angold, 2006; Zachar, 2000). However, syndromes may still be treated as dimensional in statistical models even if ultimately categorical treatment decisions will be made. In fact, dimensional models of psychopathology can have advantages in terms of *statistical power* (i.e., the chance of detecting an effect when there is one) and in terms of prediction accuracy (e.g., Bergman, von Eye, & Magnusson, 2006; MacCallum, Zhang, Preacher, & Rucker, 2002; Markon, Chmielewski, & Miller, 2011). On the flip side, syndromes may still be treated as categorical in statistical models even if ultimately theory considers them as continuous constructs. One rationale for doing so is that assumptions imposed by dimensional models of psychopathology (e.g., that the underlying liability distribution for depression is normal) may be violated, and categorical representations of psychopathology can avoid restrictive distributional assumptions. However, preliminary empirical examinations of such latent syndrome liability distributions (van den Oord, Pickles, & Waldman, 2003) have not evidenced profound nonnormality to date (see also Schmitt, Mehta, Aggen, Kubarych, & Neale, 2006; Sterba, Baldasaro, & Bauer, 2012).

In sum, there may be, but does not need to be, an exact match between how the psychopathological construct is conceptualized theoretically (as a discrete or continuous syndrome) and how the psychopathological construct is treated in statistical models. In statistical models, it may be treated as categorical—a binary depression diagnosis variable or a nominal depression class membership variable—versus continuous—a continuous score on a depression factor or a sum of depression items, or a combination.

Are We Measuring the Same Syndrome Construct Over Time?

There were relatively few explicit developmental modifications of DSM-IV Axis I psychiatric syndromes for particular age groups (see

Costello & Angold, 2006, for review). This was a topic of discussion in the revisions for DSM-V (e.g., Pine et al., 2011; Rutter, 2011) resulting in several more modifications for DSM-V (see Regier et al. (2013) for a review.) Historically, there has been an assumption that psychiatric syndromes manifest similarly across developmental time, though they may differ in rate (e.g., tendency for higher levels of a disruptive behavior latent construct in toddlers, higher levels of an anxiety latent construct in middle childhood, and higher levels of a depression latent construct in adolescence). In fact, in order to assess *quantitative* longitudinal change in a behavior or syndrome (a topic considered in detail shortly), we must be able to make this assumption that we are measuring the same thing over time—i.e., that our construct displays *measurement invariance*. Specifically, in the context of psychiatric syndromes, this means each symptom should relate to the underlying latent syndrome in the same way, regardless of age.

The popular theoretical concept of *developmental pathways* of psychopathological behavior (Loeber, Keenan, & Zhang, 1997; Pickles & Hill, 2006) is not inconsistent with the existence of measurement invariance of psychiatric constructs. For instance, in one common example of such pathways, some children with oppositional defiant behavior in middle childhood desist by adolescence. However, among the children with persistent oppositionality, some develop conduct disorder problems in adolescence. This phenomenon is also called successive comorbidity (Angold, Costello, & Erkanli, 1999). So long as oppositional defiant symptoms consistently represent that syndrome over time and so long as conduct disorder symptoms consistently represent that syndrome over time, measurement invariance could still hold. An example of a theory that suggests violation of measurement invariance is that of Patterson (1993) who suggests that there is one underlying liability for antisocial behavior that he likens to a chimera; it manifests qualitatively differently over time depending on the cognitive level and developmental milestones of a given developmental

period. Whereas biting could be an indicator of the antisocial behavior construct in toddlerhood, it would not be an equally valid indicator in adolescence. Another theory that suggests violation of measurement invariance posits developmental differentiation of psychopathology (Knapp & Jensen, 2006; Lilienfeld, Waldman, & Israel, 1994) in which psychiatric syndromes are thought to be undifferentiated in early childhood. With advances in cognitive and emotional capacity, distinct syndromes like those described in the DSM are thought to be eventually capable of manifesting.

It is possible to statistically evaluate whether measurement invariance holds, presuming the availability of multivariate, longitudinal, symptom-level data. The particular statistical method for doing so will depend on whether psychopathology is being represented dimensionally (i.e., using syndrome factors) or categorically (using discrete classes with differing symptom patterns). Using the dimensional representation, measurement invariance can be evaluated using a longitudinal factor analysis framework (e.g., Tisak & Meredith, 1990). A factor analysis model is specified at every time point, and increasingly restrictive constraints are tested regarding the stability of the relationship between symptom indicators and syndrome factors across time points. Instead of using the categorical representation, measurement invariance can be evaluated using a latent transition model framework (Collins & Wugalter, 1992). In this framework, a latent class model is specified at every time point, and classes at times $t-1$ and t are related; increasingly restrictive constraints are tested regarding the stability of symptom endorsement probabilities within-class across-time (see Collins & Lanza, 2010 for an example).

One possible manifestation of measurement *non*invariance in the form of developmental differentiation would be if the number of factors or number of classes representing a construct increased over time. In one illustrative analysis that used a dimensional representation of Axis I DSM-IV syndromes, the factor structure representing these syndromes in preschoolers (Sterba,

Egger & Angold, 2007; see also Strickland et al., 2011) remained largely similar in a separate sample across middle childhood to adolescence, with little evidence of developmental differentiation except with respect to generalized anxiety and depression in later adolescence (Sterba et al., 2010). If measurement invariance is partially supported (e.g., most but not all items retain the same relationship to their respective construct over time), longitudinal change in the construct can still be quantified so long as (a) some items display measurement invariance (called anchor items) and (b) a longitudinal model is chosen that explicitly allows for noninvariant symptom-to-syndrome relationships over time. Quantifying change with partially invariant constructs is discussed in Edwards and Wirth (2009), and costs of assuming full invariance when only partial invariance holds are described in Wirth (2008). New Bayesian methods for more flexibly imposing partial measurement invariance are described in Muthén and Asparouhov (2013). In the subsequent sections, we assume measurement invariance of psychological constructs and focus instead on alternative approaches for quantifying change.

Describing Growth in a Psychological Construct

A common objective of developmental psychopathology applications is describing and predicting growth in a target psychopathology construct over time (e.g., Curran & Willoughby, 2003; Dougherty, Klein, & Davila, 2004; Lenzenweger, Johnson, & Willett, 2004). Later we consider quantifying multivariate change in multiple constructs at once. For simplicity, suppose that we have an observed outcome repeatedly measured for N persons ($i = 1...N$) across $t = 1...T$ time points. Our observed repeated measure itself could be categorical or continuous. In the running example in this and the next section, our repeated measure is a binary physical aggression indicator recorded at $T = 3$ time points spaced approximately one year apart.

This measure was collected from $N = 428$ young adults who were recruited in 2002 at age 17–18[1] as they were transitioning out of Midwestern state-run or foster care facilities (Courtney & Cusick, 2007). This repeated measure will exhibit a particular mean trend over time, and its scores will be correlated over time. We can also expect that there will be heterogeneity around the sample mean trend in individual patterns of change over time—these individual patterns are often called individual *trajectories* of change.

Statistically, we have alternatives for modeling this heterogeneity. As two examples, we could account for this heterogeneity by assuming that individual trajectories vary continuously around a population mean trajectory, and then we could estimate a mean trend and continuous variability around this trend. This approach is often called random coefficient growth modeling (RCGM), hierarchical linear modeling, or latent curve modeling (Bollen & Curran, 2006; Singer & Willett, 2003). Figure 6.1 Panel (a) depicts a decreasing marginal mean trajectory (bold solid line) from a RCGM for our running example, superimposed upon a continuous distribution of individual trajectories implied by the model (thin grey lines). An alternative is to account for individual heterogeneity in change over time by assuming that it can be described by a finite number of prototype trajectories and that we can statistically select an optimal number of prototype trajectories. Children following the same prototype trajectory are considered members of their own latent *trajectory class*. Specifically, *within* a class, individuals are assumed to follow the same trend apart from random noise, although the functional form of the trend can differ *between* classes. This

---

[1] Exact ages for participants in this *Crime during the Transition to Adulthood* dataset, at www.icpsr.umich.edu, were not available to the public. A physically aggressive conduct offense was considered to have occurred if an adolescent over the past 12 months participated in a group fight, shot or stabbed someone, pulled a knife or gun, badly injured someone, or threatened someone with a weapon. Other representations of this aggression construct would be possible.

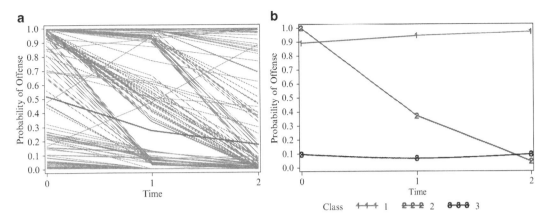

Fig. 6.1 Unconditional RCGM versus LCGM aggression trajectories for the empirical example. (**a**) RCGM mean trajectory (*bold solid line*) & 150 model-implied individual trajectories (*thin gray lines*) and (**b**) LCGM with 3 class trajectories. *Notes. RCGM* random coefficient growth model, *LCGM* latent class growth model

approach is often called latent class growth modeling (LCGM) or semiparametric group-based trajectory modeling (Muthén, 2001; Nagin, 1999); a related model not considered in detail here is called a growth mixture model (e.g., Muthén & Shedden, 1999). Figure 6.1 Panel (b) depicts the results of fitting a LCGM to the running example dataset. The best-fitting[2] 3-class solution is shown. These classes are seen to differ qualitatively in functional form (e.g., a high-chronic, low-stable, vs. decreasing shape). They also differ in probability of class membership (i.e., class proportions: 0.11 vs. 0.37 vs. 0.52, respectively).

Hundreds of applications of RCGMs and LCGMs (and closely related models) in the developmental psychopathology field have been published in the last decade alone (for reviews, see Nagin & Odgers, 2010; Sterba et al., 2012). Many of these applications have been in areas of substance abuse, delinquent behaviors, and internalizing behavior. Although there has been

some discussion of which model is best to apply under certain conditions (e.g., Maughan, 2005; Nagin & Tremblay, 2005b; Raudenbush, 2001, 2005; Sampson & Laub, 2005), this has remained unresolved because even when both models are fit to the same data, it is difficult to statistically tell if extracted LCGM trajectory classes truly exist or whether they are approximating an underlying continuous distribution of individual differences in change (Bauer & Curran, 2003a, 2003b).

Instead, there has been increasing interest in synthesizing LCGM and RCGM results across and within studies (e.g., Connell, Dishion, & Deater-Deckard, 2006; Hirsh-Pasek & Burchinal, 2006; Reinecke, 2006; Romens, Abramson, & Alloy, 2009). One obstacle to this synthesis has been the perception that a RCGM implies only one trajectory (the mean trend) and thus is not comparable to LCGM results that extract multiple class trajectories. Even efforts to synthesize LCGM results across studies have encountered obstacles. Many researchers expected that if classes literally correspond to population subgroups, the number of best-fitting class trajectories in LCGM should be replicable across studies using the same outcome

---

[2]The best-fitting number of classes was determined using Akaike's information criterion and the Lo-Mendell-Rubin adjusted likelihood ratio test.

(e.g., antisocial behavior). Such replicability has not been found (e.g., Fontaine, Carbonneau, Vitaro, Barker, & Tremblay, 2009; Horn, 2000; Nandi, Beard, & Galea, 2009; Skardhamar, 2010; van Dulmen, Goncy, Vest, & Flannery, 2009). For instance, in Fontaine et al.'s (2009) review of 21 applications of LCGM to girls' antisocial behavior, 5 % of studies had >5 classes, 29 % had 5 classes, 28 % had 4, 28 % had 3, and 10 % had 2. The proportions and shapes of these classes also differed widely [e.g., chronic (4 %), escalators (12 %), desistors (35 %), late onsetters (17 %), nonoffenders (32 %) vs. high rising (35 %), low (65 %) vs. high decreasers (4 %), low decreasers (15 %), near zero (81 %)]. Statistically, however, these findings are not surprising; the best-fitting number of LCGM trajectory classes extracted depends to some extent on N and T, just as the amount of continuous variability detectable in RCGM (e.g., continuous variation in just intercepts or also in linear and quadratic slopes of time) is known to depend on N and T (Fitzmaurice, Laird, & Ware, 2011; Hedeker & Gibbons, 2006). Other factors, such as measurement/distributional properties of the outcome and sampling characteristics, also affect the amount of heterogeneity that can be accounted for with either trajectory classes or continua (Bauer & Curran, 2003a; Eggleston, Laub, & Sampson, 2004; Jackson & Sher, 2008). Even if we could equate across-study characteristics when comparing LCGM applications within a given topic area (e.g., antisocial behavior), however, we still face the inability to integrate descriptive results across studies when LCGM is fit in one study and RCGM is fit in another study.

We can circumvent the latter impasse by shifting from focusing exclusively on description of individual change over time to focusing on the more concrete and arguably more clinically relevant objective of explaining and predicting individual patterns of change over time (Butler & Louis, 1992; Cudeck & Henly, 2003; Raudenbush, 2005; Sterba & Bauer, 2013). We will later see that considering prediction of change over time yields opportunities for comparing and synthesizing LCGM and RCGM results within and across developmental psychopathology studies.

Predicting Growth in a Psychological Construct

Both RCGM and LCGM allow prediction of growth trajectories, using either time invariant covariates (TICs, e.g., gender, race, presence of birth trauma, presence of a particular gene) that are measured once or time-varying covariates (TVCs, e.g., whether an adolescent became homeless at time t, joined a gang at time t, or was pregnant at time t) that are measured at multiple repeated time points. The effect (i.e., slope) of time may differ across values of a TIC, such as if rate of change in the antisocial behavior outcome is more positive for boys than girls. The effect of a TVC could also differ across time (e.g., if peer victimization at $t =$ age 13 had a larger effect on antisocial behavior than did peer victimization at $t =$ age 18). When the effect of a predictor differs across the levels of another predictor (here, for instance, time), this is statistically termed an interaction. Higher order interactions involve more than two variables. Nonlinear interactions imply that the effect of a predictor depends nonlinearly on the levels of another variable (see Aiken & West, 1991 for examples). It is also possible for TICs to interact with each other or to interact with particular TVCs, but our illustration here focuses on interactions involving time.

Recovery of potentially complex interactions involving person-level variables, environmental/contextual variables, and biological/neurological variables over time is central to many research traditions in the developmental psychopathology field, including the person-oriented research paradigm (Bergman & Magnusson, 1997; Cairns, Bergman, & Kagan, 1998; Muthén & Muthén, 2000; Sterba & Bauer, 2010a, 2010b; Von Eye & Bergman, 2003) and the holistic-interactional research paradigm (e.g., Gottleib & Halpern, 2002; Magnusson, 1985). The latter paradigm, for instance, calls for investigating "how person factors and environmental factors—independently and jointly in interaction—operate and influence the course of development from childhood to adolescence" (Magnusson, 1985, p. 119). Put simply, incorporating interaction relationships allows for conclusions to be made about change over time in a psychological construct with a greater degree of individual specificity. One could conclude that children with a particular constellation of characteristics may have differently shaped trajectories (with different rates of change over time in the outcome) than children with another constellation of characteristics.

Methods like LCGMs which classify children into classes or clusters are thought to have a distinct advantage for recovering complex potentially nonlinear interactions, compared to regression-based methods which do not extract classes, such as RCGM (e.g., Bergman, 2001; Bergman & Trost, 2006; Connell et al., 2006; Laursen & Hoff, 2006; Moffitt, 2006, 2008; Muthén, 2001, 2004; Nagin & Tremblay, 2005b; Segawa, Ngwe, Li, Flay, & Coinvestigators, 2005). The anticipated advantages of classification-based methods such as LCGMs may be based on the perspective that models like RCGMs can only accommodate linear predictive relationships (Hill, White, Chung, Hawkins, & Catalano, 2000; Shaw & Liang, 2012; Torppa, Poikkeus, Laakso, Eklund, & Lyytinen, 2006)—despite the fact that procedures exist for incorporating nonlinear and/or interactive predictor relationships in models such as RCGMs (Aiken & West, 1991; Curran, Bauer, & Willoughby, 2004). Anticipated advantages are also attributed to classification methods' greater flexibility in accounting for predictor relations (e.g., Laursen & Hoff, 2006; Pastor, Barron, Miller, & Davis, 2007).

However, Sterba and Bauer (2013) showed that, rather than one model being inherently superior at recovering such relationships, LCGMs and RCGMs accommodate interactions in different ways, and if specified appropriately both models can approximately equally well recover the same interactions—even higher-order nonlinear interactions. For instance, to accommodate interactions between TICs and time, RCGMs require explicitly including product terms (e.g., $TIC \times time$, $TIC \times time^2$, $TIC^2 \times time$) as predictors of the outcome. In contrast, LCGMs accommodate interactions between TICs and time by

including the TIC as a main effect predictor of class membership. The class trajectories, which differ in functional form of time, are then weighted by the probability of class membership—which is now conditional on the TIC. This specification intrinsically accommodates interactions between TIC and time. Thus, for recovering complex interactions involving TICs and time, these models require different things. RCGMs require entering higher-order product terms as covariates, whereas LCGMs require more classes, higher-order functional forms of time within class, and class-varying predictor effects (Sterba & Bauer, 2013). Yet for other kinds of interactions, both models require the same procedures. For instance, both models can account for an effect of a TVC that differs over time, by either including an explicit product term $TVC \times time$ as a covariate or by specifying different slopes of the TVC at each time point.

We now use our running example on physical aggression to illustrate how our RCGM and our 3-class LCGM each account for similar patterns of change for adolescents with particular TIC and TVC characteristics. In other words, despite the fact that marginally the RCGM implies *one mean trajectory* and the LCGM implies *3 class-specific mean trajectories*, both models will be able to recover approximately the same predicted trajectories of change conditional on chosen person-level characteristics. For our example, TICs of interest are: presence of an alcohol or substance abuse diagnosis at time 1 (alc_i), male gender ($male_i$), level of social support (sup_i, a standardized scale score from Sherbourne and Stewart's [1991] inventory), and presence of a prior arrest record (arr_i). TVCs of interest are whether an adolescent was in school at time t (sch_{it}) and whether the adolescent was selling drugs at time t ($sell_{it}$). An i subscript for a predictor denotes that it can have a unique value for every person, and an it subscript denotes that it can have a unique value for every person at every time point.

Though key results are shortly presented in graphical format, for interested readers, we briefly present the formulas for predicted trajectories—expected values of the outcome at each time point given chosen values of the covariates. For the logic behind calculating predicted trajectories to convey conditional relationships over time, see Bauer and Shanahan (2007), Curran et al. (2004), Nagin and Tremblay (2005a), or Sterba and Bauer (2013). Importantly, although predicted trajectories are not often presented in LCGM applications, Nagin and Tremblay (2005a) recommend their use because "even if the groups [i.e., latent trajectory classes] are thought of as real entities, it

is not possible to assign individuals definitively to a specific trajectory ex ante based on number of risk factors. It is possible to construct only an expected trajectory" (p. 885).

Since our outcome is binary, our focus is on the predicted probability of physically aggressing at time t (i. e., $y_{it} = 1$) given covariates, which we refer to as $\hat{p}_{it}$. For RCGM, we can calculate $\hat{p}_{it}$ for person i at time t from the following equation for the log-odds:

$$
\begin{aligned}
\log(\hat{p}_{it} / (1 - \hat{p}_{it})) = {} & \gamma_{00} + \gamma_{01}\text{alc}_i + \gamma_{02}\text{male}_i + \gamma_{03}\sup_i + \gamma_{04}\text{arr}_i + \\
& \left(\gamma_{10} + \gamma_{11}\text{alc}_i + \gamma_{12}\text{male}_i + \gamma_{13}\sup_i + \gamma_{14}\text{arr}_i \right)\text{time}_{it} + \gamma_{2t}\text{sell}_{it} + \gamma_{30}\text{sch}_{it}
\end{aligned}
\tag{6.1}
$$

γ's are estimated model coefficients. Note that the fact that time is multiplied by all quantities inside the parentheses implies interactions of time with each alc_i, male_i, $\sup_i$, and arr_i. Finally, note that sell_{it} was allowed to interact semipara-

metrically with time because it has a different effect per time point (γ_{2t} for $t = 1$–3). For LCGM, we can calculate $\hat{p}_{it}$ for person i at time t from the following equation for the log-odds:

$$
\log(\hat{p}_{it} / (1 - \hat{p}_{it})) = \sum_{k=1}^{K} \pi_i^{(k)} \left(\beta_{00}^{(k)} + \beta_{10}^{(k)}\text{time}_{it} + \beta_{2t}^{(k)}\text{sell}_{it} + \beta_{30}^{(k)}\text{sch}_{it} \right)
\tag{6.2}
$$

$$
\pi_i^{(k)} = \frac{\exp\left(\delta_0^{(k)} + \delta_1^{(k)}\text{alc}_i + \delta_2^{(k)}\text{male}_i + \delta_3^{(k)}\sup_i + \delta_4^{(k)}\text{arr}_i \right)}{\sum_{k=1}^{K} \exp\left(\delta_0^{(k)} + \delta_1^{(k)}\text{alc}_i + \delta_2^{(k)}\text{male}_i + \delta_3^{(k)}\sup_i + \delta_4^{(k)}\text{arr}_i \right)}
\tag{6.3}
$$

K is the number of classes (in our example, 3). A k superscript for a model coefficient implies that coefficient varies across latent classes $k = 1 \ldots K$. In Eq. (6.2), β s are estimated coefficients for time and for TVCs in the within-class trajectory. Note that sell_{it} is again allowed to interact with time as in Eq. (6.1) via a different effect per time point ($\beta_{2t}^{(k)}$ for $t = 1 \ldots 3$). $\pi_i^{(k)}$ is person i's probability of membership in class k. In Eq. (6.3), person i's probability of class membership is shown to be predicted by the TICs using a multinomial logistic specification. δ 's are multinomial logistic coefficients and are fixed to 0 in the last class for identification.

For illustrative purposes, we chose to plot predicted trajectories of physical aggression

propensity from each fitted model (RCGM and LCGM) at four chosen combinations of covariate values. Figure 6.2 depicts predicted trajectories for males with no baseline alcohol diagnosis, low social support, and a prior arrest record who quit school at time 2; these males either did (dashed line) or did not (solid line) begin to deal drugs. We can see that both the RCGM and LCGM predict that males with such multiple risk factors will likely start with high aggression at age 17–18 but rapidly decrease over time in their probability of physical aggression even if they quit school without a college degree. However, starting to deal drugs at approximately age 18–19 (time 2) stabilizes the probability of continued clinically meaningful aggression. Correspondingly, there

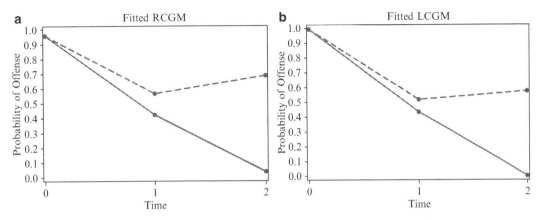

Fig. 6.2 Predicted aggression trajectories for males with no baseline alcohol diagnosis, low social support, and a prior arrest record who drop out of school at time 2. At time 2 these males start dealing drugs (*dotted line*) versus do not start dealing drugs (*solid line*)

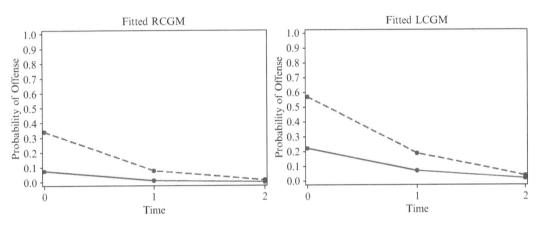

Fig. 6.3 Predicted aggression trajectories for participants who have a baseline alcohol diagnosis but stay in school, do not deal drugs, have no arrest record, have high social support, and are female (*dotted line*) versus male (*solid line*)

was statistically significant evidence of a drug dealing by time interaction in both models. Figure 6.3 depicts predicted trajectories for both fitted models at a different combination of covariates: adolescents who have a baseline alcohol diagnosis, stay in school, do not deal drugs, have no arrest record, have high social support, and are either female (dashed line) or male (solid line). These adolescents have multiple contextual protective factors such as strong social support, though they do still have the risk factor of a prior substance abuse disorder. Nonetheless, particularly for females with these characteristics, we see

a relatively low probability of physical aggression over time; for males we see a moderate and decreasing propensity.

In sum, when we only talk about *describing* change over time with categorical versus continuous variation growth models (Fig. 6.1 Panels a vs. b), it is difficult to reconcile results across models. Nevertheless, when we move on to talk about *predicting* and explaining individual change over time using covariates, similar predictive patterns can emerge from both kinds of models given equivalently flexible specification of both. Still, flexible specifications of either model can potentially run into practical problems recovering interactions of TICs or TVCs and time, particularly in small samples. For RCGMs, many product terms could induce estimation problems due to multicollinearity; for LCGMs, a sufficient number of classes to allow full variation of the predictor effect across time may not be estimable. Additionally, each kind of model presents unique conceptual challenges involving interpretation. Because TICs predict the entire trajectory as a whole in the LCGM (Eq. 6.3), we lack information about whether a TIC's effect entails a main effect or interaction with time. On the other hand, although the RCGM conveys whether particular main or interaction effects of predictors are statistically significant, the researcher is tasked with conceptually reintegrating this information to obtain a holistic understanding of predictive relations (Magnussan, 1998). For instance, from the running example LCGM, we learn that gender significantly differentiated class membership between each class 1 versus 3 and 2 versus 3, whereas from the RCGM we learn that there was a significant main effect of gender on intercepts, but not an interaction of gender with time.

Other interactions could have been investigated in our running example; for instance, if we posited that the amount by which predicted trajectories change across levels of social support differs by gender, RCGM would require inclusion of a three-way product term $male_i \times sup_i \times time_{it}$ predictor, whereas LCGM would require inclusion of a two-way product $male_i \times sup_i$ predicting class membership, with its effect allowed to vary across class. This empirical dataset was limited in the kinds of nonlinear interactions with time that could be investigated due to the relatively small number of time points ($T = 3$); to see examples of recovery of higher-order nonlinear predictive relationships recovered with both RCGM and LCGM, see Sterba and Bauer (2013). Finally, note that predicted trajectories can be calculated, plotted, and compared using estimates from already-published RCGM and LCGM applications (regardless of the number of classes) so long as similar predictor sets were used. Doing so would facilitate refining of

theories about longitudinal predictor-outcome relationships, in the context of methodological pluralism.

Modeling Psychopathology Across Developmental Time: Extension Topics

The earlier sections "Describing Growth in a Psychological Construct" and "Predicting Growth in a Psychological Construct" of this chapter focused on methods for describing and predicting change in univariate models for one behavioral or psychiatric construct over time. Many extensions are possible, a few of which are highlighted here. Addressing questions about whether the course of one behavior or syndrome (e.g., depression) concurrently or sequentially affects the course of another behavior or syndrome (e.g., separation anxiety) requires multivariate longitudinal models (e.g., Farrell, Sullivan, Esposito, Meyer, & Valois, 2005). *Multivariate* extensions of LCGM models that relate class membership on multiple behaviors are reviewed in Nagin and Tremblay (2001) and Nagin (2005). Multivariate extensions of RCGMs that relate aspects of change on multiple behaviors are reviewed in MacCallum, Kim, Malarkey, and Kiecolt-Glaser (1997) and Duncan, Duncan, and Stryker (2006). If repeated measures on behavior A were collected before repeated measures on behavior B, these models can capture sequential relations among the behaviors' patterns of change. If repeated measures on behavior A were collected simultaneously with repeated measures on behavior B, these models capture parallel relations among each behavior's pattern(s) of change. Using such models, it may be of interest to examine whether the effects of TICs (say, treatment) on the slopes of one syndrome are *mediated* by the intercept (or slope) of the other syndrome (e.g., von Soest & Hagtvet, 2011). Also, in the case of *multiple-informant data* (e.g., parent, child, teacher report), it would be possible to specify a parallel process RCGM or LCGM, interrelating change in maternal report (process A), child report (process B), and teacher report (process C), for example (e.g., Kobor,

Takacs, Urban, & Csepe, 2012; Obrien & Fitzmaurice, 2005). Other options for modeling change in multiple-informant data include fitting one change trajectory to a superordinate latent construct that is itself defined by repeated measures from multiple informants (Hancock, Kuo, & Lawrence, 2001; Petersen et al., 2012).

Additionally, although prior sections have focused on the description and prediction of change, another common goal is to use aspects of change themselves to predict a *distal outcome*, such as whether at a follow-up assessment a hospitalization, suicide attempt, psychiatric diagnosis, college graduation, employment, or incarceration had occurred (e.g., Rudolph, Troop-Gordon, Hessel, & Schmidt, 2011). LCGMs and RCGMs can be extended to include distal outcomes which are often predicted, in the former case, by class membership and, in the latter case, by the continuously distributed aspects of change, i.e., intercepts and/or slopes of time (see, e.g., Bollen & Curran, 2006; Muthén, 2004). For instance, if two latent trajectory classes of markedly different initial levels and functional forms had equivalent rates of a psychiatric diagnosis distal outcome, this would be an example of *equifinality* (Cicchetti & Rogosch, 1996).

Design and Data Considerations for Longitudinal Modeling of Psychopathology

We have thus far focused on alternative model specifications that may be of use in answering particular research questions in developmental psychopathology. New design and data collection features can expand these modeling possibilities. For instance, developmental psychopathology research is enriched by increasingly multimodal data collection methodologies. Neuroimaging data and/or DNA sequencing data collected on existing longitudinal samples provides new predictors of psychopathology trajectories and new avenues for investigating gene-environment interactions (for methodological reviews, see Dodge & Rutter, 2011; Lindquist, 2008). Developmental psychopathologists also have increasing possibilities for individual-specific

number, spacing, and timing of data collection occasions using technology developed for intensive longitudinal designs, also called daily diary studies (see Walls & Schafer, 2008 for review; see also Mehta & West, 2000; Sterba, 2013).

Additionally, it is now more feasible for developmental psychopathologists to conduct secondary data analyses of large-scale, and often publicly available, *complex probability samples* involving clustering, stratification, and known but unequal probabilities of selection (e.g., the National Comorbidity Survey). The use of such probability samples has long been recommended by developmental epidemiologists (e.g., Costello & Angold, 2006), and recent statistical developments allow for their complex design features to be accommodated in popular statistical models (Muthén & Satorra, 1995; Sterba, 2009; Wu & Kwok, 2012). New statistical developments in the area of integrative data analysis (IDA), involving pooling more than one sample in a single analysis (Curran, 2009), can help to alleviate persistent problems involving underpowered studies in the field. See Bauer and Hussong (2009) for an IDA application in the area of internalizing behavior. Finally, recent advances in statistical estimation involving nonnormal and categorical data in latent variable modeling frameworks (Bandalos, 2013; Wirth & Edwards, 2007) provide new possibilities for the analysis of symptom-level data using more complex models than were feasible even 10 years ago.

Summary

The increasing availability of repeated measures data and rapidly advancing statistical modeling techniques suitable for addressing longitudinal research questions present exciting opportunities for developmental psychopathologists. We began by identifying background conceptual and statistical issues involving the representation of *individual differences in psychopathological constructs* as continuous or discrete (using multiple symptom indicators at a single time point). This topic has received increased attention in DSM-V with respect to representing not only individual sysndromes but also relations among them (as higher-order dimensions and/or categories; Regier et al. 2013). Then, in the second section we discussed preconditions necessary for studying quantitative change in such constructs. In the third section we discussed alternative models (namely, RCGMs and LCGMs) for describing and predicting change; these models posit that *individual differences in change* are continuous or discrete (using repeated measures of a single construct). It was illustrated in the fourth section that, even when LCGMs and RCGMs give fundamentally different results regarding the description of change, they can provide convergent results regarding the prediction of change—which is often of ultimate interest to developmental psychopathologists. As such, the fourth section described new opportunities for investigating substantive convergence of published findings on prediction of individual change across studies using very different statistical modeling strategies. Finally, we concluded with modeling extension topics as well as several data collection and design considerations particularly relevant to developmental psychopathologists. Developmental psychopathologists are encouraged to seek models suited to emerging research questions and designs—while at the same time remaining familiar with the assumptions, limitations, and interconnections among new and existing models.

References

Aiken, L. S., & West, S. G. (1991). *Multiple regression: Testing and interpreting interactions.* Newbury Park, CA: Sage.

American Psychiatric Association. (2000). *Diagnostic and statistical manual of mental disorder IV text revision.* Washington, DC: American Psychiatric Association.

American Psychiatric Association. (2013). *Diagnostic and statistical manual of mental disorders* (5th ed.). Washington, DC: American Psychiatric Association.

Angold, A., Costello, J., & Erkanli, A. (1999). Comorbidity. *Journal of Child Psychology and Psychiatry, 40,* 57–87.

Bandalos, D. (2013). Performance of the ML, MLMV, WLSMV, and WLS estimators under model misspecification, nonnormality, and coarse categorization. *Structural Equation Modeling* (in press).

Bauer, D. J., & Curran, P. J. (2003a). Distributional assumptions of growth mixture models: Implications for overextraction of latent trajectory classes. *Psychological Methods, 8,* 338–363.

Bauer, D. J., & Curran, P. J. (2003b). Over-extraction of latent trajectory classes: Much ado about nothing? Reply to Rindskopf (2003), Muthén (2003), and Cudeck and Henly (2003). *Psychological Methods, 8,* 384–393.

Bauer, D. J., & Hussong, A. M. (2009). Psychometric approaches for developing commensurate measures across independent studies: Traditional and new models. *Psychological Methods, 14,* 101–125.

Bauer, D. J., & Shanahan, M. J. (2007). Modeling complex interactions: Person-centered and variable-centered approaches. In T. D. Little, J. A. Bovaird, & N. A. Card (Eds.), *Modeling contextual effects in longitudinal studies* (pp. 255–284). Mahwah, NJ: Lawrence Erlbaum.

Bergman, L. R. (2001). A person approach in research on adolescence: Some methodological challenges. *Journal of Research on Adolescence, 16,* 28–53.

Bergman, L. R., & Magnusson, D. (1997). A person-oriented approach in research on developmental psychopathology. *Developmental Psychopathology, 9,* 291–319.

Bergman, L. R., & Trost, K. (2006). The person-oriented versus variable-oriented approach: Are they complementary, opposites, or exploring different worlds? *Merrill-Palmer Quarterly, 52,* 601–632.

Bergman, L., von Eye, A., & Magnusson, D. (2006). Person-oriented research strategies in developmental psychopathology. In D. Cicchetti & D. Cohen (Eds.), *Developmental psychopathology* (2nd ed., Vol. 1, pp. 850–888). Hoboken, NJ: Wiley.

Bollen, K. A. (1989). *Structural equations with latent variables.* New York: Wiley.

Bollen, K. A., & Curran, P. J. (2006). *Latent curve models: A structural equation approach.* Hoboken, NJ: Wiley.

Brown, T., & Barlow, D. (2005). Dimensional versus categorical classification of mental disorders in the fifth edition of the Diagnostic and statistical manual of mental disorders and beyond: Comment on the special section. *Journal of Abnormal Psychology, 114,* 551–556.

Butler, S. M., & Louis, T. A. (1992). Random effects models with non-parametric priors. *Statistics in Medicine, 11,* 1981–2000.

Cairns, R. B., Bergman, L. R., & Kagan, J. (1998). *Methods and models for studying the individual.* London: Sage.

Cicchetti, D., & Rogosch, F. A. (1996). Equifinality and multifinality in developmental psychopathology. *Development and Psychopathology, 8,* 597–600.

Collins, L., & Lanza, S. (2010). *Latent class and latent transition analysis.* Hoboken, NJ: Wiley.

Collins, L., & Wugalter, S. (1992). Latent class models for stage-sequential dynamic latent variables. *Multivariate Behavioral Research, 27,* 131–157.

Connell, A. M., Dishion, T. J., & Deater-Deckard, K. (2006). Variable- and person-centered approaches to the analysis of early adolescent substance use: Linking peer, family, and intervention effects with developmental trajectories. *Merrill-Palmer Quarterly, 52,* 421–448.

Conway, C., Hammen, C., & Brennan, P. (2012). A comparison of latent class, latent trait, and factor mixture models of DSM-IV borderline personality disorder criteria in a community setting: Implications for DSM-V. *Journal of Personality Disorders, 26,* 793–803.

Costello, E., & Angold, A. (2006). Developmental epidemiology. In D. Cicchetti & D. Cohen (Eds.), *Developmental psychopathology* (2nd ed., Vol. 1, pp. 41–75). Hoboken, NJ: Wiley.

Courtney, M., & Cusick, G. (2007). Crime during the transition to adulthood: How youth fare as they leave out-of-home care in Illinois, Iowa and Wisconsin. [Computer file].

Cudeck, R., & Henly, S. (2003). A realistic perspective on pattern representation in growth data: Comment on Bauer and Curran (2003). *Psychological Methods, 8,* 378–383.

Curran, P. J. (2009). The seemingly quixotic pursuit of a cumulative psychological science: Introduction to the special issue. *Psychological Methods, 14,* 77–80.

Curran, P., Bauer, D., & Willoughby, M. (2004). Testing and probing main effects and interactions in latent curve analysis. *Psychological Methods, 9,* 220–237.

Curran, P., & Willoughby, M. (2003). Implications of latent trajectory models for the study of developmental psychopathology. *Development and Psychopathology, 15,* 581–612.

Dodge, K., & Rutter, M. (2011). *Gene-environmental interactions in developmental psychopathology.* New York, NY: Guilford Press.

Dougherty, L., Klein, D., & Davila, J. (2004). A growth curve analysis of the course of dysthymic disorder: The effects of chronic stress and moderation by adverse parent–child relationships and family history. *Journal of Consulting and Clinical Psychology, 72,* 1012–1021.

Duncan, T., Duncan, S., & Stryker, L. (2006). *An introduction to latent variable growth curve modeling* (2nd ed.). Mahwah, NJ: Erlbaum.

Edwards, M. C., & Wirth, R. J. (2009). Measurement and the study of change. *Research in Human Development, 6,* 74–96.

Eggleston, E. P., Laub, J. H., & Sampson, R. J. (2004). Methodological sensitivities to latent class analysis of long-term criminal trajectories. *Journal of Quantitative Criminology, 20,* 1–26.

Farrell, A., Sullivan, T., Esposito, L., Meyer, A., & Valois, R. (2005). A latent growth curve analysis of the structure of aggression, drug use, and delinquent behaviors and their interrelations over time in urban and rural adolescents. *Journal of Research on Adolescence, 15,* 179–204.

Fitzmaurice, G., Laird, N., & Ware, J. (2011). *Applied longitudinal analysis* (2nd ed.). Hoboken, NJ: Wiley.

Fontaine, N., Carbonneau, R., Vitaro, F., Barker, E. D., & Tremblay, R. E. (2009). Research review: A critical review of studies on the developmental trajectories of antisocial behavior in females. *Journal of Child Psychology and Psychiatry, 50,* 363–385.

Gillespie, N., Neale, M., Legrand, L., Iacono, W., & McGve, M. (2011). Are the symptoms of cannabis use disorder best accounted for by dimensional, categorical, or factor mixture models? A comparison of male and female young adults. *Psychology of Addictive Behaviors, 26,* 68–77.

Gottlieb, G., & Halpern, C. T. (2002). A relational view of causality in normal and abnormal development. *Development and Psychopathology, 14,* 421–435.

Hallquist, M., & Pilkonis, P. (2012). Refining the phenotype of borderline personality disorder: Diagnostic criteria and beyond. *Personality disorders: Theory, research, and treatment, 3,* 228–246.

Hancock, G., Kuo, W.-L., & Lawrence, F. (2001). An illustration of second-order latent growth curve models. *Structural Equation Modeling, 8,* 470–489.

Haslam, N., Holland, E., & Kuppens, P. (2012). Categories versus dimensions in personality and psychopathology: A quantitative review of taxometric research. *Psychological Medicine, 42,* 903–920.

Hedeker, D., & Gibbons, R. D. (2006). *Longitudinal data analysis.* New York: Wiley.

Hill, K., White, H., Chung, I.-J., Hawkins, J., & Catalano, R. (2000). Early adult outcomes of adolescent binge drinking: Person- and variable-centered analyses of binge drinking trajectories. *Alcoholism, Clinical and Experimental Research, 24,* 892–901.

Helzer, J., van den Brink, W., & Guth, S. (2006). Should there be both categorical and dimensional criteria for the substance use disorders in DSM-V? *Addition, 101,* 17–22.

Hirsh-Pasek, K., & Burchinal, M. (2006). Mother and caregiver sensitivity over time: Predicting language and academic outcomes with variable- and person-centered approaches. *Merrill Palmer Quarterly, 52,* 449–485.

Horn, J. L. (2000). Comments on integrating person-centered and variable-centered research on problems associated with the use of alcohol. *Alcoholism, Clinical and Experimental Research, 24,* 924–930.

Jackson, K. M., & Sher, K. J. (2008). Comparison of longitudinal phenotypes based on alternate heavy drinking cut scores: A systematic comparison of trajectory approaches III. *Psychology of Addictive Behaviors, 22,* 198–209.

Knapp, P., & Jensen, P. S. (2006). Recommendations for DSM-V. In P. S. Jensen, P. Knapp, & D. Mrazek (Eds.), *Toward a new diagnostic system for child psychopathology: Moving beyond the DSM* (pp. 162–182). New York: Guilford Press.

Kobor, A., Takacs, A., Urban, R., & Csepe, V. (2012). The latent classes of subclinical ADHD symptoms:

Convergences of multiple informant reports. *Research in Developmental Disabilities, 33,* 1677–1689.

Kraemer, H. C., Shrout, P. E., & Rubio-Stipec, M. (2007). Developing the diagnostic and statistical manual V: What will "statistical" mean in DSM-V? *Social Psychiatry and Psychiatric Epidemiology, 42,* 259–267.

Krueger, R., Markon, K., Patrick, C., & Iacono, W. (2005). Externalizing psychopathology in adulthood: A dimensional-spectrum conceptualization and its implications for DSM-V. *Journal of Abnormal Psychology, 114,* 537–550.

Laursen, B., & Hoff, E. (2006). Person-centered and variable-centered approaches to longitudinal data. *Merrill-Palmer Quarterly, 52,* 377–389.

Lenzenweger, M., Johnson, M., & Willett, J. (2004). Individual growth curve analysis illuminates stability and change in personality disorder features. *Archives of General Psychiatry, 61,* 1015–1024.

Lilienfeld, S., Waldman, I., & Israel, A. (1994). A critical examination of the use of the term and concept of comorbidity in psychopathology research. *Clinical Psychology: Science and Practice, 1,* 71–83.

Lindquist, M. (2008). The statistical analysis of fMRI data. *Statistical Science, 23,* 439–464.

Loeber, R., Keenan, K., & Zhang, Q. (1997). Boys' experimentation and persistence in developmental pathways toward serious delinquency. *Journal of Child and Family Studies, 6,* 321–357.

Lubke, G. (2012). Old issues in a new jacket: Power and validation in the context of mixture modeling. *Measurement, 10,* 212–216.

Lubke, G., Muthén, B., Moilanen, I., McGovgh, J., Loo, S., Swanson, J. et al. (2007). Subtypes versus severity differences in attention-deficit/hyperactivity disorder in the Northern Finnish Birth Cohort. *American Academy of Child and Adolescent Psychiatry, 46,* 1584–1593.

Lubke, G., & Neale, M. (2006). Distinguishing between latent classes and continuous factors: Resolution by maximum likelihood? *Multivariate Behavioral Research, 41,* 499–532.

Lubke, G., & Neale, M. (2008). Distinguishing between latent classes and continuous factors with categorical outcomes: Class invariance of parameters of factor mixture models. *Multivariate Behavioral Research, 43,* 592–620.

Lubke, G., & Tueller, S. (2010). Latent class detection and class assignment: A comparison of the MAXEIG taxometric procedure and factor mixture modeling approaches. *Structural Equation Modeling, 17,* 605–628.

MacCallum, R. C., Kim, C., Malarkey, W. B., & Kiecolt-Glaser, J. K. (1997). Studying multivariate change using multilevel models and latent curve models. *Multivariate Behavioral Research, 32,* 215–253.

MacCallum, R., Zhang, S., Preacher, K., & Rucker, D. (2002). On the practice of dichotomization of quantitative variables. *Psychological Methods, 7,* 19–40.

Magnusson, D. (1985). Implications of an interactional paradigm for research on human development. *International Journal of Behavioral Development, 8,* 115–137.

Magnussan, D. (1998). The logic and implications of a person-oriented approach. In R. Cairns, L. Bergman & J. Kagan (Eds.), Methods and models for studying the individual. London, Sage.

Markon, K., Chmielewski, M., & Miller, C. (2011). The reliability and validity of discrete and continuous measures of psychopathology: A quantitative review. *Psychological Bulletin, 137,* 856–879.

Maughan, B. (2005). Developmental trajectory modeling: A view from developmental psychopathology. *Annals of the American Academy of Political and Social Science, 602,* 118–130.

Mehta, P. D., & West, S. G. (2000). Putting the individual back into individual growth curves. *Psychological Methods, 5,* 23–43.

Moffitt, T. (2006). Life-course persistent versus adolescent-limited antisocial behavior. In D. Cicchetti & D. Cohen (Eds.), *Developmental psychopathology* (Vol. 3). New York: Wiley.

Moffitt, T. E. (2008). A review of research on the taxonomy of life-course persistent versus adolescence-limited antisocial behavior. In F. T. Cullen, J. P. Wright, & K. R. Blevins (Eds.), *Taking stock–The status of criminological theory: Advances in criminological theory* (Vol. 15). New Brunswick, NJ: Transaction Publishers.

Muthén, B. (2001). Latent variable mixture modeling. In G. A. Marcoulides & R. E. Schumacker (Eds.), *New developments and techniques in structural equation modeling* (pp. 1–33). Mahwah, NJ: Lawrence Erlbaum.

Muthén, B. (2004). Latent variable analysis: Growth mixture modeling and related techniques for longitudinal data. In D. Kaplan (Ed.), *Handbook of quantitative methodology for the social sciences* (pp. 345–368). Newbury Park, CA: Sage.

Muthén, B. O. (2006). Should substance use disorders be considered as categorical or dimensional? *Addiction, 101,* 6–16.

Muthén, B., & Asparouhov, T. (2013). *BSEM measurement invariance analysis.* Retrieved from http://www.statmodel.com

Muthén, B., & Muthén, L. (2000). Integrating person-centered and variable-centered analyses: Growth mixture modeling with latent trajectory classes. *Alcoholism, Clinical and Experimental Research, 24,* 882–891.

Muthén, B. O., & Satorra, A. (1995). Complex sample data in structural equation modeling. *Sociological Methodology, 25,* 267–316.

Muthén, B., & Shedden, K. (1999). Finite mixture modeling with mixture outcomes using the EM algorithm. *Biometrics, 55,* 463–469.

Nagin, D. S. (1999). Analyzing developmental trajectories: A semi-parametric, group-based approach. *Psychological Methods, 4,* 139–157.

Nagin, D. S. (2005). *Group-based modeling of development.* Cambridge: Harvard University Press.

Nagin, D. S., & Odgers, C. (2010). Group-based trajectory modeling in clinical research. *Annual Reviews of Clinical Psychology, 6*, 109–138.

Nagin, D. S., & Tremblay, R. E. (2001). Analyzing developmental trajectories of distinct but related behaviors: A group-based method. *Psychological Methods, 6*, 18–34.

Nagin, D. S., & Tremblay, R. E. (2005a). Developmental trajectory groups: Fact or a useful statistical fiction? *Criminology, 43*, 873–904.

Nagin, D. S., & Tremblay, R. E. (2005b). From seduction to passion: A response to Sampson and Laub. *Criminology, 43*, 915–918.

Nandi, A., Beard, J., & Galea, S. (2009). Epidemiologic heterogeneity of common mood and anxiety disorders over the lifecourse in the general population: A systematic review. *BMC Psychiatry, 9*, 31.

O'brien, L., & Fitzmaurice, G. (2005). Regression models for the analysis of longitudinal Gaussian data from multiple sources. *Statistics in Medicine, 24*, 1725–1744.

Pastor, D., Barron, K., Miller, B., & Davis, S. (2007). A latent profile analysis of college students' achievement goal orientation. *Contemporary Educational Psychology, 32*, 8–47.

Patterson, G. (1993). Orderly change in a stable world: The antisocial trait as a chimera. *Journal of Consulting and Clinical Psychology, 61*, 911–919.

Petersen, I., Bates, J., Goodnight, J., Dodge, K., Lansford, J., Pettit, G., et al. (2012). Interaction between serotonin transporter polymorphism (5-HTTLPR) and stressful life events in adolescents' trajectories of anxious/depressed symptoms. *Developmental Psychology, 48*, 1463–1475.

Pickles, A., & Hill, J. (2006). Developmental pathways. In D. Cicchetti & D. Cohen (Eds.), *Developmental psychopathology* (2nd ed., Vol. 1, pp. 211–243). Hoboken, NJ: Wiley.

Pine, D., Costello, J., Dahl, R., James, R., Leckman, J., Leibenluft, E., et al. (2011). Increasing the developmental focus in DSM-V: Broad issues and specific potential applications in anxiety. In D. Rogier, W. Narrow, E. Kuhl, & D. Kumpfer (Eds.), *The conceptual evolution of DSM-5* (pp. 305–321). Washington, DC: American Psychiatric Publishing.

Raudenbush, S. W. (2001). Comparing-personal trajectories and drawing causal inferences from longitudinal data. *Annual Review of Psychology, 52*, 501–525.

Raudenbush, S. W. (2005). How do we study "what happens next?". *Annals of the American Academy of Political and Social Science, 602*, 131–144.

Regier, D., Kuhl, E., & Kupfer, D. (2013). The DSM-5: Classification and cnteria changes. *World Psychiatry, 12*, 92–98.

Reinecke, J. (2006). Longitudinal analysis of adolescents' deviant and delinquent behavior: Applications of latent class growth curves and growth mixture models. *Methodology, 2*, 100–112.

Romens, S., Abramson, L., & Alloy, L. B. (2009). High and low cognitive risk for depression: Stability from late adolescence to early adulthood. *Cognitive Therapy and Research, 33*, 480–498.

Rudolph, K., Troop-Gordon, W., Hessel, E., & Schmidt, J. (2011). A latent growth curve analysis of early and increasing peer victimization as predictors of mental health across elementary school. *Journal of Clinical Child & Adolescent Psychology, 40*, 111–122.

Rutter, M. (2011). Research review: Child psychiatric diagnosis and classification: Concepts, findings, challenges and potential. *Journal of Child Psychology and Psychiatry, 52*, 647–660.

Sampson, R. J., & Laub, J. H. (2005). Seductions of method: Rejoinder to Nagin and Tremblay's "Developmental Trajectory Groups: Fact or Fiction?". *Criminology, 43*, 905–913.

Schmitt, J., Mehta, P., Aggen, S., Kubarych, T., & Neale, M. (2006). Semi-nonparametric methods for detecting latent non-normality: A fusion of latent trait and ordered latent class modeling. *Multivariate Behavioral Research, 47*, 427–443.

Segawa, E., Ngwe, J. E., Li, Y., Flay, B., & Aban Aya Coinvestigators. (2005). Evaluation of the effects of the Aban Aya Youth Project in reducing violence among African American adolescent males using latent class growth mixture modeling techniques. *Evaluation Review, 29*, 128–148.

Shaw, B., & Liang, J. (2012). Growth models with multilevel regression. In J. Newsom, R. Jones, & S. Hofer (Eds.), *Longitudinal data analysis: A practical guide for researchers in aging, health, and social sciences* (pp. 217–242). New York: Routledge.

Sherbourne, C., & Stewart, A. (1991). The MOS social support survey. *Social Science & Medicine, 32*(6), 705–714.

Singer, J., & Willett, J. (2003). *Applied longitudinal data analysis: Modeling change and event occurrence.* New York: Oxford University Press.

Skardhamar, T. (2010). Distinguishing facts and artifacts in group-based modeling. *Criminology, 48*, 295–320.

Sterba, S. K. (2009). Alternative model-based and design-based frameworks for inference from samples to populations: From polarization to integration. *Multivariate Behavioral Research, 44*, 711–740.

Sterba, S. K. (2013). Fitting nonlinear latent growth models with individually-varying time points. *Structural Equation Modeling* (in press).

Sterba, S. K., Baldasaro, R. E., & Bauer, D. J. (2012). Factors affecting the adequacy and preferability of semiparametric groups-based approximations of continuous growth trajectories. *Multivariate Behavioral Research, 40*, 590–634.

Sterba, S. K., & Bauer, D. J. (2010a). Statistically evaluating person-oriented principles revisited: Reply to Molenaar (2010), von Eye (2010), Ialongo (2010) and Mun, Bates and Vaschillo (2010). *Development and Psychopathology, 22*, 287–294.

Sterba, S. K., & Bauer, D. J. (2010b). Matching method with theory in person-oriented developmental psychopathology research. *Development and Psychopathology, 22*, 239–254.

Sterba, S. K., & Bauer, D. J. (2013). Predictions of individual change recovered with latent class or random coefficient growth models. *Structural Equation Modeling* (in press).

Sterba, S. K., Copeland, W., Egger, H., Costello, J., Erkanli, A., & Angold, A. (2010). Longitudinal dimensionality of adolescent psychopathology: Testing the differentiation hypothesis. *Journal of Child Psychology and Psychiatry, 51*, 871–884.

Sterba, S. K., Egger, H. L., & Angold, A. (2007). Diagnostic specificity and non-specificity in the dimensions of preschool psychopathology. *Journal of Child Psychology and Psychiatry, 48*, 1005–1013.

Strickland, J., Keller, J., Lavigne, J., Gouze, K., Hopkins, J., & LeBailly, S. (2011). The structure of psychopathology in a community sample of preschoolers. *Journal of Abnormal Child Psychology, 39*, 601–610.

Tisak, J., & Meredith, W. (1990). Longitudinal factor analysis. In A. von Eye (Ed.), *Statistical methods in longitudinal research* (Vol. 1, pp. 125–149). Boston, MA: Academic.

Torppa, M., Poikkeus, A., Laakso, M., Eklund, K., & Lyytinen, H. (2006). Predicting delayed letter knowledge development and its relation to grade 1 reading achievement among children with and without familial risk for dyslexia. *Developmental Psychology, 42*, 1128–1142.

Trull, T., & Durrett, C. (2005). Categorical and dimensional models of personality disorder. *Annual Review of Clinical Psychology, 1*, 355–380.

van den Oord, E., Pickles, A., & Waldman, I. D. (2003). Normal variation and abnormality: An empirical study of the liability distributions underlying depression and delinquency. *Journal of Child Psychology and Psychiatry, 44*, 180–192.

van Dulmen, M., Goncy, E., Vest, A., Flannery, D. (2009). Group-based trajectory modeling of externalizing behavior problems from childhood through adulthood: Exploring discrepancies in the empirical findings. In J. Savage (Ed.), *The development of persistent criminology*. Oxford Scholarship Online Monographs

von Eye, A., & Bergman, L. R. (2003). Research strategies in developmental psychopathology: Dimensional identity and the person-oriented approach. *Development and Psychopathology, 15*, 553–580.

von Soest, T., & Hagtvet, K. (2011). Mediation analysis in a latent growth curve modeling framework. *Structural Equation Modeling, 18*, 289–314.

Waller, N., & Meehl, P. (1998). *Multivariate taxometric procedures: Distinguishing types from continua.* Thousand Oaks, CA: Sage.

Walls, T., & Schafer, J. (2008). *Models for intensive longitudinal data.* New York: Oxford University Press.

Walton, K., Ormel, J., & Krueger, R. (2011). The dimensional nature of externalizing behaviors in adolescence: Evidence from a direct comparison of categorical, dimensional, and hybrid models. *Journal of Abnormal Child Psychology, 39*, 553–561.

Widiger, T., & Samuel, D. (2005). Diagnostic categories or dimensions? A question for the diagnostic and statistical manual of mental disorders–Fifth edition. *Journal of Abnormal Psychology, 114*, 494–504.

Wirth, R. J. (2008). *The effects of measurement non-invariance on parameter estimation in latent growth models.* Unpublished dissertation, University of North Carolina at Chapel Hill.

Wirth, R. J., & Edwards, M. E. (2007). Item factor analysis: Current approaches and future directions. *Psychological Methods, 12*, 58–79.

Witkiewitz, K., King, K., McMahon, R., Wu, J., Luk, J., Bierman, K., et al. (2013). Evidence for a multidimensional latent structural model of externalizing disorders. *Journal of Abnormal Child Psychology, 41*, 223–237.

Wu, J., & Kwok, O. (2012). Using SEM to analyze complex survey data: A comparison between design-based single-level and model-based multilevel approaches. *Structural Equation Modeling, 19*, 16–35.

Zachar, P. (2000). Psychiatric disorders are not natural kinds. *Philosophy, Psychiatry, Psychology, 7*, 167–182.

Resilience and Positive Psychology

7

Suniya S. Luthar, Emily L. Lyman,
and Elizabeth J. Crossman

Since its introduction to the scientific literature in the mid-1990s, developmental science has seen incremental refinements in research on resilience, which is a process or phenomenon reflecting positive child adjustment despite conditions of risk. In this chapter, we describe accumulated evidence on this construct in the field of developmental psychopathology and appraise critical directions for future work. We begin by briefly describing the history of work in this area through contemporary times, defining core constructs, and summarizing major findings on factors associated with resilience. In the second half of the chapter, we examine commonalities and differences between the resilience framework and a related, relatively new area of scientific inquiry: positive psychology. Our objective is to elucidate

ways in which progress in each of these areas might most usefully inform efforts in the other, collectively maximizing the promotion of well-being among individuals, families, and society.

Historical Overview of Childhood Resilience Research

The roots of resilience research can be traced back to pioneering research with children of schizophrenics during the 1960s and 1970s. Garmezy (1974), along with Anthony (1974) and Rutter (1979), found that among these children at high risk for psychopathology was a subset of children who had surprisingly healthy patterns. Their scientific interest in the positive outcomes of these children reflected a notable departure from the symptom-based medical models of the time.

Expanding the research on resilience beyond children of mentally ill parents, Murphy and Moriarty (1976) examined vulnerability and coping patterns in children exposed to naturally occurring stressors such as deaths or injuries in the family. Shortly after, Emmy Werner published the first of many articles on the birth cohort from 1954 from the Hawaiian island of Kauai (Werner & Smith, 1982, 1992, 2001). Werner observed a number of protective factors that distinguished well-functioning at-risk youth from those faring more poorly, including strong, supportive ties with the family, informal support systems outside the home, and dispositional attributes such as sociability.

S.S. Luthar, Ph.D. (✉)
Department of Psychology, Arizona State University, 900S. McAllister Rd. Tempe, AZ 85287-1104, USA
e-mail: Suniya.Luthar@asu.edu

E.L. Lyman, M.A.
Department of Counseling and Clinical Psychology, Teachers College, Columbia University,
New York, NY 10027, USA

E.J. Crossman, M.A.
Department of Human Development,
Teachers College, Columbia University, New York, NY 10027, USA

M. Lewis and K.D. Rudolph (eds.), *Handbook of Developmental Psychopathology*,
DOI 10.1007/978-1-4614-9608-3_7, © Springer Science+Business Media New York 2014

The 1980s and early 1990s brought several changes in conceptual approaches to studying resilience, two of which were particularly salient. The first concerned perspectives on the locus of resilience. In early studies in this area, the effort had been to identify personal qualities of resilient children, such as autonomy or belief in oneself. As work in the area evolved, however, researchers acknowledged that resilient adaptation often may derive from factors external to the child. Thus, three sets of factors came to be commonly cited as central to the development of resilience: attributes of the children themselves, aspects of their families, and characteristics of their wider social environments (Garmezy & Masten, 1986; Rutter, 1987; Werner & Smith, 1982).

The second change involved conceptions of resilience as potentially fluctuating over time rather than fixed. In some early writings, those who did well despite multiple risks were labeled "invulnerable" (Anthony, 1974). Recognizing that this term implied that risk evasion was absolute and unchanging, researchers gradually began to use the more qualified term "resilience" instead. Implicit in this change of terminology was the recognition that positive adaptation despite adversity is never permanent; rather, it is a developmental progression with new vulnerabilities and strengths emerging with changing life circumstances (Garmezy & Masten, 1986; Werner & Smith, 1992).

Another critical qualifier rested in the recognition that resilience is never an across-the-board phenomenon, but can be, and often is, domain specific. Much as children in general do not manifest uniformly positive or negative adaptation across different areas of adjustment, researchers cautioned that at-risk children too can display remarkable strengths in some areas while showing notable deficits in others (Luthar, Doernberger, & Zigler, 1993).

Most importantly, children under stress could seem resilient in terms of their behaviors while still struggling with inner distress in the form of problems, such as depression and anxiety (Farber & Egeland, 1987; Luthar, 1991). Recognizing the heterogeneity in adjustment levels across domains, scientists now tend to use more circumspect terms that specify domains in which resilience is manifest, referring, for example, to academic resilience (Obradović et al., 2009), emotional resilience (Jain, Buka, Subramanian, & Molnar, 2012), or external (behavioral) resilience (Yates & Grey, 2012).

Research on Resilience: Defining Critical Constructs

As noted earlier, resilience is defined as a phenomenon or process reflecting relatively positive adaptation despite experiences of significant adversity or trauma. Because resilience is a superordinate construct subsuming two distinct dimensions—significant *adversity* and *positive adaptation*—it is never directly measured, but rather is indirectly inferred based on evidence of the two subsumed constructs.

Adversity

In developmental psychopathology research on resilience, risk or adversity is defined in terms of statistical probabilities: A high-risk condition is one that carries high odds for measured maladjustment in critical domains (Luthar, 2006; Masten, 2001). Exposure to community violence or to maternal depression, for example, constitutes high risk given that children experiencing each of these factors reflect significantly greater maladjustment than those who do not. Aside from discrete risk dimensions such as community violence or parent psychopathology, researchers have also examined composites of multiple risk indices, such as parents' low income and education, histories of mental illness, and disorganization in neighborhoods. Seminal research by Rutter (1979) demonstrated that when risks such as these coexist (as they often do, in the real world), effects tend to be synergistic, with child outcomes being far poorer than when any of these risks exists in isolation.

Positive Adaptation

The second component in the construct of resilience is positive adjustment: outcomes that are substantially better than what would be expected, given exposure to a specific identified risk. In many studies of resilience across diverse risk circumstances, this concept has been defined in terms of behaviorally manifested social competence or success at meeting stage-salient developmental tasks (Luthar, Cicchetti, & Becker, 2000; Masten & Tellegen, 2012). Among young children, for example, competence is often operationally defined in terms of manifest secure attachment with caregivers, and among older children, in terms of aspects of school-based functioning.

In addition to being developmentally appropriate, indicators used to define "positive adaptation" must also be conceptually of high relevance to the risk examined in terms of both domains assessed and stringency of criteria used (Luthar, 2006; Vanderbilt-Adriance & Shaw, 2008). When communities carry many risks for antisocial problems, for example, it makes sense to assess the degree to which children are able to maintain socially conforming behaviors (Jain et al., 2012), whereas among children of depressed parents, the absence of depressive diagnoses would be of special significance (Beardslee, Gladstone, & O'Connor, 2012). With regard to stringency of criteria, similarly, decisions must depend on the seriousness of the risks under consideration. In studying children facing major traumas, it is entirely appropriate to define risk evasion simply in terms of the absence of serious psychopathology rather than superiority or excellence in everyday adaptation (Luthar et al., 2000; Rutter, 2012).

Whereas approaches to measuring risk can involve one negative circumstance, competence must necessarily be defined across multiple spheres, for overly narrow definitions can convey a misleading picture of success in the face of adversity [for a more in-depth discussion, see Luthar (2006)]. Furthermore, it should be noted that in some situations, competence is most appropriately operationalized in terms of better than expected functioning of families or communities, rather than the children themselves. To illustrate, toddlers are still too young to reliably be judged as manifesting resilience because their functioning is largely regulated by others; thus, it is more logical to operationalize positive adjustment in terms of the mother–child dyad or

family unit. In a similar vein, the label resilience can sometimes be most appropriate for communities of well-functioning at-risk youth. Research on neighborhoods, for example, has demonstrated that some low-income urban neighborhoods reflect far higher levels of cohesiveness, organization, and social efficacy than others (Jain et al., 2012; Leventhal & Brooks-Gunn, 2000), with the potential, therefore, to serve as important buffers against negative socializing influences.

As positive adaptation does not necessarily occur as part of a continuous trajectory, an important area of resilience research is concerned with those who "bounce back" from earlier dysfunction (Luthar & Brown, 2007; Masten, 2001; Rutter, 2012). Long-term prospective studies have been invaluable in identifying critical turning points not only in childhood but also across the life span, illuminating instances where apparently negative adjustment trajectories were transformed into positive, healthy ones (Hauser, Allen, & Golden, 2006; Sampson & Laub, 1993; Vaillant, 2012).

As we define terms, it is important to distinguish resilience from two related—and, in error, often conflated—constructs: competence and ego resiliency. Competence and resilience may be described as closely related subconstructs as both represent positive adaptation, but there are four major differences (Luthar, 2006; Yates & Masten, 2004). First, resilience, but not competence, presupposes risk. Second, resilience encompasses both negative and positive adjustment indices (absence of disorder and presence of health), and competence chiefly reflects the latter. Third, resilient outcomes are defined in terms of emotional and behavioral indices, whereas competence usually involves only manifest, observable behaviors. Finally, resilience is a superordinate construct that subsumes aspects of competence (along with high levels of risk).

A second overlapping construct—and one with which resilience is frequently confused (Luthar et al., 2000)—is *ego resiliency*, a construct developed by Block and Block (1980) that refers to a personal trait reflecting general resourcefulness, sturdiness of character, and flexibility in response to environmental circumstances. Commonalities with resilience are that both involve strengths. Differences are that (a) only resilience presupposes conditions of risk and (b) resilience is a phenomenon, not a personality trait. Finally, just as competence is subsumed within resilience, ego resiliency has been examined as a potential predictor of resilient adaptation, that is, as a trait that could protect individuals against stressful experiences (Cicchetti & Rogosch, 1997; Eisenberg et al., 2010).

In developmental psychopathology research, it is critical that scientists proactively guard against any suggestions that resilience is essentially a personal trait, as this can foster perspectives that blame the victim (Luthar & Brown, 2007; Yates & Masten, 2004). Toward this end, several precautions have been noted for future studies (Luthar et al., 2000; Rutter, 2012). Most importantly, all reports should include clear definitions of resilience, unequivocally stating that it refers to a process or phenomenon and *not* a trait. Additionally, it is best to avoid using the term *resiliency*, which carries the connotation of a personality characteristic even more so than does *resilience*. Furthermore, it is prudent to avoid using the term resilient as an adjective for individuals and apply it instead to profiles or trajectories because phrases such as "resilient adaptation" carry no suggestion of who (the child or others) is responsible for manifest risk evasion.

Vulnerability and Protective Processes

The central objective of resilience researchers is to identify *vulnerability* and *protective factors* that might *modify* the negative effects of adverse life circumstances, and then to identify *mechanisms* or *processes* that might underlie associations found. Vulnerability factors or markers encompass those indices that exacerbate the ill effects of the adverse condition (e.g., poverty) on child outcomes, such as alienation from parents or a negative school climate. Promotive or protective factors are those that modify the effects of risk in a positive direction. Examples include support from caregivers and peers and strong social-emotional skills.

In the resilience literature, there have been two major approaches to identifying protective or vulnerability factors (or risk modifiers): variable-based and person-based statistical analyses.

Variable-based analyses such as multivariate regressions allow researchers to look at continuous scales of (a) adversity and (b) risk modifiers in relation to outcomes, examining how the latter are directly related (as main effects), and in interaction effects with the former. One of the first efforts to use this variable-based approach was the groundbreaking paper by Garmezy, Masten, and Tellegen (1984), demonstrating that high IQ was protective: Increases in life stress seemed to affect intelligent children far less than their low IQ peers. Person-based analyses in resilience research, on the other hand, involve comparisons between a group of children who are categorized according to their outcome and risk profiles. For example, comparisons of two groups of at-risk youth, manifesting high and low competence respectively, can illuminate critical factors that confer protection against adversity.

In both variable- and person-based analyses, a hallmark of the current generation of resilience research is attention to process: If studies are truly to be informative to interventions, they must move beyond simply identifying variables linked with competence toward understanding the specific underlying mechanisms (Luthar, 2006; Masten & Cicchetti, 2012). This need to unravel underlying processes applies to risk, vulnerability, and protective factors at multiple levels. With regard to risk transmission, for example, maternal depression can affect children through various environmental processes including negative family interactions and routines, and child behavioral and emotional problems (Valdez, Mills, Barrueco, Leis, & Riley, 2011). Similarly, protective factors such as high-quality caregiver–child relationships could benefit a child through multiple pathways including feelings of being supported, a sense of being cherished as an individual, and a strong set of personal values (Werner, 2012).

What Promotes or Mitigates Resilient Adaptation? Evidence on Salient Risk Modifiers

The science of resilience is, fundamentally, applied in nature with the central goal of informing efficacious interventions (Garmezy &

Masten, 1986; Luthar, 2006); accordingly, in reviewing evidence on risk modifiers, it makes sense to prioritize domains in terms of overall likelihood of yielding benefits in interventions (Luthar & Brown, 2007). In other words, it is most useful to focus primarily on risk modifiers that are (a) the most *influential*, with effects that are relatively enduring or robust, and (b) relatively *modifiable* (as are aspects of caregivers' functioning, as opposed to intrinsic characteristics, such as IQ or genetic vulnerability).

With this prioritization in mind, we present, in sequence, findings on risk modifiers within the domains of the family—the most proximal and the most enduring of children's environments—followed by the community, which can affect children directly, as well as indirectly through their parents. Children's own characteristics are presented third, recognizing that many of these risk modifiers can and often do promote resilient adaptation, but they are often, themselves, malleable to potent forces in the proximal and distal environments (cf. Luthar, 2006).

Family Processes

Of the many factors that affect the trajectories of at-risk individuals, among the most powerful is maltreatment by primary caregivers. Maltreatment co-occurs with many high-risk circumstances including parent mental illnesses, parental conflict, community violence, and poverty (Mersky, Berger, Reynolds, & Gromoske, 2009; Rogosch, Dackis, & Cicchetti, 2011), thus serving as a widespread vulnerability factor. Maltreated children show deficits spanning multiple domains including interpersonal relationships, emotional regulation, cognitive processing, and even linguistic development (Cicchetti, 2002). This degree of dysfunction is not surprising, given that maltreatment connotes serious disturbances in the most proximal level of the child's ecology, with the caregiving environment failing to provide typical experiences essential for normal development (Cicchetti, 2002).

Despite the inimical effects of maltreatment, profiles of adjustment are not homogeneous. Pronounced deficits are most likely to be associated with greater severity and chronicity of maltreatment, as well as early age of onset (Cicchetti & Rogosch, 1997; Kim, Cicchetti, Rogosch, & Manly, 2009). In terms of protective processes, positive relationships with peers and high school engagement can mitigate the deleterious effects of maltreatment (Afifi & MacMillan, 2011; Williams & Nelson-Gardell, 2012). At the same time, research has suggested that even when maltreated children function well at some critical periods in time, this successful adaptation tends to be unstable across development (Thompson & Tabone, 2010).

As maltreatment thwarts resilient adaptation, conversely, positive, supportive family relationships are vital in maintaining good adjustment in the face of adversities. The critical importance of family relationships is recurrently emphasized in reviews of the literature (e.g., Luthar & Brown, 2007; Masten, 2001; Shonkoff & Phillips, 2000; Vanderbilt-Adriance & Shaw, 2008), resonant with early reports that the presence of a close relationship with at least one parent figure constitutes a potent protective factor (Garmezy, 1974; Rutter, 1979; Werner & Smith, 1982). Furthermore, the protective potential of positive parenting is evident not only in early childhood but in later years as well, through adolescence and even emerging adulthood (Burt & Paysnick, 2012; Steinberg, 2001).

Although maternal nurturance is widely discussed as critical for positive child development, high-quality relationships with other family members can also significantly modify the effects of adversity. For example, studies have established the protective potential of strong attachment relationships with fathers and father figures (Coley, 2001; Martin, Ryan, & Brooks-Gunn, 2010). Older siblings may often serve as critical role models, with younger siblings mirroring their profiles of high behavioral competence (e.g., Brody, Kim, Murry, & Brown, 2004) and, conversely, emulating their negative behavior patterns involving delinquency and substance use (Stormshak, Comeau, & Shepard, 2004). Finally, support from extended kin can be important in protecting at-risk youth. Among children exposed to harsh maternal parenting, for example, high levels of grandmother involvement can reduce the risk of maladjustment in grandchildren (Barnett, Scaramella, Neppl, Ontai, & Conger, 2010).

Going beyond the general importance of strong attachments with parent figures, there are also contextually salient vulnerability and protective processes, or those that are important within particular family and cultural contexts. To illustrate, upper-middle class American youth, in general, are at considerably elevated risk for substance use, and perceived parental leniency on this front is a potent vulnerability factor for these teens' frequent use of alcohol, marijuana, and other substances (Luthar & Barkin, 2012). Among immigrant families, second-generation children's revocation of traditional family values and mores can be linked with elevated adjustment problems (García Coll & Marks, 2009). Among families affected by mental illnesses such as depression, unique protective processes include the child's understanding of the illness (including its potential causes), as well as the ability to maintain healthy psychological boundaries from the affected parent (Beardslee, 2002).

Recent years have seen an explosion of research on family genetic factors in adjustment and in particular, on G×E interactions (Grigorenko & Cicchetti, 2012; Kim-Cohen & Turkewitz, 2012); while clearly invaluable for basic science, these findings are unlikely to inform psychological interventions to foster resilience in the foreseeable future [for a detailed discussion, see Luthar and Brown (2007)]. Genetics research might suggest, for some, the potential to guide treatment as an understanding of biological pathways can inform pharmacotherapy. However, any such knowledge about "indicated pharmacotherapies" does not readily generalize to treating psychological problems (Luthar & Brown, 2007). In a recent review of relevant evidence, Dodge and Rutter (2011) concluded, explicitly, that the most direct practical implication of the G×E revolution belongs to the field of personalized medicine. Furthermore, the authors reaffirmed that any such personalized medicine is unlikely to reduce individual psychopathologies as (a) G×E interactions, even if replicated, tend to be very small, and (b) there is inevitably a plethora of other unmeasured risks generated by both genes and environments (Dodge & Rutter, 2011; Rutter, 2012).

Community Processes

As with maltreatment in the family, chronic exposure to violence in the community can have overwhelming deleterious effects that are difficult for other positive forces to override. Exposure to violence substantially exacerbates risks for a range of problems, encompassing internalizing symptoms such as anxiety, depression, and post-traumatic stress disorders (Herrenkohl, Sousa, Tajima, Herrenkohl, & Moylan, 2008; Walsh, 2007), as well as externalizing problems such as delinquent, antisocial behaviors (Aisenberg & Herrenkohl, 2008) and attenuated academic competence, social skills, and self-concept (Cedeno, Elias, Kelly, & Chu, 2010).

With regard to risk modifiers, support from parents can serve protective functions but, unfortunately, parents themselves are also highly vulnerable to the stresses of chronic community violence (Jain et al., 2012), experiencing high distress themselves and even, sometimes, displaying elevated maltreatment of children (Herrenkohl et al., 2008). Overall, the variability in children's responses to community violence is likely to be least pronounced if exposure is sporadic rather than chronic, and if it does not involve personally witnessing violent events or experiencing the loss of a friend or family member (Gorman-Smith & Tolan, 2003).

Whereas exposure to prolonged serious community violence is rarely overcome by other protective processes, there certainly are exosystemic forces that can attenuate the ill effects of other types of adversities. In particular, studies have documented the benefits of early exposure to high-quality childcare, where caregivers have positive personal characteristics and offer emotionally supportive caregiving (Maggi, Roberts, MacLennan, & D'Angiulli, 2011). In later years as well, supportive relationships with teachers in K-12 can be protective (Ebersöhn & Ferreira, 2011). To illustrate, when teachers identify the function of problem behaviors among at-risk youth and, in response, provide positive support strategies, there are significant benefits for adaptive behaviors (Stoiber & Gettinger, 2011).

Aside from teachers, relationships with informal mentors also can promote resilient adaptation

(Rhodes & Lowe, 2008). Examining the frequently stressful transition from elementary to middle school, Van Ryzin (2010) found that 40 % of the children named their advisor as a secondary attachment figure. Furthermore, those who did so reported greater engagement in middle school, and manifested greater gains in achievement and adjustment as compared to those who did not. With regard to mediators and moderators, mentoring effects tend to be mediated by improved family relations, while the duration and closeness of the relationship serve as significant moderators (DuBois, Portillo, Rhodes, Silverthorn, & Valentine, 2011).

Finally, positive relationships with peers can serve important ameliorative functions for at-risk children. Peer-assisted learning can result in significant increases in achievement (Neal, Neal, Atkins, Henry, & Frazier, 2011), and affiliation with peers who model responsible behavior (e.g., good students and good citizens) can mitigate, to some degree, the effects of violence exposure (Jain et al., 2012). At the same time, close friendships can confer vulnerability as well, particularly when they entail deviant behaviors. Youth who affiliate with deviant peers can engage in mutual "deviancy training" (Dishion, McCord, & Poulin, 1999), resulting in poor outcomes across multiple domains including conduct disturbances, substance use, and academic problems (Tiet, Huizinga, & Byrnes, 2010; Véronneau & Dishion, 2010).

Moving from the relatively proximal extrafamilial contexts of school, mentors, and peers to those more distal, aspects of the neighborhood may also play an important role in buffering risk for children. Particularly important are social organization processes in the neighborhood, which involve features such as high levels of cohesion, a sense of belonging to the community, supervision of youth by community adults, and high participation in local organizations (Rios, Aiken, & Zautra, 2012; Zimmerman & Brenner, 2010). Such social processes can help buffer the impact of structural characteristics of the community such as poverty or violence (Jain et al., 2012), by providing, for example, opportunities for structured and supervised extracurricular activities (Peck, Roeser, Zarrett, & Eccles, 2008).

In a similar vein, support gleaned from involvement in religious communities can be beneficial (Pargament & Cummings, 2010), with the buffering effects of religiosity on adolescent maladjustment often operating by increasing social resources and promoting prosocial behaviors (Sherman, Duarte, & Verdeli, 2011).

Individual Attributes

Intelligence is perhaps the most commonly mentioned personal asset in promoting resilient adaptation. Studies on diverse risk groups find that individuals with high IQs tend to fare better than others, with the underlying mechanisms potentially entailing superior problem-solving skills as well as a history of successes (e.g., at school or work) over time (Luthar, 2006; Masten, 2001). At the same time, there is much evidence that continuing adversities in the proximal environment can mitigate this personal asset. Young children exposed to chronic adversities such as domestic violence in the home or institutionalized care show significantly lower IQ scores than their counterparts who are not exposed to these risks (Koenen, Moffitt, Caspi, Taylor, & Purcell, 2003; Rutter, 1998; Sameroff & Rosenblum, 2006).

One might argue that the protective potential of high IQ would be more "fixed" later in development; although probably true, the evidence is not unequivocal, even at older ages. Among multiple samples of low-income adolescents (see Luthar, 2006), intelligence was not found to be protective; on the contrary, there were suggestions that bright youth may be more sensitive than others to negative environmental forces. Among adults, Fiedler (1995) reported that high-IQ people showed leadership success under conditions of low stress, but that when stress was high, IQ was inversely correlated with leadership success. Findings such as these have been viewed as suggesting that the manifest "benefits" of innate intelligence can vary substantially, depending on the potency and chronicity of risks in the proximal environment.

The previously described evidence on intelligence is paralleled by similar evidence on temperament, also shown to confer protection against stress, with benefits found in relation to diverse adjustment outcomes (e.g., Eisenberg et al., 2010; Murry, Bynum, Brody, Willert, & Stephens, 2001). Temperamental differences can be seen as early as 4 months of age and they show continuity over early childhood (e.g., Kagan, Snidman, & Arcus, 1998). At the same time, the manifestation of temperament can be modified by environmental features. As Rutter (2000) has underscored, scientists have long moved past the point of assuming that "constitutional" factors are unalterable; whereas some children may tend to be more impulsive or oppositional than others, their interactions with the world contribute to determining the behavioral conformity they display in everyday life.

Similar cautions apply to inferences about the positive personality traits. Shiner and Masten (2012) have demonstrated significant long-term beneficial effects for childhood conscientiousness, agreeableness, and openness, as well as low neuroticism, even after controlling for childhood adversity. Whereas these findings undoubtedly indicate that personal strengths can help individuals overcome the effects of childhood life stressors, it is important to note also that even among adults, positive personal attributes are typically maximized only in the scaffolding of supportive interpersonal contexts. Kashdan and Steger (2011) have presciently emphasized that across the life span, individuals can possess strengths without necessarily using them: Context is critical in maximizing their use. We discuss this issue in depth in the section that follows.

Resilience and Positive Psychology

In terms of central research questions and constructs, the scientific study of resilience has much in common with other disciplines including the long-standing fields of risk research and prevention science [for a more in-depth discussion, see Luthar (2006)]. In this chapter, we focus specifically on differences and similarities with the relatively new but burgeoning field of positive psychology, with an emphasis, specifically, on useful directions for future work in both areas.

As resilience research began over 60 years ago with a focus on strengths and not just disorder, the field of positive psychology, christened in the early 1990s, was established to address the negative bias and medicalization that suffused psychological research since the end of the Second World War (Peterson & Park, 2003). As its name suggests, positive psychology is the study of positive emotions (e.g., joy and hope), positive character (e.g., creativity and kindness), and positive institutions (e.g., family, communities, and the workplace; Seligman & Csikszentmihalyi, 2000). In the decade since its inception, positive psychology has witnessed impressive refinements in both theory and research, as exemplified most recently in a seminal edited volume designed to "take stock, and move forward" (Sheldon, Kashdan, & Steger, 2011).

Differences

At this stage in the ontogenesis of the two fields, there are some substantive differences between positive psychology and resilience research, among the most prominent of which is the consideration of life adversities. As noted before, studies of resilience presuppose exposure to extreme adversity, whereas positive psychology concerns all individuals, not just those who have experienced major risks [although there are now increasing inroads into studies in the context of adversity, such as those of stress-related growth (Park, 2010) and those showing that character strengths can protect against major illness (Peterson, Park, & Seligman, 2006)].

The second difference concerns the centrality of developmental issues, which are at the very core of resilience research (Luthar, 2006; Masten, 2001), not only during childhood and adolescence, but also across adulthood (Collishaw, Maughan, Goodman, & Pickles, 2004; Hauser et al., 2006; Sampson & Laub, 1993; Staudinger, Freund, Linden, & Maas, 1999; Vaillant, 2012). Positive psychology by contrast has been focused largely on adults, although there are now increasing calls for attention to developmental variations, critically examining whether findings on particular adult samples might generalize to children and to adults at different stages of the life span (see Oishi & Kurtz, 2011; Roberts, Brown, Johnson, & Reinke, 2002).

Third, studies of resilience, grounded firmly in the discipline of developmental psychopathology, adhere to a core, defining feature of this field: that studies of normal development aid our understanding of atypical processes and, conversely, studies of the atypical inform our understanding of normative development (Luthar, 2003; Yates & Masten, 2004). Thus far, in positive psychology, the tendency has been to "use the normal as a base from which to understand the abnormal, rather than *also* [emphasis added] using the abnormal to illuminate the normal" (Hames & Joiner, 2011, p. 314).

The fourth difference pertains to operationalization of positive outcomes, and in this regard, there are two distinctions. First, resilience researchers have considered both the presence of competent, healthy adjustment, as well as the evasion of psychopathology (when individuals are exposed to severe or chronic stressors; cf. Luthar & Brown, 2007; Rutter, 2012). In its early years, positive psychology was concerned only with positive aspects of adjustment and health promotion. Again, recent appraisals of the first decade of this science (Sheldon et al., 2011) have led to exhortations to consider negative dimensions as well, because some of these aspects can be beneficial. Anger, for example, mobilizes us to defend ourselves, and sadness is linked with critical and detail-focused thinking, which is important for certain kinds of problem solving (Oishi & Kurtz, 2011). More broadly, Ryff (1989) has noted that from a lifespan developmental perspective, psychological health results from active engagement of all that life has to offer—the positive, as well as the negative, just as Wong (2007) has argued, if positive psychology is to address the full potential of human beings, it must do so by addressing the challenges brought by life along with the successes.

The second difference in operationalizing positive outcomes concerns the parameters used to define healthy or optimal development. When studying children, resilience researchers have, tra-ditionally, emphasized overt behavioral success as judged by proximal others—adaptive behaviors as rated by teachers, friends, parents, or others. In positive psychology, by contrast, there do not seem to be efforts to ascertain *others'* opinions on whether the individual is doing well—as a good spouse or parent, for example, or as a colleague at work. In fact, even when there are constructs tapping into interpersonal themes, these largely involve the individual's own reports, with social acceptance defined in terms of individuals having positive attitudes toward others and social integration as individuals' feelings of being supported by their communities (Keyes & Lopez, 2002). Heavy reliance on self-reports can be a particularly salient source of bias in positive psychology, because many of the constructs studied are socially desirable and people tend to want to portray themselves favorably (Lambert, Fincham, Gwinn, & Ajayi, 2011). Thus, there is a pressing need for greater consideration of indicators not based in self-reports (Noftle, Schnitker, & Robins, 2011).

Conversely, there is an important lesson that those of us seeking to maximize childhood resilience could learn from positive psychology, and that is that we need to consider positive subjective experiences. Developmental studies commonly include assessments of children's feelings of depression, anxiety, or low self-worth, but we rarely ask youth about their own feelings of happiness or life satisfaction. In the future, it will be important for childhood resilience researchers to consider not only the degree to which young people conform to adults' expectations and evade distress but also the degree to which they themselves subjectively experience feelings of happiness, hope, and optimism.

Similarities

Despite these areas of difference, it should be emphasized that resilience research has many similarities to positive psychology. First, as both disciplines have matured, there have been ongoing critical appraisals of the scientific integrity of the corpus of work, examining issues of operational definitions, methodological approaches, and veridicality of conclusions (e.g., Lopez & Snyder, 2009; Luthar et al., 2000; Rutter, 1987, 2000; Sheldon et al., 2011; Synder & Lopez, 2002; Vanderbilt-Adriance & Shaw, 2008). In both cases, for example, there have been in-depth discussions about whether and why the field warrants a distinct identity as opposed to representing just a new term for other, long-established spheres of inquiry, such as competence (Luthar et al., 2000; Yates & Masten, 2004) or positive emotions (Oishi & Kurtz, 2011). Both fields have witnessed an emphasis on ensuring that research that is grounded in a set of strong organizing theory, with specific suggestions proffered in this regard (Lambert et al., 2011; Luthar et al., 2000; Sheldon et al., 2011; Vanderbilt-Adriance & Shaw, 2008).

In terms of central goals of research, Michael Rutter's seminal 1987 paper spawned concerted efforts among resilience researchers to understand the underlying processes or mechanisms via which a given promotive or vulnerability factor may operate, and we are now witnessing similar exhortations in positive psychology. For example, Oishi and Kurtz (2011) noted that random acts of kindness make people happier, but we need to disentangle the major underlying mechanisms, illuminating whether these feelings occur because people see themselves in a positive light, or because they build a sense of trust and social capital. As emphasized earlier, disentangling these mechanisms is particularly critical when designing interventions.

Another parallel is that both disciplines entail concerted attention to interlinked, mutually beneficial salutary constructs. Rutter (1987, p. 57, 316–331) described "chain" effects, wherein, for example, the quality of family relationships affects children's sense of self-worth and attachment security, which, in turn, promotes openness to other potentially supportive relationships. Resonant with this premise is Fredrickson's (1998, p. 300) "broaden and build" conceptualization, where positive emotions—of joy, engagement, meaning, and, perhaps most importantly, love—"serve to broaden an individual's momentary thought-action repertoire, which in turn has the effect of building that individual's physical, intellectual, and social resources."

Researchers in both fields have faced the complexities of defining "doing well," given that meaningful variations exist across domains of adjustment. Just as childhood resilience has long been recognized as being a non-unidimensional construct (Luthar et al., 1993), increasingly, vicissitudes in adjustment are noted in the positive psychology literature. To illustrate, McCrae (2011) has argued that people have different personal strengths, some of which can work against each other, wherein high levels of conscientiousness, for example, can run counter to personal growth. In broadly defining the life well lived, similarly, Little (2011) has cautioned that an individual's exuberant pursuit of personally meaningful life goals can create problems for family members.

In the field of resilience, we have long grappled with these complexities of varying profiles of competence, compelled, eventually, to confront the fact that choices must be made in prioritizing particular domains—and that such prioritization must be made on strong theoretical grounds (Luthar et al., 2000). As noted in the first half of this chapter, our operationalizations of doing well are always conceptually related, first, to the nature and severity of the particular risk experienced (e.g., emotional resilience among children of depressed parents, or behavioral resilience among youth at risk for conduct disorder). Currently, there is a plethora of constructs subsumed in the field of positive psychology, ranging from happiness [with various connotations; see Algoe, Fredrickson, and Chow (2011)] to meaning making, altruism, selflessness, gratitude, and wisdom. As the field moves forward, an important scientific task will be to derive, consensually, some prioritization or hierarchy of dimensions that are deemed most central to operationally defining whether a life has, indeed, been lived well (see Sheldon et al., 2011), as opposed to other dimensions that are potentially informative, but not cardinal.

At a substantive level, both fields are fundamentally applied in nature, seeking to make a difference. In both cases, an initial scientific interest in uncovering basic psychological processes has led to acknowledgements that the central goals are to benefit humanity (Csikszentmihalyi & Nakamura, 2011; Luthar & Brown, 2007; Sheldon et al., 2011; Yates & Masten, 2004). And with this applied focus in mind, scientists in both fields explicitly highlight the charge of proactively and responsibly disseminating our work. Acknowledging early and often well-deserved criticisms of research on resilience (and the inherent appeal of this notion to the lay public), Luthar and Cicchetti (2000) underscored the need for the highest possible standards of evidence and self-scrutiny in dissemination. In a similar vein, Kashdan and Steger (2011) cautioned against the rush of excitement to share new knowledge in positive psychology, noting that it is critical to obtain replications and seek alternative explanations, with the onus of responsibility doubled when research offers directions for interventions (see also Biswas-Diener, Kashdan, & King, 2009).

Perhaps most importantly, the core findings derived from accumulated work in both areas are strikingly similar. A review of 50 years of research on resilience—among children as well as adults—led to the simple conclusion that "Resilience rests, fundamentally, on relationships" (Luthar, 2006, p. 780). Strikingly resonant is Zautra's (2014) assertion, "Resilience is social, after all," and Peterson's (2006) "three-word summary of positive psychology: *Other people matter*" (p. 249). Reis and Aron (2008) noted that human love is part of a constellation of evolved regulatory mechanisms with enormous significance for positive adjustment, as Lambert et al. (2011) note the recurrent acknowledgement in the positive psychology literature that close relationships are essential to individuals' well-being (Diener & Oishi, 2005).

In terms of how our science can best benefit humanity, cognizance of the fundamental importance of relationships has led resilience researchers to emphasize attention to proximal contexts in any efforts to improve personal strengths. As long as individuals remain in interpersonal settings that are damaging to their psychological adjustment, any pull-out, short-term efforts to promote particular skills will have limited value (Luthar & Brown, 2007; Pianta & Walsh, 1998). Increasingly,

there is explicit emphasis on context within positive psychology interventions as well, as seen in Gillham, Brunwasser, and Freres (2008) school-based program to promote positive child attributes (e.g., empathy and self-control), while developing these skills within the teachers themselves. As the fields of resilience and positive psychology continue to delineate key principles for future interventions, we hope that there will be a steadfast attention, in both cases, to individuals' contexts. Kashdan and Steger's (2011, p. 13) words of caution must be heeded by scientists in both fields, equally: "If positive psychology is going to progress at the scientific and applied level, context can no longer be underappreciated, ignored, and untreated" (Kashdan & Steger, 2011, p. 13).

Future Directions

In concluding, we present two themes that we believe merit much greater attention by positive psychologists and resilience researchers alike, in formulating future theories, research, and practice implications. The first is despite our shared emphasis on the positive and salutary, we must explicitly recognize that "bad is stronger than good" (Baumeister, Bratslavsky, Findenauer, & Vohs, 2001, p. 323): People are generally much more deeply affected by negative feedback such as rejection than by positive ones such as praise. For positive psychologists, this would imply the need for explicit recognition that if individuals are to flourish, experiences of positive emotions (e.g., joy or hope) must collectively outnumber experiences of negative ones (such as fear, sadness, or guilt)—by a ratio as high as three to one (Fredrickson & Losada, 2005). In parallel, even as resilience researchers urge attention to strengths of families and communities, our first order of business must be to attend to known potent toxins. Research has established incontrovertibly, for example, that chronic maltreatment is insidious and rarely overcome by other protective processes; yet, such forces are not always identified as *primary and essential targets* for at-risk populations. With survival threatened, positive attributes cannot flourish.

Second, in operationalizing optimal outcomes in both fields, the notions of generativity, or doing for the greater good, must be given much greater priority with these attributes rated by others and not just by the self. In positive psychology, the most compelling definition of "a life well lived," arguably, would be not just self-reported health and happiness but when adults are judged as committed to doing for others, with positive contributions to society (Bermant, Talwar, & Rozin, 2011; Little, 2011). Similarly, generativity can (and should) be considered a core positive outcome in operationalizing resilience among children and youth. We need to move beyond social conformity and academic grades to focusing on behavioral manifestations of kindness, generosity, and self-lessness. If the shared goal of these two scientific disciplines is, ultimately, to promote the well-being of humanity, then humanitarian acts must be central in our own scholarly efforts—in our theories, research foci, and above all, in the messages disseminated to the public and policy makers.

In summary, resilience research and positive psychology have much in common. As both fields continued to mature—retaining the highest standards of scientific inquiry—we face many of the same challenges. We each will need to arrive at some prioritization of which, among dozens of criteria, must be treated as integral in defining the "life well lived," and must critically appraise this question at different developmental stages across the life span. Notwithstanding our shared conceptual commitment to strengths and assets, we must be attentive to coexisting inimical influences that can powerfully thwart these. And beyond the thriving of individuals, we must focus on what individuals do to benefit others including family, friends, and society, and on how such generativity might best be fostered. Such a focus will keep us true to what has been emphasized by past presidents of the American Psychological Association across many decades (Zigler, 1998): that a central aim of psychology, as a broad discipline, must be to serve the public good and to promote the welfare of humankind.

Acknowledgements We gratefully acknowledge funding from the National Institutes of Health (R01DA014385, R13 MH082592, R01 DA010726). Our sincere thanks to Sasha Heinz for valuable input on prior drafts and to Nina L. Kumar for assistance in background research.

References

Afifi, T. O., & MacMillan, H. L. (2011). Resilience following maltreatment: A review of protective factors. *Canadian Journal of Psychiatry, 56,* 266–272. Retrieved from http://publications.cpa-apc.org/

Aisenberg, E., & Herrenkohl, T. (2008). Community violence in context: Risk and resilience in children and families. *Journal of Interpersonal Violence, 23,* 296–315. doi:10.1177/0886260507312287.

Algoe, S. B., Fredrickson, B. L., & Chow, S. M. (2011). The future of emotions research within positive psychology. In K. M. Sheldon, T. B. Kashdan, & M. F. Steger (Eds.), *Designing positive psychology: Taking stock and moving forward* (pp. 115–132). New York, NY: Oxford University Press.

Anthony, E. J. (1974). The syndrome of the psychologically invulnerable child. In E. J. Anthony & C. Koupernik (Eds.), *The child in his family: Children at psychiatric risk* (pp. 3–10). New York, NY: Wiley.

Barnett, M. A., Scaramella, L. V., Neppl, T. K., Ontai, L. L., & Conger, R. D. (2010). Grandmother involvement as a protective factor for early childhood adjustment. *Journal of Family Psychology, 24,* 635–645. doi:10.1037/a0020829.

Baumeister, R. F., Bratslavsky, E., Findenauer, C., & Vohs, K. D. (2001). Bad is stronger than good. *Review of General Psychology, 5,* 323–370. doi:10.1037/1089-2680.5.4.323.

Beardslee, W. R. (2002). *When a parent is depressed: How to protect your children from the effects of depression in the family.* Boston, MA: Little, Brown.

Beardslee, W., Gladstone, T. R. G., & O'Connor, E. E. (2012). Transmission and prevention of mood disorders among children of affectively ill parents: A review. *Journal of the American Academy of Child and Adolescent Psychiatry, 50,* 1098–1109.

Bermant, G., Talwar, C., & Rozin, P. (2011). To celebrate positive psychology and extend its horizons. In K. M. Sheldon, T. B. Kashdan, & M. F. Steger (Eds.), *Designing positive psychology: Taking stock and moving forward* (pp. 430–438). New York, NY: Oxford University Press.

Biswas-Diener, R., Kashdan, T. B., & King, L. A. (2009). Two traditions of happiness research, not two distinct types of happiness. *Journal of Positive Psychology, 4,* 408–211. doi:10.1080/17439760902844400.

Block, J. H., & Block, J. (1980). The role of ego-control and ego-resiliency in the organization of behavior. In W. A. Collins (Ed.), *Development of cognition, affect, and social relations: Minnesota Symposia on Child Psychology* (Vol. 13, pp. 39–101). Hillsdale, NJ: Erlbaum.

Brody, G. H., Kim, S., Murry, V. M., & Brown, A. C. (2004). Protective longitudinal paths linking child competence to behavioral problems among African

American siblings. *Child Development, 75*, 455–467. doi:10.1111/j.1467-8624.2004.00686.x.

Burt, K. B., & Paysnick, A. A. (2012). Resilience in the transition to adulthood. *Development and Psychopathology, 24*, 493–505. doi:10.1017/S0954579412000119.

Cedeno, L. A., Elias, M. J., Kelly, S., & Chu, B. C. (2010). School violence, adjustment, and the influence of hope on low-income, African American youth. *American Journal of Orthopsychiatry, 80,* 213–226. doi:10.1111/j.1939-0025.2010.01025.x.

Cicchetti, D. (2002). The impact of social experience on neurobiological systems: Illustration from a constructivist view of child maltreatment. *Cognitive Development, 17,* 1407–1428. doi:10.1016/S0885-2014(02)00121-1.

Cicchetti, D., & Rogosch, F. A. (1997). The role of self-organization in the promotion of resilience in maltreated children. *Development and Psychopathology, 9*, 797–815. doi:10.1017/S0954579497001442.

Coley, R. L. (2001). (In)visible men: Emerging research on low-income, unmarried, and minority fathers. *American Psychologist, 56*, 743–753. doi:10.1037/0003-066X.56.9.743.

Collishaw, S., Maughan, B., Goodman, R., & Pickles, A. (2004). Time trends in adolescent mental health. *Journal of Child Psychology and Psychiatry, 45*, 1350–1362. doi:10.1111/j.1469-7610.2004.00842.x.

Csikszentmihalyi, M., & Nakamura, J. (2011). Positive psychology: Where did it come from, where is it going? In K. M. Sheldon, T. B. Kashdan, & M. F. Steger (Eds.), *Designing positive psychology: Taking stock and moving forward* (pp. 3–8). New York, NY: Oxford University Press.

Diener, E., & Oishi, S. (2005). The nonobvious social psychology of happiness. *Psychological Inquiry, 16*, 162–167. doi:10.1207/s15327965pli1604_04.

Dishion, T. J., McCord, J., & Poulin, F. (1999). When interventions harm: Peer groups and problem behavior. *American Psychologist, 54*, 755–764. doi:10.1037/0003-066X.54.9.755.

Dodge, K. A., & Rutter, M. (Eds.). (2011). *Gene-environment interactions in developmental psychopathology.* New York, NY: Guilford Press.

DuBois, D. L., Portillo, N., Rhodes, J. E., Silverthorn, N., & Valentine, J. C. (2011). How effective are mentoring programs for youth? A systematic assessment of the evidence. *Psychological Science in the Public Interest, 12*, 57–91. doi:10.1177/1529100611414806.

Ebersöhn, L., & Ferreira, R. (2011). Coping in an HIV/AIDS-dominated context: Teachers promoting resilience in schools. *Health Education Research, 26*, 596–613. doi:10.1093/her/cyr016.

Eisenberg, N., Rg, H., Spinrad, T. L., Hofer, C., Chassin, L., Zhou, Q., et al. (2010). Relations of temperament to maladjustment and ego resiliency in at-risk children. *Social Development, 19*, 577–600. doi:10.1111/j.1467-9507.2009.00550.x.

Farber, E. A., & Egeland, B. (1987). Invulnerability in abused and neglected children. In E. J. Anthony & B. J. Cohler (Eds.), *The invulnerable child* (pp. 253–288). New York, NY: Guilford Press.

Fiedler, F. E. (1995). "Cognitive resources and leadership performance": A rejoinder. *Applied Psychology, 44*, 50–56. doi:10.1111/j.1464-0597.1995.tb01386.x.

Fredrickson, B. L. (1998). What good are positive emotions? *Review of General Psychology, 2*, 300–319. doi:10.1037/1089-2680.2.3.300.

Fredrickson, B. L., & Losada, M. F. (2005). Positive Affect and the Complex Dynamics of Human Flourishing. *American Psychologist, 60*, 678–686. doi:10.1037/0003-066X.60.7.678.

García Coll, C. T., & Marks, A. K. (Eds.). (2009). *Immigrant stories: Ethnicity and academics in middle childhood.* New York, NY: Oxford University Press.

Garmezy, N. (1974). The study of competence in children at risk for severe psychopathology. In E. J. Anthony & C. Koupernik (Eds.), *The child in his family: Vol. 3: Children at psychiatric risk* (pp. 77–97). New York, NY: Wiley.

Garmezy, N., & Masten, A. S. (1986). Stress, competence, and resilience: Common frontiers for therapist and psychopathologist. *Behavior Therapy, 17*, 500–521. doi:10.1016/S0005-7894(86)80091-0.

Garmezy, N., Masten, A. S., & Tellegen, A. (1984). The study of stress and competence in children: A building block for developmental psychopathology. *Child Development, 55*, 97–111. doi:10.1111/j.1467-8624.1984.tb00276.x.

Gillham, J. E., Brunwasser, S. M., & Freres, D. R. (2008). Preventing depression in early adolescence: The Penn Resiliency Program. In J. R. Z. Abela & B. L. Hankin (Eds.), *Handbook of depression in children and adolescents* (pp. 309–332). New York, NY: Guilford Press.

Gorman-Smith, D., & Tolan, P. H. (2003). Positive adaptation among youth exposed to community violence. In S. S. Luthar (Ed.), *Resilience and vulnerability: Adaptation in the context of childhood adversities* (pp. 392–413). New York, NY: Cambridge University Press.

Grigorenko, E. L., & Cicchetti, D. (2012). The contribution of genetic/genomic sciences to developmental psychopathology [Special issue]. *Development and Psychopathology, 24*(4).

Hames, J. L., & Joiner, T. E., Jr. (2011). The dog woman, Addie Bundren, and the ninth circle: Positive psychology should be more open to the negative. In K. Sheldon, T. Kashdan, & M. Steger (Eds.), *Designing the future of positive psychology: Taking stock and moving forward* (pp. 313–323). New York, NY: Oxford University Press.

Hauser, S. T., Allen, J. P., & Golden, E. (2006). *Out of the woods: Tales of resilient teens.* Cambridge, MA: Harvard University Press.

Herrenkohl, T. I., Sousa, C., Tajima, E. A., Herrenkohl, R. C., & Moylan, C. A. (2008). Intersection of child abuse and children's exposure to domestic violence. *Trauma, Violence, and Abuse, 9*, 84–99. doi:10.1177/1524838008314797.

Jain, S., Buka, S. L., Subramanian, S. V., & Molnar, B. E. (2012). Protective factors for youth exposed to violence: Role of developmental assets in building emotional resilience. *Youth Violence and Juvenile Justice, 10*, 107–129. doi:10.1177/1541204011424735.

Kagan, J., Snidman, N., & Arcus, D. (1998). Childhood derivatives of reactivity in infancy. *Child Development, 69*, 1483–1493. doi:10.1111/j.1467-8624.1998.tb06171.x.

Kashdan, T. B., & Steger, M. F. (2011). Challenges, pitfalls, and aspirations for positive psychology. In K. M. Sheldon, T. B. Kashdan, & M. F. Steger (Eds.), *Designing positive psychology: Taking stock and moving forward* (pp. 9–21). New York, NY: Oxford University Press.

Keyes, C. L. M., & Lopez, S. J. (2002). Toward a science of mental health: Positive directions in diagnosis and interventions. In C. R. Synder & S. J. Lopez (Eds.), *The handbook of positive psychology* (pp. 45–59). New York, NY: Oxford University Press.

Kim, J., Cicchetti, D., Rogosch, F. A., & Manly, J. T. (2009). Child maltreatment and trajectories of personality and behavioral functioning: Implications for the development of personality disorder. *Development and Psychopathology, 21*, 889–912. doi:10.1017/S0954579409000480.

Kim-Cohen, J., & Turkewitz, R. (2012). Resilience and measured gene-environment interactions. *Development and Psychopathology, 24*, 1297–1306. doi:10.1017/S0954579412000715.

Koenen, K. C., Moffitt, T. E., Caspi, A., Taylor, A., & Purcell, S. (2003). Domestic violence is associated with environmental suppression of IQ in young children. *Development and Psychopathology, 15*, 297–311. doi:10.1017/S0954579403000166.

Lambert, N. M., Fincham, F. D., Gwinn, A. M., & Ajayi, C. A. (2011). Positive relationship science: A new frontier for positive psychology? In K. M. Sheldon, T. B. Kashdan, & M. F. Steger (Eds.), *Designing positive psychology: Taking stock and moving forward* (pp. 280–292). New York, NY: Oxford University Press.

Leventhal, T., & Brooks-Gunn, J. (2000). The neighborhoods they live in: The effects of neighborhood residence on child and adolescent outcomes. *Psychological Bulletin, 126*, 309–337. doi:10.1037/0033-2909.126.2.309.

Little, B. R. (2011). Personality science and the northern tilt: As positive as possible under the circumstances. In K. M. Sheldon, T. B. Kashdan, & M. F. Steger (Eds.), *Designing positive psychology: Taking stock and moving forward* (pp. 228–248). New York, NY: Oxford University Press.

Lopez, S. J., & Snyder, C. R. (Eds.). (2009). *Oxford handbook of positive psychology*. New York, NY: Oxford University Press.

Luthar, S. S. (1991). Vulnerability and resilience: A study of high-risk adolescents. *Child Development, 62*, 600–616. doi:10.1111/j.1467-8624.1991.tb01555.x.

Luthar, S. S. (Ed.). (2003). *Resilience and vulnerability: Adaptation in the context of childhood adversities*. New York: Cambridge University Press.

Luthar, S. S. (2006). Resilience in development: A synthesis of research across five decades. In D. Cicchetti & D. J. Cohen (Eds.), *Developmental psychopathology, Vol. 3: Risk, disorder, and adaptation* (2nd ed., pp. 739–795). Hoboken, NJ: Wiley.

Luthar, S. S., & Barkin, S. H. (2012). Are affluent youth truly "at risk"? Vulnerability and resilience across three diverse samples. *Development and Psychopathology, 24*, 429–449. doi:10.1017/S0954579412000089.

Luthar, S. S., & Brown, P. J. (2007). Maximizing resilience through diverse levels of inquiry: Prevailing paradigms, possibilities, and priorities for the future. *Development and Psychopathology, 19*, 931–955. doi:10.1017/S0954579407000454.

Luthar, S., & Cicchetti, D. (2000). The construct of resilience: Implications for interventions and social policies. *Development and Psychopathology, 12*, 857–885.

Luthar, S. S., Cicchetti, D., & Becker, B. (2000). The construct of resilience: A critical evaluation and guidelines for future research. *Child Development, 71*, 543–562. doi:10.1111/1467-8624.00164.

Luthar, S. S., Doernberger, C. H., & Zigler, E. (1993). Resilience is not a unidimensional construct: Insights from a prospective study of inner-city adolescents. *Development and Psychopathology, 5*, 703–717. doi:10.1017/S0954579400006246.

Maggi, S., Roberts, W., MacLennan, D., & D'Angiulli, A. (2011). Community resilience, quality childcare, and preschoolers' mental health: A three-city comparison. *Social Science and Medicine, 73*, 1080–1087. doi:10.1016/j.socscimed.2011.06.052, 10.1016%2Fj.socscimed.2011.06.052.

Martin, A., Ryan, R. M., & Brooks-Gunn, J. (2010). When fathers' supportiveness matters most: Maternal and paternal parenting and school readiness. *Journal of Family Psychology, 24*, 145–155. doi:10.1037/a0018073.

Masten, A. S. (2001). Ordinary magic: Resilience processes in development. *American Psychologist, 56*, 227–238. doi:10.1037/0003-066X.56.3.227.

Masten, A. S., & Cicchetti, D. (2012). Risk and resilience in development and psychopathology: The legacy of Norman Garmezy. *Development and Psychopathology, 24*, 333–334. doi:10.1017/S0954579412000016.

Masten, A. S., & Tellegen, A. (2012). Resilience in developmental psychopathology: Contributions of the Project Competence Longitudinal Study. *Development and Psychopathology, 24*, 345–361. doi:10.1017/S095457941200003X.

McCrae, R. (2011). Personality traits and the potential of positive psychology. In K. M. Sheldon, T. B. Kashdan, & M. F. Steger (Eds.), *Designing positive psychology: Taking stock and moving forward* (pp. 192–206). New York, NY: Oxford University Press.

Mersky, J. P., Berger, L. M., Reynolds, A. J., & Gromoske, A. N. (2009). Risk factors for child and adolescent maltreatment: A longitudinal investigation of a cohort of inner-city youth. *Child Maltreatment, 14*, 73–88. doi:10.1177/1077559508318399.

Murphy, L. B., & Moriarty, A. E. (1976). *Vulnerability, coping, and growth: From infancy to adolescence*. New Haven, CT: Yale University Press.

Murry, V., Bynum, M. S., Brody, G. H., Willert, A., & Stephens, D. (2001). African American single mothers and children in context: A review of studies on risk and resilience. *Clinical Child and Family Psychology Review, 4*, 133–155. doi:10.1023/A:1011381114782.

Neal, J. W., Neal, Z. P., Atkins, M. S., Henry, D. B., & Frazier, S. L. (2011). Channels of change: Contrasting network mechanisms in the use of interventions. *American Journal of Community Psychology, 47*, 277–286. doi:10.1007/s10464-010-9403-0.

Noftle, E. E., Schnitker, S. A., & Robins, R. W. (2011). Character and personality: Connections between positive psychology and personality psychology. In K. M. Sheldon, T. B. Kashdan, & M. F. Steger (Eds.), *Designing the future of positive psychology: Taking stock and moving forward* (pp. 207–227). New York: Oxford University Press.

Obradović, J., Long, J. D., Cutuli, J. J., Chan, C., Hinz, E., Heistad, D., et al. (2009). Academic achievement of homeless and highly mobile children in an urban school district: Longitudinal evidence on risk, growth, and resilience. *Development and Psychopathology, 21*, 493–518. doi:10.1017/S0954579409000273.

Oishi, S., & Kurtz, J. L. (2011). The positive psychology of positive emotions: An avuncular view. In K. M. Sheldon, T. B. Kashdan, & M. F. Steger (Eds.), *Designing positive psychology: Taking stock and moving forward* (pp. 101–114). New York, NY: Oxford University Press.

Pargament, K. I., & Cummings, J. (2010). Anchored by faith: Religion as a resilience factor. In J. W. Reich, A. J. Zautra, & J. S. Hall (Eds.), *Handbook of adult resilience* (pp. 193–210). New York, NY: Guilford Press.

Park, C. L. (2010). Stress-related growth and thriving through coping: The roles of personality and cognitive processes. *Journal of Social Issues, 54*, 267–277. doi:10.1111/j.1540-4560.1998.tb01218.x.

Peck, S. C., Roeser, R. W., Zarrett, N., & Eccles, J. S. (2008). Exploring the roles of extracurricular activity quantity and quality in the educational resilience of vulnerable adolescents: Variable- and pattern-centered approaches. *Journal of Social Issues, 64*, 135–155. doi:10.1111/j.1540-4560.2008.00552.x.

Peterson, C. (2006). *A primer in positive psychology*. New York, NY: Oxford University Press.

Peterson, C., & Park, N. (2003). Positive psychology as the evenhanded positive psychologist views it. *Psychological Inquiry, 14*, 141–146. doi:10.1207/S15327965PLI1402_03.

Peterson, C., Park, N., & Seligman, M. E. P. (2006). Greater strengths of character and recovery from illness. *The Journal of Positive Psychology, 1*, 17–26. doi:10.1080/17439760500372739.

Pianta, R. C., & Walsh, D. I. (1998). Applying the construct of resilience in schools: Cautions from a developmental systems perspective. *School Psychology Review, 27*, 407–417. Retrieved from http://www.nasponline.org/publications/spr.

Reis, H. T., & Aron, A. (2008). Love: What is it, why does it matter, and how does it operate? *Psychological Science, 3*, 80–86. doi:10.1111/j.1745-6916.2008.00065.x.

Rhodes, J., & Lowe, S. R. (2008). Youth mentoring and resilience: Implications for practice. *Child Care in Practice, 14*, 9–17. doi:10.1080/13575270701733666.

Rios, R., Aiken, L. S., & Zautra, A. J. (2012). Neighborhood contexts and the mediating role of neighborhood social cohesion on health and psychological distress among Hispanic and non-Hispanic residents. *Annals of Behavioral Medicine, 43*, 50–61. doi:10.1007/s12160-011-9306-9.

Roberts, M. C., Brown, K. J., Johnson, R. J., & Reinke, J. (2002). Positive psychology for children: Development, prevention, and promotion. In C. R. Snyder & S. J. Lopez (Eds.), *Handbook of positive psychology* (pp. 663–671). New York, NY: Oxford University Press.

Rogosch, F. A., Dackis, M. N., & Cicchetti, D. (2011). Child maltreatment and allostatic load: Consequences for physical and mental health in children from low-income families. *Development and Psychopathology, 23*, 1107–1124. doi:10.1017/S0954579411000587.

Rutter, M. (1979). Protective factors in children's responses to stress and disadvantage. In M. W. Kent & J. E. Rolf (Eds.), *Primary prevention in psychopathology, Vol. 3: Social competence in children* (pp. 49–74). Hanover, NH: University Press of New England.

Rutter, M. (1987). Psychosocial resilience and protective mechanisms. *American Journal of Orthopsychiatry, 57*, 316–331. doi:10.1111/j.1939-0025.1987.tb03541.x.

Rutter, M. (1998). Developmental catch-up, and deficit, following adoption after severe early privation. *Journal of Child Psychology and Psychiatry, 39*, 465–476. doi:10.1111/1469-7610.00343.

Rutter, M. (2000). Resilience reconsidered: Conceptual considerations, empirical findings, and policy implications. In J. P. Shonkoff & S. J. Meisels (Eds.), *Handbook of early childhood intervention* (2nd ed., pp. 651–682). New York, NY: Cambridge University Press.

Rutter, M. (2012). Resilience as a dynamic concept. *Development and Psychopathology, 24*, 335–344. doi:10.1017/S0954579412000028.

Ryff, C. D. (1989). Happiness is everything, or is it? Explorations on the meaning of psychological well-being. *Journal of Personality and Social Psychology, 57*, 1069–1081. doi:10.1037/0022-3514.57.6.1069.

Sameroff, A. J., & Rosenblum, K. L. (2006). Psychosocial constraints on development of resilience. *Annals of the New York Academy of Science, 1094*, 116–124. doi:10.1196/annals.1376.010.

Sampson, R. J., & Laub, J. H. (1993). *Crime in the making: Pathways and turning points through life*. Cambridge, MA: Harvard University Press.

Seligman, M. E. P., & Csikszentmihalyi, C. (2000). Positive psychology: An introduction. *American Psychologist, 55*, 5–14. doi:10.1037/0003-066X.55.1.5.

Sheldon, K. M., Kashdan, T. B., & Steger, M. F. (Eds.). (2011). *Designing positive psychology: Taking stock and moving forward*. New York, NY: Oxford University Press.

Sherman, B. J., Duarte, C. S., & Verdeli, H. (2011). Internalizing and externalizing problems in adolescents from Bahia, Brazil: Sociodemographic correlates and family environment in boys and girls. *International Journal of Mental Health, 40*(3), 55–76. doi:10.2753/IMH0020-7411400304.

Shiner, R. L., & Masten, A. S. (2012). Childhood personality as a harbinger of competence and resilience in adulthood. *Development and Psychopathology, 24*, 507–528. doi:10.1017/ S0954579412000120.

Shonkoff, J. P., & Phillips, D. A. (Eds.). (2000). *From neurons to neighborhoods: The science of early childhood development*. Washington, DC: National Academy Press.

Staudinger, U. M., Freund, A. M., Linden, M., & Maas, I. (1999). Self, personality and life regulation: Facets of psychological resilience in old age. In P. B. Baltes & K. U. Mayer (Eds.), *The Berlin aging study: Aging from 70 to 100* (pp. 302–328). New York, NY: Cambridge University Press.

Steinberg, L. (2001). We know some things: Adolescent-parent relationships in retrospect and prospect. *Journal of Research on Adolescence, 11*, 1–19. doi:10.1111/1532-7795.00001.

Stoiber, K. C., & Gettinger, M. (2011). Functional assessment and positive support strategies for promoting resilience: Effects on teachers and high-risk children. *Psychology in the Schools, 48*, 686–706. doi:10.1002/pits.20587.

Stormshak, E. A., Comeau, C. A., & Shepard, S. A. (2004). The relative contribution of sibling deviance and peer deviance in the prediction of substance use across middle childhood. *Journal of Abnormal Child Psychology, 32*, 635–649. doi:10.1023/B:JACP.0000047212.49463.c7.

Synder, C. R., & Lopez, S. J. (Eds.). (2002). *The handbook of positive psychology*. New York, NY: Oxford University Press.

Thompson, R., & Tabone, J. K. (2010). The impact of early alleged maltreatment on behavioral trajectories. *Child Abuse and Neglect, 34*, 907–916. doi:10.1016/j.chiabu.2010.06.006.

Tiet, Q. Q., Huizinga, D., & Byrnes, H. F. (2010). Predictors of resilience among inner city youths. *Journal of Child and Family Studies, 19*, 360–378. doi:10.1007/s10826-009-9307-5.

Vaillant, G. E. (2012). *Triumphs of experience: The men of the Harvard Grant Study*. Cambridge, MA: Harvard University Press.

Valdez, C. R., Mills, C. L., Barrueco, S., Leis, J., & Riley, A. W. (2011). A pilot study of a family-focused intervention for children and families affected by maternal depression. *Journal of Family Therapy, 33*, 3–19. doi:10.1111/j.1467-6427.2010.00529.x.

Van Ryzin, M. (2010). The secondary school advisor as mentor and secondary attachment figure. *Journal of Community Psychology, 38*, 131–154. doi:10.1002/jcop.20356.

Vanderbilt-Adriance, E., & Shaw, D. S. (2008). Conceptualizing and re-evaluating resilience across levels of risk, time, and domains of competence. *Clinical Child and Family Psychology Review, 11*, 30–58. doi:10.1007/s10567-008-0031-2.

Véronneau, M.-H., & Dishion, T. J. (2010). Predicting change in early adolescent problem behavior in the middle school years: A mesosystemic perspective on parenting and peer experiences. *Journal of Abnormal Child Psychology, 38*, 1125–1137. doi:10.1007/s10802-010-9431-0.

Walsh, F. (2007). Traumatic loss and major disasters: Strengthening family and community resilience. *Family Process, 46*, 207–227. doi:10.1111/j.1545-5300.2007.00205.x.

Werner, E. E. (2012). Children and war: Risk, resilience, and recovery. *Development and Psychopathology, 24*, 553–558. doi:10.1017/S0954579412000156.

Werner, E. E., & Smith, R. (1982). *Vulnerable but invincible: A longitudinal study of resilient children*. New York, NY: McGraw-Hill.

Werner, E. E., & Smith, R. S. (1992). *Overcoming the odds: High risk children from birth to adulthood*. Ithaca, NY: Cornell University Press.

Werner, E. E., & Smith, R. S. (2001). *Journeys from childhood to midlife: Risk, resilience, and recovery*. Ithaca, NY: Cornell University Press.

Williams, J., & Nelson-Gardell, D. (2012). Predicting resilience in sexually abused adolescents. *Child Abuse and Neglect, 36*, 53–63. doi:10.1016/j.chiabu.2011.07.004.

Wong, P. T. P. (2007). *The promises and perils of positive psychology*. PsycCRITIQUES, Contemporary Psychology: APA Review of Books.

Yates, T., & Grey, I. K. (2012). Adapting to aging out: Profiles of risk and resilience among emancipated foster youth. *Development and Psychopathology, 24*, 475–492. doi:10.1017/S0954579412000107.

Yates, T. M., & Masten, A. S. (2004). Fostering the future: Resilience theory and the practice of positive psychology. In P. A. Linley & S. Joseph (Eds.), *Positive psychology in practice* (pp. 521–539). Hoboken, NJ: Wiley.

Zautra, A. J. (2014). Resilience is social, after all. In M. Kent, M. C. Davis, & J. W. Reich (Eds.), *The resilience handbook: Approaches to stress and trauma* (pp. 185–196). New York: Rutledge.

Zigler, E. (1998). A place of value for applied and policy studies. *Child Development, 69*, 1467–8624.

Zimmerman, M. A., & Brenner, A. B. (2010). Resilience in adolescence: Overcoming neighborhood disadvantage. In J. W. Reich, A. J. Zautra, & J. S. Hall (Eds.), *Handbook of adult resilience* (pp. 283–308). New York, NY: Guilford Press.

Family Context in the Development of Psychopathology

Patrick T. Davies and Melissa L. Sturge-Apple

High public health significance is attached to understanding how family relationships impact child psychopathology. Decades of research have established that a wide array of family characteristics serve as pivotal precursors of children's mental health outcomes (Morris, Silk, Steinberg, Myers, & Robinson, 2007; Repetti, Taylor, & Seeman, 2002). Reviews of the literature within the framework of "risky" family environments have specifically documented that aggression, conflict, and disengagement in the whole family, parent–child, interparental, and sibling contexts qualify as risk factors for the emergence and persistence of psychological problems throughout childhood and adulthood (Repetti, Robles, & Reynolds, 2011; Repetti et al., 2002). Since the last edition of this book over 10 years ago, significant headway has been made in elucidating the processes and conditions underlying the variability in outcomes of children exposed to these specific family characteristics. By the same token, significant gaps remain in understanding how and why family processes affect children's mental health within a developmental framework. Accordingly, the overarching objective of this chapter is to describe the progress, potential, and challenges

in characterizing the unfolding cascade of developmental processes underlying links between risky family contexts and child psychopathology.

Figure 8.1 illustrates our organizational framework for addressing the central conceptual and empirical themes for research on family processes and developmental psychopathology. To provide a bridge between the existing family risk research and our developmental perspective, the first section of the chapter provides a brief synopsis of the primary family relationship characteristics that serve as proximal risk factors for the development of psychopathology. Next, we illustrate some of the advances that have been made in contextualizing these risk factors within the broader dynamics of the family. Building on the analysis of risk factors, the following sections of the paper examine the question of how and why these family risk factors increase children's risk for psychopathology. Toward the goal of more deeply characterizing the diversity of trajectories of adaptation, we demonstrate the utility of identifying the regulatory conditions and contexts that underlie the sources of heterogeneity in the developmental pathways children follow. In closing the chapter, we briefly summarize the progress in relation to the next generation of research.

Patrick T. Davies was supported by the James McKeen Cattell Fund Sabbatical Fellowship during the writing of this chapter.

P.T. Davies, Ph.D. (✉) • M.L. Sturge-Apple, Ph.D.
Department of Clinical and Social Sciences
in Psychology, University of Rochester,
Rochester 14627, NY, USA
e-mail: patrick.davies@rochester.edu

Family Risk Factors

In the terminology of developmental psychopathology, risk factors are defined as characteristics that probabilistically increase the likelihood of

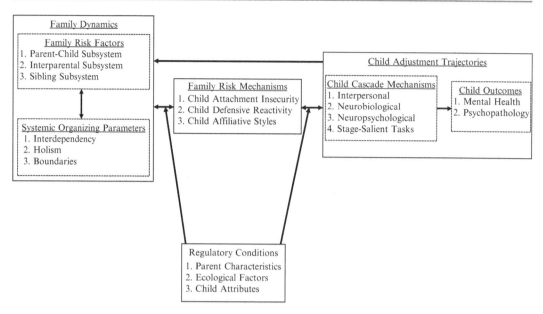

Fig. 8.1 A graphical depiction of our organizational framework for understanding the developmental pathways, mechanisms, and conditions underlying associa- tions among family characteristics and children's developmental psychopathology

child maladjustment. For the sake of parsimony, we selectively focus on the more heavily investigated classes of family risk factors as a way to concisely summarize key findings in the literature (see Fig. 8.1). Consistent with key subsystems identified in family systems theory, the following sections summarize the primary attributes of the parent–child, interparental, and sibling relationships that are associated with individual differences in children's psychopathology.

Parent–Child Subsystem

One of the most proximal developmental contexts for children is the parent–child subsystem. Although family systems theory emphasizes the transactional nature of subsystem relationships (Cox & Paley, 1997), theoretical conceptualizations of the dynamics of the parent–child subsystem have predominantly elaborated on the unidirectional effects by which parenting influences children's developing capacities. Thus, the behaviors and strategies used by parents toward socializing children have historically been dimensionalized across two primary

axes including sensitivity/responsiveness and demandingness/control (Barber, 1996; Maccoby & Martin, 1983), out of which arise a tripartite classification of parental behavior including warmth/support, behavioral control, and psychological control (Barber, 1996). Parental warmth/ support has been conceptualized as parental behaviors that convey positive affect and emotional availability, are sensitively responsive to the emotional needs of the child, and suggest a supportive presence on the part of the caregiver. Parental behavioral control refers to the regulation or structure of children's behavior through monitoring and discipline, whereas psychological control involves parental attempts to control and constrain a child's psychological world through guilt induction, love withdrawal, and manipulation of feelings (e.g., Barber, 1996).

Over several decades, empirical research has examined how diminished caretaking across different parenting practices increases children's vulnerability to mental health difficulties and socioemotional maladjustment (Borkowski, Ramey, & Bristol-Power, 2002). Although a full accounting of the multitude of research examining these parenting behaviors and child psychopathology is beyond the scope of this chapter, empirical work has delineated associations between these constructs and children's depressive symptoms (McLeod, Weisz, & Wood, 2007), externalizing problems (Hoeve et al., 2009), and peer relationships (Clark & Ladd, 2000). Some specificity between parenting practices and developmental outcomes has been reported. Specifically, research suggests that poor behavioral control is primarily related to externalizing symptomatology whereas psychological control and warmth/support may be more strongly associated with poor self-esteem, low agency, and internalizing symptomatology (e.g., Barber, Olsen, & Shagle, 1994; Gray & Steinberg, 1999).

Toward achieving greater precision in delineating how these wide constellations of parenting behaviors may differentially influence children's development, theorists have utilized pattern-based conceptualizations of parenting and parent–child relationship dynamics. Using the original dimensions of parenting behaviors, four broad parenting profiles have been demarcated in the literature including authoritative, authoritarian, permissive/indulgent, and rejecting/neglecting (Maccoby & Martin, 1983), and findings suggest some specificity of effects on children's adjustment. Authoritarian parenting styles characterized by high levels of both demandingness and responsiveness have been associated with the highest levels of adjustment in children (Lamborn, Mounts, Steinberg, & Dornbusch, 1991). However, findings suggest that lax/permissive (low demandingness/high responsiveness) and rejecting/neglecting (low demandingness/ low responsiveness) parenting styles are linked to a plethora of adverse outcomes including insecure forms of attachment, difficulties in peer relationships, higher levels of misconduct and externalizing symptomatology, lower self-regulation, and lower academic achievement and school competence (e.g., Luyckx et al., 2011). In contrast, research examining authoritarian parenting styles has produced mixed outcomes with some studies suggesting either a risk or protective effect of authoritarian parenting within certain ecological niches (Steinberg & Silk, 2002).

Interparental Relationship Characteristics

Due to the prevalence of divorce, cohabitation, remarriage, and premarital childbearing, children in contemporary society vary widely in their experience of different relationship arrangements between parents. Research examining different family structures has documented that the experience of interparental relationship instability in the form of separations, the establishment of new romantic relationships, and single parenthood place children at risk for psychological problems, including academic difficulties, poor social competence, emotional problems, and delinquency (Amato, 2010; Cavanagh & Huston, 2008). Nevertheless, it is important not to overpathologize the risk associated with these forms of interparental relationship instability. Structural changes in the interparental relationship are generally modest risk factors for psychopathology. Moreover, research has shown that the emotional tenor and quality of the interparental relationship is a more potent risk factor and a primary mechanism that explains why interparental transitions take a psychological toll on children (Grych & Fincham, 2001).

Interparental relationship quality is, itself, a broad construct consisting of multiple dimensions. Initial empirical efforts to more precisely identify the risk properties underlying interparental relationship quality underscored the developmental significance of how parents manage stress, conflict, and challenges. For example, conflict between parents is a better predictor of a wide range of child problems than general distress or dissatisfaction between parents (Jouriles et al., 1991). However, because disputes and disagreements between parents are common occurrences in homes, it is important to distinguish between the properties of conflict that are harmful and benign for children. Constructive forms of conflict involving calm, rational disagreements that end in resolution are associated with better psychological adjustment in children (Cummings & Davies, 2010). In fact, constructive conflict may have a positive effect, teaching children important conflict management strategies that they can subsequently use when interacting with siblings and peers (Davies, Martin, & Cicchetti, 2013; McCoy, Cummings, & Davies, 2009). Conversely, high levels of hostile, escalating, and unresolved forms of interparental conflict are consistent predictors of a wide array of child problems, including social difficulties, behavioral problems, emotional symptoms, academic setbacks, and physical troubles (e.g., illness, sleep problems). Research has further shown that physical violence, psychological abuse (i.e., name-calling, threats), and disagreements over child-rearing constitute particularly damaging forms of interparental conflict that incrementally predict children's vulnerability to psychopathology beyond the risk conferred by global discord and hostility between parents (Fergusson & Horwood, 1998; Jouriles et al., 1991; McHale & Fivaz-Depeursinge, 1999).

Sibling Relationship Quality

Family scholars have increasingly turned their attention to the dynamics of the sibling relationship as a context for children's development (Dunn, 1991). Attesting to the importance of sibling relationships, an estimated 80% of children will grow up with a sibling (Cicirelli, 1995), and children spend more time on average interacting with their siblings than with parents or other family members in the household (e.g., McHale & Crouter, 1996). Given the more egalitarian nature of siblings with respect to power and dominance within a family hierarchy, research examining the impact of siblings on individual's socioemotional development has primarily focused on the two parameters of sibling relationships: conflict and cohesion. With respect to conflict between sibling dyads, studies have linked aversive, chronic, and physical conflict to a host of adjustment difficulties including internalizing symptoms (Milevsky & Levitt, 2005), lower social competence (Stormshak, Bellanti, & Bierman, 1996), and externalizing problems (Ensor, Marks, Jacobs, & Hughes, 2010). In terms of relational

cohesion and warmth, sibling relationships may provide an opportunity to express emotions, communicate wants and needs, as well as provide a context for emotional support. Sibling warmth has been linked with positive self-worth (Stocker, 1994), reduced externalizing behavior (Branje, van Lieshout, van Aken, & Haselager, 2004), and more resilient functioning in the context of environmental adversity (e.g., Jenkins, 1992).

Systemic Organizing Parameters

Although identifying characteristics of specific family relationships that serve as risk factors is a valuable approach in developmental psychopathology, a complementary objective in family process research is to better understand how each specific family characteristic operates in the context of the larger fabric of the family system. Within the open system conceptualization of family systems theory, any one subsystem or individual is regarded as inextricably embedded within the family unit. Systemic processes operating at the broader family level play a critical role in regulating how family characteristics operate together to influence children's psychological maladjustment. Open system frameworks are instantiated more precisely in several key principles. For the sake of illustration, Figure 8.1 depicts the role of three concepts in advancing the field of developmental psychopathology: interdependency, holism, and boundaries.

Interdependency

Interdependency refers to the existence of the reciprocal influences among subsystems and individuals in the family (Cox & Paley, 1997; Minuchin, 1985). Each family relationship (e.g., parent–child subsystem) and its members are conceptualized as both causes and products of one another. Thus, perturbations in any one subsystem are posited to reverberate through other family relationships in a negative reciprocal cycle. Since Patricia Minuchin (1985) broadly introduced the concept of circularity to a large audience of developmental scientists, developmental psychopathology models of family process have increasingly acknowledged the operation of bidirectional influences between multiple family subsystems (McHale, 2007). Consistent with these assumptions, interparental animosity and distress predicts subsequent coparenting difficulties characterized by lack of mutual support in child-rearing, active undermining of each other's parenting goals, and greater discrepancies between parents in their levels of involvement with their children (Paley, O'Connor, Kogan, & Findlay, 2005). Interparental conflict is also associated with ensuing decrements in parenting (e.g., warmth, involvement, discipline) and parent–child relationship qualities across an array of temporal spans (i.e., days, months, and years) and methodological designs (Almeida, Wethington, & Chandler, 1999; Jouriles & Farris, 1992; Sturge-Apple, Davies, & Cummings, 2006a). In demonstrating bidirectionality among subsystems, other studies have indicated that coparenting relationship qualities are key prognosticators of subsequent increases in interparental discord (e.g., Schoppe-Sullivan, Mangelsdorf, Frosch, & McHale, 2004).

Documentation of transactions among family subsystems begs the question of how multiple risk factors in the family operate together in understanding the development of psychopathology. In integrating this systemic principle into family risk models of child psychopathology, researchers have gained a fuller appreciation of the multitude and complexity of mediational pathways among family risk factors and child psychopathology. For example, many family theories postulate that interparental hostility increases children's vulnerability to psychological problems by undermining parenting practices and the parent–child relationship (e.g., Davies & Cummings, 1994; Grych & Fincham, 1990). Supporting this hypothesis, there is now empirical evidence indicating that the association between interparental conflict and child psychopathology is partially accounted for by a wide array of parenting difficulties, including low warmth, disengagement, inconsistent and harsh discipline, hostility, and psychological

control (Gerard, Krishnakumar, & Buehler, 2006; Sturge-Apple, Davies, & Cummings, 2006b). Likewise, coparenting difficulties have also been delineated as key explanatory processes underlying the heightened vulnerability of children exposed to destructive interparental conflict (Cui, Donnellan, & Conger, 2007; Katz & Low, 2004).

Holism

According to the principle of holism, the family as a unit is not simply reducible to an additive aggregation of functioning within each family subsystem (Cox & Paley, 1997). In the field of developmental psychopathology, a primary corollary is that the collective adjustment of the whole family unit will have distinct implications for children's development even after considering the additive contributions of each family subsystem. Empirical tests of this hypothesis are difficult to conduct due to the challenges of ensuring that targeted dimensions of functioning with each family subsystem are assessed in a comparably comprehensive way as the "holistic" or family-level forms of functioning. In spite of these challenges, studies have supported the distinctive developmental advantages of capturing family-level functioning above and beyond the analysis of the family subsystems (e.g., Ackerman, Kogos, Youngstrom, Schoff, & Izard, 1999; Katz & Low, 2004; McHale & Rasmussen, 1998). For example, McHale and Rasmussen (1998) reported that observations of family-level dynamics (i.e., hostility, harmony, discrepancies in parent involvement) in triadic interactions involving mothers, fathers, and infants predicted child psychological problems 3 years later even after controlling for parental characteristics and marital quality.

The significance of holism is also evident at dyadic or individual levels of analysis in the family as it assumes that any aspect of functioning in a subsystem gains critical meaning and purpose from other parts of the family unit. Thus, any attempt to disaggregate specific family risk factors from the broader constellation of family processes must be balanced by complementary efforts to understand how family characteristics may have different implications for children depending on characteristics in the larger family context. For example, according to the compensatory hypothesis, some parents who are facing high levels of discord may defy the odds of experiencing parenting difficulties and even devote substantial efforts to offset children's vulnerability to this adversity by increasing their warmth, engagement, and responsiveness in interactions with children (e.g., Cox, Paley, & Harter, 2001). As McHale (2007) notes, high levels of warmth and engagement are commonly interpreted as beneficial for children and families. However, family systems theory cautions against interpreting increases in positive parenting in high-conflict homes at face value. Under some family conditions, warmth is part of a broader pattern of parent–child triangulation, emotional entanglement, and intrusiveness (Kretchmar & Jacobvitz, 2002; Marvin & Stewart, 1990). In other words, associations among a focal family predictor (e.g., warmth) and children's psychopathology are assumed to be moderated by (or vary as a function of) the broader organization of the family climate (e.g., triangulation, entanglement). Thus, understanding diversity and underlying meaning of patterns of relations between family characteristics and child psychopathology will require progressively holistic accounts of the family system.

Boundaries

In building on the notion of holism, family systems frameworks underscore the usefulness of analyzing interpersonal boundaries in fully deciphering the meaning of interaction patterns in family subsystems. Boundaries within and across relationships in the family are defined by characteristic ways of exchanging resources, information, and materials in the family unit. Although theory and research on family systems has identified a number of different configurations of emotional and relational functioning in the family, cohesive, disengaged, enmeshed, and triangulated patterns of communication have been most consistently delineated in empirical work (Davies, Cummings, & Winter, 2004; Johnson, 2010; Kerig, 1995; Kretchmar & Jacobvitz, 2002; Minuchin, 1974). Flexible, well-defined boundaries characteristic of cohesive families provide children with ready access to resources (e.g., warmth, support, guidance) while respecting their autonomy and individuality. Conflict and distress among family members tend to be mild, well-managed, and encapsulated within interparental, parent–child, and sibling relationships and are substantially outweighed by warmth, affection, and autonomy support. Thus, children in these families tend to develop along healthy psychological trajectories.

Children growing up in families with the other types of boundaries have been shown to fare significantly worse than children in cohesive families. Overly rigid, thick, and inflexible boundaries in disengaged families block access to support, protection, and other resources across family subsystems. Consequently, high levels of emotional detachment, apathy, and alienation are commonly accompanied by bouts of hostility and collectively serve to increase or maintain psychological distance between family members. As a result, children growing up in these homes evince a heightened risk for developing patterns of maladjustment characterized by high interpersonal disregard, social withdrawal, and externalizing problems (Jacobvitz, Hazen, Curran, & Hitchens, 2004; Sturge-Apple, Davies, & Cummings, 2010). In contrast, enmeshed families are characterized by weak metaphorical boundaries in families in which children's access to resources commonly comes at a price of a loss of autonomy and undue exposure to discord and turmoil. Thus, any displays of warmth and support commonly occur in a larger context of family expressions of psychological control, intrusiveness, and hostility that tend to proliferate seamlessly across individuals and relationships. By emotionally drawing or coaxing children into family difficulties, theory and research support the notion that diffuse boundaries in enmeshed families increase children's risk for anxiety, emotional distress, and interpersonal dependency (Davies et al., 2004; Jacobvitz et al., 2004; Kerig, 1995).

Likewise, triangulation in families reflects various complex blends of enmeshment and disengagement across family subsystems and individuals in which family members form defensive alliances (i.e., enmeshed component) against another individual or subsystem (i.e., disengaged component). For example, in detouring families, children's psychological symptoms progressively intensify as they serve to increase closeness between parents who are in an otherwise unhappy relationship. Conversely, the psychological burdens of serving as caretaker, confidante, or guardian in parent–child coalitions may pose its own unique set of risks for children (Johnson, 2010; Kerig, 1995).

Mechanisms of Family Risk

Further progress in understanding family processes in the development of psychopathology hinges on identifying the risk mechanisms underlying the family risk factors. Risk in family socialization pathways does not operate in an instantaneous way; rather, it is part of an unfolding cascade of mechanisms that ultimately explain why family relationship parameters are associated with child psychopathology. Thus, a pressing goal is to address the questions of how and why family risk factors increase the likelihood of child psychopathology. Within these process-oriented frameworks, exposure to family risk is conceptualized as setting in motion dynamic risk mechanisms or processes that serve as more proximal agents in the development of child psychopathology. In statistical terminology, risk mechanisms are regarded as the mediators or the intermediary, explanatory processes that link risk factors to specific child outcomes. In our account of transactions among family characteristics (see the Interdependency section), it is evident that some family factors may actually serve as risk mechanisms that mediate or explain the risk posed by another family factor. For example, coparenting and parenting difficulties have been identified as risk mechanisms that account, in part, for the association between interparental conflict and child psychopathology. However,

fully charting the risk mechanisms also requires understanding how these more proximal family risk factors engender changes in children's adaptation and coping processes that ultimately coalesce, intensify, and crystallize into more intractable patterns of child maladjustment. Contemporary work on family risk mechanisms has produced a complex, multilayered array of potential processes (e.g., Grusec & Davidov, 2010). To illustrate the value of identifying risk mechanisms, we selectively describe some of the processes that are consistently implicated in the genesis of child psychopathology (Davies, Sturge-Apple, & Martin, 2013).

Child Attachment Insecurity

Attachment theory proposes that the quality of family relationships impact children's success in maximizing sensitivity and protection of caregivers in times of distress and threat (Bowlby, 1988). Children's histories of successfully procuring supportive resources from primary caregivers are theorized to be a primary determinant of individual differences in parent–child security. Thus, displays of sensitivity, warmth, and availability by caregivers, particularly under conditions of distress, foster children's confidence in their ability to access caregivers. The end result is the very efficient operation of the attachment system characterized overtly by patterns of behavior that reflect assertive, direct bids for support and, in turn, effectively reduce fear and distress (McElwain & Booth-LaForce, 2006). In contrast, prolonged experiences with harsh, inconsistent or diminished levels of caregiver availability are key processes that undermine children's ability to reliably use parents as safe bases of security (Belsky & Fearon, 2004).

Although natural selection likely equipped children with many ways of coping with inaccessible attachment figures, specific stimuli and cues in the caregiving environment may engender different strategies for coping with insecurity. Within the attachment literature, studies have distinguished between two specific types of strategies based on whether they serve to deactivate or hyperactivate the natural output of the attachment system (Ainsworth, Blehar, Waters, & Wall, 1978). Whereas avoidant attachment styles reflect deactivating strategies for minimizing children's overt expression of negative effect, bids for support, and the processing of attachment-relevant information, resistant or ambivalent patterns of attachment are hyperactivating approaches that serve to amplify and inflate overt distress, dependency, and the processing of attachment cues (Cassidy, 2008; Kobak, Cole, Ferenz-Gillies, Fleming, & Gamble, 1993). Deactivation or avoidance is specifically regarded as an adaptive strategy for limiting exposure to the negative consequences of repeatedly approaching chronically inaccessible, rejecting caregivers. Conversely, hyperactivation of the attachment system may be a functional strategy for eliciting more reliable responsiveness and sensitivity from a caregiver who is inconsistent in supporting the child's needs (Cassidy, 2008). Patterns of insecure attachment, in turn, have been documented to be predictors of a wide array of child mental health problems (e.g., Thompson, 2008; Sroufe, Egeland, Carlson, & Collins, 2005) (see Cascade Mechanisms section for an account of how attachment insecurity may increase psychopathology).

However, risk factors for attachment insecurity may not simply be limited to parental sensitivity and support under stressful conditions. At the level of risk mechanisms, it is not uncommon for children to develop more extensive attachment hierarchies that go beyond relationships with parents. For example, children may rely on their siblings as attachment figures in many families (Ainsworth, 1989; Howes, 1999). Although the sibling attachment relationship may assume a more subsidiary role in the lives of children than the parent–child attachment relationship, the sparse studies on sibling emotional relationships suggest that children do utilize siblings as bases of security (Gass, Jenkins, & Dunn, 2007; Stewart & Marvin, 1984). However, more research is sorely needed as we still know very little about the specific family precursors and psychological sequelae of sibling attachment quality.

At the level of risk factors, researchers have expanded their search for family precursors and pathways of insecure attachment beyond the delimited set of caregiving (e.g., sensitivity responsiveness) antecedents (Davies, Harold, Goeke-Morey, & Cummings, 2002). For example, in reflecting a more indirect pathway, parental distress, preoccupation, and anger stemming from interparental conflict may ultimately impact children's attachment insecurity and psychopathology by undermining their abilities to provide sensitive and responsive care to their children. In reflecting a more direct pathway, witnessing frightening (e.g., hostile, aggressive), vulnerable (e.g., distressing, fearful), or volatile (e.g., emotionally labile) parental behaviors during interparental conflict may directly undermine children's confidence in parents as figures who can competently allay their distress. Studies using a variety of methods and designs support each of these pathways (Davies et al., 2002; Frosch, Mangelsdorf, & McHale, 2000; Sturge-Apple, Davies, Winter, Cummings, & Schermerhorn, 2008).

Child Defensive Reactivity

In complementing the primary focus of attachment theory on how children use family relationships as resources for *regaining or preserving* of security, several family process models share the assumption that family characteristics can also serve as a *source of threat* that undermine children's sense of safety and well-being (Davies & Sturge-Apple, 2007; Grych & Fincham, 1990; Repetti et al., 2011). Children's experiences as indirect bystanders or direct targets of family discord are specifically proposed to alter the ways in which children process and react behaviorally and emotionally to threat. According to the sensitization hypothesis, repeated exposure to interparental disharmony, parental rejection and hostility, and sibling conflict in high-conflict homes may progressively increase the salience of survival or self-protective strategies in subsequent family contexts and, in the process, increase children's risk for psychopathology (Davies, Sturge-Apple, et al., 2013; Monroe & Harkness, 2005). Behavioral manifestations of the heightened operation of survival or self-protective strategies include greater perceptual sensitivity to threat cues, prolonged fear, distress, and vigilance, flight and camouflaging (e.g., avoidance, inhibiting overt emotions) activities, and fight (e.g., triangulation or alliance formation) behaviors (Davies & Sturge-Apple, 2007).

Consistent with the sensitization hypothesis, studies have indicated that witnesses and targets of various forms of family hostility (e.g., interparental conflict, physical abuse) exhibit greater sensitivity and reactivity to subsequent signs of interpersonal and family adversity (Davies, Martin, et al., 2013; Shackman, Shackman, & Pollak, 2007). In further reflecting the operation of mediational pathways, these predispositions to respond in guarded, hypervigilant ways to family stressors have been empirically identified as precursors to later psychological problems (Davies, Sturge-Apple, et al., in press; Repetti et al., 2011). Although identifying the cascade of processes underpinning the pathogenic effects of defensive responding in the family remains a critical research direction, conceptual models offer promising guides in achieving this objective. For example, prolonged concerns for security would be expected to tip the balanced allocation of psychobiological resources toward investing in immediate personal safety at the cost of sufficient investment in the mastery of the physical and social environment (Davies, Sturge-Apple, et al., 2013; Ford, 2009) (see Cascade Mechanisms section for more details).

However, it is important to note that the sensitization process does not appear to be readily applicable across all developmental and family risk conditions. From a developmental standpoint, children's distress cannot increase in an incremental, graduated way following each episode of family discord over time. If sensitization operated in a uniform way across long temporal spans of family risk exposure, then children from chronically discordant homes would respond in exceedingly distressing ways to virtually every family event, be it supportive, benign, or threatening. Working from a biological framework, the stress autonomy and attenuation models postulate that sensitization to family adversity is only evident in the early stages of exposure (Monroe

& Harkness, 2005; Susman, 2006). Over long periods of time, recurrent family adversity may set in motion other mechanisms that supersede the initial risk posed by family processes. For example, in the attenuation model, the tendency of systems to maintain an internal state of equilibrium is proposed to dampen stress-sensitive physiological reactivity in the face of chronic family adversity. Inhibition of these physiological systems (e.g., sympathetic nervous system, hypothalamic–pituitary–adrenocortical axis) may reflect the activation of processes designed to thwart the toxic effects of chronic physiological arousal to threat (Susman, 2006). Social-experiential models of canalization further propose that children's patterns of adapting to risky family environments may become increasingly intractable and resistant to subsequent family influences as they increasingly select out stressful niches or evoke negative responses from others (Davies & Windle, 2001; Sroufe, 1997). Thus, the relationship between family stress and children's heightened reactivity may be curvilinear in form, reaching an asymptote that signifies progressively weaker associations between family adversity and children's defensive responses. In spite of the rich, theoretically guided hypotheses, little is known empirically about the conditions and mechanisms underlying the potential changes in sensitization over time.

Specific configurations of family risk may also result in diminished reactivity in specific domains or levels of responding. At a physiological level, the attenuation hypothesis postulates that family conflict manifested in emotional instability and unpredictability may actually dampen physiological stress responses to threatening events by disrupting the capacity of the limbic system to process and acquire information on the interpersonal consequences of emotional events in the family (Susman, 2006). Resulting difficulties in neurobiological processing of emotion and fear-relevant parameters may be particularly likely to be manifested in aggressogenic attributes such as fearlessness, sensation seeking, and callousness. At a psychological level, the reformulated emotional security theory has proposed that children may experience diminished displays of distress to family difficulties following exposure to specific patterns of family risk (Davies & Sturge-Apple, 2007). For example, tendencies to progressively inhibit feelings of fear and distress in the service of directly and aggressively engaging family threat is proposed to be an adaptive solution to coping with recurrent family conflict that is accompanied by parental displays of vulnerability (e.g., depression, anxiety), disengagement, and collapses in the family power hierarchy. Tendencies to exhibit this dominant pattern of responding to family threat, in turn, are proposed to specifically coalesce into externalizing symptoms by breeding hostile views of the social world, interpersonal disenfranchisement, callousness, and the rigid, reflexive use of aggressive behaviors.

Child Affiliative Styles

Many process models rooted in social learning and information processing theories posit that children's elevated vulnerability to psychological problems in high-conflict homes results from exposure to pathogenic learning contingencies in the family. Observational and enactive learning processes are two primary classes of learning mechanisms that are regarded as shaping children's patterns of affiliating in the family (Eron, Huesmann, & Zelli, 1991). According to the observational learning component of the theory, witnessing distraught family members (e.g., parents, siblings) provides children with opportunities to master new ways of enacting distressing behaviors through (a) imitation, (b) acquisition of generalized scripts or abstract rules, and (c) reduction of inhibitions for engaging in behaviors (Cox et al., 2001; Margolin, Oliver, & Medina, 2001). The articulation of specific vicarious (i.e., observational) learning processes generates a more precise articulation of specific linkages between risk factors, risk mechanisms, and outcomes. For example, subsequent increases in displays of anger and hostility by children in family settings are theorized to emerge through their emulation of hostile family behaviors (Hyde, Shaw, & Moilanen, 2010). In turn, increasing

tendencies to display hostility are proposed to intensify and proliferate into externalizing difficulties. Conversely, witnessing recurrent bouts of anxiety, social disengagement, and dysphoria by family members are postulated to magnify children's vulnerability to internalizing symptoms by fostering their vicarious displays of distress and social withdrawal (Morris et al., 2007).

Within the enactive component of social learning theory, reinforcement contingencies are primary mechanisms underpinning the development of psychopathology in risky family environments, particularly in the context of parental management of children's behavior (Restifo & Bogels, 2009). From a social learning perspective, perturbations in parental abilities to regulate child behavior as manifested in inadequate supervision, vague communication of expectations for appropriate child conduct, and lax, harsh, or inconsistent discipline in response to child transgressions have two major consequences. On the one hand, the lax or hostile parental behaviors do not positively reinforce children's prosocial behaviors by providing rewarding consequences for appropriate child conduct. On the other hand, these same parenting difficulties preclude the ability to dispense effective punishments that serve to impose negative consequences following bouts of child misbehavior (Patterson, 1982; Snyder, Schrepferman, McEachern, & Suarez, 2010). The resulting intensification of children's tendencies to adopt coercive, hostile styles of affiliation is, in turn, proposed to be a central risk mechanism in the development of broader behavioral problems (Forgatch, Patterson, DeGarmo, & Beldavs, 2009).

Greater dispositions to exhibit significant behavior problems among the children from high-conflict homes also substantially increase the probability of coercive parent–child exchanges that may further intensify children's behavior problems. In social learning theory, coercive process is defined as a specific set of transactional influences between parental and child behavior that create, maintain, or intensify inept parenting and child problems through reinforcement contingencies (Patterson & Yoerger, 1997; Snyder et al., 2010). In many cases, this process begins with parents responding to bouts of child complaints and mild misbehavior with threats or dismissive statements. This results in a mutually escalating cycle of negativity and hostility between parents and children. Children specifically respond to parents by "stepping up" their misbehavior and parents react to children by further intensifying their threats and negativity. Over time, however, parents in these coercive cycles trend toward capitulating to the demands of their children without enforcing any negative consequences for children (i.e., no discipline). The mutual influence of parent and child negative behaviors is theorized to result in negative reinforcement processes that spur more inept, volatile parenting behaviors and child negative behaviors in the future. Through this negative reinforcement process, the children learn that escalating tantrums and misbehavior results in the elimination of an aversive and negative stimulus in the form of parental negativity. Likewise, because abdicating power to the child during these conflicts commonly results in a reduction of child tantrums and misconduct, surrendering to the demands of the child is also negatively reinforcing to the parent. Thus, parents are postulated to be more likely to submit to children's demands in the future (Snyder, Edwards, McGraw, Kilgore, & Holton, 1994; Stoolmiller, Patterson, & Snyder, 1997).

Developmental Pluralism

Consistent with the concept of developmental pluralism, our characterization of the multiplicity of family risk factors, family risk mechanisms, and child outcomes underscores the diverse pathways children experience in the development of psychological problems. By the same token, a myopic focus on these specific pathways offers an incomplete picture of the complexity and array of children's trajectories of adjustment. To address this gap, the following sections examine three main themes in developmental psychopathology that serve as valuable tools for advancing an understanding of children's adaptation to adverse family contexts.

Cascade Mechanisms

The characterization of children's developmental trajectories does not end with the identification of family risk mechanisms as mediators of links among risky family environments. Rather, it raises a new set of questions revolving around how family risk mechanisms produce a cascade of broader processes that ultimately proliferate beyond the family unit and develop into trait-like forms of psychopathology. We refer to these intermediary processes in the pathways among risk mechanisms and children's mental health outcomes as cascade mechanisms (see Fig. 8.1). Thus, in our selective account of family risk mechanisms, attachment insecurity, defensive reactivity, and malevolent affiliative patterns in the family may serve as blueprints for cascade mechanisms that reflect specific ways of filtering, interpreting, and responding to subsequent interpersonal events outside the family. Several theoretical frameworks share the premise that the highly reflexive and automatic algorithms for processing and responding to stressful family events are later used as guides in novel or challenging settings to simplify, evaluate, and adapt to social experiences (e.g., Cassidy, 2008; Davies & Cummings, 1994; Dodge, 2006; Johnston Roseby, & Kuehnle, 2009). Consistent with this hypothesis, research has indicated that parent–child attachment insecurity predicts children's internalizing and externalizing symptoms through its association with more hostile, inflexible patterns of processing and responding to challenging peer problems (Cassidy, Kirsh, Scolton, & Parke, 1996; Dodge, 2006; Granot & Mayesless, 2012). Likewise, as a potential cascade mechanism, hostile processing of peer transgressions has been shown to mediate associations between children's negative representations of interparental relationships and increases in their school maladjustment over a 1-year period (Bascoe, Davies, Sturge-Apple, & Cummings, 2009).

Multiple-levels-of-analysis conceptualizations of developmental cascades have also stimulated new research directions in understanding the neurobiological underpinnings of linkages between family risk mechanisms and child psychopathology (Cicchetti & Walker, 2001; Mead, Beauchaine, & Shannon, 2010). Risky family environment models have posited that family risk mechanisms produce neuropsychological and psychological problems by changing stress-sensitive biological systems, including the hypothalamic-pituitary-adrenocortical (HPA) axis and the sympathetic nervous system (SNS) (Repetti et al., 2002, 2011). Through the process of allostasis, the SNS and HPA axis are designed to respond adaptively to environmental stress and challenge by generating physiological resources necessary to effectively protect individuals. In the immediate wake of stress, the SNS primes the body for fight-or-flight responses in the face of threat through increases in cardiac output, oxygen flow, and blood glucose levels (Porges, 2006). As a subsequent response to threat and challenge (Gunnar & Vazquez, 2006), the HPA axis and its end product of cortisol prime defense mechanisms by mobilizing energy (e.g., glucose, oxygen) and modulating the processing, encoding, and memory consolidation of emotionally significant events. However, successive cycles of allostasis engendered by prolonged coping with family adversity are theorized to alter the set points of the physiological systems by amplifying or attenuating their sensitivity (Repetti et al., 2011; Susman, 2006). For example, some forms of attachment insecurity have been linked with high arousal of the HPA axis (e.g., Spangler & Grossman, 1993). Likewise, research has documented that deviations in the set points of the physiological systems predict an array of difficulties in the form of emotion dysregulation, social impairments, mental health problems, immune suppression, and neurotoxicity (McEwen, 1998; Sapolsky, 2000; Turnbull & Rivier, 1999).

As a final illustration of a developmental cascade, evaluating children's mastery of stage-salient tasks may prove useful in understanding the processes whereby family risk mechanisms crystallize into psychological problems. Stage-salient tasks refer to challenges that become prominent at a given developmental period and remain important throughout the individual's lifetime (Cicchetti, 1993). Because these tasks are already challenging even under benign developmental conditions, their successful resolution may be particularly difficult in the context of family risk mechanisms. Moreover, mastery of new developmental challenges and the probability of following healthy trajectories depend, in part, on adequate differentiation and integration of prior stage-salient tasks. For example, the transition to toddlerhood is characterized by the challenges of effectively exploring the social and physical worlds, achieving a sense of mastery and autonomy, and regulating emotions (Cole, Zahn-Waxler, Fox, Usher, & Welsh, 1996; Sroufe et al., 2005). Acquiring these skills, in turn, provides important building blocks for subsequent developmental challenges of establishing self-control, self-reliance, and harmonious peer relations in preschool. Thus, children's successful negotiation of developmental tasks is posited to mediate pathways among family risk mechanisms and their psychopathology. Supporting this prediction, children's fearful reactivity to interparental conflict increased the likelihood of disruptive behavior problems during preschool by undermining their mastery of stage-salient tasks during toddlerhood (Davies, Manning, & Cicchetti, 2013).

Regulating Conditions

Even with the increasing integration of cascade mechanisms into the study of family risk, the resulting family models typically account for only modest to moderate proportions of the individual differences in children's adjustment. In some cases, children who are resilient are able to develop along adaptive developmental trajectories by successfully weathering the burdens associated with family adversity. Conversely, other children exhibit disproportionately high susceptibility to psychopathology in the context of minimal or moderate stress in the family. This observation raises a central question: Why do children who experience similar family and developmental circumstances often develop differently? As illustrated in Fig. 8.1, a primary approach to addressing this question is to identify the regulatory conditions that alter the mediational cascade of processes in associations between family adversity and child psychopathology. From a developmental psychopathology perspective, individual development is regarded as operating within an open system characterized by the ongoing transactional interplay between an actively changing organism and a dynamic context (Granic & Hollenstein, 2003). It follows, then, that developmental pathways set in motion by family risk factors will lawfully vary as a function of the broader matrix of contextual or regulatory conditions. Regulatory conditions are commonly identified as moderators that alter the magnitude or direction of family risk pathways. Although it is important to note that more fine-grained forms of moderating effects exist (Belsky & Pluess, 2009; Luthar, Cicchetti, & Becker, 2000), two of the more common classes of moderation in developmental psychopathology consist of (1) vulnerability" or "potentiating" factors that amplify links in the family risk pathways and (2) "protective" factors or buffers that reduce or offset the deleterious impact of family risk factors or mechanisms. Moreover, as Fig. 8.1 outlines, these potentiating and protective factors may be usefully organized into a diverse array of substantive domains including child dispositional attributes (e.g., temperament, personality, history of coping, gender, age), family characteristics (e.g., parent personality and psychopathology), and ecological or extrafamilial characteristics (e.g., community characteristics, culture) (Garmezy, 1985).

Although a comprehensive review of studies on the moderating conditions of family processes is beyond the scope of this chapter, even a brief sampling of the empirical work highlights the value of searching for these types of moderators in understanding heterogeneity in child outcomes. For example, within the domain of family characteristics, research has shown that the potency of some family risk factors (e.g., hostile or overprotective child-rearing) in the prediction of children's psychological problems is amplified in the context of parental psychopathology (e.g., Guimond et al., 2012). Furthermore, some family characteristics may serve multiple functions in roles as both predictors of child psychopathology and moderators of other family risk factors. For example, in models predicting children's peer adjustment, parent–child attachment security and low levels of parent–child negative reciprocity served as protective factors that offset the risk posed by marital conflict (Lindsey, Caldera, & Tankersley, 2009).

As another illustration in the domain of child attributes, children's difficult temperament has been shown to potentiate associations between several family risk factors (e.g., interparental conflict, child-rearing difficulties) and child psychopathology (Davies & Windle, 2001; Rothbart & Bates, 2006). Until recently, findings on the moderating effects of child temperament and personality were commonly interpreted within diathesis-stress models (Belsky & Pluess, 2009). Difficult temperamental characteristics were specifically designated as "diatheses" or constitutional predispositions to experience disorder that were amplified in the context of family risk factors. However, emerging evidence suggests that many of these moderating effects of difficult or reactive temperamental attributes reflect dispositions of children to exhibit greater sensitivity or plasticity to family processes for better or for worse. According to this relatively new differential susceptibility theory, children with higher levels of temperamental negative emotionality should fare significantly worse in highly discordant homes as the diathesis-stress model posits. However, unlike the diathesis-stress model, differential susceptibility models propose that children with difficult temperaments will also fare significantly better in supportive homes than children without difficult temperaments (see Belsky & Pluess, 2009). Evidence of greater sensitivity or plasticity of child characteristics has also been identified at other levels of analysis, including genetic, epigenetic, and biological functioning (Ellis, Boyce, Belsky, Bakermans-Kranenburg, & van Ijzendoorn, 2011).

Transactional Models

A complementary goal in developmental psychopathology is to better understand children's mental health and disorder as an evolving product of mutual, reciprocal influences between children and dynamic family processes over time (Sameroff, 2009). In these transactional models, the family not only influences children's adjustment but is also influenced by children's development in a continuous cycle of actions and reactions. Moreover, these transactions occur at multiple points along the cascade of family processes. First, at the level of family risk mechanisms, children's reaction patterns in family relationships reflect transactions between their own attributes and family characteristics that occur over relatively short developmental spans of minutes, days, or weeks. For example, in the Affiliative Patterns section of the chapter, children's hostile patterns of relating to parents emerge from escalating cycles of aversive dyadic exchanges that conclude with parents surrendering to stop the disciplinary bout (Patterson, 1982; Snyder et al., 2010). In applying similar negative reinforcement principles to understanding children's reactions to interparental conflict, Emery (1989) proposed a model of the transactional effects between children and the interparental subsystem. In the initial series of unfolding processes, interparental conflict is hypothesized to be an aversive event that produces distress in children. In the subsequent series of interactions, children's dysregulated expressions of distress (e.g., aggression, temper tantrums) reduce their exposure to aversive interparental stimuli by distracting parents from engaging in ongoing conflicts. In turn, children's disruptive patterns are more likely to be enacted by the child in subsequent conflicts because it reduces or eliminates the aversive stimulus (i.e., conflict).

Second, because family risk mechanisms are defined by children's adaptation in the context of specific family relationships, recurrent behaviors of children in family settings may progressively alter the dynamics of the family over longer periods of months and years. Thus, as shown in Fig. 8.1, family risk mechanisms (e.g., affiliative behaviors or defense responses) can feedback to alter family processes. For example, in a rigorous cross-lagged longitudinal design over a 2-year period, Reuter and Conger (1998) showed that hostile, erratic parenting practices were both predictors and sequelae of adolescent inflexibility and hostility during parent–child conflicts. It is important to note that the effects of risk mechanisms may also be qualitatively different across these longer developmental spans. For example, although Emery (1989) noted that disruptive behavioral reactions to interparental conflict may temporarily reduce bouts of discord between parents over the period of minutes or hours, these dysregulated reactions may take a cumulative toll on parents and their relationships over months and years. Supporting this hypothesis, research has found that children's disruptive behavioral reactions to interparental conflict predicted increases in interparental conflict 1 year later even after controlling for prior levels of interparental conflict (Schermerhorn, Cummings, DeCarlo, & Davies, 2007).

Third, at yet another level of the model in Fig. 8.1, transactional processes have also been identified between family risk dynamics and children's adjustment (e.g., psychopathology). Findings from the Child Development Project have repeatedly demonstrated bidirectional relationships between parenting and child maladjustment. In a study by Laird, Petti, Bates, and Dodge (2003), decreases in parental monitoring predicted subsequent increases in adolescent delinquency over a 1-year period. Adolescent delinquency, in turn, was associated with further decreases in parental monitoring 1 year later. In addition, another study showed that physical discipline was related to increases in externalizing behavior and greater externalizing behavior was associated with higher physical discipline over 1-year autoregressive lags (Lansford et al., 2011). Furthermore, in one of the strongest tests of transactional processes involving children and the interparental subsystem to date, Cui et al. (2007) examined the reciprocal interplay between interparental conflict and adolescent symptomatology in a series of cross-lagged autoregressive analyses across three annual measurement occasions. Consistent with transactional models, adolescent depressive and delinquency problems served as both outcomes and predictors of interparental conflict.

Conclusions

In conclusion, the growth of developmental psychopathology since the last edition of this handbook has been accompanied by significant advances in identifying the pathways among family risk factors, risk mechanisms, and children's adjustment trajectories in the broader constellation of family and ecological settings. Armed with an array of guiding concepts and principles (e.g., risk mechanisms, cascade processes, potentiating and protective frameworks), developmental psychopathologists have made considerable progress in identifying the mediating mechanisms and moderating conditions underlying the vulnerability of children from discordant homes within frameworks that consider dynamical transactional processes (e.g., Repetti et al., 2011). The end result is a level of greater acknowledgement and identification of the complexity underlying children's development that more closely approximates the open system assumptions of developmental psychopathology.

Although paying tribute to these advances is important, it is also critical to take stock of the research landscape and consider future research directions. In the spirit of moving the field forward, we assert that the scientific pendulum is swinging dangerously close to translating open system assumptions into excessively vague, expansive, and dispersive conceptual models and hypotheses. As a case in point, Thompson (2008) noted in his review of attachment that "One might wonder whether there is anything with which attachment security is *not* associated (p. 348)." As the quote implies, continuing to expand the substantive scope without conceptual checks and empirical balances runs the risk of producing unwieldy and dispersive bodies of knowledge. It does not take a huge inferential leap to conclude that a similar state of affairs exists in the study of a wider range of family risk factors, risk mechanisms, and cascade processes (e.g., Davies, Sturge-Apple, et al., 2013). Our cautionary note is that this direction, if unfettered, will make it difficult to deduce anything more than the relatively unremarkable conclusion that inherently

positive and negative experiences (or coping) will, respectively, beget healthy and unhealthy outcomes. Thus, although open system paradigms will remain critical tools in contextualizing our understanding of developmental psychopathology, we are advocating that these approaches be complemented by the formulation of models that achieve greater precision and novelty in predictions and interpretations (Richters, 1997). In closing, we hope that the next generation of research makes significant headway in formulating hypotheses, interpretations of existing findings, and heuristics for future research by increasing (a) exactness and specificity (i.e., precision) and (b) bold efforts to account for what would otherwise be unexplainable in existing scientific frames (i.e., novelty).

References

Ackerman, B. P., Kogos, J., Youngstrom, E., Schoff, K., & Izard, C. E. (1999). Family instability and the problem behaviors of children from economically disadvantaged families. *Developmental Psychology, 35*, 258–268.

Ainsworth, M. D. S. (1989). Attachments beyond infancy. *American Psychologist, 44*, 709–716.

Ainsworth, M. S., Blehar, M. C., Waters, E., & Wall, S. (1978). *Patterns of attachment: A psychological study of the strange situation*. Oxford: Lawrence Erlbaum.

Almeida, D. M., Wethington, E., & Chandler, A. L. (1999). Daily transmission of tensions between marital dyads and parent–child dyads. *Journal of Marriage & the Family, 61*, 49–61.

Amato, P. R. (2010). Research on divorce: Continuing trends and new developments. *Journal of Marriage and the Family, 3*, 650–666.

Barber, B. (1996). Parental psychological control: Revisiting a neglected construct. *Child Development, 67*, 3296–3319.

Barber, B. K., Olsen, J. E., & Shagle, S. C. (1994). Associations between parental psychological and behavioral control and youth internalized and externalized behavior. *Child Development, 65*, 1116–1132.

Bascoe, S. M., Davies, P. T., Sturge-Apple, M. L., & Cummings, E. M. (2009). Children's insecure interparental representations and school maladjustment: Children's peer information processing as an explanatory mechanism. *Developmental Psychology, 45*, 1740–1751.

Belsky, J., & Fearon, R. M. P. (2004). Exploring marriage-parenting typologies: Their contextual antecedents and developmental sequelae. *Development and Psychopathology, 16*, 501–523.

Belsky, J., & Pluess, M. (2009). Beyond diathesis stress: Differential susceptibility to environmental influences. *Psychological Bulletin, 135*, 885–908. doi:10.1037/a0017376.

Borkowski, J. G., Ramey, S., & Bristol-Power, M. (2002). *Parenting and the child's world: Influences on intellectual, academic, and social-emotional development.* Mahwah, NJ: Lawrence Erlbaum.

Bowlby, J. (1988). *A secure base: Parent–child attachment and healthy human development.* New York: Basic Books.

Branje, S. J. T., van Lieshout, C. F. M., van Aken, M. A. G., & Haselager, G. J. T. (2004). Perceived support in sibling relationships and adolescent adjustment. *Journal of Child Psychology and Psychiatry, and Allied Disciplines, 45*, 1385–1396.

Cassidy, J. (2008). The nature of the child's ties. In J. Cassidy & P. R. Shaver (Eds.), *Handbook of attachment: Theory, research, and clinical applications* (2nd ed.). New York: Guilford Press.

Cassidy, J., Kirsh, S. J., Scolton, K. L., & Parke, R. D. (1996). Attachment and representations of peer relationships. *Developmental Psychology, 32*, 892–904.

Cavanagh, S. E., & Huston, A. C. (2008). The timing of family instability and children's social development. *Journal of Marriage and Family, 5*, 1258–1270.

Cicchetti, D. (1993). Developmental psychopathology: Reactions, reflections, projections. *Developmental Review, 13*, 471–502.

Cicchetti, D., & Walker, E. F. (2001). Stress and development: Biological and psychological consequences. *Development and Psychopathology, 13*, 413–753.

Cicirelli, V. G. (1995). Sibling influence throughout the lifespan. In M. E. Lamb & B. Sutton-Smith (Eds.), *Sibling relationships: Their nature and significance across the lifespan* (pp. 267–284). Hillsdale, NJ: Lawrence Erlbaum.

Clark, K. E., & Ladd, G. W. (2000). Connectedness and autonomy support in parent–child relationships: Links to children's socioemotional orientation and peer relationships. *Developmental Psychology, 36*, 485–498.

Cole, P. M., Zahn-Waxler, C., Fox, N. A., Usher, B. A., & Welsh, J. D. (1996). Individual differences in emotion regulation and behavior problems in preschool children. *Journal of Abnormal Psychology, 105*, 518–529.

Cox, M. J., & Paley, B. (1997). Families as systems. *Annual Review of Psychology, 48*, 243–267.

Cox, M. J., Paley, B., & Harter, K. (2001). Interparental conflict and parent–child relationships. In J. Grych & F. Fincham (Eds.), *Child development and interparental conflict* (pp. 249–272). New York: Cambridge University Press.

Cui, M., Donnellan, M. B., & Conger, R. D. (2007). Reciprocal influences between parents' marital problems and adolescent internalizing and externalizing behavior. *Developmental Psychology, 43*, 1544–1552.

Cummings, E. M., & Davies, P. T. (2010). *Marital conflict and children: An emotional security perspective.* New York: Guilford Press.

Davies, P. T., & Cummings, E. M. (1994). Marital conflict and child adjustment: An emotional security hypothesis. *Psychological Bulletin, 116*, 387–411.

Davies, P. T., Cummings, E. M., & Winter, M. A. (2004). Pathways between profiles of family functioning, child security in the interparental subsystem, and child psychological problems. *Development and Psychopathology, 16*, 525–550.

Davies, P. T., Harold, G. T., Goeke-Morey, M., & Cummings, E. M. (2002). Children's emotional security and interparental conflict. *Monographs of the Society for Research in Child Development, 67*, 1–129.

Davies, P. T., Manning, L. G., & Cicchetti, D. (2013). Tracing the developmental cascade of children's insecurity in the interparental relationship: The role of stage-salient tasks. *Child Development, 84*, 297–312.

Davies, P. T., Martin, M. J., & Cicchetti, D. (2013). Delineating the sequelae of destructive and constructive interparental conflict for children within an evolutionary framework. *Developmental Psychology, 48*, 939–955.

Davies, P. T., & Sturge-Apple, M. L. (2007). Advances in the formulation of emotional security theory: An ethologically-based perspective. *Advances in Child Behavior and Development, 35*, 87–137.

Davies, P. T., Sturge-Apple, M. L., & Martin, M. J. (2013). Family discord and child health: An emotional security formulation. In A. Booth, N. Landale, & S. M. McHale (Eds.), *Families and child health* (pp. 45–74). New York: Springer.

Davies, P. T., & Windle, M. (2001). Interparental discord and adolescent adjustment trajectories: The potentiating and protective role of intrapersonal attributes. *Child Development, 72*, 1163–1178.

Dodge, K. A. (2006). Translational science in action: Hostile attributional style and the development of aggressive behavior problems. *Development and Psychopathology, 18*, 791–814.

Dunn, J. (1991). The developmental importance of siblings' experiences within the family. In K. McCartney & K. Pillemer (Eds.), *Parent–child relationships through the lifespan* (pp. 113–124). Hillsdale, NJ: Lawrence Erlbaum.

Ellis, B. J., Boyce, W. T., Belsky, J., Bakermans-Kranenburg, M. J., & van Ijzendoorn, M. H. (2011). Differential susceptibility to the environment: An evolutionary neurodevelopmental theory. *Development and Psychopathology, 23*, 7–28.

Emery, R. E. (1989). Family violence. *American Psychologist, 44*, 321–328.

Ensor, R., Marks, A., Jacobs, L., & Hughes, C. (2010). Trajectories of antisocial behaviour towards siblings predict antisocial behaviour towards peers. *Journal of Child Psychiatry and Psychology, 51*, 1208–1216.

Eron, L. D., Huesmann, L. R., & Zelli, A. (1991). The role of parental variables in the learning of aggression. In D. Pepler & K. Rubin (Eds.), *The development and treatment of childhood aggression* (pp. 169–188). Hillsdale, NJ: Lawrence Erlbaum.

Fergusson, D. M., & Horwood, L. J. (1998). Exposure to interparental violence in childhood and psychosocial adjustment in young adulthood. *Child Abuse and Neglect, 22*, 339–357.

Ford, J. D. (2009). Neurobiological and developmental research: Clinical implications. In C. A. Courtois & J. D. Ford (Eds.), *Treating complex traumatic stress disorders: An evidenced-based guide* (pp. 31–58). New York: Guildford Press.

Forgatch, M. S., Patterson, G. R., DeGarmo, D. S., & Beldavs, Z. G. (2009). Testing the Oregon delinquency model with nine-year follow-up of the Oregon divorce study. *Development and Psychopathology, 21*, 637–660.

Frosch, C. A., Mangelsdorf, S. C., & McHale, J. L. (2000). Marital behavior and the security of the preschooler–parent attachment relationships. *Journal of Family Psychology, 14*, 144–161.

Garmezy, N. (1985). Stress-resistant children: The search for protective factors. In J. E. Stevenson (Ed.), Recent research in developmental psychopathology. *Journal of Child Psychology and Psychiatry Book* (Suppl. 4, pp. 213–233). Oxford: Pergamon Press.

Gass, K., Jenkins, J., & Dunn, J. (2007). Are sibling relationships protective? A longitudinal study. *Journal of Child Psychology and Psychiatry, 48*, 167–175.

Gerard, J. M., Krishnakumar, A., & Buehler, C. (2006). Marital conflict, parent–child relations, and youth maladjustment: A longitudinal investigation of spillover effects. *Journal of Family Issues, 27*, 951–975.

Granic, I., & Hollenstein, T. (2003). Dynamic systems methods for models of developmental psychopathology. *Development and Psychopathology, 15*, 641–669.

Granot, D. & Mayseless, O. (2012). Representations of mother-child attachment relationships and social information processing of peer relationships in early adolescence. *Journal of Early Adolescence, 32*, 537–564.

Gray, M., & Steinberg, L. (1999). Unpacking authoritative parenting: Reassessing a multidimensional construct. *Journal of Marriage and the Family, 61*, 574–587.

Grusec, J. E., & Davidov, M. (2010). Integrating different perspectives on socialization theory and research: A domain-specific approach. *Child Development, 81*, 687–709.

Grych, J. H., & Fincham, F. D. (1990). Marital conflict and children's adjustment: A cognitive-contextual framework. *Psychological Bulletin, 108*, 267–290.

Grych, J. H., & Fincham, F. D. (2001). Interparental conflict and child adjustment: An overview. In J. H. Grych & F. D. Fincham (Eds.), *Interparental conflict and child development: Theory, research, and application* (pp. 1–6). New York: Cambridge University Press.

Guimond, F. A., Brendgen, M., Forget-Dubois, N., Dionne, G., Vitaro, F., Tremblay, R. E., et al. (2012). Associations of mother's and father's parenting practices with children's observed social reticence in a competitive situation: A monozygotic twin difference study. *Journal of Abnormal Child Psychology, 40*, 391–402.

Gunnar, M., & Vazquez, D. (2006). Stress neurobiology and developmental psychopathology. In D. Cicchetti & D. Cohen (Eds.), *Developmental psychopathology: Developmental neuroscience* (pp. 533–577). New York: Wiley.

Hoeve, M., Dubas, J. S., Eichelsheim, V. I., Van der Laan, P. H., Smeenk, W. H., & Gerris, J. R. M. (2009). The relationship between parenting and delinquency: A meta-analysis. *Journal of Abnormal Child Psychology, 37*, 749–775.

Howes, C. (1999). Attachment relationships in the context of multiple caregivers. In J. Cassidy & P. R. Shaver (Eds.), *Handbook of attachment: Theory, research, and clinical applications* (pp. 671–687). New York: Guilford Press.

Hyde, L. W., Shaw, D. S., & Moilanen, K. (2010). Developmental precursors of moral disengagement and the role of moral disengagement in the development of antisocial behavior. *Journal of Abnormal Child Psychology, 38*, 197–209.

Jacobvitz, D., Hazen, N., Curran, M., & Hitchens, K. (2004). Observations of triadic family interactions: Boundary disturbances in the family predict depressive, anxious, and ADHD symptoms in middle childhood. *Development and Psychopathology, 16*, 577–592.

Jenkins, J. M. (1992). Sibling relationships in disharmonious homes. In F. Boer & J. Dunn (Eds.), *Sibling relationships: Developmental and clinical issues*. Hove: Lawrence Erlbaum.

Johnson, V. K. (2010). Marital interaction, family organization, and differences in parenting behavior: Explaining variations across family interaction contexts. *Family Relations, 59*, 313–325.

Johnston, J., Roseby, V., & Kuehnle, K. (2009). *In the Name of the Child*. New York: Springer.

Jouriles, E. N., & Farris, A. M. (1992). Effects of marital conflict on subsequent parent-son interactions. *Behavior Therapy, 23*, 355–374.

Jouriles, E. N., Murphy, C., Farris, A. M., Smith, D. A., Richters, J. E., & Waters, E. (1991). Marital adjustment, childrearing disagreements, and child behavior problems: Increasing the specificity of the marital assessment. *Child Development, 62*, 1424–1433.

Katz, L. F., & Low, S. M. (2004). Marital violence, coparenting and family-level processes, and children's adjustment. *Journal of Family Psychology, 18*, 372–382.

Kerig, P. K. (1995). Triangles in the family circle: Effects of family structure on marriage, parenting, and child adjustment. *Journal of Family Psychology, 9*, 28–43.

Kobak, R. R., Cole, H. E., Ferenz-Gillies, R., Fleming, W. S., & Gamble, W. (1993). Attachment and emotion regulation during mother-teen problem solving: A control theory analysis. *Child Development, 64*, 231–245.

Kretchmar, M. D., & Jacobvitz, D. B. (2002). Observing mother-child relationships across generations: Boundary patterns, attachment, and the transmission of caregiving. *Family Process, 41*, 351–374.

Laird, R. D., Petit, G. S., Bates, J. E., & Dodge, K. A. (2003). Parents' monitoring-relevant knowledge and adolescents' delinquent behavior: Evidence of correlated developmental changes and reciprocal influences. *Child Development, 74*, 752–768.

Lamborn, S. D., Mounts, N. S., Steinberg, L., & Dornbusch, S. M. (1991). Patterns of competence and adjustment among adolescents from authoritative, authoritarian, indulgent, and neglectful families. *Child Development, 62*, 1049–1065.

Lansford, J. E., Criss, M. M., Laird, R. D., Shaw, D. S., Pettit, G. S., Bates, J. E., et al. (2011). Reciprocal relations between parents' physical discipline and children's externalizing behavior during middle childhood and adolescence. *Development and Psychopathology, 23*, 225–238.

Lindsey, E. W., Calder, Y. M., & Tankersley, L. (2009). Marital conflcit and the quality of young children's peer play behavior: The mediating and moderating role of parent-child emotional reciprocity and attachment security. *Journal of Family Psychology, 23*, 130–145.

Luthar, S. S., Cicchetti, D., & Becker, B. (2000). The construct of resilience: A critical evaluation and guidelines for future work. *Child Development, 71*, 543–562.

Luyckx, K., Tildesley, E. A., Soenens, B., Andrews, J. A., Hampson, S. E., Peterson, M., et al. (2011). Parenting and trajectories of children's maladaptive behaviors: A 12-year prospective community study. *Journal of Clinical Child and Adolescent Psychology, 40*, 468–478.

Maccoby, E. E., & Martin, J. A. (1983). Socialization in the context of the family: Parent–child interaction. In P. H. Mussen (Series Ed.) & E. M. Hetherington (Vol. Ed.), *Handbook of child psychology: Vol 4. Socialization, personality, and social development* (4th ed., pp. 1–101). New York: Wiley.

Margolin, G., Oliver, P., & Medina, A. (2001). Conceptual issues in understanding the relation between interparental conflict and child adjustment: Integrating developmental psychopathology and risk/resilience perspectives. In J. Grych & F. Fincham (Eds.), *Child development and interparental conflict* (pp. 9–38). New York: Cambridge University Press.

Marvin, R. S., & Stewart, R. B. (1990). A family systems framework for the study of attachment. In M. Greenberg, D. Cicchetti, & E. M. Cummings (Eds.), *Attachment in the preschool years: Theory, research, and intervention* (pp. 51–86). Chicago: University of Chicago.

McCoy, K., Cummings, E. M., & Davies, P. T. (2009). Constructive and destructive marital conflict, emotional security, and children's prosocial behavior. *Journal of Child Psychology and Psychiatry, 50*, 270–279.

McElwain, N. L., & Booth-LaForce, C. (2006). Maternal sensitivity to infant distress and nondistress as predictors of infant-mother attachment security. *Journal of Family Psychology, 20*, 247–255.

McEwen, B. S. (1998). Stress, adaptation, and disease: Allostasis and allostatic load. In S. McCann & J. M. Lipton (Eds.), *Annals of the New York Academy of Sciences. Neuroimmunomodulation: Molecular aspects, integrative systems, and clinical advances* (Vol. 840, pp. 33–44). New York: New York Academy of Sciences.

McHale, J. P. (2007). When infants grow up in multiperson relationship systems. *Infant Mental Health Journal, 28*, 370–392.

McHale, S. M., & Crouter, A. C. (1996). The family contexts of children's sibling relationships. In G. H. Brody (Ed.), *Sibling relationships: Their causes and consequences* (pp. 173–195). Westport, CT: Ablex.

McHale, J., & Fivaz-Depeursinge, E. (1999). Understanding triadic and family group process during infancy and early childhood. *Clinical Child and Family Psychology Review, 2*, 107–127.

McHale, J. P., & Rasmussen, J. L. (1998). Coparental and family group-level dynamics during infancy: Early family precursors of child and family functioning during preschool. *Development & Psychopathology, 10*, 39–59.

McLeod, B. D., Weisz, J. R., & Wood, J. J. (2007). Examining the association between parenting and childhood depression: A meta-analysis. *Clinical Psychology Review, 27*, 986–1003.

Mead, H. K., Beauchaine, T. P., & Shannon, K. E. (2010). Neurobiological adaptations to violence across development. *Development and Psychopathology, 22*, 1–22.

Milevsky, A., & Levitt, M. J. (2005). Sibling support in early adolescence: Buffering and compensation across relationships. *European Journal of Developmental Psychology, 2*, 299–320.

Minuchin, S. (1974). *Families and family therapy.* Cambridge, MA: Harvard University Press.

Minuchin, P. (1985). Families and individual development: Provocations from the field of family therapy. *Child Development, 56*, 289–302.

Monroe, S. M., & Harkness, K. L. (2005). Life stress, the "kindling" hypothesis, and the recurrence of depression: Considerations from a life stress perspective. *Psychological Review, 112*, 417–445.

Morris, A. S., Silk, J. S., Steinberg, L., Myers, S. S., & Robinson, L. R. (2007). The role of the family context in the development of emotion regulation. *Social Development, 16*, 361–388.

Paley, B., O'Connor, M. J., Kogan, N., & Findlay, R. (2005). Prenatal alcohol exposure, child externalizing behavior, and maternal stress. *Parenting: Science and Practice, 5*, 29–56.

Patterson, G. R. (1982). *Coercive family process.* Eugene, OR: Castalia Press.

Patterson, G. R., & Yoerger, K. (1997). A developmental model for late-onset delinquency. In D. W. Osgood (Ed.), *Motivation and delinquency* (pp. 119–177). Lincoln, NE: University of Nebraska Press.

Porges, S. W. (2006). Asserting the role of biobehavioral sciences in translational research: The behavioral neurobiology revolution. *Developmental Psychopathology, 18*, 923–933.

Repetti, R. L., Taylor, S. E., & Seeman, T. E. (2002). Risky families: Family social environments and the mental and physical health of offspring. *Psychological Bulletin, 128*, 330–366.

Repetti, R. S., Robles, T. F., & Reynolds, B. R. (2011). Allostatic processes in the family. *Development and Psychopathology, 23*, 921–938.

Restifo, K., & Bogels, S. (2009). Family processes in the development of youth depression: Translating the evidence to treatment. *Clinical Psychology Review, 4*, 294–316.

Reuter, M., & Conger, R. (1998). Reciprocal influences between parenting and adolescent problem-solving behavior. *Developmental Psychology, 34*, 1470–1482.

Richters, J. E. (1997). Toward a developmental perspective on conduct disorder. *Development and Psychopathology, 9*, 193–229.

Rothbart, M. K., & Bates, J. E. (2006). Temperament. In N. Eisenberg & W. Damon (Eds.), *Social, emotional, and personality development: Handbook of child psychology, Vol. 3* (5th ed., pp. 105–176). New York: Wiley.

Sameroff, A. J. (2009). Conceptual issues in studying the development of self-regulation. In S. L. Olson & A. J. Sameroff (Eds.), *Regulatory processes in the development of behavior problems: Biological, behavioral, and social-ecological perspectives.* Cambridge: Cambridge University Press.

Sapolsky, R. M. (2000). The possibility of neurotoxicity in the hippocampus in major depression: A primer on neuron death. *Biological Psychiatry, 48*, 755–765.

Schermerhorn, A. C., Cummings, E. M., DeCarlo, C. A., & Davies, P. T. (2007). Children's influence in the marital relationship. *Journal of Family Psychology, 21*, 259–269.

Schoppe-Sullivan, S. J., Mangelsdorf, S. C., Frosch, C. A., & McHale, J. L. (2004). Associations between coparenting and marital behaviors from infancy to the preschool years. *Journal of Family Psychology, 18*, 194–207.

Shackman, J. E., Shackman, A. J., & Pollak, S. D. (2007). Physical abuse amplifies attention to threat and increases anxiety in children. *Emotion, 7*, 838–852.

Snyder, J., Edwards, P., McGraw, K., Kilgore, K., & Holton, A. (1994). Escalation and reinforcement in mother-child conflict: Social processes associated with the development of physical aggression. *Development and Psychopathology, 6*, 305–321.

Spangler, G., & Grossman, K. E., (1993). Biobehavioral organization in securely and insecurely attached infants. *Child Development, 64*, 1439–1450.

Snyder, J., Schrepferman, L., McEachern, A., & Suarez, M. (2010). Early covert conduct problems: Phenomenology, prevalence, cross-setting diffusion, growth and consequences. *Journal of Behavior Analysis Offender and Victim: Treatment and Prevention, 2*, 4–19.

Sroufe, L. A. (1997). Psychopathology as an outcome of development. *Development and Psychopathology, 9*, 251–268.

Sroufe, L. A., Egeland, B., Carlson, E., & Collins, W. A. (2005). *The development of the person: The Minnesota study of risk and adaptation from birth to adulthood.* New York: Guilford Publications.

Steinberg, L., & Silk, J. (2002). Parenting adolescents. In M. Bornstein (Ed.), *Handbook of parenting: Volume 1: Children and parenting* (pp. 103–133). Mahwah, NJ: Lawrence Erlbaum.

Stewart, R. B., & Marvin, R. S. (1984). Sibling relations: The role of conceptual perspective-taking in the ontogeny of sibling caregiving. *Child Development, 55*, 1322–1332.

Stocker, C. M. (1994). Children's perceptions of relationships with siblings, friends, and mothers: Compensatory processes and links with adjustment. *Journal of Child Psychology and Psychiatry, 8*, 1447–1459.

Stoolmiller, M., Patterson, G. R., & Snyder, J. (1997). Parental discipline and child antisocial behavior: A contingency-based theory and some methodological refinements. *Psychological Inquiry, 3*, 223–229.

Stormshak, E. A., Bellanti, C. J., & Bierman, K. L. (1996). The quality of sibling relationships and the development of social competence and behavioral control in aggressive children. *Developmental Psychology, 32*, 79–89.

Sturge-Apple, M. L., Davies, P. T., & Cummings, E. M. (2006a). The impact of interparental hostility and withdrawal on parental emotional unavailability and children's adjustment difficulties. *Child Development, 77*, 1623–1641.

Sturge-Apple, M. L., Davies, P. T., & Cummings, E. M. (2006b). Hostility and withdrawal in marital conflict: Effects on parental emotional unavailability and inconsistent discipline. *Journal of Family Psychology, 20*, 227–238.

Sturge-Apple, M. L., Davies, P. T., & Cummings, E. M. (2010). Typologies of family functioning: Implications for children's adjustment during the early school years. *Child Development, 81*, 1320–1335.

Sturge-Apple, M. L., Davies, P. T., Winter, M. A., Cummings, E. M., & Schermerhorn, A. (2008). Interparental conflict and children's school adjustment: The explanatory role of children's internal representations of interparental and parent–child relationships. *Developmental Psychology, 44*, 1678–1690.

Susman, E. J. (2006). Psychobiology of persistent antisocial behavior: Stress, early vulnerabilities, and the attenuation hypothesis. *Neuroscience and Biobehavioral Reviews, 30*, 376–389.

Thompson, R. A. (2008). Early attachment and later development: Familiar questions, new answers. In J. Cassidy & P. R. Shaver (Eds.), *Handbook of attachment: Theory, research, and clinical applications* (2nd ed., pp. 348–365). New York: Guilford Press.

Turnbull, A. V., & Rivier, C. L. (1999). Regulation of the hypothalamic-pituitary-adrenal axis by cytokines: Actions and mechanisms of action. *Physiological Reviews, 79*, 1–71.

Schooling and the Mental Health of Children and Adolescents in the United States

9

Robert W. Roeser and Jacquelynne S. Eccles

Schools are a central cultural context of child and adolescent development. Children spend more time in schools than in any other context outside their homes (Eccles & Roeser, 2010, 2011). Success in school is associated with both current mental health status and future life opportunities (NAS, 2006; NCES, 2006). Yet research shows that not everyone in the USA either thrives in or completes K–12 schooling. Poor children (a disproportionately high percentage of whom are African-, Mexican-, and Native American), as well as those with significant emotional/behavioral problems (Kessler, Foster, Saunders & Stang, 1995), are much less likely to complete high school or enroll in and graduate from college (Aud, KewalRamani, & Frohlich, 2011). This leaves many young people unprepared to participate and prosper fully in the changing US economy (Duncan & Murane, 2011). In addition, many children, particularly but not only those living in poverty, come to school unprepared to deal with the demands of schooling and with unmet health and mental health needs (Adelman & Taylor,

2009; Greenberg et al., 2003). Lack of readiness and untreated problems can contribute to academic failure at school and growing social and behavioral problems across the school years.

Under the right circumstances, schools and teachers can help two broad categories of children and adolescents to learn and thrive emotionally and socially at school: those who are or have been exposed to multiple developmental risks outside of school, and those who are exposed to new developmental risks at school because they either have great difficulty mastering the curriculum or experience social difficulties with peers. To address the needs of these two broad categories of students, schools today offer both targeted intervention services for vulnerable children, adolescents, and their families (Christener, Mennuti, & Whitaker, 2009), as well as school-wide reforms and universal prevention programs aimed at cultivating academic and social-emotional skills and prosocial behavior among all students (Hawkins et al., 2008; Zins, Weissberg, Wang, & Walberg, 2004).

In this chapter, we discuss schooling in relation to the mental health of children and adolescents using a developmental systems framework. The chapter is divided into four main sections. First, we describe the demographic characteristics of the current US school-aged population, the educational progress and problems characteristic of this population, and the fact that poverty disproportionately affects different racial/ethnic groups in the school-aged population in ways that

R.W. Roeser, Ph.D. (✉)
Department of Psychology, Portland State University,
Portland, OR 97207, USA
e-mail: rroeser@pdx.edu

J.S. Eccles, Ph.D.
School of Education, University of California,
Irvine, CA 92697-5500, USA

M. Lewis and K.D. Rudolph (eds.), *Handbook of Developmental Psychopathology*,
DOI 10.1007/978-1-4614-9608-3_9, © Springer Science+Business Media New York 2014

create and exacerbate gaps in school readiness and mental health before children even begin schooling (Duncan & Murane, 2011). We document the prevalence, co-occurrence, and reciprocal influence of physical, social-emotional, and academic development among the school-aged population. We discuss how school-based mental health efforts can comprise an integral part of a national investment strategy in human health and development that targets poor children and their families, begins early, and is part of an ongoing system of investments that stretch from cradle to career (Heckman, 2007). Second, we describe malleable self-system factors associated with co-occurring patterns of emotional/ behavioral and academic problems in school-aged children and youth, including (1) self-regulatory processes (e.g., executive function and emotion regulation), (2) self-representations (e.g., autobiographical self-narrative), and (3) social-cognitive processes (e.g., empathy and perspective-taking). We propose these malleable factors are key *psychological targets* of school-based interventions and prevention programs aimed at students' mental health (Roeser, Peck, & Nasir, 2006). Third, we outline four roles that elementary and secondary schools can play in the social-emotional development of students and their families, including crisis intervention, service provision, use of social-emotional learning programs, and school-wide reform. In this section, we conceptualize schools as multilevel contexts of human development that can be designed to run in ways that foster children's and adolescents' healthy social-emotional development and, at the same time, prevent emotional/ behavioral problems from arising or worsening by fostering students' belonging in and bonding to the aims of the school (Catalano, Haggerty, Oesterle, Fleming, & Hawkins, 2004). Fourth, we highlight several malleable school system factors associated with the prevention of problems and the cultivation of social-emotional learning and prosocial behavior that represent key *ecological targets* of school reform efforts aimed at improving students' academic success and mental health.

Characteristics of the US School Population

Demographic Characteristics of US School Population

There are approximately 49 million school-aged children and adolescents (ages 5–18 years) in the USA today (Sable & Garofano, 2007). One in five in this population is either the child of recent immigrants or an immigrant himself/herself (Garcia, Jensen, & Cuellar, 2006) and speaks a language other than English (most frequently Spanish) in their homes (NCES, 2006). Overall, the school-aged population today is approximately 57 % European-American, 20 % Latin- American, 17 % African-American, 5 % Asian-American/ Pacific Islander, and 1 % Native American/ American Indian (Sable & Garofano, 2007).

Educational Characteristics of US School Population

By the 12th grade, African-American and Latino students are, on average, approximately 4 years behind Asian- and European-American students in school achievement (NCES, 2006). In addition, dropout rates in 2010 were highest among Latin Americans (15%), Native Americans/ Native Alaskans (12%), and African-Americans (8%) and lowest among European (5%) and Asian-Americans (4%) (Aud et al., 2011). The dropout rate of immigrant Mexicans and their children is particularly high and troubling given the size of this population of students (Slavin & Calderon, 2001) and reflects the effects of diverse factors, including poverty, under--resourced schools, discrimination, early childbearing among females, the need to work to support one's family, and long-standing difficulties in school (Lopez, 2009). Mexican-American youth are also the least likely to attend college, as well as the most likely to attend 2-year community colleges rather than 4-year undergraduate colleges (Slavin & Calderon, 2001). By age 25 years, approximately

32% of Asian-Americans/Pacific Islanders, 20% of European-Americans, 13% of African-Americans, 9% of Latin Americans, and 10% of Native Americans/Alaskan Natives have attained a 4-year college degree (Aud et al., 2011).

Poverty and Achievement Gaps in US School Population

The cumulative stress of poverty exerts significant detrimental influences on children's health, mental health, and readiness to learn in school—contributing to achievement gaps during elementary and secondary school (Blair & Diamond, 2008; Gunnar & Quevedo, 2007). Poor children begin kindergarten 2 or more years behind their classmates academically, and these differences persist or increase over time due to various ecological risk factors in neighborhoods, school, and families (Ramey & Ramey, 2004). The precursors to later achievement gaps between Asian- and European-Americans and their African-, Latin- and Native American peers begin before school entry and differences in achievement between Asian-and European-American students and their African-, Latin- and Native-American counterparts are at least partially a function of greater poverty rates (and associated ecological risk factors) among the latter groups (Duncan & Murane, 2011; Sameroff, Seifer, Baldwin & Baldwin, 1993). Over 33% of Latin-American and between 25 and 33% of all African- and Native American/Native Alaskan students grow up in poverty (NCES, 2006).

Physical Health Problems in the US School Population

Chronic health problems in the US school population are now quite prevalent, especially among those living in poverty. Low-income students, including disproportionate numbers of African-, Latin, and Native Americans, are at greater risk for dental, health, and mental health issues and are less likely to receive services for such issues compared to their Asian- and European-American counterparts (Flores & Tomany-Korman, 2008). Health problems in the school population include those associated with breathing (e.g., asthma; Akinbami, Moorman, Garbe, & Sondik, 2009), eating (e.g., obesity; Datar, Sturm, & Magnabosco, 2004), and sleeping (e.g., fatigue; Stein, Mendelsohn, Obermeyer, Amronmin, & Benca, 2001)—all of which are negatively associated with school attendance, attention, and engagement and learning. It was estimated that school children with asthma, for instance, collectively missed about 10.5 million days of school due to their illness in 2008 (Akinbami, Moorman, & Liu, 2011). Young people today also report considerably higher levels of daily stress than members of older generations (Pew Research, 2010)—yet another health problem that can undermine school learning and emotional well-being (Blair & Diamond, 2008).

Mental Health Problems in the US School Population

Approximately 25 % of the US school population is characterized by mental health problems that impair students' daily functioning in and out of school (Costello, Copeland, & Angold, 2011; Merikangas et al., 2010). Many never receive services for these problems in or outside the schools (Adelman & Taylor, 2009). Fiscally, the costs of these problems are enormous: The "annual quantifiable cost of such disorders among young people was estimated in 2007 to be $247 billion" (Institute of Medicine, 2009, p. 1).

Internalizing problems. The median ages of onset for anxiety and depression are 6 and 13 years of age, respectively (Merikangas et al., 2010), with girls showing more internalizing problems than boys beginning in early adolescence (Garber, 2006). Internalizing problems are associated with poorer school functioning and peer difficulties during both childhood and adolescence (Nolen-Hoeksema, Girgus, & Seligman, 1986; Roeser, Strobel, & Quihuis, 2002). A pessimistic or helpless explanatory style is hypothesized to be a central feature of co-occurring internalizing and school/achievement-related problems in childhood and adolescence (Dweck, 2008; Joiner & Wagner, 1995; Roeser et al., 2006).

Across both childhood and adolescence, males are more likely than females to manifest externalizing problems (Merikangas et al., 2010). The predictive relation between externalizing problems in childhood, especially those involving inattention and school failure, and school withdrawal later during adolescence, is well-documented (Cairns, Cairns, & Neckerman, 1989; Hinshaw, 1992). Males are more likely to have co-occurring school, peer, and externalizing problems than females (Merikangas et al., 2010). Rejection sensitive and hostile attributional styles may underlie co-occurring externalizing and school/achievement-related problems (Dodge, 2006; Fontaine, 2010).

Violence is a prevalent form of externalizing problem in US schools. In 2009–2010, approximately 75% of US public schools recorded one or more incidents of violent crime (rape, physical attack, robbery) and approximately 33% of students in grades 9–12 reported "being in a physical fight during the past year" (Robers, Zhang, & Truman, 2012). Physical fights and fears of physical attack peak after the transition to secondary school and decline thereafter (Robers et al., 2012). Bullying (repeated, aggressive behavior intended to harm or disturb a person or group who is less powerful) is also prevalent in US schools (Nansel et al., 2001). Bullying includes physical threats and harm, name-calling, teasing, spreading of rumors, social rejection, and theft of personal property. It can occur either face to face or online. In a nationally representative study of US students in grades 6–10, 31% reported moderate to frequent bullying and 4% reported being cyberbullied at or outside of school (NCES, 2011). Bullying (as both a perpetrator and a target) is more prevalent among males than females (Nansel et al., 2001). Lesbian, gay, bisexual, and transgender (LGBT) adolescents are at particular risk for homophobic forms of bullying. Among self-identified LGBT youth, adolescent males, adolescents who attend rural schools in isolated communities, and younger adolescents are at greatest risk of exposure to homophobic language or other forms of victimization in school (Russell, Seif, &Truong, 2001). Frequent exposure to bullying is a risk factor for depression, suicidal ideation and attempts, and diminished academic achievement among heterosexual and LGBT youth, especially gay males (King et al., 2008; Poteat & Espelage, 2007; Swearer, Espelage, Vaillancourt, & Hymel, 2010). Bullies do worse in school and engage in more problem behavior (drinking, smoking) than their non-bully peers (Nansel et al., 2001). Bullying, like other forms of school violence, peaks after the transition to secondary school and declines thereafter (Neiman, 2011). Clearly, the transition to secondary school is a key time for school violence prevention efforts.

Co-occurring Patterns of Problems in US School Population

Internalizing and externalizing problems co-occur with each other (Merikangas et al., 2010) and with academic problems in a substantial minority (25%) of the US school population. In an effort to bring together research on mental health and school problems among the US school population, we have proposed the existence of at least three patterns of academic and emotional/behavioral functioning (Roeser & Eccles, 2000). The first pattern is characterized by an academically helpless classroom motivational style (i.e., worry, anxiety, and internalizing blame for school failure), achievement and social difficulties with peers (loneliness, neglect), and internalizing emotional/behavioral problems. The second pattern is characterized by an academically helplessness and defiant motivational style (anger, frustration, and externalizing blame for school failure), achievement and social difficulties with peers (aggression, rejection), and externalizing emotional/behavioral problems. The third and most adaptive pattern is that of educational resilience characterized by a mastery-oriented, malleability-focused classroom motivational style despite internalizing and/or externalizing problems (Aunola, Stattin, & Nurmi, 2000; Lau & Roeser, 2007; Roeser, Eccles, & Sameroff, 2000; Roeser et al., 2002). These three hypothesized subgroups closely resemble the three personality types described as "over-controllers," "under-controllers," and "resilients," respectively (Asendorpf, Borkenau, Ostendorf, & van Aken, 2001; Block & Block, 1980; Rammstedt, Riemann, Angleitner, & Borkenau, 2004; Robins, John, Caspi, Moffitt, & Stouthamer-Loeber, 1996).

Of particular interest are students who manifest *educational resilience*—school success despite significant emotional/behavioral problems and exposure to developmental risks (Becker & Luthar, 2002; Roeser et al., 2006). Roeser and Peck (2003) examined unexpected processes of educational resilience (defined as enrollment in college after completion of high school) among young people who faced exposure to multiple personal and family, school, and peer risks in early adolescence. Results showed that participation in positive out-of-school activities during high school was a key factor predicting which at-risk youth completed high school and enrolled in college by age 25. In follow-up studies, results showed that educational resilience among these at-risk youth was predicted by specific kinds of structured after-school activities, those that bonded high-risk adolescents to their school (e.g., athletics), church (e.g., volunteering), or other community-based institutions (Peck, Roeser, Zarrett, & Eccles, 2008). By age 30, results showed it was a combination of such bonding activities in high school and greater self-regulation during early adulthood that predicted which high-risk individuals graduated from a 4-year college by age 30 (Peck, Malanchuk, Roeser, & Eccles, 2012). This work highlights the important roles of self-regulation (Moffitt et al., 2011) and community settings and other extracurricular activities that foster self-regulation in promoting *educational resilience* among high-risk children and adolescents (Eccles & Gootman, 2002; McLaughlin, 2000). It may prove beneficial for future research to focus on co-occurring patterns of risk and resilience across the domains of physical health, mental health, and school functioning in different subgroups of students. This work could inform the next generation of school-based programs by accurately targeting maladaptive processes and fostering protective factors among students facing developmental risks (Becker & Luthar, 2002).

Malleable Psychological Processes

Advances have been achieved in identifying key psychological self-system processes associated with co-occurring patterns of academic, social, and emotional/behavioral functioning such as those just described. Such processes represent key psychological targets of school-based mental health programs (Roeser et al., 2006; Snow, Corno, & Jackson, 1996). Here we describe three key domains of such processes characteristic of the self-system, including (a) self-regulation or executive function; (b) self-representation; and (c) social cognition. We briefly discuss how each domain is relevant to students' academic and social-emotional development and cite basic evidence suggesting such processes are amenable to intervention.

Self-Regulation

The domain of self-regulation (SR) refers to individual factors such as self-awareness, self-control, resilience following setbacks, resisting temptations, cognitive flexibility, planning, and meta-cognition related to learning. SR is heavily implicated in academic and social-emotional competence across development (Blair & Razza, 2007). Individual differences in SR early in life predict subsequent differences in school readiness, mastery of basic literacy and numeracy skills, and externalizing behavior problems in childhood (Blair & Razza, 2007), academic and social-emotional problems in adolescence (Cairns et al., 1989), and physical health, economic security, and social functioning in adulthood (Moffitt et al., 2011). In a recent review in *Science* on interventions designed to cultivate executive functioning (EF) across development, Diamond and Lee (2011) concluded that diverse activities can be used to improve children's executive functioning, including computerized training, non-computerized games, aerobics, martial arts, yoga, mindfulness, and school curricula. Central to all of these activities is repeated practice with intrinsically motivating, increasingly challenging tasks. Diamond and Lee (2011) suggest that in efforts to improve executive functions, "focusing narrowly on them may not be as effective as also addressing emotional and social development (as do curricula that improve executive functions) and physical development (shown by positive effects of aerobics, martial arts, and yoga)." These ways of fostering EF may be especially important for children whose out-of-school environments are stressful, chaotic, and less likely to be characterized by structured out-of-school opportunities for physical, social, and emotional development (Grantham-McGregor et al., 2007). Results from randomized trials have shown that social-emotional learning programs such as the PATHS curriculum are effective ways that schools can cultivate SR in students (Greenberg et al., 2003). In addition, research shows that when teachers impart self-regulatory strategies to students that they can use to learn content more effectively, especially strategies involving meta-cognition (e.g., asking oneself if one understands what one is reading while reading to monitor comprehension) and planning (e.g., setting aside a specific time in a quiet space for homework), they learn more effectively (Hattie, Biggs, & Purdie, 1996).

Self-Representation

Psychological representations of self in terms of perceived competence and worth, attributional styles for personally relevant events, and goals are also implicated in patterns of academic and emotional/behavioral risk and resilience (Wigfield, Eccles, Roeser, & Schiefele, 2008). Self representations and attributional styles represent a second domain that can be positively influenced through school-based prevention, intervention, and health promotion efforts (Dweck & London, 2004). Students' self-perceived academic competence, for instance, interacts reciprocally and negatively with depressive symptoms (Roeser et al., 2000; Uhrlass, Schofield, Coles, & Gibb, 2009). Educational and developmental research has confirmed the following key determinants of school engagement and disengagement, as well as mentally healthy responses to school failure and academic difficulties: (1) attributional processes concerning the causes of success and failure at school, (2) belief in one's (or lack of) ability to influence academic competence

and intelligence, (3) valuing of different subjects, and (4) mastery goal orientation when learning in the classroom. After controlling for students' cognitive ability, the more students believe that they are academically competent and can develop their abilities or intelligence through effort (e.g., Bandura, 1997; Dweck, 2008), and the more students attribute the causes of academic difficulty to malleable factors rather than to an internal stable deficit in ability or intelligence (Graham, 1997), the more likely they are to approach, persist at, and master academic tasks and persist through difficulties. Similarly, the more students find an academic subject intrinsically interesting and important with respect to other goals or values, the more likely they are to invest in learning the subject, to choose related courses and activities in the future, and to stay engaged in school, even if they otherwise show elevated levels of distress (Wigfield et al., 2008). Finally, the more that students pursue goals of mastery and self-improvement, in contrast to pursuing goals such as trying to demonstrate one's superior relative ability or hide one's perceived relative inability, the more resilient they are in the face of inevitable academic setbacks (Meece, Anderman, & Anderman, 2005). These phenomena representational processes underlying co-occurring academic and emotional/behavioral problems and educational resilience despite emotional/behavioral problems (Roeser & Eccles, 2000).

Blackwell and colleagues showed that early adolescent students randomly assigned to a condition in which they were taught about the malleability of intelligence showed positive change in classroom motivation and less of a decline in grades after the transition to secondary school compared to controls (Blackwell, Trzesniewski, & Dweck, 2007). Similarly, in intervention studies aimed at reducing the detrimental effects of stereotype threats on the achievement of African-American students, Aronson and colleagues (2009) identified three vital components of effective interventions: (1) reinforcement of the idea that intelligence is malleable and, like a muscle, grows stronger when exercised; (2) reinforcement of the idea that difficulties in school are often part of a normal learning curve or adjustment process, rather than something unique to a particular students' abilities, social identity, or sociocultural background; and (3) provisions of opportunities for students to reflect on sources of their self-worth beyond school achievement. In sum, self-representations represent key targets for school-based interventions targeting students with academic problems, social-emotional/behavioral problems, or both (Dweck & London, 2004).

Social Cognition

Social cognitive processes represent a third domain of psychological targets for school-based mental health efforts. Social cognition (SC) refers to information processing about the social environment and other people (Fiske & Taylor, 1991). Social cognitive processes such as empathy and perspective taking are important psychological features of individuals with emotional/behavioral problems (Lansford et al., 2006; Rood, Roelofs, Bogels, Nolen-Hoeksema, & Schouten, 2009). Research on social information processing styles like rejection sensitivity suggests a malleable set of schemas (beliefs, images, feelings) that are rather automatically applied in social situations and that generate perceived social threat, anxiety, and behaviors that can fuel social rejection (Romero-Canyas, Downey, Berenson, Ayduk, & Kang, 2010). Social cognition also includes the skills of empathy and perspective taking. The development of empathy is relatively plastic during childhood and adolescence (e.g., MLERN, 2012), and school-based efforts such as the Roots of Empathy program (Gordon, 2007) or conflict resolution/peer mediating programs may aid in the promotion of healthier interpersonal appraisal processes and empathic and socially responsible behavior. For instance, meta-analyses show that the school-wide use of conflict resolution education (CRE) programs and peer mediation programs reduces antisocial behavior, especially during early and middle adolescence as compared to childhood (Burrell, Zirbel, & Allen, 2003; Garrard & Lipsey, 2007).

In sum, school-based efforts that target these kinds of malleable psychological processes that are common to health, mental health, and school functioning in different subgroups of students are one way to build more efficacious and effective school-based interventions in the future. In the next section, we address in greater detail the roles that schools can play in fostering social-emotional development in all students and meeting the needs of those who face significant health and mental health-related barriers to success in school.

Investing in Human Health and Development From "Cradle to Career"

The long-term educational costs of ignoring or inadequately addressing physical and mental health problems among those in the school-aged population are substantial (Institute of Medicine, 2009). Kessler, Foster, Saunders, and Stang (1995) estimated that early-onset psychiatric disorders (especially conduct disorders in males and anxiety disorders in females) are related to truncated educational attainments in approximately 7.2 million Americans. There are significant losses in earnings for the individual, loss of productivity for society, and increased burdens on social welfare and criminal justice systems for those who develop serious mental illnesses (Kessler et al., 2008). The costs of early-onset problems to society are so large that they have spurred economists to develop models of the potential return on investments to a society that are possible if governments invested in human health in an early and ongoing way.

In one approach, Heckman (2007) outlined his human capital (HC) approach to health economics—an approach with the goal of maximizing human health through governmental investments in empirically validated programs that stretch from cradle to career (Kania & Kramer, 2011). Heckman (2007) outlined nine empirically supported propositions of the human capital investment model: (1) health and life success are strongly reliant upon human abilities, and it is the lack of abilities such as self-control that leads to educational failure, lower earnings, and greater involvement in the criminal justice and healthcare systems; (2) human abilities are manifold in nature and include both cognitive and noncognitive (social-emotional) abilities; (3) the promotion of a focus on prevention/intervention requires an understanding of human abilities as produced in development through gene–epigenome–environment transactions; (4) gaps in cognitive and non-cognitive abilities implicated in human health, education, and well-being arise and widen between individuals and socioeconomic status groups early in human development well before individuals arrive to school; (5) there are critical and sensitive periods in the development of various cognitive (e.g., language) and noncognitive (e.g., emotion regulation) abilities; (6) despite low returns on investment for interventions targeting disadvantaged adolescents, the empirical literature shows high economic returns for remedial investments targeting disadvantaged young children; (7) early investments in disadvantaged children's health and well-being need to be followed with later investments or the effects of early investment will fade; (8) the effects of poverty on child development depend on timing, with family economic hardship having the most detrimental impacts on young children; and (9) noncognitive social-emotional skills promote cognitive skills, healthy behaviors, and school readiness and are an important product of successful families and successful interventions in socioeconomically disadvantaged families. On the basis of this summary, Heckman proposed that governments should invest in the "health stocks" of young citizens in a particular way. Specifically, governments should invest in empirically validated programs that cultivate early social-emotional abilities in young children and their families as a way of supporting the development of future cognitive abilities necessary for school readiness and life success (e.g., Ramey & Ramey, 2004). Heckman (2007) estimated an 8–to–1 return on investment to governments that focus their efforts in a scientifically-validated, intense and on-going way on human health, early childhood, and families in poverty. His basic message is clear: abilities are necessary for human health, school achievement, and life success. To maximize these goods in society, abilities must be invested in as early as possible with particular attention on children in disadvantaged families; with sustained support

at later periods in children's and adolescent's lives through the collective and developmentally cumulative impact of government investments in family, school- and community-based programs (Kania & Kramer, 2011).

Four Roles for Schools in the Mental Health of Students

A developmental social policy such as Heckman's human capital (HC) approach to health economics seems particularly important for helping schools to successfully educate students by sharing the burden of addressing health and mental health problems in the school-aged population. The poverty-linked vulnerabilities that characterize a significant minority of the school-aged population today, as well as the lack of community-based services that are available to address these vulnerabilities, create enormous challenges for school administrators and teachers who are charged with educating all students to higher standards of academic proficiency. These challenges are especially formidable in poor urban school districts where significant family and emotional/behavioral problems characterize a large proportion of the student population (Adelman & Taylor, 2009). In the context of these various societal demands, we see four main roles that schools can play in the mental health of children and adolescents—ranging from intervention to prevention to health promotion approaches (Institute of Medicine, 1994; 2009). These roles include (1) crisis intervention; (2) provision of school-based health, mental health, and educational services; (3) provision of universal social-emotional learning programs for students and professional development for educators in this regard; and (4) the creation and maintenance of school environments that are safe, supportive, and focused on academic and social-emotional learning.

Crisis Intervention in Schools

In the aftermath of 9/11 and numerous school shootings, the role of schools in crisis intervention is recognized as an efficient means of helping students and their families deal with tragedy and trauma (Christner et al., 2009; Love & Cobb, 2012). School-aged children are exposed to trauma at significant rates, especially but not only children in poor urban environments, with predictable negative consequences on their school attendance, ability to sustain attention on learning, and school performance (Hurt, Malmud, Brodsky, & Giannetta, 2001; Thompson & Rippey Massat, 2005). For instance, between 20 and 25% of America's children report having directly experienced or witnessed violence by the age of 13 (Koenen, Roberts, Stone, & Dunn, 2010).

Crisis intervention involves planning for crises and providing services aimed at stabilizing and enhancing students' resilience and coping in the aftermath of community tragedy or personal trauma. Preparing for crisis intervention services requires school leadership. A recent survey of public school superintendents showed that (1) most school leaders have an evacuation plan for emergencies but rarely practice it, (2) plans for special needs students and post-disaster counseling services are lacking in about 25% of surveyed schools, and (3) urban schools are better prepared for disasters than rural ones (Graham, Shirm, Liggin, Aitken, & Dick, 2006). Program evaluation research has demonstrated that professional development activities can enhance school personnel's crisis planning and intervention-related attitudes and knowledge (Brock, Nickerson, Reeves, Savage, & Woitaszewski, 2011).

School-Linked Services

The untreated health and mental health problems that characterize a substantial minority of the school-aged population necessitate that schools attempt to address such issues through direct service provision as part of their broader mandate (Adelman & Taylor, 2009; Dryfoos, 1994). Today, approximately 50% of US middle and high schools have mental health counseling services available on-site. Approximately 11% have mental health counseling, physical examinations, and substance abuse counseling available on-site. Rural schools, small schools, and schools in the Midwest and the South are most likely to have no services (Slade, 2003). A few schools deliver mental health and social services through school-based health centers. Arrangements with providers not located on school property are more common (Brener, Weist, Adelman, Taylor, & Vernon-Smiley, 2007). There remains relatively little research on the effectiveness of so-called full service schools (Evans, 1999), though pilot studies have shown some promising results for student mental health (e.g., Walter et al., 2011).

What about school-based counseling and psychotherapy services? Several groups have concluded that group-oriented, cognitive–behavioral programs aimed at preventing internalizing and externalizing problems show success only if a specific set of implementation criteria is met (Rones & Hoagwood, 2000). These include (1) consistent program implementation; (2) inclusion of parents, teachers, or peers; (3) use of multiple modalities (e.g., the combination of psychoeducation with cognitive–behavioral skill training); (4) integration of program content into classroom curriculum; (5) developmentally appropriate program components; and (6) a focus on specific processes related to self-regulation, self-representation, and social cognition (Conduct Disorder Prevention Research Group, 1999; Rones, & Hoagwood, 2000). Unfortunately, research shows a general scarcity of such systemic efforts. Instead, there is evidence that the delivery of evidence-based intervention services of any kind in schools is challenging, constrained by many barriers, and often marginalized from everyday school routines and structures (Adelman & Taylor, 2009; Langley, Nadeem, Kataoka, Stein, & Jaycox, 2010).

Academic tutoring or mentoring programs, especially those that target children struggling to learn basic literacy skills, are empirically validated ways schools can prevent failure among vulnerable students (Eby, Allen, Evans, Ng, & DuBois, 2008; Ritter, Barnett, Denny, & Albin, 2009). Tutors can be trained volunteers, paraprofessionals, or even students themselves (McLaughlin, 2000). In the Valued Youth Partnership program in Texas, for instance, secondary school students at risk of dropping out were given an opportunity to serve as tutors of younger children. Researchers found that of the

100 at-risk adolescents who joined the program, 94 remained in school, while only six dropped out (see Roth & Brooks-Gunn, 2003).

Another role schools can play in the mental health of children and adolescents involves using buildings during after-school hours to host safe after-school activities (Eccles & Gootman, 2002). A recent meta-analysis showed "small but statistically significant positive effects of out-of-school time (OST) on both reading and mathematics student achievement and larger positive effect sizes for programs with specific characteristics such as tutoring in reading" (Lauer, Akiba, Wilkerson, Snow, & Martin-Glenn, 2006, p. 275). Mahoney and Cairns (1997) found that participation in extracurricular activities is related to lower rates of school dropout, particularly for high-risk youth. By and large, organized activities and service-learning settings are good for adolescents because (1) doing good things with one's time takes time away from opportunities to get involved in risky activities; (2) one can learn good things (like specific competencies and prosocial values) while engaged in constructive and/or service-learning activities; and (3) involvement in organized activity settings increases the possibility of establishing positive social networks and values (Mahoney, Larson, & Eccles, 2005).

The provision of organized summer activities in schools (not just remedial summer school) is another role for schools in the academic and social-emotional development of students. Alexander, Entwistle, and colleagues showed that much of the social class differential in school achievement reflects differences that already exist when the students enter kindergarten and those that accumulate over summer vacations. On average, children living in poor families learn less and forget more over the summer vacation, in part because wealthier families are able to provide their children with a variety of structured learning experiences over the summer that poorer families cannot (Alexander, Entwisle, & Olson, 2007; Duncan & Murane, 2011). Research on effective summertime programs provides a blueprint for how schools can offer such programs in communities where they are unavailable (Bell & Carrillo, 2007).

Social-Emotional Learning

A third approach to mental health in the schools involves provision of universal social-emotional learning programs. Over the past three decades, scholars have been developing the scientific and practical case for the notion that schools are most successful when they integrate universal efforts to promote children's academic, social, and emotional learning (Zins et al., 2004). Social and emotional learning (SEL) has been defined as "the process through which children enhance their ability to integrate thinking, feeling, and behaving to achieve important life tasks. Those competent in SEL are able to recognize and manage their emotions, establish healthy relationships, set positive goals, meet personal and social needs, and make responsible and ethical decisions" (Zins et al., 2004, p. 6). SEL aims at "teaching children to be self-aware, socially cognizant, able to make responsible decisions, and competent in self-management and relationship-management skills so as to foster their academic success" (Zins et al., 2004, p. 6). Furthermore, SEL aims to transform the totality of school and classroom learning environments to make them safe, supportive, and conducive to learning *and* well-being, knowledge *and* ethical conduct, and achievement *and* harmonious and caring social relationships (Zins et al., 2004).

Reviews and meta-analyses of SEL programs delivered in classrooms provide evidence that they can reduce substance abuse (Gottfredson & Wilson, 2003), antisocial behavior (Wilson, Gottfredson, & Najaka, 2001), and mental health problems (Durlak & Wells, 1997). A recent meta-analysis (Durlak, Weissberg, Taylor, & Dymnicki, 2011) examined the outcomes of over 250 experimental studies of SEL programs for all students. Of the 27 programs that examined indicators of academic achievement at the post-intervention period, student receiving SEL programs showed significant and meaningful improvements on achievement test performance—the effect was equivalent to an approximately 10% point gain. Further, program students were significantly more likely to attend school, less likely to be disciplined for misbehavior, and received better grades. The incorporation of cultural issues into SEL programs, and a focus not just on self-regulation and well-being but also on ethical responsibilities to others in these programs, represents important future directions in SEL programs in US schools (Hoffman, 2009; Waterhouse, 2006). Work on how the social-emotional competence (SEC) of the teacher may affect SEL program implementation and effectiveness is also beginning (Brown, Jones, LaRusso, & Aber, 2010; Jennings & Greenberg, 2009).

A novel approach to cultivating social-emotional competence among educators has been the introduction of mindfulness training for teachers and school leaders (Roeser, Skinner, Beers, & Jennings, 2012). Mindfulness has been described as a mental state or trait characterized by focused attention, a calm and clear awareness of what is happening in the present moment, and an attitude of openness, curiosity, and acceptance in place of emotional reactivity, conceptual elaboration, or denial or rejection of what is actually happening (Kabat-Zinn, 2003). Evidence suggests that mindfulness is a trainable habit of mind that may contribute to the improvement of leadership, teaching, and learning in the schools (MLERN, 2012). Only a handful of such studies exist, however. Winzelberg and Luskin (1999) found that preservice teachers who participated in a 4-week, 3-h mindfulness training reported significant reductions in somatic, emotional, and behavioral indicators of stress. Kemeny and colleagues (2012) found that teachers' randomization to an eight-week, 42-h meditation/emotion regulation training was associated with declines in depression and anxiety, increases in positive affect, and improvement in a behavioral task requiring recognition of emotions. Benn, Akiva, Arel, and Roeser (2012) found that randomization to a five-week, 35-h mindfulness/emotion regulation training for teachers and parents of children with special needs was associated with reductions in emotional distress and increases in well-being. Jennings, Snowberg, Coccia, and Greenberg (2011) reported positive, though less consistent, results with respect to training-related changes in teachers' mindfulness and stress reduction. More research on potential educational benefits of mindfulness training for educators is needed (Meiklejohn et al., 2012).

Mindfulness and yoga programs for students are also beginning to form part of the array of SEL and other universal programs that schools offer directly to students in efforts to foster well-being and prevent problems (Block-Lerner, Holston, & Messing, 2009). The scientific investigation of the effects of mindfulness or yoga practice on child and adolescent development is also just beginning, however (Greenberg & Harris, 2012; MLERN, 2012; Zelazo & Lyons, 2012). In one study, children randomly assigned to a brief mindfulness training curriculum (administered in small groups in bi-weekly sessions over the course of five weeks) showed improved sustained attention and perspective taking but not cognitive flexibility (Johnson, Forston, Gunnar, & Zelazo, 2011). Flook and her colleagues (2010) found that children identified by teachers and parents as having problems with self-regulation showed significant improvement in teacher and parent ratings of self-regulation following an eight-week mindfulness program. In a study of 9- to 11-year-old boys and girls, a mindful yoga program was associated with decreases in youth self-reports of rumination, intrusive thoughts, and emotional arousal to stressful events (Mendelson et al., 2010). In a study of 8- to 12-year-old boys and girls in Canada, Schonert-Reichl and Lawlor (2010) found increases in student-reported optimism and reductions in teacher reports of students' aggressive and oppositional behavior in the classroom. Broderick and Metz (2009) found a significant reduction in negative affect and a significant increase in feelings of relaxation, calm, and self-acceptance among 12th grade high school girls following a mindfulness program. In summarizing this emerging body of research, Greenberg and Harris (2012) noted "meditation and yoga may be associated with beneficial outcomes for children and youth, but the generally limited quality of research tempers the allowable conclusions" (p. 161).

School-Wide Reform

The fourth key role we see schools playing in students' mental health is supporting the success of all students through school-wide reforms aimed at creating safe, respectful, orderly, emotionally supportive, and motivating school climates for student learning. There is considerable evidence that everyday practices of leadership and teaching in the schools, as well as supportive relationships between educators and students contribute to the prevention of emotional/behavioral problems and the cultivation of positive academic and social-emotional development in students (Catalano et al., 2004; Hawkins, Kosterman, Catalano, Kill, & Abbott, 2008).

The context of schooling can be described as a complex social system ranging from macro- and distal (e.g., national educational policies) to micro- and proximal (design of particular academic task) levels of analysis and socialization processes that both indirectly and directly influence students' development in school (Eccles & Roeser, 2010). A depiction of the various levels of analysis that constitute schools as a context of child and adolescent development is presented in Fig. 9.1. Regarding the role of schooling in the mental health of children and adolescents, we make five basic assumptions derived from developmental systems thinking: (1) the study of student mental health in the context of schooling in the USA necessitates a focus on the unique barriers to health, mental health, and school success facing students living in poverty and those from different racial/ethnic and linguistic family backgrounds; (2) the context of schooling is characterized by multiple levels of structure and organization, each of which is further characterized by specific socialization processes (e.g., schools and principal leadership styles, classrooms and teaching styles) that can influence students' social and emotional/behavioral development; (3) it is in complex causal chains of socialization processes operating within and across levels of the school system that so-called school influences on children's social-emotional and behavioral development are located; (4) the kinds of structures and processes associated with contexts of schooling "develop" as the growing child moves through the various institutions that comprise the school system (elementary, middle, and high schools), with contextual changes providing either a "fit" or a "mismatch" with the

growing child's stage-relevant and cultural needs; and (5) school socialization effects on students' academic and social-emotional outcomes are mediated to a significant degree by students' agency and subjective perceptions of their school contexts as either fitting with or being mismatched with their developmental and cultural needs. School environments that actually and subjectively "fit" stage- and culture-relevant needs of students are hypothesized to promote school bonding, learning, well-being, and prosocial behavior, whereas those that are "mismatched" with such needs are hypothesized to promote school alienation, disengagement, acting out, and dropping out (see Eccles & Roeser, 2010, 2011; Rutter & Maughan, 2002). In the next section, we briefly discuss particular malleable school system factors depicted in Fig. 9.1 that represent key targets for intervention because they address key student needs.

Malleable Ecological Factors as Targets for School-Wide Reform

School Scheduling

The regulation of time in schools and classrooms can affect the quality of students' attention, engagement, behavior, and learning. Learning requires periods of mental activity and rest in alternation (Snow et al., 1996). Long periods of work with few breaks for physical activity can fuel student inattention. The use of frequent recess breaks has a salutary effect on children's concentration and learning (Ramstetter, Murray, & Garner, 2010).

During adolescence, research shows puberty causes an increased need for sleep (Carskadon, 1990; Sadeh, Dahl, Shahar, & Rosenblat-Stein, 2009). Preferred diurnal patterns of sleep and wake cycles shift such that youth prefer to stay up later at night and to sleep later in the morning. During this same period, secondary schools typically begin earlier in the morning, necessitating earlier rise times for adolescent students (Carskadon, 1990). This creates a "developmental mismatch" that promotes adolescents' daytime

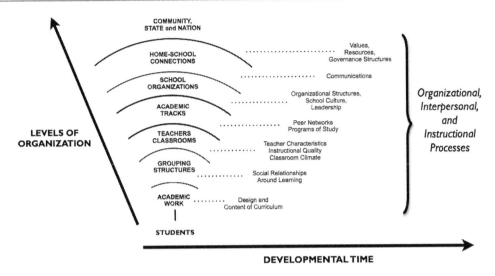

Fig. 9.1 School as a central cultural context of child and adolescent development: structures and processes

sleepiness and undermines their ability to make it to school on time and ready to learn (Dewald, Meijer, Oort, Kerkhof, & Bögels, 2010). Sleep fatigue, created by early school start times that are mismatched with adolescent sleep needs, has been linked to poor concentration in school, symptoms of depression, aggression, and negative perceptions of classes (Wolfson & Carskadon, 1998). Schools should reconsider start times in light of this evidence.

The time at which school ends also has implications for adolescents' mental health. In communities where few structured after-school opportunities exist, adolescents are more likely to be involved in high-risk behaviors such as substance use, crime, and sexual activity between 2 and 8 pm when parents are still working (Carnegie Corporation, 1992). Keeping schools open later for activities is one prevention strategy indicated here.

Teacher Quality

Teachers' educational qualifications are associated with the amount their students learn across their development (Rowan, Correnti, & Miller, 2002). Unfortunately, poor children and English language learners (ELLs) are disproportionately exposed to unqualified teachers across their development (Darling-Hammond, 1997). Beyond

teacher qualifications, the quality of teachers' instruction is also linked to student achievement gains (Pianta & Hamre, 2009). Instructional quality is often mediocre in US public schools, however, especially if schools have a high proportion of poor students (Pianta, Belsky, Houts, & Morrison, 2007). Chetty, Friedman, and Rockoff (2011) found that students assigned to a high-quality teacher were more likely to attend college, attended higher-ranked colleges, earned higher salaries, lived in higher SES neighborhoods, and saved more for retirement. They were also less likely to have children as teenagers. Replacing a relatively poor-quality teacher with an average-quality teacher was estimated to increase lifetime earnings by more than $250,000 for the average classroom in the study. Improving teacher qualifications and the quality of teaching through reforms in teacher education, mentorship programs for new teachers, high-quality teacher professional development, and teacher licensure are several teacher-focused approaches to improving schools and reducing student failure and dropout (Darling-Hammond & Bransford, 2005).

Teacher–Student Relationships

Emotionally supportive teachers are a critical foundation for students' motivation to learn, and especially for poor and ethnic minority youth who often experience " belonging uncertainty" in schools that can undermine their motivation and achievement (e.g., Walton & Cohen, 2007). The promotion of positive teacher-student relationships is an essential ingredient for all school reform and universal school-based prevention strategies (Catalano et al., 2004; Schaps, 2003). Individualized interventions designed to foster positive dyadic relationships between teachers and challenging students have proven effective (Pianta, Stuhlman, & Hamre, 2011). Intervention work done by the Child Development Project (CDP) in California takes a school-level approach to fostering relationships and student bonding to school. Central to this approach are practices that directly engage students in community-building activities, including cooperative learning projects, classroom management strategies that rely on student participation in norm setting and decision making, teaching of conflict resolution skills, and curricula that focus on themes of care. Evidence shows such practices foster a "community of care" that positively influences students' motivation to learn, belonging, and prosocial behavior (Schaps, 2003).

School Climate

The overarching social climate of the school also matters for students' motivation, learning, and prosocial vs. antisocial behavior. Both the Seattle Social Development Project (SSDP) and the Raising Healthy Children (RHC) Project used a school-based universal prevention program aimed at promoting student mental health and academic success through the creation of a healthy social climate in the school and positive school-family connections. Randomized trials of these programs showed that changes in the school social climate promoted changes to students' school bonding, which, in turn, increased their engagement in prosocial behavior and decreased their engagement in antisocial behavior over time (Catalano et al., 2004; Hawkins et al., 2008).

Such preventative approaches can be contrasted with relatively more punitive ones. For instance, many US schools have adopted Zero

Tolerance policies with regard to violence—do they work? In 2008, the American Psychological Association released its report that concluded the evidence for the effectiveness of Zero Tolerance policies is weak at best (APA, 2008). Furthermore, such policies were found often to result in higher rates of suspension, particularly for minority students, poor students, and students with disabilities, without leading to improvements in school safety. The report suggests alternative approaches for intervention aimed at changing the school culture, reconnecting alienated students, increasing school bonding, developing a planned continuum of steps to be followed with at-risk students, and increasing the collaboration between the various community, school, and family stakeholders. Research on anti-bullying programs has come to the same conclusions: the most promising programs involve multilevel, school-wide approaches in which the existence of rules and consequences for bullying are salient, where conflict resolution strategies are in place, and where teachers are trained on bullying issues (Vreeman & Carroll, 2007). In both cases, recommendations to reduce violence and bullying point towards the kind of school-wide preventative programs described above by the Child Development Center and Seattle Social Development and Raising Healthy Children (RHC) projects (Catalano et al., 2004; Hawkins et al., 2008).

Part of a safe school culture that is being discussed more and more in relation to US schools today concerns the norms and practices that exist (or do not) in a school with regard to respect for cultural and sexual diversity and the unacceptability of discrimination in any form. Treuba (1988) outlined five key issues for schools in this regard, including (1) a school-wide recognition of the significance of culture in student learning; (2) the development of policies and practices that prevent stereotyping of minorities; (3) the resolution of disputes around cultural diversity in an open, fair, and caring manner; (4) improvement of home-school connections; and (5) a focus on the development of students' linguistic competencies so that all students could participate meaningfully in classroom learning. Relatedly, others have argued that the sexual diversity climate of secondary schools can be improved for all students through inclusive policies, the education of students and staff on sexual diversity issues, and the establishment of and support for gay-straight alliances (e.g., Szalacha, 2003).

School Physical Environment

The physical environment of the school also can affect students' emotional/behavioral development. Rutter and colleagues in their London study found that observer ratings of building cleanliness and the presence of plants, pictures, the display of student work and other decorations inside the school buildings predicted less student misconduct (after accounting for their social background—Rutter & Maughan, 2002). The "broken windows" theory of delinquency and crime (Wilson & Kelling, 1982) posits that unmaintained or abandoned physical spaces connote a message of a lack of ownership and, in a sense, a lack of moral structure. Such spaces may therefore become tacit seedbeds for misconduct and antisocial activity. Astor, Meyer, and Behre (1999) found that most violent events reported by students occurred in "undefined public spaces" of the school—spaces such as parking lots, bathrooms, and hallways where no adults assumed supervisory jurisdiction. These spaces were undefined in terms of adult monitoring of student behavior, and thus were the frequent sites for fights, unwanted sexual attention, and other negative interactions. Maintaining the physical environment of schools and reclaiming so-called undefined spaces represent strategies for improving school safety.

School Size

Barker and Gump (1964) theorized that smaller secondary schools affect young people's social and academic development by providing various opportunities not available in larger schools—opportunities that include (a) closer relationships between teachers and students, (b) greater adult monitoring of and responsibility for student progress, and (c) a particularly favorable roles-to-people ratio with respect to school extracurricular activities and the need for many students in the school to participate to fulfill those roles. By affecting these mediating processes, school size was hypothesized to affect student outcomes. Research has consistently verified these hypotheses (e.g., Crosnoe, Johnson, & Elder, 2004). The creation of smaller learning communities is implicated by these findings. However, studies on school size agree that although smaller learning communities provide a student with benefits around belonging and participation, they must also provide high-quality instruction if increased student learning is to flourish as well in such schools (Ready & Lee, 2008).

Family–School Connections

Parent involvement in their child's schooling has consistently emerged as a positive factor in students' academic achievement and social-emotional well-being. Parent involvement also helps to establish a "safety net" of concerned adults (parents and teachers) that can support children's academic and social-emotional development and assist children if adjustment problems should arise (cf. NRC/IOM, 2004). Evidence suggests that home-school connections are relatively infrequent during the elementary school years and become almost nonexistent during the middle and high school years (NRC/IOM, 2004). Nonetheless, a recent meta-analysis confirmed the continuing importance of parental involvement in school even during adolescence (Hill & Tyson, 2009). Specifically, these authors found that parents' academic socialization of their child, including the communication of their valuing of education, their expectations for their child's grades, strategies for learning, and the necessity of their child thinking about and planning for future educational and occupational goals were key aspects of parental support. Improving parental involvement is a key strategy in school-based mental health efforts, and research shows that when implemented faithfully, school-wide reforms can improve parent involvement and student outcomes (Cook, Murphy, & Hunt, 2000).

Community-Based Service Learning

Structured opportunities for service learning in community settings outside of school can positively influence students' development. In 1989, the Turning Points report (Carnegie, 1989) recommended that every middle school include supervised youth service in the community or school as part of the core academic curriculum. Today 25% of elementary schools, 38% of middle schools, and 46% of all high schools have students participating in either mandatory or voluntary service-learning activities (NCES, 2006). Students who participate in well-designed service-learning programs do better than comparison groups on measures of problem solving, reading and mathematics achievement, social responsibility, and attitudes toward diverse groups in society (Eccles & Roeser, 2010). Service learning has also been related to reductions in academic and behavior problems and pregnancy (Kirby, 2002).

School Transitions

School transitions provide unique opportunities for school-based mental health efforts. Normative school transitions in early childhood, early adolescence, and middle adolescence are times of heightened risk for children and adolescents due to predictable and often temporary declines in felt safety and belonging, motivation to learn, and academic achievement (cf. Eccles & Roeser, 2011). For students with long-term academic and emotional/behavioral problems, the transitions to middle and high school are times of increasing disengagement and accelerating pathways towards school dropout (Rumberger, 2011). Ensuring that students who are older due to grade retention or other factors do not decide to drop out of school during secondary school transitions is

essential for decreasing dropout (Neild, 2009). In addition, facilitating successful school transitions for all students requires attention to both (a) preparing students and their families for these transitions through outreach efforts, information sharing, and school tours and (b) ensuring that schools have reception and peer-support programs for welcoming new students and teaching them the routines of daily life in school (Anderson, Jacobs, Schramm, & Splittgerber, 2000; Benner, 2011).

In summary, malleable school system processes that affect students' social and emotional/behavioral development exist at the various levels of the subcontexts of schooling depicted in Fig. 9.1. Focusing on these as key ecological targets in future school reform efforts may prove fruitful not only in improving academic success but also in preventing emotional/behavioral problems and promoting well-being and prosociality (Greenberg et al., 2003).

Conclusion

In this chapter, we have summarized the many ways in which schools can influence child and adolescent development and their mental health in particular. We described the current US school-aged population demographically, educationally, and in relation to health and mental health problems. We concluded that at least 25 % of the school population suffers from health and mental health problems that interfere with readiness to learn, and we suggested that processes of self-regulation, self-representation, and social cognition represent key malleable psychological factors underlying co-occurring patterns of school, social, and emotional/behavioral problems. We suggested that these psychological factors represent key targets of school-based interventions. We described how poverty plays a role in these findings, disproportionately affects different racial/ethnic groups, and fuels achievement gaps well before students even begin schooling. We then outlined four roles that elementary and secondary schools can play in preventing emotional/behavioral problems and fostering the academic and social-emotional development of students and their families, including (1) crisis intervention, (2) service provision, (3) provisions of social-emotional learning programs and educator professional development, and (4) school reform. The challenges facing the US school population due to poverty and other developmental risks necessitate that schools play a role in not only the education of students, but also in their mental health. Schools cannot address the problems of the school-aged population alone, but represent a key cultural institution that can, in conjunction with reforms in health care, immigration, and social welfare policy, assist all children and their families in achieving a better future.

References

Adelman, H., & Taylor, L. (2009). Ending the marginalization of mental health in schools: A comprehensive approach. In R. Christener & R. Mennuti (Eds.), *School-based mental health: A practitioner's guide to comparative practices* (pp. 25–54). New York: Routledge.

Akinbami, L. J., Moorman, J. E., Garbe, P. L., & Sondik, E. J. (2009). Status of childhood asthma in the United States, 1980–2007. *Pediatrics, 123*, 131–145.

Akinbami L. J., Moorman, J. E., & Liu, X. (2011). *Asthma prevalence, health care use, and mortality: United States, 2005–2009*. National Health Statistics Reports No. 32. Hyattsville, MD: National Center for Health Statistics.

Alexander, K. L., Entwisle, D. R., & Olson, L. S. (2007). Lasting consequences of the summer learning gap. *Sociology of Education, 72*, 167–180.

American Psychological Association Zero Tolerance Task Force. (2008). Are zero tolerance policies effective in the schools? *American Psychologist, 63*, 852–862.

Anderson, L. W., Jacobs, J., Schramm, S., & Splittgerber, F. (2000). School transitions: Beginning of the end or a new beginning? *International Journal of Educational Research, 33*, 325–339.

Aronson, J., Cohen, G., McColskey, W., Montrosse, B., Lewis, K., & Mooney, K. (2009). *Reducing stereotype threat in classrooms*. Washington, DC: U.S. Department of Education, Institute of Education Sciences, National Center for Education Evaluation and Regional Assistance, Regional Educational Laboratory Southeast. Retrieved from http://ies.ed.gov/ncee/edlabs

Asendorpf, J. B., Borkenau, P., Ostendorf, F., & van Aken, M. A. G. (2001). Carving personality description at its

joints: Confirmation of three replicable personality prototypes for both children and adults. *European Journal of Personality, 15*, 169–198.

Astor, R. A., Meyer, H. A., & Behre, W. J. (1999). Unowned places and times: Maps and interviews about violence in high schools. *American Educational Research Journal, 36*, 3–42.

Aud, S., KewalRamani, A., & Frohlich, L. (2011). *America's youth: Transitions to adulthood* (NCES 2012-026). U.S. Department of Education, National Center for Education Statistics. Washington, DC: U.S. Government Printing Office.

Aunola, K., Stattin, H., & Nurmi, J. E. (2000). Adolescents' achievement strategies, school adjustment, and externalizing and internalizing problem behaviors. *Journal of Youth and Adolescence, 29*, 289–306.

Bandura, A. (1997). *Self-efficacy: The exercise of control*. New York: Freeman.

Barker, R., & Gump, P. (1964). *Big school, small school: High school size and student behavior*. Stanford, CA: Stanford University Press.

Becker, B. E., & Luthar, S. S. (2002). Social–emotional factors affecting achievement outcomes among disadvantaged students: Closing the achievement gap. *Educational Psychologist, 37*, 197–214.

Bell, S. R., & Carrillo, N. (2007). Characteristics of effective summer learning programs in practice. *New Directions for Youth Development, 114*, 45–63.

Benn, R., Akiva, T., Arel, S., & Roeser, R. W. (2012). Mindfulness training effects for parents and educators of children with special needs. *Developmental Psychology, 48*, 1476.

Benner, A. D. (2011). The transition to high school: Current knowledge, future directions. *Educational Psychology Review, 23*, 299–328.

Blackwell, L. S., Trzesniewski, K. H., & Dweck, C. S. (2007). Implicit theories of intelligence predict achievement across an adolescent transition: A longitudinal study and an intervention. *Child Development, 78*, 246–263.

Blair, C., & Diamond, A. (2008). Biological processes in prevention and intervention: The promotion of self-regulation as a means of preventing school failure. *Development and Psychopathology, 20*, 899–911.

Blair, C., & Razza, R. P. (2007). Relating effortful control, executive function, and false belief understanding to emerging math and literacy ability in kindergarten. *Child Development, 78*, 647–663.

Block, J. H., & Block, J. (1980). The role of ego-control and ego-resiliency in the organization of behavior. In W.A. Collins, (Ed.), *Symposium on Child Psychology 13*, 39–101. New York: Erlbaum.

Block-Lerner, J., Holston, M. A., & Messing, M. (2009). Seeing through clearer eyes: Mindfulness and acceptance-based behavioral interventions in the school. In R. W. Christener & R. B. Mennuti (Eds.), *School-based mental health: A practitioner's guide to comparative practices* (pp. 373–404). New York: Routledge.

Brener, N. D., Weist, M., Adelman, H., Taylor, L., & Vernon-Smiley, M. (2007). Mental health and social services: Results from the school health policies and programs study 2006. *Journal of School Health, 77*, 486–499.

Brock, S. E., Nickerson, A. B., Reeves, M. A., Savage, T. A., & Woitaszewski, S. A. (2011). Development, evaluation, and future directions of the PREP a RE school crisis prevention and intervention training curriculum. *Journal of School Violence, 10*, 34–52.

Broderick, P. C., & Metz, S. (2009). Learning to BREATHE: Pilot trial of a mindfulness curriculum for adolescents. *Advances in School Mental Health Promotion, 2*, 35–46.

Brown, J. L., Jones, S. M., LaRusso, M. D., & Aber, J. L. (2010). Improving classroom quality: Teacher influences and experimental impacts of the 4Rs program. *Journal of Educational Psychology, 102*, 153–167.

Burrell, N. A., Zirbel, C. S., & Allen, M. (2003). Evaluating peer mediation outcomes in educational settings: A meta-analytic review. *Conflict Resolution Quarterly, 21*, 7–26.

Cairns, R. B., Cairns, B. D., & Neckerman, H. J. (1989). Early school dropout: Configurations and determinants. *Child Development, 60*, 1437–1452.

Carnegie Corporation of New York. (1992). *A matter of time: Risk and opportunity in the nonschool hours.* New York: Carnegie Corporation of New York.

Carnegie Council on Adolescent Development. (1989). *Turning points: Preparing American youth for the 21st century.* New York: Carnegie Corporation.

Carskadon, M. A. (1990). Patterns of sleep and sleepiness in adolescents. *Pediatrician, 17*, 5–12.

Catalano, R. F., Haggerty, K. P., Oesterle, S., Flemings, C. B., & Hawkins, J. D. (2004). The importance of bonding to school for healthy development: Findings from the social development research group. *Journal of School Health, 74*, 252–261.

Chetty, R., Friedman, J. N., & Rockoff, J. E. (2011). *The long-term impacts of teachers: Teacher value-added and student outcomes in adulthood* (Working Paper No. w17699). Washington, DC: National Bureau of Economic Research.

Christener, R. W., Mennuti, R. B., & Whitaker, J. S. (2009). An overview of school-based mental health practice: From systems service to crisis intervention. In R. Christener & R. Mennuti (Eds.), *School-based mental health: A practitioner's guide to comparative practices* (pp. 3–22). New York: Routledge.

Conduct Problems Prevention Research Group. (1999). Initial impact of the fast track prevention trial for conduct problems: II. Classroom effects. *Journal of Consulting and Clinical Psychology, 67*, 648–657.

Cook, T. D., Murphy, R. F., & Hunt, H. D. (2000). Comer's school development program in Chicago: A theory-based evaluation. *American Educational Research Journal, 37*, 535–597.

Costello, E. J., Copeland, W., & Angold, A. (2011). Trends in psychopathology across the adolescent years: What changes when children become adolescents, and when adolescents become adults? *Journal of Child Psychology and Psychiatry, 52*, 1015–1025.

Crosnoe, R., Johnson, M. K., & Elder, G. H. (2004). School size and the interpersonal side of education: An examination of race/ethnicity and organizational context. *Social Science Quarterly, 85*, 1259–1274.

Darling-Hammond, L. (1997). *The right to learn: A blueprint for creating schools that work.* San Francisco, CA: Jossey-Bass.

Darling-Hammond, L., & Bransford, J. (Eds.). (2005). *Preparing teachers for a changing world: What teachers should learn and be able to do.* San Francisco: Wiley.

Datar, A., Sturm, R., & Magnabosco, J. L. (2004). Childhood overweight and academic performance: National study of kindergartners and first-graders. *Obesity Research, 12*, 58–68.

Dewald, J. F., Meijer, A. M., Oort, F. J., Kerkhof, G. A., & Bögels, S. M. (2010). The influence of sleep quality, sleep duration and sleepiness on school performance in children and adolescents: A meta-analytic review. *Sleep Medicine Reviews, 14*, 179–189.

Diamond, A., & Lee, K. (2011). Interventions shown to aid executive function development in children 4–12 years old. *Science, 333*, 959–964.

Dodge, K. A. (2006). Translational science in action: Hostile attributional style and the development of aggressive behavior problems. *Development and Psychopathology, 18*, 791–814.

Dryfoos, J. G. (1994). *Full service schools: A revolution in health and social services for children, youth, and families.* San Francisco, CA: Jossey-Bass.

Duncan, G. J., & Murane, R. (Eds.). (2011). *Whither opportunity? Rising inequality, schools and children's life chances.* New York: Russell Sage Foundation.

Durlak, J. A., Weissberg, R. P., Dymnicki, A. B., Taylor, R. D., & Schellinger, K. B. (2011). The impact of enhancing students' social and emotional learning: A meta-analysis of school-based universal interventions. *Child Development, 82*, 405–432.

Durlak, J. A., & Wells, A. M. (1997). Primary prevention mental health programs for children and adolescents: A meta-analytic review. *American Journal of Community Psychology, 25*, 115–152.

Dweck, C. (2008). Can personality be changed? The role of beliefs in personality and change. *Current Directions in Psychological Science, 17*, 391–394.

Dweck, C. S., & London, B. E. (2004). The role of mental representation in social development. *Merrill-Palmer Quarterly, 50*, 428–444.

Eby, L. T., Allen, T. D., Evans, S. C., Ng, T., & DuBois, D. L. (2008). Does mentoring matter? A multidisciplinary meta-analysis comparing mentored and non-mentored individuals. *Journal of Vocational Behavior, 72*, 254–267.

Eccles, J. S., & Gootman, J. A. (Eds.). (2002). *Community programs to promote youth development.* Washington, DC: National Academy Press.

Eccles, J. S., & Roeser, R. W. (2010). School and community influences on human development. In M.

Boorstein & M. Lamb (Eds.), *Developmental psychology: An advanced textbook* (6th ed.). Hillsdale, NJ: Erlbaum.

Eccles, J. S., & Roeser, R. W. (2011). School as developmental contexts during adolescence. *Journal of Research on Adolescence, 21*, 225–241.

Evans, S. W. (1999). Mental health services in schools: Utilization, effectiveness and consent. *Clinical Psychology Review, 19*, 165–178.

Fiske, S. T., & Taylor, S. E. (1991). *Social cognition.* New York: McGraw-Hill Book Company.

Flook, L., Smalley, S. L., Kitil, M. J., Galla, B. M., Kaiser Greenland, S., Locke, J., et al. (2010). Effects of mindful awareness practices on executive functions in elementary school children. *Journal of Applied School Psychology, 26*, 70–95.

Flores, G., & Tomany-Korman, S. C. (2008). Racial and ethnic disparities in medical and dental health, access to care, and use of services in US children. *Pediatrics, 113*, 286–298.

Fontaine, R. G. (2010). New developments in developmental research on social information processing and antisocial behavior. *Journal of Abnormal Child Psychology, 38*, 569–573.

Garber, J. (2006). Depression in children and adolescents: Linking risk research and prevention. *American Journal of Preventative Medicine, 31*, 104–125.

Garcia, E. E., Jensen, B., & Cuellar, D. (2006). Early academic achievement of Hispanics in the United States: Implications for teacher preparation. *The New Educator, 2*, 123–147.

Garrard, W. M., & Lipsey, M. W. (2007). Conflict resolution education and antisocial behavior in U.S. schools: A meta-analysis. *Conflict Resolution Quarterly, 25*, 9–38.

Gordon, M. (2007). *Roots of empathy: Changing the world child by child.* Toronto: Thomas Allen.

Gottfredson, D. C., & Wilson, D. B. (2003). Characteristics of effective school-based substance abuse prevention. *Prevention Science, 4*, 27–38.

Graham, S. (1997). Using attribution theory to understand social and academic motivation in African American youth. *Educational Psychologist, 32*, 21–34.

Graham, J., Shirm, S., Liggin, R., Aitken, M. E., & Dick, R. (2006). Mass-casualty events at schools: A national preparedness survey. *Pediatrics, 117*, 8–15.

Grantham-McGregor, S. Cheung, Y. B., Cueto, S., Glewwe, P., Richter, L., Strupp, B., & the International Child Development Steering Group. (2007). Child development in developing countries: Developmental potential in the first 5 years for children in developing countries. *Lancent, 369*, 60–70.

Greenberg, M. T., & Harris, A. R. (2012). Nurturing mindfulness in children and youth: Current state of research. *Child Development Perspectives, 6*, 161–166.

Greenberg, M. T., Weissberg, R. P., Utne O'Brien, M., Zins, J. E., Fredericks, L., & Resnik, H. (2003). Enhancing school-based prevention and youth development through coordinated social, emotional, and academic learning. *American Psychologist, 58*, 466–474.

Gunnar, M., & Quevedo, K. (2007). The neurobiology of stress and development. *Annual Review of Psychology, 58*, 145–173.

Hattie, J., Biggs, J., & Purdie, N. (1996). Effects of learning skills interventions on student learning: A meta-analysis. *Review of Educational Research, 66*, 99–136.

Hawkins, J. D., Kosterman, R., Catalano, R. F., Kill, K. G., & Abbott, R. D. (2008). Effects of social development intervention in childhood 15 years later. *Archives of Pediatrics and Adolescent Medicine, 162*, 1133–1141.

Heckman, J. J. (2007). The economics, technology and neuroscience of human capability formation. *Proceedings of the National Academic of Sciences, 104*, 13250–13255.

Hill, N. E., & Tyson, D. F. (2009). Parental involvement in middle school: A meta-analytic assessment of strategies that promote achievement. *Developmental Psychology, 45*, 740–763.

Hinshaw, S. P. (1992). Externalizing behavior problems and academic underachievement in childhood and adolescence: Causal relationships and underlying mechanisms. *Psychological Bulletin, 111*, 127–155.

Hoffman, D. M. (2009). Reflecting on social emotional learning: A critical perspective on trends in the United States. *Review of Educational Research, 79*, 533–556.

Hurt, H., Malmud, E., Brodsky, N. L., & Giannetta, J. (2001). Exposure to violence: Psychological and academic correlates in child witnesses. *Archives of Pediatrics & Adolescent Medicine, 155*, 1351–1356.

Institute of Medicine. (1994). *Reducing risks for mental disorders: Frontiers for preventive intervention research.* Washington, DC: National Academy Press.

Institute of Medicine. (2009). *Preventing mental, emotional, and behavioral disorders among young people: Progress and possibilities.* Washington, DC: National Academy Press.

Jennings, P. A., & Greenberg, M. (2009). The prosocial classroom: Teacher social and emotional competence in relation to child and classroom outcomes. *Review of Educational Research, 79*, 491–525.

Jennings, P. A., Snowberg, K. E., Coccia, M. A., & Greenberg, M. T. (2011). Improving classroom learning environments by cultivating awareness and resilience in education (CARE): Results of two pilot studies. *Journal of Classroom Interaction, 46*, 37–48.

Johnson, A. E., Forston, J. L., Gunnar, M. R., & Zelazo, P. D. (2011, April). *A randomized controlled trial of mindfulness meditation training in preschool children.* Poster presented at the Society for Research in Child Development Biennial Meeting in Montreal, QC.

Joiner, T. E., & Wagner, K. D. (1995). Attributional style and depression in children and adolescents: A meta-analytic review. *Clinical Psychology Review, 15*, 777–798.

Kabat-Zinn, J. (2003). Mindfulness-based interventions in context: Past, present and future. *Clinical Psychology: Science and Practice, 10*, 144–156.

Kania, J., & Kramer, M. (2011). Collective impact. *Stanford Social Innovation Review, 36–41*.

Kemeny, M. E., Foltz, C., Cullen, M., Jennings, P., Gillath, O., Wallace, B. A., et al. (2012). Contemplative/emotion training reduces negative emotional behavior and promotes prosocial responses. *Emotion, 12*, 338–350.

Kessler, R. C., Foster, C. L., Saunders, W. B., & Stang, P. E. (1995). Social consequences of psychiatric disorders, I: Educational attainment. *American Journal of Psychiatry, 152*, 1026–1032.

Kessler, R. C., Heeringa, S., Lakoma, M. D., Petukhova, M., Rupp, A. E., Schoenbaum, M., et al. (2008). The individual-level and societal-level effects of mental disorders on earnings in the United States: Results from the National Comorbidity Survey Replication. *American Journal of Psychiatry, 15*, 703–711.

King, M., Semlyen, J., Tai, S. S., Killaspy, H., Osborn, D., Popelyuk, D., et al. (2008). A systematic review of mental disorder, suicide and deliberate self-harm in lesbian, gay and bisexual people. *BioMed Central Psychiatry, 8*, 70.

Kirby, D. B. (2002). Effective approaches to reducing adolescent unprotected sex, pregnancy, and childbearing. *Journal of Sex Research, 39*, 51–57.

Koenen, K. C., Roberts, A., Stone, D., & Dunn, E. (2010). The epidemiology of childhood trauma. In R. Lanius, E. Vermetten, & C. Pain (Eds.), *The impact of early life trauma on health and disease: The hidden epidemic* (pp. 13–24). Cambridge: Cambridge University Press.

Langley, A. K., Nadeem, E., Kataoka, S. H., Stein, B. D., & Jaycox, L. H. (2010). Evidence-based mental health programs in schools: Barriers and facilitators of successful implementation. *School Mental Health, 2*, 105–113.

Lansford, J. E., Malone, P. S., Dodge, K. A., Crozier, J. C., Pettit, G. S., & Bates, J. E. (2006). A 12-year prospective study of patterns of social information processing problems and externalizing behaviors. *Journal of Abnormal Child Psychology, 34*, 709–718.

Lau, S., & Roeser, R. W. (2007). Cognitive abilities and motivational processes in science achievement and engagement: A person-centered analysis. *Learning and Individual Differences, 18*, 497–504.

Lauer, P. A., Akiba, M., Wilkerson, S. B., Snow, D., & Martin-Glenn, M. L. (2006). Out-of-school-time programs: A meta-analysis of effects for at-risk students. *Review of Educational Research, 76*, 275–313.

Lopez, M. H. (2009). *Latinos and education: Explaining the attainment gap*. Washington, DC: Pew Hispanic Center.

Love, R. A., & Cobb, N. (2012). Developing schools' capacities to respond to community crisis: The Tennessee initiative. *Journal of Child and Adolescent Psychiatric Nursing, 25*, 158–163.

Mahoney, J. L., & Cairns, R. B. (1997). Do extracurricular activities protect against early school dropout? *Developmental Psychology, 33*, 241–253.

Mahoney, J. L., Larson, R., & Eccles, J. (Eds.). (2005). *Organized activities as contexts of development: Extracurricular activities, after-school and community programs*. Hillsdale, NJ: Lawrence Erlbaum.

McLaughlin, M. W. (2000). *Community counts: How youth organizations matter for youth development*. Washington, DC: Public Education Network.

Meece, J. L., Anderman, E. M., & Anderman, L. H. (2005). Classroom goal structure, student motivation and academic achievement. *Annual Review of Psychology, 57*, 487–503.

Meiklejohn, J., Phillips, C., Freedman, M. L., Griffin, M. L., Biegel, G., Roach, A., et al. (2012). Integrating mindfulness training into K-12 education: Fostering the resilience of teachers and students. *Mindfulness, 3*, 291–307.

Mendelson, T., Greenberg, M. T., Dariotis, J., Gould, L. F., Rhoades, B., & Leaf, P. J. (2010). Feasibility and preliminary outcomes of a school-based mindfulness intervention for urban youth. *Journal of Abnormal Child Psychology, 38*, 985–994.

Merikangas, K. R., He, J., Burstein, M., Swanson, S. A., Avenevoli, S., Cui, L., et al. (2010). Lifetime prevalence of mental disorders in US adolescents: Results from the national co-morbidity survey replication—Adolescent supplement (NCS-A). *Journal of American Academy of Child and Adolescent Psychiatry, 49*, 980–989.

Mind and Life Education Research Network. (2012). Contemplative practices and mental training: Prospects for American education. *Child Development Perspectives, 6*, 146–153.

Moffitt, T. E., Arseneault, L., Belsky, D., Dickson, N., Hancox, R. J., Harrington, H., et al. (2011). A gradient of childhood self-control predicts health, wealth, and public safety. *Proceedings of the National Academy of Sciences, 108*, 2693–2698.

Nansel, T. R., Overpeck, M., Pilla, R. S., Ruan, W. J., Simons-Morton, B., & Scheidt, P. (2001). Bullying behaviors among US youth: Prevalence and association with psychosocial adjustment. *Journal of the American Medical Association, 285*, 2094–2100.

National Academy of Sciences. (2006). *Rising above the gathering storm: Energizing and employing America for a brighter economic future*. Washington, DC: National Academies Press.

National Center for Education Statistics. (2006). *The condition of education*. Washington, DC: U.S. Department of Education.

National Center for Educational Statistics. (2011). *Web tables: Student reports of bullying and cyber-bullying: Results from the 2007 school crime supplement to the national crime victimization survey*. Washington, DC.

National Research Council and Institute of Medicine (NRC/IOM). (2004). *Engaging schools*. Washington, DC: National Academies Press.

Neild, R. C. (2009). Falling off track during the transition to high school: What we know and what can be done. *The Future of Children, 19*, 53–76.

Neiman, S. (2011). *Crime, violence, discipline, and safety in U.S. public schools: Findings from the school survey on crime and safety: 2009–10*. U.S. Department of Education, National Center for Education Statistics. Washington, DC: U.S. Government Printing Office.

Nolen-Hoeksema, S., Girgus, J. S., & Seligman, M. E. P. (1986). Learned helplessness in children: A longitudinal study of depression, achievement, and explanatory style. *Journal of Personality and Social Psychology, 51*, 435–442.

Peck, S. C., Malanchuk, O., Roeser, R. W., & Eccles, J. S. (2012, October). *The effects of self-regulation on educational pathways for high-risk youth.* Poster presented at the special meeting of the Society for Research on Child Development, Tampa, FL.

Peck, S., Roeser, R. W., Zarrett, N. R., & Eccles, J. S. (2008). Exploring the role of extracurricular activity involvement in the educational resilience of vulnerable adolescents: Pattern- and variable-centered approaches. *Journal of Social Issues, 64*, 135–156.

Pew Research Center. (2010). Millenials: Confident, connected, open to change. Downloaded Jan 2013. http://www.pewresearch.org/millennials.

Pianta, R. C., Belsky, J., Houts, R., & Morrison, F. (2007). Opportunities to learn in America's elementary classrooms. *Science, 5820*, 1795–1796.

Pianta, R. C., & Hamre, B. K. (2009). Conceptualization, measurement and improvement of classroom processes. *Educational Researcher, 38*, 109–119.

Pianta, R. C., Stuhlman, M. W., & Hamre, B. K. (2011). How schools can do better: Fostering stronger connections between teachers and students. *New Directions for Mental Health Services, 2002*(93), 91–107.

Poteat, V. P., & Espelage, D. L. (2007). Predicting psychosocial consequences of homophobic victimization in middle school students. *Journal of Early Adolescence, 27*, 175–191.

Ramey, C. T., & Ramey, S. L. (2004). Early learning and school readiness: Can early intervention make a difference? *Merrill-Palmer Quarterly, 50*, 471–491.

Rammstedt, B., Riemann, R., Angleitner, A., & Borkenau, P. (2004). Resilients, overcontrollers, and undercontrollers: The replicability of the three personality prototypes across informants. *European Journal of Personality, 18*, 1–14.

Ramstetter, C. L., Murray, R., & Garner, A. S. (2010). The crucial role of recess in schools. *Journal of School Health, 80*, 517–526.

Ready, D. D., & Lee, V. E. (2008). Choice, equity, and schools-within-schools reform. *Teachers College Record, 110*, 1930–1958.

Ritter, G. W., Barnett, J. H., Denny, G. S., & Albin, G. R. (2009). The effectiveness of volunteer tutoring programs for elementary and middle school students: A meta-analysis. *Review of Educational Research, 79*, 3–38.

Robers, S., Zhang, J., & Truman, J. (2012). *Indicators of school crime and safety.* Washington, DC: National Center for Education Statistics, U.S. Department of Education, and Bureau of Justice Statistics, Office of Justice Programs, U.S. Department of Justice.

Robins, R. W., John, O. P., Caspi, A., Moffitt, T. E., & Stouthamer-Loeber, M. (1996). Resilient, overcontrolled, and undercontrolled boys: Three replicable personality types. *Journal of Personality and Social Psychology, 70*, 157–171.

Roeser, R. W., & Eccles, J. S. (2000). Schooling and mental health. In A. Sameroff, M. Lewis, & S. Miller (Eds.), *Handbook of developmental psychopathology* (2nd ed., pp. 135–156). New York: Plenum.

Roeser, R. W., Eccles, J. S., & Sameroff, A. J. (2000). School as a context of social-emotional development: A summary of research findings. *Elementary School Journal, 100*, 443–471.

Roeser, R. W., & Peck, S. C. (2003). Patterns and pathways of educational achievement across adolescence: A holistic-developmental perspective. In W. Damon (Series Ed.), S. Peck, & R. Roeser (Vol. Eds.), *New directions for child and adolescent development: Vol. 101. Person-centered approaches to studying development in context* (pp. 39–62). San Francisco, CA: Jossey-Bass.

Roeser, R. W., Peck, S. C., & Nasir, N. S. (2006). Self and identity processes in school motivation, learning, and achievement. In P. Alexander & P. Winne (Eds.), *Handbook of educational psychology* (2nd ed., pp. 391–424). Mahwah, NJ: Lawrence Erlbaum.

Roeser, R. W., Skinner, E., Beers, J., & Jennings, P. A. (2012). Mindfulness training and teachers' professional development: An emerging area of research and practice. *Child Development Perspectives, 6*, 167–173.

Roeser, R. W., Strobel, K. R., & Quihuis, G. (2002). Studying early adolescents' academic motivation, social-emotional functioning, and engagement in learning: Variable- and person-centered approaches. *Anxiety, Stress, and Coping, 15*, 345–368.

Romero-Canyas, R., Downey, G., Berenson, K., Ayduk, O., & Kang, N. J. (2010). Rejection sensitivity and the rejection–hostility link in romantic relationships. *Journal of Personality, 78*, 119–148.

Rones, M., & Hoagwood, K. (2000). School-based mental health services: A research review. *Clinical Child and Family Psychology Review, 3*, 223–241.

Rood, L., Roelofs, J., Bogels, S. M., Nolen-Hoeksema, S., & Schouten, E. (2009). The influence of emotion-focused rumination and distraction on depressive symptoms in non-clinical youth: A meta-analytic review. *Clinical Psychology Review, 29*, 607–616.

Roth, J. L., & Brooks-Gunn, J. (2003). Youth development programs: Risk, prevention and policy. *Journal of Adolescent Health, 32*, 170–182.

Rowan, B., Correnti, R., & Miller, R. J. (2002). What large-scale, survey research tells us about teacher effects on student achievement: Insights from the prospects study of elementary schools. *Teachers College Record, 104*, 1525–1567.

Rumberger, R. W. (2011). *Dropping out: Why students drop out of high school and what can be done about it.* Cambridge: Harvard University Press.

Russell, S. T., Seif, H., & Truong, N. L. (2001). School outcomes of sexual minority youth in the United States: Evidence from a national study. *Journal of Adolescence, 24*, 111–127.

Rutter, M., & Maughan, B. (2002). School effectiveness findings 1979–2002. *Journal of School Psychology, 40*, 451–475.

Sable, J., & Garofano, A. (2007). Public elementary and secondary school student enrollment, high school completions, and staff from the common core of data: School year 2005–06 (NCES 2007-352).

Sadeh, A., Dahl, R. E., Shahar, G., & Rosenblat-Stein, S. (2009). Sleep and the transition of adolescence. *Sleep, 1*, 1602–1609.

Sameroff, A. J., Seifer, R., Baldwin, A., & Baldwin, C. (1993). Stability of intelligence from preschool to adolescence: The influence of social and family risk factors. *Child Development, 64*, 80–97.

Schaps, E. (2003). The heart of a caring school. *Educational Leadership, 60*, 31–33.

Schonert-Reichl, K. A., & Lawlor, M. S. (2010). The effects of a mindfulness-based education program on pre- and early adolescents' wellbeing and social and emotional competence. *Mindfulness, 1*, 137–151.

Slade, E. (2003). The relationship between school characteristics and the availability of mental health and related health services in middle and high schools in the United States. *The Journal of Behavioral Health Services and Research, 30*, 382–392.

Slavin, R. E., & Calderon, M. (2001). *Effective programs for Latino students*. Mahwah, NJ: Erlbaum.

Snow, R. E., Corno, L., & Jackson, D. (1996). Individual differences in affective and conative functions. In D. C. Berliner & R. C. Calfee (Eds.), *Handbook of educational psychology* (pp. 243–310). New York: Simon & Schuster Macmillan.

Stein, M. A., Mendelsohn, J., Obermeyer, W. H., Amronmin, J., & Benca, R. (2001). Sleep and behavior problems in school-aged children. *Pediatrics, 107*.

Swearer, S. M., Espelage, D. L., Vaillancourt, T., & Hymel, S. (2010). What can be done about school bullying? Research to educational practice. *Educational Researcher, 39*, 38–47.

Szalacha, L. A. (2003). Safer sexual diversity climates. *American Journal of Education, 110*, 58–88.

Thompson, T., & Rippey Massat, C. (2005). Experiences of violence, post-traumatic stress, academic achievement, and behavior problems of urban African-American children. *Child and Adolescent Social Work Journal, 22*, 367–393.

Treuba, H. T. (1988). *Raising silent voices: Educating the linguistic minorities for the 21st Century*. New York: Harper & Row.

Uhrlass, D. J., Schofield, C. A., Coles, M. E., & Gibb, B. E. (2009). Self-perceived competence and prospective changes in symptoms of depression and social anxiety. *Journal of Behavior Therapy and Experimental Psychiatry, 40*, 329–337.

Vreeman, R. C., & Carroll, A. E. (2007). A systematic review of school-based interventions to prevent bullying. *Archives of Pediatrics & Adolescent Medicine, 161*, 78–88.

Walter, H. J., Gouze, K., Cicchetti, C., Arend, R., Mehta, T., Schmidt, J., et al. (2011). A pilot demonstration of comprehensive mental health services in inner-city public schools. *Journal of School Health, 81*, 185–193.

Walton, G. M., & Cohen, G. L. (2007). A question of belonging: Race, social fit, and achievement. *Journal of Personality and Social Psychology, 92*, 82–96.

Waterhouse, L. (2006). Inadequate evidence for multiple intelligences, Mozart effect, and emotional intelligence theories. *Educational Psychologist, 41*, 247–255.

Wigfield, A., Eccles, J. S., Roeser, R. W., & Schiefele, U. (2008). Development of achievement motivation. In W. Damon & R. M. Lerner (Eds.), *Developmental psychology: An advanced coursebook*. New York: Wiley.

Wilson, D. B., Gottfredson, D. C., & Najaka, S. S. (2001). School-based prevention of problem behaviors: A meta-analysis. *Journal of Quantitative Criminology, 17*, 247–272.

Wilson, J. Q., & Kelling, G. L. (1982, March). Broken windows, *Atlantic Monthly*. Downloaded May 2008. http://www.theatlantic.com/doc/198203/broken-windows

Winzelberg, A. J., & Luskin, F. M. (1999). The effects of a meditation training on stress levels in secondary school teachers. *Stress Medicine, 15*, 69–77.

Wolfson, A. R., & Carskadon, M. A. (1998). Sleep schedules and daytime functioning in adolescents. *Child Development, 69*, 875–887.

Zelazo, P. D., & Lyons, K. E. (2012). The potential benefits of mindfulness training in early childhood: A developmental social cognitive neuroscience perspective. *Child Development Perspectives, 6*, 154–160.

Zins, J. E., Weissberg, R. P., Wang, M. C., & Walberg, H. J. (2004). *Building academic success on social and emotional learning*. New York: Teachers College Press.

Peer Relationships and the Development of Psychopathology

10

Sophia Choukas-Bradley and Mitchell J. Prinstein

Merely a half century ago, research examining contextual correlates of youth psychopathology focused almost exclusively on parental factors (Hartup, 1970). Several influential initial studies revealed that children and young adults experiencing significant emotional difficulties could be identified by their troubling experiences with peers earlier in childhood (e.g., Roff, 1961). Soon after, follow-forward studies revealed that children who were disliked by their peers appeared to be at greater risk for a host of later negative outcomes, including delinquent or criminal activity and various symptoms of psychopathology (e.g., Coie, Terry, Lenox, Lochman, & Hyman, 1995). These findings contributed to an emphasis on understanding how children's peer status, or acceptance/rejection among peers, may be associated with later psychopathology. Over time, researchers began to take interest in developmental antecedents or determinants of children's peer status and in more broadly understanding the nature of early childhood peer experiences. Soon, an awareness of other types of peer relationships began to dominate researchers' interest. For instance, studies revealed that Youths' success in dyadic relationships was orthogonal to their status within the overall peer group (Hartup, 1996). Children's formation, maintenance, and quality of friendships soon became a focus of research; associations among aspects of friendships and adjustment also proliferated.

In recent years, studies of peer relationships have included a wide variety of additional constructs. This work has demonstrated that interactions with peers include a broad range of peer behaviors (e.g., prosocial, aggression, withdrawal, victimization), relationships (e.g., dyadic friendships, cliques, networks), statuses and reputations (e.g., peer acceptance/rejection, popularity, crowd membership), and developmental processes (e.g., peer support, influence/socialization). Moreover, these experiences occur in a variety of formats (e.g., in-person, online) and vary in presentation and function across development. Of course, the peer context is only one of several environmental systems (e.g., family, school, neighborhood, and cultural contexts) in which Youths' development is embedded. Moreover, numerous other developmental domains (e.g., biological, cognitive) continually transact with the environment (Magnusson & Stattin, 1998).

Symptoms of psychopathology likely are the consequence of multiple interacting systems that may occur in development shortly before, or even years prior to the presentation of a symptom that could be classified as psychopathology (Sameroff, 2009). Developmental psychopathologists conceptualize maladjustment as the product of interactions between multiple systems of development that alter trajectories; changes in developmental trajectories themselves may implicate new responses from the environment, or even dormant

S. Choukas-Bradley, M.A. (✉)
M.J. Prinstein, Ph.D., A.B.P.P.
Department of Psychology, University of North Carolina at Chapel Hill, Chapel Hill, NC 27599, USA
e-mail: sccb@unc.edu; mitch.prinstein@unc.edu

biological characteristics that further alter the ever-changing mosaic of developmental adaptation (Cole, 2009).

Unfortunately, as a relatively new area of inquiry in developmental psychopathology research, studies of peer relations have predominantly focused on "main effects" models of peer predictors that may be relevant for understanding psychological symptoms. Indeed, most research of the past several decades has offered important descriptive results regarding the myriad of constructs relevant for understanding Youths' experiences within the peer context and the types of psychopathology correlated with each one.

The current chapter offers a brief review of three broad domains of peer relations that have received substantial attention within the literature: peer status, peer victimization, and friendship processes (including friend behaviors and friend influence). These constructs include aspects of peer interaction that involve the broader peer group context, as well as peer experiences that occur within smaller groups of peers, often at the dyadic level. Our review is brief, focusing on definitional issues, highlighting select research linking peer experiences to psychopathology, and when possible, reviewing research that has adopted a developmental psychopathology approach to putative mechanisms. True to a developmental psychopathology approach, the chapter begins with a brief review of the normative trajectory of peer experiences, to provide a context for understanding maladaptation.

Normative Peer Experiences: A Brief Developmental Overview

An understanding of potentially maladaptive peer experiences can be aided by a brief overview of typical expectations and developmental competencies. Children's interest in peers first is evident in infancy, beginning with an interest in mutual eye contact, touching, and vocalizing with peers, and soon evolving to include more sophisticated social play over the first 2 years of life (Vandell, Wilson, & Buchanan, 1980). Interactions grow rapidly in sophistication

throughout toddlerhood. Children aged 2–3 years engage in reciprocal turn-taking with peers, express empathy, and engage in some conflict regulation skills (Mueller & Brenner, 1977). By age 3, children are able to identify a peer's distress and have knowledge about appropriate ways to comfort distressed peers (Caplan & Hay, 1989). Additionally, by age 3 children have developed social preferences and can provide reports of the peers they like and dislike (Denham, McKinley, Couchoud, & Holt, 1990). As verbal and other cognitive competencies progress, the complexities of children's peer interactions and relationships also evolve. Within the preschool years, children participate in extended conversations with peers and can engage in reciprocal play interactions. Many of these play interactions involve pretend-play scenarios or rules, which children can effectively communicate to each other and agree to within a play-bout (Fein, 1981). By age 4, some children develop reciprocated friendships that involve a clear preference for mutual companionship and increased levels of positive behavior. Children express different types of affect among friends compared to nonfriend peers (Gershman & Hayes, 1983).

By school age (i.e., 5–12 years), children's experiences with peers often involve school-based activities as well as after-school contexts that offer further opportunities for peer interaction. During these years, children demonstrate notable variability in their capacity to successfully engage in mutual, cooperative peer interactions, characterized by positive affect. Difficulties developing reciprocated interest among peers, regulating emotions with peers (e.g., aggression), or maintaining extended positive interactions become more stable features of some children's peer interactions, and appear to present risks for successful future peer relations (for a review, see La Greca & Prinstein, 1999). Variability in children's social competencies is associated with the formation of stable levels of status or reputation within the overall peer group, as well as the formation of clearly defined friendships.

The adolescent period is accompanied by increasing cognitive ability, striving for autonomy, and rapid identity development.

Peer experiences further increase in frequency during this period, accompanied by concomitant decreases in parent–child interaction. Adolescents experiment with new social behaviors, their friendships involve more sophisticated interactions (e.g., greater disclosure, emotional intimacy), and peers become a primary source of social support for many distressed youth. Friendships, previously limited to mostly same-gender peers in earlier years, begin to include a greater number of cross-gender friends for many in early adolescence. Cross-gender friendships originate in larger groups of peers; early adolescents then experiment with cross-gender dyadic interactions and slowly form more exclusive partnerships that can include romantic components (Furman, 1989). As a marker of identity, peer statuses and reputations become especially salient in adolescence (for a review, see Prinstein, Rancourt, Guerry, & Browne, 2009). Adolescents rely on peer feedback as a primary determinant for their own self-worth (Harter, Stocker, & Robinson, 1996). Consequently, peer influence becomes especially powerful in adolescence. Stressors within the peer context (e.g., peer rejection, victimization, absence of friendship) also have the potential to be especially damaging for adolescents, contributing to the development of psychopathology.

Peer Status and Developmental Psychopathology

Difficulties with peers are exhibited in numerous ways and may reflect challenges within the broader peer group or within specific dyadic peer relationships. The broader peer group, and Youths' overall peer status in particular, arguably has been examined most frequently as a predictor of developmental outcomes, including symptoms of psychopathology. Originally referred to as "sociometric popularity," but more recently referred to as "peer acceptance/rejection" or "social preference," this construct represents the degree to which children are accepted or rejected (i.e., liked or disliked) by their peers. Peer acceptance/rejection typically is assessed using a peer nomination procedure; peer nominators are asked to nominate those whom they "like the most" and "like the least." Data can be used either to derive a continuous score of peer acceptance/rejection (i.e., a standardized difference score between each participant's standardized tally of "like most" and "like least" nominations), referred to as "social preference," or to compute sociometric status categories (i.e., "popular," "rejected," "neglected," "controversial," and "average"; Coie & Dodge, 1983). Sociometric nomination procedures are considered the most valid and reliable measures of peer status (Coie & Dodge, 1983). Peer acceptance/rejection is remarkably stable across development (Coie & Dodge, 1983) and across contexts; for example, children's sociometric status among familiar peers has been replicated in groups of unfamiliar peers within a short period of time (Coie & Kupersmidt, 1983).

Children's peer acceptance/rejection consistently is associated prospectively with externalizing behavior, including aggressive, delinquent, oppositional, and illegal behaviors (e.g., Coie et al., 1995). This association appears to be robust across reporters of youth externalizing problems, as well as when externalizing symptoms are measured based on symptom checklists, externalizing diagnoses, or public records of criminal offenses (for a review, see Prinstein, Rancourt, et al., 2009). In addition, the association between peer rejection and later externalizing symptoms is revealed consistently across developmental stages (e.g., Coie et al., 1995; Lansford, Malone, Dodge, Pettit, & Bates, 2010; Prinstein & Cillessen, 2003). Peer rejection also is associated longitudinally with social and relational aggression (i.e., forms of aggression in which social relationships or reputations are targeted) among both girls and boys (e.g., Prinstein & Cillessen, 2003).

Not all peer-rejected youth are at increased risk for externalizing symptoms, however. Cillessen, Van Ijzendoorn, Van Lieshout, and Hartup (1992) revealed that peer-rejected youth can be classified reliably into subgroups of rejected-aggressive, rejected-withdrawn, and other rejected youth. Subsequent research has suggested that rejected-aggressive youth are at substantially greater risk of increasing trajectories of externalizing behavior as compared to youth who are aggressive only, rejected only, or neither aggressive nor rejected (Bierman & Wargo, 1995; Prinstein & La Greca, 2004).

Although studied far less frequently, results from some longitudinal studies indicate that peer rejection also is associated with later health risk behaviors. For example, peer-rejected youth are more likely to engage in cigarette use, heavy episodic drinking, and marijuana use, even a decade later (e.g., Dishion, Capaldi, Spracklen, & Li, 1995; Zettergren, Bergman, & Wångby, 2006). However, some studies have failed to find significant longitudinal associations between peer rejection and substance use (e.g., Lochman & Wayland, 1994), and others suggest that peer *acceptance* may be associated with longitudinal increases in substance use (e.g., Allen, Porter, McFarland, Marsh, & McElhaney, 2005; Feldman, Rosenthal, Brown, & Canning, 1995) and sexual intercourse (Feldman et al., 1995) when measured in adolescence. Results suggest that the timing in the measurement of peer rejection, and the heterogeneity of youth who engage in adolescent health risk behaviors, may be especially important to consider. Rejection in early childhood may reflect gross social incompetencies and may be associated with early engagement in health risk behaviors. However, both low- and high-status adolescents engage in health risk behaviors by mid-adolescence (Prinstein, Choukas-Bradley, Helms, Brechwald, & Rancourt, 2011).

Researchers also have examined associations between peer status and internalizing disorders. Studies using broad measures of internalizing symptoms (e.g., symptom checklists) generally have found that peer rejection is associated with increases in internalizing symptoms (e.g., Lochman & Wayland, 1994), with particularly robust and consistent effects revealed in the prediction of loneliness (e.g., Hymel, Rubin, Rowden, & LeMare, 1990).

Potential Mechanisms and Moderators

Recently, research has focused less on *whether* peer acceptance/rejection is associated with later indices of psychopathology and more on the potential mechanisms that could explain this link. Substantial work has implicated social-cognitive processes that may develop atypically among youth who are rejected by peers. Specifically, Crick and Dodge's (1994) social information processing model suggests that social stimuli require individuals' encoding and interpretation (i.e., attributions of causes and intentions), followed by the perceiver's selection of social goals, generation of behavioral response options, selection of a specific behavioral strategy, and finally, enacting that behavior. Peer-rejected youth may develop a specific type of bias that confers future risk for subsequent maladaptive peer interactions and symptoms of psychopathology.

Theory and research suggest that as compared to non-rejected youth, rejected children lack sufficient opportunities to learn skills for processing social information (Dodge et al., 2003). Instead of experiencing social situations that facilitate the development of appropriate social skills and competencies, rejected children may be faced with social experiences that teach them that their peers are hostile. Indeed, findings indicate that some youth have a tendency to interpret benign or ambiguous social cues as having hostile intent. This *hostile attribution bias* may be related to hypervigilance to hostile cues, failure to attend to nonhostile cues, or both (Dodge, Bates, & Pettit, 1990). Peer-rejected youth, especially rejected-aggressive youth, are more likely than others to exhibit a hostile attribution bias (e.g., Dodge & Coie, 1987). This is manifested as deficits in several social-cognitive processes, such as problems encoding relevant social cues, interpreting ambiguous or benign cues as hostile, generating fewer social responses, and generating more aggressive responses to hypothetical social situations (e.g., Dodge et al., 2003). Additionally, a hostile attribution bias is associated with an increased risk for externalizing symptoms (Dodge et al., 2003; Lansford et al., 2010). In one recent study, a "cascade effect" was successfully demonstrated, suggesting that peer rejection in early elementary school is associated with increases in maladaptive social information processing, which in turn predicts increased youth aggression, with compounding effects occurring in iterative cycles across a 4-year period (Lansford et al., 2010).

In addition to the role of social-cognitive processes, an association between peer rejection and externalizing symptoms may be explained by the tendency for rejected youth to develop friendships with others who have had difficulties with peers, forming deviant peer groups. The social augmentation hypothesis proposes that when children and adolescents have had limited positive experiences in a specific social context (e.g., peer rejection in the classroom), the reinforcing value of other peer relationships (e.g., friendships with deviant peers) is augmented (e.g., Dishion, Véronneau, & Myers, 2010). Peer rejection is associated longitudinally with deviant peer affiliation in adolescence (e.g., Dishion, Patterson, Stoolmiller, & Skinner, 1991), which subsequently is associated with increased risk for externalizing symptoms and other health risk behaviors, such as substance use (e.g., Dishion & Owen, 2002).

The mediating roles of social-cognitive deficits and deviant peer group affiliation may become especially relevant among youth with other known risk factors for externalizing and health risk behaviors. Exclusion from the normative peer context, combined with school failure and poor parental management, contributes to these Youths' later affiliation with deviant peers in adolescence (e.g., Dishion, Patterson, & Griesler, 1994). Additionally, early family disadvantage and maladaptive parenting practices statistically predict social-cognitive deficits (including a hostile attribution bias), which further combine with peer rejection, conduct problems, and academic failure to predict adolescent deviant peer affiliation and violence (Dodge, Greenberg, Malone, & The Conduct Problems Prevention Research Group, 2008). Similar processes have been revealed for youth diagnosed with ADHD, involving bidirectional, cascading associations across middle childhood and adolescence between academic difficulties and peer rejection (Murray-Close et al., 2010). Collectively, such results offer compelling evidence of how developmental systems dynamically transact with each other over the course of childhood and adolescence, contributing to maladaptive developmental trajectories. Peer status in childhood appears to be an important component of these models and an integral aspect of development that interacts with other risks to alter developmental trajectories over time.

Mechanisms explaining associations between peer rejection and internalizing symptoms have received less empirical attention, but extant research suggests that peer rejection may interact with children's behavioral competencies (e.g., aggression; Coie et al., 1995) and social information processing styles (e.g., depressogenic attributional styles; Prinstein, Cheah, & Guyer, 2005) to predict longitudinal increases in internalizing symptoms. Additionally, *chronic* rejection may be especially associated with internalizing symptoms over time among boys (Burks, Dodge, & Price, 1995). Last, recent work suggests that peer rejection may be associated with specific social behaviors that alienate friends, contributing to depressive symptoms (Prinstein, Borelli, Cheah, Simon, & Aikins, 2005). Continued work is needed to examine mechanisms of the link between peer rejection and internalizing symptoms.

Peer-Perceived Popularity and the Development of Psychopathology

While developmental psychologists examined peer status based on children's and adolescents' personal preferences for (i.e., liking) one another, human ethologists and sociologists were interested in understanding social dominance, influence, prestige, centrality, and visibility in the peer hierarchy (e.g., Eder, 1985). Although developmental psychologists long believed that these qualities aptly described the sociometrically "popular" youth identified using traditional methods for assessing children's peer acceptance/rejection, researchers examining adolescents determined that older youth are increasingly capable of distinguishing between their own personal liking *preferences* and their peers' overall *reputations* of high status or "popularity" in the peer group. Parkhurst and Hopmeyer (1998) were among the first to ask youth to directly nominate peers who are "most popular" and "least popular," yielding a reputation-based construct of "peer-perceived popularity." With this construct, youth may nominate peers as "popular" whom they do not personally like, and peer-perceived popularity and sociometric popularity are only moderately correlated (Parkhurst & Hopmeyer, 1998). Furthermore, the association between peer-perceived and sociometric popularity declines steadily across the adolescent transition, especially among girls (Cillessen & Mayeux, 2004).

Compared to sociometric popularity, peer-perceived popularity is differentially associated with psychosocial outcomes. For example, in contrast to the previously discussed association between *lower* levels of social preference and higher levels of aggression, research suggests an association between *high* peer-perceived popularity and aggression. Higher levels of peer-perceived popularity in middle childhood and adolescence are associated with longitudinal increases in both overt and relational aggression over time (e.g., Prinstein & Cillessen, 2003). Research also suggests a curvilinear association, in which adolescents low in peer-perceived popularity as well as those high in peer-perceived popularity may use relational aggression (Prinstein & Cillessen, 2003). Several studies in the past decade also have revealed longitudinal associations between high peer-perceived popularity and health risk behaviors, including substance use (Mayeux, Sandstrom, & Cillessen, 2008; Prinstein et al., 2011), sexual behavior (Mayeux et al., 2008; Prinstein et al., 2011), and weight-related behaviors (Rancourt & Prinstein, 2010). However, results are mixed and suggest the importance of considering curvilinear effects and gender moderation in analyses. Very few studies have examined associations between peer-perceived popularity and internalizing symptoms, but preliminary work suggests that low levels of popularity may be associated concurrently with loneliness (Gorman, Schwartz, Nakamoto, & Mayeux, 2011). Additionally, low levels of popularity may predict increases in suicidal ideation over time (Heilbron & Prinstein, 2010). Thus, preliminary work suggests that higher levels of peer-perceived popularity may be associated with externalizing symptoms, whereas

lower levels of peer-perceived popularity may be associated with internalizing symptoms. This is an area ripe for further research. It may be that high peer-perceived popularity is a marker for access to greater deviant or health risk behaviors, particularly if popularity is associated with dominance and access to resources, as has been found in studies of nonhuman species (Hawley & Geldhof, 2012); in contrast, low peer-perceived popularity may be a marker for broader psychosocial difficulties that are associated with internalizing symptoms.

Peer Victimization and Developmental Psychopathology

Peer victimization experiences have been of great interest to teachers, parents, and policy makers for many years. For many decades, however, research on peer victimization was somewhat sparse. More recently, research has revealed that peer victimization experiences are an important, unique correlate and predictor of maladjustment. Victimization is related to peer rejection, but these two constructs differ conceptually and empirically: Whereas peer rejection reflects broad group-level processes (e.g., amalgamated preferences among an entire peer context) and involves peers' attitudes rather than behaviors, peer victimization typically involves a child's exposure to negative behaviors perpetrated by a single or small number of peers. Although both overt and relational victimization are associated with peer rejection (e.g., Crick & Grotpeter, 1996) and low rates of friendship (e.g., Boulton, Trueman, Chau, Whitehand, & Amatya, 1999), which in turn are associated with maladjustment, victimization explains variance not shared with peer rejection and friendship participation (e.g., Ladd, Kochenderfer, & Coleman, 1997). Peer victimization occurs in different forms. Initially researchers defined peer victimization exclusively as physical acts of aggression or verbal threats of physical aggression. Findings suggested that as compared to girls, boys more frequently were perpetrators and victims of aggression (e.g., Boulton & Underwood, 1992).

However, researchers later expanded the definition of victimization to include relational or social forms of victimization (e.g., when relationship status or social reputation is targeted through social exclusion or gossip), resulting in increased estimates of victimization among girls (e.g., Crick & Bigbee, 1998). In recent years, an overlapping but new form of victimization has emerged in the lives of youth: cyber-victimization, in which overt or relational aggression is perpetrated electronically through text messages, social media sites (e.g., Facebook), email, blogs, chat rooms, and other Internet forums. In spite of media interest in cyberbullying following well-publicized adolescent suicides, few empirical studies have examined associations between cyber-victimization and psychopathology.

It is important to note that researchers have used various definitions of "victimization," at times conflating it with "Being bullied"; conflicting results across studies may be related to differences in how bullying/victimization is measured, such as whether a power differential between perpetrator and victim is necessary (Salmivalli & Peets, 2009). Additionally, researchers have relied on various methods of measuring victimization. Many studies use children's self-reports, which may be confounded with a child's psychopathology (De Los Reyes & Prinstein, 2004). However, children's own reports of their victimization may provide important information not captured by parent, peer, or teacher reports; in particular, self-reports have been shown to be more strongly associated with children's intrapersonal adjustment difficulties (Graham & Juvonen, 1998). Peer nominations typically are utilized to measure peer victimization, allowing the aggregation of reports from multiple witnesses across a range of situations to identify victims. However, peer reports of victimization are likely not reliable, valid, and stable until late elementary school (Goodman, Stormshak, & Dishion, 2001). Victimization stabilizes by late elementary or middle school, with a small subset of children chronically targeted by peers (e.g., Perry, Kusel, & Perry, 1988).

Extensive work has identified internalizing symptoms as important correlates and outcomes of peer victimization. Overt victimization is concurrently associated with internalizing symptoms (e.g., Prinstein, Boergers, & Vernberg, 2001) and also predicts longitudinal increases in internalizing symptoms (e.g., Vernberg, 1990). Relational victimization also has been linked with internalizing symptoms and psychological distress (e.g., Crick & Grotpeter, 1996; Prinstein et al., 2001). A recent meta-analytic review revealed small to moderate effect sizes in the longitudinal association between peer victimization and increases in internalizing symptoms (Reijntjes, Kamphuis, Prinzie, & Telch, 2010). Additionally, peer victimization is associated with higher levels of suicidal ideation and engagement in nonsuicidal self-injury (Heilbron & Prinstein, 2010). There may be gender differences in the associations between victimization and internalizing symptoms. For example, one study found that relational victimization was associated with internalizing symptoms among both boys and girls, whereas overt victimization was associated with depressive symptoms among boys only (Prinstein et al., 2001). Recent work suggests that experiencing multiple types of victimization (e.g., overt, relational, cyber) is associated with higher levels of depression (Wang, Iannotti, Luk, & Nansel, 2010).

Researchers also have been interested in examining associations between victimization and externalizing symptoms. A recent meta-analytic review revealed small to moderate effect sizes in the association between victimization and longitudinal increases in externalizing symptoms (Reijntjes et al., 2011). Perhaps especially interesting has been work suggesting that victimization and aggression often co-occur. Olweus (1978) identified a small subset of victims who were also aggressive themselves. Showing distinct behavioral patterns compared to their more passive, nonaggressive victim peers, aggressive victims appear to be at greater risk for maladjustment, including peer rejection, externalizing symptoms, and internalizing symptoms (e.g., Schwartz, 2000).

Research increasingly has revealed reciprocal associations among symptom domains and peer victimization, suggesting likely bidirectional and perhaps cascading associations between victimization and psychopathology (Reijntjes et al., 2010, 2011). As noted above, aggressive behavior, particularly reactive aggression, is a consistent predictor of victimization by peers (Card & Little, 2006). This idea has been supported in clinical populations as well; as compared to normative peers, children with externalizing symptoms, and especially those with ADHD, are victimized more frequently (e.g., Cardoos & Hinshaw, 2011). Additionally, various markers of internalizing distress (e.g., depressive symptoms, anxiety, withdrawal, passivity) predict later peer victimization (e.g., Hodges & Perry, 1999). Some work has indicated cyclical associations between symptoms and peer victimization; for example, a longitudinal study of middle childhood and preadolescent youth revealed that low self-regard predicted increases in victimization above and beyond behavioral predictors, as well as reciprocal associations between victimization and later increases in low self-regard (Egan & Perry, 1998). Models testing longitudinal, transactional associations between peer victimization and psychopathology may provide important and fruitful lines of future research.

Potential Mechanisms and Moderators

Surprisingly little work has examined *why* peer victimization may predict later internalizing and externalizing symptoms. Some conceptualize peer victimization as a chronic stressor. An influential theory proposed by Repetti, Taylor, and Seeman (2002) proposes that the longitudinal association between chronic stress and negative health outcomes is mediated by poor social competence and emotion dysregulation. Indeed, one study found that emotion dysregulation mediated the longitudinal association between peer victimization and internalizing symptoms (McLaughlin, Hatzenbuehler, & Hilt, 2009). Global self-worth (Grills & Ollendick, 2002) and self-esteem (Lopez & DuBois, 2005) also mediate associations between peer victimization and internalizing

symptoms. In contrast, it is likely that the association between victimization and subsequent externalizing symptoms is mediated by social information processing biases—specifically, the hostile attribution bias, discussed previously; however, this has not been examined empirically.

Given that peer victimization typically is conceptualized as an especially troubling and salient stressor among youth, there has been some surprise that the associations between peer victimization and maladaptive outcomes are not stronger. However, many have noted that peer victimization is a remarkably common phenomenon. Thus, links with adjustment may depend on joint effects of peer victimization, perhaps especially chronic victimization, and other maladaptive developmental systems.

As previously noted, a small subset of victims also is aggressive. Aggressive victims have more significant behavioral impairments (e.g., hyperactive and impulsive behaviors) and emotional impairments (e.g., emotion dysregulation, internalizing symptoms) compared to nonaggressive victims, as well as problems with academic failure (e.g., Schwartz, 2000). Additionally, early aggression predicts more chronic trajectories of victimization (Kochenderfer-Ladd, 2003), and genetic risk may interact with gender and victimization to predict aggression (Brendgen et al., 2008). Peer victimization is associated longitudinally with depressive symptoms when combined with maladaptive attributional styles (Graham, Bellmore, Nishina, & Juvonen, 2009; Prinstein, Cheah, et al., 2005), poor coping strategies (Kochenderfer-Ladd & Skinner, 2002), dysfunctional temperament (Sugimura & Rudolph, 2012), or maladaptive physiological stress responses (Rudolph, Troop-Gordon, & Granger, 2011). Consistent with dynamic systems theories, research also supports environmental factors as moderators of associations between victimization and greater maladjustment, including low parental or school support (Stadler, Feifel, Rohrmann, Vermeiren, & Poustka, 2010) and a lack of mutual friendships (e.g., Hodges, Boivin, Vitaro, & Bukowski, 1999). Chronic or increasing victimization may be a more potent predictor of internalizing symptoms than is a high frequency of victimization identified at a single time point (e.g., Kochenderfer-Ladd & Wardrop, 2001; Rudolph, Troop-Gordon, Hessel, & Schmidt, 2011). Collectively, research suggests that the role of victimization in children's development is complex, with children's various competencies, as well as other contextual systems, contributing to the development of adaptive or maladaptive trajectories.

Friendship, Friendship Behaviors, Friend Influence, and Developmental Psychopathology

Children's dyadic relationships with specific peers offer distinct contributions to Youths' typical and atypical developmental trajectories (Berndt & McCandless, 2009). Multiple types of dyadic relationships have been examined (e.g., antipathies, romantic relationships, acquaintanceships). Prior research has focused most closely on friendships. Characterized by more intense affective and affiliative features (Newcomb & Bagwell, 1996), friendships vary considerably in quality, and youth vary in their number of mutual (i.e., reciprocated) friendships. In this chapter we will consider both the protective benefits afforded by friendships and also the risks that they may confer for Youths' developmental outcomes.

Unfortunately, friendships can be very difficult to study, in part because the concept of friendship (e.g., vs. acquaintanceship), the identification of best (i.e., most important) friendships, and the duration of friendships can elude specific, consistent operationalization. Most commonly, youth are asked to identify friends using traditional peer nomination techniques. However, issues regarding the best source of information about Youths' friendships (e.g., youth themselves, parents, teachers), how many nominations should be permitted, and whether nominations must be reciprocated vary considerably across development, and each involves trade-offs (Berndt & McCandless, 2009). Generally, researchers agree that during the toddler and preschool years, children's self-reports are not a valid measure of their friendships, but are preferred over parent and

teacher reports beginning in the early elementary school years (c.f., Berndt & McCandless, 2009; Ladd, 2009). Data from a single youth regarding his/her friendships offer valid information about his/her *perceptions* of those friendships, but not necessarily accurate information about actual friendship dynamics or processes (Ladd, 2009). Reciprocated data from peers regarding friendship status or quality are especially useful but are often difficult to obtain within large samples and especially among clinically referred samples.

Nevertheless, research has accumulated to suggest that Youths' participation in friendships can offer numerous developmental advantages and is likely to interact with other types of peer experiences. For instance, reciprocated friendships protect children from peer victimization (Hodges et al., 1999). It may be that children prefer to victimize friendless peers because they are more socially isolated and are thus safer targets (Hodges, Malone, & Perry, 1997). Additionally, it is possible that friendships provide opportunities for children to practice social skills that discourage peers from victimizing them (Reavis, Keane, & Calkins, 2010).

Unfortunately, some of the children who might most be in need of the protective effects of friendships are less likely to have friends. For example, in addition to being more likely to be rejected and victimized compared to normative peers, children with ADHD have fewer friendships, less stable friendships, and lower friendship quality (e.g., Blachman & Hinshaw, 2002). Depressed youth also are more likely to have significant interpersonal problems, including difficulty forming high-quality friendships (for a review, see Hammen & Rudolph, 2003). Additionally, depressed youth may be more likely to elicit negative reactions from peers, including their friends (e.g., Prinstein, Borelli, et al., 2005; Rudolph, Hammen, & Burge, 1994).

Friendship as a Buffer Against the Development of Psychopathology

Friendships appear to offer developmental advantages, particularly as a source of support for youth experiencing stressors. Perhaps the most consistent findings in the study of friendships suggest that participation in a reciprocated friendship, particularly one characterized by high levels of positive friendship qualities (e.g., support), serves as a moderator of the association between various types of risk factors or stressors (e.g., negative peer and family experiences, behavioral or genetic risk factors, negative life events, chronic illness, disaster exposure) and later maladjustment or further negative peer experiences (e.g., Laursen, Bukowski, Aunola, & Nurmi, 2007; Wasserstein & La Greca, 1996). For instance, the presence of a reciprocated friendship is a significant protective factor for depression among youth with heightened genetic risk (Brendgen et al., 2013).

The "Dark Sides" of Friendships

In spite of these benefits, some friendships may fail to provide protective effects and may even confer risk. Research examining depression-related social behaviors has revealed a variety of experiences within dyadic relationships (e.g., excessive reassurance-seeking, negative feedback-seeking) that are associated with positive friendship quality but also are associated longitudinally with negative outcomes (Borelli & Prinstein, 2006; Prinstein, Borelli, et al., 2005). Rose (2002) identified a particularly unique phenomenon, referred to as "co-rumination" (i.e., extensive discussion, rumination, and speculation about problems among peers) that is associated with adolescent girls' elevated risk for depression, relative to adolescent boys and younger girls. Whereas co-rumination predicts increases in friendship quality among both boys and girls, it predicts increases in internalizing symptoms among girls only (Rose, Carlson, & Waller, 2007), and it mediates the gender difference in onset of depressive episodes (Stone, Hankin, Gibb, & Abela, 2011). Additionally, cascading cycles have been revealed, involving reciprocal longitudinal associations among co-rumination, interpersonal stressors, and internalizing symptoms among both boys and girls (Hankin, Stone, & Wright, 2010).

In addition to potentially maladaptive social behaviors within dyadic interactions, the friendship context also provides potential for peer socialization. Although peer socialization processes can be associated with adaptive outcomes, the vast majority of research has focused on deleterious peer influence processes. More specifically, the majority of research on peer influence in adolescence has focused on the socialization of antisocial, deviant, and health risk behaviors (for a review, see Brechwald & Prinstein, 2011). Extensive research indicates that peers' actual behaviors, as well as adolescents' perceptions of their peers' behaviors, are associated with adolescents' own engagement in such behaviors, including alcohol use, smoking, and aggressive and/or illegal behaviors. Peer influence also is relevant for internalizing symptoms, including depressive symptoms and nonsuicidal self-injury (for a review, see Prinstein, Guerry, Browne, Rancourt, & Nock, 2009). Additionally, initial research suggests possible peer influence on eating problems and body image concerns among preadolescents (e.g., Rancourt, Conway, Burk, & Prinstein, 2013), and studies in samples of college women have highlighted the role of friends' "fat talk" (i.e., negative body talk) in body dissatisfaction (e.g., Stice, Maxfield, & Wells, 2003).

Potential Mechanisms and Moderators

Research examining mechanisms of peer socialization is relatively scarce, but at least two possibilities have been discussed. Consistent with a social learning perspective, Dishion and colleagues have revealed that social reinforcement of adolescents' deviant talk within dyadic interactions is an important predictor of increased deviance (e.g., Dishion, Eddy, Haas, Li, & Spracklen, 1997). Whereas deviant talk is a mechanism that helps explain the transmission of antisocial attitudes and behaviors, co-rumination mediates the contagion of internalizing symptoms (Schwartz-Mette & Rose, 2012). Peer socialization may be most likely when youth believe their behaviors match the behaviors of valued or admired peers. Consistent with social psychological theories (e.g., prototype/willingness model; e.g., Gibbons, Gerrard, Blanton, & Russell, 1998), adolescents estimate the behaviors of high-status peers (i.e., perceived social norms) and adjust behavior to more closely match these norms (Cohen & Prinstein, 2006). As discussed earlier, adolescents' affiliation with deviant peers is associated with longitudinal increases in delinquent and health risk behaviors (e.g., Dishion & Owen, 2002), and these associations are likely explained by complex, cascading influences across multiple environmental systems (e.g., peer, family, school) as well as individuals' competencies (e.g., cognitive, behavioral; e.g., Dodge et al., 2008).

Limited work has examined moderators of peer socialization, but adolescents' social anxiety, the level of peer influence sources' popularity, and measures of closeness between influence sources and targets each increases the likelihood of peer socialization effects (e.g., Cohen & Prinstein, 2006; Dishion, Nelson, Winter, & Bullock, 2004; Prinstein, 2007).

Summary and Future Directions

Over the past decade, significant advances have been made in understanding the complex, dynamic associations between children and their peer contexts that contribute to the development of psychopathology. Collectively, research on peer relations and adjustment indicates that peer status (and especially peer rejection), victimization, friendlessness, maladaptive friendship behaviors, deviant peer affiliation, and peer contagion all represent risk factors for the development of psychopathology. Moreover, research suggests that associations among peer processes and children's symptoms are bidirectional and that they transact with other domains (e.g., academic performance, emotion regulation) and systems (e.g., parents' behaviors). It is expected that future work will involve increased attention to complex statistical models (e.g., developmental cascade models) and methods (e.g., social network analysis); biological processes and markers (e.g., genetic influences on peer relations; physiological

responses to peer stressors); the roles of race, ethnicity, and cultural influences in children's peer relations; and the increasingly central role of technology in children's peer interactions.

Developmental Cascade Models

One important development in the field of peer relations over the past decade has involved the use of increasingly complex statistical models capable of capturing dynamic, longitudinal transactions. For example, recent statistical advances have begun to bridge the gap between theory and research regarding the important role of peer experiences in developmental cascades. Cascade models allow an examination of the mutually influential transactions among evolving constructs over time, controlling for prior levels of each construct. Cascade studies typically employ complex longitudinal designs and statistical approaches capable of capturing nonlinear increases and decreases in variables of interest, with attention to the bidirectional influences and "spillover effects" across domains or levels of functioning (Masten & Cicchetti, 2010). In the past decade, researchers have used cascade models to test complex, longitudinal, dynamic interactions among children, their levels and domains of functioning (e.g., emotional, academic), and other systems (e.g., peers, parents). For example, research supports a developmental cascade in which neighborhood disadvantage and maladaptive parenting practices (e.g., coercive styles, low monitoring) transact with children's social-cognitive styles (e.g., hostile attribution biases) and early conduct problems; collectively, these factors predict peer experiences that reinforce children's cognitive biases, resulting in cascades of peer difficulties and exclusion from mainstream peer groups—all of which increase likelihood of affiliation with deviant peers in adolescence and contribute to longitudinal increases in externalizing problems, academic problems, health risk behaviors, and violence (Dodge et al., 2008). Although developmental cascade models and other complex statistical models of longitudinal transactions require the tracking and retention of large samples over time, studies utilizing this approach are likely to increase in frequency, yielding more nuanced models of peer relationships' putative effects on development.

Social Network Analysis

Another important recent statistical advance is the use of complex modeling to identify friendship networks, which has greatly improved the ability to examine peer contagion. More specifically, advances in social network analysis have allowed more rigorous and sophisticated analyses of processes that account for similarity of behaviors in friendship dyads or groups. Social network analyses using large longitudinal datasets can parse effects of friendship socialization (i.e., when friends' behaviors become more similar to each other's over time) from friendship selection (i.e., when youth similar in behaviors initially select each other as friends). Programs such as SIENA (Simulation Investigation for Empirical Network Analyses; Snijders, Steglich, Schweinberger, & Huisman, 2006) differentiate between selection and socialization effects by modeling changes in individuals' behaviors as well as changes in the structure of the social network, while also taking into account a friendship dyad's position in a wider network of peers (Burk, Steglich, & Snijders, 2007). Recent studies using social network analysis have indicated that selection processes may be more predictive than socialization processes of adolescents' substance use (e.g., for alcohol, Burk, Van der Vorst, Kerr, & Stattin, 2012; for cigarettes, Mercken, Steglich, Sinclair, Holliday, & Moore, 2012), whereas socialization appears to be more important than selection in explaining similar depressive levels in girls' friendships (Giletta et al., 2011). Research using programs such as SIENA is likely to increase, furthering our understanding of complex friendship dynamics and the transmission of behaviors within peer networks. Studies examining reciprocal effects within friendships remain rare at this time, and social network analysis methods may facilitate this line of inquiry.

Biological Mechanisms and Moderators

Research over the next decade also will likely involve increased attention to the role of biologically based mechanisms and moderators in associations between peer experiences and psychopathology. For example, researchers are beginning to investigate the role of physiological responses to stress (e.g., cortisol levels) in children's reactions to peer rejection and victimization (e.g., Rudolph, Troop-Gordon, & Granger, 2010, 2011). The role of genetics in associations between children's peer experiences and the development of psychopathology has also been a recent focus of inquiry. Behavioral-genetics research facilitates a greater understanding of genetic and environmental influences on children's peer relationships, as well as of genetic moderators of associations between peer experiences and developmental outcomes (Brendgen & Boivin, 2009). Such research, for example, allows an investigation of genetic contributions to popularity and victimization, although thus far findings are mixed (Brendgen & Boivin, 2009). Recent research indicates that genetic vulnerability interacts with exposure to peer influence to predict substance use (Harden, Hill, Turkheimer, & Emery, 2008) and aggression (van Lier et al., 2007). Additionally, genetic vulnerability interacts with peer victimization and gender in the prediction of aggression (Brendgen et al., 2008). In general, behavioral-genetics research on peer relations is in its infancy (Brendgen & Boivin, 2009). A promising additional area of work for future years is molecular genetics; advances in DNA collection (e.g., cheek swabs) now allow researchers a relatively inexpensive method of analyzing the interaction between environmental factors and specific genes, although the contribution of any one gene to peer relations is expected to be small (Brendgen & Boivin, 2009).

Race and Ethnicity

Research sorely is needed on the roles of race and ethnicity in children's peer relations. Graham, Taylor, and Ho (2009) noted that of the peer relations articles published over the 20-year period from 1986 to 2006, only 7 % focused on ethnicity. Little is known about racial or ethnic differences in peer processes. Moreover, studies that treat race or ethnicity as an independent variable, with the peer experiences of different groups then compared, can confound race with social class, frame behaviors of ethnic minorities as deviations from the (Caucasian) norm, or emphasize between-group differences over within-group variability (Garcia-Coll et al., 1996).

However, an increasing number of studies (including many referenced in this paper) are using ethnically and racially diverse samples. One robust finding of these studies is that children and adolescents seem to have a preference for same-race/ethnicity friendships (Graham, Taylor, et al., 2009). Extant studies are mixed regarding the role of race and ethnicity in children's experiences of peer influence processes (Padilla-Walker & Bean, 2009). As for peer status, extant research suggests that when in the numerical minority of a specific context (e.g., African American youth in a predominately Caucasian classroom), children receive fewer and poorer sociometric nominations, resulting in distorted estimates of peer status and other peer-nominated constructs (Rock, Cole, Houshyar, Lythcott, & Prinstein, 2011). As for peer victimization, Graham, Taylor, and Ho (2009) note that the racial composition of a classroom may affect findings regarding ethnically based differences in peer victimization; victimized students are more likely to be in the numerical minority of a particular school context, but students from the numerical *majority* group who are victimized may be at higher risk for internalizing symptoms. Overall, researchers have called for further studies of moderation and mediation, using sophisticated statistical methods, to test theories about the roles of race and ethnicity in children's peer relations and adjustment (Graham, Taylor, et al., 2009).

Cross-Cultural Considerations

Researchers have also emphasized the need for studies of peer relations in cultural context; many studies have indicated that children's experiences with peers, their interpretations of those experiences, and peers' responses to specific behaviors all are substantially influenced by cultural norms and values. Chen, Chung, and Hsiao (2009) offer a review of peer interactions and relationships from a cross-cultural perspective. They highlight different values placed by self- and group-oriented cultures on social initiative and behavioral control in peer relationships, reviewing how cultural values influence the ways in which different social behaviors are socialized in children and rewarded by adults and peers. For example, the authors note that whereas aggressive behaviors are sometimes encouraged by peers in Western cultures, Chinese youth who exhibit aggressive behaviors typically have widespread social and psychological problems. The authors emphasize the need for cross-cultural research on peer relations from a developmental perspective. Additionally, far more cross-cultural research is needed regarding associations between peer relations and the development of psychopathology.

Electronic Peer Interactions

Arguably one of the most important areas of needed growth in the field of peer relations involves technology. With every year, an increasing proportion of Youths' peer interactions occur electronically. In particular, the surge in recent years of adolescents' (and even children's) use of increasingly advanced cellular phones (with Internet capabilities), and the now ubiquitous presence of social media sites such as Facebook and Twitter in Youths' lives, are transforming the nature of peer interactions. Many children and adolescents now can communicate with each other at any hour of the day, from virtually any location, and the nature of this communication ranges from dyadic (e.g., text messaging through cellular phones, individual Internet messaging) to wide scale (e.g., posting messages on one's own or someone else's public social media webpage, which may be viewed by hundreds or even thousands of peers). Although current knowledge about the frequency of various types of electronic interactions is very limited, Underwood and colleagues recently completed a study in which adolescents were provided with BlackBerries and phone service plans, and the researchers found that adolescents exchanged an average of more than 100 text messages per day (i.e., sent more than 50 and received more than 50 messages; Underwood, Rosen, More, Ehrenreich, & Gentsch, 2012).

With this dramatic change in the nature and frequency of peer interactions, it is the responsibility of peer relations researchers to identify and understand the impact of these changes on children's and adolescents' relationships with peers and their overall well-being. There is strong overlap between adolescents' "online" and "offline" interactions with peers, with a primary interest in strengthening offline peer relationships through online interactions (Reich, Subrahmanyam, & Espinoza, 2012). However, online peer interactions may pose unique risks. For example, cyber-victimization increases an adolescent's longitudinal risk of face-to-face victimization, controlling for previous levels of face-to-face victimization (Jose, Kljakovic, Scheib, & Notter, 2012). Basic research is sorely needed on the frequency with which children and adolescents engage in electronic interactions of various types, the types of relationships in which interactions commonly occur (e.g., friendships, acquaintanceships, romantic relationships, antipathies), the content and quality of the interactions, and the psychological impact of such interactions. Additionally, some researchers have called for the use of new technologies, such as daily diary or experience-sampling methods using children's mobile phones, to facilitate large-scale longitudinal studies of trajectories of specific friendship processes and their reciprocal associations with the development of psychopathology (e.g., Fabes, Martin, & Hanish, 2009).

Conclusion

In summary, this chapter offers a brief review of research on peer status, victimization, and friendship processes, and their associations with children's competencies and the development of

psychopathology, with a focus on externalizing and internalizing symptoms, as well as health risk behaviors. Collectively, studies of peer relations and psychopathology suggest that peers play an important role in children's and adolescents' developmental trajectories. Peer experiences transact with developmental processes and multiple domains of functioning, contributing to adaptive and maladaptive trajectories. Future work should continue to examine transactions among domains and systems that contribute to children's development of psychopathology, with a focus on methodological approaches capable of capturing the complex associations that contribute to children's and adolescents' developmental trajectories. Further studies are needed to measure peer relations constructs, symptoms of psychopathology, and other competencies at multiple time points, with variation in the time between data collections to help capture both immediate and more enduring associations. Furthermore, process-oriented studies are needed to elucidate mechanisms through which such associations develop, and research should continue to examine the complex roles of race and ethnicity, culture, genetics, and technology in these developmental processes. Research thus far has documented consistent reciprocal associations between Youths' peer experiences and their psychological adjustment. Peers provide a context that can facilitate adaptive and maladaptive developmental trajectories. Elucidating the processes by which peer experiences influence development will be a focus of additional research efforts for decades to come.

References

Allen, J. P., Porter, M. R., McFarland, F. C., Marsh, P., & McElhaney, K. (2005). The two faces of adolescents' success with peers: Adolescent popularity, social adaptation, and deviant behavior. *Child Development, 76*(3), 747–760. doi:10.1111/j.1467-8624.2005.00875.x.

Berndt, T. J., & McCandless, M. A. (2009). Methods for investigating children's relationships with friends. In K. H. Rubin, W. M. Bukowski, & B. Laursen (Eds.), *Handbook of peer interactions, relationships, and groups* (pp. 63–81). New York, NY: Guilford Press.

Bierman, K., & Wargo, J. B. (1995). Predicting the longitudinal course associated with aggressive-rejected, aggressive (nonrejected), and rejected (non-aggressive) status. *Development and Psychopathology, 7*(4), 669–682. doi:10.1017/S0954579400006775.

Blachman, D. R., & Hinshaw, S. P. (2002). Patterns of friendship among girls with and without attention-deficit/hyperactivity disorder. *Journal of Abnormal Child Psychology, 30*(6), 625–640. doi:10.1023/A:1020815814973.

Borelli, J. L., & Prinstein, M. J. (2006). Reciprocal, longitudinal associations among adolescents' negative feedback-seeking, depressive symptoms, and peer relations. *Journal of Abnormal Child Psychology, 34*(2), 159–169. doi:10.1007/s10802-005-9010-y.

Boulton, M. J., Trueman, M., Chau, C., Whitehand, C., & Amatya, K. (1999). Concurrent and longitudinal links between friendship and peer victimization: Implications for befriending interventions. *Journal of Adolescence, 22*(4), 461–466. doi:10.1006/jado.1999.0240.

Boulton, M. J., & Underwood, K. (1992). Bully/victim problems among middle school children. *British Journal of Educational Psychology, 62*(1), 73–87. doi:10.1111/j.2044-8279.1992.tb01000.x.

Brechwald, W. A., & Prinstein, M. J. (2011). Beyond homophily: A decade of advances in understanding peer influence processes. *Journal of Research on Adolescence, 21*(1), 166–179. doi:10.1111/j.1532-7795.2010.00721.x.

Brendgen, M., & Boivin, M. (2009). Genetic factors in children's peer relations. In K. H. Rubin, W. M. Bukowski, & B. Laursen (Eds.), *Handbook of peer interactions, relationships, and groups* (pp. 455–472). New York, NY: Guilford Press.

Brendgen, M., Boivin, M., Vitaro, F., Girard, A., Dionne, G., & Pérusse, D. (2008). Gene-environment interaction between peer victimization and child aggression. *Development and Psychopathology, 20*(2), 455–471. doi:10.1017/S0954579408000229.

Brendgen, M., Vitaro, F., Bukowski, W. M., Dionne, G., Tremblay, R., & Boivin, M. (2013). Can friends protect genetically vulnerable children from depression? *Development and Psychopathology., 25,* 277–289. doi:10.1017/S0954579412001058.

Burk, W. J., Steglich, C. E. G., & Snijders, T. A. B. (2007). Beyond dyadic interdependence: Actor-oriented models for co-evolving social networks and individual behaviors. *International Journal of Behavioral Development, 31*(4), 397–404. doi:10.1177/0165025407077762.

Burk, W. J., Van der Vorst, H., Kerr, M., & Stattin, H. (2012). Alcohol use and friendship dynamics: Selection and socialization in early-, middle-, and late-adolescent peer networks. *Journal of Studies on Alcohol and Drugs, 73*(1), 89–98. Retrieved from http://www.jsad.com/.

Burks, V., Dodge, K. A., & Price, J. M. (1995). Models of internalizing outcomes of early rejection. *Development and Psychopathology, 7*(4), 683–695. doi:10.1017/S0954579400006787.

Card, N. A., & Little, T. D. (2006). Proactive and reactive aggression in childhood and adolescence: A meta-analysis of differential relations with psychosocial adjustment. *International Journal of Behavioral Development, 30*(5), 466–480. doi:10.1177/0165025406071904.

Caplan, M. Z., & Hay, D. F. (1989). Preschoolers' responses to peers' distress and beliefs about bystander intervention. *Journal of Child Psychology and Psychiatry, 30*(2), 231-242. doi: 10.1111/j.1469-7610.1989.tb00237.x.

Cardoos, S. L., & Hinshaw, S. P. (2011). Friendship as protection from peer victimization for girls with and without ADHD. *Journal of Abnormal Child Psychology, 39*(7), 1035–1045. doi:10.1007/s10802-011-9517-3.

Chen, X., Chung, J., & Hsiao, C. (2009). Peer interactions and relationships from a cross-cultural perspective. In K. H. Rubin, W. M. Bukowski, & B. Laursen (Eds.), *Handbook of peer interactions, relationships, and groups* (pp. 432–451). New York, NY: Guilford Press.

Cillessen, A. H., & Mayeux, L. (2004). From censure to reinforcement: Developmental changes in the association between aggression and social status. *Child Development, 75*(1), 147–163. doi:10.1111/j.1467-8624.2004.00660.x.

Cillessen, A. H., Van Ijzendoorn, H. W., Van Lieshout, C. F., & Hartup, W. W. (1992). Heterogeneity among peer-rejected boys: Subtypes and stabilities. *Child Development, 63*(4), 893–905. doi:10.2307/1131241.

Cohen, G. L., & Prinstein, M. J. (2006). Peer contagion of aggression and health-risk behavior among adolescent males: An experimental investigation of effects on public conduct and private attitudes. *Child Development, 77*(4), 967–983. doi:10.1111/j.1467-8624.2006.00913.x.

Coie, J. D., & Dodge, K. A. (1983). Continuities and changes in children's social status: A five-year longitudinal study. *Merrill-Palmer Quarterly, 29*(3), 261–282. Retrieved from http://muse.jhu.edu/journals/mpq/.

Coie, J. D., & Kupersmidt, J. B. (1983). A behavioral analysis of emerging social status in boys' groups. *Child Development, 54*(6), 1400–1416. doi:10.2307/1129803.

Coie, J. D., Terry, R., Lenox, K., Lochman, J. E., & Hyman, C. (1995). Childhood peer rejection and aggression as predictors of stable patterns of adolescent disorder. *Development and Psychopathology, 7*(4), 697–713. doi:10.1017/S0954579400006799.

Cole, S. W. (2009). Social regulation of human gene expression. *Current Directions in Psychological Science, 18*(3), 132–137. doi:10.1111/j.1467-8721.2009.01623.x.

Crick, N. R., & Bigbee, M. A. (1998). Relational and overt forms of peer victimization: A multiinformant approach. *Journal of Consulting and Clinical Psychology, 66*(2), 337–347. doi:10.1037/0022-006X.66.2.337.

Crick, N. R., & Dodge, K. A. (1994). A review and reformulation of social information processing mechanisms in children's social adjustment. *Psychological Bulletin, 115*(1), 74–101. doi:10.1037/0033-2909.115.1.74.

Crick, N. R., & Grotpeter, J. K. (1996). Children's treatment by peers: Victims of relational and overt aggression. *Development and Psychopathology, 8*(2), 367–380. doi:10.1017/S0954579400007148.

De Los Reyes, A., & Prinstein, M. J. (2004). Applying depression-distortion hypotheses to the assessment of peer victimization in adolescents. *Journal of Clinical Child and Adolescent Psychology, 33*(2), 325–335. doi:10.1207/s15374424jccp3302_14.

Denham, S. A., McKinley, M. J., Couchoud, E. A., & Holt, R. (1990). Emotional and behavioral predictors of preschool peer ratings. *Child Development, 61*(4), 1145–1152. doi:10.2307/1130882.

Dishion, T. J., Capaldi, D., Spracklen, K. M., & Li, F. (1995). Peer ecology of male adolescent drug use. *Development and Psychopathology, 7*, 803–824. doi:10.1017/S0954579400006854.

Dishion, T. J., Eddy, M. J., Haas, E., Li, F., & Spracklen, K. (1997). Friendships and violent behavior during adolescence. *Social Development, 6*, 207–223. doi:10.1111/j.1467-9507.1997.tb00102.x.

Dishion, T. J., Nelson, S. E., Winter, C. E., & Bullock, B. (2004). Adolescent friendship as a dynamic system: Entropy and deviance in the etiology and course of male antisocial behavior. *Journal of Abnormal Child Psychology, 32*(6), 651–663. doi:10.1023/B:JACP.0000047213.31812.21.

Dishion, T. J., & Owen, L. D. (2002). A longitudinal analysis of friendships and substance use: Bidirectional influence from adolescence to adulthood. *Developmental Psychology, 38*(4), 480–491. doi:10.1037/0012-1649.38.4.480.

Dishion, T. J., Patterson, G. R., & Griesler, P. C. (1994). Peer adaptations in the development of antisocial behavior: A confluence model. In L. Huesmann (Ed.), *Aggressive behavior: Current perspectives* (pp. 61–95). New York, NY: Plenum Press.

Dishion, T. J., Patterson, G. R., Stoolmiller, M. M., & Skinner, M. L. (1991). Family, school, and behavioral antecedents to early adolescent involvement with antisocial peers. *Developmental Psychology, 27*(1), 172–180. doi:10.1037/0012-1649.27.1.172.

Dishion, T. J., Véronneau, M., & Myers, M. W. (2010). Cascading peer dynamics underlying the progression from problem behavior to violence in early to late adolescence. *Development and Psychopathology, 22*(3), 603–619. doi:10.1017/S0954579410000313.

Dodge, K. A., Bates, J. E., & Pettit, G. S. (1990). Mechanisms in the cycle of violence. *Science, 250*(4988), 1678–1683. doi:10.1126/science.2270481.

Dodge, K. A., & Coie, J. D. (1987). Social-information-processing factors in reactive and proactive aggression in children's peer groups. *Journal of Personality and Social Psychology, 53*(6), 1146–1158. doi:10.1037/0022-3514.53.6.1146.

Dodge, K. A., Greenberg, M. T., Malone, P. S., & The Conduct Problems Prevention Research Group. (2008). Testing an idealized dynamic cascade model of the development of serious violence in adolescence. *Child Development, 79*(6), 1907–1927. doi:10.1111/j.1467-8624.2008.01233.x.

Dodge, K. A., Lansford, J. E., Burks, V., Bates, J. E., Pettit, G. S., Fontaine, R., et al. (2003). Peer rejection and social information processing factors in the development of aggressive behavior problems in children. *Child Development, 74*(2), 374–393. doi:10.1111/1467-8624.7402004.

Eder, D. (1985). The cycle of popularity: Interpersonal relations among female adolescents. *Sociology of Education, 58*(3), 154–165. doi:10.2307/2112416.

Egan, S. K., & Perry, D. G. (1998). Does low self-regard invite victimization? *Developmental Psychology, 34*(2), 299–309. doi:10.1037/0012-1649.34.2.299.

Fabes, R. A., Martin, C., & Hanish, L. D. (2009). Children's behaviors and interactions with peers. In K. H. Rubin, W. M. Bukowski, & B. Laursen (Eds.), *Handbook of peer interactions, relationships, and groups* (pp. 45–62). New York, NY: Guilford Press.

Fein, G. G. (1981). Pretend play in childhood: An integrative review. *Child Development, 52*(4), 1095–1118. doi:10.2307/1129497.

Feldman, S., Rosenthal, D. R., Brown, N. L., & Canning, R. D. (1995). Predicting sexual experience in adolescent boys from peer rejection and acceptance during childhood. *Journal of Research on Adolescence, 5*(4), 387–411. doi:10.1207/s15327795jra0504_1.

Furman, W. (1989). The development of children's social networks. In D. Belle (Ed.), *Children's social networks and social supports* (pp. 151–172). Oxford: Wiley.

Garcia-Coll, C., Lamberty, G., Jenkins, R., McAdoo, H. P., Crnic, K., Wasik, B. H., et al. (1996). An integrative model for the study of developmental competencies in minority children. *Child Development, 67*(5), 1891–1914. doi:10.2307/1131600.

Gershman, E. S., & Hayes, D. S. (1983). Differential stability of reciprocal friendships and unilateral relationships among preschool children. *Merrill-Palmer Quarterly, 29*(2), 169–177. Retrieved from http://muse.jhu.edu/journals/mpq/.

Gibbons, F. X., Gerrard, M., Blanton, H., & Russell, D. W. (1998). Reasoned action and social reaction: Willingness and intention as independent predictors of health risk. *Journal of Personality and Social Psychology, 74*, 1164–1180. doi:10.1037/0022-3514.74.5.1164.

Giletta, M., Scholte, R. J., Burk, W. J., Engels, R. E., Larsen, J. K., Prinstein, M. J., et al. (2011). Similarity in depressive symptoms in adolescents' friendship dyads: Selection or socialization? *Developmental Psychology, 47*(6), 1804–1814. doi:10.1037/a0023872.

Goodman, M., Stormshak, E. A., & Dishion, T. J. (2001). The significance of peer victimization at two points in development. *Journal of Applied Developmental Psychology, 22*(5), 507–526. doi:10.1016/S0193-3973(01)00091-0.

Gorman, A., Schwartz, D., Nakamoto, J., & Mayeux, L. (2011). Unpopularity and disliking among peers: Partially distinct dimensions of adolescents' social experiences. *Journal of Applied Developmental Psychology, 32*(4), 208–217. doi:10.1016/j.appdev.2011.05.001.

Graham, S., Bellmore, A., Nishina, A., & Juvonen, J. (2009). "It must be me": Ethnic diversity and attributions for peer victimization in middle school. *Journal of Youth and Adolescence, 38*(4), 487–499. doi:10.1007/s10964-008-9386-4.

Graham, S., & Juvonen, J. (1998). Self-blame and peer victimization in middle school: An attributional analysis. *Developmental Psychology, 34*(3), 587–599. doi:10.1037/0012-1649.34.3.587.

Graham, S., Taylor, A. Z., & Ho, A. Y. (2009). Race and ethnicity in peer relations research. In K. H. Rubin, W. M. Bukowski, & B. Laursen (Eds.), *Handbook of peer interactions, relationships, and groups* (pp. 394–413). New York, NY: Guilford Press.

Grills, A. E., & Ollendick, T. H. (2002). Peer victimization, global self-worth, and anxiety in middle school children. *Journal of Clinical Child and Adolescent Psychology, 31*(1), 59–68. doi:10.1207/153744202753441675.

Hammen, C., & Rudolph, K. D. (2003). Childhood mood disorders. In E. J. Mash & R. A. Barkley (Eds.), *Child psychopathology* (2nd ed., pp. 233–278). New York, NY: Guilford Press.

Hankin, B. L., Stone, L., & Wright, P. (2010). Corumination, interpersonal stress generation, and internalizing symptoms: Accumulating effects and transactional influences in a multiwave study of adolescents. *Development and Psychopathology, 22*(1), 217–235. doi:10.1017/S0954579409990368.

Harden, K., Hill, J. E., Turkheimer, E., & Emery, R. E. (2008). Gene-environment correlation and interaction in peer effects on adolescent alcohol and tobacco use. *Behavior Genetics, 38*(4), 339–347. doi:10.1007/s10519-008-9202-7.

Harter, S., Stocker, C., & Robinson, N. S. (1996). The perceived directionality of the link between approval and self-worth: The liabilities of a looking glass self-orientation among young adolescents. *Journal of Research on Adolescence, 6*(3), 285–308. Retrieved from http://www.blackwellpublishing.com/journal.asp?ref=1050-8392.

Hartup, W. W. (1970). Peer interaction and social organization. In P. H. Mussen (Ed.), *Manual of child psychology* (3rd ed., Vol. 2). New York, NY: Wiley.

Hartup, W. W. (1996). The company they keep: Friendships and their developmental significance. *Child Development, 67*(1), 1–13. doi:10.2307/1131681.

Hawley, P. H., & Geldhof, G. (2012). Preschoolers' social dominance, moral cognition, and moral behavior: An evolutionary perspective. *Journal of Experimental Child Psychology, 112*(1), 18–35. doi:10.1016/j.jecp.2011.10.004.

Heilbron, N., & Prinstein, M. J. (2010). Adolescent peer victimization, peer status, suicidal ideation, and non-suicidal self-injury. *Merrill-Palmer Quarterly, 56*(3), 388–419. doi:10.1353/mpq.0.0049.

Hodges, E. E., Boivin, M., Vitaro, F., & Bukowski, W. M. (1999). The power of friendship: Protection against an escalating cycle of peer victimization. *Developmental Psychology, 35*(1), 94–101. doi:10.1037/0012-1649.35.1.94.

Hodges, E. E., Malone, M. J., & Perry, D. G. (1997). Individual risk and social risk as interacting determinants of victimization in the peer group. *Developmental Psychology, 33*(6), 1032–1039. doi:10.1037/0012-1649.33.6.1032.

Hodges, E. E., & Perry, D. G. (1999). Personal and interpersonal antecedents and consequences of victimization by peers. *Journal of Personality and Social Psychology, 76*(4), 677–685. doi:10.1037/0022-3514.76.4.677.

Hymel, S., Rubin, K. H., Rowden, L., & LeMare, L. (1990). Children's peer relationships: Longitudinal prediction of internalizing and externalizing problems from middle to late childhood. *Child Development, 61*(6), 2004–2021. doi:10.1111/j.1467-8624.1990.tb03582.x.

Jose, P. E., Kljakovic, M., Scheib, E., & Notter, O. (2012). The joint development of traditional bullying and victimization with cyber bullying and victimization in adolescence. *Journal of Research on Adolescence, 22*(2), 301–309. doi:10.1111/j.1532-7795.2011.00764.x.

Kochenderfer-Ladd, B. (2003). Identification of aggressive and asocial victims and the stability of their peer victimization. *Merrill-Palmer Quarterly, 49*, 401–425. Retrieved from: http://muse.jhu.edu/journals/mpq/.

Kochenderfer-Ladd, B., & Skinner, K. (2002). Children's coping strategies: Moderators of the effects of peer victimization? *Developmental Psychology, 38*(2), 267–278. doi:10.1037/0012-1649.38.2.267.

Kochenderfer-Ladd, B., & Wardrop, J. L. (2001). Chronicity and instability of children's peer victimization experiences as predictors of loneliness and social satisfaction trajectories. *Child Development, 72*(1), 134–151. doi:10.1111/1467-8624.00270.

La Greca, A. M., & Prinstein, M. J. (1999). Peer group. In W. K. Silverman & T. H. Ollendick (Eds.), *Developmental issues in the clinical treatment of children* (pp. 171–198). Needham Heights, MA: Allyn & Bacon.

Ladd, G. W. (2009). Trends, travails, and turning points in early research on children's peer relationships: Legacies and lessons for our time? In K. H. Rubin, W. M. Bukowski, & B. Laursen (Eds.), *Handbook of peer interactions, relationships, and groups* (pp. 20–41). New York, NY: Guilford Press.

Ladd, G. W., Kochenderfer, B. J., & Coleman, C. C. (1997). Classroom peer acceptance, friendship, and victimization: Distinct relational systems that contribute uniquely to children's school adjustment? *Child Development, 68*(6), 1181–1197. doi:10.2307/1132300.

Lansford, J. E., Malone, P. S., Dodge, K. A., Pettit, G. S., & Bates, J. E. (2010). Developmental cascades of peer rejection, social information processing biases, and aggression during middle childhood. *Development and Psychopathology, 22*(3), 593–602. doi:10.1017/S0954579410000301.

Laursen, B., Bukowski, W. M., Aunola, K., & Nurmi, J. (2007). Friendship moderates prospective associations between social isolation and adjustment problems in young children. *Child Development, 78*(4), 1395–1404. doi:10.1111/j.1467-8624.2007.01072.x.

Lochman, J. E., & Wayland, K. K. (1994). Aggression, social acceptance, and race as predictors of negative adolescent outcomes. *Journal of the American Academy of Child and Adolescent Psychiatry, 33*(7), 1026–1035. doi:10.1097/00004583-199409000-00014.

Lopez, C., & DuBois, D. L. (2005). Peer victimization and rejection: Investigation of an integrative model of effects on emotional, behavioral, and academic adjustment in early adolescence. *Journal of Clinical Child and Adolescent Psychology, 34*(1), 25–36. doi:10.1207/s15374424jccp3401_3.

Magnusson, D., & Stattin, H. (1998). Person-context interaction theories. In W. Damon & R. M. Lerner (Eds.), *Handbook of child psychology* (Theoretical models of human development 5th ed., Vol. 1, pp. 685–759). Hoboken, NJ: Wiley.

Masten, A. S., & Cicchetti, D. (2010). Developmental cascades. *Development and Psychopathology, 22*(3), 491–495. doi:10.1017/S0954579410000222.

Mayeux, L., Sandstrom, M. J., & Cillessen, A. N. (2008). Is being popular a risky proposition? *Journal of Research on Adolescence, 18*(1), 49–74. doi:10.1111/j.1532-7795.2008.00550.x.

McLaughlin, K. A., Hatzenbuehler, M. L., & Hilt, L. M. (2009). Emotion dysregulation as a mechanism linking peer victimization to internalizing symptoms in adolescents. *Journal of Consulting and Clinical Psychology, 77*(5), 894–904. doi:10.1037/a0015760.

Mercken, L., Steglich, C., Sinclair, P., Holliday, J., & Moore, L. (2012). A longitudinal social network analysis of peer influence, peer selection, and smoking behavior among adolescents in British schools. *Health Psychology, 31*(4), 450–459. doi:10.1037/a0026876.

Mueller, E., & Brenner, J. (1977). The origins of social skills and interaction among playgroup toddlers. *Child Development, 48*(3), 854–861. doi:10.2307/1128334.

Murray-Close, D., Hoza, B., Hinshaw, S. P., Arnold, L., Swanson, J., Jensen, P. S., et al. (2010). Developmental processes in peer problems of children with Attention-Deficit/Hyperactivity Disorder in The Multimodal Treatment Study of Children With ADHD: Developmental cascades and vicious cycles. *Development and Psychopathology, 22*(4), 785–802. doi:10.1017/S0954579410000465.

Newcomb, A. F., & Bagwell, C. L. (1996). The developmental significance of children's friendship relations. In W. M. Bukowski, A. F. Newcomb, & W. W. Hartup (Eds.), *The company they keep: Friendship in childhood and adolescence* (pp. 289–321). New York, NY: Cambridge University Press.

Olweus, D. (1978). *Aggression in the schools: Bullies and whipping boys.* Oxford: Hemisphere.

Padilla-Walker, L. M., & Bean, R. A. (2009). Negative and positive peer influence: Relations to positive and negative behaviors for African American, European American, and Hispanic adolescents. *Journal of Adolescence, 32*(2), 323–337. doi:10.1016/j.adolescence.2008.02.003.

Parkhurst, J. T., & Hopmeyer, A. (1998). Sociometric popularity and peer-perceived popularity: Two distinct dimensions of peer status. *The Journal of Early Adolescence, 18*(2), 125–144. doi:10.1177/0272431698018002001.

Perry, D. G., Kusel, S. J., & Perry, L. C. (1988). Victims of peer aggression. *Developmental Psychology, 24*(6), 807–814. doi:10.1037/0012-1649.24.6.807.

Prinstein, M. J. (2007). Moderators of peer contagion: A longitudinal examination of depression socialization between adolescents and their best friends. *Journal of Clinical Child and Adolescent Psychology, 36*(2), 159–170. doi:10.1037/0022-3514.92.6.1040.

Prinstein, M. J., Boergers, J., & Vernberg, E. M. (2001). Overt and relational aggression in adolescents: Social-psychological adjustment of aggressors and victims. *Journal of Clinical Child Psychology, 30*(4), 479–491. doi:10.1207/S15374424JCCP3004_05.

Prinstein, M. J., Borelli, J. L., Cheah, C. L., Simon, V. A., & Aikins, J. (2005). Adolescent girls' interpersonal vulnerability to depressive symptoms: A longitudinal examination of reassurance-seeking and peer relationships. *Journal of Abnormal Psychology, 114*(4), 676–688. doi:10.1037/0021-843X.114.4.676.

Prinstein, M. J., Cheah, C. L., & Guyer, A. E. (2005). Peer victimization, cue interpretation, and internalizing symptoms: Preliminary concurrent and longitudinal findings for children and adolescents. *Journal of Clinical Child and Adolescent Psychology, 34*(1), 11–24. doi:10.1207/s15374424jccp3401_2.

Prinstein, M. J., Choukas-Bradley, S. C., Helms, S. W., Brechwald, W. A., & Rancourt, D. (2011). High peer popularity longitudinally predicts adolescent health risk behavior, or does it? An examination of linear and quadratic associations. *Journal of Pediatric Psychology, 36*(9), 980–990. doi:10.1093/jpepsy/jsr053.

Prinstein, M. J., & Cillessen, A. N. (2003). Forms and functions of adolescent peer aggression associated with high levels of peer status. *Merrill-Palmer Quarterly, 49*(3), 310–342. doi:10.1353/mpq.2003.0015.

Prinstein, M. J., Guerry, J. D., Browne, C. B., Rancourt, D., & Nock, M. K. (2009). Interpersonal models of nonsuicidal self-injury. In M. K. Nock (Ed.), *Understanding nonsuicidal self-injury: Origins, assessment, and treatment* (pp. 79–98). Washington, DC: American Psychological Association. doi:10.1037/11875-005.

Prinstein, M. J., & La Greca, A. M. (2004). Childhood peer rejection and aggression as predictors of adolescent girls' externalizing and health risk behaviors: A 6-year longitudinal study. *Journal of Consulting and Clinical Psychology, 72*(1), 103–112. doi:10.1037/0022-006X.72.1.103.

Prinstein, M. J., Rancourt, D., Guerry, J. D., & Browne, C. B. (2009). Peer reputations and psychological adjustment. In K. H. Rubin, W. M. Bukowski, & B. Laursen (Eds.), *Handbook of peer interactions, relationships, and groups* (pp. 548–567). New York, NY: Guilford Press.

Rancourt, D., Conway, C. C., Burk, W. J., & Prinstein, M. J. (2013). Gender composition of preadolescents' friendship groups moderates peer socialization of body change behaviors. *Health Psychology., 32*, 283–292. doi:10.1037/a0027980.

Rancourt, D., & Prinstein, M. J. (2010). Peer status and victimization as possible reinforcements of adolescent girls' and boys' weight-related behaviors and cognitions. *Journal of Pediatric Psychology, 35*(4), 354–367. doi:10.1093/jpepsy/jsp067.

Reavis, R. D., Keane, S. P., & Calkins, S. D. (2010). Trajectories of peer victimization: The role of multiple relationships. *Merrill-Palmer Quarterly, 56*(3), 303–332. doi:10.1353/mpq.0.0055.

Reich, S. M., Subrahmanyam, K., & Espinoza, G. (2012). Friending, IMing, and hanging out face-to-face: Overlap in adolescents' online and offline social networks. *Developmental Psychology, 48*(2), 356–368. doi:10.1037/a0026980.

Reijntjes, A., Kamphuis, J. H., Prinzie, P., Boelen, P. A., van der Schoot, M., & Telch, M. J. (2011). Prospective linkages between peer victimization and externalizing problems in children: A meta-analysis. *Aggressive Behavior, 37*(3), 215–222. doi:10.1002/ab.20374.

Reijntjes, A., Kamphuis, J. H., Prinzie, P., & Telch, M. J. (2010). Peer victimization and internalizing problems in children: A meta-analysis of longitudinal studies. *Child Abuse and Neglect, 34*(4), 244–252. doi:10.1016/j.chiabu.2009.07.009.

Repetti, R. L., Taylor, S. E., & Seeman, T. E. (2002). Risky families: Family social environments and the mental and physical health of offspring. *Psychological Bulletin, 128*(2), 330–366. doi:10.1037/0033-2909.128.2.330.

Rock, P. F., Cole, D. J., Houshyar, S., Lythcott, M., & Prinstein, M. J. (2011). Peer status in an ethnic context: Associations with African American adolescents' ethnic identity. *Journal of Applied Developmental Psychology, 32*, 163–169. doi:10.1016/j.appdev.2011.03.002.

Roff, M. M. (1961). Childhood social interactions and young adult bad conduct. *The Journal of Abnormal and Social Psychology, 63*(2), 333–337. doi:10.1037/h0041004.

Rose, A. J. (2002). Co-rumination in the friendships of girls and boys. *Child Development, 73*(6), 1830–1843. doi:10.1111/1467-8624.00509.

Rose, A. J., Carlson, W., & Waller, E. M. (2007). Prospective associations of co-rumination with friendship and emotional adjustment: Considering the socioemotional trade-offs of co-rumination. *Developmental Psychology, 43*(4), 1019–1031. doi:10.1037/0012-1649.43.4.1019.

Rudolph, K. D., Hammen, C., & Burge, D. (1994). Interpersonal functioning and depressive symptoms in childhood: Addressing the issues of specificity and comorbidity. *Journal of Abnormal Child Psychology, 22*(3), 355–371. doi:10.1007/BF02168079.

Rudolph, K. D., Troop-Gordon, W., & Granger, D. A. (2010). Peer victimization and aggression: Moderation by individual differences in salivary cortisol and alpha-amylase. *Journal of Abnormal Child Psychology, 38*(6), 843–856. doi:10.1007/s10802-010-9412-3.

Rudolph, K. D., Troop-Gordon, W., & Granger, D. A. (2011). Individual differences in biological stress responses moderate the contribution of early peer victimization to subsequent depressive symptoms.

Psychopharmacology, 214(1), 209–219. doi:10.1007/s00213-010-1879-7.

Rudolph, K. D., Troop-Gordon, W., Hessel, E. T., & Schmidt, J. D. (2011). A latent growth curve analysis of early and increasing peer victimization as predictors of mental health across elementary school. *Journal of Clinical Child and Adolescent Psychology, 40*(1), 111–122. doi:10.1080/15374416.2011.533413.

Salmivalli, C., & Peets, K. (2009). Bullies, victims, and bully-victim relationships in middle childhood and early adolescence. In K. H. Rubin, W. M. Bukowski, & B. Laursen (Eds.), *Handbook of peer interactions, relationships, and groups* (pp. 322–340). New York, NY: Guilford Press.

Sameroff, A. (2009). *The transactional model of development: How children and contexts shape each other.* Washington, DC: American Psychological Association. doi:10.1037/11877-000.

Schwartz, D. (2000). Subtypes of victims and aggressors in children's peer groups. *Journal of Abnormal Child Psychology, 28*(2), 181–192. doi:10.1023/A:1005174831561.

Schwartz-Mette, R. A., & Rose, A. J. (2012). Co-rumination mediates contagion of internalizing symptoms within youth's friendships. *Developmental Psychology, 48*, 1355–1365. doi:10.1037/a0027484.

Snijders, T. A. B., Steglich, C. E. G., Schweinberger, M., & Huisman, M. (2006). *Manual for SIENA, version 3.* Groningen: University of Groningen.

Stadler, C., Feifel, J., Rohrmann, S., Vermeiren, R., & Poustka, F. (2010). Peer-victimization and mental health problems in adolescents: Are parental and school support protective? *Child Psychiatry and Human Development, 41*(4), 371–386. doi:10.1007/s10578-010-0174-5.

Stice, E., Maxfield, J., & Wells, T. (2003). Adverse effects of social pressure to be thin on young women: An experimental investigation of the effects of 'fat talk'. *International Journal of Eating Disorders, 34*(1), 108–117. doi:10.1002/eat.10171.

Stone, L. B., Hankin, B. L., Gibb, B. E., & Abela, J. Z. (2011). Co-rumination predicts the onset of depressive disorders during adolescence. *Journal of Abnormal Psychology, 120*(3), 752–757. doi:10.1037/a0023384.

Sugimura, N., & Rudolph, K. D. (2012). Temperamental differences in children's reactions to peer victimization. *Journal of Clinical Child and Adolescent Psychology, 41*(3), 314–328. doi:10.1080/15374416.2012.656555.

Underwood, M. K., Rosen, L. H., More, D., Ehrenreich, S. E., & Gentsch, J. K. (2012). The BlackBerry project: Capturing the content of adolescents' text messaging. *Developmental Psychology, 48*(2), 295–302. doi:10.1037/a0025914.

van Lier, P., Boivin, M., Dionne, G., Vitaro, F., Brendgen, M., Koot, H., et al. (2007). Kindergarten children's genetic variabilities interact with friends' aggression to promote children's own aggression. *Journal of the American Academy of Child & Adolescent*

Psychiatry, *46*(8), 1080–1087. doi:10.1097/ CHI.0b013e318067733e.

Vandell, D. L., Wilson, K. S., & Buchanan, N. R. (1980). Peer interaction in the first year of life: An examination of its structure, content, and sensitivity to toys. *Child Development, 51*(2), 481–488. doi:10.2307/1129282.

Vernberg, E. M. (1990). Psychological adjustment and experiences with peers during early adolescence: Reciprocal, incidental, or unidirectional relationships? *Journal of Abnormal Child Psychology, 18*(2), 187–198. doi:10.1007/BF00910730.

Wang, J., Iannotti, R. J., Luk, J. W., & Nansel, T. R. (2010). Co-occurrence of victimization from five subtypes of bullying: Physical, verbal, social exclusion, spreading rumors, and cyber. *Journal of Pediatric Psychology, 35*(10), 1103–1112. doi:10.1093/jpepsy/ jsq048.

Wasserstein, S. B., & La Greca, A. M. (1996). Can peer support buffer against behavioral consequences of parental discord? *Journal of Clinical Child Psychology, 25*(2), 177–182. doi:10.1207/s15374424jccp2502_6.

Zettergren, P., Bergman, L. R., & Wångby, M. (2006). Girls' stable peer status and their adulthood adjustment: A longitudinal study from age 10 to age 43. *International Journal of Behavioral Development, 30*(4), 315–325. doi:10.1177/0165025406072793.

The Influence of Stressors on the Development of Psychopathology

11

Kathryn E. Grant, Susan Dvorak McMahon, Jocelyn Smith Carter, Russell A. Carleton, Emma K. Adam, and Edith Chen

Stressful life experiences represent the most well-established environmental predictor of psychopathology across the life-span. Research focused on children and adolescents, in particular, has documented a predictive relation between stressors and both internalizing psychological symptoms (such as depression and anxiety) and externalizing psychological problems (such as aggression and delinquency) (Grant, Compas, Thurm, McMahon, & Gipson, 2004). There is also growing recognition that exposure to some degree of stress may be necessary for the development of problem-solving abilities and adaptive coping strategies (Hetherington, Parke, Gauvain, & Locke, 2005). Nonetheless, many basic questions remain about stress processes and effects on mental health and psychopathology. These include the following: (1) Which types and what magnitude of stress exposure are associated with positive and negative mental health outcomes for most individuals of a given age? (2) Do specific types of stressors predict specific types of mental health problems? (3) Are there types of stress exposure that promote positive outcomes in some mental health domains (e.g., internalizing) but negative outcomes in others (e.g., externalizing)? (4) What biological, cognitive, and emotional processes mediate associations between stressors and mental health problems? (5) What factors moderate those relations? (6) How do specific stressors, moderators, mediators, and mental health problems relate to one another reciprocally and dynamically across development?

In this chapter, we will summarize the progress that has been made toward answering those questions, conceptualization and measurement issues that have limited that progress, and recommendations for the next steps with stress research. The chapter is informed by findings from the most recent reviews on stress and child and adolescent psychopathology as well as new developments that have occurred since those reviews.

Conceptualizing Stress for Child and Adolescent Research

Historically, stress conceptualization and measurement has represented stimulus, response, and transactional perspectives (Grant & McMahon, 2005; Schwarzer & Schulz, 2002). Stimulus approaches focus on external, environmental threat (Holmes and Rahe, 1967); response approaches focus on physiological or emotional

Preparation of this chapter was supported by a grant from the National Institute on Alcohol Abuse and Alcoholism through the National Institutes of Health Basic Behavioral and Social Science Opportunity Network (OppNet) (5R21AA021073-02).

K.E. Grant, Ph.D. (✉) • S.D. McMahon, Ph.D.
J.S. Carter, Ph.D. • R.A. Carleton, Ph.D.
Department of Psychology, DePaul University,
Chicago, IL 60614, USA
e-mail: kgrant@depaul.edu

E.K. Adam, Ph.D. • E. Chen, Ph.D.
Department of Psychology, Institute for Policy
Research, Northwestern University,
Evanston, IL 60208, USA

responses to external threat (e.g., McEwen & Seeman, 1999; Romero, 2004); and transactional approaches emphasize interactions between external threat and appraisal processes (Lazarus & Folkman, 1984).

The field of developmental psychopathology has been dominated by stimulus (or objective threat) approaches and by transactional perspectives (Grant & McMahon, 2005). Thus, prevailing definitions of stress used in child and adolescent research include an environmental component. Definitions of stress differ, however, in the degree to which they emphasize psychological processes that occur in response to the environment. One approach has focused on exposure to environmental events (e.g., loss of a loved one, natural disaster) and chronic conditions (e.g., poverty) that represent objective measurable changes in, or characteristics of, individuals' environmental conditions, in the tradition originally outlined by Holmes and Rahe (1967). This perspective emphasizes the importance of objectively documenting the occurrence and effects of environmental events and conditions independent of the potential confounds of cognitive appraisals (e.g., Brown, 1993; Cohen, Kessler, & Gordon, 1995; Dohrenwend, 2006).

In contrast, a second approach is reflected in transactional models, which posit that stress is dependent on the degree to which individuals appraise environmental demands as threatening, challenging, or harmful (Lazarus & Folkman, 1984). Although the transactional theory that Lazarus and Folkman (1984) proposed has been seminal in advancing our understanding of stress processes, there are some inherent problems with including appraisal in the definition of stress, particularly for research with children and adolescents (Grant et al., 2003). Results of research on stress during infancy indicate there are clear negative effects of maternal separation, abuse, and neglect on infants (e.g., Goldberg et al., 2003) which occur, presumably, without the cognitive appraisal component that is central to the transactional definition. In addition, preliminary research indicates that cognitive appraisal processes that play a significant role later in development do not play the same

role for young children exposed to stressors (Nolen-Hoeksema, Girgus, & Seligman, 1992).

Further, in recent years, theoretical models of the etiology of developmental psychopathology have become more sophisticated with a greater emphasis on moderating and mediating processes that influence or explain the relation between stressors and psychopathology across development (Pearlin, 1999). Reliance on a definition of stress that "lumps" together potential mediating or moderating processes, such as cognitive appraisal processes, with stressors is conceptually unclear and empirically problematic (Reiss & Oliveri, 1991). To understand fully how stressful experiences, moderating factors, and mediating processes relate to one another in the prediction of psychopathology, it is important to discretely define and measure each of these variables (Aneshensel, 1999). This is particularly true in child and adolescent research, because the role of specific mediating and moderating processes is likely to shift across development (Grant et al., 2003).

A final reason for moving beyond a transactional definition of stress is that the individually based focus of such an approach may accentuate confounding of genetic and environmental contributions to mental health problems in stress research (Grant & McMahon, 2005). From a transactional perspective, whether an experience is defined as a stressor is based on whether the individual appraises it as such. Appraisal processes, however, may reflect genetic or other vulnerability contributions to risk, thereby exacerbating potential confounding of vulnerabilities and environmental contributions to symptomatology (Dohrenwend, 2006).

The single essential element of stress research—distinct from moderators and mediators, psychological symptoms, and other sources of risk or vulnerability—is external, environmental threat to the individual (Cohen et al., 1995). For this reason, we have proposed that *stress* be defined as "environmental events or chronic conditions that objectively threaten the physical and/ or psychological health or well-being of individuals of a particular age in a particular society" (Grant et al., 2003, p. 449). Such a definition is consistent with traditional "stimulus-based" definitions of stress (Holmes & Rahe, 1967) and with more recent definitions of *objective stress* (e.g., Brown, 1993; Dohrenwend, 2006; Hammen & Rudolph, 1999. UCLA child and adolescent life stress interview. Unpublished manuscript).

Given the historical association of the term *stress* with a wide array of psychological phenomena and definitions, we have recommended the use of the word *stressor* to refer to the environmental experiences that should be the defining feature of stress research (Grant et al., 2003). The broader term *stress* is more useful as an inclusive term that refers not only to the environmental stressors themselves but also to the range of processes set in motion by exposure to environmental stressors. Thus, *stress research* refers to the body of literature that examines environmental stressors as well as reciprocal and dynamic processes among stressors, mediators, moderators, and psychological symptoms.

Conceptualizing the Role of Stressors in the Development of Psychopathology

More than 2,000 studies have examined the association between stressors and mental health problems affecting children and adolescents. Although important discoveries have been made, progress has not been commensurate with the sheer volume of investigation. A primary reason for this lack of progress is that most studies of the relation between stressors and psychological problems in children and adolescents have not been theory-driven (Grant et al., 2003).

To address this problem, we have proposed a general conceptual model of the role of stressors in the etiology of child and adolescent psychopathology (Grant et al., 2003). This model builds on previously proposed specific models of psychopathology (e.g., Albano, Chorpita, & Barlow, 1996; Hammen & Rudolph, 2003) and includes five central propositions (see Fig. 11.1): (a) stressors contribute to psychopathology; (b) moderators influence the relation between stressors and psychopathology; (c) mediators explain the relation between stressors and psychopathology; (d) there is specificity in the relations among stressors, moderators, mediators, and psychopathology; and (e) relations among stressors, moderators, mediators, and psychopathology are reciprocal and dynamic. None of these propositions is mutually exclusive. All may operate at once or in dynamic interactions.

To organize extant findings and to promote incremental research, we conducted a series of four reviews of the literature on stressors and developmental psychopathology, which we

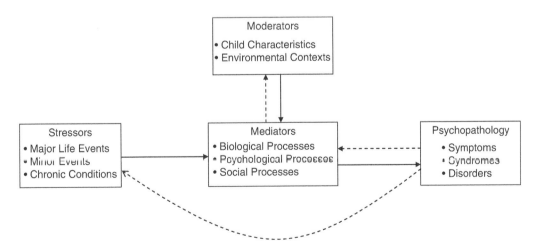

Fig. 11.1 General conceptual model of the role of stressors in the etiology of child and adolescent psychopathology. From Grant, K. E., Compas, B. E., & Stuhlmacher, A. F., Thurm, A. E., McMahon, S. D., & Halpert, J. A. (2003). Stressors and child and adolescent psychopathology: Moving from markers to mechanisms of risk. *Psychological Bulletin, 129,* 447–466

published between 2003 and 2006 (Grant et al., 2003, 2004, 2006; McMahon, Grant, Compas, Thurm, & Ey, 2003). Across the four reviews, we evaluated the evidence in support of each proposition of our general conceptual model. Summaries of findings from those reviews, along with more recent updates and directions for future research in each area are provided below.

Empirical Findings on the Role of Stressors in the Development of Psychopathology

Prospective Findings

The first proposition of this conceptual model, that stressors contribute to psychopathology, provides the most basic hypothesis for studies in the field. Evidence for this proposition for adults has been established for some time (e.g., Monroe, 1982). In our 2004 review (Grant et al., 2004), we found consistent support for this proposition with young people. Across 60 prospective studies conducted with children and adolescents, evidence that stressful life experiences predict psychological problems in children and adolescents (controlling for prior symptom levels) was consistently found (Grant et al., 2004). Cumulative measures of stressors and particular stressful experiences (e.g., poverty, divorce) were both found to predict psychological symptoms. In addition, stressful events were found to predict both internalizing symptoms, such as depression and anxiety, and externalizing problems, such as aggression and delinquency, though the associations were typically stronger with internalizing than externalizing problems and externalizing symptoms were examined less frequently. As a result of this work, investigations designed solely to test the hypothesis that stressors predict mental health problems in children, adolescents, or adults are no longer needed. Nonetheless, much additional research is needed to test for mediation, moderation, specificity, and reciprocal and dynamic relations over time and across development.

Additional prospective research is also needed to understand associations between particular types and magnitudes of stress exposure and potential positive mental health outcomes. Findings in this area are important for the development of effective coping interventions to prevent psychopathology and promote positive mental health in youth exposed to stressors. For example, it is likely that exposure to mild to moderate stressors within the context of neighborhood, school, family, and peer protective factors provide youth with the opportunity to learn adaptive coping strategies (Del Giudice, Ellis, & Shirtcliff, 2011; Katz, Liu, Schaer, Parker, Ottet, Epps, & Lyons, 2009).

Further, some youths are able to demonstrate growth even when faced with stress levels that have been shown to predict psychological problems (Kilmer & Gil-Rivas, 2010). Paradoxically, emerging work in the area of posttraumatic growth in children and adolescents suggests that youth must experience psychological distress in order to experience psychological growth in response to trauma (Meyerson, Grant, Carter, & Kilmer, 2011). Provocative findings such as these highlight how much remains to be learned about relations among stressors, psychological symptomatology, and positive mental health across development.

Finally, multilevel models can be used to better understand the complexities and patterns in the relations between stressors and psychopathology in longitudinal studies, and they have the advantage of taking into account the dependency in the data due to repeated assessments across time. Lagged models allow exploration of prospective effects, and within- and between-person models enable assessment of intraindividual change and interindividual differences (Curran & Bauer, 2011). For example, with regard to within-person effects, McMahon and colleagues (2013) found that greater exposure to community violence at one point in time, as compared to one's average exposure to community violence across time, was associated with higher self-reported aggressive behavior, but not teacher- or peer-reported behavior. This association highlights the meaningful connections between variations in exposure to community stressors and aggressive behaviors as well as how setting and context may lead to reporter differences. Multilevel models can also be used effectively to take into account nesting effects to better account for environmental context, such as when students are nested within classrooms, schools, and neighborhoods (Luke, 2005).

Moderation Findings

The notion that moderators influence the relation between stressors and psychopathology has been examined in numerous studies of children, adolescents, and adults. Moderators may be conceptualized as vulnerabilities or protective factors, because they represent preexisting characteristics (in existence prior to exposure to the stressor) that increase or decrease the likelihood that stressors will lead to psychopathology (Baron & Kenny, 1986; Holmbeck, 1997). Moderators may also be viewed as the mechanisms that explain variability in processes and outcomes ranging from equifinality to multifinality (i.e., the mechanisms that explain why varying processes may lead to similar outcomes, and similar processes may lead to varying outcomes; Sameroff, Lewis, & Miller, 2000).

In our 2006 review of the literature on moderators of the association between stressors and psychological problems in young people (Grant et al., 2006), few consistent moderating effects emerged. However, most studies simply included variables, such as age or sex, in more general analyses without reference to conceptual models of developmental psychopathology. Those that tested a specific theory-based hypothesis were more likely to report positive findings, although few studies examined analogous constructs, limiting analysis of patterns across studies. One simple, expected pattern of results was that boys were more likely to exhibit externalizing symptoms, and girls were more likely to exhibit internalizing symptoms, in association with stressors.

Since the 2006 review of the literature, many studies have focused on testing theoretically driven hypotheses using sophisticated designs. Significant moderating effects of social support (Auerbach, Bigda-Peyton, Eberhart, Webb, & Ho, 2011; Flouri, Buchanan, Tan, Griggs, & Attar-Schwartz, 2010; Rueger & Malecki, 2011), cognitions (Bohon, Stice, Burton, Fudell, & Nolen-Hoeksema, 2008; Carter & Garber, 2011; Morris, Ciesla, & Garber, 2008; Skitch & Abela, 2008; Stein, Gonzalez, & Huq, 2012), and coping (Carpenter, Laney, & Mezulis, 2012; Sontag, Graber, Brooks-Gunn, & Warren, 2008; Wadsworth, Raviv, Santiago, & Etter, 2011) on the relations between stressors and internalizing and externalizing symptoms have been found. For example, Wadsworth et al. (2011) found that disengagement coping exacerbated the effects of poverty-related stress on both internalizing and externalizing symptoms while secondary control coping buffered the effects of poverty-related stress on internalizing symptoms.

In addition to advances in the conceptualization and testing of theoretically driven moderators, additional trends in the literature include (1) a focus on biological factors, (2) the inclusion of diverse samples, and (3) statistical and methodological advances. Recent research has focused on understanding the moderating role of biological factors such as the 5-HTTLPR gene in the prediction of depressive symptoms (e.g., Hammen, Brennan, Keenan-Miller, Hazel, & Najman, 2010) and respiratory sinus arrhythmia in the prediction of externalizing symptoms (Obradović, Bush, Stamperdahl, Adler, & Boyce, 2010). For example, a notable study found that the youth with higher levels of stress over time who had two short copies of the 5-HTTLPR gene were more likely to experience depressive symptoms (Hankin, Jenness, Abela, & Smolen, 2011). This effect showed specificity as well, such that the moderating effects were not found in the prediction of anxious symptoms and were still present when controlling for anxious symptoms.

Recent studies have also focused on testing moderation models in culturally diverse samples both within the USA with Latino adolescents (e.g., Stein et al., 2012) and internationally with Chinese adolescents (e.g., Abela, Stolow, Mineka, Yao, Zhu, & Hankin, 2011). Studies like these show that there are particular types of stressors, such as economic stressors, that are more likely to interact with negative cognitions to predict depressive symptoms in specific samples of youth (Stein et al., 2012).

Methodological improvements also characterize many recent studies. Given the inherent difficulty in detecting moderation effects (McClelland & Judd, 1993), investigators have begun to incorporate statistical methods such as structural equation modeling, which reduces measurement error and increases the likelihood of finding moderation, and multilevel modeling, which takes into account dependency in the data due to nesting and repeated measures. In addition, more studies are following up on significant interaction effects with post hoc probing to determine whether simple slopes are statistically different from zero (e.g., Abaied & Rudolph, 2010; Skitch & Abela, 2008) as recommended by Holmbeck (2002). The use of multi-wave approaches that allow for the testing of interaction effects over multiple data points and allow idiographic approaches to the measurement of stress (e.g., Skitch & Abela, 2008) and the examination of three-way interactions (e.g., Rueger & Malecki, 2011) represent additional methodological improvements.

Mediation Findings

Although some variables may serve either a moderating or mediating function (e.g., cognitive attributions, coping), mediators are conceptually distinct from moderators in that they are "activated," "set off," or "caused by" the current stressful experience and serve to account, conceptually and statistically, for the relation between stressors and psychopathology (Baron & Kenny, 1986; Holmbeck, 1997). Mediators become characteristics of the individual or his or her social network in response to the stressor. In some cases, the individual may possess some of the mediating characteristic prior to exposure, but the characteristic increases (or decreases) substantially in response to the stressor. Mediators, conceptually and empirically, explain how and why stressors are predictive of

psychopathology. Broadly conceptualized, mediators include biological processes, psychological processes, and social processes.

Our 2006 review of the literature on mediators of the association between stressors and psychological problems in young people reported promising evidence of mediating effects (Grant et al., 2006). The most frequently examined and validated conceptual model has been one in which negative parenting mediates the relation between poverty/economic stressors and child and adolescent psychopathology (see Grant et al., 2003, 2006). Recent studies have provided further support for this conceptual model (e.g., Doan, Fuller-Rowell, & Evans, 2012; Reising et al., 2012).

More recent trends in the literature include the examination of additional mediators such as emotion regulation, proximal stressors, psychopathology, and coping responses. For example, emotion regulation was found to prospectively mediate the relation between peer victimization and internalizing symptoms (McLaughlin, Hatzenbuehler, & Hilt, 2009). Another study found evidence suggestive of emotion regulation explaining the relation between children's maltreatment and internalizing symptoms (Alink, Cicchetti, Kim, & Rogosch, 2009), although formal tests for mediation were not performed (e.g., Cole & Maxwell, 2003).

Evidence for proximal stressors as mediators of the effects of more distal stressors has also been reported (e.g., Flouri & Tzavidis, 2008). For example, Hazel, Hammen, Brennan, and Najman (2008) found that cumulative stress measured at age 15 mediated the relation between early adversity (including financial hardship, childhood illness, and maternal life events) experienced in the first 5 years of life and adolescent depressive diagnoses. Similarly, stressful life events and exposure to violence were found to mediate the effects of neighborhood-level poverty and segregation on adolescent internalizing and externalizing symptoms (Katz, Esparza, Carter, Grant, & Meyerson, 2012). Several studies have also found that continued stressors mediate the relations between childhood stressors and externalizing, but not internalizing, symptoms (e.g., Bakker, Ormel, Verhulst, & Oldehinkel, 2012; Turner &

Butler, 2003). The stress generation (Connolly, Eberhart, Hammen, & Brennan, 2010; Hammen, 1991) and stress sensitization (Hammen, Henry, & Daley, 2000) models provide frameworks for further delineating the mechanisms through which proximal stressors mediate the relation between distal stressors and psychological outcomes.

Recent work has also begun focusing on the mediating effects of one type of psychological symptom on other types of psychological symptoms. For example, externalizing symptoms measured in young adulthood mediated the relation between stressors measured in adolescence and drug dependence disorders in young adulthood (King & Chassin, 2008). Further, negative mood, but not total depressive symptoms, mediated the relation between stressors and substance abuse (Skitch & Abela, 2008). More mediational work of this nature is critical for better understanding the developmental psychopathology mechanisms of comorbidity (e.g., Drabick & Kendall, 2010; Sheidow et al., 2008).

Finally, preliminary evidence that particular types of coping responses mediate the relation between stressors and symptoms has been found (e.g., Sontag & Graber, 2010) since the publication of the 2006 review (Grant et al., 2006). Sontag and colleagues (2008) examined different types of coping strategies as mediators of the relation between peer stress and internalizing symptoms in adolescent girls. While higher levels of peer stress predicted decreased use of primary and secondary control coping responses and increased use of involuntary coping responses, only primary and secondary control coping significantly mediated the relation between peer stress and internalizing symptoms. Another study that used a different method of conceptualizing coping did not find evidence that avoidant coping mediated the relation between stressors and depressed mood even though stressors significantly predicted increased use of avoidant coping (Martyn-Nemeth, Penckofer, Gulanick, Velsor-Friedrich, & Bryant, 2009). These studies provide preliminary evidence that lower levels of adaptive coping strategies, rather than higher levels of maladaptive coping

strategies, mediate the relation between stressors and internalizing symptoms.

Future research on mediation models would benefit from the use of multi-wave designs and direct tests of the significance of mediation paths using recommended approaches (e.g., Cole & Maxwell, 2003; Hayes, 2009). Researchers should also formally test for mediation effects when they find evidence that there are several variables that predict outcomes, such as the longitudinal findings that acculturation stress and relationship problems both predicted internalizing symptoms (Smokowski, Bacallo, & Buchanan, 2009). Future research should also explicitly examine moderated mediation (Preacher, Rucker, & Hayes, 2007), given that studies reviewed here have found mediation paths for girls, but not boys (e.g., Sontag et al., 2008). Finally, additional research on biological mediators (e.g., cortisol reactivity) of stress effects on mental health is needed. Despite growing interest (Del Giudice et al., 2011), few tests of these variables have been conducted using recommended approaches for testing mediation (Cole & Maxwell, 2003; Hayes, 2009).

Specificity Findings

The fourth proposition of our broad conceptual model is that there is specificity in relations among particular stressors, moderators, mediators, and psychological outcomes. According to this proposition, a particular type of stressor (e.g., interpersonal rejection) is linked with a particular type of psychological problem (e.g., depression) via a particular mediating process (e.g., ruminative coping) in the context of a particular moderating variable (e.g., female gender, adolescent age).

Findings from our 2003 review of the literature on specificity in the relation between particular stressors and particular psychological problems in children and adolescents (McMahon et al., 2003) revealed that, with a few notable exceptions (e.g., Eley & Stevenson, 2000; Sandler, Reynolds, Kliewer, & Ramirez, 1992), these studies did not define themselves as "specificity" studies, nor did they test a specificity theory. Further, a consistent pattern of specific effects failed to emerge, with the exception of findings for sexual abuse. Several studies demonstrated that sexual abuse was specifically associated with internalizing outcomes, posttraumatic stress disorder (PTSD), and sexual acting out.

Since our 2003 review on specificity (McMahon et al., 2003), there has been significant growth in the number of self-identified specificity studies, and this particular review has been cited 164 times to date according to Google Scholar. Further, specificity is increasingly being investigated internationally (e.g., Bancila & Mittelmark, 2005; Benjet, Borges, Mendez, Fleiz, & Medina-Mora, 2011; Davis & Humphrey, 2012; Gustafsson, Larsson, Nelson, & Gustafsson, 2009; Lee et al., 2011; Phillips, Hammen, Brennan, Najman, & Bor, 2005). However, there are still relatively few studies that identify as specificity studies and test theory-based hypotheses with multiple stressors and multiple outcomes using rigorous methods across time.

Recent large-scale international studies have found some evidence for specificity as well as evidence for equifinality (varying processes lead to similar outcomes) and multifinality (similar processes lead to varying outcomes), consistent with our previous review (McMahon et al., 2003). For example, Benjet and colleagues (2011) found that family dysfunction adversities (e.g., abuse and violence) were consistently associated with many types of disorders among Mexican adolescents but also found evidence of specificity with regard to parental loss and adolescent anxiety disorders. Phillips and colleagues (2005) also found some evidence of specificity among low-income Australian adolescents. In particular, the youth with an anxiety disorder were significantly more likely to have been exposed to mothers' partner changes, prenatal marital dissatisfaction, and mothers' partners' troubles with the law. More generally, adolescents with anxiety disorders were more likely to have experienced a greater number of adversities than adolescents with depressive disorders. Studies such as these examined many stressors and many outcomes,

but did not test specific, comprehensive models based on theory.

Here we highlight two studies that demonstrate progress in testing for specificity using comprehensive theory-based hypotheses. First, Hankin, Wetter, Cheely, and Oppenheimer (2008) tested specificity of mediation and moderation processes based on Beck's (1987) cognitive theory of depression in a racially diverse, predominantly middle-class sample of youth and found that dysfunctional attitudes combined with negative life events predicted anhedonic depressive symptoms but not general depressive, anxious, or externalizing symptoms over time. Bidirectional effects were evident and moderated by sex, showing initial depressive symptoms and stressors predicted changes in dysfunctional attitudes over time more strongly for girls than boys.

Flynn and Rudolph (2011) also provide an excellent illustration of theory-based specificity research using a longitudinal design. They examined specificity by pitting noninterpersonal versus interpersonal stressors and anxiety versus depression and also examined models that proposed alternative directions of effects. They found that time two self-generated interpersonal stressors mediated the relation between time one ineffective stress responses and time three depression. These studies provide illustrations of progress in the field toward theory-based analysis of comprehensive specificity hypotheses (McMahon et al., 2003).

Although there has been growth in specificity research and advances in the rigor of studies that test specific theory-based hypotheses, this field of study is still in its infancy. Part of the reason for this is that there are so many combinations of variables that can be examined that it will take a long time to accumulate evidence on any given pattern of findings. Furthermore, much of the recent self-identified specificity literature has focused on depression and/or anxiety, suggesting a need to examine a more diverse set of outcomes. In addition, there has been little work examining specificity of stressors in relation to positive outcomes. Finally, there are still relatively few studies that include diverse samples (e.g., Hankin, 2008). Thus, we recommend that researchers test theory-based models using rigorous, longitudinal designs and examine multiple stressors in relation to multiple outcomes with diverse samples. Such research is needed to reveal complex patterns that may exist for specific populations. In addition, another review of the literature is warranted to establish current patterns in specificity research.

Reciprocal and Dynamic Findings

The final proposition, that relations among stressors, moderators, mediators, and psychopathology are reciprocal and dynamic, broadly encompasses the following specific hypotheses: (a) Each variable in the model influences the other (with some exceptions, e.g., fixed moderators such as age will not be influenced by other variables); (b) the role of specific variables within the model may vary across specific stressors and shift over time (e.g., a mediator that developed in response to a particular stressor may become a fixed pattern of responding and may thus interact as a moderator with subsequent stressors); and (c) reciprocal and dynamic relations among stressors, moderators, and mediators will predict not only the onset of psychological problems but also the exacerbation of symptoms and the movement along a continuum from less to more severe forms of psychopathology (e.g., shifts from depressive symptoms to depressive disorder).

The proposition that relations among stressors, moderators, mediators, and psychopathology are reciprocal and dynamic has received the least research attention. Extant research has generally focused on psychopathology predicting additional stressful experiences (Hammen, 1991). Our 2004 review (Grant et al., 2004) suggests that symptoms do predict increased exposure to stressors, indicating that at least some children and adolescents are caught in a continuing cycle in which stressful experiences contribute to increases in internalizing or externalizing symptoms, which contribute to other problems and stressors. Some findings also suggest that cognitive variables may serve initially as mediators in

young children but later crystalize, as children become adolescents, to function as moderators in relation to later stress exposure (e.g., Grant et al., 2004; Nolen-Hoeksema et al., 1992).

Since the publication of our 2004 review, new evidence has emerged that psychological symptoms and stressors predict each other in a reciprocal fashion using designs with two time points (Kercher, Rapee, & Schniering, 2009; Yang, Chiu, Soong, & Chen, 2008). In addition, more researchers are collecting multi-wave data that include more than two time points (e.g., Carter et al., 2006; Cole et al., 2006; Rudolph et al., 2009). Multi-wave studies allow more complex relations among variables to be examined (e.g., Auerbach et al., 2011; Flynn & Rudolph, 2011; Hankin, Stone, & Ann Wright, 2010; McLaughlin et al., 2009) and allow researchers to test changes in relations among variables across development. For example, in a 3-year study of adolescents, stressors predicted rumination at one wave, but not the other (Hankin et al., 2010). More researchers are also using structural equation modeling, which is well suited for tests of these types of models as they allow researchers to test multiple relations among multiple variables (Hankin et al., 2010; McLaughlin et al., 2009).

An emerging area of research has demonstrated the role that stressors can play as moderators of other variables (i.e., potential protective factors) typically viewed as moderators of stress effects. In particular, Luthar, Cicchetti, and Becker (2000) introduced the concept of a protective reactive effect, in which protective moderators lose their power at the highest level of stress exposure. In other words, stressors may change the relation between protective factors and outcomes. Several studies have documented such an effect (e.g., Gerard, & Buehler, 2004; Formoso, Gonzales, & Aiken, 2000; Seidman, Lambert, Allen, & Aber, 2003). For example, in some of our work (Grant, 2011), we found evidence that stress exposure moderated the association between protective factors and psychological symptoms, such that protective factors were associated with fewer symptoms under conditions of low stress but with more symptoms under conditions of high stress in a sample of low-income urban youth. Consistent with this pattern, cluster analyses with this sample revealed stronger prospective associations between stressors and psychological symptoms among the youth who relied on individually based coping strategies than the youth who reported not using any coping strategies at all. Supplemental analyses indicated, however, that even highly stressed youth could benefit from individually based coping strategies if they were used in the context of supportive interpersonal relationships and protective settings (i.e., family, school, church, community organization). Additional research is needed to replicate findings such as these, as they suggest the potential for iatrogenic or protective reactive effects for individually based programs targeting highly stressed youth unless sufficient interpersonal and setting support is ensured (Farahmand, Grant, Polo, Duffy, & Dubois, 2011).

More generally, much additional research is needed to test reciprocal and dynamic relations among stressors, moderators, mediators, and outcomes. Only one general pattern has been established to date in this area and that is that psychopathology also predicts exposure to stressors. Some promising trends suggest that cognitive variables may initially serve as mediators early in development but progress to become moderators as children become adolescents (e.g., Grant et al., 2004; Nolen-Hoeksema et al., 1992), and that stressors can change the association between protective moderators and mental health outcomes (Grant, 2011; Luthar et al., 2000). But, much remains to be learned and established. The creation and examination of specific models and hypotheses related to reciprocal and dynamic relations among stressors, moderators, mediators, and mental health outcomes across development are needed.

Remaining Barriers to Progress in Stress Research

In addition to the findings emanating from our reviews summarized above, we also concluded that measurement issues have negatively affected progress in the field. In fact, our reviews of the literature led us to conclude that the single most important barrier to progress in the field has been inadequate and inconsistent measurement of stressful life experiences (Grant et al., 2003, 2004, 2006; McMahon et al., 2003). To illustrate, we found that fewer than 10 % of stress researchers used a well-validated measure, and no single measure was used in more than 3 % of studies (Grant et al., 2004). Nonetheless, concurrent with the execution of thousands of studies examining the association between stressors and psychopathology, a small rigorous body of research has focused on stressor measurement. We summarize results of that research to date, measurement issues that continue to plague the field, and strategies for addressing remaining issues.

Progress and Barriers in Stressor Measurement

As noted toward the beginning of this chapter, there has been growing agreement that stressors should be defined as environmentally based events or circumstances that are "objectively threatening" (i.e., independent raters agree they would pose threat to the average individual) (e.g., Cohen & Hamrick, 2003; Monroe, 2008). The most commonly used measures (i.e., stressor checklists), however, have not been empirically developed to assess objective threat (Dohrenwend, 2006; Grant et al., 2004).

Stressor Checklists

The most widely used method for assessing stressors is the self-report checklist. Checklists are relatively easy to administer and allow investigators to collect data on large samples, thus increasing statistical power to detect relations among stressors, mediating and moderating variables, and psychological outcomes. Data have established the test-retest reliability and concurrent validity of several stress checklists for adolescents, in particular (for a review, see Grant et al., 2004). Nonetheless, many problems with these measures remain. Most notably, the items have been selected by researchers based on focus groups or authors' opinion, without empirical evaluation of the objective threat level associated with each item/stressor (Grant et al., 2004). Furthermore, as checklists include a list of brief items (e.g., death of a grandparent), it is unclear to what degree each stressor assesses the same experience for different adolescents (Dohrenwend, 2006). For example, death of a grandparent who has had little contact with a young person is less threatening than death of a grandparent who has served as that youth's primary caregiver (Hammen & Rudolph, 1999. UCLA child and adolescent life stress interview. Unpublished manuscript). Stressor checklists have also been critiqued for not requiring respondents to provide information about the timing, frequency, or chronicity of events (e.g., Grant et al., 2004; Hammen & Rudolph, 1999. UCLA child and adolescent life stress interview. Unpublished manuscript).

Stressor Interviews

Stressor interviews were developed to address the methodological shortcomings of stressor checklists and to provide relatively objective indices of contextual threat. Interviews are used to generate a list of stressful events experienced and the surrounding conditions, including a description of what happened, when it happened, who was involved, and the consequences of the event (Rudolph & Hammen, 1999; Rudolph & Flynn, 2007). External raters then evaluate the level of threat and severity of impact of each event and objectives indices are formed (e.g., Garber, Keiley, & Martin, 2002; Rudolph & Flynn, 2007). Inter-rater reliability of objective threat ratings has typically been quite high (e.g., Garber et al., 2002; Rudolph & Flynn, 2007), and, in the adult literature, stress interviews have generally proven superior to checklist measures in accuracy and ability to predict negative outcomes (e.g., Dohrenwend, 2006). There have been far fewer published comparisons of the two approaches with adolescents, and the results of these comparisons have been less conclusive (e.g., Duggal et al., 2000; Wagner, Abela, & Brozina, 2006). One possible reason for weaker effects for adolescents is that interviews may be less likely to elicit information that is embarrassing or have potential negative consequences if reported (Singleton & Straits, 1999), and these concerns may be especially salient for younger samples. In addition, personnel and time demands associated with stressor interviews have limited their use with researchers (Grant et al., 2004).

Stress interviews are limited in several other important ways. For example, although existing interviews capture some minor stressors (e.g., failing a test, argument with a friend), they do not comprehensively measure minor stressors, which may also predict negative outcomes (e.g., Miller, Webster, & MacIntosh, 2002). Nor do they comprehensively assess stressors at the opposite of the continuum (i.e., broad and pervasive systemic stressors such as racism or classism), perhaps because the very nature of these stressors increases the likelihood that they will go unrecognized by individuals who experience them. For example, interviews developed for young people have not included questions about exposure to discrimination, and researchers who have added discrimination questions or have assessed for discrimination using checklist methods have found that the youth report relatively few events (Gee & Walsemann, 2009; Flores, Tschann, Dimas, Pasch, & de Groat, 2010; Seaton, 2009). This finding stands in contrast to growing evidence that health disparities associated with race/ethnicity and class may be largely attributable to differences in stress exposure (Adler, 2009; Goodman, McEwen, Dolan, Schafer-Kalkhoff, & Adler, 2005; Jackson, Knight, & Rafferty, 2010) and suggests the need for new approaches to the assessment of systems-level stressors. Another problem with the stress interview is its retrospective approach, which limits the linking of stressful experiences with mediating processes that are immediately activated.

Physiologically Focused Laboratory Measures of Stress

During a period in which developmental psychopathologists have worked to conceptualize stressors objectively and measure them using narrative interviews, stress researchers in other disciplines took a different approach. Biologists and neurologists interested in understanding stress effects on physical health developed measures that focused on physiological responses to stressors (e.g., McEwen & Seeman, 1999; Romero, 2004). This approach is most consistent with a response definition of stress (Grant & McMahon, 2005). Studies conducted using this approach have revolutionized stress research by revealing proximal physiological responses to stressors and linking those responses to long-term physical health outcomes (McEwen & Seeman, 2006). Nonetheless, conceptualization and measurement of stress in this area also remains incomplete. In particular, response definitions of stress confound external stressors with stress responses, making it difficult to examine these variables discretely or to test responses as mediators and moderators of long-term stressor effects (Grant et al., 2003). Additionally, such approaches can suffer from circular logic by defining a stressor as any experience that produces a stress response (Monroe, 2008). Finally, although frequently conceptualized as acute responses, physiological processes change in response to stressors over different time spans (i.e., chronic versus acute stressors elicit different, sometimes opposite, responses; Adam, 2012; Miller, Chen, & Zhou, 2007) highlighting the need to examine the role of stressor chronicity in biological responses to stress.

Beyond critiques of checklist, interview, and physiologically focused laboratory measurement approaches lies a central problem affecting each method: a lack of standardization of stressor measurement. As noted above, our reviews revealed that fewer than 10 % of stress researchers used a well-validated measure, and no single measure was used in more than 3 % of studies (Grant et al., 2004). Lack of standardization highlights a central difference between the state of the field of stressor conceptualization and measurement compared to psychopathology conceptualization and measurement. Specifically, taxonomies of psychopathology (e.g., the *DSM-5*; APA, 1994; the Achenbach System of Empirically Based Assessment; ASEBA; Achenbach & Rescorla, 2001) have been developed, but no such taxonomy exists for stressors. In order to foster incremental research, we need to agree upon a common conceptualization of stressors and to develop and utilize valid and reliable measures of stressors that capture their breadth and complexity.

Strategies for Addressing Measurement Barriers

The development of reliable and valid narrative stressor interviews indicates that it is possible to achieve agreement about events and conditions that pose threat to youth in our society. Evidence for the reliability and validity of stressor checklists has also emerged in spite of the fact that these measures have been developed independently from empirically based objective threat ratings. In addition, advances in theory and measurement of physiological responses to stress provide models for examining mediators of stress effects on developmental psychopathology in real time. These achievements suggest that a standardized system of stress measurement, which builds on the strengths of each of those methodologies, could be developed. Members of our research group have been working to do just that with a particular focus on adolescents, given their heightened exposure to stressors, greater risk for mental health problems, and capacity to report on their own stress exposure (Grant et al., 2004).

Our goal is to create a series of advanced checklist measures that offer the increased confidentiality and reduced time demands of checklists while preserving the strengths of interviews, including contextual indicators of objective threat and assessment of stressor duration and frequency. We also are working to develop novel laboratory-based stress challenges that mimic minor stressors identified by youth themselves (through daily diary studies) and rated as objectively threatening by independent coders (perhaps by virtue of exposure to multiple minor events or exposure to minor events linked with major or systems-level stressors). These stressor challenges will facilitate collection of biological, cognitive, and affective response data in real time.

In addition, we are working to empirically examine possible taxonomic organizations based on conceptual hypotheses. For example, we will test the hypothesis that particular types of minor stressors (e.g., achievement frustration tasks) will be consistently rated as objectively threatening when they are experienced within the context of major events (e.g., academic failure) and/or systemic stressors (e.g., racist stereotypes) within the same meaning domain (e.g., agency/achievement). Through empirical analysis of conceptually based hypotheses such as these, we hope to develop a stressor taxonomy that will guide, and be refined through longitudinal and life-span research, and, ultimately, be standardized for use across multiple studies. Standardization (on a large, nationally representative sample) would establish stressor base rates, norms, and risk cut points relative to clinically significant symptomatology as well as competence cut points, highlighting levels of stress exposure ideal for the development of adaptive coping strategies.

Summary and Conclusion

Thousands of studies have examined the association between stressful life experiences and mental health problems affecting children and adolescents. Although important discoveries have been made, progress has not been commensurate with the sheer volume of investigation. A primary reason for this lack of progress is that most studies of the relation between stressors and developmental psychopathology have not been theory-driven.

To address this problem, we have proposed a general conceptual model of the role of stressors in the etiology of child and adolescent psychopathology. This model builds on previously proposed specific models of psychopathology and includes five central propositions (see Fig. 11.1): (a) stressors contribute to psychopathology; (b) moderators influence the relation between stressors and psychopathology; (c) mediators explain the relation between stressors and psychopathology; (d) there is specificity in the relations among stressors, moderators, mediators, and

psychopathology; and (e) relations among stressors, moderators, mediators, and psychopathology are reciprocal and dynamic. In a series of four reviews, we evaluated evidence for each proposition of the model.

Results indicate the field has unequivocally established that stressful life experiences prospectively predict mental health problems in young people (consistent with well-established patterns for adults), and there is growing evidence that mental health problems, in turn, predict stress exposure. Evidence has also emerged that gender influences the type of distress associated with stress exposure and that sexual abuse specifically predicts internalizing problems. These two latter patterns, however, highlight the need for further analysis and integration across stress research areas, as sexual abuse is much more common for girls (i.e., moderation and specificity findings are confounded). Finally, there is solid evidence that compromised parenting behavior and disrupted family relationships mediate the association between poverty/economic stressors and mental health problems affecting young people.

Exciting new patterns to emerge since our reviews were completed (i.e., between 2003 and 2006) include findings on positive mental health effects associated with mild to moderate stress exposure and the possibility of posttraumatic growth even in the face of more severe exposure. Research on moderators of stress effects has become more sophisticated with greater use of theory-driven hypotheses, longitudinal designs, multilevel modeling, rigorous post hoc probing, tests for three-way interactions, inclusion of culturally diverse samples, and examination of genetic moderators of stress effects. New findings in the area of mediation suggest that emotion regulation, proximal stressors, specific types of psychopathology, and coping responses also mediate stress effects on mental health problems in young people. Additional integrative research is needed to test for moderated mediation.

There has been growth in the number of studies, as well as quality and rigor of designs that allow for comprehensive tests of specificity. Researchers are now recognizing the importance of understanding the context in which specific types of stressors lead to specific outcomes among particular populations and beginning to test for alternative plausible models that clarify the reach of their findings. Additional longitudinal, theory-based research with diverse samples is needed in this area.

In the area of reciprocal and dynamic relations among stressors, moderators, mediators, and psychopathology, emerging research suggests that stressors can moderate the association between protective factors/processes and mental health outcomes. Despite findings such as these, research in this area is the least developed of all. The creation and examination of specific models and hypotheses related to reciprocal and dynamic relations among stressors, moderators, mediators, and mental health outcomes across development are needed.

Beyond establishing points of progress in the field, our reviews also highlight methodological problems, particularly with stressor measurement, that have impeded progress. There has been growing agreement that stressors should be defined as environmentally based events or circumstances that are "objectively threatening" (i.e., independent raters can agree they would pose threat to the average individual); yet, only the most labor-intensive narrative interviews are capable of assessing such threat, and such interviews have been used by only a small minority of stress researchers. Furthermore, narrative interviews are limited in their assessment of minor stressors, which may also predict negative outcomes, due to challenges in achieving agreement about what constitutes objective threat with minor events. Narrative interviews are also limited in their capacity to assess stressors at the opposite end of the continuum: systemic stressors that are so broad and pervasive they may not be recognized as stressors by individuals who experience them (e.g., racism, classism). Finally, stressor interviews are limited by their retrospective approach, which does not allow for the linking of stressful experiences with mediating processes in real time.

To address current limitations with conceptualization and measurement of stressful life experiences, we recommend the creation of an empirically based series of measures capable of (a) assessing stressful experiences across multiple levels ranging from minor stressors to broad systemic pressures and (b) linking those stressors, individually and in combination, with the biological, cognitive, and emotional processes that mediate their effects on developmental psychopathology. Constructing such a system will require integration of the strengths of existing approaches to stress measurement including checklists, narrative interviews, and physiologically focused laboratory measures. We also recommend that measurement advances are used to develop a taxonomy of stressors that organizes stressor subtypes in ways that are theoretically and empirically meaningful.

In conclusion, if the field of stress research were an architectural drawing, it would present a strange-looking picture. On the one hand, many architects have contributed numerous structures to the drawing including multiple simple structures (many of these redundant in function) and also some amazingly creative and complex ones. All the while, the foundation to support these structures remains incompletely drawn. If we, as stress research architects, could complete our foundation drawings, we could consolidate our basic structures and integrate our beautiful ones and, ultimately, build an impressive cathedral of knowledge. In this way, the potential for stress theory and research to substantially influence basic and applied understanding of processes leading to developmental psychopathology would be realized.

References

Abaied, J. L., & Rudolph, K. D. (2010). Mothers as a resource in times of stress: Interactive contributions of socialization of coping and stress to youth psychopathology. *Journal of Abnormal Child Psychology, 38,* 273–289.

Abela, J. Z., Stolow, D., Mineka, S., Yao, S., Zhu, X., & Hankin, B. L. (2011). Cognitive vulnerability to depressive symptoms in adolescents in urban and rural Hunan, China: A multiwave longitudinal study. *Journal of Abnormal Psychology, 120,* 765–778.

Achenbach, T. M., & Rescorla, L. A. (2001). *Manual for the ASEBA school-age forms and profiles.* Burlington:

University of Vermont, Research Center for Children, Youth, and Families.

Adam, E. K. (2012). Emotion-cortisol transactions occur over multiple time scales in development: Implications for research on emotion and the development of emotional disorders. In T. A. Dennis, K. A. Buss, & P. D. Hastings (Eds). *Physiological Measures of Emotion from a Developmental Perspective: State of the Science. Monographs of the Society for Research in Child Development, 77* (2), 17–27.

Adler, N. (2009). Health disparities through a psychological lens. *American Psychologist, 663–673.*

Albano, A. M., Chorpita, B. F., & Barlow, D. H. (1996). Childhood anxiety disorders. In E. J. Mash & R. A. Barkley (Eds.), *Child psychopathology* (pp. 196–241). New York: Guilford Press.

Alink, L. A., Cicchetti, D., Kim, J., & Rogosch, F. A. (2009). Mediating and moderating processes in the relation between maltreatment and psychopathology: Mother-child relationship quality and emotion regulation. *Journal of Abnormal Child Psychology, 37,* 831–843.

American Psychiatric Association. (1994). *Diagnostic and statistical manual of mental disorders* (4th ed.). Washington, DC: Author.

Aneshensel, C. S. (1999). Outcomes of the stress process. In A. V. Horwitz & T. L. Scheid (Eds.), *A handbook for the study of mental health: Social contexts, theories, and systems* (pp. 211–227). New York: Cambridge University Press.

Auerbach, R., Bigda-Peyton, J. S., Eberhart, N. K., Webb, C. A., & Ho, M. (2011). Conceptualizing the prospective relationship between social support, stress, and depressive symptoms among adolescents. *Journal of Abnormal Child Psychology, 39,* 475–487.

Bakker, M. P., Ormel, J., Verhulst, F. C., & Oldehinkel, A. J. (2012). Childhood family instability and mental health problems during late adolescence: A test of two mediation models—The TRAILS study. *Journal of Clinical Child and Adolescent Psychology, 41,* 166–176.

Bancila, D., & Mittelmark, M. B. (2005). Specificity in the relationships between stressors and depressed mood among adolescents: The roles of gender and self-efficacy. *The International Journal of Mental Health Promotion, 7,* 4–14.

Baron, R., & Kenny, D. (1986). The moderator-mediator variable distinction in social psychological research: Conceptual, strategic, and statistical considerations. *Journal of Personality and Social Psychology, 51,* 1173–1182.

Beck, A. T. (1987). Cognitive models of depression. *Journal of Cognitive Psychotherapy, 1,* 5–37.

Benjet, C., Borges, G., Méndez, E., Fleiz, C., & Medina-Mora, M. E. (2011). The association of chronic adversity with psychiatric disorder and disorder severity in adolescents. *European Child & Adolescent Psychiatry, 20,* 459–468.

Bohon, C., Stice, E., Burton, E., Fudell, M., & Nolen-Hoeksema, S. (2008). A prospective test of cognitive vulnerability models of depression with adolescent girls. *Behavior Therapy, 39,* 79–90.

Brown, G. W. (1993). The role of life events in the aetiology of depressive and anxiety disorders. In C. S. Stanford & P. Salmon (Eds.), *Stress: From synapse to syndrome* (pp. 23–50). San Diego, CA: Academic.

Carpenter, T. P., Laney, T., & Mezulis, A. (2012). Religious coping, stress, and depressive symptoms among adolescents: A prospective study. *Psychology of Religion And Spirituality, 4,* 19–30.

Carter, J., & Garber, J. (2011). Predictors of the first onset of a major depressive episode and changes in depressive symptoms across adolescence: Stress and negative cognitions. *Journal of Abnormal Psychology, 120,* 779–796.

Carter, J. S., Garber, J., Ciesla, J. A., & Cole, D. A. (2006). Modeling relations between hassles and internalizing and externalizing symptoms in adolescents: A four-year prospective study. *Journal of Abnormal Psychology, 115*(3), 428.

Cohen, S., & Hamrick, N. (2003). Stable individual differences in physiological response to stressors: Implications for stress-elicited changes in immune related health. *Brain, Behavior, and Immunity, 17,* 407–414.

Cohen, S., Kessler, R. C., & Gordon, L. U. (1995). Strategies for measuring stress in studies of psychiatric and physical disorders. In S. Cohen, R. C. Kessler, & L. U. Gordon (Eds.), *Measuring stress: A guide for health and social scientists* (pp. 3–26). New York: Oxford University Press.

Cole, D. A., & Maxwell, S. E. (2003). Testing mediational models with longitudinal data: Questions and tips in the use of structural equation modeling. *Journal of Abnormal Psychology, 112,* 558–577.

Cole, D. A., Nolen-Hoeksema, S., Girgus, J., & Paul, G. (2006). Stress exposure and stress generation in child and adolescent depression: A latent trait-state-error approach to longitudinal analyses. *Journal of Abnormal Psychology, 115*(1), 40.

Connolly, N. P., Eberhart, N. K., Hammen, C. L., & Brennan, P. A. (2010). Specificity of stress generation: A comparison of adolescents with depressive, anxiety, and comorbid diagnoses. *International Journal of Cognitive Therapy, 3,* 368–379.

Curran, P. J., & Bauer, D. J. (2011). The disaggregation of within-person and between-person effects in longitudinal models of change. *Annual Review of Psychology, 62,* 583–619.

Davis, S. K., & Humphrey, N. (2012). Emotional intelligence as a moderator of stressor-mental health relations in adolescence: Evidence for specificity. *Personality and Individual Differences, 52,* 100–105.

Del Giudice, M., Ellis, B. J., & Shirtcliff, E. A. (2011). The Adaptive Calibration Model of stress reactivity. *Neuroscience and Biobehavioral Reviews, 35,* 1562–1592.

Doan, S. N., Fuller-Rowell, T. E., & Evans, G. W. (2012). Cumulative risk and adolescent's internalizing and externalizing problems: The mediating roles of maternal responsiveness and self-regulation. *Developmental Psychology, 48*, 1529–1539.

Dohrenwend, B. (2006). Inventorying stressful life events as risk factors for psychopathology: Toward resolution of the problem of intracategory variability. *Psychological Bulletin, 132*, 477–495.

Drabick, D. G., & Kendall, P. C. (2010). Developmental psychopathology and the diagnosis of mental health problems among youth. *Clinical Psychology: Science and Practice, 17*, 272–280.

Duggal, S., Malkoff-Schwartz, S., Birmaher, B., Anderson, B. P., Matty, M. K., Houck, P. R., et al. (2000). Assessment of life stress in adolescents: Self-report versus interview methods. *Journal of the American Academy of Child & Adolescent Psychiatry, 39*, 445–452.

Eley, T. C., & Stevenson, J. (2000). Specific life events and chronic experiences differentially associated with depression and anxiety in young twins. *Journal of Abnormal Psychology, 28*, 383–394.

Farahmand, F. K., Grant, K. E., Polo, A., Duffy, S. N., & Dubois, D. L. (2011). School-based mental health programs for low-income urban youth: A systematic and meta-analytic review. *Clinical Psychology: Science and Practice, 18*, 372–390.

Flores, E., Tschann, J., Dimas, J., Pasch, L., & de Groat, C. (2010). Perceived racial/ethnic discrimination, posttraumatic stress symptoms, and health risk behaviors among Mexican American adolescents. *Journal of Counseling Psychology, 57*, 264–273.

Flouri, E., Buchanan, A., Tan, J., Griggs, J., & Attar-Schwartz, S. (2010). Adverse life events, area socioeconomic disadvantage, and adolescent psychopathology: The role of closeness to grandparents in moderating the effect of contextual stress. *Stress: The International Journal on the Biology of Stress, 13*, 402–412.

Flouri, E., & Tzavidis, N. (2008). Psychopathology and prosocial behavior in adolescents from socioeconomically disadvantaged families: The role of proximal and distal adverse life events. *European Child & Adolescent Psychiatry, 17*, 498–506.

Flynn, M., & Rudolph, K. D. (2011). Stress generation and adolescent depression: Contribution of interpersonal stress responses. *Journal of Abnormal Child Psychology, 39*, 1187–1198.

Formoso, D., Gonzales, N. A., & Aiken, L. S. (2000). Family conflict and children's internalizing and externalizing behavior: Protective factors. *American Journal of Community Psychology, 28*, 175–199.

Garber, J., Keiley, M. K., & Martin, N. C. (2002). Developmental trajectories of adolescents' depressive symptoms: Predictors of change. *Journal of Consulting and Clinical Psychology, 70*, 79–95.

Gee, G., & Walsemann, K. (2009). Does health predict the reporting of racial discrimination or do reports of discrimination predict health? Findings from the national longitudinal study of youth. *Social Science & Medicine, 68*, 1676–1684.

Gerard, J. M., & Buehler, C. (2004). Cumulative environmental risk and youth maladjustment: The role of youth attributes. *Child Development, 75*, 1832–1849.

Goldberg, S., Levitan, R., Leung, E., Masellis, M., Basile, V. S., Nemeroff, C. B., et al. (2003). Cortisol concentrations in 12- to 18-month-old infants: Stability over time, location and stressor. *Biological Psychiatry, 54*(7), 719–726.

Goodman, E., McEwen, B., Dolan, L., Schafer-Kalkhoff, T., & Adler, N. (2005). Social disadvantage and adolescent stress. *Journal of Adolescent Health, 37*, 484–492.

Grant, K. E. (2011). *Stressors and developmental psychopathology: Conceptualization issues, empirical findings, and translation into intervention*. Colloquium presented to the Psychology Department at the University of North Carolina at Charlotte.

Grant, K. E., Compas, B. E., Stuhlmacher, A. F., Thurm, A. E., McMahon, S. D., & Halpert, J. A. (2003). Stressors and child and adolescent psychopathology: Moving from markers to mechanisms of risk. *Psychological Bulletin, 129*, 447–466.

Grant, K. E., Compas, B. E., Thurm, A. E., McMahon, S. D., & Gipson, P. Y. (2004). Stressors and child and adolescent psychopathology: Measurement issues and prospective effects. *Journal of Clinical Child & Adolescent Psychology, 334*, 412–425.

Grant, K. E., Compas, B. E., Thurm, A. E., McMahon, S. D., Gipson, P., Campbell, A., et al. (2006). Stressors and child and adolescent psychopathology: Evidence of moderating and mediating effects. *Clinical Psychology Review, 26*, 257–283.

Grant, K. E., & McMahon, S. D. (2005). Conceptualizing the role of stressors in the development of psychopathology. In B. L. Hankin & J. R. Z. Abela (Eds.), *Development of psychopathology: A vulnerability-stress perspective* (pp. 3–31). Thousand Oaks, CA: Sage.

Gustafsson, P. E., Larsson, I., Nelson, N., & Gustafsson, P. A. (2009). Sociocultural disadvantage, traumatic life events, and psychiatric symptoms in preadolescent children. *American Journal of Orthopsychiatry, 79*, 387–397.

Hammen, C. (1991). Generation of stress in the course of unipolar depression. *Journal of Abnormal Psychology, 100*, 555–561.

Hammen, C., Brennan, P. A., Keenan-Miller, D., Hazel, N. A., & Najman, J. M. (2010). Chronic and acute stress, gender, and serotonin transporter gene environment interactions predicting depression symptoms in youth. *Journal of Child Psychology and Psychiatry, 51*, 180–187.

Hammen, C., Henry, R., & Daley, S. E. (2000). Depression and sensitization to stressors among young women as a function of childhood adversity. *Journal of Consulting and Clinical Psychology, 68*, 782–787.

Hammen, C., & Rudolph, K. D. (2003). Childhood mood disorders. In E. J. Mash & R. A. Barkley (Eds.), *Child psychopathology* (2nd ed., pp. 233–278). New York: Guilford Press.

Hankin, B. L. (2008). Cognitive vulnerability-stress model of depression during adolescence: Investigating depressive symptom specificity in a multi-wave prospective study. *Journal of Abnormal Child Psychology, 36*, 999–1014.

Hankin, B. L., Jenness, J., Abela, J. Z., & Smolen, A. (2011). Interaction of 5-HTTLPR and idiographic stressors predicts prospective depressive symptoms specifically among youth in a multiwave design. *Journal of Clinical Child and Adolescent Psychology, 40*, 572–585.

Hankin, B. L., Stone, L., & Ann Wright, P. (2010). Corumination, interpersonal stress generation, and internalizing symptoms: Accumulating effects and transactional influences in a multiwave study of adolescents. *Development and Psychopathology, 22*, 217–235.

Hankin, B. L., Wetter, E., Cheely, C., & Oppenheimer, C. W. (2008). Beck's cognitive theory of depression in adolescence: Specific prediction of depressive symptoms and reciprocal influences in a multi-wave prospective study. *International Journal of Cognitive Therapy, 1*, 313–332.

Hayes, A. F. (2009). Beyond Baron and Kenny: Statistical mediation analysis in the new millennium. *Communication Monographs, 76*, 408–420.

Hazel, N. A., Hammen, C. C., Brennan, P. A., & Najman, J. J. (2008). Early childhood adversity and adolescent depression: The mediating role of continued stress. *Psychological Medicine: A Journal of Research in Psychiatry and the Allied Sciences, 38*, 581–589.

Hetherington, E. M., Parke, R. D., Gauvain, M., & Locke, V. (2005). *Child psychology: A contemporary viewpoint*. New York: McGraw-Hill.

Holmbeck, G. N. (1997). Toward terminological, conceptual, and statistical clarity in the study of mediators and moderators: Examples from the child-clinical and pediatric psychology literatures. *Journal of Consulting & Clinical Psychology, 65*, 599–610.

Holmbeck, G. N. (2002). Post-hoc probing of significant moderational and mediational effects in studies of pediatric populations. *Journal of Pediatric Psychology, 27*, 87–96.

Holmes, T., & Rahe, T. (1967). The social readjustment rating scale. *Journal of Psychosomatic Research, 11*, 213–218.

Jackson, J., Knight, K., & Rafferty, J. (2010). Race and unhealthy behaviors: Chronic stress, the HPA axis, and physical and mental health disparities over the life course. *American Journal of Public Health, 100*, 933–939.

Katz, B. N., Esparza, N. P., Carter, J. S., Grant, K. E., & Meyerson, D. A. (2012). Intervening processes in the relation between neighborhood characteristics and psychological symptoms in urban youth. *Journal of Early Adolescence, 32*, 649–679.

Katz, M., Liu, C., Schaer, M., Parker, K. J., Ottet, M., Epps, A., et al. (2009). Prefrontal plasticity and stress inoculated-induced resilience. *Developmental Neuroscience, 31*, 293–299.

Kercher, A. J., Rapee, R. M., & Schniering, C. A. (2009). Neuroticism, life events and negative thoughts in the development of depression in adolescent girls. *Journal of Abnormal Child Psychology, 37*, 903–915.

Kilmer, R. P., & Gil-Rivas, V. (2010). Exploring posttraumatic growth in children impacted by Hurricane Katrina: Correlates of the phenomenon and developmental considerations. *Child Development, 81*, 1211–1227.

King, K. M., & Chassin, L. (2008). Adolescent stressors, psychopathology, and young adult substance dependence: A prospective study. *Journal of Studies on Alcohol and Drugs, 69*, 629–638.

Lazarus, R. S., & Folkman, S. (1984). *Stress, appraisal, and coping*. New York: Springer Publishing Company.

Lee, S., Guo, W. J., Tsang, A., He, Y. L., Huang, Y. Q., Zhang, M. Y., et al. (2011). The prevalence of family childhood adversities and their association with first onset of DSM-IV disorders in metropolitan China. *Psychological Medicine: A Journal of Research in Psychiatry and the Allied Sciences, 41*, 85–96.

Luke, D. (2005). Getting the big picture in community science: Methods that capture context. *American Journal of Community Psychology, 35*(3/4), 185–200.

Luthar, S. S., Cicchetti, D., & Becker, B. (2000). The construct of resilience: A critical evaluation and guidelines for future work. *Child Development, 71*, 543–562.

Martyn-Nemeth, P., Penckofer, S., Gulanick, M., Velsor-Friedrich, B., & Bryant, F. B. (2009). The relationships among self-esteem, stress, coping, eating behavior, and depressive mood in adolescents. *Research in Nursing & Health, 32*(1), 96–109.

McClelland, G. H., & Judd, C. M. (1993). Statistical difficulties of detecting interactions and moderator effects. *Psychological Bulletin, 114*, 376–390.

McEwen, B. S., & Seeman, T. (1999). Protective and damaging effects of mediators of stress: Elaborating and testing the concepts of allostasis and allostatic load. In N. E. Adler, M. Marmot, B. S. McEwen, & J. Stewart (Eds.), *Socioeconomic status and health in industrial nations: Social, psychological, and biological pathways* (pp. 30–47). New York: New York Academy of Sciences.

McEwen, B. S., & Seeman, T. (2006). Protective and damaging effects of mediators of stress: Elaborating and testing the concepts of allostasis and allostatic load. *Annals of the New York Academy of Sciences, 896*, 30–47.

McLaughlin, K. A., Hatzenbuehler, M. L., & Hilt, L. M. (2009). Emotion dysregulation as a mechanism linking peer victimization to internalizing symptoms in adolescents. *Journal of Consulting And Clinical Psychology, 77*, 894–904.

McMahon, S. D., Grant, K. E., Compas, B. E., Thurm, A. E., & Ey, S. (2003). Stress and psychopathology in children and adolescents: Is there evidence of specificity? *Journal of Child Psychology & Psychiatry & Allied Disciplines, 44*, 107–133.

McMahon, S. D., Todd, N. R., Martinez, A., Coker, C., Sheu, C.F., Shah, S., & Washburn, J.J. (2013)

Aggressive and prosocial behavior: Community violence, cognitive, and behavioral predictors among urban African American youth. *American Journal of Community Psychology, 51*, 407–421.

Meyerson, D. A., Grant, K. E., Carter, J. S., & Kilmer, R. (2011). Posttraumatic growth among children and adolescents: A systematic review. *Clinical Psychology Review, 31*, 949–964.

Miller, G. E., Chen, E., & Zhou, E. S. (2007). If it goes up, must it come down? Chronic stress and the hypothalamic-pituitary-adrenocortical axis in humans. *Psychological Bulletin, 133*, 25–45.

Miller, D. B., Webster, S. E., & MacIntosh, R. (2002). What's there and what's not: Measuring daily hassles in urban African American adolescents. *Research on Social Work Practice, 12*, 375–388.

Monroe, S. M. (1982). Life events and disorders: Event-symptom association and the course of disorders. *Journal of Abnormal Psychology, 91*, 14–24.

Monroe, S. M. (2008). Modern approaches to conceptualizing and measuring human life stress. *Annual Review of Clinical Psychology, 4*, 33–52.

Morris, M. C., Ciesla, J. A., & Garber, J. (2008). A prospective study of the cognitive-stress model of depressive symptoms in adolescents. *Journal of Abnormal Psychology, 117*(4), 719.

Nolen-Hoeksema, S., Girgus, J. S., & Seligman, M. E. P. (1992). Predictors and consequences of childhood depressive symptoms: A 5-year longitudinal study. *Journal of Abnormal Psychology, 101*, 405–422.

Obradović, J., Bush, N. R., Stamperdahl, J., Adler, N. E., & Boyce, W. (2010). Biological sensitivity to context: The interactive effects of stress reactivity and family adversity on socioemotional behavior and school readiness. *Child Development, 81*, 270–289.

Pearlin, L. I. (1999). Stress and mental health: A conceptual overview. In A. V. Horwitz & T. L. Scheid (Eds.), *A handbook for the study of mental health: Social contexts, theories, and systems* (pp. 161–175). Cambridge: Cambridge University Press.

Phillips, N. K., Hammen, C. L., Brennan, P. A., Najman, J. M., & Bor, W. (2005). Early adversity and the prospective prediction of depressive and anxiety disorders in adolescents. *Journal of Abnormal Child Psychology, 33*, 13–24.

Preacher, K. J., Rucker, D. D., & Hayes, A. F. (2007). Addressing moderated mediation hypotheses: Theory, methods, and prescriptions. *Multivariate Behavioral Research, 42*, 185–227.

Reising, M. M., Watson, K. H., Hardcastle, E. J., Merchant, M. J., Roberts, L., Forehand, R., et al. (2012). Parental depression and economic disadvantage: The role of parenting in associations with internalizing and externalizing symptoms in children and adolescents. *Journal of Child and Family Studies, 1–9*.

Reiss, D., & Oliveri, M. E. (1991). The family's conception of accountability and competence: A new approach to the conceptualization and assessment of family stress. *Family Process, 30*, 193–214.

Romero, L. M. (2004). Physiological stress in ecology: Lessons from biomedical research. *Trends in Ecology & Evolution, 19*, 249–255.

Rudolph, K. D., & Hammen, C. (1999). Age and gender as determinants of stress exposure, generation and reactions in youngsters: A transactional perspective. *Child Development, 70*, 660–677.

Rudolph, K. D., & Flynn, M. (2007). Childhood adversity and youth depression: The role of gender and pubertal status. *Development and Psychopathology, 19*, 497–521.

Rudolph, K. D., Flynn, M., Abaied, J. L., Groot, A., & Thompson, R. (2009). Why is past depression the best predictor of future depression? Stress generation as a mechanism of depression continuity in girls. *Journal of Clinical Child & Adolescent Psychology, 38*(4), 473–485.

Rueger, S., & Malecki, C. (2011). Effects of stress, attributional style and perceived parental support on depressive symptoms in early adolescence: A prospective analysis. *Journal Of Clinical Child And Adolescent Psychology, 40*, 347–359.

Sameroff, A. J., Lewis, M., & Miller, S. M. (2000). *Handbook of developmental psychopathology*. Dordrecht: Kluwer.

Sandler, I. N., Reynolds, K. D., Kliewer, W., & Ramirez, R. (1992). Specificity of the relation between life events and psychological symptomatology. *Journal of Clinical Child Psychology, 21*, 240–248.

Schwarzer, R., & Schulz, U. (2002). Stressful life events. In A. M. Nezu, C. M. Nezu, & P. A. Geller (Eds.), *Comprehensive handbook of psychology* (Health psychology, Vol. 9, pp. 27–49). New York: Wiley.

Seaton, E. (2009). Perceived racial discrimination and racial identity profiles among African American adolescents. *Cultural Diversity and Ethnic Minority Psychology, 15*, 137–144.

Seidman, E., Lambert, L. E., Allen, L., & Aber, J. (2003). Urban adolescents' transition to junior high school and protective family transactions. *The Journal of Early Adolescence, 23*, 166–193.

Sheidow, A. J., Strachan, M. K., Minden, J. A., Henry, D. B., Tolan, P. H., & Gorman-Smith, D. (2008). The relation of antisocial behavior patterns and changes in internalizing symptoms for a sample of inner-city youth: Comorbidity within a developmental framework. *Journal of Youth and Adolescence, 37*, 821–829.

Singleton, R. A., & Straits, B. C. (1999). *Approaches to social research*. London: Oxford University Press.

Skitch, S. A., & Abela, J. Z. (2008). Rumination in response to stress as a common vulnerability factor to depression and substance misuse in adolescence. *Journal of Abnormal Child Psychology, 36*, 1029–1045.

Smokowski, P. R., Bacallao, M., & Buchanan, R. L. (2009). Interpersonal mediators linking acculturation stressors to subsequent internalizing symptoms and self-esteem in Latino adolescents. *Journal of Community Psychology, 37*, 1024–1045.

Sontag, L. M., & Graber, J. A. (2010). Coping with perceived peer stress: Gender-specific and common pathways to symptoms of psychopathology. *Developmental Psychology, 46*, 1605–1620.

Sontag, L. M., Graber, J. A., Brooks-Gunn, J., & Warren, M. P. (2008). Coping with social stress: Implications for psychopathology in young adolescent girls. *Journal of Abnormal Child Psychology, 36*, 1159–1174.

Stein, G. L., Gonzalez, L. M., & Huq, N. (2012). Cultural Stressors and the Hopelessness Model of Depressive Symptoms in Latino Adolescents. *Journal of Youth and Adolescence, 1–11*.

Turner, H. A., & Butler, M. J. (2003). Direct and indirect effects of childhood adversity on depressive symptoms in young adults. *Journal of Youth and Adolescence, 32*, 89–103.

Wadsworth, M. E., Raviv, T., Santiago, C., & Etter, E. M. (2011). Testing the adaptation to poverty-related stress model: Predicting psychopathology symptoms in families facing economic hardship. *Journal of Clinical Child and Adolescent Psychology, 40*, 646–657.

Wagner, C., Abela, J., & Brozina, K. (2006). A comparison of stress measures in children and adolescents: A self-report checklist versus an objectively rated interview. *Journal of Psychopathology and Behavioral Assessment, 28*, 251–261.

Yang, H. J., Chiu, Y. J., Soong, W. T., & Chen, W. J. (2008). The roles of personality traits and negative life events on the episodes of depressive symptoms in nonreferred adolescents: a 1-year follow-up study. *Journal of Adolescent Health, 42*, 378–385.

Culture and Developmental Psychopathology

12

Xinyin Chen, Rui Fu, and Lingli Leng

Human development is a complex phenomenon that must be understood with cultural context taken into account (e.g., Vygotsky, 1978). Culture may affect development through various processes such as facilitation and suppression of specific behaviors (Weisz, Weiss, Suwanlert, & Chaiyasit, 2006). Cultural norms and values may also provide a frame of reference for social evaluations of behaviors and thus give "meaning" to the behaviors. As a result, whether and to what extent a behavior is adaptive or maladaptive depend largely on cultural context.

In this chapter, we focus on how culture is involved in the development of social, behavioral, and psychological problems. We first discuss some conceptual issues in the study of culture and developmental psychopathology. Then, we review research on the prevalence and developmental patterns of major socioemotional and behavioral problems among children in different cultures. In our discussion, we pay particular attention to how macro-level social and cultural conditions play a role in defining functional meanings of specific behaviors and in promoting or impeding their development through socialization and social interaction processes.

The chapter concludes with a discussion of future directions in cross-cultural research on developmental psychopathology.

Culture and Adaptive and Maladaptive Development: Theoretical Perspectives

Two of the most prominent theories of culture and human development are the socioecological theory (Bronfenbrenner & Morris, 2006) and the sociocultural theory (Vygotsky, 1978). Both theories contend that culture influences socialization practices, which in turn contribute, independently or in interaction with personal and social factors, to developmental outcomes. In addition to the broadband theories, a cultural anthropological perspective (Benedict, 1934), which is particularly relevant to developmental psychopathology, focuses on how culture affects the judgment of normality of behaviors. These theoretical perspectives have guided work on culture and developmental psychopathology for the past 50 years.

Traditional Perspectives

According to the socioecological theory (Bronfenbrenner & Morris, 2006), the cultural beliefs and practices that are endorsed within a society, community, or group are a part of the socioecological environment that shapes the development of children's socioemotional

X. Chen, Ph.D. (✉) • R. Fu, M.S.
Graduate School of Education, University of Pennsylvania, Philadelphia, PA 19104, USA
e-mail: xinyin@gse.upenn.edu

L. Leng, M.Ed.
Department of Social Work and Social Administration, Hong Kong University, Hong Kong, China

M. Lewis and K.D. Rudolph (eds.), *Handbook of Developmental Psychopathology*,
DOI 10.1007/978-1-4614-9608-3_12, © Springer Science+Business Media New York 2014

characteristics and cognitive abilities. Whereas culture is considered in the earlier writings a distal influence in the outermost layer of the environment in which the child does not directly participate, in more recent socioecological conceptualizations, cultural factors have been integrated with proximal setting conditions such as community services, child care practices, and family activities (Tietjen, 2006). Thus, culture may affect development through organizing social settings including child-rearing conditions and interpersonal relationships. From the socioecological perspective, providing constructive cultural conditions is important for promoting adaptive development and preventing developmental problems. In a developmental niche model, which is consistent with the socioecological perspective, Super and Harkness (1986) propose that culture may be linked with individual development through three interacting "developmental niches": the physical and social settings, the historically constituted customs and practices of child care and child rearing, and the psychology of the caretakers, particularly parental ethnotheories shared with the community. Disadvantageous settings, disorganized child-rearing practices, and socially inappropriate socialization beliefs may constitute main sources of risk for developing problems.

The sociocultural theory is primarily concerned with the internalization of external cultural systems from the interpersonal level to the intrapersonal level (Vygotsky, 1978). Participation in social and cultural practices determines, to a large extent, human development. Changes in sociocultural structures or social practices are likely to result in reorganization of mental processes and formation of new mental systems. Consistent with the sociocultural perspective, the results of cross-cultural studies indicate that relative to their counterparts who participated in sophisticated social activities, children and adults who lived in traditional lifestyles in rural villages (Greenfield, Maynard, & Childs, 2000; Rogoff, 2003) displayed lower levels of cognitive performance that was constrained by the immediate physical features of the circumstances. The mental processes of individuals in these societies became more abstract, decontextualized, and logical as they engaged in more commercial and social activities and school learning.

An important and long-held perspective in psychopathology, proposed mainly by cultural anthropologists, Benedict (1934) and Mead (1928), emphasizes cultural relativity in the judgment of normal and abnormal behaviors. The relativist perspective asserts that normality is defined by culture; a behavior viewed as abnormal in one culture may be viewed normal in another. Due to historical, socioeconomic, and other reasons, different societies may place different values on specific behaviors. Normality is characterized by a segment of human behaviors that are approved and encouraged within a culture, and abnormality represents the segment that is incompatible with the societal norm. Thus, normal behaviors are the ones that fall within the limits of the society, and those beyond the limits are typically considered problematic or psychopathological. Accordingly, individuals whose behaviors are not congenial to those selected in the society are regarded as deviant and abnormal, even though these behaviors may be valued in other cultures.

The relativist perspective (Benedict, 1934) is not necessarily incompatible with the universalist view, which indicates that psychological disorders have universal and core symptoms and that cultures vary on the presentations or perceptions of the disorders. The basic assumption of the universalist view is that the underlying internal disorder or psychopathology is the same, but what varies across cultures is the symptomatic manifestation of the disorder or the threshold of what is judged as normal or abnormal (e.g., Roberts & Roberts, 2007). A more thorough relativist point of view (e.g., Kleinman & Kleinman, 1991) claims that culture can affect not only the manifestation and perceptions of a behavior but also the nature and development of the behavior per se. Cultural environments determine the occurrence, magnitude, and form of the behavior as well as social responses to the behavior.

Between the relativist and universalist views, many researchers hold a position that disorders based mostly on neural pathology (e.g., autism, schizophrenia) are more likely to be universal and unreceptive to contextual influence, whereas common problems are more likely to be affected by social and cultural conditions (see Canino & Alegría, 2008). To what extent a specific behavior or problem occurs and how it is viewed in a culture may depend on the nature of the behavior or problem. Our discussion of cultural influence on developmental psychopathology in the following sections focuses mainly on relatively common behaviors such as aggression, defiance, and social anxiety, although they may be biologically or dispositionally rooted.

The Contextual-Developmental Perspective

Chen and colleagues (e.g., Chen, 2012; Chen & French, 2008) have recently proposed a contextual-developmental perspective on relations between cultural values and children's socioemotional functioning and the role of social interactions in mediating the relations. This perspective focuses on social initiative and self-control as two fundamental dimensions of socioemotional functioning (Rothbart & Bates, 2006). *Social initiative* refers to the tendency to spontaneously initiate and maintain social participation, especially in stressful settings. A major indication of low social initiative is the display of internalizing behaviors such as inhibition, shyness, and withdrawal in social situations, accompanied with anxious and fearful emotions. *Self-control* represents the regulatory ability to modulate behavioral and emotional reactivity for maintaining appropriate behavior during interactions. The dimension of control, which is indicated mostly by the exhibition of cooperative-compliant and aggressive-defiant behaviors, is concerned with "fit in with others" and thus is important for achieving interpersonal and group harmony.

Different societies may emphasize social initiative and norm-based behavioral control in children to different extents. In Western individualistic cultures where acquiring self-expressive and assertive skills is an important socialization goal, a low level of social initiative is viewed as indicating incompetence. In group-oriented or collectivistic cultures, social initiative is less appreciated because it may not have clear benefits for group well-being. To maintain interpersonal and group harmony, however, individuals need to restrain personal desires in order to address the needs and interests of others. The lack of control, which is often manifested in externalizing behaviors such as aggression and defiance, is viewed as highly unacceptable.

According to the contextual-developmental perspective, social evaluation and response processes in interactions play a crucial role in building and facilitating the links between culture and adaptive and maladaptive development. Specifically, during interactions, adults and peers evaluate children's behaviors in manners that are consistent with cultural beliefs and values in the society, community, or group. Moreover, adults and peers in different cultures may respond differently and express different attitudes (e.g., acceptance, rejection) toward children who display these behaviors. To acquire acceptance, children need to understand social expectations and maintain or modify their behavior according to the expectations. Thus, evaluation and response processes in social interactions serve to regulate children's behaviors and ultimately their developmental patterns (Chen, 2012). The extent to which children can maintain or modify their behaviors in keeping with culturally directed social evaluations is associated with adjustment outcomes. Children who are sensitive to social expectations and adjust their behaviors accordingly may obtain approval and support, which promotes adaptive development. However, children who fail to do so may experience unfavorable treatment, which may elicit distress, frustrations, anger, and other negative emotions. These negative emotional reactions in turn may lead to internalizing problems such as negative self-feelings if directed toward the self, externalizing problems such as aggressive and antisocial behaviors if directed toward others, or both.

The Display of Internalizing and Externalizing Behaviors Across Cultures

Cross-cultural researchers have conducted a number of studies of children's and adolescents' behaviors in different societies (e.g., Chen, Chung, Lechcier-Kimel, & French, 2011; Whiting & Edwards, 1988). These studies have relied mostly on adult or youth self-reports, which suffer from methodological problems such as judgment biases, response style biases, and reference group biases (e.g., Schneider, French, & Chen, 2006). Despite the methodological problems, some interesting patterns of cross-cultural differences have emerged among Asian, Latino, European, and North American children and adolescents.

Depression, Anxiety, and Somatic Complaints Across Cultures

Based on the Child Behavior Checklist (CBCL) data collected from multiple countries such as Australia, Belgium, China, Germany, Jamaica, the Netherlands, Puerto Rico, Thailand, and the USA, Achenbach and his colleagues (e.g., Rescorla et al., 2011) found some similar cross-cultural gender differences: girls had higher scores than boys on internalizing behaviors such as somatic complaints and anxiety. Higher scores of girls on fear, anxiety, and depression have been found in other studies of Asian, Latino, and Euro-American children (e.g., Austin & Chorpita, 2004; Céspedes & Huey, 2008). Nevertheless, different results have been reported on sex differences. Kistner, David, and White (2003) found that whereas girls had higher scores than boys on depression among Euro-American children, boys reported higher depression than girls among African American children. Chen, Cen, Li, and He (2005) also found that boys reported higher levels of depression than girls in China.

Concerning cultural or ethnic differences, it has been found that Latino children and adolescents report more depression, anxiety, and other internalizing symptoms than some other ethnic groups. Twenge and Nolen-Hoeksema (2002), for example, found that among diverse ethnic girls at 12–19 years in the USA, Latino girls had a higher prevalence of depression, alcohol use, and suicidal attempts. Kelder et al. (2001) found that Latino middle school students were more susceptible than other ethnic groups to depression and substance use. Compared with Euro-Americans, African Americans and Native Americans tended to have a higher prevalence of anxiety disorder and posttraumatic stress (Grant et al., 2006; Lambert, Cooley, Campbell, Benoit, & Stansbury, 2004), although inconsistent findings were reported (Austin & Chorpita, 2004).

Asian youths also tend to report higher levels of depression than Euro-American youths. Choi, Stafford, Meininger, Roberts, and Smith (2002) found that depression scores of Korean teenagers were higher than those of their European counterparts. Similarly, Chen, Rubin, and Li (1995a) found that Chinese children had higher depression scores than Western children. Within the USA, Austin and Chorpita (2004) found that Chinese American, Filipino American, and Japanese American children and adolescents reported higher levels of social anxiety and fear than their Euro-American counterparts. According to Janssen et al. (2004), the cross-cultural differences are likely to be associated with parental child-rearing practices. Parents in many Asian cultures often use verbal criticism, punishment, and threat to socialize their children, which may induce high anxiety and depression (e.g., Chao, 1994; Lin & Fu, 1990).

In an interesting cross-cultural experimental study (Norasakkunkit & Kalick, 2009), Japanese and US undergraduate students were primed to access an independent mode of thought by instructing them to write down as many examples as they could remember from their personal experiences that represented this situation—"I enjoy being unique and different from others in many respects." Then, the students were asked to complete measures of social anxiety and fear of negative social evaluations. The results indicated that the Japanese scored higher than the

Americans on social anxiety and fear. Moreover, independent priming caused social anxiety and fear scores to decrease. The results suggest that the cultural orientation of independence at the individual level is negatively related to negative emotions in social situations.

A behavioral characteristic in early childhood that is associated with, and predictive of, social anxiety, fear, and withdrawal is behavioral inhibition or reactivity to stressful situations (Kagan, 1997). Children who are inhibited or display fearful reactions to stressful situations are likely to develop shy, anxious, and solitary behaviors and thus are considered at risk for internalizing problems. There is cumulative evidence indicating cross-cultural differences in children's reactivity. For example, Chinese, Japanese, Vietnamese, and Haitian mothers rated their children as more anxious and fearful in challenging settings and less likely to approach unfamiliar situations than did American parents (e.g., Gartstein et al., 2006). Rubin et al. (2006) found that Korean and Chinese toddlers exhibited more anxious reactions than Italian and Australian toddlers in novel situations. Chen, Hastings, et al. (1998) found that Chinese toddlers stayed closer to their mothers and were less likely to explore the environment than Canadian toddlers. When interacting with a stranger, Chinese toddlers displayed more inhibited and anxious behaviors, as reflected in their higher scores on the latency to approach the stranger and to touch the toys when they were invited to do so.

A salient cross-cultural difference that researchers have found is that emotional distress is more strongly associated with somatic complaints in Asian, Latino, African, and Native American youths than in Euro-American youths (e.g., Gureje, Simon, Ustun, & Goldberg, 1997). Somatic complaints generally refer to complaints about, or the presence of, physical symptoms such as headaches, stomach pains, chronic fatigue, and sleep problems that may have a strong psychological basis. It was found that complaints of headaches, insomnia, and dizziness were common symptoms of Chinese and Vietnamese depressive patients (Kleinman & Kleinman, 1985; Lin, Ihle, & Tazuma, 1985;

Ryder et al., 2008). South Asian Hindu preschoolers were also somatically oriented in their expression of distress (Raval, Martini, & Raval, 2010). In addition, Turkish immigrants in Belgium (Beirens & Fontaine, 2011) and Greek Americans (Christoforidou, 2004) reported more somatic complaints than the majority of a European origin in the countries.

Culture may affect the rate as well as the content of somatic complaints. A common feature of somatic complaints in Latin Americans and the Caribbeans is ataque de nervios ("attack of nerves"), categorized as a culture-bound syndrome that is indicated by episodic, dramatic outbursts of negative emotions in response to stress such as uncontrollable screaming, trembling, heart palpitations, and other intense somatic reactions (Hinton, Chong, Pollack, Barlow, & McNally, 2008). However, for Africans, "feeling of heat," "peppery and crawling sensations," and "numbness" are frequently mentioned, and for Indians, "burning hands and feet" and "hot, peppery sensations in head" are included in descriptions of somatic reactions (Escobar, 1995). In addition, Koreans often report their somatic complaints as Hwabyung, a feeling of chest pain and respiratory stuffiness.

Researchers have attempted to explain somatic complaints of youths and adults in non-Western, particularly East Asian, societies in terms of display rules, stigmatization of mental illness, and cultural conceptualization of health. In Asian cultures, mental illness may carry with it serious social stigma indicating weak will and spirit (Chung & Wong, 2004). Moreover, the social stigma associated with mental problems is believed to damage the reputation of the family, whereas physical illness may not bring humiliation and shame to the individual or the family. It has also been suggested that the collectivistic orientation requires individuals to suppress the expression of their negative emotions, which may in turn lead to somatic dysfunctions of the body system (e.g., Traue & Pennebaker, 1993). Finally, the tendency to somatize emotional distress may be related to cultural conceptualizations of health. In traditional Chinese medicine, the mind and body are viewed as inherently connected in the holistic system; the imbalance of yin and yang is seen to simultaneously affect psychological and physical functions of the body.

Aggressive and Antisocial Behaviors Across Cultures

Researchers have found cross-cultural differences in children's aggressive, antisocial, and other externalizing behaviors. Cultures that value competitiveness and the pursuit of personal goals seem to allow for more externalizing behaviors, whereas cultures that emphasize group harmony and personal control tend to inhibit externalizing behaviors. Relative to their North American counterparts, for example, children in some Asian countries such as China, Korea, and Thailand, Australia, and some European nations such as Sweden and the Netherlands tend to exhibit lower levels of aggression and oppositional defiance (e.g., Bergeron & Schneider, 2005; Liu, Cheng, & Leung, 2011; Weisz et al., 1988).

Cultural differences have also been demonstrated in children's reactions to provocations in social situations. Zahn-Waxler, Friedman, Cole, Mizuta, and Hiruma (1996), for example, found that Japanese children showed less anger and less aggressive behavior than US children in their responses to hypothetical situations involving conflict and distress. Cole, Tamang, and Shrestha (2006) examined children's reactions to provocative social situations such as peer conflict in two villages in Nepal: Brahmans who were high-caste Hindus and valued hierarchy and dominance and Tamangs who valued social equality, compassion, modesty, and nonviolence. The researchers found that, consistent with the general cultural orientations, Brahman children were more likely than Tamang children to endorse aggressive behavior and react to difficult social situations with anger and other negative emotions.

Farver, Welles-Nystrom, Frosch, Wimbarti, and Hoppe-Graff (1997) conducted a cross-cultural study of preschool children's aggression using narrative stories in the USA, Sweden, Germany, and Indonesia. The children were asked to tell two stories with toys that facilitated imaginative play. Children's stories were coded according to aggressive words such as guns, kill, shoot, punch, kick, and hit and sounds made when characters in the story harmed or injured themselves or another figure (e.g., Ouch! Pow! Bang! Crash!). Story contents were coded for the description of the characters' behaviors such as engaging in aggression with the intent to harm and destroy or mastering situation or conflict with or without aggression. The results indicated that American children had more aggressive themes and words, physical aggression, and mastery of situations with aggression than did German, Swedish, and Indonesian children. Indonesian children's narratives contained fewer aggressive figures and features of mastering situations or conflicts without aggression. According to Farver et al. (1997), the differences between the American and Indonesian children's narratives reflect different norms with regard to conflict resolution and different levels of intolerance of interpersonal aggression. American children are often socialized to be assertive and to fight back in response to physical assault, insult, or attack on one's possessions. In contrast, Indonesian children are trained to avoid conflicts with others and to settle disputes through negotiation rather than physical or verbal aggression.

Cross-cultural differences in aggressive and antisocial behaviors also exist between Southeast Asian and North American adolescents. Greenberger, Chen, Beam, Whang, and Dong (2000) found that US adolescents had higher scores than Korean adolescents, who in turn had higher scores than Chinese adolescents on risk-taking, physical aggression toward others, property violation, and school misconduct. Moreover, US adolescents reported more aggressive behaviors among family members, friends, and school peers than did either of the two Asian groups.

In Western nations, researchers found that children in Nordic countries (e.g., Norway, Denmark) displayed fewer aggressive behaviors than children in the USA (Heiervang, Goodman, & Goodman, 2008; Obel et al., 2004). Within the

USA, native Hawaiian/Pacific Islanders tended to display a higher prevalence of antisocial behavior and drug addiction than Euro-Americans (e.g., Le, 2002; Sakai, Risk, Tanaka, & Price, 2007). It has also been reported that, compared with their Euro-American counterparts, a higher proportion of African American male high school students engaged in physical fights and carried weapons (e.g., guns, knives) (Centers for Disease Control and Prevention, 2000; Hawkins, Laub, Lauritsen, & Cothern, 2000). In a within-culture study of Dutch youth, Weenink (2011) found that urban adolescents, particularly girls, were more likely to engage in delinquent behavior than were rural counterparts. The results suggested that more traditional value orientations in rural societies seemed to be associated with fewer antisocial behaviors.

Cultural variations have been found on the levels of self-regulation and control in early childhood, which is a reliable developmental predictor of aggressive, disruptive, and antisocial behaviors. East Asian infants are often rated by their mothers as displaying higher levels of control than Western infants, and the differences tend to increase with age (e.g., Gartstein et al., 2006). East Asian preschoolers also seem to perform more competently than their US counterparts on executive function tasks assessing self-control abilities (e.g., Oh & Lewis, 2008). Interestingly, Gartstein, Peleg, Young, and Slobodskaya (2009) recently reported that Russian infants in Israel demonstrated higher regulatory ability than Russian infants in the USA. Gartstein et al. (2009) argued that this might be due to the fact that coping with stress was an inherent component of everyday life in Israel and that effective regulation, including recovery from minor distress, was critical to adjustment in the Israeli environment. Moreover, for the Russian immigrants in Israel, parental involvement in the Israeli (host) culture was related to greater infants' regulatory capacity.

In summary, empirical research has revealed relatively consistent cross-cultural differences in major aspects of socioemotional functioning including social anxiety, depression, somatic complaints, reactivity to stressful situations, aggression, delinquency, and self-control. To understand the cross-cultural differences, it is necessary to explore how culturally directed socialization processes play a role in development and, more specifically, how cultural values serve as guidance for social evaluations of, and responses to, children's behaviors.

Cultural Values, Social Attitudes, and Children's Behaviors

Individuals in different societies may hold different attitudes toward behaviors that children display, particularly in social situations. These attitudes constitute a part of the general cultural belief system that is critical to understanding the normal or psychopathological nature of children's behaviors.

Parental Attitudes and Socialization Practices

Parental attitudes toward children's behaviors are determined, to a large extent, by socialization goals and expectations, which often reflect the demands of the society. In Western societies, parents tend to have negative attitudes toward children who display higher levels of social anxiety and fear. Hudson and Rapee (2001) compared clinic-referred anxiety-disordered children with normal children on observed maternal negative behaviors and found that mothers of anxious children were more negative (i.e., less accepting) in mother-child interactions than mothers of control children. Similarly, Dumas, LaFreniere, and Serketich (1995) identified anxious and non-anxious preschool children based on teacher-ratings and found that mothers of anxious children displayed more negative and rejecting behaviors during a mother-child problem-solving task. Rubin and Mills (1992) also found that parents of socially wary and withdrawn children were more concerned about their children's behavior and used more power-assertive and directive parenting, which in turn reinforced the child's feelings of insecurity and anxiety.

Chen, Hastings, et al. (1998) investigated the relations between parental attitudes and toddlers' anxious reactivity to novel situations in Canada and China. The results indicated that child reactivity was positively associated with mothers' negative attitudes, such as punishment orientation and rejection, toward the child in Canada but positively associated with maternal warm and accepting attitudes in China. Shy-anxious behavior in Chinese children and adolescents was also associated with parental positive attitudes (e.g., Chen, Dong, and Zhou (1997).

Pina and Silverman (2004) suggested that the relatively high rate of somatic complaints in Latino youth might be related to parents' attitudes. When Latino children expressed the somatic complaints, their parents might give them positive feedbacks such as extra attention, special foods, get-well gifts, and allowing them to stay home from school, which could reinforce the behavior of somatic complaints. Nevertheless, there have been no empirical data supporting the argument.

Parents across cultures may also react differently to children's aggressive, disruptive, and defiant behaviors. In a study of caregivers' attitudes and reactions to children's anger and under-controlled behavior in Nepal, Cole et al. (2006) found that the majority of active responses (i.e., not ignoring) by Tamang caregivers involved rebuking the angry youngster, whereas most of active responses by Brahman caregivers involved supporting the angry child to feel better. Brahman parents were more likely than Tamang parents to indicate to the child that anger and under-controlled behavior were acceptable. The results might be due to the fact that whereas Brahmans were high-caste Hindus who valued hierarchy and power, Tamangs valued social equality and compassion.

Hackett and Hackett (1993) conducted interviews about attitudes toward various behaviors with samples of Gujarati and English parents of 4- to 7-year-old children in England. The Gujarati community consisted of groups based on Hinduism and the Gujarati language. It was found that Gujarati parents were less tolerant of their children's aggression than English parents.

When they were told that their child was hit by a peer in the school playground, 19 % of Gujarati parents and 51 % of English parents would tell their children to retaliate. When their child was involved in a fight with a peer, 51 % of Gujarati parents and 20 % of English parents stopped such fights immediately and punished their children. If a peer grabbed a toy from their child when playing outside, 5 % of Gujarati parents and 51 % of English parents expected their child to get the toy back by force.

Peer Evaluations and Responses

With age, peer interactions become an increasingly important socialization context. To investigate cultural differences in peer evaluations, Chen and colleagues conducted a series of studies concerning shy-anxious behavior and peer interactions and relationships in Canadian and Chinese children. In an observational study, Chen, DeSouza, Chen, and Wang (2006) found that when shy-anxious children in Canada showed a behavior to initiate social interaction, peers were likely to make negative responses such as overt refusal, disagreement, and intentional ignoring of the initiation. However, peers tended to respond in a more positive manner in China by controlling their negative actions and by showing approval and support. Apparently, the passive and wary behaviors displayed by shy-anxious children were regarded by peers as deviant in Canada, but appropriate or even desirable in China.

Cultural values are reflected in general peer attitudes such as acceptance and rejection. There is evidence that shy-anxious children tend to experience fewer problems in peer acceptance in societies where assertiveness and autonomy are not valued or encouraged. Eisenberg, Pidada, and Liew (2001) found that shyness in Indonesian children was negatively associated with peer nominations of dislike. Chen, Rubin, and Li (1995b) found that shyness was associated with peer rejection in Canadian children, but with peer acceptance in Chinese children in the early 1990s. Moreover, as urban China is changing toward a competitive market-oriented society with the introduction of more individualistic values, shyness is increasingly associated with negative peer attitudes (Chen et al., 2005).

Heinrichs et al. (2006) investigated perceived cultural norms and their relations to youth's social anxiety. The results first indicated that youths in Japan, Korea, and Spain reported greater levels of social anxiety and more fear of blushing than youths in Australia, Canada, Germany, the Netherlands, and the USA. Moreover, youths in collectivistic, especially East Asian, countries were more accepting of socially reticent behaviors than their counterparts in individualistic countries. The level of social anxiety or fear of blushing symptoms was positively associated with the acceptance of socially wary and vigilant behavior at both the individual and cultural levels. In another study with adolescents in Western (Australia, Canada, Germany, the Netherlands, and the USA) and East Asian (China, Japan, and Korea) countries, Rapee et al. (2011) presented a series of vignettes describing individuals who displayed shy and reserved behaviors or outgoing and socially confident behaviors and then asked the participants to indicate the extent to which they would expect the individuals in the vignettes to be socially liked and to succeed in their career. It was found that adolescents in Western groups viewed shy and anxious behaviors as having a more negative impact on social and life adjustment than their counterparts in East Asia.

Compared with shyness and social anxiety, aggressive, antisocial, and other externalizing behaviors seem to be associated with negative peer evaluations more consistently across cultures. Nevertheless, some cultural differences have been found. In cultures such as that of the Yanoamo Indians where aggressive and violent behaviors are considered socially acceptable, children, especially boys, who display these behaviors may be regarded as "heroes" by their peers (Chagnon, 1983). In some central and southern Italian communities, aggressive and defiant behaviors may be perceived by children as reflecting social assertiveness and competence (Casiglia, Lo Coco, & Zappulla, 1998; Schneider

& Fonzi, 1996). In North America, although aggression is generally discouraged, aggressive children and adolescents may receive social support from their peers (e.g., Rodkin, Farmer, Pearl, & van Acker, 2000). In peer groups that approve violence, being able to engage in fighting and display aggressive acts is related to the maintenance of one's social identity and personal "honor" in the group (Bernburg & Thorlindsson, 2005).

Positive evaluations of antisocial behaviors in certain peer groups in the USA are clearly demonstrated by the work of Dishion and colleagues (e.g., Boislard, Poulin, Kiesner, & Dishion, 2009). In a longitudinal project on the development of delinquent behavior, the researchers asked adolescents to discuss topics such as planning a joint activity and solving a social problem. The results indicated that delinquent youth engaged in four times the amount of talk about rule-breaking than nondelinquent youth. Moreover, delinquent youths were likely to display contingent positive reactions to deviant talk such as laughter and expression of attention and interest, whereas nondelinquent youths often ignored deviant talk.

Children's aggressive, antisocial, and violent behaviors tend to be regarded as more problematic and abnormal in collectivistic cultures. In Chinese schools, these behaviors are strictly prohibited, and many strategies are applied to support this prohibition. A major practice to help children control their aggressive and disruptive behavior is the public evaluation in which students are required to evaluate themselves and each other in the class in terms of whether their behaviors are in accord with school standards. Children who display aggressive and disruptive behaviors are likely to be criticized and humiliated by others (e.g., Chen et al., 2005).

In a cross-cultural study of correlates of adolescent misconduct, Chen, Greenberger, Lester, Dong, and Guo (1998) examined perceptions of peer approval and disapproval of a series of behaviors in four samples of junior high school students: Euro-Americans, Chinese Americans, Chinese in Taipei, and Chinese in Beijing. Students reported their peers' attitudes toward their behaviors such as talking back to teacher or principal, doing something dangerous for excitement, cheating on a test, stealing, lying to parents, and smoking and drinking. Students were asked whether their peers would "admire" or "think badly of" them if they were to engage in these behaviors. The results indicated that Euro-American adolescents had higher scores on peer approval for these behaviors than did Chinese adolescents in Beijing and Taipei. Chinese American adolescents fell between Euro-Americans and the two Chinese groups. These results were replicated in another study conducted with adolescents in different samples in the USA, China, and Korea (Greenberger et al., 2000).

In short, research findings have indicated different cultural norms and values with regard to children's behaviors and problems. These norms and values are often manifested in adults' and peers' attitudes and responses in interactions, which constitute social environments for the development of children who display the behaviors and problems. Culture is involved in adaptive and maladaptive development through organizing socialization environments.

Adjustment Outcomes of Internalizing and Externalizing Behaviors: The Imprint of Culture

Although culture provides guidance for social evaluations of, and responses to, children's behaviors, social evaluation and response processes in interactions may regulate children's behaviors and their developmental patterns (Chen, 2012). The regulatory function of these social processes occurs as children attempt to maintain or modify their behaviors according to cultural expectations and standards in the society or group. Although little research has been conducted to directly examine social interaction processes in the development of psychopathology, some studies suggest that social interaction context may enhance or weaken children's and adolescents' adaptive and maladaptive behaviors.

Prinstein (2007), for example, found that youth in socially active groups such as Populars

and Jocks experienced significant declines in social anxiety and depression, whereas youth in academically oriented groups such as Brains exhibited increases in emotional distress from childhood to adolescence. Van Zalk, Van Zalk, and Kerr (2011) found that Radical crowds (Punks and Goths) that included adolescents who were shy and socially fearful with extremely eye-catching or shocking appearance facilitated the group socialization of individual social anxiety. Dishion and his colleagues (e.g., Piehler & Dishion, 2007) found that interactions among adolescents such as talk about rule-breaking and positive reactions to the talk about externalizing behaviors led to increased substance use, delinquency, violence, and high-risk sexual behavior in subsequent years. Moreover, peer groups with more salient norms and more intensive norm-based social evaluations and responses may exert greater influence on youth, and group effects seem to be magnified for those who are more discrepant from their peers (Boxer, Guerra, Huesmann, & Morales, 2005).

Shyness-Inhibition and Social Anxiety and Adjustment

Research evidence has indicated that adjustment outcomes of internalizing behaviors, particularly shyness-inhibition and social anxiety, may vary across cultures. In Western societies, children who display shy, inhibited, and anxious behaviors are likely to develop school problems, negative self-perceptions, and other psychological problems such as loneliness, depression, and emotion disorders (e.g., Coplan, Prakash, O'Neil, & Armer, 2004; Rubin, Coplan, & Bowker, 2009; Schwartz, Snidman, & Kagan, 1999). In a longitudinal study, Gest, Sesma, Masten, and Tellegen (2006) found that peer-assessed shy-withdrawn behavior in childhood negatively predicted the quality of overall social life (overall social acceptance, formation of friendships and networks) and the establishment of romantic relationships 10 years later, with gender, IQ, SES, and stability of adjustment controlled. Similarly, Asendorpf, Denissen, and van Aken (2008) found that shy-anxious behavior, particularly in boys, predicted adjustment problems such as career instability in adulthood. Shy-inhibited, withdrawn, and anxious behaviors were also associated with adulthood affective disorders, suicidal behaviors, and poor marital relationships (Clark, Rodgers, Caldwell, Power, & Stansfeld, 2007; Fergusson, Horwood, & Ridder, 2005). These results generally support the argument that shyness and social anxiety represent a risk factor in development in Western societies (Rubin et al., 2009).

Shy-inhibited and anxious behaviors appear to be related to less negative outcomes societies where social assertiveness and self-expression are less valued. Chen, Chen, Li, and Wang (2009) found in Chinese children that toddlerhood inhibition as observed in the laboratory setting positively predicted peer liking, perceived social integration, positive school attitudes, and school competence 5 years later. Extreme group analysis further indicated that children who were inhibited in toddlerhood were more competent in social and school performance and had fewer behavioral and learning problems in middle childhood than "average" and uninhibited children. Chen, Rubin, Li, and Li (1999) found in China that shyness in middle childhood was not associated with adjustment problems, either externalizing or internalizing, in adolescence. Moreover, shyness was positively associated with adolescent adjustment including leadership, academic achievement, and self-perceptions of competence. As urban China has been changing in recent years toward a market-oriented society, behavioral qualities such as social initiative, competitiveness, and self-expression are increasingly valued and encouraged. Consequently, shyness has been associated with adjustment difficulties such as negative self-perceptions and depression in urban Chinese children (Chen et al., 2005; Chen, Wang, & Wang, 2009).

Relatively positive outcomes of shyness have been found in other societies. Kerr, Lambert, and Bem (1996) followed a sample of children born in a suburb of Stockholm in the mid-1950s to adulthood and found that although shyness predicted later marriage and parenthood, it did not affect adulthood careers including occupational stability, education, or income among Swedish men. Kerr et al. (1996) argued that the results were due to the social welfare and support systems in Sweden, which assured that people did not need to display competitiveness and assertiveness to achieve career success.

Taken together, relative to what has been found in North America, shyness-inhibition, social anxiety, and other internalizing behaviors in some cultures such as Chinese and Northern European cultures may lead to less maladaptive outcomes. In these cultures, social support and assistance that shy, inhibited, and anxious children receive likely enhance their confidence and ability to participate in social activities which, in turn, provides the opportunity for these children to learn skills to manage challenges in different situations. At the same time, social relationships that these children establish may help them cope with psychological difficulties.

Aggression, Self-Control, and Adjustment

Research in the West has revealed that aggressive and other externalizing behaviors are associated with a wide range of adjustment problems such as crime, substance use, school dropout, unemployment, and mental health problems (e.g., Timmermans, van Lier, & Koot, 2008). Evidence from longitudinal research programs has consistently demonstrated the link between childhood aggression and adolescent and adulthood problems, particularly of a high-risk, violent, and antisocial nature (Dodge, Coie, & Lynam, 2006; Tremblay, 2010).

The adjustment outcomes of aggressive behavior in non-Western societies appear to be largely similar to those in Western societies. Nevertheless, there are findings indicating that children who display aggressive behavior in group-oriented cultures may report more negative self-perceptions and self-feelings (e.g., Chen, He, et al., 2004). In the Western literature, the results concerning the relations between aggressive behavior and psychological problems are generally mixed. Whereas some researchers found that aggression was related to internalizing symptoms (e.g., Holt & Espelage, 2007), others failed to find significant relations (e.g., Mercer & DeRosier, 2008). It has been argued that perhaps due to social support received from their peers, aggressive children tend to develop biased self-perceptions of social competence (Dodge et al., 2006). Indeed, in North America, aggression has been found to be positively associated with perceived social competence (e.g., Chen, Zappulla, et al., 2004); aggressive children are more likely than their nonaggressive counterparts to report that they are socially competent.

In Asian group-oriented societies such as those of China, Japan, Korea, and Taiwan, children who display aggressive and disruptive behaviors are often criticized and shamed by others in the public setting. As argued by Fung (2006), negative social evaluations such as shaming are based on a strong group concern because the experience of these evaluations may lead to self-examination, which may promote the internalization of rules and social responsibility. This evaluation process likely makes aggressive, disruptive, and antisocial children develop psychological difficulties such as depression. Consistent with this argument, Chen, He, et al. (2004) found that aggression was positively associated with feelings of loneliness through the mediation of peer relationships in Chinese children, but not in Brazilian, Canadian, or Italian children. Chen et al. (2003) also found in a Chinese sample that externalizing behaviors negatively predicted perceived self-worth and positively predicted emotional problems including depression 2 years later.

Crick and colleagues (Kawabata, Crick, & Hamaguchi, 2010a, 2010b) recently examined how overt and relational aggression was associated with adjustment problems in American and Japanese elementary school children. The results first indicated that in both samples, physical aggression was associated with delinquency and relational aggression was associated with depression. Further analyses indicated that the association between relational aggression and depressive symptoms was stronger in Japanese children than in American children. The results suggested that Japanese children were more vulnerable to negative interpersonal experiences. It is possible that, relative to their counterparts in the West, children who use relational aggression in Japan are viewed as more aversive and are more ostracized by peers because these children act against cultural beliefs and values. As a result, these children may feel so estranged from peer groups that they lack of a sense of belonging.

The cross-cultural results concerning the emotional problems of aggressive children are consistent with findings on relations between self-control and adjustment in American and Asian cultures. Several studies conducted with American children indicated virtually no or positive associations between self-control, such as the suppression of one's behavior or a dominant response to achieve certain goals, and emotional problems (Eisenberg et al., 2007; Murray & Kochanska, 2002). However, Eisenberg et al. (2007) and Chen, Zhang, Chen, and Li (2012) found that self-control was *negatively* associated with, and predictive of, symptoms of fearfulness and anxiety in Chinese children. Similarly, Cheung and Park (2010) found that the suppression of negative emotions such as anger was positively associated with depression in Euro-Americans, but the associations were significantly weaker in Asian Americans. Moreover, a stronger interdependent self-construal attenuated the relation between anger suppression and depressive symptoms.

Conclusions and Future Directions

Cultural norms and values determine, to a large extent, the functional "meanings" of children's and adolescents' behaviors in development. Consequently, the exhibition of specific behaviors and their relations with adjustment outcomes may vary across cultures. The social evaluation and response processes in interactions play a significant role in mediating cultural influence on adaptive and maladaptive behaviors and their developmental patterns.

Research on culture and developmental psychopathology has relied heavily on direct or indirect comparisons of samples of children and adolescents in different cultures. Although cross-cultural similarities and differences from the comparisons are interesting, this approach provides little information about how culture is involved in individual development. We discussed in this chapter the role of social interaction in mediating cultural influence on adaptive and maladaptive development from a contextual-developmental perspective (Chen, 2012). However, many issues in the framework need to be clarified. For example, it will be important to examine how parent–child interaction and peer interaction affect each other in their joint contributions to the development of psychopathological functioning. In addition, according to the contextual-developmental perspective, cultural influence on individual behavior is a dynamic process in which children play an increasingly active role during development. It is virtually unknown how children in different cultures actively participate in constructing their developmental patterns. Continuous exploration of children's social interaction in different societies will be necessary to achieve an in-depth understanding of culture and developmental psychopathology.

Cross-cultural researchers are often interested in comparing children in Western individualistic societies with those in non-Western collectivistic societies. It is important to note that dramatic social and cultural changes are occurring in most countries in the world, both Western and non-Western, due to globalization and technological development. The rapid increase in cross-border trade, integration of cultural systems, and massive movements of populations have made the exposure to different beliefs and lifestyles a part of the experience of children and adults today. A distinct feature of the recent social change is that heightened cultural exchange and interaction has created a context of diverse values for human development. Adapting to a changing environment with mixed social and cultural requirements may be challenging and stressful. At the same time, social, economic, and cultural changes also provide opportunities for young people to develop sophisticated skills that allow them to function effectively in different circumstances. It will be interesting to investigate youth

experiences of social and cultural changes and personal and social factors that may moderate their effects on development.

References

Asendorpf, J. B., Denissen, J. J. A., & van Aken, M. A. G. (2008). Inhibited and aggressive preschool children at 23 years of age: Personality and social transition into adulthood. *Developmental Psychology, 44*, 997–1011.

Austin, A. A., & Chorpita, B. F. (2004). Temperament, anxiety, and depression: Comparisons across five ethnic groups of children. *Journal of Clinical Child and Adolescent Psychology, 33*, 216–226.

Beirens, K., & Fontaine, J. (2011). Somatic complaint differences between Turkish immigrants and Belgians: Do all roads lead to Rome? *Ethnicity & Health, 16*, 73–88.

Benedict, R. (1934). *Patterns of culture*. New York, NY: Houghton Mifflin.

Bergeron, N., & Schneider, B. H. (2005). Explaining cross-national differences in peer-directed aggression: A quantitative synthesis. *Aggressive Behavior, 31*, 116–137.

Bernburg, J., & Thorlindsson, T. (2005). Violent values, conduct norms, and youth aggression: A multilevel study in Iceland. *The Sociological Quarterly, 46*, 457–478.

Boislard, P., Poulin, F., Kiesner, J., & Dishion, T. J. (2009). A longitudinal examination of risky sexual behaviors among Canadian and Italian adolescents: Considering individual, parental, and friend characteristics. *International Journal of Behavioral Development, 33*, 265–276.

Boxer, P., Guerra, N. G., Huesmann, L. R., & Morales, J. (2005). Proximal peer-level effects of a small-group selected prevention on aggression in elementary school children: An investigation of the peer contagion hypothesis. *Journal of Abnormal Child Psychology, 33*, 325–338.

Bronfenbrenner, U., & Morris, P. A. (2006). The bioecological model of human development. In W. Damon (Series Ed.) & R. M. Lerner (Vol. Ed.), *Handbook of child psychology: Vol 1. Theoretical models of human development* (pp. 793–828). New York, NY: Wiley.

Canino, G., & Alegría, M. (2008). Psychiatric diagnosis – is it universal or relative to culture? *Journal of Child Psychology and Psychiatry, 49*, 237–250.

Casiglia, A. C., Lo Coco, A., & Zappulla, C. (1998). Aspects of social reputation and peer relationships in Italian children: A cross-cultural perspective. *Developmental Psychology, 34*, 723–730.

Centers for Disease Control and Prevention. (2000). Youth risk behavior surveillance – United States, 1999. *Morbidity and Mortality Weekly Report, 49*(SS05), 1–96.

Céspedes, Y. M., & Huey, S. J., Jr. (2008). Depression in Latino adolescents: A cultural discrepancy perspective. *Cultural Diversity and Ethnic Minority Mental Health, 14*, 168–172.

Chagnon, N. A. (1983). *Yanomamo: The fierce people*. New York, NY: Holt, Rinehart and Winston.

Chao, R. K. (1994). Beyond parental control and authoritarian parenting style: Understanding Chinese parenting through the cultural notion of training. *Child Development, 65*, 1111–1119.

Chen, X. (2012). Culture, peer interaction, and socioemotional development. *Child Development Perspectives, 6*, 27–34.

Chen, X., Cen, G., Li, D., & He, Y. (2005). Social functioning and adjustment in Chinese children: The imprint of historical time. *Child Development, 76*, 182–195.

Chen, X., Chen, H., Li, D., & Wang, L. (2009). Early childhood behavioral inhibition and social and school adjustment in Chinese children: A 5-year longitudinal study. *Child Development, 80*, 1692–1704.

Chen, X., Chung, J., Lechcier-Kimel, R., & French, D. (2011). Culture and children's social development. In P. Smith & C. Hart (Eds.), *Wiley Blackwell handbook of childhood social development* (2nd ed., pp. 141–160). Malden, MA: Wiley-Blackwell.

Chen, X., DeSouza, A., Chen, H., & Wang, L. (2006). Reticent behavior and experiences in peer interactions in Canadian and Chinese children. *Developmental Psychology, 42*, 656–665.

Chen, X., Dong, Q., & Zhou, H. (1997). Authoritative and authoritarian parenting practices and social and school performance in Chinese children. *International Journal of Behavioral Development, 21*, 855–873.

Chen, X., & French, D. (2008). Children's social competence in cultural context. *Annual Review of Psychology, 59*, 591–616.

Chen, C., Greenberger, E., Lester, J., Dong, Q., & Guo, M. (1998). A cross-cultural study of family and peer correlates of adolescent misconduct. *Developmental Psychology, 34*, 770–781.

Chen, X., Hastings, P., Rubin, K. H., Chen, H., Cen, G., & Stewart, S. L. (1998). Childrearing attitudes and behavioral inhibition in Chinese and Canadian toddlers: A cross-cultural study. *Developmental Psychology, 34*, 677–686.

Chen, X., He, Y., De Oliveira, A., Lo Coco, A., Zappulla, C., Kaspar, V., et al. (2004). Loneliness and social adaptation in Brazilian, Canadian, Chinese and Italian children: A multi-national comparative study. *Journal of Child Psychology and Psychiatry, 45*, 1373–1384.

Chen, X., Rubin, K. H., & Li, B. (1995a). Depressed mood in Chinese children: Relations with school performance and family environment. *Journal of Consulting and Clinical Psychology, 63*, 938–947.

Chen, X., Rubin, K. H., & Li, Z. (1995b). Social functioning and adjustment in Chinese children: A longitudinal study. *Developmental Psychology, 31*, 531–539.

Chen, X., Rubin, K. H., Li, B., & Li, Z. (1999). Adolescent outcomes of social functioning in Chinese children. *International Journal of Behavioral Development, 23*, 199–223.

Chen, X., Rubin, K. H., Liu, M., Chen, H., Wang, L., Li, D., et al. (2003). Compliance in Chinese and Canadian toddlers. *International Journal of Behavioral Development, 27*, 428–436.

Chen, X., Wang, L., & Wang, Z. (2009). Shyness-sensitivity and social, school, and psychological adjustment in rural migrant and urban children in China. *Child Development, 80*, 1499–1513.

Chen, X., Zappulla, C., Coco, A. L., Schneider, B., Kaspar, V., De Oliveira, A., et al. (2004). Self-perceptions of competence in Brazilian, Canadian, Chinese and Italian children: Relations with social and school adjustment. *International Journal of Behavioral Development, 28*, 129–138.

Chen, X., Zhang, G., Chen, H., & Li, D. (2012). Performance on delay tasks in early childhood predicted socioemotional and school adjustment nine years later: A longitudinal study in Chinese children. *International Perspectives in Psychology: Research, Practice, Consultation, 1*, 3–14.

Cheung, R. Y. M., & Park, I. J. K. (2010). Anger suppression, interdependent self-construal, and depression among Asian American and European American college students. *Cultural Diversity and Ethnic Minority Psychology, 16*, 517–525.

Choi, H., Stafford, L., Meininger, J. C., Roberts, R. E., & Smith, D. P. (2002). Psychometric properties of the DSM scale for depression (DSD) with Korean-American youths. *Issues of Mental Health Nursing, 23*, 735–756.

Christoforidou, A. (2004). Prevalence of psychosomatic disorders among Greeks, Americans and Greek-Americans. *Dissertation Abstracts International: Section B: The Sciences and Engineering 64* (8B).

Chung, K. F., & Wong, M. C. (2004). Experience of stigma among Chinese mental health patients in Hong Kong. *Psychiatric Bulletin, 28*, 451–454.

Clark, C., Rodgers, B., Caldwell, T., Power, C., & Stansfeld, S. (2007). Childhood and adulthood psychological ill health as predictors of midlife affective and anxiety disorders: The 1958 British birth cohort. *Archives of General Psychiatry, 64*, 668–678.

Cole, P. M., Tamang, B. L., & Shrestha, S. (2006). Cultural variations in the socialization of young children's anger and shame. *Child Development, 77*, 1237–1251.

Coplan, R. J., Prakash, K., O'Neil, K., & Armer, M. (2004). Do you 'want' to play? Distinguishing between conflicted-shyness and social disinterest in early childhood. *Developmental Psychology, 40*, 244–258.

Dodge, K. A., Coie, J. D., & Lynam, D. R. (2006). Aggression and antisocial behavior in youth. In W. Damon (Series Ed.) & N. Eisenberg (Vol. Ed.), *Handbook of child psychology: Vol. 3. Social, emotional, and personality development* (6th ed.) (pp. 719–788). New York, NY: Wiley.

Dumas, J. E., LaFreniere, P. J., & Serketich, W. J. (1995). "Balance of power": A transactional analysis of control in mother-child dyads involving socially competent, aggressive, and anxious children. *Journal of Abnormal Psychology, 104*, 104–113.

Eisenberg, N., Ma, Y., Chang, L., Zhou, Q., West, S. G., & Aiken, L. (2007). Relations of effortful control, reactive undercontrol, and anger to Chinese children's adjustment. *Development and Psychopathology, 19*, 385–409.

Eisenberg, N., Pidada, S., & Liew, J. (2001). The relations of regulation and negative emotionality to Indonesian children's social functioning. *Child Development, 72*, 1747–1763.

Escobar, J. I. (1995). Transcultural aspects of dissociative and somatoform disorders. *Psychiatric Clinics of North America, 18*, 555–569.

Farver, J., Welles-Nystrom, B., Frosch, D. L., Wimbarti, S., & Hoppe-Graff, S. (1997). Toy stories: Aggression in children's narratives in the U.S., Sweden, Germany, and Indonesia. *Journal of Cross-Cultural Psychology, 28*, 393–420.

Fergusson, D. M., Horwood, L. J., & Ridder, E. M. (2005). Partner violence and mental health outcomes in a New Zealand birth cohort. *Rejoinder Journal of Marriage and Family, 67*, 1131–1136.

Fung, H. (2006). Affect and early moral socialization: Some insights and contributions from indigenous psychological studies in Taiwan. In U. Kim, K. S. Yang, & K. K. Hwang (Eds.), *Indigenous and cultural psychology: Understanding people in context* (pp. 175–196). New York, NY: Springer.

Gartstein, M. A., Gonzalez, C., Carranza, J. A., Ahadi, S. A., Ye, R., Rothbart, M. K., et al. (2006). Studying cross-cultural differences in the development of infant temperament: People's Republic of China, the United States of America, and Spain. *Child Psychiatry & Human Development, 37*, 145–161.

Gartstein, M. A., Peleg, Y., Young, B. N., & Slobodskaya, H. R. (2009). Infant temperament in Russia, United States of America, and Israel: Differences and similarities between Russian-speaking families. *Child Psychiatry and Human Development, 40*, 241–256.

Gest, S. D., Sesma, A., Masten, A. S., & Tellegen, A. (2006). Childhood peer reputation as a predictor of competence and symptoms 10 years later. *Journal of Abnormal Child Psychology, 34*, 509–526.

Grant, B. F., Hasin, D. S., Stinson, F. S., Dawson, D. A., Goldstein, R. B., Smith, S., et al. (2006). The epidemiology of DSM-IV panic disorder and agoraphobia in the United States: Results from the national epidemiologic survey on alcohol and related conditions. *Journal of Clinical Psychiatry, 67*, 363–374.

Greenberger, E., Chen, C., Beam, M., Whang, S.-M., & Dong, Q. (2000). The perceived social contexts of adolescents' misconduct: A comparative study of youths in three cultures. *Journal of Research on Adolescence, 10*, 369–392.

Greenfield, P. M., Maynard, A. E., & Childs, C. P. (2000). History, culture, learning, and development. *Cross-Cultural Research, 34*, 351–374.

Gureje, O., Simon, G. E., Ustun, T. B., & Goldberg, D. P. (1997). Somatization in cross-cultural perspective: A World Health Organization study in primary care. *The American Journal of Psychiatry, 154*, 989–995.

Hackett, L., & Hackett, R. J. (1993). Parental ideas of normal and deviant child behaviour: A comparison of two ethnic groups. *British Journal of Psychiatry, 162*, 353–357.

Hawkins, D., Laub, J., Lauritsen, J., & Cothern, L. (2000). *Race, ethnicity, and serious and violent juvenile offending*. Washington, DC: Office of Juvenile Justice and Delinquency Prevention.

Heiervang, E., Goodman, A., & Goodman, R. (2008). The Nordic advantage in child mental health: Separating health differences from reporting style in a cross-cultural comparison of psychopathology. *Journal of Child Psychology and Psychiatry, 49*, 678–685.

Heinrichs, N., Rapee, R. M., Alden, L. A., Bögels, S., Hofmann, S. G., Oh, K. J., et al. (2006). Cultural differences in perceived social norms and social anxiety. *Behaviour Research and Therapy, 44*, 1187–1197.

Hinton, D. E., Chong, R., Pollack, M., Barlow, D., & McNally, R. (2008). Ataque de nervios: Relationship to anxiety sensitivity and dissociation predisposition. *Depression and Anxiety, 25*, 489–495.

Holt, M. K., & Espelage, D. L. (2007). Perceived social support among bullies, victims, and bully-victims. *Journal of Youth and Adolescence, 36*, 984–994.

Hudson, J. L., & Rapee, R. M. (2001). Parent–child interactions and anxiety disorders: An observational study. *Behaviour Research and Therapy, 39*, 1411–1427.

Janssen, M. M., Verhulst, F. C., Bengi-Arslan, L., Erol, N., Salter, C. J., & Crijnen, A. A. (2004). Comparison of self-reported emotional and behavioral problems in Turkish immigrant, Dutch and Turkish adolescents. *Social Psychiatry and Psychiatric Epidemiology, 39*, 133–140.

Kagan, J. (1997). Temperament and the reactions to unfamiliarity. *Child Development, 68*, 139–143.

Kawabata, Y., Crick, N. R., & Hamaguchi, Y. (2010a). Forms of aggression, social-psychological adjustment, and peer victimization in a Japanese sample: The moderating role of positive and negative friendship quality. *Journal of Abnormal Child Psychology, 38*, 471–484.

Kawabata, Y., Crick, N. R., & Hamaguchi, Y. (2010b). The role of culture in relational aggression: Associations with social-psychological adjustment problems in Japanese and US school-aged children. *International Journal of Behavioral Development, 34*, 354–362.

Kelder, S. H., Murray, N. G., Orpinas, P., Prokhorov, A., McReynolds, L., Zhang, Q., et al. (2001). Depression and substance use in minority middle-school students. *American Journal of Public Health, 91*, 761–766.

Kerr, M., Lambert, W. W., & Bem, D. J. (1996). Life course sequelae of childhood shyness in Sweden: Comparison with the United States. *Developmental Psychology, 32*, 1100–1105.

Kistner, J. A., David, C. F., & White, B. A. (2003). Ethnic and sex differences in children's depressive symptoms: Mediating effects of perceived and actual competence. *Journal of Clinical Child & Adolescent Psychology, 32*, 341–351.

Kleinman, A., & Kleinman, J. (1985). Somatization: The interconnections among culture, depressive experiences, and the meanings of pain. A study in Chinese society. In A. Kleinman & B. Good (Eds.), *Culture and depression* (pp. 132–167). Berkeley, CA: University of California Press.

Kleinman, A., & Kleinman, J. (1991). Suffering and its professional transformation: Toward an ethnography of interpersonal experience. *Culture, Medicine and Psychiatry, 15*, 275–301.

Lambert, S. F., Cooley, M. R., Campbell, K. D. M., Benoit, M. Z., & Stansbury, R. (2004). Assessing anxiety sensitivity in inner-city African American children: Psychometric properties of the childhood anxiety sensitivity index. *Journal of Clinical Child and Adolescent Psychology, 33*, 248–259.

Le, T. (2002). Delinquency among Asian/Pacific islanders: Review of literature and research. *The Justice professional, 15*, 57–70.

Lin, C. C., & Fu, V. R. (1990). A comparison of child-rearing practices among Chinese, immigrant Chinese, and Caucasian-American parents. *Child Development, 61*, 429–433.

Lin, E., Ihle, L., & Tazuma, L. (1985). Depression among Vietnamese refugees in a primary care clinic. *The American journal of Medicine, 78*, 41–44.

Liu, J., Cheng, H., & Leung, P. (2011). The application of the Preschool Child Behavior Checklist and the Caregiver–Teacher Report Form to mainland Chinese children: Syndrome structure, gender differences, country effects, and inter-informant agreement. *Journal of Abnormal Child Psychology, 39*, 251–264.

Mead, M. (1928). *Coming of age in Samoa*. New York, NY: Morrow.

Mercer, S. H., & DeRosier, M. E. (2008). Teacher preference, peer rejection, and student aggression: A prospective study of transactional influence and independent contributions to emotional adjustment and grades. *Journal of School Psychology, 46*, 661–685.

Murray, K. T., & Kochanska, G. (2002). Effortful control: Factor structure and relation to externalizing and internalizing behaviors. *Journal of Abnormal Child Psychology, 30*, 503–514.

Norasakkunkit, V., & Kalick, S. (2009). Experimentally detecting how cultural differences on social anxiety measures misrepresent cultural differences in emotional well-being. *Journal of Happiness Studies, 10*, 313–327.

Obel, C., Heiervang, E., Rodriguez, A., Heyerdahl, S., Smedje, H., Sourander, A., et al. (2004). The strengths and difficulties questionnaire in the Nordic countries. *European Child and Adolescent Psychiatry, 13*(Suppl 2), II32–II39.

Oh, S., & Lewis, C. (2008). Korean preschoolers' advanced inhibitory control and its relation to other executive skills and mental state understanding. *Child Development, 79*, 80–99.

Piehler, T. F., & Dishion, T. J. (2007). Interpersonal dynamics within adolescent friendships: Dyadic mutuality, deviant talk, and patterns of antisocial behavior. *Child Development, 78*, 1611–1624.

Pina, A. A., & Silverman, W. K. (2004). Clinical phenomenology, somatic symptoms, and distress in Hispanic/Latino and European American youths with anxiety disorders. *Journal of Clinical Child and Adolescent Psychology, 33*, 227–236.

Prinstein, M. J. (2007). Assessment of adolescents' preference- and reputation-based peer status using sociometric experts. *Merrill-Palmer Quarterly, 53*, 243–261.

Rapee, R. M., Kim, J., Wang, J., Liu, X., Hofmann, S. G., Chen, J., et al. (2011). Perceived impact of socially anxious behaviors on individuals' lives in Western and East Asian countries. *Behavior Therapy, 42*(3), 485–492.

Raval, V., Martini, T. S., & Raval, P. (2010). Methods of, and reasons for, emotional expression and control in children with internalizing, externalizing, and somatic problems in urban India. *Social Development, 19*, 93–112.

Rescorla, L. A., Achenbach, T. M., Ivanova, M. Y., Harder, V. S., Otten, L., Bilenberg, N., et al. (2011). International comparisons of behavioral and emotional problems in preschool children: Parents' reports from 24 societies. *Journal of Clinical Child & Adolescent Psychology, 40*, 456–467.

Roberts, R. E., & Roberts, C. R. (2007). Ethnicity and risk of psychiatric disorder among adolescents. *Research in Human Development, 41*, 89–117.

Rodkin, P. C., Farmer, T. W., Pearl, R., & van Acker, R. (2000). Heterogeneity of popular boys: Antisocial and prosocial configurations. *Developmental Psychology, 36*, 14–24.

Rogoff, B. (2003). *The cultural nature of human development*. New York, NY: Oxford University Press.

Rothbart, M. K., & Bates, J. E. (2006). Temperament. In N. Eisenberg (Ed.), *Handbook of child psychology* (Social, emotional, and personality development, Vol. 3, pp. 99–166). New York, NY: Wiley.

Rubin, K. H., Coplan, R., & Bowker, J. (2009). Social withdrawal in childhood. *Annual Review of Psychology, 60*, 141–171.

Rubin, K. H., Hemphill, S. A., Chen, X., Hastings, P., Sanson, A., Coco, A., et al. (2006). Across-cultural study of behavioral inhibition in toddlers: East–West–North–South. *International Journal of Behavioral Development, 30*, 219–226.

Rubin, K. H., & Mills, R. S. L. (1992). Parents' thoughts about children's socially adaptive and maladaptive behaviors: Stability, change, and individual differences. In I. Sigel, A. McGillicuddy-DeLisi, & J. Goodnow (Eds.), *In parental belief systems: The psychological consequences for children* (2nd ed., pp. 41–69). Hillsdale, NJ: Erlbaum.

Ryder, A. G., Yang, J., Zhu, X., Yao, S., Yi, J., Heine, S. J., et al. (2008). The cultural shaping of depression: Somatic symptoms in China, psychological symptoms in North America? *Journal of Abnormal Psychology, 117*, 300–313.

Sakai, J., Risk, N., Tanaka, C., & Price, R. (2007). Conduct disorder among Asians and Native Hawaiian/Pacific Islanders in the USA. *Psychological Medicine, 37*, 1013–1025.

Schneider, B. H., & Fonzi, A. (1996). La stabilita dell'amicizia: Unostudio cross-culturale Italia-Canada [Friendship stability: A cross-cultural study in Italy-Canada]. *Eta Evolutiva, 3*, 73–79.

Schneider, B., French, D., & Chen, X. (2006). Peer relationships in cultural perspective: Methodological reflections. In X. Chen, D. French, & B. Schneider (Eds.), *Peer relationships in cultural context* (pp. 489–500). New York, NY: Cambridge University Press.

Schwartz, C. E., Snidman, N., & Kagan, J. (1999). Adolescent social anxiety as an outcome of inhibited temperament in childhood. *Journal of the American Academy of Child & Adolescent Psychiatry, 38*, 1008–1015.

Super, C. M., & Harkness, S. (1986). The developmental niche: A conceptualization at the interface of child and culture. *International Journal of Behavioral Development, 9*, 545–569.

Tietjen, A. M. (2006). Cultural influences on peer relations: An ecological perspective. In X. Chen, D. C. French, & B. H. Schneider (Eds.), *Peer relationships in cultural context* (pp. 52–74). New York, NY: Cambridge University Press.

Timmermans, M., van Lier, P. A., & Koot, H. M. (2008). Which forms of child/adolescent externalizing behaviors account for late adolescent risky sexual behavior and substance use? *Journal of Child Psychology and Psychiatry, 49*, 386–394.

Traue, H., & Pennebaker, J. W. (Eds.). (1993). *Emotion, inhibition, and health*. Seattle, WA: Hogrefe & Huber Publishers.

Tremblay, R. E. (2010). Developmental origins of disruptive behavior problems: The original sin hypothesis, epigenetics and their consequences for prevention. *Journal of Child Psychology and Psychiatry, 51*, 341–367.

Twenge, J. M., & Nolen-Hoeksema, S. (2002). Age, gender, race, socioeconomic status, and birth cohort differences on the Children's Depression Inventory: A meta-analysis. *Journal of Abnormal Psychology, 111*, 578–588.

Van Zalk, N., Van Zalk, M. H. W., & Kerr, M. (2011). Socialization of social anxiety in adolescent crowds. *Journal of Abnormal Child Psychology, 39*, 1239–1249.

Vygotsky, L. S. (1978). *Mind in society*. Cambridge, MA: Harvard University Press.

Weenink, D. (2011). Delinquent behavior of Dutch rural adolescents. *Journal of youth and adolescence, 40*, 1132–1146.

Weisz, J. R., Suwanlert, S., Chaiyasit, W., Weiss, B., Walter, B. R., & Anderson, W. W. (1988). Thai and American perspectives on over-and undercontrolled child behavior problems: Exploring the threshold model among parents, teachers, and psychologists. *Journal of Consulting and Clinical Psychology, 56*, 601–609.

Weisz, J. R., Weiss, B., Suwanlert, S., & Chaiyasit, W. (2006). Culture and youth psychopathology: Testing the syndromal sensitivity model in Thai and American adolescents. *Journal of Consulting and Clinical Psychology, 74*, 1098–1107.

Whiting, B. B., & Edwards, C. P. (1988). *Children of different worlds*. Cambridge, MA: Harvard University Press.

Zahn-Waxler, C., Friedman, R. J., Cole, P. M., Mizuta, I., & Hiruma, N. (1996). Japanese and United States preschool children's responses to conflict and distress. *Child Development, 67*, 2462–2477.

Developmental Behavioral Genetics

13

Thomas G. O'Connor

Progress in understanding genetic influences on health and development continues to be swift and substantial, both resolving and raising core questions for clinical and developmental science. That general point would have been predicted from the last edition of this *Handbook*. What might not have been obvious at the time of the previous volume is the degree of methodological migration away from traditional behavioral genetic approaches using of sibling, twin, and adoption designs to molecular, genetic, and particularly epigenetic approaches; indeed, molecular and epigenetic approaches have since become the more attention-getting, if not the more dominant, methods for testing genetic hypotheses. As a result, the understanding and tracking the field of developmental behavioral genetics now requires a good deal of appreciation for technical laboratory procedures as well as the quantitative sophistication and grounding in behavioral science. Alongside this shift in methods has been a concomitant shift in research questions; that is a theme of this chapter. After a brief review of some of the basic concepts in behavioral genetics, this chapter seeks to present a current overview of the field of developmental behavioral genetics that attends to the changing methods and questions that drive the field. The latter section of the chapter considers the new ideas and applications of developmental behavioral genetic research, particularly to treatment.

Several preliminary organizational points are in order. The first concerns the scope of research that might be considered for a chapter on behavioral genetics. The term "behavioral genetics" came to be synonymous with the family (e.g., twin, sibling, adoption, parent–offspring) study methods that led to an inference about genetic influence based on quantitative analyses. In contrast, molecular genetic research adopted the different approach in which a candidate genetic target (or an index of one) is measured and examined in relation to behavioral phenotypes and/or as a moderator of environmental factors in relation to a behavioral phenotype. At the time of the previous version of this volume, the former was pervasive and the latter was in a chrysalis stage. Things have changed. Currently, molecular genetic approaches are not only ascendant but arguably dominant, and it would be impossible to discuss the impact of genetic research on developmental outcomes without considerable emphasis on molecular genetic findings. Moreover, as discussed below, key concepts for studying gene–environment interplay vary somewhat between behavioral genetic and molecular genetic approaches, and these require consideration. Thus, it is more relevant to define behavioral genetics according to the phenotype under study than according to a research design. Accordingly, the current chapter considers behavioral genetic research that tests hypotheses about genetic

T.G. O'Connor, Ph.D. (✉)
Department of Psychiatry, Wynne Center for Family Research, University of Rochester Medical Center, Rochester, NY 14642, USA
e-mail: tom_oconnor@urmc.rochester.edu

M. Lewis and K.D. Rudolph (eds.), *Handbook of Developmental Psychopathology*, DOI 10.1007/978-1-4614-9608-3_13, © Springer Science+Business Media New York 2014

influence indirectly via a genetically informative research design (e.g., comparing MZ and DZ twins) as well as directly by measuring specific genes. A second organizational point concerns the term "developmental." Development is a process (e.g., the carrying forward of effects) rather than a stage in life (e.g., childhood), as so the chapter covers research throughout the life span. Lastly, this volume includes other chapters on epigenetics and gene–environment interplay; the current chapter seeks to complement rather than overlap with those chapters.

Behavioral Genetic Strategies for Estimating Genetic Influence and Testing Genetic Hypotheses

A first strategy for estimating genetic influence and for testing genetic hypotheses is what is often referred to as an "inferred" strategy. That is, genetic influence is not directly measured, but is instead inferred from capitalizing on a genetically informative research design. Twin and adoptee research designs are fundamental to this inferred approach because they are "natural experiments"—an "experiment" by nature (rather than by experimental design) that offers leverage for inferring genetic influence. The simplest case is the study of monozygotic (MZ) and dizygotic (DZ) twins. Because we know that MZ twins are genetically identical and that DZ twins share, on average 50 % of their segregating genes, it would be expected on genetic basis alone that MZ twins would be more alike than DZ twins. If that is found to the case, then is it reasonable to suppose that the greater similarity of MZ twins on a particular phenotype is attributable in part to their greater genetic similarity, even without having measured genes?

Genetic influence in a twin study is inferable because of the research design and not because genes have been measured directly. The twin design is a major paradigm in research, but there is actually a reasonable controversy and about how much twin studies can say about genetic influence on behavioral or biological measures of adjustment and health. That is because there may

be confounding factors that make inferences about genetic influence more complex than is implied by the calculations used to estimate genetic influence (see below). Critiques of the twin method, and behavioral genetics more broadly, are biological and conceptual and methodological (Meaney, 2010). At least the methodological concerns have been tackled extensively. One of the better-known examples is concerned about the equal environmental assumption—the notion that greater environmental similarity of MZ twins confounds conclusions the impact of greater genetic resemblance. A more complex concern is that chorion type that could influence resemblance in prenatal nutrition, which could confound genetic resemblance because this may vary among MZ twins. Empirical analyses have tended to show that neither of these particular threats is likely to present a major problem for the twin method, (e.g., see Kendler, Neale, Kessler, Heath, & Eaves, 1993) for analyses of the equal environmental assumptions and (Wichers et al., 2002) for chorion type.

Nonetheless, in principle, natural experiments, as any research design, are not without their limits. Fortunately, then, as noted in the previous volume, there are a host of other designs that are genetically informative; all have relative strengths and weaknesses for ascertaining genetic influence. So, for example, if there were sizable gene–gene interactions or epistasis, then they would be captured in the MZ-DZ design but might not be detected in a design that compares resemblance of full siblings with adopted (biologically unrelated) siblings. There are solid reasons why, from a purely genetic perspective, estimates of genetic influence might differ across designs that compare MZ-DZ twins with designs that compare full and adoptive siblings, or designs that compare biologically related parents and children with adoptive parents and children. However, rather than devote substantial space in this chapter to what are now very familiar issues in behavioral genetics, readers can consult the prior version of this chapter of one of several textbooks. A key point is that no single design should be considered adequate for inferring genetic influence and that studies that incorporate a mixture of genetically informative approaches (Deater-Deckard & O'Connor, 2000; O'Connor, Hetherington, Reiss, & Plomin, 1995) may yield the most generalizable effects. A concluding point on this issue, which anticipates the subsequent discussion, is that understanding genetic influence also requires careful attention to environmental factors and the range of environments in particular. Studies that fail to obtain genetically informative samples across a wide range of environmental conditions will likely mis-specify the impact of genetic influence on a phenotype (e.g., Stoolmiller, 1999).

Behavioral Genetic Studies Provide Insight into Genetic and Environmental "Effects"

Genetically informative designs do not separate the influence of genes and environments; instead, they simply make it possible to test the hypothesis that outcomes or processes are partly genetically influenced. The term "genetic influence" is admittedly vague, but it may not have quite the degree of misunderstanding that is associated with the term "heritability"—the variance of a phenotype thought to be genetically influenced. One of the problems in the discussion and translation of behavioral genetic findings was that they were sometimes interpreted (occasionally with encouragement from an overly casual writing style) to suggest that heritability could be considered independent of environmental input. That was an unfortunate side effect of a variance-partitioning approach in behavioral genetic studies that separated variance into genetic and shared (environmental factors making, e.g., siblings similar to one another) and non-shared environment (environmental factors making, e.g., siblings dissimilar to one another). The variance partitioning exercise was sometimes taken too literally to imply that the genetic component in these models could separate the "genetic" effects from the "environmental" effect. It cannot. There are many concrete reasons for that. The most obvious and compelling is that the genetic component in the variance partitioning models

included many forms of gene–environment interplay, including genotype–environment correlation and interaction. Accordingly, broader terms such as "genetic influence" and "gene–environment interplay" are quite inclusive terms that inevitably need clarification, but may be preferable to variance-partitioning terms such as heritability that are often misunderstood and misapplied.

Two other core concepts in the traditional behavioral genetic literature are shared and non-shared environment. Shared and non-shared environments are parameter estimates in traditional behavioral genetic designs and are specific to behavioral genetic research designs. Their existence is driven by the behavioral genetic model, which seeks to examine why, for example, siblings are similar or different from one another. According to the model, there are two sources of similarity: genetic factors (typically referred to as "A," which stands for additive genetic influence) and shared environmental factors (typically referred to as "C," which stands for common environment). The third parameter is non-shared environment (typically referred to as "E," which stands for unique environment) which indexes environmental factors that make siblings different from one another. Estimating these parameters can be quite complex, and there are many books and research papers available that amply demonstrate this analytic complexity. And, measurement error is a major confound, which could elevate the magnitude of non-shared environment (in the case of poor measurement or response bias particular to each sibling) or elevate shared environment (e.g., in the case of a parent providing data on both siblings). But, a simple illustration is possible. The basis for the simplicity is that, because MZ twins are on average twice as similar as are DZ twins, doubling the difference in correlations between MZ and DZ twins is a ballpark estimate of heritability (the actual story is obviously a bit more complicated than this, and other designs require additional considerations). So, if, for example, MZ twins are correlated 0.60 and DZ twins are correlated 0.40 for a measure of depression, then the calculation is that genetic influence or "heritability" is $2 \times (0.60-0.40)$, or

40 %. Estimating C or shared environmental influence is the difference between the heritability and the difference between the MZ and DZ correlations, or 0.40–0.20, or 0.20, i.e., 20 %. Furthermore, we observe that MZ are not identical despite their identical genes, by an amount of 1–0.60. This estimate, 0.40 or 40 % is referred to as non-shared environmental influence. We note that A, C, and E sum to 100 %; this is a necessity as A, C, and E are portions of total variance for a phenotype.

The unit of analysis in traditional behavioral genetic designs is an index of similarity; measures of similarity are compared to make conclusions about the likely role of genetic, shared environment, and non-shared environment. In the classic MZ–DZ twin design, investigators consider not a child depression score as such, but rather the correlation between MZ twins on a measure of depression and compare that with a correlation between DZ twins on that same measure. Mean or absolute levels of depression of each individual MZ or DZ twin can be included in the models but rarely are and in any event seem to matter little in shaping the estimates of genetic and environmental parameters. Of course, most socialization theories—the model that was often set as a counterweight to the genetic models—did not take as its focus sibling similarity. That inevitably meant that it would be difficult to reconcile behavioral genetic concepts and findings with those in traditional developmental psychology. Nonetheless, it was certainly a challenge for traditional socialization theory to account for why, despite living in the same household, non-related siblings show little resemblance to each other and why identical twins who were reared apart were so similar to one another (Bouchard, Lykken, McGue, Segal, & Tellegen, 1990). More broadly, why it is that siblings (perhaps especially genetically related siblings) are so different from one another persists as an important observation, with lessons for understanding both genetics and environment (Plomin & Daniels, 2011), and theories of family process.

There are all sorts of qualifications and footnotes that would be needed to interpret this ACE tripartite analytic model. So, for example, genes

also make nonidentical twins different from one another, but this is not well captured in the model. And, as noted elsewhere (but is still worth repeating), the genetic component "A" includes many different kinds of gene–environment interplay, including genotype–environment correlation and interaction; in other words, the genetic component, A, incorporates environment influence. Also, more complex genetic factors such as gene–gene interactions and nonadditive genetic effects (e.g., random mutations and rare variants) are not well configured. Aside from particular concerns about the ACE parameters, there are other limits of traditional behavioral genetic designs. One is that they offer no clues about the particular genes involved. That is not necessarily a major limitation, however, as it may be better to see behavioral genetic approaches as a first step in research to test genetic hypotheses; nevertheless, it does signal behavioral genetics as at best a midpoint in research in understanding genes, genetic mechanisms, and gene–environment interplay. Second, traditional behavioral genetic designs do not imply anything particular about how or if genetic influences increase or decrease the likelihood of a phenotype. Rather, the traditional behavioral genetic design, because of its focus on similarity (e.g., between MZ and DZ twins), is agnostic about genes for vulnerability or resilience. This latter point may turn out to be important given recent studies that suggest that there may be genetic influences on susceptibility to environmental influence; see below van Ijzendoorn, Belsky, and Bakermans-Kranenburg (2012).

Criticisms of the behavioral genetic ACE model need to be put in context, however. Behavioral genetic designs have very many useful features that have had a major impact on etiological models of health and development. Just a few of these impacts are noted here. One is the pervasive impact of genetic influence. Twin studies have documented genetic influence on a remarkable number of phenotypes, from core constructs of psychological disturbance to subtle, dynamic, and presumably cultural factors, such as parent–child interaction quality (O'Connor, Deater-Deckard, Fulker, Rutter, & Plomin, 1998; Lytton, 1978; O'Connor et al., 1995), exposure to stressful life events (Kendler, Neale, Kessler, Heath, & Eaves, 1993), and religiosity (Bradshaw & Ellison, 2008).

Second, behavioral genetic studies have substantially influenced how we understand gene–environment interplay (see also below). In the first instance, those same ACE models that were criticized for partitioning variance into "genetic" and "environmental" effects were instrumental in showing that there are genetic influences on environmental measures (Plomin, 1995). Moreover, bivariate genetic analyses, which decompose the covariation between measures into genetic and environmental influence, have shown that, for example, the association between family conflict or quality of parent–child relationships and child behavioral adjustment is partly genetically mediated (Burt, Krueger, McGue, & Iacono, 2003; Neiderhiser, Reiss, Hetherington, & Plomin, 1999; O'Connor, Deater-Deckard, et al., 1998). Adoption studies have demonstrated the same idea in demonstrating that the covariation between measures of family risk and child outcome is reliably stronger in parent–child dyads that are biologically related than in nongenetically related adoptive parent–child dyads (McGue, Sharma, & Benson, 1996). Many other examples of bivariate behavioral genetic analyses have identified genetic components of associations that were held to be examples of environmental causation (Kendler & Gardner, 2010). Perhaps the most important legacy of behavioral genetic studies is the way in which it constructed how genes and environment coalesced in developmental models of psychopathology. That is a fundamental concept, and it is a bit ironic that the models that had been criticized for "separating" genes and environment are now appreciated for how they put genes and environment together into causal hypotheses. This issue is getting special attention elsewhere in this volume, so only a very brief discussion is offered here. Perhaps the most obvious point is that, given the pervasive influence of genetic influence on behavioral phenotypes, behavioral genetics in recent years has focused its attention on examining how genetic factors may be involved in the mediation of psychological adjustment and psychosocial risk.

This shift toward testing genetic-environment hypotheses is as strong in research on family process (Reiss et al., 1995) as it is in research on major mental disorder (Wynne et al., 2006).

Several specific forms of gene–environment interplay have been underscored by behavioral genetic research. One basic notion is that the genetic and environmental factors are not independent from one another, that is, they are correlated. Genotype–environment correlations come in a variety of forms; different research designs are needed to assess their presence and magnitude (Plomin, DeFries, & Loehlin, 1977). "Passive" genotype–environment correlations exist because parents provide genes and environments for their children. The term "passive" implies that the child plays no direct role in creating this overlap of genetic and environmental factors. A fundamental implication of passive genotype–environment correlations means that studies of biologically related parents and children cannot draw conclusions about the "effects" of environment because it is confounded with genetics. Confounds introduced by passive genotype–environment surface in virtually all developmental studies in the psychological and psychiatric literature because of the reliance on biologically related families. A second type of genotype–environment correlation is referred to as evocative or active. Evocative or active genotype–environment correlations arise because individuals are active agents in seeking out and evoking experiences and reactions from their families, peer groups, and social settings. Here again, the key notion is that environments and experiences are not randomly distributed in the population, but are correlated with genetically influenced traits. That idea builds on and extends the "child effects" hypothesis that challenged cause–effect thinking in developmental studies (e.g., Bell, 1968).

The pervasive and confounding presence of genotype–environment correlations in developmental and clinical studies meant that many of the presumed environmental effects needed reconsideration and reanalysis in a genetically informative design. Many examples of this have now been reported. One of the more interesting is the case of parental divorce and children's adjustment. Although decades of studies had suggested that parental divorce is associated with increased adjustment problems in children, they were limited by the reliance on biologically related families. Accordingly, they could not rule out the alternative hypothesis that genetic influences on personality and adjustment problems in the parent that may have led to parental divorce were transmitted to the child to increase the likelihood of child adjustment problems. Under that scenario, the parental divorce was an epiphenomenon with no causal impact on the child's adjustment difficulties. Fortunately, this research question has now been tackled by several studies using a mixture of genetically informed designs (Burt, Barnes, McGue, & Iacono, 2008; D'Onofrio et al., 2007; O'Connor, Caspi, DeFries, & Plomin, 2000). The results indicate that environmental mediation of the divorce effect is substantiated, even if there is also some modest genetic mediation as well. This is but one of several examples of how developmental scientists have needed to retest, in a genetically informative design, a hypothesis that was thought to be settled prior to the behavioral genetic "revolution."

A further approach to test genetic hypotheses is to examine genotype–environment interaction. Although marginalized in some early studies using traditional behavioral genetic designs, genotype–environment interactions have moved to the forefront of research in developmental psychology and mental illness. And, as noted below, they have occupied much of the more recent research on molecular genetics. A general concept of the interaction is that there is genetic control over sensitivity to the environment and/or environmental moderation of heritable characteristics (Kendler & Eaves, 1986). Genetically influenced vulnerabilities are herein thought to influence how the individual responds to environmental exposures. To date, there are several empirical examples of genotype–environment interaction in which the genetic measure is inferred from a genetically informative design (Cadoret, Cain, & Crowe, 1983; Tienari et al., 2004). Other examples of genotype–environment interactions are those demonstrating that the amount of genetic influence on a trait varies across environmental conditions. One recent example provides further evidence for greater genetic influence on cognitive ability in higher SES homes but low/minimal genetic influence in low-SES homes (Tucker-Drob, Rhemtulla, Harden, Turkheimer, & Fask, 2011). In an important way, the current focus on genotype–environment interaction and movement away from "main effects" models mimics other areas of developmental studies that consider not so much the main effects of parenting influence but how the presumed effects of parenting are moderated by child characteristics (Kochanska, 1997) or the social setting (Pettit, Bates, Dodge, & Meece, 1999). Searching for interactions simply reflects the growing appreciation of the complexity of developmental processes.

A Next Stage of Research on Genetic Influences

A typical approach for a revised chapter in an updated handbook would be to update the findings and reconsider the core debates in the field in light of the new findings. That approach does not seem adequate in this case because there has not been a very substantial change in the research findings from twin, adoption, and sibling designs as regards the role of genetic or environmental influences on behavioral phenotypes. That is, recent behavioral genetic findings have not overturned or even substantially qualified results from some years ago. Indeed, one of the most important take-home messages is the persistence of the lessons from behavioral genetic research a decade ago, including the near omnipotence of genetic influence on a variety of phenotypes and the prevalence of gene–environment interplay such as genotype–environment correlation. Furthermore, recent reviews of the non-shared environmental literature (Plomin & Daniels, 2011) can make nearly identical claims to reviews published two decades earlier (Dunn & Plomin, 1991): siblings even in the same family exhibit diverse outcomes on a range of behavioral phenotypes and are exposed to disparate environmental conditions, whether the focus is on within-family factors such as parent–child relationships or external factors such as peer relationships.

However, some new trends in behavioral genetic studies are evident, and these are worth noting. One is the increasing use of multivariate strategies to test the hypothesis that disorders and dimensions of psychopathology arise because of a common or shared genetic liability (Huizink, van den Berg, van der Ende, & Verhulst, 2007; Kendler, Neale, Kessler, Heath, & Eaves, 1992; Lahey, Van Hulle, Singh, Waldman, & Rathouz, 2011; O'Connor, McGuire, Reiss, Hetherington, & Plomin, 1998). The key concept underlying these studies is pleiotropy, which is the notion that one gene may be associated with multiple phenotypic traits. Behavioral genetic studies showing that multiple dimensions of psychopathology or disorders are associated with a common underlying genetic risk are not a recent phenomenon. However, recent studies of this kind are interesting in the contemporary context because the results conform nicely with work from nongenetic studies on the structure of psychopathologies (Krueger, 1999; Vollebergh et al., 2001) and with the changing approaches for studying genetics from a molecular perspective, from SNPs to microarrays and genome-wide scans.

Another trend in more recent behavioral genetic work has been a reconsideration of the nongenetic sources of similarity between siblings ("shared environment") and intergenerational transmission (e.g., Burt, 2009). The concepts of shared environment—environmental experiences having similar effects on siblings to make them similar to one another—had been fairly marginal, as the similarity between siblings was, in many cases, attributable largely or even entirely to their genetic similarity. In fact, that helped explain why adoptive siblings who share no genes were so dissimilar to one another on so many behavioral measures.

More recent research suggests a modest change to that conclusion, as there is increasing evidence in behavioral genetic studies to suggest that shared environment may play a more important role in development. In one study

based on the Sibling Interaction and Behavior Study (Burt, McGue, & Iacono, 2010), the authors found that there were sizable effects of shared environment on antisocial behavior and that there was substantial stability of this shared environmental effect over a 4-year period. Antisocial behavior is phenotype for which shared environmental effects have been consistently reported. But there are others. One of the most interesting is child–parent attachment (Bokhorst et al., 2003; O'Connor & Croft, 2001). In contrast to many developmental phenotypes—including other measures of parent–child relationship quality—child–parent attachment appears to be influenced by environmental factors. That, of course, was the hypothesis put forward by attachment theory: child–parent attachment was shaped largely or even entirely by caregiving sensitivity. Nonetheless, decades of research on caregiving and attachment could not rule out an alternative hypothesis that attachment was a behavioral phenotype that, like so many other phenotypes such as temperament, was under genetic influence. Twin studies of attachment were needed. Conclusions from twin studies about the primary role of the caregiving environment rather than genetics in shaping attachment insecurity have since been reinforced by data in foster care sample (Dozier, Stovall, Albus, & Bates, 2001) which, from a genetic perspective, is notable because parents and foster children do not have genes in common, i.e., it is a quasi-adoption study design. Interestingly, the lack of genetic influence on attachment from behavioral genetic studies is consistent with a lack of robust genetic influence from a number of target genes (Luijk et al., 2011). Rather than being under direct genetic influence, there has now been a shift toward assessing child–parent attachment in gene–environment studies (Gervai, 2009). A further example of research emphasizing shared environmental effects indicated that a sizable portion of the link between caregiving quality and academic and social competence in young children might be environmental rather than genetic in origin (Roisman & Fraley, 2012). Finally, other instances of a reemergence of a more broadly defined environmental influence on phenotypes with a recognized strong genetic influence are evident in recent years. One such example is the work showing elevated rates of schizophrenia in migrant groups (Fearon & Morgan, 2006).

Analytic advances and novelties are also evident in recent behavioral genetic research. For example, strategies for testing genetic hypotheses using multilevel modeling, which may have some particular advantages, have been reported (Guo & Wang, 2002; Rasbash, Jenkins, O'Connor, Tackett, & Reiss, 2011). Advances in modeling genotype–environment interactions have also been described (Wong, Day, Luan, Chan, & Wareham, 2003; Wong, Day, Luan, & Wareham, 2004). Also, although not new, meta-analysis is an analytic practice that has been used extensively in the field of developmental behavioral genetics to tackle the wave of research reports on main effects of genes, genotype–environment interactions, and genetic influences on response to drug treatment (Porcelli, Fabbri, & Serretti, 2012; Risch et al., 2009).

Probably the most novel hypothesis concerning genetic influences on behavioral development to emerge in recent years is that there are genetic influences on susceptibility of the environment. There is an important difference between this model and the now familiar hypothesis that there is genetic control over sensitivity to the environment. The hypothesis that there are susceptibility genes (Bakermans-Kranenburg & van Ijzendoorn, 2007; van Ijzendoorn et al., 2012) means that the *same* gene may be associated with better outcomes in the case of positive environmental conditions *and* more negative outcomes in the case of environmental adversity. One example with the dopamine system indicated that children with the 7-repeat DRD4 allele exhibited more externalizing behaviors when raised by insensitive caregivers than children of insensitive caregivers without the 7-repeat allele; however, children with the 7-repeat allele with sensitive caregivers exhibited the lowest levels of externalizing behaviors, compared with children with sensitive caregivers without the 7-repeat allele (Bakermans-Kranenburg & van Ijzendoorn, 2006). A recent meta-analysis (van Ijzendoorn et al., 2012) indicated some support for the hypothesis that the serotonin transporter gene may show this susceptibility pattern rather than merely the genetic vulnerability pattern. More work in this area is expected, and the list of susceptibility genes may lengthen.

Epigenetic research is another novel area with implications for behavioral genetics. This topic is covered elsewhere in this volume, but two points are particularly pertinent to this behavioral genetic chapter. One is that the epigenetic work, which is as impressive as it is complicated, places a clear and decisive and causal role for the environment in behavioral and brain development. Importantly, the epigenetic work does this in an especially compelling matter, that is, from a biological mechanism's perspective. Specifically, the basic notion in epigenetic work is that environmental signals may alter gene expression. Gene expression can be modulated by methylation, which creates a more tightly coiled structure that silences the expression of genes, and acetylation, which opens the coiled structure of the DNA molecule to facilitate the expression of genes. Epigenetic work in animals now makes clear that caregiving experience can alter gene expression, particularly involving those genes in the stress response system (Champagne et al., 2006; Szyf, Weaver, Champagne, Diorio, & Meaney, 2005; Weaver et al., 2004, 2005). Human studies that employ these ideas and models are beginning to be reported, with some intriguing findings (Essex et al., 2011; Oberlander et al., 2008; Poulter et al., 2008). There are sizable challenges in translating the animal findings to humans, including the tissue-specific nature of the genetic effects which implies that gene expression changes in the brain may not be accessible from peripheral samples. There is no question, however, that this kind of human research will proliferate in the near future. In any event, what is now clear is that the epigenetic work shows underscore careful assessments of the environment which may alter gene expression (Cole et al., 2007). The idea that careful measures of the environment are needed to study the interplay between genetics and the environment is not new, of course, but the epigenetic work underscores how powerful environmental "effects" might be.

Aside from emphasizing the need for careful assessments of the (early) caregiving environment, as well as other exposures, a second key implication of the epigenetic work is that it further extinguishes the "nature-nurture" debate (Bagot & Meaney, 2010; Kappeler & Meaney, 2010; Meaney, 2010; Zhang & Meaney, 2010). That may sound trivial, and it certainly is for those who have conducted genetic work within the animal model. But, it is an important statement insofar as it further rejects the notion that genetic influence can be distinguished empirically from environmental influence. Moreover, these studies show that knowing that an individual has a gene is not adequate for understanding likely risk or resilience. That is because it is not clear if the gene is or will be expressed. Accordingly, molecular genetic studies that focus on the presence of, for example, a risk allele in a particular gene might not be targeting the key feature: epigenetic work shows that it is the expression of the gene (and not its mere presence) which needs to be assessed in studies of health and development.

Greater appreciation epigenetics and gene expression is one area in which understanding of genetic mechanisms underlying behavioral phenotypes has increased in recent years, but there are others. Several examples are worth highlighting. One is the recent observation of the passing on of random mutations from fathers, which is positively associated with paternal age at the child's conception (Kong et al., 2012). That is an important finding insofar as certain conditions, including autism, have been linked to new mutations (O'Roak et al., 2012), and that paternal age at the child's conception has been linked with autism, among other conditions (Reichenberg et al., 2006). Another factor needing consideration is the possibility that rare genetic variants may have a sizable influence on disorder and disease (e.g., Cirulli & Goldstein, 2010).

There is then basic discoveries in genetics, including the realization that "junk DNA" actually plays a significant role in regulating the activity of genes, as recently reported by the ENCODE project. These examples of genetic influence are not the kinds that are searched for in the twin or adoption studies or the molecular genetic studies. It is not yet clear what if any role they have to play in resolving the vanishing heritability issue (see below). Nonetheless, what is important is that these kinds of studies are a further reminder that "genetic influence" comes in many forms and that no particular research design is likely to be adequate for operationalizing genetic influence.

Linking Molecular and Behavioral Genetic Approaches to Studying Development and Psychopathology

It is not longer feasible to consider behavioral genetic findings apart from those from molecular genetic approaches. There are obvious reasons for this. The first is that behavioral and molecular genetic approaches are both seeking to test the common hypotheses about genes, environment, and their influence on behavioral health and development. The second is that behavioral genetic research—which seeks to identify *any* genetic influence—is generally viewed as a preamble to the molecular genetic research—which seeks to examine *which* genetic factors account for that influence, once an influence has been established. The third is that it is important to consider the degree to which behavioral genetic findings converge with findings from molecular genetics, insofar as that is possible. Interestingly, a core theme emerging from the molecular work is that influential molecular approaches to study genetic influences have not supplanted the behavioral genetic approaches that use research design to infer genetic influence. One reason is what has been termed the "missing heritability" problem (Plomin, 2012): traditional behavioral genetic findings consistently suggest strong genetic influences on psychological and psychiatric outcomes, but the molecular genetic work so far has been inconclusive and inconsistent and rarely has been able to account for anything but trivial variance in a phenotype.

Molecular genetic studies have numerous advantages over the twin/sibling/adoption designs. The main feature is that they shift from a behavioral genetic design in which typically neither the environment nor genetics is assessed to a model in which there are measured genes and measured environments. There is therefore greater leverage for deriving findings that are specific enough to shape developmental theory and clinical practice. There is then the matter of practicality. No doubt one of the reasons for the expansion of molecular genetic work in developmental science is the comparative ease of obtaining the necessary samples. Buccal swabs obtained by minimally intrusive measures can yield a high rate of genetic success (although there is some debate on that) and are easily collected, stored, and analyzed in commercial and academic labs ("easily" is, of course, a relative term). In short, that means that any study with ongoing contact with the sample can be retrofitted for molecular genetics—something that has not been lost on developmental investigators. Compared to the complex and typically onerous process of gathering sizable twin and adoption samples, the molecular genetic design requirements seem simple. Moreover, although there remains some variation in how the collection and particularly storage of DNA is considered by Institutional Review Boards, there is now a substantial track record for developing an ethical "best practice."

Molecular genetic approaches also have a particular set of limitations, as least as regards common (current) practice. The most troublesome is the tendency to focus on a single genetic focus or allelic pattern. As widely noted, studies seeking to link a specific gene with a specific outcome such as psychiatric disorder have not yielded consistent findings and have led to reconsiderations of both methods and biology (Hamer, 2002; Insel & Collins, 2003). Additionally, some of the lessons derived from behavioral genetic research have not yet been widely incorporated into molecular genetic approaches. For example, behavioral genetic models are based on the assumption that a phenotype is influenced by multiple genes, each having small and additive effects. Whether or not that assumption is actually true is unclear, but it is notable that the behavioral genetic models that adopt this assumption have proved to be robust, which at least suggests that

that assumption is not wildly off base. However, as noted, much of the molecular genetic research tends to focus on a single gene and by assessing single nucleotide polymorphisms (SNPs). There are a host of technical issues in linking allelic identity to genetic influence, but perhaps an even bigger concern is conceptual: if most phenotypes of interest are influenced by a multitude of genes each having a small effect, then linking a phenotype with a single SNP to index a single gene would seem to be an unsuccessful strategy. This is presumed to be the basis for the missing heritability problem mentioned above.

Another example concerns pleiotropy, which has been robustly supported in behavioral genetic work. Molecular genetic approaches continue to imply a "single gene, single disorder" model because a single SNP is linked with a singular dimension or disorder. That is changing somewhat, but clearly the bulk of recently published studies focuses on a single gene or single index of a gene rather than gene systems that are almost certainly playing modulating effects. In current research, for example, it would be very difficult to justify focus only on the serotonin transporter promoter region in a study of serious behavioral or emotional disturbance because the biological argument for many other gene systems would be as substantial. Indeed, numerous psychological and psychiatric outcomes could easily be argued to involve the many genes involved in the stress response; neurotrophic factors; sympathetic nervous system response, plus serotonin; and other usual suspects. The list of molecular genetic candidates with a powerful influence on brain and behavioral development is long and growing (Cirulli et al., 2009, 2011) and underscores the need for genetic research that models genetic complexity and biological mechanisms. A recent exception is the work using microarrays, which do not specify a specific genetic marker but gene systems. On the other hand, microarray studies have few of the advantages of standard molecular genetic studies: they are very expensive, densely complex as regards bioinformatics, and not as widely accessible.

Like behavioral genetic research, molecular genetic research has penetrated deeply into what was purely developmental psychology terrain that went no deeper than psychological and behavioral phenotypes. And, many genotype–environment interactions have been reported that could alter groundwork in psychological theory. Attachment theory is one example that has been targeted by numerous molecular genetic studies. For example, Kochanska and her colleagues reported that children possessing the short variant of the 5-HTTLPR gene were more likely to exhibit insecure attachments in infancy, but only if they had insensitive caregivers (Barry, Kochanska, & Philibert, 2008b). They also showed that young children with the short variant of the serotonin transporter and an insecure attachment exhibited poorer emotion regulation compared with securely attached children or those with the long variant of the allele (Kochanska, Philibert, & Barry, 2009); see also Pauli-Pott, Friedel, Hinney, and Hebebrand (2009). Dopamine genes have also been examined in relation to attachment and genotype–environment interactions (Bakermans-Kranenburg & van Ijzendoorn, 2006; Propper, Willoughby, Halpern, Carbone, & Cox, 2007).

Questions about *which* genetic mechanisms were at work could not be answered by behavioral genetic designs. It was perhaps inevitable, then, that there was a move toward molecular genetics. The change in design signals a corresponding alteration in the kinds of hypotheses being tested or, at a minimum, emphasized in research. Most notably, molecular genetic research is characterized by a much greater emphasis on genotype–environment interaction. It is also worth noting that the move to molecular genetic designs also means a move away from the types of environmental hypotheses that were ushered in with the behavioral genetic design. Specifically, the "shared" and "non-shared" environmental parameters, which were essential components of the analytic model in behavioral genetics, do not register in molecular genetic studies. Given the profound impact of the non-shared environmental findings that characterized the early (as well as current) behavioral genetic research, it is striking that this concept is ignored in molecular genetic work.

Developmental Timing and Developmental Programming

Genetics is inherently developmental. That is, our understanding of genetic influence is through a complex process whereby genes and gene products unfold in development or ontogeny (Meaney, 2010). More concretely, it is obvious that many strongly genetically influenced conditions (Parkinson's disease, Alzheimer's disease, Huntington's disease, schizophrenia) are not apparent until comparatively late in development. It is not that the individual does not have the genetic vulnerability, but rather that the genetic vulnerability is not expressed until late in development. This is one of several obvious examples of developmental genetics. Alongside these not fully understood biological mechanisms that modulate gene expression in development is a psychological theory of developmental behavioral genetics (Plomin, 1983; Scarr & McCartney, 1983). Among the hypotheses proposed in these models is that genotype–environment correlations—and consequently genetic influence—may become stronger in development (Scarr & McCartney, 1983).

Human studies have only begun to try to translate the animal work on developmental timing of genetic effects and timing effects of environmental influence on gene expression. Of particular interest is the impressive body of experimental animal data referenced above that demonstrates that early maternal care is associated with substantial and apparently lasting genetic changes in the offspring. It remains unclear if the plasticity of gene expression in animals can be conceptually or methodologically extended to human development. In light of the data showing that there are some conditions leading to persisting effects of early exposures and experiences (O'Donnell, O'Connor, & Glover, 2009; Vorria et al., 2006; Wiik et al., 2011), there seem to be several kinds of opportunities to examine how the timing of an environmental influence such as stress exposure would affect individuals according to genetic vulnerability (or resilience). Many questions remain about, for example, which periods of development and which gene systems are may be especially sensitive to environmental input.

One way in which behavioral genetic studies have already contributed to developmental models is the assessment of genetic influences on stability and change in behavioral phenotypes. One set of studies shows that behavioral stability may be strongly genetically mediated; many of the same studies also provide evidence the there may be genetic influences on change in behavioral phenotypes (Hopwood et al., 2011; O'Connor, Neiderhiser, Reiss, Hetherington, & Plomin, 1998; Trzaskowski, Zavos, Haworth, Plomin, & Eley, 2012). It remains to be seen if findings from longitudinal behavioral genetic analyses can be integrated with those from molecular genetic and epigenetic work.

Molecular genetic research that has adopted a developmental framework is now quite limited. There are some interesting longitudinal connections, however. Some of the examples of genotype–environment interaction predict changes over time, so that the developmental trajectories of those who experienced early poor care might be thought to differ according to genetic risk (Barry, Kochanska, & Philibert, 2008a; Caspi et al., 2002; Propper et al., 2008).

Applications for Psychopathology and Treatment

One striking change since the last volume in research on developmental behavioral genetics is the availability of data on genetic influences on treatment for mental disorder. The possibility that there would be genetic influences on treatment response is a natural extension to the finding that there are genetic influences on susceptibility to the environment, a core framework for studying genotype interaction. Of course, rather than focus on genetic vulnerabilities that lead to psychopathology when paired with stress exposure, the kind of interaction relevant for treatment would suggest that there are genetic influences on benefitting from a positive or enhanced environment. Whether or not the traditional treatment context and its dose of

environmental manipulation (which is still quite modest in most cases, e.g., <15 h of treatment sessions) is adequate for detecting a genotype–environment interaction that is not obvious. By comparison, where there have been robust genotype environments implying vulnerability for psychopathology, the environmental stress exposure has been chronic and severe (Cicchetti, Rogosch, & Oshri, 2011; Kaufman et al., 2006; Uher et al., 2011)—hardly comparable to the kind of environmental exposure associated with modern-day psychological treatments. The counterargument is that a successful treatment could yield a sizable change in behavioral adjustment, as effect sizes of 0.5 or greater have been reported in many forms of treatment for many disorders. If large behavioral (or biochemical) changes are possible, then that might auger well for finding genetic response to treatment.

The proliferation of studies assessing genetic influences on response to drug and psychological therapies in recent years is no doubt due in large measure to the relative ease and modest cost of collecting and analyzing DNA from buccal swabs. Testing treatment hypotheses using the twin or sibling study methods that were the foundation of behavioral genetics was clearly unwieldy, as it would have required random assignment of, for example, affected MZ and DZ twins to treatment and comparison condition; practical and perhaps even ethical concerns would be difficult to resolve. Of course, molecular approaches to studying response to treatment also have challenges. Probably the most pressing is that if, as is widely presumed, depression and virtually all other mental disorders are a product of very many genes each having a very small effect (and genetic vulnerability may vary across depressed individuals), then there are clearly going to be problems in identifying genetic influences on treatment response. Multiple gene systems would have to be canvassed, and either very large samples (which is challenging) or very large individual gene effects (which may be unlikely) would be required to detect an effect. As noted below, most of the current examples focus on a single gene or a very small number of genes. It is to be anticipated that greater use of more powerful genetic strategies such as microarrays will be incorporated into treatment designs.

The same genetic candidates that have been used in nontreatment studies of psychopathology might also be relevant for assessing genetic response to treatment. The recent work on susceptibility genes (Morey et al., 2011; van Ijzendoorn et al., 2012) may offer one way forward insofar as they would be expected to influence response to both negative (e.g., stress) and salutary (e.g., treatment) conditions. However, evidence supporting this pattern has not been consistent (Nederhof, Belsky, Ormel, & Oldehinkel, 2012), and the identity of genes that might show the differential susceptibility pattern is unresolved, as discussed previously.

Empirical demonstrations that show genetic moderation of psychological treatments are beginning to appear in the literature. For example, in a study of childhood anxiety, Lester and colleague (2012) found that a marker of the nerve growth factor (NGF) gene but not BDNF was associated with reduction in anxiety in response to CBT. If this finding is replicated, then it may be positioned to influence treatment decisions. Other examples of how genetic influences may alter response to psychological treatment have been reported (Beach et al., 2009; Brody, Beach, Philibert, Chen, & Murry, 2009).

Many more studies have investigated the impact of genetic influence on drug treatment response, as noted. To be sure, there are some positive findings, although there is considerable complexity as variation in the genetic influence on treatment response may be related to the course of the disorder, drug treatment applied, comorbid conditions, ethnicity, or a host of other factors (Kim et al., 2006; Porcelli et al., 2012).

There is now a robust debate about the viability of personalized medicine (Collins, 2010; Nebert & Zhang, 2012). Although the promise is clear, so is the basic problem: if most diseases and disorders are a product of many genetic factors each with a small effect and each also under genetic or environmental regulation, then the genetic lab test—even if one were made affordable—could only offer a small glimpse into the

risk for disease. Whether or not that would compare favorably with other clinical data such as blood glucose or cortisol levels is unclear. In other words, although studies of genetic influence on response to treatment are encouraging, there are a host of questions that remain: is the genetic moderation effect sizably larger than other treatment moderators? Is incorporating genetic information cost effective? At least for now, the current wave of genotype-treatment interaction research may best be viewed as "proof of principle" studies rather than studies that can yet shape clinical decisions.

In the meantime, it is important to continue to note the role of nongenetically informative treatment studies in research on environmental causality. The capability to make claims about environmental mediation in treatment studies derives not from the controlling for genetic influence, but from the randomized clinical trial design. The impact of randomized clinical trials for understanding environmental causality is not sufficiently attended to in genetic studies and reviews. So, for example, parent training programs can lead to a reduction in disruptive child behavior by changing parenting behavior and not actually treating the child (Scott et al., 2010; Webster-Stratton, Hollinsworth, & Kolpacoff, 1989). The "trickle-down" of treatment benefits is a form of environmental causality that cannot be explained by genetics—although factors that moderate response to treatment might be (e.g., see Scott & O'Connor, 2012). On this basis, it would not be plausible for genetic studies to suggest that virtually all of the variation in disruptive behavior is genetic (of course, very few do).

Conclusions and Future Directions

Several fundamental contributions of behavioral genetic research to developmental and clinical science have had and will continue to have a legacy on subsequent research design and theory. These include the observations that studies of biologically related families are unable to identify environmentally causal connections; that there are sizable genetic influences on some of the most studied "environmental risks"; that siblings growing up in the same home show marked differences in psychological outcomes despite the presumed "shared" family environment; that there may be genetic control over sensitivity to the environment; and that there are pervasive genotype–environment correlations, meaning that an individual's genetic makeup may influence the environment that he/she elicits. It is noteworthy that findings supporting these basic lessons had been reported well more than a decade ago; none of the recent papers from behavioral genetic or other lines of research has fundamentally challenged any of these notions.

Many future research avenues are apparent from this review. One area that is sure to grow—and needs to grow—is the research on whether or not, and how, genetic influences alter response to psychoactive drugs or psychological therapies. The treatment applications of developmental behavioral genetics have, to date, been sizable conceptually but practically minimal. To be sure, there has been progress in the development and application of psychological treatments for a range of disorders in recent years; however, it is not obvious that this has been coordinated with or influenced by findings in developmental behavioral genetics.

It is too soon to tell if there are robust genetic moderation effects on treatment, and so the import of this work for the clinic is uncertain, if promising. That is not so much of a surprise given the generally slow translation of research findings to the clinic.

Another conclusion pointing to a future direction for research is the need to resolve the contradiction or paradox apparent in the genotype–environment interaction research. On the one hand, there are very many examples of interactions (e.g., Cicchetti & Rogosch, 2012; Fergusson, Boden, Horwood, Miller, & Kennedy, 2011), highlighting the likely robust model of genotype–environment interactions that are evident in most models and research programs. On the other hand, there remain concerns about methodological strategies and the formidable nature of the task of identifying moderation effects given the multitude of genetic and environmental candidates (Bookman et al., 2011; Young-Wolff, Enoch, &

Prescott, 2011). Indeed, three recent meta-analyses of the genotype–environment interaction between stress exposure the serotonin transporter gene in leading to depression have yielded contrary findings, or at least led to contrary conclusions (Karg, Burmeister, Shedden, & Sen, 2011; Munafo, Durrant, Lewis, & Flint, 2009; Risch et al., 2009). And, most of that debate has focused on moderation involving a target genetic focus (or gene system) and a specific environmental risk; interactions involving complex disease are almost certain to be more complex than a two-way interaction. Although the field has clearly moved away from variance partitioning as a research strategy, there are formidable challenges in addressing the methodological, data analytic, and biological challenges raised by the flurry of genotype–environment interaction studies.

There are other important and influential hypotheses in health and development that have not yet been systematically integrated with genetic hypotheses. Examples include the pervasive social class gradient of health (Steptoe et al., 2010) and developmental programming (Bale et al., 2010). The next series of studies will no doubt integrate these sociological and biological observations into genetically informed investigations. Finally, genetic research has only fairly recently begun to integrate biomarkers alongside the genes that presumably underlie them. So, for example, of all the numerous studies of the serotonin transporter gene, it is interesting to note how many (hardly any) also include a biomarker of serotonergic function. On the other hand, genetic studies that also include brain measures such as EEG and imaging are now being reported. It is certain that the next steps of genetic research will attempt to fill the sizable gap between a genetic finding and a biologically active product of that gene as it functions in the brain and body.

References

Bagot, R. C., & Meaney, M. J. (2010). Epigenetics and the biological basis of gene x environment interactions. *Journal of the American Academy of Child and Adolescent Psychiatry, 49*(8), 752–771.

Bakermans-Kranenburg, M. J., & van Ijzendoorn, M. H. (2006). Gene-environment interaction of the dopamine

D4 receptor (DRD4) and observed maternal insensitivity predicting externalizing behavior in preschoolers. *Developmental Psychobiology, 48*(5), 406–409.

Bakermans-Kranenburg, M. J., & van Ijzendoorn, M. H. (2007). Research review: Genetic vulnerability or differential susceptibility in child development: The case of attachment. *Journal of Child Psychology and Psychiatry, 48*(12), 1160–1173.

Bale, T. L., Baram, T. Z., Brown, A. S., Goldstein, J. M., Insel, T. R., McCarthy, M. M., et al. (2010). Early life programming and neurodevelopmental disorders [Research Support, N.I.H., Extramural Research Support, Non-U.S. Gov't Review]. *Biological Psychiatry, 68*(4), 314–319.

Barry, R. A., Kochanska, G., & Philibert, R. A. (2008a). G x E interaction in the organization of attachment: Mothers' responsiveness as a moderator of children's genotypes. *Journal of Child Psychology and Psychiatry, 49*(12), 1313–1320.

Barry, R. A., Kochanska, G., & Philibert, R. A. (2008b). G x E interaction in the organization of attachment: Mothers' responsiveness as a moderator of children's genotypes [Research Support, N.I.H., Extramural Research Support, Non-U.S. Gov't]. *Journal of Child Psychology and Psychiatry, and Allied Disciplines, 49*(12), 1313–1320.

Beach, S. R., Brody, G. H., Kogan, S. M., Philibert, R. A., Chen, Y. F., & Lei, M. K. (2009). Change in caregiver depression in response to parent training: Genetic moderation of intervention effects [Research Support, N.I.H., Extramural]. *Journal of Family Psychology, 23*(1), 112–117.

Bell, R. Q. (1968). A reinterpretation of the direction of effects in studies of socialization [Review]. *Psychological Review, 75*(2), 81–95.

Bokhorst, C. L., Bakermans-Kranenburg, M. J., Fearon, R. M., van Ijzendoorn, M. H., Fonagy, P., & Schuengel, C. (2003). The importance of shared environment in mother-infant attachment security: A behavioral genetic study [Twin Study]. *Child Development, 74*(6), 1769–1782.

Bookman, E. B., McAllister, K., Gillanders, E., Wanke, K., Balshaw, D., Rutter, J., et al. (2011). Gene-environment interplay in common complex diseases: Forging an integrative model-recommendations from an NIH workshop. *Genetic Epidemiology.* doi: 10.1002/gepi.20571.

Bouchard, T. J., Jr., Lykken, D. T., McGue, M., Segal, N. L., & Tellegen, A. (1990). Sources of human psychological differences: The Minnesota Study of Twins Reared Apart [Research Support, Non-U.S. Gov't Research Support, U.S. Gov't, Non-P.H.S. Research Support, U.S. Gov't, P.H.S.]. *Science, 250*(4978), 223–228.

Bradshaw, M., & Ellison, C. G. (2008). Do genetic factors influence religious life? Findings from a behavior genetic analysis of twin siblings. *Journal for the Scientific Study of Religion, 47*, 529–544.

Brody, G. H., Beach, S. R., Philibert, R. A., Chen, Y. F., & Murry, V. M. (2009). Prevention effects moderate the association of 5-HTTLPR and youth risk behavior initiation: Gene x environment hypotheses tested via a randomized prevention design [Randomized Controlled Trial Research Support, N.I.H., Extramural]. *Child Development, 80*(3), 645–661.

Burt, S. A. (2009). Rethinking environmental contributions to child and adolescent psychopathology: A meta-analysis of shared environmental influences [Meta-Analysis]. *Psychological Bulletin, 135*(4), 608–637.

Burt, S. A., Barnes, A. R., McGue, M., & Iacono, W. G. (2008). Parental divorce and adolescent delinquency: Ruling out the impact of common genes. *Developmental Psychology, 44*(6), 1668–1677.

Burt, S. A., Krueger, R. F., McGue, M., & Iacono, W. (2003). Parent-child conflict and the comorbidity among childhood externalizing disorders [Research Support, U.S. Gov't, P.H.S. Twin Study]. *Archives of General Psychiatry, 60*(5), 505–513.

Burt, S. A., McGue, M., & Iacono, W. G. (2010). Environmental contributions to the stability of antisocial behavior over time: Are they shared or nonshared? [Research Support, N.I.H., Extramural]. *Journal of Abnormal Child Psychology, 38*(3), 327–337.

Cadoret, R. J., Cain, C. A., & Crowe, R. R. (1983). Evidence for gene-environment interaction in the development of adolescent antisocial behavior [Research Support, Non-U.S. Gov't]. *Behavior Genetics, 13*(3), 301–310.

Caspi, A., McClay, J., Moffitt, T. E., Mill, J., Martin, J., Craig, I. W., et al. (2002). Role of genotype in the cycle of violence in maltreated children. *Science, 297*(5582), 851–854.

Champagne, F. A., Weaver, I. C., Diorio, J., Dymov, S., Szyf, M., & Meaney, M. J. (2006). Maternal care associated with methylation of the estrogen receptor-alpha1b promoter and estrogen receptor-alpha expression in the medial preoptic area of female offspring. *Endocrinology, 147*(6), 2909–2915.

Cicchetti, D., & Rogosch, F. A. (2012). Gene x Environment interaction and resilience: Effects of child maltreatment and serotonin, corticotropin releasing hormone, dopamine, and oxytocin genes [Research Support, N.I.H., Extramural Research Support, Non-U.S. Gov't]. *Development and Psychopathology, 24*(2), 411–427.

Cicchetti, D., Rogosch, F. A., & Oshri, A. (2011). Interactive effects of corticotropin releasing hormone receptor 1, serotonin transporter linked polymorphic region, and child maltreatment on diurnal cortisol regulation and internalizing symptomatology [Research Support, N.I.H., Extramural Research Support, Non-U.S. Gov't]. *Development and Psychopathology, 23*(4), 1125–1138.

Cirulli, F., Francia, N., Berry, A., Aloe, L., Alleva, E., & Suomi, S. J. (2009). Early life stress as a risk factor for mental health: Role of neurotrophins from rodents to non-human primates [Research Support, N.I.H., Extramural Research Support, N.I.H., Intramural

Research Support, Non-U.S. Gov't Review].
Neuroscience and Biobehavioral Reviews, 33(4),
573–585.

Cirulli, E. T., & Goldstein, D. B. (2010). Uncovering the
roles of rare variants in common disease through
whole-genome sequencing [Review]. *Nature Reviews
Genetics, 11*(6), 415–425.

Cirulli, F., Reif, A., Herterich, S., Lesch, K. P., Berry, A.,
Francia, N., et al. (2011). A novel BDNF polymor-
phism affects plasma protein levels in interaction with
early adversity in rhesus macaques [Research Support,
N.I.H., Extramural Research Support, N.I.H.,
Intramural Research Support, Non-U.S. Gov't].
Psychoneuroendocrinology, 36(3), 372–379.

Cole, S. W., Hawkley, L. C., Arevalo, J. M., Sung, C. Y.,
Rose, R. M., & Cacioppo, J. T. (2007). Social regula-
tion of gene expression in human leukocytes. *Genome
Biology, 8*(9), R189.

Collins, F. S. (2010). *The language of life: DNA and the
revolution in personalized medicine.* New York:
Harper Collins.

D'Onofrio, B. M., Turkheimer, E., Emery, R. E., Maes, H.
H., Silberg, J., & Eaves, L. J. (2007). A children of
twins study of parental divorce and offspring psycho-
pathology [Research Support, N.I.H., Extramural
Twin Study]. *Journal of Child Psychology and
Psychiatry, and Allied Disciplines, 48*(7), 667–675.

Deater-Deckard, K., & O'Connor, T. G. (2000). Parent-
child mutuality in early childhood: Two behavioral
genetic studies. *Developmental Psychology, 36*(5),
561–570.

Dozier, M., Stovall, K. C., Albus, K. E., & Bates, B.
(2001). Attachment for infants in foster care: The role
of caregiver state of mind [Research Support, U.S.
Gov't, P.H.S.]. *Child Development, 72*(5),
1467–1477.

Dunn, J., & Plomin, R. (1991). Why are siblings so differ-
ent? The significance of differences in sibling experi-
ences within the family [Research Support, Non-U.S.
Gov't Research Support, U.S. Gov't, Non-P.H.S.
Research Support, U.S. Gov't, P.H.S. Review]. *Family
Process, 30*(3), 271–283.

Essex, M. J., Thomas Boyce, W., Hertzman, C., Lam, L.
L., Armstrong, J. M., Neumann, S. M., et al. (2011).
Epigenetic vestiges of early developmental adversity:
Childhood stress exposure and DNA methylation in
adolescence. *Child Development, 84*(1), 58–75.

Fearon, P., & Morgan, C. (2006). Environmental factors in
schizophrenia: The role of migrant studies.
Schizophrenia Bulletin, 32(3), 405–408.

Fergusson, D. M., Boden, J. M., Horwood, L. J., Miller,
A. L., & Kennedy, M. A. (2011). MAOA, abuse expo-
sure and antisocial behaviour: 30-year longitudinal
study [Research Support, N.I.H., Extramural Research
Support, Non-U.S. Gov't]. *The British Journal of
Psychiatry, 198*(6), 457–463.

Gervai, J. (2009). Environmental and genetic influences
on early attachment. *Child Adolescent Psychiatry
Mental Health, 3*(1), 25.

Guo, G., & Wang, J. (2002). The mixed or multilevel
model for behavior genetic analysis [Research
Support, Non-U.S. Gov't Research Support, U.S.
Gov't, Non-P.H.S. Twin Study]. *Behavior Genetics,
32*(1), 37–49.

Hamer, D. (2002). Genetics. Rethinking behavior genetics. *Science, 298*(5591), 71–72.

Hopwood, C. J., Donnellan, M. B., Blonigen, D. M.,
Krueger, R. F., McGue, M., Iacono, W. G., et al.
(2011). Genetic and environmental influences on personality trait stability and growth during the transition
to adulthood: A three-wave longitudinal study
[Research Support, N.I.H., Extramural Twin Study].
Journal of Personality and Social Psychology, 100(3),
545–556.

Huizink, A. C., van den Berg, M. P., van der Ende, J., &
Verhulst, F. C. (2007). Longitudinal genetic analysis
of internalizing and externalizing problem behavior in
adopted biologically related and unrelated sibling
pairs [Comparative Study Research Support, Non-
U.S. Gov't]. *Twin Research and Human Genetics,
10*(1), 55–65.

Insel, T. R., & Collins, F. S. (2003). Psychiatry in the
genomics era [Historical Article]. *The American
Journal of Psychiatry, 160*(4), 616–620.

Kappeler, L., & Meaney, M. J. (2010). Epigenetics and
parental effects [Research Support, N.I.H., Extramural
Research Support, Non-U.S. Gov't Review].
Bioessays, 32(9), 818–827.

Karg, K., Burmeister, M., Shedden, K., & Sen, S. (2011).
The serotonin transporter promoter variant
(5-HTTLPR), stress, and depression meta-analysis
revisited: Evidence of genetic moderation [Meta-
Analysis Research Support, N.I.H., Extramural
Research Support, Non-U.S. Gov't]. *Archives of
General Psychiatry, 68*(5), 444–454.

Kaufman, J., Yang, B. Z., Douglas-Palumberi, H., Grasso,
D., Lipschitz, D., Houshyar, S., et al. (2006). Brain-
derived neurotrophic factor-5-HTTLPR gene interac-
tions and environmental modifiers of depression in
children [Comparative Study Research Support,
N.I.H., Extramural Research Support, Non-U.S. Gov't
Research Support, U.S. Gov't, Non-P.H.S.]. *Biological
Psychiatry, 59*(8), 673–680.

Kendler, K. S., & Eaves, L. J. (1986). Models for the joint
effect of genotype and environment on liability to psychiatric illness [Research Support, Non-U.S. Gov't
Research Support, U.S. Gov't, P.H.S.]. *The American
Journal of Psychiatry, 143*(3), 279–289.

Kendler, K. S., & Gardner, C. O. (2010). Dependent
stressful life events and prior depressive episodes in
the prediction of major depression: The problem of
causal inference in psychiatric epidemiology
[Comparative Study Research Support, N.I.H.,
Extramural Research Support, Non-U.S. Gov't Twin
Study]. *Archives of General Psychiatry, 67*(11),
1120–1127.

Kendler, K. S., Neale, M. C., Kessler, R. C., Heath, A. C.,
& Eaves, L. J. (1992). Major depression and

generalized anxiety disorder. Same genes, (partly) different environments? [Research Support, U.S. Gov't, P.H.S.]. *Archives of General Psychiatry, 49*(9), 716–722.

Kendler, K. S., Neale, M., Kessler, R., Heath, A., & Eaves, L. (1993a). A twin study of recent life events and difficulties [Research Support, U.S. Gov't, P.H.S.]. *Archives of General Psychiatry, 50*(10), 789–796.

Kendler, K. S., Neale, M. C., Kessler, R. C., Heath, A. C., & Eaves, L. J. (1993b). A test of the equal-environment assumption in twin studies of psychiatric illness [Research Support, U.S. Gov't, P.H.S.]. *Behavior Genetics, 23*(1), 21–27.

Kim, H., Lim, S. W., Kim, S., Kim, J. W., Chang, Y. H., Carroll, B. J., et al. (2006). Monoamine transporter gene polymorphisms and antidepressant response in koreans with late-life depression [Research Support, Non-U.S. Gov't]. *JAMA, 296*(13), 1609–1618.

Kochanska, G. (1997). Multiple pathways to conscience for children with different temperaments: From toddlerhood to age 5. *Developmental Psychology, 33*(2), 228–240.

Kochanska, G., Philibert, R. A., & Barry, R. A. (2009). Interplay of genes and early mother-child relationship in the development of self-regulation from toddler to preschool age. *Journal of Child Psychology and Psychiatry, 50*(11), 1331–1338.

Kong, A., Frigge, M. L., Masson, G., Besenbacher, S., Sulem, P., Magnusson, G., et al. (2012). Rate of de novo mutations and the importance of father's age to disease risk [Research Support, N.I.H., Extramural Research Support, Non-U.S. Gov't]. *Nature, 488*(7412), 471–475.

Krueger, R. F. (1999). The structure of common mental disorders [Research Support, Non-U.S. Gov't Research Support, U.S. Gov't, P.H.S.]. *Archives of General Psychiatry, 56*(10), 921–926.

Lahey, B. B., Van Hulle, C. A., Singh, A. L., Waldman, I. D., & Rathouz, P. J. (2011). Higher-order genetic and environmental structure of prevalent forms of child and adolescent psychopathology [Research Support, N.I.H., Extramural Twin Study]. *Archives of General Psychiatry, 68*(2), 181–189.

Lester, K. J., Hudson, J. L., Tropeano, M., Creswell, C., Collier, D. A., Farmer, A., et al. (2012). Neurotrophic gene polymorphisms and response to psychological therapy [Research Support, Non-U.S. Gov't]. *Translational Psychiatry, 2*, e108.

Luijk, M. P., Roisman, G. I., Haltigan, J. D., Tiemeier, H., Booth-Laforce, C., van Ijzendoorn, M. H., et al. (2011). Dopaminergic, serotonergic, and oxytonergic candidate genes associated with infant attachment security and disorganization? In search of main and interaction effects [Research Support, N.I.H., Extramural Research Support, Non-U.S. Gov't]. *Journal of Child Psychology and Psychiatry, and Allied Disciplines, 52*(12), 1295–1307.

Lytton, H. (1978). Genetic analysis of twins' naturalistically observed behavior. *Progress in Clinical and Biological Research, 24A*, 43–48.

McGue, M., Sharma, A., & Benson, P. (1996). Parent and sibling influences on adolescent alcohol use and misuse: Evidence from a U.S. adoption cohort [Research Support, U.S. Gov't, P.H.S.]. *Journal of Studies on Alcohol, 57*(1), 8–18.

Meaney, M. J. (2010). Epigenetics and the biological definition of gene x environment interactions [Review]. *Child Development, 81*(1), 41–79.

Morey, R. A., Hariri, A. R., Gold, A. L., Hauser, M. A., Munger, H. J., Dolcos, F., et al. (2011). Serotonin transporter gene polymorphisms and brabin function during emotional distraction from cognitive processing in posttraumatic stress disorder [Research Support, N.I.H., Extramural Research Support, Non-U.S. Gov't Research Support, U.S. Gov't, Non-P.H.S.]. *BMC Psychiatry, 11*, 76.

Munafo, M. R., Durrant, C., Lewis, G., & Flint, J. (2009). Gene X environment interactions at the serotonin transporter locus [Meta-Analysis Research Support, Non-U.S. Gov't]. *Biological Psychiatry, 65*(3), 211–219.

Nebert, D. W., & Zhang, G. (2012). Personalized medicine: Temper expectations [Comment Letter]. *Science, 337*(6097), 910. author reply 910–911.

Nederhof, E., Belsky, J., Ormel, J., & Oldehinkel, A. J. (2012). Effects of divorce on Dutch boys' and girls' externalizing behavior in gene x environment perspective: Diathesis stress or differential susceptibility in the Dutch Tracking Adolescents' Individual Lives Survey study? [Research Support, Non-U.S. Gov't]. *Development and Psychopathology, 24*(3), 929–939.

Neiderhiser, J. M., Reiss, D., Hetherington, E. M., & Plomin, R. (1999). Relationships between parenting and adolescent adjustment over time: Genetic and environmental contributions [Research Support, Non-U.S. Gov't Research Support, U.S. Gov't, P.H.S. Twin Study]. *Developmental Psychology, 35*(3), 680–692.

O'Connor, T. G., Caspi, A., DeFries, J. C., & Plomin, R. (2000). Are associations between parental divorce and children's adjustment genetically mediated? An adoption study. *Developmental Psychology, 36*(4), 429–437.

O'Connor, T. G., & Croft, C. M. (2001). A twin study of attachment in preschool children. *Child Development, 72*(5), 1501–1511.

O'Connor, T. G., Deater-Deckard, K., Fulker, D., Rutter, M., & Plomin, R. (1998). Genotype-environment correlations in late childhood and early adolescence: Antisocial behavioral problems and coercive parenting. *Developmental Psychology, 34*(5), 970–981.

O'Connor, T. G., Hetherington, E. M., Reiss, D., & Plomin, R. (1995). A twin-sibling study of observed parent-adolescent interactions [Research Support, Non-U.S. Gov't Research Support, U.S. Gov't, P.H.S.]. *Child Development, 66*(3), 812–829.

O'Connor, T. G., McGuire, S., Reiss, D., Hetherington, E. M., & Plomin, R. (1998). Co-occurrence of depressive symptoms and antisocial behavior in adolescence: A common genetic liability. *Journal of Abnormal Psychology, 107*(1), 27–37.

O'Connor, T. G., Neiderhiser, J. M., Reiss, D., Hetherington, E. M., & Plomin, R. (1998). Genetic contributions to continuity, change, and co-occurrence of antisocial and depressive symptoms in adolescence. *Journal of Child Psychology and Psychiatry, 39*(3), 323–336.

O'Donnell, K., O'Connor, T. G., & Glover, V. (2009). Prenatal stress and neurodevelopment of the child: Focus on the HPA axis and role of the placenta. *Developmental Neuroscience, 31*(4), 285–292.

O'Roak, B. J., Vives, L., Girirajan, S., Karakoc, E., Krumm, N., Coe, B. P., et al. (2012). Sporadic autism exomes reveal a highly interconnected protein network of de novo mutations [Research Support, N.I.H., Extramural Research Support, Non-U.S. Gov't]. *Nature, 485*(7397), 246–250.

Oberlander, T. F., Weinberg, J., Papsdorf, M., Grunau, R., Misri, S., & Devlin, A. M. (2008). Prenatal exposure to maternal depression, neonatal methylation of human glucocorticoid receptor gene (NR3C1) and infant cortisol stress responses. *Epigenetics, 3*(2), 97–106.

Pauli-Pott, U., Friedel, S., Hinney, A., & Hebebrand, J. (2009). Serotonin transporter gene polymorphism (5-HTTLPR), environmental conditions, and developing negative emotionality and fear in early childhood [Research Support, Non-U.S. Gov't]. *Journal of Neural Transmission, 116*(4), 503–512.

Pettit, G. S., Bates, J. E., Dodge, K. A., & Meece, D. W. (1999). The impact of after-school peer contact on early adolescent externalizing problems is moderated by parental monitoring, perceived neighborhood safety, and prior adjustment [Research Support, U.S. Gov't, P.H.S.]. *Child Development, 70*(3), 768–778.

Plomin, R. (1983). Developmental behavioral genetics [Research Support, Non-U.S. Gov't Research Support, U.S. Gov't, Non-P.H.S. Research Support, U.S. Gov't, P.H.S.]. *Child Development, 54*(2), 253–259.

Plomin, R. (1995). Genetics and children's experiences in the family [Research Support, Non-U.S. Gov't Research Support, U.S. Gov't, Non-P.H.S. Research Support, U.S. Gov't, P.H.S. Review]. *Journal of Child Psychology and Psychiatry, and Allied Disciplines, 36*(1), 33–68.

Plomin, R. (2012). Child development and molecular genetics: 14 years later. *Child Development, 84*(1), 104–120.

Plomin, R., & Daniels, D. (2011). Why are children in the same family so different from one another? [Research Support, N.I.H., Extramural Research Support, Non-U.S. Gov't Review]. *International Journal of Epidemiology, 40*(3), 563–582.

Plomin, R., DeFries, J. C., & Loehlin, J. C. (1977). Genotype-environment interaction and correlation in the analysis of human behavior. *Psychological Bulletin, 84*(2), 309–322.

Porcelli, S., Fabbri, C., & Serretti, A. (2012). Meta-analysis of serotonin transporter gene promoter polymorphism (5-HTTLPR) association with antidepressant efficacy [Meta-Analysis Research Support, Non-U.S. Gov't Review]. *European Neuropsychopharmacology, 22*(4), 239–258.

Poulter, M. O., Du, L., Weaver, I. C., Palkovits, M., Faludi, G., Merali, Z., et al. (2008). GABAA receptor promoter hypermethylation in suicide brain: Implications for the involvement of epigenetic processes [Research Support, Non-U.S. Gov't]. *Biological Psychiatry, 64*(8), 645–652.

Propper, C., Moore, G. A., Mills-Koonce, W. R., Halpern, C. T., Hill-Soderlund, A. L., Calkins, S. D., et al. (2008). Gene-environment contributions to the development of infant vagal reactivity: The interaction of dopamine and maternal sensitivity [Research Support, U.S. Gov't, Non-P.H.S.]. *Child Development, 79*(5), 1377–1394.

Propper, C., Willoughby, M., Halpern, C. T., Carbone, M. A., & Cox, M. (2007). Parenting quality, DRD4, and the prediction of externalizing and internalizing behaviors in early childhood [Research Support, U.S. Gov't, Non-P.H.S.]. *Developmental Psychobiology, 49*(6), 619–632.

Rasbash, J., Jenkins, J., O'Connor, T. G., Tackett, J., & Reiss, D. (2011). A social relations model of observed family negativity and positivity using a genetically informative sample. *Journal of Personality and Social Psychology, 100*(3), 474–491.

Reichenberg, A., Gross, R., Weiser, M., Bresnahan, M., Silverman, J., Harlap, S., et al. (2006). Advancing paternal age and autism [Comparative Study]. *Archives of General Psychiatry, 63*(9), 1026–1032.

Reiss, D., Hetherington, E. M., Plomin, R., Howe, G. W., Simmens, S. J., Henderson, S. H., et al. (1995). Genetic questions for environmental studies. Differential parenting and psychopathology in adolescence. *Archives of General Psychiatry, 52*(11), 925–936.

Risch, N., Herrell, R., Lehner, T., Liang, K. Y., Eaves, L., Hoh, J., et al. (2009). Interaction between the serotonin transporter gene (5-HTTLPR), stressful life events, and risk of depression: A meta-analysis [Meta-Analysis Research Support, N.I.H., Extramural Research Support, N.I.H., Intramural]. *JAMA, 301*(23), 2462–2471.

Roisman, G. I., & Fraley, R. C. (2012). A behavior-genetic study of the legacy of early caregiving experiences: Academic skills, social competence, and externalizing behavior in kindergarten [Research Support, U.S. Gov't, Non-P.H.S. Twin Study]. *Child Development, 83*(2), 728–742.

Scarr, S., & McCartney, K. (1983). How people make their own environments: A theory of genotype greater than environment effects [Research Support, Non-U.S. Gov't Research Support, U.S. Gov't, P.H.S.]. *Child Development, 54*(2), 424–435.

Scott, S., & O'Connor, T. G. (2012). An experimental test of differential susceptibility to parenting among emotionally dysregulated children in a randomized controlled trial for oppositional behavior. *Journal of Child Psychology and Psychiatry, 53*(11), 1184–1193.

Scott, S., Sylva, K., Doolan, M., Price, J., Jacobs, B., Crook, C., et al. (2010). Randomised controlled trial of parent groups for child antisocial behaviour targeting multiple risk factors: The SPOKES project.

Journal of Child Psychology and Psychiatry, 51(1), 48–57.

Steptoe, A., Hamer, M., O'Donnell, K., Venuraju, S., Marmot, M. G., & Lahiri, A. (2010). Socioeconomic status and subclinical coronary disease in the Whitehall II epidemiological study. *PLoS One, 5*(1), e8874.

Stoolmiller, M. (1999). Implications of the restricted range of family environments for estimates of heritability and nonshared environment in behavior-genetic adoption studies [Research Support, U.S. Gov't, P.H.S. Review]. *Psychological Bulletin, 125*(4), 392–409.

Szyf, M., Weaver, I. C., Champagne, F. A., Diorio, J., & Meaney, M. J. (2005). Maternal programming of steroid receptor expression and phenotype through DNA methylation in the rat [Review]. *Frontiers in Neuroendocrinology, 26*(3–4), 139–162.

Tienari, P., Wynne, L. C., Sorri, A., Lahti, I., Laksy, K., Moring, J., et al. (2004). Genotype-environment interaction in schizophrenia-spectrum disorder. Long-term follow-up study of Finnish adoptees [Research Support, Non-U.S. Gov't Research Support, U.S. Gov't, P.H.S.]. *The British Journal of Psychiatry, 184*, 216–222.

Trzaskowski, M., Zavos, H. M., Haworth, C. M., Plomin, R., & Eley, T. C. (2012). Stable genetic influence on anxiety-related behaviours across middle childhood [Research Support, Non-U.S. Gov't Twin Study]. *Journal of Abnormal Child Psychology, 40*(1), 85–94.

Tucker-Drob, E. M., Rhemtulla, M., Harden, K. P., Turkheimer, E., & Fask, D. (2011). Emergence of a Gene x socioeconomic status interaction on infant mental ability between 10 months and 2 years [Research Support, N.I.H., Extramural Twin Study]. *Psychological Science, 22*(1), 125–133.

Uher, R., Caspi, A., Houts, R., Sugden, K., Williams, B., Poulton, R., et al. (2011). Serotonin transporter gene moderates childhood maltreatment's effects on persistent but not single-episode depression: Replications and implications for resolving inconsistent results. *Journal of Affective Disorders, 135*(1–3), 56–65.

van Ijzendoorn, M. H., Belsky, J., & Bakermans-Kranenburg, M. J. (2012). Serotonin transporter genotype 5HTTLPR as a marker of differential susceptibility? A meta-analysis of child and adolescent gene-by-environment studies. *Translational Psychiatry, 2*, e147.

Vollebergh, W. A., Iedema, J., Bijl, R. V., de Graaf, R., Smit, F., & Ormel, J. (2001). The structure and stability of common mental disorders: The NEMESIS study [Research Support, Non-U.S. Gov't]. *Archives of General Psychiatry, 58*(6), 597–603.

Vorria, P., Papaligoura, Z., Sarafidou, J., Kopakaki, M., Dunn, J., Van Ijzendoorn, M. H., et al. (2006). The development of adopted children after institutional care: A follow-up study. *Journal of Child Psychology and Psychiatry, 47*(12), 1246–1253.

Weaver, I. C., Cervoni, N., Champagne, F. A., D'Alessio, A. C., Sharma, S., Seckl, J. R., et al. (2004). Epigenetic programming by maternal behavior. *Nature Neuroscience, 7*(8), 847–854.

Weaver, I. C., Champagne, F. A., Brown, S. E., Dymov, S., Sharma, S., Meaney, M. J., et al. (2005). Reversal of maternal programming of stress responses in adult offspring through methyl supplementation: Altering epigenetic marking later in life [Research Support, Non-U.S. Gov't]. *The Journal of Neuroscience, 25*(47), 11045–11054.

Webster-Stratton, C., Hollinsworth, T., & Kolpacoff, M. (1989). The long-term effectiveness and clinical significance of three cost-effective training programs for families with conduct-problem children. *Journal of Consulting and Clinical Psychology, 57*(4), 550–553.

Wichers, M. C., Danckaerts, M., Van Gestel, S., Derom, C., Vlietink, R., & van Os, J. (2002). Chorion type and twin similarity for child psychiatric symptoms [Letter Twin Study]. *Archives of General Psychiatry, 59*(6), 562–564.

Wiik, K. L., Loman, M. M., Van Ryzin, M. J., Armstrong, J. M., Essex, M. J., Pollak, S. D., et al. (2011). Behavioral and emotional symptoms of post-institutionalized children in middle childhood. *Journal of Child Psychology and Psychiatry, 52*(1), 56–63.

Wong, M. Y., Day, N. E., Luan, J. A., Chan, K. P., & Wareham, N. J. (2003). The detection of gene-environment interaction for continuous traits: Should we deal with measurement error by bigger studies or better measurement? [Research Support, Non-U.S. Gov't]. *International Journal of Epidemiology, 32*(1), 51–57.

Wong, M. Y., Day, N. E., Luan, J. A., & Wareham, N. J. (2004). Estimation of magnitude in gene-environment interactions in the presence of measurement error [Research Support, Non-U.S. Gov't]. *Statistics in Medicine, 23*(6), 987–998.

Wynne, L. C., Tienari, P., Nieminen, P., Sorri, A., Lahti, I., Moring, J., et al. (2006). I. Genotype-environment interaction in the schizophrenia spectrum: Genetic liability and global family ratings in the Finnish Adoption Study [Research Support, N.I.H., Extramural Research Support, Non-U.S. Gov't]. *Family Process, 45*(4), 419–434.

Young-Wolff, K. C., Enoch, M. A., & Prescott, C. A. (2011). The influence of gene-environment interactions on alcohol consumption and alcohol use disorders: A comprehensive review [Research Support, N.I.H., Extramural Research Support, Non-U.S. Gov't Review]. *Clinical Psychology Review, 31*(5), 800–816.

Zhang, T. Y., & Meaney, M. J. (2010). Epigenetics and the environmental regulation of the genome and its function [Research Support, N.I.H., Extramural Research Support, Non-U.S. Gov't Review]. *Annual Review of Psychology, 61*, 439–466. C431–433.

Functional Magnetic Resonance Imaging in Developmental Psychopathology: The Brain as a Window into the Development and Treatment of Psychopathology

14

Johnna R. Swartz and Christopher S. Monk

Rather than resolving the classic debate of nature versus nurture, advances in developmental psychopathology have illuminated the complex interactions between nature and nurture across development. The transactional model of development highlights the interdependent nature of these interactions; the model proposes that development is the product of reciprocal interacting influences between the child and environment over time (Sameroff, 2010). The complexity of these interactions at the biopsychosocial level is delineated in Gottlieb's theory of probabilistic epigenesis (Gottlieb, 2007a, 2007b). Rejecting the traditional notion that genes lead to psychological or behavioral outcomes in a unidirectional fashion, Gottlieb argued that the environment also alters gene expression and that gene–environment interactions are fundamental to understanding development.

Within this framework, the field that encompasses the neuroscience of developmental psychopathology must consider the bidirectional influences between genes, brain, behavior, and environment. Genes code for the synthesis of proteins that then influence brain development, organization, structure, and function. However, the environment also influences neural development and alters the influence of genes through epigenetics (Meaney, 2010), a set of biological mech-

anisms that permit the environment to modify gene expression. Importantly, the brain is at the intersection of many of these genetic and environmental influences on mental health outcomes and, as a mediator of these reciprocal interacting influences, provides a unique window into the development and treatment of psychopathology (Cicchetti & Dawson, 2002; Hariri & Weinberger, 2003; Hyde, Bogdan, & Hariri, 2011; Monk, 2008).

Throughout this chapter, we emphasize that the inclusion of the brain as a level of analysis in conjunction with genetic, epigenetic, and environmental measures can provide important insights into the development of psychopathology and contribute to the development and testing of novel treatments. In order to illustrate the importance of considering brain function in developmental psychopathology research, we focus our review on two types of psychopathology: anxiety disorders and autism spectrum disorder (ASD). These disorders share common abnormalities in emotion processing and are both associated with alterations in neural circuitry related to emotion processing and regulation (Monk, 2008). Anxiety disorders encompass a range of conditions characterized by excessive fears or anxiety such as social anxiety disorder, which involves excessive anxiety in social situations. ASD is characterized by social interaction deficits, language and communication impairment, and stereotyped or repetitive behaviors. As we will discuss, some evidence suggests it may also be associated with heightened anxiety in response to social stimuli. We begin with a brief

J.R. Swartz, M.S. (✉) • C.S. Monk, Ph.D.
Department of Psychology, University of Michigan,
Ann Arbor, MI 48109, USA
e-mail: jrswartz@umich.edu; csmonk@umich.edu

M. Lewis and K.D. Rudolph (eds.), *Handbook of Developmental Psychopathology*,
DOI 10.1007/978-1-4614-9608-3_14, © Springer Science+Business Media New York 2014

review of the current state of knowledge regarding abnormalities in brain function in anxiety disorders and ASD. We then discuss how this knowledge of brain abnormalities can be combined with genetic, epigenetic, and treatment research to increase progress in our understanding of the development and treatment of these disorders.

The Role of the Amygdala and Ventral Prefrontal Cortex in Anxiety Disorders and ASD

Anxiety disorders and ASD are associated with abnormal activity in multiple neural regions, including the amygdala and ventral prefrontal cortex. These two regions are implicated in face processing, social cognition, and emotion processing (Adolphs, 2010). The amygdala is a bilateral structure located deep inside the brain, and the ventral prefrontal cortex encompasses the lower portion of the prefrontal cortex (above it is the dorsal prefrontal cortex). The amygdala is involved in the experience of anxiety and fear and may be more broadly involved in detecting any positively or negatively valenced social stimuli in the environment. The ventral prefrontal cortex is associated with a range of functions related to receiving and interpreting signals from other brain regions about conditions in the external environment and internal psychological states. In addition, the ventral prefrontal cortex can modify or inhibit responses in other regions in order to allow an individual to flexibly respond to current contextual or task demands.

The amygdala and ventral prefrontal cortex communicate with one another through reciprocal connections that allow for neural signaling between the regions. Signals from the amygdala to the ventral prefrontal cortex can communicate information regarding the emotional significance of stimuli, whereas signals from the ventral prefrontal cortex to the amygdala can modify amygdala activation (Ghashghaei, Hilgetag, & Barbas, 2007; Sarter & Markowitsch, 1984; Ray & Zald, 2012). Research from animal models and human

neuroimaging data suggests that the ventral prefrontal cortex plays an important role in emotion regulation by regulating amygdala activity via signals to the amygdala that inhibit activation. The dorsolateral prefrontal cortex may also be involved in emotion regulation, but because it has fewer direct connections to the amygdala, its role in emotion regulation is likely mediated through the ventral prefrontal cortex (Ray & Zald, 2012). The ventral prefrontal cortex can be further divided into subregions including the orbitofrontal cortex, the ventromedial prefrontal cortex, the ventral anterior cingulate cortex, and the ventrolateral prefrontal cortex. These regions can be associated with different cognitive functions depending on the tasks that participants perform while undergoing scanning, but frameworks have suggested that medial regions (the ventromedial prefrontal cortex, the subgenual anterior cingulate cortex, and the medial orbitofrontal cortex) may be involved in more automatic processes (e.g., generating expectations of reward or punishment, fear extinction) whereas lateral regions (the ventrolateral prefrontal cortex and lateral orbitofrontal cortex) may be more involved in voluntary processes (e.g., inhibiting prepotent responses, voluntarily controlling attention) (Phillips, Ladouceur, & Drevets, 2008; Ray & Zald, 2012). Because both automatic and voluntary emotion regulation processes involve regulation of the amygdala by the ventral prefrontal cortex, abnormalities in this circuitry likely play an important role in psychopathology characterized by disturbances in emotion regulation such as anxiety disorders and ASD. It has been proposed that there exists a further subdivision within the ventromedial prefrontal cortex: the posterior region of the ventromedial prefrontal cortex is posited to be involved in amplifying negative affect and amygdala response, whereas more anterior regions are involved in inhibiting amygdala response and reducing anxiety (Myers-Schulz & Koenigs, 2012). Thus, psychopathology characterized by disturbances in emotion regulation may reflect a combination of under-regulation of negative affect and amplification of negative affect by different prefrontal regions.

Examining Neural Activation and Functional Connectivity with fMRI

Functional magnetic resonance imaging (fMRI) is a tool to probe brain function in vivo and can be used to relate neural function to specific cognitive and emotional tasks performed during scanning. FMRI relies on measuring changes in oxygenated blood flow as an indirect measure of neural activity in the brain. In addition to the advantage of providing indirect measurement of neural activity, fMRI has good spatial resolution and the ability to examine activation in subcortical regions that cannot be localized through other methods such as electroencephalography (EEG).

One analytic approach of fMRI is functional connectivity, which is used to examine the correlation in activation across regions. If two regions show correlated increases and decreases in activity across a task, it is said that they demonstrate functional connectivity. Such findings would be consistent with the concept that the regions are interacting during the performance of the task. As highlighted in the conceptual framework above, understanding how neural regions communicate with one another will likely be crucial to fully understanding abnormal neural function in psychopathology. However, it is important to note that functional connectivity is limited in that it does not directly assess neural signaling and cannot be used to determine whether signals between regions are excitatory or inhibitory. Additionally, as with all correlational research, direction of causation (i.e., whether one region is modifying activity in the other or vice versa) cannot be determined. Despite these limitations, functional connectivity analyses can provide important information regarding differences in the strength of connectivity between regions such as the ventral prefrontal cortex and amygdala in patient and typically developing populations. This knowledge can be used in the context of research with animal models that can more invasively examine structural and functional connectivity, and in the context of the tasks performed in fMRI experiments, in order to draw inferences regarding the functional consequences of differences in connectivity strength between patients and controls. In the following sections we briefly discuss fMRI research that has characterized prefrontal cortex-amygdala circuitry in anxiety disorders and ASD. For more extended reviews, see Monk (2008), Pine (2007), and Philip et al. (2012).

Theoretical Considerations for Developmental Neuroimaging Research

Three general theoretical principles have been put forth for examining development with fMRI (Johnson, Halit, Grice, & Karmiloff-Smith, 2002). First, rather than the notion that development may reflect the maturation of one area specialized for one cognitive process, current research suggests that development also reflects the reorganization and integration of activity across distributed networks of regions. Thus, it is necessary for researchers to examine how the connectivity across different regions changes over development.

Second, the regions associated with a cognitive task in adults may not correspond to the regions recruited by children or adolescents during the same task, either because the participants use different strategies or because the functional organization of neural networks differs from that of adults. Therefore, rather than extrapolating findings from fMRI studies in clinical adult samples, it is necessary to conduct research with pediatric samples if we are interested in answering questions about how psychopathology develops.

Third, in line with Gottlieb's probabilistic epigenesis, theoretical views of the role of neural development in psychopathology must move beyond a unidirectional influence from brain to psychopathology and consider that the environment and behavior (such as symptoms or abnormal cognitive patterns) can also influence the neural activity observed when scanning clinical populations.

Prefrontal-Amygdala Function in Anxiety Disorders

One of the most consistent findings in clinical neuroimaging is that anxiety disorders are associated with heightened amygdala activation to threatening stimuli, such as fearful or angry faces, both in children and adolescents (Guyer et al., 2008; McClure, Monk, et al., 2007; Monk et al., 2008; Thomas et al., 2001) and in adults (Etkin & Wager, 2007). Moreover, there is increasing evidence for altered ventral prefrontal cortex activation and connectivity with the amygdala in youth with anxiety disorders (Guyer et al., 2008; McClure, Monk, et al., 2007; Monk et al., 2006, 2008) and adults with anxiety disorders (e.g., Etkin, Prater, Hoeft, Menon, & Schatzberg, 2010), consistent with the hypothesis that ventral prefrontal regulation of the amygdala may be weaker and amplification of negative affect may be stronger in anxiety disorder patients. Because the amygdala is associated with arousal and the experience of fear, reduced regulation from the prefrontal cortex to the amygdala may relate to the cognitive and emotional biases posited to contribute to the development and maintenance of anxiety disorders, including increased fear conditioning and difficulty extinguishing conditioning, heightened attention to threat, and interpretation of ambiguous stimuli as threatening (Britton, Lissek, Grillon, Norcross, & Pine, 2011; Daleiden & Vasey, 1997).

Developmental frameworks suggest that the transition to adolescence and the adolescent period may involve heightened risk for the development of affective disorders because the balance between amygdala and prefrontal cortex activity is still in flux (Casey, Jones, & Hare, 2008; Steinberg et al., 2006). Specifically, research examining the function and the structure of the prefrontal cortex (including both the volume of gray matter and the volume of white matter, representing long-range connections with other regions) has indicated that this region and its connections may develop along a relatively protracted time course across the period of childhood through adolescence and into adulthood (Giedd & Rapoport, 2010; Gogtay et al., 2004; Hare et al., 2008; Monk et al., 2003; Rubia et al., 2000; Yurgelon-Todd & Killgore, 2006). During this time, the amygdala may be relatively under-regulated, creating a risk for disturbances in emotion processing. An important point for

developmental psychopathologists is that this may also be a sensitive period for environmental influences on the development of this circuitry and potentially a window for intervention. Understanding genetic and epigenetic influences on this neural circuitry across the child and adolescent developmental periods as well as how treatments during these periods alter this circuitry may have the potential to improve preventions and treatments for these disorders, with potentially long-lasting results.

Prefrontal-Amygdala Function in Autism Spectrum Disorders

Although many have suggested that the socioemotional impairments of ASD are related to abnormal amygdala function (Dawson et al., 2005; Schultz, 2005), the results of fMRI studies have been inconsistent regarding the nature of this dysfunction. Many studies have found decreased amygdala activation in individuals with ASD relative to controls (e.g., Ashwin, Baron-Cohen, Wheelwright, O'Riordan, & Bullmore, 2007; Baron-Cohen et al., 1999), whereas others have found evidence for amygdala hyperactivation in ASD (Dalton et al., 2005; Kliemann, Dziobek, Hatri, Baudewig, & Heekeren, 2012; Kleinhans et al., 2009; Monk et al., 2010; Weng et al., 2011).

Whether individuals with ASD exhibit amygdala hypo-activation or hyperactivation to social stimuli relative to controls may depend on the type of task used during fMRI scanning. Studies that found amygdala hypo-activation in ASD generally used relatively long presentation times of face stimuli. In contrast, those utilizing brief presentation times and behavioral tasks to verify that subjects were attending to the stimuli produced evidence for amygdala hyperactivation in ASD (Monk et al., 2010; Weng et al., 2011). Because individuals with ASD attend away from faces (Klin, Jones, Schultz, Volkmar, & Cohen, 2002), studies with long presentation times afford participants the opportunity to attend away from faces in the scanner, resulting in amygdala hypo-activation due to reduced attention toward the stimuli. In contrast, studies with brief stimulus presentation times minimize differences in attention between participants with ASD and controls, producing evidence of amygdala hyperactivation to faces. In line with this, an fMRI investigation that incorporated eye tracking found a correlation between the amount of time spent fixating on eyes and amygdala activation in individuals with ASD (Dalton et al., 2005). Similarly, in a study that manipulated participants' initial fixations on either the eye or mouth region, participants with ASD showed heightened amygdala response when fixating the eyes relative to controls (Kliemann et al., 2012). Based on these results, we suggest that individuals with ASD avoid social stimuli because these stimuli induce over-arousal, indexed by amygdala hyperactivation (Dalton et al., 2005; Joseph, Ehrman, McNally, & Keehn, 2008; Kliemann et al., 2012; Kliemann, Dziobek, Hatri, Steimke, & Heekeren, 2010; Monk et al., 2010; Neumman, Spezio, Piven, & Adolphs, 2006; Weng et al., 2011). Reduced attention to social stimuli over the course of development could prevent infants and young children with ASD from acquiring the same level of social experiences as typically developing children, which could lead to a cascade of abnormal development of regions associated with social processing.

Some research has also detected abnormal ventral prefrontal cortex activity or ventral prefrontal cortex-amygdala connectivity in individuals with ASD (Dalton, et al., 2005; Monk et al., 2010; Swartz, Wiggins, Carrasco, Lord, & Monk, 2013). For example, Swartz et al. (2013) found evidence for reduced ventromedial prefrontal connectivity with the amygdala while youth with ASD viewed sad faces, as well as heightened amygdala response in the ASD group. Therefore, initial evidence suggests that amygdala hyperactivation in ASD may be the result of or compounded by altered prefrontal connectivity.

ASD emerges much earlier than anxiety disorders, typically before age 3, sparking increased interest in examining neural development across infancy and early childhood as well

as at later ages (Giedd & Rapoport, 2010; Courchesne et al., 2007). However, because very young children cannot typically perform task-based fMRI studies, much of this research has examined changes in brain structure. Overall, there is evidence for an altered trajectory of brain development characterized by increased brain volume, including the amygdala and prefrontal cortex, in infancy and early childhood compared to typically developing controls and then decreases in volume later in development, often resulting in smaller volumes of brain structures such as the amygdala in adolescents and adults with ASD compared to controls (Courchesne et al., 2007; Schumann et al., 2004). A key theme emerging from this research is that ASD is associated with differences in the timing and trajectory of brain development. For example, Carmody and Lewis (2010) found that young children with ASD showed overdevelopment of white matter in the medial prefrontal cortex and underdevelopment of white matter in the left temporoparietal junction, a region associated with the development of self-representation in typically developing children (Lewis & Carmody, 2008). Moreover, degree of deviation from typical levels of development associated with ASD symptoms. In older children and adolescents, fMRI research has suggested that amygdala activation to emotional faces may decrease with age (Weng et al., 2011). Further research will be necessary to examine how prefrontal cortex-amygdala connectivity changes with age and whether this developmental pattern relates to changes in ASD symptoms across childhood and adolescence.

Having outlined the current state of research on brain function in anxiety disorders and ASD, we now consider how neuroimaging may be used to further our understanding of the development and treatment of psychopathology. We focus on three specific examples: imaging genetics, imaging epigenetics, and treatment studies. These examples are not meant to be exhaustive, but rather to illustrate various areas in which neuroimaging research can help achieve advances in this field.

The Brain as a Mediator of Genetic and Epigenetic Influence on the Development of Anxiety Disorders and ASD

Genes and Gene × Environment Interactions in Anxiety Disorders

Investigators have examined the relation between a number of different gene variants and anxiety disorders, but some of the most studied genes are those regulating serotonin (5-hydroxytryptamine; 5-HT) levels in the brain. Serotonin-related genes have been considered important candidates when investigating anxiety disorders for several reasons. First, serotonin is a neurotransmitter involved in signaling and modulating the signals between different neural regions, including the ventral prefrontal cortex and amygdala (Nordquist & Oreland, 2010; Pinto & Sesack, 2003) which, as we have discussed above, have been shown to function abnormally in anxiety disorders. Second, a first-line pharmacological treatment for anxiety disorders is a class of medications called selective serotonin reuptake inhibitors (SSRIs), which affect serotonin levels in the brain. Thus, serotonin may play a key role in the development of anxiety disorders.

Serotonin levels within the brain are influenced by genetic variation. Serotonin is released into the synapse to signal other neurons and afterwards must be cleared from the synapse by serotonin transporters, which reuptake serotonin back into the presynaptic neuron. The rate at which serotonin is cleared from the synapse can influence the strength and duration of serotonin signaling (Daws & Gould, 2011). The amount of serotonin transporters available for this process is regulated by the serotonin transporter gene. Genetic variation in the promoter region for this gene, referred to as the serotonin transporter-linked polymorphic region (5-HTTLPR), results in two common functional variants. The variant with the short allele leads to less efficient transcription and therefore reduced availability of the serotonin transporter, whereas the long allele is associated with increased transcriptional

efficiency. There are also two variants of the long allele, one of which appears to behave similarly to the short allele (Hu et al., 2006). Therefore, we will use the terms *low-expressing* allele to refer to the variants that result in decreased serotonin transporter expression and *high-expressing* allele to refer to the variant associated with increased serotonin transporter expression. Although we focus on the 5-HTTLPR in our review, other genes implicated in serotonin signaling, such as genes regulating serotonin receptor levels, have also been implicated in the development of anxiety disorders.

Some research has linked the low-expressing alleles of the 5-HTTLPR to increased risk for being high on anxiety-related personality traits such as neuroticism (Lesch et al., 1996), although this link is not always consistent (Munafo et al., 2009). A meta-analysis also revealed a moderate effect size for the low-expressing allele on attention bias for threat, which is a cognitive pattern frequently associated with anxiety disorders (Pergamin-Hight, Bakermans-Kranenburg, van Ijzendoorn, & Bar-Haim, 2012).

There has also been support for the involvement of the 5-HTTLPR in gene × environment interactions on the development of anxiety disorders or anxiety-related traits including the interaction between 5-HTTLPR and low social support on the development of PTSD after a hurricane (Kilpatrick et al., 2007), low family social support on behavioral inhibition in middle childhood (a temperamental pattern associated with anxiety disorders) (Fox et al., 2005), and child maltreatment on anxiety sensitivity (Stein, Schork, & Gelernter, 2008). In all of these cases, the risk allele of the genotype (the low-expressing allele) is only associated with the development of psychopathology or personality traits associated with risk for psychopathology under conditions of environmental risk. In contrast, proponents of a differential susceptibility theory have suggested that the low-expressing allele of the 5-HTTLPR and other "risk-related" gene variants are better conceptualized as conveying increased susceptibility to environmental context, so that susceptible children raised in risky environments are at heightened risk for developing psychopathology but susceptible children raised in positively enriched environments benefit more from these environments than less susceptible children (Ellis, Boyce, Belsky, Bakermans-Kranenburg, & van Ijzendoorn, 2011). Understanding the neural mediators of gene × environment interactions will help to clarify the mechanisms through which genes such as the 5-HTTLPR confer increased risk or susceptibility to environmental context.

It should be noted that, as in main effect analyses of genetic risk factors, gene–environment interaction studies have produced mixed results as well. For example, one study found that the high-expressing allele of the 5-HTTLPR interacted with environmental risk factors to predict depression and anxiety in 19-year-olds (Laucht et al., 2009). Because many of these contrary gene–environment interaction results have been found in adolescent or young adult samples, it has been argued that gene–environment interactions may vary at different stages of development (although methodological issues such as the relevance of stressful life event questionnaires for young participants may also underlie variation in findings; Uher & McGuffin, 2010).

Genes and Gene × Environment Interactions in ASD

Although studies examining the heritability of ASD suggest a strong genetic component, the search for genes associated with ASD has yielded inconsistent results. As with anxiety disorders, serotonin-related genes are important potential candidates because a relatively consistent finding has been that ASD is associated with increased blood platelet serotonin levels, or hyperserotonemia (Veenstra-VanderWeele & Blakely, 2012). Some evidence suggests that increased serotonin blood platelet levels may be associated with faster rates of serotonin reuptake and reduced availability of serotonin in the synapse (Daws & Gould, 2011). However, despite the similarities in altered neural function across anxiety disorders and ASD and the consistent finding of altered serotonin levels in ASD, the relation

between 5-HTTLPR variation and risk for ASD is less clear than for anxiety disorders. A meta-analysis of association studies found no main effect of the low-expressing allele of the 5-HTTLPR on autism status, although there was a relation in studies with mixed ethnicity American populations (versus European or Asian) (Huang & Santengelo, 2008).

One complication that arises in genetic research is that ASD encompasses a heterogeneous set of disorders that vary greatly in terms of severity and type of symptoms (e.g., from little language impairment to severely language impaired) across individuals. Given this level of heterogeneity, it is perhaps not surprising that genetic association studies have been inconsistent. Several investigators have suggested that the low-expressing allele may not in fact be associated with greater risk for ASD, but that variation in the 5-HTTLPR may be associated with specific ASD symptoms (Mundy, Henderson, Inge, & Coman, 2007). For example, the low-expressing allele is associated with greater impairment in the social/communication domain, including nonverbal communication, whereas the high-expressing allele is associated with greater severity of restricted and repetitive behaviors in children with ASD (Brune et al., 2006; Tordjman et al., 2001). The results of these studies suggest that variation in the 5-HTTLPR may influence the severity or type of symptoms in ASD, indicating the need to examine potential neural correlates that may mediate this relation.

Environmental interactions with the 5-HTTLPR may also play a role in the emergence of ASD symptoms. For example, maternal smoking during pregnancy and low birth weight interacted with the 5-HTTLPR to predict ASD symptoms in children with attention-deficit/hyperactivity disorder (Nijmeijer et al., 2010). In this case, the low-expressing allele led to more ASD symptoms with exposure to environmental risk factors.

Although these studies suggest a relation between genetic variation in the 5-HTTLPR, environmental risk factors, and anxiety disorders or ASD, they are subject to some limitations. First, as illustrated through the inconsistent findings in gene association studies, it can be difficult to find direct links between specific genes and mental disorders (Caspi & Moffitt, 2006; Geschwind, 2011). Second, these studies cannot address the underlying neural processes whereby genes and gene × environment interactions influence the development of psychopathology. FMRI has been useful in addressing both of these limitations of previous research by providing more consistent correlations between 5-HTTLPR variation and neural function and providing a potential neural mechanism linking this gene to anxiety disorder and ASD symptoms.

Imaging Genetics, Imaging Gene × Environment Interactions, and Imaging Epigenetics

Some of the difficulty involved in finding direct associations between genes and mental disorders may be due in part to the complexity that arises from probabilistic epigenesis (Gottlieb, 2007a, 2007b), as it is likely that there is not a one-to-one correspondence between genotype and phenotype due to gene-gene and gene–environment interactions over the course of development. fMRI can help to clarify the role of genes in the development of psychopathology. Because genes are distal from the behavioral phenotypes and symptoms observed for a clinical diagnosis, using fMRI to consider brain function as a more proximal mediating step between genes and psychiatric outcomes may improve our ability to pinpoint important genes involved in the development of psychopathology (Hariri & Weinberger, 2003). This approach of using neural activity as a more proximal phenotype to examine genes' contributions to psychopathology is termed imaging genetics (Hariri & Weinberger, 2003).

Investigators have also proposed methods for examining the neural underpinnings of gene × environment interactions using fMRI. One approach is to examine a mediation model in which neural function mediates the interaction of genes and environment on the development of

psychopathology, which has been called imaging gene–environment interactions (Hyde et al., 2011). This approach can be thought of as an extension of imaging genetic research that incorporates both genetic and environmental predictors to examine whether their interaction relates to neural function, which in turn mediates behavioral symptoms or disorders.

Another approach involves incorporating epigenetics into fMRI designs. Consistent with the predictions of probabilistic epigenesis, it has been shown that the environment can alter the way that genes are expressed through processes that fall under the category of epigenetics (Meaney, 2010). Epigenetic regulation encompasses modifications to the structure of DNA without changes to the DNA sequence. Modifications to the structure of the DNA can alter its accessibility to transcription factors, either preventing or increasing the transcription of genes into proteins, which could in turn lead to changes in the structure or function of the brain. This occurs through many different mechanisms. One of the most commonly studied is DNA methylation of promoter regions, which occurs when methyl groups attach to cytosines at cytosine-phosphate-guanosine (CpG) sites on the DNA. This epigenetic modification makes the promoter region less accessible to transcription factors, decreasing the expression of the gene (for more extended reviews on this topic see Bagot & Meaney, 2010; Meaney, 2010; van Ijzendoorn, Bakermans-Kranenburg, & Ebstein, 2011). Importantly, DNA methylation can be altered by environmental influences such as quality of parenting during development (McGowan et al., 2009; Meaney, 2010; Weaver et al., 2004). Thus, methylation represents a potentially important pathway for the influence of the environment on gene expression, neural function, and the development of psychopathology. FMRI can be used to examine the functional consequences of these epigenetic influences in an extension of imaging genetic research termed imaging epigenetics (Wiers, 2012), in which methylation levels of genes of interest are related to neural function.

Imaging Genetics in Anxiety Disorders

The first imaging genetic studies examining the 5-HTTLPR were performed in adults and demonstrated that the low-expressing allele is associated with increased amygdala activation (Hariri et al., 2002; Munafo, Brown, & Hariri, 2008) during processing of emotional stimuli. Additional research suggested that the low-expressing allele predicted decreased connectivity between prefrontal regulatory regions and the amygdala (Pezawas et al., 2005), suggesting that the low-expressing allele may lead to decreased prefrontal regulation, which in turn results in heightened amygdala response. Further research in adults replicated these findings (Surguladze et al., 2012; but see Heinz et al. (2005) and O'Nions, Dolan, and Roiser (2011) for inconsistent results).

In typically developing children and adolescents, the low-expressing allele of the 5-HTTLPR is also related to increased amygdala activation (Battaglia et al., 2012; Furman, Hamilton, Joormann, & Gotlib, 2011; Lau et al., 2009) and increased activation in frontal and parietal regions associated with attention to threat (Thomason et al., 2010). These imaging genetic studies demonstrate the utility of fMRI in producing more consistent links between genes and neural function than can be found between genes and behavioral phenotypes. In addition, they suggest a potential mechanism through which genetic variation may lead to risk for psychopathology: low-expressing alleles of the 5-HTTLPR are associated with reduced coupling between the prefrontal cortex and amygdala; this reduced connectivity may interrupt important feedback and regulatory processes that maintain adaptive levels of amygdala activation. Importantly, this is the same pattern of activation that has already been observed in anxiety disorder patients, as described earlier.

An apparent paradox in the serotonin transporter literature has been noted (Sibille & Lewis, 2006). The low-expressing allele of the 5-HTTLPR may confer risk for anxiety disorders, but an effective treatment for adults is the administration of selective serotonin reuptake inhibitors (SSRIs), which function similarly to the low-expressing allele of the 5-HTTLPR by reducing serotonin transporter availability. Results from animal models suggest that developmental processes may underlie these seemingly contradictory results. In mice, SSRIs administered during early childhood (which reduce serotonin transporter availability, similar to being a carrier of the low-expressing alleles of the 5-HTTLPR) lead to increased anxiety-related behaviors when these mice reach adulthood (Ansorge, Zhou, Lira, Hen, & Gingrich, 2004), whereas administering SSRIs chronically to adult mice has an anxiolytic effect (Troelsen, Nielsen, & Mirza, 2005). One potential explanation for this discrepancy is that serotonin is involved in guiding neural development in addition to its role as a neurotransmitter (Nordquist & Oreland, 2010). Therefore, reduced reuptake of serotonin early in development may affect neurodevelopmental processes and produce different results on brain function than reduced reuptake of serotonin later in development, once neurodevelopmental processes are complete (Daws & Gould, 2011; Sibille & Lewis, 2006).

Furthermore, several fMRI studies have suggested that 5-HTTLPR variation may relate to neural function differently depending on developmental stage. For example, fMRI research with typically developing children and adolescents has demonstrated an age x genotype interaction in which 5-HTTLPR genotype influences the cross-sectional association between age and amygdala activation, as well as functional connectivity (Wiggins et al., 2012, in press). Although these results are cross-sectional, they suggest that the 5-HTTLPR may alter the trajectory of changes in connectivity across childhood and adolescence, such that the relation between 5-HTTLPR and brain function will depend on the developmental stage assessed. Indeed, Lau et al. (2009) found that, contrary to the adult literature, children and adolescents with anxiety disorders with the *high-expressing* allele of the 5-HTTLPR had increased amygdala activation compared to carriers of the low-expressing allele. This illustrates one of the principles of developmental neuroscience that findings from adults cannot necessarily be extrapolated to pediatric populations, as there may be important differences in the gene-brain interplay across development. Consideration of developmental timing will be critical moving forward in imaging genetic research.

Despite the promise of imaging genetic studies, there are also limitations that should be acknowledged. For example, although neural function is more proximal to genetic influence than behavioral phenotypes, there still exists a complex path from gene expression to protein synthesis to neural function, which may lead to weaker relations between genes and neural function than originally anticipated. Additionally, the psychological context or task chosen for investigation may have a large impact on neural function, such that there will be no straightforward relation between genetic variation and neural function across every condition, requiring more nuanced approaches to task design and careful consideration of psychological context.

Imaging Gene–Environment Interactions and Epigenetics in Anxiety Disorders

Although not testing a mediation model, several studies have approximated an imaging gene–environment interaction approach by demonstrating that 5-HTTLPR genotype interacts with life stress on amygdala responsiveness or amygdala activation at rest (Canli et al., 2006; Lemogne et al., 2011; Williams et al., 2009). This could provide support for Hyde et al.'s (2011) synergistic model suggesting that the low-expressing allele of the 5-HTTLPR may interact with environmental stress in a cumulative manner to lead to increased amygdala activity, which mediates heightened vulnerability for anxiety disorders. An additional potential mechanism that may underlie or interact with the mediation pathway proposed is that environmental stress may lead to epigenetic changes that alter gene expression and neural function.

Preliminary evidence suggests that DNA methylation of CpG sites in the promoter region of the 5-HTT gene may play a role in the previously observed gene × environment interactions in anxiety disorders. A series of publications from the Iowa Adoption Studies have examined the association between 5-HTTLPR genotype, history of child abuse, methylation of the serotonin transporter gene, and risk for developing depression. They found that a history of child abuse is associated with increased methylation in the promoter region of the 5-HTT gene (Beach, Brody, Todorov, Gunter, & Philibert, 2010). In another paper, investigators found that the influence of methylation of a CpG island in the 5-HTT gene on serotonin transporter expression (as measured through serotonin transporter mRNA levels) was only significant when 5-HTTLPR genotype was controlled (Philibert et al., 2007). Follow-up analyses revealed a trend for greater methylation associated with the low-expressing allele compared to the high-expressing allele, suggesting that methylation status may interact with 5-HTTLPR variation, although it should be noted this was marginally significant and not replicated with a larger sample (Philibert et al., 2008). Finally, greater methylation of the serotonin transporter promoter is marginally associated with a lifetime history of depression (Philibert et al., 2008).

Similar results have been reported in research on nonhuman primates. For example, Kinnally et al. (2010) found that the low-expressing allele of the 5-HTTLPR was associated with increased methylation of CpG sites on the 5-HTT gene in macaques, which in turn was associated with decreased levels of serotonin transporter mRNA, suggesting that higher methylation leads to reduced serotonin transporter expression. Additionally, increased methylation interacted with early life stress (separation from mother or unpredictable food availability) to predict higher scores on a behavioral measure of stress reactivity (Kinnally et al., 2010, 2011). This initial work suggests a potential pathway for epigenetic influences on the development of psychopathology: early environmental stress (e.g., child abuse) leads to increased methylation of the serotonin transporter promoter region, but this is stronger for individuals with a low-expressing allele of the 5-HTTLPR (Beach et al., 2010; Kinnally et al., 2010; Philibert et al., 2007). Increased methylation of the 5-HTT gene leads to reduced transcription of the serotonin transporter (Kinnally et al., 2010), and is associated with increased risk for affective disorders such as major depression (Philibert et al., 2008) or heightened stress reactivity in nonhuman primates (Kinnally et al., 2011). This could be one potential mechanism for a gene × environment interaction in which individuals with the low-expressing allele who are exposed to stressful life events are at increased risk for developing psychopathology.

In contrast to the results reported above, others have found that methylation is protective and associated with decreased likelihood of developing PTSD after trauma (Koenen et al., 2011) or experiencing unresolved loss of an attachment figure (in low-expressing 5-HTTLPR allele carriers; van IJzendoorn, Caspers, Bakermans-Kranenburg, Beach, & Philibert, 2010). Indeed, Koenen et al. (2011) reported an interaction in which high methylation levels predicted higher rates of PTSD when individuals were exposed to a low number of traumatic events whereas when individuals were exposed to a high number of traumatic events, high methylation levels decreased the likelihood of developing PTSD. There are many differences in methodology across these studies that could underlie the differences in results including the methods used to assess DNA methylation levels and the CpG sites on the DNA where significant methylation differences were observed. Nevertheless, the finding that increased methylation levels may be protective in some cases raises this intriguing possibility proposed by Meaney (2010): methylation has an adaptive function of preparing the organism for whatever environment the organism is raised in. However, caution must be taken in interpreting results with cross-sectional designs such as those discussed above. Although we can assume that DNA sequences assessed in adulthood have not changed from early development, the same may not necessarily be true for epigenetic modifications, given that they are subject to environ-

mental influence (Houston et al., 2012). Thus, prospective longitudinal designs assessing DNA methylation levels early in development will be necessary in order to examine methylation levels preceding the development of psychopathology in adulthood.

Although the research reviewed above provides a biologically plausible model for gene–environment interactions, we are still restricted in the conclusions that can be drawn due to several limitations. First, these studies reported on peripheral levels of DNA methylation, which may not be reflective of methylation levels in the brain, as research has shown that methylation levels vary by cell type (Houston et al., 2012). Incorporating fMRI measures of brain activity, although not a substitute for directly measuring DNA methylation in brain tissue, could offer a complementary approach to help determine whether methylation levels measured peripherally alter neural activity in the predicted direction. This will be an important direction for research, as it is not possible to obtain levels of DNA methylation in neural cells from human participants except in postmortem studies. Second, the mechanisms linking increased methylation of the 5-HTT gene to increased risk for psychopathology need to be further delineated. Although studies have shown that methylation of the 5-HTT gene alters mRNA transcription of the serotonin transporter gene, the effect of 5-HTT methylation on brain function needs to be examined. An important candidate for investigation is that 5-HTT methylation levels may influence the development of prefrontal-amygdala circuitry, which in turn could lead to decreased emotion regulatory abilities and vulnerability to psychopathology. In order to test this hypothesis, however, imaging epigenetic studies incorporating fMRI assessments with measures of peripheral DNA methylation will need to be conducted. So far, with the exception reported below, relatively little work has been done in this area.

Although not reporting on the 5-HTTLPR, a recent imaging epigenetic study provides an example of how fMRI can help to elucidate the mechanisms of gene–environment interactions and represents what we believe is an important direction for future research. This study examined a common functional variant in the gene regulating Catechol-O-methyltransferase (COMT), an enzyme that breaks down dopamine in the prefrontal cortex (Ursini et al., 2011). The COMT gene has two functional variants: the Val allele, which is associated with greater COMT activity and reduced prefrontal efficiency, and the Met allele, which is associated with less COMT expression. This gene may be an important candidate for gene × environment interactions because methylation at the region investigated in this study is possible on the Val allele, where there is a CpG site, but not on the Met allele (Wiers, 2012). In this case, unlike with the 5-HTT gene, methylation of the Val allele is associated with better function, because it reduces expression of COMT; reduced expression of COMT increases available dopamine levels and prefrontal cortex efficiency. Ursini et al. found that environmental stress predicted reduced methylation in Val/Val participants. Moreover, reduced methylation was associated with reduced working memory performance and reduced prefrontal cortex efficiency. Importantly, because methylation can only occur on the Val allele, there was a gene × environment interaction: greater stress and reduced methylation predicted less efficient prefrontal cortex function in Val/Val participants only. In contrast, this effect was not seen for Val/Met or Met/Met allele carriers. The results of this study nicely illustrate a potential gene × environment interaction mechanism similar to what we have proposed for the 5-HTTLPR: because Val allele carriers are the high expressers of COMT, methylation has a buffering influence which leads the COMT gene to function more like that of a Met allele carrier. However, when environmental stress is introduced, methylation is reduced, which leads to increased COMT expression, decreased prefrontal cortex efficiency (theoretically through reduced dopamine levels) and decreased working memory performance. However, we only see this effect when environmental stress and the Val/Val alleles are both present, leading to a gene–environment interaction. Future imaging epigenetic studies such as these will help to clarify the mediating neural mechanisms involved in these interactions.

Imaging Genetics in ASD

One example of how imaging genetic research may shed light on the relation between 5-HTTLPR variation and symptomatology in ASD is the use of proton magnetic resonance spectroscopy (measuring levels of certain brain chemicals) in children and adolescents with ASD. Endo et al. (2010) found that the low-expressing allele of the 5-HTTLPR was associated with altered chemical metabolism in the medial prefrontal cortex, possibly reflecting reduced neuronal development. Because the medial prefrontal cortex plays an important role both in communicating with the amygdala and in coordinating signals from the amygdala to aid in social cognition, this could be a neural pathway through which the low-expressing allele of the 5-HTTLPR leads to greater severity of social/communication symptoms in ASD. Therefore, imaging genetic approaches such as these may help us identify how genetic variation contributes to the development of ASD symptoms and could help disentangle the complications associated with a heterogeneous spectrum of disorders by identifying subtypes that share common developmental pathways.

Further complicating the genetic picture for ASD development, rare genetic mutations such as copy number variants (either deletion or extra copy of a chromosomal region) may have a stronger contribution to the development of ASD than common genetic variation (such as the 5-HTTLPR) observed in the general population; although rare genetic mutations and common genetic variation may interact to influence developmental outcomes (Geschwind, 2011). Given that there appears to be a large amount of rare *de novo* (not seen in the parent, but occurring in the gamete or fertilized egg) mutations that may contribute to the development of ASD (Gilman et al., 2011), Geschwind (2011) and others have argued that it will be necessary to identify common developmental pathways at the neural systems level whereby a wide array of genetic variation may lead to specific symptom and behavioral phenotypes. For example, a key neural feature of ASD may be disruption in functional connectivity such as the connections between the prefrontal cortex and the amygdala. Imaging genetic studies may therefore help link a range of rare mutations in genes involved in axonal development and synaptic formation with the development of ASD through systems-level neural mechanisms observable with fMRI.

Epigenetics in ASD

There are a few lines of evidence suggesting that epigenetic regulation may be important to consider when examining genetic influences on ASD. Investigators have demonstrated altered epigenetic profiles of neuronal cells in postmortem brains of individuals with ASD (Shulha et al., 2012) and several candidate genes linked to ASD that regulate neuronal development are regulated by DNA methylation or other epigenetic mechanisms (Grafodatskaya, Chung, Szatmari, & Weksberg, 2010). Moreover, environmental risk factors that may be linked to the development of ASD may operate by altering methylation levels (LaSalle, 2011). Indeed, epigenetic influences on the development of ASD could help explain why it has been difficult to identify genes linked to ASD through genetic association approaches.

One example of a potential epigenetic influence on ASD is methylation of the oxytocin receptor gene. Oxytocin is a neuropeptide that increases social behaviors such as trust, empathy, emotion recognition, and eye gaze when administered to healthy controls (particularly men) (Meyer-Lindenberg, Domes, Kirsch, & Heinrichs, 2011). FMRI in adults has demonstrated that the effects of oxytocin on social behaviors may be mediated through a decrease in amygdala response to social stimuli (Kirsch et al., 2005). Recent research examining both peripheral DNA methylation levels and DNA methylation in post-mortem human brain tissue has provided evidence of increased methylation of CpG sites on the promoter region of the oxytocin receptor gene in ASD, which is associated with decreased expression of the oxytocin receptor in temporal cortex (Gregory et al., 2009). Coupled with what

we know from fMRI about the influence of oxytocin on amygdala function in healthy adults and abnormalities in amygdala function in ASD, this work is suggestive of a potential pathway for epigenetic influence on ASD development: methylation of the promoter region for the oxytocin receptor gene reduces expression of the oxytocin receptor. This could in turn result in heightened amygdala activation to social stimuli, as has been observed in ASD (Dalton et al., 2005; Monk et al., 2010; Weng et al., 2011). Imaging epigenetic approaches such as those we described above could be used to test this hypothesis, which illustrates the utility of leveraging knowledge of brain function in typically developing and atypical populations in order to understand processes of genetic and epigenetic influences on the development of psychopathology.

The Brain as a Biomarker for Treatment Response in Anxiety Disorders and ASD

In addition to examining pathways through which psychopathology develops, fMRI can be a useful tool for developing novel treatments and understanding their effects on the brain. Neural activation probed through fMRI may be used as a biomarker for examining the effects of pharmacological and behavioral treatments as well as measuring their efficacy (Paulus & Stein, 2007). This could be used, for example, as a preliminary examination of novel potential therapies to test whether they alter neural activity in a predicted direction in a small number of participants before conducting multisite large-scale clinical trials that are costly and time-consuming. In addition, by allowing examination of changes in activation in neural circuitry known to relate to specific disorders, fMRI has the capability to characterize how a particular pharmacological agent has a therapeutic effect, compare the effects of different classes of drugs on neural activity, and potentially predict therapeutic response or select the best pharmacological intervention for a particular individual based on their pretreatment patterns of neural activity (Paulus & Stein, 2007). Thus, the potential applications of fMRI for developing new treatments and predicting treatment response are promising.

Treatment Studies in Anxiety Disorders

Although there are currently treatments available for anxiety disorders including selective serotonin reuptake inhibitors (SSRIs) and cognitive behavioral therapy, these treatments are not effective for many patients, and SSRIs may have adverse side effects. Therefore, fMRI could play an important role in identifying new potential treatments and in helping to select which treatments are most likely to result in positive treatment response for individual patients.

Using fMRI, investigators have demonstrated that currently available treatments for anxiety disorders alter activity in the same neural regions (prefrontal cortex and amygdala) that have been shown to function abnormally in anxiety disorder patients (Murphy, 2010; Strawn, Wehry, DelBello, Rynn, & Strakowski, 2012). FMRI research in healthy adult participants demonstrated that administration of SSRIs results in decreased amygdala activation to emotional faces (Harmer, Mackay, Reid, Cowen, & Goodwin, 2006). Moreover, treatment of anxiety disorder patients (either pharmacological or with cognitive behavioral therapy) results in decreased amygdala activation (Furmark et al., 2002) and increased activation in the ventrolateral prefrontal cortex (Maslowksy et al., 2010). In depressed patients, SSRIs have also been shown to increase connectivity between the amygdala and prefrontal regions, suggesting that SSRIs may increase communication between the amygdala and prefrontal cortex (Chen et al., 2008). Given the established role of altered ventral prefrontal cortex-amygdala circuit function in anxiety disorder patients, these results suggest that therapeutic effects may occur through some combination of decreasing amygdala activation and increasing prefrontal regulation. It is important to note, however, that when changes in neural activity occur in the context of symptom improvement in

patients, we cannot necessarily attribute a causal role in symptom improvement to changes in neural function; instead, it could be that other changes (e.g., changes in cognitive processing patterns or behavior) cause both changes in symptoms and neural activity (Murphy, 2010).

These results have important implications for the development and testing of new medications by providing a potential biomarker for measuring treatment effectiveness. For example, several recent fMRI studies have suggested that pharmacological agents not currently prescribed for the treatment of anxiety disorders may have similar influences on neural activity as SSRIs. These medications alter the release or reception of neurotransmitters other than serotonin and have been demonstrated to affect prefrontal cortex-amygdala circuitry, for instance, by decreasing amygdala activation or increasing anterior cingulate cortex activation (Aupperle et al., 2011; Furmark et al., 2005). Additional fMRI studies such as these have the potential to help identify new treatments for anxiety disorders that may be prescribed to individuals who are nonresponsive or have adverse side effects to SSRIs. Moreover, these studies show that the influence of medications on brain response can be detected with relatively small samples (less than 40 participants in each case), supporting Paulus and Stein's (2007) argument that preliminary fMRI studies of treatment response will be a more cost-effective and less time-consuming method of identifying promising new treatments before they reach the clinical trial phase.

Furthermore, it may be possible to use pretreatment neural function assessed through fMRI as a tool to choose the best treatment for an individual. For example, greater pretreatment amygdala activation predicted better response to SSRI or cognitive behavioral therapy treatment in pediatric anxiety disorder patients (McClure, Adler, et al., 2007), and greater pretreatment anterior cingulate cortex activation predicted better response to pharmacological treatment in adult generalized anxiety disorder patients (Nitschke et al., 2009). Future studies such as these have the potential to help target treatments for patients by predicting which drugs or therapies they will respond to best. For instance, two related SSRIs (citalopram and escitalopram) both reduced amygdala activation to emotional faces in healthy controls, but had different effects on activation in the ventromedial prefrontal cortex (Windischberger et al., 2010). Although this type of research is still in its infancy, understanding the differences in effects on neural activation of different types of SSRIs could help in choosing the best one to prescribe based on a patient's neural activation.

Treatment Studies in ASD

Unlike anxiety disorders, there is currently no pharmacological treatment available for the core symptoms of ASD. Based on the neuroimaging data pointing to the influence of oxytocin on amygdala function and social behavior, investigators have proposed a potential translational application of oxytocin as a treatment for the social symptoms of ASD (Meyer-Lindenberg et al., 2011). Indeed, intranasal administration of oxytocin improved emotion recognition in children and adolescents with ASD (Guastella et al., 2010), suggesting a promising potential for the treatment of social symptoms. An important question for investigation with fMRI is whether the effect of oxytocin on improvement in ASD symptoms is mediated through decreased amygdala response to social stimuli and whether the effect of oxytocin on amygdala activity varies in strength at different stages of development. FMRI could also play an important role in helping determine which individuals will respond to oxytocin and in identifying other pharmacological agents that have similar effects on neural activation.

Future Directions for fMRI Research in Developmental Psychopathology

Throughout this review we have highlighted areas in need of further investigation through imaging genetics, imaging epigenetics, and imaging treatment approaches. In the final section, we discuss methodological considerations for this research.

External Validity of fMRI Tasks

FMRI requires close attention to task design in order to ensure that the cognitive processes of interest are isolated as much as possible and that the same cognitive processes are being elicited in each participant during scanning. Along these lines, further attention to the external validity of fMRI tasks will also improve our ability to examine neural activation in the context of cognitive and emotional processes that are more likely to represent what occurs in day-to-day life and importantly during the experience of symptoms. For example, Guyer et al. (2008) used a chat room task in which adolescents were asked to rate their desire to have an Internet chat with other peers and in which they were informed that other peers would be rating their desire to chat with the participant. While undergoing fMRI scanning, participants were asked to rate how interested they thought other peers would be in chatting with them. Due to the greater external validity of this task, the cognitive processes elicited by this task may more closely approximate the social anxiety symptoms related to peer evaluation that adolescents experience in everyday life. Future research that can better model the complex social contexts and relationships characteristic of the adolescent period may thus improve the strength of relations between fMRI measures and behavioral or self-report measures of symptoms that are influenced by these social contexts.

Longitudinal Designs in fMRI and the Use of Younger Samples

Structural MRI studies have plotted longitudinal changes in gray and white matter volumes over development. Similar longitudinal work is needed with fMRI in order to examine functional changes across development. One potential concern with longitudinal research in fMRI is that it is difficult to find a task that can be performed equally well and elicits the same cognitive strategies at all age levels. A second related concern is that infants and very young children generally cannot perform task-based fMRI. Resting-state or task-free fMRI (in which participants simply lie or sleep in the scanner while imaging data is acquired) has the potential to address both of these limitations. Because it requires no task, it removes the concern that participants of different ages may be performing a cognitive task differently, and it allows for participation of very young children who cannot perform tasks.

Analysis of resting-state fMRI usually involves a functional connectivity approach that examines the correlation of low-frequency spontaneous fluctuations in BOLD signal across different neural regions, which is sometimes referred to as intrinsic connectivity (Fox & Raichle, 2007). Importantly, regions that demonstrate intrinsic connectivity at rest also tend to demonstrate functional connectivity while participants perform a task (Smith et al., 2009), suggesting that intrinsic connectivity can provide similar information regarding the strength of integration across neural regions or networks related to specific cognitive or emotional processes. The ability to collect longitudinal data starting with infants or potentially even prenatally is especially important in light of the research mentioned earlier suggesting that genetic and epigenetic influences on psychopathology may occur very early in development. Thus, the ability to examine neural function at these earlier developmental stages with resting-state fMRI could be used as a complementary approach to task-based fMRI in order to gain a more complete picture of the developmental trajectories of neural networks and to examine this development prospectively before symptoms of psychopathology may be apparent.

Large-Scale fMRI Studies

Recognition of the complexity of gene–environment interactions indicates the requirement of large samples to yield the statistical power necessary to examine these effects in imaging gene–environment interaction designs (Hyde et al., 2011). Resting-state fMRI data could be useful in this regard because it allows for the combination of data sets across different research groups without the requirement that participants all performed the same task (Biswal et al., 2010). Another example of a large-scale fMRI approach is the IMAGEN group's multisite collaborative prospective longitudinal study designed to have sufficient power to examine imaging gene–environment interactions (Schumann et al., 2010). By collecting genotype and fMRI data on an estimated 2,000 participants, this study will have increased power to detect gene–gene and gene–environment interactions and their relation to neural function compared to previous studies with smaller sample sizes.

Conclusion

Current fMRI research in developmental psychopathology has helped establish patterns of altered neural function in pediatric psychopathology and linked dysfunction in these regions with cognitive and emotional processes related to the symptoms and behavioral profiles of specific disorders. These studies have highlighted the role of prefrontal cortex-amygdala circuitry in both anxiety disorders and ASD. Imaging genetic studies have linked variation in genes regulating serotonin levels to altered functioning of this circuit, indicating a potential developmental pathway for the influence of genetic variation on neural function and laying the foundation for examination of epigenetic influences on this circuitry. Treatment studies have suggested that currently available treatments and potential novel treatments for anxiety disorders and ASD alter activity in this same neural circuitry, either by increasing prefrontal regulation or dampening amygdala responsiveness. These studies have paved the way for future imaging genetic and imaging epigenetic studies to examine how prefrontal-amygdala cortex circuitry (and, through extension of these methods, other neural circuitry and networks implicated in these disorders) is involved in the development of psychopathology and is influenced through genetic and epigenetic factors. This will help establish critical knowledge necessary to develop novel preventions and treatments, one of the major goals of the field of developmental psychopathology.

References

Adolphs, R. (2010). What does the amygdala contribute to social cognition? *Annals of the New York Academy of Sciences, 1191*, 42–61.

Ansorge, M. S., Zhou, M., Lira, A., Hen, R., & Gingrich, J. A. (2004). Early-life blockade of the 5-HT transporter alters emotional behavior in adult mice. *Science, 306*, 879–881.

Ashwin, C., Baron-Cohen, S., Wheelwright, S., O'Riordan, M., & Bullmore, E. T. (2007). Differential activation of the amygdala and the 'social brain' during fearful face-processing in Asperger Syndrome. *Neuropsychologia, 45*(1), 2–14.

Aupperle, R. L., Ravindran, L., Tankersley, D., Flagan, T., Stein, N. R., Simmons, A. N., et al. (2011). Pregabalin influences insula and amygdala activation during anticipation of emotional images. *Neuropsychopharmacology, 36*(7), 1466–1477.

Bagot, R. C., & Meaney, M. J. (2010). Epigenetics and the biological basis of gene x environment interactions. *Journal of the American Academy of Child & Adolescent Psychiatry, 49*(8), 752–771.

Baron-Cohen, S., Ring, H. A., Wheelwright, S., Bullmore, E. T., Brammer, M. J., Simmons, A., et al. (1999). Social intelligence in the normal and autistic brain: An fMRI study. *European Journal of Neuroscience, 11*, 1891–1898.

Battaglia, M., Zanoni, A., Taddei, M., Giorda, R., Bertoletti, E., Lampis, V., et al. (2012). Cerebral responses to emotional expressions and the development of social anxiety disorder: A preliminary longitudinal study. *Depression and Anxiety, 29*(1), 54–61.

Beach, S. R., Brody, G. H., Todorov, A. A., Gunter, T. D., & Philibert, R. A. (2010). Methylation at SLC6A4 is linked to family history of child abuse: An examination of the Iowa Adoptee sample. *American Journal of Medical Genetics Part B: Neuropsychiatric Genetics, 153B*(2), 710–713.

Biswal, B., Mennes, M., Zuo, X., Gohel, S., Kelly, C., Smith, S. M., et al. (2010). Toward discovery science of human brain function. *Proceedings of the National Academy of Sciences of the United States of America, 107*(10), 4734–4739.

Britton, J. C., Lissek, S., Grillon, C., Norcross, M. A., & Pine, D. S. (2011). Development of anxiety: The role of threat appraisal and fear learning. *Depression and Anxiety, 28*(1), 5–17.

Brune, C. W., Kim, S., Salt, J., Levanthal, B. L., Lord, C., & Cook, E. H., Jr. (2006). 5-HTTLPR genotype-specific phenotype in children and adolescents with autism. *The American Journal of Psychiatry, 163*(12), 2148–2156.

Canli, T., Qiu, M., Omura, K., Congdon, E., Haas, B. W., Amin, Z., et al. (2006). Neural correlates of epigenesis. *Proceedings of the National Academy of Sciences of the United States of America, 103*(43), 16033–16038.

Carmody, D. P., & Lewis, M. (2010). Regional white matter development in children with autism spectrum disorders. *Developmental Psychobiology, 52*(8), 755–763.

Casey, B. J., Jones, R. M., & Hare, T. A. (2008). The adolescent brain. *Annals of the New York Academy of Sciences, 1124*, 111–126.

Caspi, A., & Moffitt, T. E. (2006). Gene-environment interactions in psychiatry: Joining forces with neuroscience. *Nature Reviews. Neuroscience, 7*, 583–590.

Chen, C. H., Suckling, J., Ooi, C., Fu, C. H., Williams, S. C., Walsh, N. D., et al. (2008). Functional coupling of the amygdala in depressed patients treated with antidepressant medication. *Neuropsychopharmacology, 33*(8), 1909–1918.

Cicchetti, D., & Dawson, G. (2002). Multiple levels of analysis. *Development and Psychopathology, 14*, 417–420.

Courchesne, E., Pierce, K., Schumann, C. M., Redcay, E., Buckwalter, J. A., Kennedy, D. P., et al. (2007). Mapping early brain development in autism. *Neuron, 56*, 399–413.

Daleiden, E. L., & Vasey, M. W. (1997). An information-processing perspective on childhood anxiety. *Clinical Psychology Review, 17*(4), 407–429.

Dalton, K. M., Nacewicz, B. M., Johnstone, T., Schaefer, H. S., Gernsbacher, M. A., Goldsmith, H. H., et al. (2005). Gaze fixation and the neural circuitry of face processing in autism. *Nature Neuroscience, 8*(4), 519–526.

Daws, L. C., & Gould, G. G. (2011). Ontogeny and regulation of the serotonin transporter: Providing insights into human disorders. *Pharmacology & Therapeutics, 131*(1), 61–79.

Dawson, G., Webb, S. J., Wijsman, E., Schellenberg, G., Estes, A., Munson, J., et al. (2005). Neurocognitive and electrophysiological evidence of altered face processing in parents of children with autism: Implications for a model of abnormal development of social brain circuitry in autism. *Development and Psychopathology, 17*, 679–697.

Ellis, B. J., Boyce, W. T., Belsky, J., Bakermans-Kranenburg, M. J., & van Ijzendoorn, M. H. (2011). Differential susceptibility to the environment: An evolutionary-neurodevelopmental theory. *Development and Psychopathology, 23*, 7–28.

Endo, T., Kitamura, H., Tamura, R., Egawa, J., Sugai, T., Fukui, N., et al. (2010). 5-HTTLPR polymorphism influences prefrontal neurochemical metabolites in autism spectrum disorder. *Psychiatry Research, 183*(2), 170–173.

Etkin, A., Prater, K. E., Hoeft, F., Menon, V., & Schatzberg, A. F. (2010). Failure of anterior cingulate activation and connectivity with the amygdala during implicit regulation of emotional processing in generalized anxiety disorder. *The American Journal of Psychiatry, 167*, 545–554.

Etkin, A., & Wager, T. D. (2007). Functional neuroimaging of anxiety: A meta-analysis of emotional processing in PTSD, social anxiety disorder, and specific phobia. *The American Journal of Psychiatry, 164*, 1476–1488.

Fox, M. D., & Raichle, M. E. (2007). Spontaneous fluctuations in brain activity observed with functional magnetic resonance imaging. *Nature Reviews. Neuroscience, 8*, 700–711.

Fox, N. A., Nichols, K. E., Henderson, H. A., Rubin, K., Schmidt, L., Hamer, D., et al. (2005). Evidence for a gene-environment interaction in predicting behavioral inhibition in middle childhood. *Psychological Science, 16*(12), 921–926.

Furman, D. J., Hamilton, J. P., Joormann, J., & Gotlib, I. H. (2011). Altered timing of amygdala activation during sad mood elaboration as a function of 5-HTTLPR. *Social Cognitive and Affective Neuroscience, 6*(3), 270–276.

Furmark, T., Appel, L., Michelgard, A., Wahlstedt, K., Ahs, F., Zancan, S., et al. (2005). Cerebral blood flow changes after treatment of social phobia with the neurokinin-1 antagonist GR205171, citalopram, or placebo. *Biological Psychiatry, 58*(2), 132–142.

Furmark, T., Tillfors, M., Marteinsdottir, I., Fischer, H., Pissiota, A., Langstrom, B., et al. (2002). Common changes in cerebral blood flow in patients with social phobia treated with citalopram or cognitive-behavioral therapy. *Archives of General Psychiatry, 59*, 425–433.

Geschwind, D. H. (2011). Genetics of autism spectrum disorders. *Trends in Cognitive Sciences, 15*(9), 409–416.

Ghashghaei, H. T., Hilgetag, C. C., & Barbas, H. (2007). Sequence of information processing for emotions based on the anatomic dialogue between prefrontal cortex and amygdala. *NeuroImage, 34*(3), 905–923.

Giedd, J. N., & Rapoport, J. L. (2010). Structural MRI of pediatric brain development: What have we learned and where are we going? *Neuron, 67*, 728–734.

Gilman, S. R., Iossifov, I., Levy, D., Ronemus, M., Wigler, M., & Vitkup, D. (2011). Rare de novo variants associated with autism implicate a large functional network of genes involved in formation and function of synapses. *Neuron, 70*(5), 898–907.

Gogtay, N., Giedd, J. N., Lusk, L., Hayashi, K. M., Greenstein, D., Vaituzis, A. C., et al. (2004). Dynamic mapping of human cortical development during childhood through early adulthood. *Proceedings of the National Academy of Sciences of the United States of America, 101*(21), 8174–8179.

Gottlieb, G. (2007a). Developmental neurobehavioral genetics: Development as explanation. In B.C. Jones & P. Mormede (Eds.), *Neurobehavioral Genetics* (2nd ed., pp. 17–27). Boca Raton, FL: CRC Taylor & Francis.

Gottlieb, G. (2007b). Probabilistic epigenesis. *Developmental Science, 10*(1), 1–11.

Grafodatskaya, D., Chung, B., Szatmari, P., & Weksberg, R. (2010). Autism spectrum disorders and epigenetics. *Journal of the American Academy of Child & Adolescent Psychiatry, 49*(8), 794–809.

Gregory, S. G., Connelly, J. J., Towers, A. J., Johnson, J., Biscocho, D., Markunas, C. A., et al. (2009). Genomic and epigenetic evidence for oxytocin receptor deficiency in autism. *BMC Medicine, 7*, 62.

Guastella, A. J., Einfeld, S. L., Gray, K. M., Rinehart, N. J., Tonge, B. J., Lambert, T. J., et al. (2010). Intranasal oxytocin improves emotion recognition for youth with autism spectrum disorders. *Biological Psychiatry, 67*(7), 692–694.

Guyer, A. E., Lau, J. Y. F., McClure-Tone, E. B., Parrish, J. M., Shiffrin, N. D., Reynolds, R. C., et al. (2008). Amygdala and ventrolateral prefrontal cortex function during anticipated peer evaluation in pediatric social anxiety. *Archives of General Psychiatry, 65*(11), 1303–1312.

Hare, T. A., Tottenham, N., Galvan, A., Voss, H. U., Glover, G. H., & Casey, B. J. (2008). Biological substrates of emotional reactivity and regulation in adolescence during an emotional go-nogo task. *Biological Psychiatry, 63*, 927–934.

Hariri, A. R., Mattay, V. S., Tessitore, A., Kolachana, B., Fera, F., Goldman, D., et al. (2002). Serotonin transporter genetic variation and the response of the human amygdala. *Science, 297*, 400–403.

Hariri, A. R., & Weinberger, D. R. (2003). Functional neuroimaging of genetic variation in serotonergic neurotransmission. *Genes, Brain, and Behavior, 2*, 341–349.

Harmer, C. J., Mackay, C. E., Reid, C. B., Cowen, P. J., & Goodwin, G. M. (2006). Antidepressant drug treatment modifies the neural processing of nonconscious threat cues. *Biological Psychiatry, 59*(9), 816–820.

Heinz, A., Braus, D. F., Smolka, M. N., Wrase, J., Puls, I., Hermann, D., et al. (2005). Amygdala-prefrontal coupling depends on a genetic variation of the serotonin transporter. *Nature Neuroscience, 8*(1), 20–21.

Houston, I., Peter, C. J., Mitchell, A., Straubhaar, J., Rogaev, E., & Akbarian, S. (2012). Epigenetics in the human brain. *Neuropsychopharmacology, 37*, 1–15.

Hu, X. Z., Lipsky, R. H., Zhu, G., Akhtar, L. A., Taubman, J., Greenberg, B. D., et al. (2006). Serotonin transporter promoter gain-of-function genotypes are linked to obsessive-compulsive disorder. *American Journal of Human Genetics, 78*(5), 815–826.

Huang, C. H., & Santengelo, S. L. (2008). Autism and serotonin transporter gene polymorphisms: A systematic review and meta-analysis. *American Journal of Medical Genetics Part B: Neuropsychiatric Genetics, 147B*, 903–913.

Hyde, L. W., Bogdan, R., & Hariri, A. R. (2011). Understanding risk for psychopathology through imaging gene-environment interactions. *Trends in Cognitive Sciences, 15*(9), 417–427.

Johnson, M. H., Halit, H., Grice, S. J., & Karmiloff-Smith, A. (2002). Neuroimaging of typical and atypical development: A perspective from multiple levels of analysis. *Development and Psychopathology, 14*, 521–536.

Joseph, R. M., Ehrman, K., McNally, R., & Keehn, B. (2008). Affective response to eye contact and face recognition ability in children with ASD. *Journal of the International Neuropsychological Society, 14,* 947–955.

Kilpatrick, D., Koenen, K., Ruggiero, K., Acierno, R., Galea, S., & Resnick, H. (2007). The serotonin transporter genotype and social support and moderation of posttraumatic stress disorder and depression in hurricane-exposed adults. *American Journal of Psychiatry, 164*(11), 1693–1699.

Kinnally, E. L., Capitanio, J. P., Leibel, R., Deng, L., LeDuc, C., Haghighi, F., et al. (2010). Epigenetic regulation of serotonin transporter expression and behavior in infant rhesus macaques. *Genes, Brain, and Behavior, 9*(6), 575–582.

Kinnally, E. L., Feinberg, C., Kim, D., Ferguson, K., Leibel, R., Coplan, J. D., et al. (2011). DNA methylation as a risk factor in the effects of early life stress. *Brain, Behavior, and Immunity, 25*(8), 1548–1553.

Kirsch, P., Esslinger, C., Chen, Q., Mier, D., Lis, S., Siddhanti, S., et al. (2005). Oxytocin modulates neural circuitry for social cognition and fear in humans. *The Journal of Neuroscience, 25*(49), 11489–11493.

Kleinhans, N. M., Johnson, L. C., Richards, T., Mahurin, R., Greenson, J., Dawson, G., et al. (2009). Reduced neural habituation in the amygdala and social impairments in autism spectrum disorders. *The American Journal of Psychiatry, 166,* 467–475.

Kliemann, D., Dziobek, I., Hatri, A., Steimke, R., & Heekeren, H. R. (2010). Atypical reflexive gaze patterns on emotional faces in autism spectrum disorders. *The Journal of Neuroscience, 30*(37), 12281–12287.

Kliemann, D., Dziobek, I., Hatri, A., Baudwig, J., & Heekeren, H. R. (2012). The role of the amygdala in atypical gaze on emotional faces in autism spectrum disorders. *The Journal of Neuroscience, 32*(28), 9469–9476.

Klin, A., Jones, W., Schultz, R., Volkmar, F., & Cohen, D. (2002). Visual fixation patterns during viewing of naturalistic social situations as predictors of social competence in individuals with autism. *Archives of General Psychiatry, 59,* 809–816.

Koenen, K. C., Uddin, M., Chang, S. C., Aiello, A. E., Wildman, D. E., Goldmann, E., et al. (2011). SLC6A4 methylation modifies the effect of the number of traumatic events on risk for posttraumatic stress disorder. *Depression and Anxiety, 28*(8), 639–647.

LaSalle, J. M. (2011). A genomic point-of-view on environmental factors influencing the human brain methylome. *Epigenetics, 6,* 862–869.

Lau, J. Y. F., Goldman, D., Buzas, B., Fromm, S. J., Guyer, A. E., Hodgkinson, C., et al. (2009). Amygdala function and 5-HTT gene variants in adolescent anxiety and major depressive disorder. *Biological Psychiatry, 65*(4), 349–355.

Laucht, M., Treutlein, J., Blomeyer, D., Buchmann, A. F., Schmid, B., Becker, K., et al. (2009). Interaction between the 5-HTTLPR serotonin transporter polymorphism and environmental adversity for mood and anxiety psychopathology: Evidence from a high-risk community sample of young adults.

International Journal of Neuropsychopharmacology, 12, 737–747.

Lemogne, C., Gorwood, P., Boni, C., Pessiglione, M., Lehericy, S., & Fossati, P. (2011). Cognitive appraisal and life stress moderate the effects of the 5-HTTLPR polymorphism on amygdala reactivity. *Human Brain Mapping, 32*(11), 1856–1867.

Lesch, K. P., Bengel, D., Heils, A., Sabol, S. Z., Greenberg, B. D., Petri, S., et al. (1996). Association of anxiety-related traits with a polymorphism in the serotonin transporter gene regulatory region. *Science, 274,* 1527–1531.

Lewis, M., & Carmody, D. P. (2008). Self-representation and brain development. *Developmental Psychology, 44*(5), 1329–1334.

Maslowsky, J., Mogg, K., Bradley, B. P., McClure-Tone, E. B., Ernst, M., Pine, D. S., et al. (2010). A preliminary investigation of neural correlates of treatment in adolescents with generalized anxiety disorder. *Journal of Child and Adolescent Psychopharmacology, 20*(2), 105–111.

McClure, E. B., Adler, A., Monk, C. S., Cameron, J., Smith, S., Nelson, E. E., et al. (2007). fMRI predictors of treatment outcome in pediatric anxiety disorders. *Psychopharmacology, 191*(1), 97–105.

McClure, E. B., Monk, C. S., Nelson, E. E., Parrish, J. M., Adler, A., Blair, J. R., et al. (2007). Abnormal attention modulation of fear circuit function in pediatric generalized anxiety disorder. *Archives of General Psychiatry, 64,* 97–106.

McGowan, P. O., Sasaki, A., D'Alessio, A. C., Dymov, S., Labonte, B., Szyf, M., et al. (2009). Epigenetic regulation of the glucocorticoid receptor in human brain associates with childhood abuse. *Nature Neuroscience, 12*(3), 342–348.

Meaney, M. J. (2010). Epigenetics and the biological definition of gene x environment interactions. *Child Development, 81*(1), 41–79.

Meyer-Lindenberg, A., Domes, G., Kirsch, P., & Heinrichs, M. (2011). Oxytocin and vasopressin in the human brain: Social neuropeptides for translational medicine. *Nature Reviews. Neuroscience, 12,* 524–538.

Monk, C. S. (2008). The development of emotion-related neural circuitry in health and psychopathology. *Development and Psychopathology, 20*(4), 1231–1250.

Monk, C. S., McClure, E. B., Nelson, E. E., Zarahn, E., Bilder, R. M., Leibenluft, E., et al. (2003). Adolescent immaturity in attention-related brain engagement to emotional facial expressions. *NeuroImage, 20,* 420–428.

Monk, C. S., Nelson, E. E., McClure, E. B., Mogg, K., Bradley, B. P., Leibenluft, E., et al. (2006). Ventrolateral prefrontal cortex activation and attentional bias in response to angry faces in adolescents with generalized anxiety disorder. *The American Journal of Psychiatry, 163,* 1091–1097.

Monk, C. S., Telzer, E. H., Mogg, K., Bradley, B. P., Mai, X., Louro, H. M. C., et al. (2008). Amygdala and ventrolateral prefrontal cortex activation to masked angry faces in children and adolescents with generalized anxiety disorder. *Archives of General Psychiatry, 65*(5), 568–576.

Monk, C. S., Weng, S. J., Wiggins, J. L., Kurapati, N., Louro, H. M. C., Carrasco, M., et al. (2010). Neural circuitry of emotional face processing in autism spectrum disorders. *Journal of Psychiatry and Neuroscience, 35*(2), 105–114.

Munafo, M. R., Brown, S. M., & Hariri, A. R. (2008). Serotonin transporter (5-HTTLPR) genotype and amygdala activation: A meta-analysis. *Biological Psychiatry, 63*(9), 852–857.

Munafo, M. R., Freimer, N. B., Ng, W., Ophoff, R., Veijola, J., Miettunen, J., et al. (2009). 5-HTTLPR genotype and anxiety-related personality traits: A meta-analysis and new data. *American Journal of Medical Genetics Part B: Neuropsychiatric Genetics, 150B*(2), 271–281.

Mundy, P. C., Henderson, H. A., Inge, A. P., & Coman, D. C. (2007). The modifier model of autism and social development in higher functioning children. *Research & Practice for Persons with Severe Disabilities, 32*(2), 124–139.

Murphy, S. E. (2010). Using functional neuroimaging to investigate the mechanism of action of selective serotonin reuptake inhibitors (SSRIs). *Current Pharmaceutical Design, 16*, 1990–1997.

Myers-Schulz, B., & Koenigs, M. (2012). Functional anatomy of ventromedial prefrontal cortex: Implications for mood and anxiety disorders. *Molecular Psychiatry, 17*, 132–141.

Neumann, D., Spezio, M. L., Piven, J., & Adolphs, R. (2006). Looking you in the mouth: Abnormal gaze in autism resulting from impaired top-down modulation of visual attention. *Social Cognitive and Affective Neuroscience, 1*(3), 194–202.

Nijmeijer, J. S., Hartman, C. A., Rommelse, N. N. J., Altink, M. E., Buschgens, C. J. M., Fliers, E. A., & Hoekstra, P. J. (2010). Perinatal risk factors interacting with catechol O-methyltransferase and the serotonin transporter gene predict ASD symptoms in children with ADHD. *Journal of Child Psychology and Psychiatry, 51*(11), 1242–1250.

Nitschke, J. B., Sarinopoulos, I., Oathes, D. J., Johnstone, T., Whalen, P. J., Davidson, R. J., et al. (2009). Anticipatory activation in the amygdala and anterior cingulate in generalized anxiety disorder and prediction of treatment response. *The American Journal of Psychiatry, 166*, 302–310.

Nordquist, N., & Oreland, L. (2010). Serotonin, genetic variability, behaviour, and psychiatric disorders – A review. *Upsala Journal of Medical Sciences, 115*, 2–10.

O'Nions, E. J. P., Dolan, R. J., & Roiser, J. P. (2011). Serotonin transporter genotype modulates subgenual response to fearful faces using an incidental task. *Journal of Cognitive Neuroscience, 23*(11), 3681–3693.

Paulus, M. P., & Stein, M. B. (2007). Role of functional magnetic resonance imaging in drug discovery. *Neuropsychology Review, 17*(2), 179–188.

Pergamin-Hight, L., Bakermans-Kranenburg, M. J., van Ijzendoorn, M. H., & Bar-Haim, Y. (2012). Variations in the promoter region of the serotonin transporter gene and biased attention for emotional information: A meta-analysis. *Biological Psychiatry, 71*(4), 373–379.

Pezawas, L., Meyer-Lindenberg, A., Drabant, E. M., Verchinski, B. A., Munoz, K. E., Kolachana, B., et al. (2005). 5-HTTLPR polymorphism impacts human cingulate-amygdala interactions: A genetic susceptibility mechanism for depression. *Nature Neuroscience, 8*(6), 828–834.

Philibert, R., Madan, A., Andersen, A., Cadoret, R., Packer, H., & Sandhu, H. (2007). Serotonin transporter mRNA levels are associated with the methylation of an upstream CpG island. *American Journal of Medical Genetics Part B: Neuropsychiatric Genetics, 144B*(1), 101–105.

Philibert, R., Sandhu, H., Hollenbeck, N., Gunter, T., Adams, W., & Madan, A. (2008). The relationship of 5HTT (SLC6A4) methylation and genotype on mRNA expression and liability to major depression and alcohol dependence in subjects from the Iowa Adoption Studies. *American Journal of Medical Genetics Part B: Neuropsychiatric Genetics, 147B*(5), 543–549.

Philip, R. C., Dauvermann, M. R., Whalley, H. C., Baynham, K., Lawrie, S. M., & Stanfield, A. C. (2012). A systematic review and meta-analysis of the fMRI investigation of autism spectrum disorders. *Neuroscience and Biobehavioral Reviews, 36*(2), 901–942.

Phillips, M. L., Ladouceur, C. D., & Drevets, W. C. (2008). A neural model of voluntary and automatic emotion regulation: Implications for understanding the pathophysiology and neurodevelopment of bipolar disorder. *Molecular Psychiatry, 13*(9), 829, 833–857.

Pine, D. S. (2007). Research review: A neuroscience framework for pediatric anxiety disorders. *Journal of Child Psychology and Psychiatry, 48*(7), 631–648.

Pinto, A. O., & Sesack, S. R. (2003). Prefrontal cortex projections to the rat amygdala: Spatial relationships to dopamine and serotonin afferents. *Annals of the New York Academy of Sciences, 985*, 542–544.

Ray, R. D., & Zald, D. H. (2012). Anatomical insights into the interaction of emotion and cognition in the prefrontal cortex. *Neuroscience and Biobehavioral Reviews, 36*(1), 479–501.

Rubia, K., Overmeyer, S., Taylor, E., Brammer, M., Williams, S. C. R., Simmons, A., et al. (2000). Functional frontalisation with age: Mapping neurodevelopmental trajectories with fMRI. *Neuroscience and Biobehavioral Reviews, 24*, 13–19.

Sameroff, A. (2010). A unified theory of development: A dialectic integration of nature and nurture. *Child Development, 81*(1), 6–22.

Sarter, M., & Markowitsch, H. J. (1984). Collateral innervation of the medial and lateral prefrontal cortex by amygdaloid, thalamic, and brain-stem neurons. *The Journal of Comparative Neurology, 224*, 445–460.

Schultz, R. T. (2005). Developmental deficits in social perception in autism: The role of the amygdala and fusiform face area. *International Journal of Developmental Neuroscience, 23*(2–3), 125–141.

Schumann, C. M., Hamstra, J., Goodlin-Jones, B. L., Lotspeich, L. J., Kwon, H., Buonocore, M. H., et al. (2004). The amygdala is enlarged in children but not adolescents with autism; The hippocampus is enlarged at all ages. *The Journal of Neuroscience, 24*(28), 6392–6401.

Schumann, G., Loth, E., Banaschewski, T., Barbot, A., Barker, G., Buchel, C., et al. (2010). The IMAGEN study: Reinforcement-related behaviour in normal brain function and psychopathology. *Molecular Psychiatry, 15*, 1128–1139.

Şhulha, H. P., Cheung, I., Whittle, C., Wang, J., Virgil, D., Lin, C. L., et al. (2012). Epigenetic signatures of autism: Trimethylated H3K4 landscapes in prefrontal neurons. *Archives of General Psychiatry, 69*(3), 314–324.

Sibille, E., & Lewis, D. A. (2006). SERT-ainly involved in depression, but when? *The American Journal of Psychiatry, 163*(1), 8–11.

Smith, S. M., Fox, P. T., Miller, K. L., Glahn, D. C., Fox, P. M., Mackay, C. E., et al. (2009). Correspondence of the brain's functional architecture during activation and rest. *Proceedings of the National Academy of Sciences of the United States of America, 106*(31), 13040–13045.

Stein, M. B., Schork, N., & Gelernter, J. (2008). Gene-by-environment (serotonin transporter and childhood maltreatment) interaction for anxiety sensitivity, an intermediate phenotype for anxiety disorders. *Neuropsychopharmacology, 33*(2), 312–319.

Steinberg, L., Dahl, R., Keating, D., Kupfer, D. J., Masten, A. S., & Pine, D. S. (2006). The study of developmental psychopathology in adolescence: Integrating affective neuroscience with the study of context. In D. Cicchetti & D. J. Cohen (Eds.), *Developmental psychopathology, Vol 2: Developmental neuroscience* (2nd ed., pp. 710–741). Hoboken, NJ: Wiley.

Strawn, J. R., Wehry, A. M., DelBello, M. P., Rynn, M. A., & Strakowski, S. (2012). Establishing the neurobiologic basis of treatment in children and adolescents with generalized anxiety disorder. *Depression and Anxiety, 29*(4), 328–339.

Swartz, J. R., Wiggins, J. L., Carrasco, M., Lord, C., & Monk, C. S. (2013). Amygdala habituation and prefrontal functional connectivity in youth with autism spectrum disorders. *Journal of the American Academy of Child & Adolescent Psychiatry, 25*(1), 84–93.

Surguladze, S. A., Radua, J., El-Hage, W., Gohier, B., Sato, J. R., Kronhaus, D. M., et al. (2012). Interaction of catechol O-methyltransferase and serotonin transporter genes modulates effective connectivity in a facial emotion-processing circuitry. *Translational Psychiatry, 2*(1), e70.

Thomas, K. M., Drevets, W. C., Dahl, R. E., Ryan, N. D., Birmaher, B., Eccard, C. H., et al. (2001). Amygdala response to fearful faces in anxious and depressed children. *Archives of General Psychiatry, 58*, 1057–1063.

Thomason, M. E., Henry, M. L., Paul Hamilton, J., Joormann, J., Pine, D. S., Ernst, M., et al. (2010). Neural and behavioral responses to threatening emotion faces in children as a function of the short allele of the serotonin transporter gene. *Biological Psychology, 85*(1), 38–44.

Tordjman, S., Gutknecht, L., Carlier, M., Spitz, E., Antoine, C., Slama, F., et al. (2001). Role of the serotonin transporter gene in the behavioral expression of autism. *Molecular Psychiatry, 6*, 434–439.

Troelsen, K. B., Nielsen, E. O., & Mirza, N. R. (2005). Chronic treatment with duloxetine is necessary for an anxiolytic-like response in the mouse zero maze: The role of the serotonin transporter. *Psychopharmacology, 181*, 741–750.

Uher, R., & McGuffin, P. (2010). The moderation by the serotonin transporter gene of environmental adversity in the etiology of depression: 2009 update. *Molecular Psychiatry, 15*(1), 18–22.

Ursini, G., Bollati, V., Fazio, L., Porcelli, A., Iacovelli, L., Catalani, A., et al. (2011). Stress-related methylation of the catechol-O-methyltransferase Val 158 allele predicts human prefrontal cognition and activity. *The Journal of Neuroscience, 31*(18), 6692–6698.

van Ijzendoorn, M. H., Bakermans-Kranenburg, M. J., & Ebstein, R. P. (2011). Methylation matters in child development: Toward developmental behavioral epigenetics. *Child Development Perspectives, 5*(4), 305–310.

van IJzendoorn, M. H., Caspers, K., Bakermans-Kranenburg, M. J., Beach, S. R., & Philibert, R. (2010). Methylation matters: Interaction between methylation density and serotonin transporter genotype predicts unresolved loss or trauma. *Biological Psychiatry, 68*(5), 405–407.

Veenstra-VanderWeele, J., & Blakely, R. D. (2012). Networking in autism: Leveraging genetic, biomarker and model system findings in the search for new treatments. *Neuropsychopharmacology, 37*(1), 196–212.

Weaver, I. C., Cervoni, N., Champagne, F. A., D'Alessio, A. C., Sharma, S., Seckl, J. R., et al. (2004). Epigenetic programming by maternal behavior. *Nature Neuroscience, 7*(8), 847–854.

Weng, S. J., Carrasco, M., Swartz, J. R., Wiggins, J. L., Kurapati, N., Liberzon, I., et al. (2011). Neural activation to emotional faces in adolescents with autism spectrum disorders. *Journal of Child Psychology and Psychiatry, 52*(3), 296–305.

Wiers, C. E. (2012). Methylation and the human brain: Towards a new discipline of imaging epigenetics. *European Archives of Psychiatry and Clinical Neuroscience, 262*, 271–273.

Wiggins, J. L., Bedoyan, J. K., Peltier, S. J., Ashinoff, S., Carrasco, M., Weng, S., et al. (2012). The impact of serotonin transporter (5-HTTLPR) genotype on the development of resting-state connectivity in children and adolescents: A preliminary report. *NeuroImage, 59*, 2760–2770.

Wiggins, J. L., Bedoyan, J. K., Carrasco, M., Swartz, J. R., Martin, D. M., & Monk, C. S. (in press). Age-related effects of serotonin transporter-linked promoter region (5-HTTLPR) variants on amygdala and prefrontal cortex function in adolescence. *Human Brain Mapping.*

Williams, L. M., Gatt, J. M., Schofield, P. R., Olivieri, G., Peduto, A., & Gordon, E. (2009). 'Negativity bias' in risk for depression and anxiety: Brain-body fear circuitry correlates, 5-HTT-LPR and early life stress. *NeuroImage, 47*(3), 804–814.

Windischberger, C., Lanzenberger, R., Holik, A., Spindelegger, C., Stein, P., Moser, U., et al. (2010). Area-specific modulation of neural activation comparing escitalopram and citalopram revealed by pharmaco-fMRI: A randomized cross-over study. *NeuroImage, 49*(2), 1161–1170.

Yurgelon-Todd, D., & Killgore, W. D. S. (2006). Fear-related activity in the prefrontal cortex increases with age during adolescence: A preliminary fMRI study. *Neuroscience Letters, 406*, 194–199.

The Contributions of Early Experience to Biological Development and Sensitivity to Context

15

Nicole R. Bush and W. Thomas Boyce

Although long a focus of developmental psychopathology, in recent years a variety of professional disciplines and the general public have demonstrated an increased interest in the manner in which early life experience relates to the development of health outcomes. Adding to the already rich empirical evidence of early life experience effects on child development, it is now becoming common for studies of adult mental health to include indices of childhood social context. In tandem with this movement, there has been a remarkable advancement in understanding of human biology and the biological mechanisms underlying psychopathology. In combination, these advancements in the study of early experience and biology illuminate many of the etiologic complexities of mental health. This chapter will review theories and evidence for the biological embedding of early life experience and the manner in which context and biology interact to predict psychopathology. In particular, we approach this work through the lens of Biological Sensitivity to Context Theory, which allows for

examination of both phenomena and their integration, across development.

Biological Embedding of Early Life Experience

Research examining social disparities in health has played an important role in the understanding of the ways in which early life experience shapes biology. It has been well established that there is a robust graded association between socioeconomic status (SES) and health in adulthood (Adler et al., 1994; Adler & Stewart, 2010; Cohen, Janicki-Deverts, Chen, & Matthews, 2010). Differences in infant and early child development form a socioeconomic gradient as well (Adler, Bush, & Pantell, 2012; Braveman & Egerter, 2008; Chen, Matthews, & Boyce, 2002), setting young lives on trajectories toward the broader and less malleable health inequalities of adolescence and adult life. These social disparities are salient in many forms of developmental psychopathology, such that, on average, more socially and economically disadvantaged children are at increased risk for cognitive, social, emotional, and behavioral problems. Moreover, the prevalence and severity of such problems decrease with each step up the socioeconomic ladder (e.g., Keating & Hertzman, 1999; McLoyd, 1998). Social subordination in early childhood is experienced not only via family socioeconomic circumstances but also by classroom social dominance positions. Remarkably, even at age five and

N.R. Bush, Ph.D. (✉)
Department of Psychiatry,
University of California – San Francisco,
San Francisco, CA 94143, USA
e-mail: BushN@chc.ucsf.edu

W.T. Boyce, M.D.
Professor & Sunny Hill Health Centre/BC Leadership
Chair in Child Development, School of Population
and Public Health, University of British Columbia,
Vancouver, BC V6T 1Z3, Canada
e-mail: tom.boyce@ubc.ca

M. Lewis and K.D. Rudolph (eds.), *Handbook of Developmental Psychopathology*,
DOI 10.1007/978-1-4614-9608-3_15, © Springer Science+Business Media New York 2014

within groups of children from families of comparable SES, classroom social status predicts health and health risk factors (Boyce, 2004, 2007; Goldstein, Trancik, Bensadoun, Boyce, & Adler, 1999). Moreover, childhood SES and social position appear to interact so that the worst outcomes are found among subordinate children from low-SES families (Boyce et al., 2012). Social disparities in health, and the body of evidence examining them, have demanded consideration of how, when, and by what means early life social factors might exert lifelong influence on health.

Although not deterministic, lower social class is generally accompanied by an increased risk for both acute and chronic family, school, and neighborhood stressors (American Psychological Association, 2007), and most studies examining the effects of SES are interested in understanding how constellations of these adverse factors (or their absence) affect health. Using the term "biological embedding" (Hertzman & Wiens, 1996) to describe the process whereby differential human experiences systematically affect health across the life cycle, Hertzman (1999, 2012) provided an articulation of the range of potential processes for these effects. Placing special emphasis on early development, he offered a hypothesis that systematic differences in early environment quality, including emotional and physical support and stimulation, will affect the neurochemistry and shaping of the central nervous system in ways that will adversely affect cognitive, social, and behavioral development. Given the central nervous system's impact on the interpretation of the environment and its important relations with hormone, immune, and clotting systems, Hertzman and Boyce (2010) have argued that systematic differences in life experiences and circumstances will ultimately affect an organism's physiological patterns of response, the "objective" stressfulness of the experiences and circumstances, and the biological interpretation of these experiences and circumstances. Such differences have the potential to alter the long-term structure and function of biological pathways at varying levels of scale and complexity (i.e., neuroendocrine, telomeres, epigenetic marks, neural connectivity, dendritic spine pro-

duction, synaptic strength, etc.), creating socioeconomic differentials in morbidity and mortality that cut across a wide variety of disease processes.

This type of thinking has spurred considerable inquiry into how social environments and experiences "get under the skin" in ways that affect the course of human development. Although myriad biologic processes may be affected by social experience, Hertzman and Boyce (2010) identify candidate systems most likely to transduce social environmental factors into aspects of human biology with the capacity for embedding and influencing the rest of the life course. These four systems are influenced by daily experience, respond to experience throughout an organism's development, have meaningful impacts on health/learning/behavior, are known to function differentially in response to variations in early experience, and comprise the following: (1) the hypothalamic–pituitary–adrenal (HPA) axis and its expression of the glucocorticoid, cortisol; (2) the autonomic nervous system and its neurotransmitters, epinephrine and norepinephrine; (3) the prefrontal cortex, subserving memory, attention, and other executive functions; and (4) systems for social affiliation involving connections between the amygdala, locus coeruleus, and higher order cerebral connections, which are mediated by serotonin and other neurohormones. Other systems, such as the mesolimbic dopamine system, which mediates attentional processes, reward seeking, learning, and behavioral engagement, and biological processes such as epigenetic modifications of neuroregulatory genes and telomerase activity are emerging as likely processes by which biological embedding occurs.

Despite the plausibility of biological embedding and the champions behind it, and that nationally representative studies have shown that adverse experiences early in life predict nearly 45 % of childhood-onset and 30 % of adult-onset psychopathology (Green et al., 2010), there is surprisingly little research on the early life effects of social environment on biology. A recent chapter in "The Biology of Disadvantage" (Seeman, Epel, Gruenewald, Karlamangla, & McEwen, 2010) reviews a significant body of evidence linking low SES with greater risk in downstream peripheral biology in adults—however, only a few studies test those associations, or that of adversity and biology, in child samples, and even fewer examine outcomes such as children's autonomic nervous system reactivity. As is often the case, subfields and individual investigators have approached examination of this phenomenon from varying perspectives and with various measures, with a general focus on pathological outcomes; thus the evidence for biological embedding of early experience clusters around several types of adversity exposures (e.g., socioeconomic predictors for cardiovascular outcomes, rearing condition for HPA axis outcomes), each presumably activating the stress-response system to affect health. Although current understanding limits determination of the unique manner in which varying adversity types affect biology, the risk factors are correlated enough, and the principle mechanisms for how a range of adverse social experiences get under the skin are likely to be similar enough, that much is to be gained by considering the literatures together. Below, we review and highlight research from animal and human studies demonstrating biological embedding as indexed by the best documented social environmental effects on key biological systems and processes.

HPA Axis Regulation

The HPA axis system plays an important role in mammalian stress responses (Gunnar & Vazquez, 2006; Levine, 2005; Sapolsky, Romero, & Munck, 2000; Selye, 1950, 1956) and is a commonly identified biological mechanism by which chronic stress "gets under the skin" (Hertzman & Boyce, 2010; Miller, Chen, & Zhou, 2007), providing the preponderance of evidence for biological embedding thus far. Regulation of the HPA response to stress has been proposed as a vital biological intermediary in the effects of chronic stress on morbidity in general (Cohen, Kesler, & Underwood, 1995) and more specifically on psychiatric disorders such as depression (McEwen, 2000). Cortisol is the human glucocorticoid hormone secreted by the adrenal cortex. Cortisol plays a key facilitative and regulatory role in central nervous system activity, contributing to the processes of learning, memory, emotion, metabolism, and immune response (Sapolsky et al., 2000), yet persistent high concentrations of cortisol can damage or functionally alter brain structures (Sapolsky, 1994).

Research using animal models shows that variations in early rearing conditions—either naturally occurring or externally imposed—can have long-term effects on stress physiology and related behavior (Gunnar & Vazquez, 2006). In rats, even minor interventions such removing the mother for brief periods early in the rat pup's life can bring about a cascade of events that conditions HPA axis functioning over the remainder of the life course (Anisman, Zaharia, Meaney, & Merali, 1998; Meaney, Aitken, Van Berkel, Bhatnagar, & Sapolsky, 1988). These lifelong modifications to HPA axis functioning have been demonstrated to occur through increased maternal licking and grooming behavior that occurs after brief maternal–infant separations or, in some dams, as a predisposition within naturally varying maternal care giving. Such maternal behavior is capable of altering the offspring's corticosterone responses to stress, such that infants experiencing high maternal care have blunted responses to stressful conditions, while those encountering minimal care have substantially higher corticosterone responses. The stress hyporesponsive period (SHRP) in newborn rat pups is thought to stem, at least in part, from the HPA downregulatory changes induced by maternal behavior (de Kloet, Sibug, Helmerhorst, & Schmidt, 2005).

In a nonhuman primate model, an elegantly designed randomized experiment by Suomi and colleagues provides causal evidence for differential early rearing condition effects on HPA axis activity as measured by hair cortisol (Dettmer, Novak, Suomi, & Meyer, 2012). Infant rhesus monkeys exposed to early life adversity in the form of peer rearing demonstrated elevated hair cortisol in infancy and for a year after a relocation stressor, relative to monkeys reared with their mothers, and this appeared to be a biomarker for the later development of anxious behavior in response to a major life stressor. Further, corticotropin-releasing hormone (CRH), the hypothalamic secretagogue for pituitary adreno-corticotropic hormone (ACTH), is itself subject to dysregulatory changes following early stress and adversity. For example, variation in CRH expression follows exposure to early adversity in primates, and such variation can alter down-stream autonomic and behavioral responses to stressors that subserve vigilance, fear, and emotion regulation (Barr et al., 2009).

In humans, a range of adversity factors have also been found to alter the pattern of daily cortisol secretion, such that adversity exposure is associated with both up- and downregulation of HPA axis activation. In general, chronic stressors and adversity have been associated with elevated cortisol expression (see Loman & Gunnar, 2009). Maltreated children, for example, especially those who exhibit internalizing symptoms, show elevated basal cortisol levels across the day, when compared to non-mal-treated children (Cicchetti & Rogosch, 2001; Tarullo & Gunnar, 2006). Even less extreme but aversive home environments can impact HPA axis activity, however, as demonstrated by a study revealing higher cortisol (and alpha-amy-lase) reactivity in toddlers exposed to intrusive, overcontrolling parenting (Taylor et al., 2013). Ethnic minority groups often face discrimination and other social stressors that may also render them more vulnerable to disease, and not surprisingly, such groups have been found to have higher daily cortisol levels, even in adolescence (e.g., DeSantis et al., 2007).

Low SES, an important and prevalent source of adversity exposure (Evans, Chen, Miller, & Seeman, 2012), has been associated with higher cortisol levels in 6-year-old children (Lupien, King, Meaney, & McEwen, 2000) and has also been shown to predict increases in daily cortisol expression across two years within a sample of fifty 9–18-year-old children (Chen, Cohen, & Miller, 2010). Chen et al.'s emerging work provides some of the first longitudinal evidence showing that low SES can alter biological profiles among children over time.

In contrast, *blunted* early morning cortisol and flattened diurnal rhythms have been found in children raised in more extremely adverse environments, such as Romanian and Russian orphanages (Carlson & Earls, 1997; Gunnar & Vazquez, 2001) and some foster care settings in the United States (Dozier et al., 2006). However, blunted daily cortisol has also been found in more typical adverse settings, such as within low-income community kindergarten samples (Bush, Obradovic, Adler, & Boyce, 2011) and in disadvantaged preschool children whose parents' indifference and negativity accounts for the poverty effects on HPA axis blunting (Zalewski, Lengua, Kiff, & Fisher, 2012). Moreover, in a study of children living in low-income, urban areas of Mexico, exposure to maternal depression was linked to lower baseline cortisol and lower cortisol reactivity (Fernald, Burke, & Gunnar, 2008). Blunted cortisol is thought to reflect physiological toughening or steeling (Dienstbier, 1989; Gunnar & Vazquez, 2001), particularly if an individual cannot remove him- or herself from a chronic stressor, and may represent an adaptive biological response to harsh environments. Although there appears to be no direct human equivalent of the SHRP in infant rats, there is increasing evidence that sensitive and responsive parental care is critically essential to the early development of a well-regulated HPA axis (Loman & Gunnar, 2009).

As evidence accumulates, the association between early adverse environments and children's HPA axis functioning has become far more complex than first assumed and varies as a function of adversity types, chronicity, and severity and whether basal diurnal regulation or acute reactivity is examined. Further, our recent longitudinal findings (Bush, Obradovic, et al., 2011) point to the relevance of developmental timing of the exposure, with effects varying by whether cortisol is examined at the beginning or end of the kindergarten year and of racial or cultural differences in associations, with Caucasian and African American children evincing unique patterns of association. Indeed, a meta-analysis of findings from 107 studies of adult samples (Miller et al., 2007) concluded that the research linking stress and the HPA axis is contradictory in that exposure to chronic stress in adulthood was associated with both increased and decreased activation of the HPA axis, with variability in response shaped by stressor and person features as well as timing and individual differences in susceptibility to experience.

Although further clarity on these complex associations is needed, these apparent early life experiential effects on HPA function have implications for developmental psychopathology, as researchers have linked individual differences in both basal and reactive cortisol expression to indices of mental health (Gunnar & Vazquez, 2006). In general, in both clinical and community samples, elevated daily cortisol levels have been associated with internalizing symptoms (e.g., Klimes-Dougan, Hastings, Granger, Usher, & Zahn-Waxler, 2001), including social wariness and depressive symptom severity in kindergarten community samples (Essex, Klein, Cho, & Kalin, 2002; Smider et al., 2002), whereas unusually low levels of daily cortisol have been associated with externalizing symptoms (King, Barkley, & Barrett, 1998; Oosterlaan, Geurts, Knol, & Sergeant, 2005; Shirtcliff, Granger, Booth, & Johnson, 2005). Additionally, studies examining cortisol *changes* over a day in childcare or pre-school in community samples have linked elevated cortisol across the day (relative to the typical circadian decrease during the day) to impulsivity, poor effortful control, peer rejection, and aggression (Dettling, Parker, Lane, Sebanc, & Gunnar, 2000; Gunnar, Sebanc, Tout, Donzella, & van Dulmen, 2003), although, as was true above, findings sometimes suggest a more complex picture depending on timing of assessment and contextual factors such as school settings (Gunnar, Tout, de Haan, Pierce, & Stansbury, 1997; Sumner, Bernard, & Dozier, 2010). Comprehensive understandings of cortisol production view both overactivation (i.e., hypercortisolemia) and deficiency in signaling (hypocortisolemia) as potentially detrimental, with both elevations and declines pathogenic, depending upon the disease measured (Miller et al., 2007), and future models will require refinement to reflect this complexity.

Autonomic Nervous System Regulation

Reactivity within sympathetic (SNS) or parasympathetic (PNS) branches of the autonomic nervous system (ANS) has been targeted as a measure of stress susceptibility because of its role in mobilizing biological resources during "fight or flight" responses to threatening environmental events, as well as regulating recovery from arousal (Berntson, Cacioppo, & Quigley, 1993). Over the past decade, a small group of researchers has investigated associations between SES and measures of cardiovascular physiology in children, in an effort to identify social determinants of precursors to disease. Research has focused on the early life emergence of such disease risk factors, revealing a complex pattern of findings. In cross-sectional research, low SES has been found to be associated with elevated resting blood pressure in children (Chen et al., 2002), greater ambulatory heart rate in adolescents (McGrath, Matthews, & Brady, 2006), and greater blood pressure and heart rate reactivity in adolescents (Chen, Langer, Raphaelson, & Matthews, 2004). Research has also demonstrated that early life neglect and disordered attachment predict greater sympathetic reactivity, as indicated by pre-ejection period, and poorer parasympathetic regulation, as indicated by respiratory sinus arrhythmia, for children in foster care responding to the stressor of the Strange Situation (Oosterman, De Schipper, Fisher, Dozier, & Schuengel, 2010). Across these bodies of evidence, findings suggest that a variety of adverse early life contexts predict increased ANS reactivity as measured by a range of ANS measures. Yet, as was true for the HPA axis, not all evidence points to a positive association between adversity and ANS reactivity.

In a longitudinal study of the effects of SES on autonomic nervous system reactivity in children, Evans and Kim (2007) found that the longer 13-year-olds had lived in poverty, the lower their levels of cardiovascular reactivity in adolescence were, suggesting that their bodies became less efficient in handling environmental demands. Excessive exposure to poverty appeared to operate through cumulative environmental risk exposure and its damaging effects on stress regulatory mechanisms, and such damage has been implicated as the principal mechanism underlying disease etiology (McEwen, 2000, 2007). While it is intriguing that these links have been demonstrated, there are limitations to this research and its interpretation. Findings suggest that low SES is associated with higher resting blood pressure and higher blood pressure reactivity concurrently, but lower blood pressure reactivity years later—not an altogether coherent set of results. Further, each of these studies used only one time point of reactivity, and no studies have examined the relation between SES and *change* in reactivity over time, a necessary step for achieving inference about a causal relationship and establishing whether SES continues to exert effects throughout development by actually shaping physiological regulation. Further longitudinal stress reactivity work is needed to understand these relations in childhood.

Our emerging work (Bush, Adler, & Boyce, 2013) provides some such longitudinal evidence. Within a community sample of 338 ethnically and socioeconomically diverse kindergarten children, we assessed autonomic reactivity (heart rate, HR; respiratory sinus arrhythmia, RSA; and pre-ejection period, PEP) in response to four developmentally challenging tasks (social interview, cognitive recall, lemon juice, and emotional video) in the fall and spring seasons of the kindergarten year (Bush, Alkon, Stamperdahl, Obradović, & Boyce, 2011). Results revealed linkages between SES and developmental changes in children's physiology, such that lower SES children displayed lower HR and PEP reactivity than their upper SES peers. Children from higher SES families, moreover, showed increases in reactivity to challenge over the school year, whereas lower SES children showed dampened reactivity over this time. Consistent with McEwen's allostatic load theory, experiences of children residing in low-SES families appear to lead to downregulated stress physiology.

Brain Circuitry and Function

Mounting evidence from animal studies indicates that stress and environmental factors can contribute to lasting disruptions in brain development. A particularly compelling example is the finding that two weeks of post-weaning isolation in mice led to alteration in prefrontal cortex function and myelination, changes that persisted even after the mice were reintroduced into a social environment (Makinodan, Rosen, Ito, & Corfas, 2012). Evidence from human research is also accumulating, yet it is not well understood what kinds of experiences are important in the development of higher order association cortex or how fundamental aspects of brain plasticity play out in humans. Reviews of the literature indicate that SES is an important predictor of neurocognitive performance, particularly language and executive function, and that even when a group of individuals exhibit equal performance levels, SES differences in neural processing can be detected (Hackman & Farah, 2009). It is challenging, however, to find studies unconfounded by scanner task complexity that explicitly test linkages between brain function and behavioral differences in children from low- and high-adversity environments. One exception is a study involving typically developing nine- and ten-year-old children that used electroencephalography (EEG) of event-related potentials (ERPs) to assess brain function in response to a simple target detection task that could be performed easily by all children independent of SES level. Children of high SES showed more activity and greater responsivity in the prefrontal cortex than did their low-SES peers when confronted with a novel or unexpected stimulus (Kishiyama, Boyce, Jimenez, Perry, & Knight, 2009). In another study offering confirmatory results, D'Angiulli and coworkers (2012) found, in a similar sample of preadolescent children, equivalent prefrontal performance among low- and high-SES children but substantial differences in frontal ERP waveforms, suggesting that low-SES participants utilized supplementary neural resources to attend to both targeted and irrelevant stimuli. Such functional differences in prefrontal cortical responses in lower socioeconomic status may explain why children growing up in resource-poor environments have more trouble with the kinds of behavioral control that the prefrontal cortex is involved in regulating. These findings were further replicated in a study using fMRI in children aged 8–12, demonstrating an association between parental SES and PFC function (Sheridan, Sarsour, Jutte, D'Esposito, & Boyce, 2012). Using measures of language complexity in the home environment and change in salivary cortisol before and after fMRI scanning, this group of researchers demonstrated that language environment and stress reactivity were two likely mechanisms by which SES could come to affect PFC function.

Additionally, in a recent study of 249 older adults that investigated the relations between early adversity and measures of typical brain aging and Alzheimer's disease, investigators found a significant association between childhood SES and magnetic resonance imaging (MRI)-derived hippocampal volume after adjusting for mental ability at age 11 years, adult SES, gender, and education. This finding is consistent with established neurodevelopmental findings that early life conditions have an effect on structural brain development (Staff et al., 2012). Although human research is limited, neuroscientists are beginning to demonstrate that early life stress is also associated with alterations in the structure, function, and connectivity of corticolimbic neural circuits, including the amygdala and ventromedial prefrontal cortex (vmPFC), which subserve the identification of threat and responsivity to challenges and orchestrate adaptive changes in behavior and physiology (Bogdan & Hariri, 2012). The effects of early life environmental challenge on corticolimbic neural circuitry are likely mediated by stress-related alterations in HPA axis function and moderated by genetic variation (Barr et al., 2009).

Profiles of Epigenetic Modification

Epigenetic modification refers to the developmental process by which changes in gene expression or cellular phenotype, including func-

tionally relevant chromatin modifications such as DNA methylation and histone acetylation, are established and inherited without a change in DNA sequence (Meaney, 2010). As understanding of the process advances, epigenetic regulation is also emerging as a key mechanism by which early social environmental signals activate, repress, and maintain genomic responses, thereby contributing to persistent mood and behavior changes that may underlie social gradients in psychopathology (Bredy, Sun, & Kobor, 2010). Here we highlight a few lines of research as illustrations.

Suomi, Szyf, and colleagues have used rigorous randomization experiments in rhesus monkeys to study the effects of typical maternal rearing or attachment-deprived, peer-rearing contexts on DNA methylation in brain and peripheral white blood cells. These contrasting early life-rearing conditions have been shown to predict large differences in stress regulation and phenotypic mental health behaviors that are long-lasting (Conti et al., 2012; Dettmer et al., 2012), and their research demonstrates that epigenetic changes are a likely mechanism for these effects. The researchers found genome-wide absolute differences in methylation between the two rearing conditions, with higher and lower methylation levels for numerous genes in both prefrontal cortex tissue and leukocytes (Provencal et al., 2012).

Although more limited in its ability to support causal inference, human research also provides some evidence for early experience effects on epigenetic marks. For example, Essex and colleagues, in prospective analyses of data from the Wisconsin Study of Families and Work, showed robust associations between early, parent-reported stressors in the infancy and preschool periods and differential methylation of a large number of genes in buccal epithelial cells harvested in mid-adolescence (Essex et al., 2013). Further, mothers' reports of stressors during their children's infancy periods were linked to differential hypermethylation in a large number of CpG dinucleotides in both boys and girls, while fathers' reported stressors in the preschool period covaried with hypomethylation of such sites, primarily in girls. Prospective twin studies also provide compelling evidence in humans that differences in intrauterine environments can influence epigenetic profiles (Saffery et al., 2012). Such data increase confidence in the strength of other prenatal programming research, such as the reported increased methylation within the glucocorticoid (GR) promoter among cord blood samples from neonates born to depressed mothers (Oberlander et al., 2008).

Recent genome-wide methylation analyses on a subset of subjects from both ends of the socioeconomic status spectrum in the 1958 British Cohort Study demonstrated that adult blood DNA methylation profiles show more associations with childhood SES than adult SES and that patterns of association between SES and gene promoter region methylation clustered in specific genomic regions across the genome (Borghol et al., 2012). Both hypo- and hypermethylation were found to be associated with lower early childhood SES, depending upon the functional pathway examined (extracellular signaling, intracellular signaling, DNA signaling, and metabolism). Evidence from such nationally representative epidemiologic studies bolsters the credibility of the assertion that early experience "matters more" than later experiences in the programming of psychobiological response pathways and that effects on key biological processes underlying responsivity to adversity can last a lifetime.

When methylation occurs in gene promoter regions, expression can be altered, and changes in gene methylation patterns are preserved with every cell replication, making socially induced methylation differences potentially functional for long periods of time. Remarkably, animal research has even demonstrated intergenerational transmission of epigenetic changes, highlighting the great importance of early life stress on biology across generations. Our understanding of the complex biological processes examined in current studies of social disparities in epigenetic modification is decidedly nascent. Yet as the cost of measuring DNA methylation decreases and interest in assessing these processes in large, well-characterized, longitudinal samples increases, this area holds tremendous

promise for advancing the field of developmental psychopathology.

Telomeres

Telomeres are specialized nucleoprotein complexes located at the ends of chromosomes that promote chromosomal stability. Telomere shortening, a marker of biological aging that has been linked to psychopathology (Simon et al., 2006; Wolkowitz, Epel, Reus, & Mellon, 2010), may represent an additional cellular-level biomarker of adversity. Despite concerns over the direction of causation in associations between aging and telomere lengths (De Meyer, 2011), recent studies offer strong evidence that telomere and telomerase dysfunction mediate associations between stress, aging, and pathological conditions (De Meyer, 2011; Puterman & Epel, 2012; Sahin et al., 2011). Although a body of evidence within adult samples demonstrates associations between early life stress and telomere shortening (Epel et al., 2004; Shalev, 2012), even showing maternal stress levels during pregnancy predict shorter telomere length in young adulthood (Entringer et al., 2011), almost nothing is known about these processes in childhood.

In one of the first studies examining whether telomere length in childhood is associated with early life experiences, Drury, Theall, and colleagues (2012) found that Romanian children with greater lengths of exposure to institutional care had significantly shorter telomere lengths in middle childhood. Forthcoming work demonstrates an association between maternal psychosocial stress during pregnancy and newborn telomere length (Entringer et al., 2013). Such an early impact on a biomarker of cellular aging suggests its potentially great importance in the pathogenesis of developmental psychopathology. Studies also suggest that heightened biological and psychological responses to acutely stressful situations may play a role in the relation between chronic stress exposure and telomere length (Kroenke et al., 2011; O'Donovan et al., 2012; Tomiyama et al., 2012). Moreover, Puterman and Epel's (2012) review of the animal literature emphasizes that a complete understanding of the effects of experience on telomere length across the life span requires consideration of many positive buffering factors (such as exercise and quality sleep) that may promote resiliency in individuals exposed to chronic stress.

Allostatic Load

Important theoretical work has defined the "allostatic processes" by which an organism achieves stability via brain circuitry mediating continual physiological adjustment to environmental conditions (Ganzel, Morris, & Wethington, 2010; McEwen, 1998, 2007; Sterling & Eyer, 1989). The term "allostatic load" (McEwen & Stellar, 1993) has been used to represent the incurred, cumulative biological costs of homeostatic responses to stressor exposure across physical, social, and cultural contexts. Allostatic load theories posit that, although accommodations to stressors may serve an adaptive or protective function in the short term, chronic or inefficient activation of stress response systems may contribute to growing biological "wear and tear" that results in the emergence of pathogenesis and subsequent, long-term disease outcomes. The allostatic load construct has been a useful heuristic and has been shown to predict disease risk in adulthood (Seeman, Gruenewald, et al., 2010; Seeman, McEwen, Rowe, & Singer, 2001) as well as in children (Evans, Kim, Ting, Tesher, & Shannis, 2007; Theall, Drury, & Shirtcliff, 2012). Much work remains, however, to elucidate *early* life processes that contribute to allostatic load, particularly as they may relate to developmental psychopathology.

Although cumulative indices of physiologic markers may be powerful predictors of developmental and health outcomes (McEwen, 2000; Seeman, Epel, et al., 2010), they can overlook careful consideration of the nuanced manner in which those associations occur. Various biological systems mature at different rates throughout development, and accommodations in one physiologic system can have cascading or countervailing effects in other systems (McEwen,

2007; Sapolsky et al., 2000). These regulatory processes are lost in the simple aggregation of measures of multiple physiologic systems. As we have argued elsewhere (Bush, Obradovic, et al., 2011), the importance of differentiating systems is particularly salient in childhood where much remains to be understood about the way in which physiological systems refine their function and critical periods for those processes. Over time, the functioning of various biological systems may contribute to a combined cumulative biological attrition that we call allostatic load, but that maladaptive synchronization may not yet be present in early childhood.

Sensitive and Critical Periods

Biological embedding is most likely to occur within sensitive periods of development for each of these systems and their neural circuitry underpinnings. Social experiences exert influences even in the early phases of conception and the prenatal and postnatal periods of children's development (Swain, Lorberbaum, Kose, & Strathearn, 2007; Talge, Neal, & Glover, 2007). Although a large degree of maturation at the structural and functional level occurs postnatally, the success of such developmental processes is very much dependent upon the prenatal establishment of fundamental neurobiological architecture that provides the basis for complex human behavior within an ever-changing environment (Hammock & Levitt, 2006).

Sensitive periods in brain and biological development start in the prenatal period, occur frequently in the first few years of life, and are generally thought to continue at a declining rate throughout childhood, with a resurgence in adolescence (Andersen & Teicher, 2008; Fox, Levitt, & Nelson, 2010). However, increasingly, neuroscientists are demonstrating plasticity in neuronal maturation and function in adulthood in brain regions such as the hippocampus (Piatti et al., 2011). Although "critical periods" have been established for the proper formation of vision and language, little is known about critical periods within the developmental course of stress physiology systems in *Homo sapiens*. Accordingly, although concepts such as allostatic load examine cumulative biological changes in adulthood, the phenomena of critical periods or sensitivity "windows" demand careful attention to what is known about the timing of formation of biological systems and their time course of malleability across development. For example, the prefrontal cortex (PFC) shows change in grey matter volume from birth through late adolescence, and such an extended developmental trajectory provides a longtime range of opportunities for experience to shape the function of the PFC. Moreover, there may be gender-specific stress-sensitive periods, given, for example, that it seems that females' amygdala reach adult-like volume in childhood whereas males' volume grows through adolescence (Giedd et al., 1996), and there appears to be gender-specific early life epigenetic regulation of estrogen receptor-α, which has anxiogenic effects and implications for HPA axis regulation (see Bogdan & Hariri, 2012 for discussion). Later in this chapter, we discuss intervention findings that suggest sensitive periods for social effects on neurobiological systems.

Biological Sensitivity to Context

Contexts and experiences do not have universal influence across individual organisms, and psychology has paid particular attention to understanding organismic factors (e.g., impulsivity, fearfulness) that place some individuals at greater risk for development of problems in adverse environments (diathesis stress). More recently, emphasis has shifted to understanding individual difference factors that reliably allow some individuals to be anomalously resilient in the face of adversity (see Luthar, Lyman, & Crossman, 2014; Masten, 2012; Rutter, 2012; Werner, 2012). In particular, an individual's "stress reactivity" appears to be an important individual difference variable that influences the manner in which an organism responds to environmental experiences (Ellis, Boyce, Belsky, Bakermans-Kranenburg, & van Ijzendoorn,

2011; Obradović, Bush, Stamperdahl, Adler, & Boyce, 2010).

Although heightened stress reactivity has traditionally been considered to be a factor that uniformly increases risk, burgeoning empirical evidence suggests instead a "differential susceptibility" to environmental conditions among some individuals who show exaggerated sensitivity or "permeability" to both negative and positive environmental conditions (Belsky, 1997, 2005; Boyce, Chesney, Alkon, et al., 1995; Boyce & Ellis, 2005; Ellis et al., 2011). Specifically, Biological Sensitivity to Context Theory (BSCT) suggests that higher levels of physiologic stress reactivity may promote adaptation in the context of exceptionally supportive environments but exacerbate risk for maladaptive outcomes in exceptionally stressful childhood environments (Boyce, 1996, 2007; Boyce, Chesney, Alkon, et al., 1995; Boyce & Ellis, 2005; Ellis, Essex, & Boyce, 2005b). The theory is consistent with research on behavioral reactivity indicating that children with high levels of negative affectivity are particularly susceptible to both negative and positive experiences (Belsky, Bakermans-Kranenburg, & Van IJzendoorn, 2007) and also corresponds with recent research showing that genetic polymorphisms can moderate the effects of adversity on adaptive functioning (see Belsky & Pluess, 2009 for a review; Bush, Guendelman, Adler, & Boyce, 2013a).

Paralleling research on the biological embedding of adversity, a range of factors, across multiple levels of biology, have been thought to represent or subserve neurobiological sensitivity to social contexts, including genetic variation, chromatin modification, gene transcriptional control, ANS and HPA activation, and differences in brain structure and functions. The dominant lines of BSC research have tested differential susceptibility models by demonstrating interactive effects between various types of contextual stress (e.g., marital conflict, financial stress, parental psychopathology) and psychobiological reactivity in the prediction of health outcomes (e.g., Belsky & Pluess, 2009; Boyce, Chesney, Alkon–Leonard, et al., 1995; Obradović et al., 2010). Such research finds support for the claim that associations between risky and supportive environmental exposures and adaptation vary across different levels of stress reactivity.

Studies demonstrating this greater susceptibility of neurobiologically responsive children to both positive and negative aspects of their environments have now included a wide variety of the following: *stressors,* including peer victimization and aggression (Rudolph, Troop-Gordon, & Granger, 2010, 2011), parental depression and antisocial behavior (Cummings, El-Sheikh, Kouros, & Keller, 2007; Shannon, Beauchaine, Brenner, Neuhaus, & Gatzke-Kopp, 2007), marital conflict (El-Sheikh, 2005; El-Sheikh, Keller, & Erath, 2007), and overall family adversity (Obradović et al., 2010); *positive environments,* including parental warmth (Ellis, McFadyen-Ketchum, Dodge, Pettit, & Bates, 1999) and supportive interventions (Bakermans-Kranenburg, Van, Pijlman, Mesman, & Juffer, 2008); and *biological measurement levels,* including physiological reactivity (Alkon et al., 2006; Boyce, Chesney, Alkon, et al., 1995), structural and functional differences in brain circuitry (Whittle et al., 2011), and gene polymorphisms (Knafo, Israel, & Ebstein, 2011).

More recently, we have investigated the manner in which "stress-sensitive" alleles moderate the effects of early life adversity on stress physiology. Exploring the established negative association between SES and chronic cortisol arousal in children, Bush and colleagues found that 5HTTLPR and BDNF genotype moderated the effects of early life family SES on children's chronic daily cortisol arousal (Bush, Guendelman, Adler, & Boyce, 2013a; Bush, Guendelman, Adler, & Boyce, 2013b), such that children with the "l/l" genotype of the serotonin transporter or who are carriers of the BDNF met allele had the highest chronic cortisol levels when growing up in low-SES homes, but the lowest levels when growing up in high-SES homes. Strikingly, for "s" carriers and Val/val genotypes, SES did not affect chronic daily cortisol levels. Beyond providing additional examples of BSC (and contributing to the small literature demonstrating that "l/l" genotypes are most "sensitive" to some environments), this

work highlights how susceptibility via one biomarker (genes) can influence stress sensitivity in other systems (HPA axis arousal).

Within the BSCT body of work, Boyce and Ellis (2005) also argue, in the second, less extensively explored component of the theory, for the importance of considering U-shaped associations, predicted from evolutionary principles, between the stressful versus supportive character of early rearing environments and the proportion of individuals evincing highly reactive phenotypes. The second of the 2005 papers advancing the differential susceptibility theory provided provisional evidence from two studies supporting the postulated U-shaped association between adversity and the prevalence of high-reactivity phenotypes (Ellis, Essex, & Boyce, 2005a). The character of early contextual experiences likely plays a role, through conditional adaptations, in *shaping* the development of children's physiology. Those raised in stimulating and nurturing contexts may disproportionately acquire heightened biological sensitivity as a means of maximizing the advantages of resources and opportunities therein. On the other hand, children reared in harsh, threatening environments might also develop greater biological sensitivity in order to enhance vigilance to threats and other hazards. In contrast, the majority of children, raised within species-typical environments falling within these two extremes, may acquire diminished, more normative biological sensitivity, as the environments to which they are exposed are neither highly nurturing nor highly threatening (see Ellis & Boyce, 2011; Ellis et al., 2011 for the full argument in this regard). More recently, the concept of differential susceptibility has been embellished in a more detailed evolutionary framework referred to as the "Adaptive Calibration Model" (Del Giudice, Ellis, & Shirtcliff, 2011).

Boyce, Ellis, and colleagues thus suggest that high-reactivity phenotypes will be most prevalent in the contexts of low- and high-adversity exposure. In accordance with this theory, a U-shaped association between adversity and physiologic reactivity could provide for diverging trajectories of subsequent mental health over time. For example, although high reactivity may be adaptive across very low- and very high-stress contexts in the short term, as high reactivity becomes established (i.e., canalized), subsequent exposures to adversity over time would predispose the highly reactive individual to disorders of mental health. However, only longitudinal studies of the interplay between environmental effects and stress reactivity, starting with prenatal development and within broadly variable social contexts, can provide credible empirical evidence for this hypothesis. Moreover, to date, research has rarely considered U-shaped associations despite the value to be gained from understanding with greater precision the shape of associations between contextual stressors and the biological systems that contribute to psychopathology.

Three recent papers do explore curvilinear influences of early environmental stressors on the development of physiologic systems, specifically the HPA axis. Gunnar, Frenn, Wewerka, and Van Ryzin (2009) reported that children with moderate levels of early life adversity demonstrated lower cortisol reactivity to laboratory stressors than did children with either low or high levels of adversity, providing additional evidence for curvilinear associations between early life stress and HPA axis regulation. A second study, using a sample of young adults, found a curvilinear effect in the opposite direction from that proposed by BSC theory and found in Gunnar et al.'s study. Engert et al. (2010) found evidence for an inverted U-shaped relation between retrospective self-report of levels of maternal care received in childhood and young adults' cortisol stress reactivity, such that stress-induced cortisol levels for low and high maternal care groups were lower than for those in medium-care group. Such divergent patterns found between studies may result from meaningful differences in developmental timing of physiological assessment, intensity of the stressors, and factors such as retrospective reporting of stressors versus concurrent or prospective assessments. Both studies examine effects on reactivity to laboratory stressors, which may not generalize to daily levels of physiologic load that are more relevant to allo-

static load. A third paper, a review by Macri et al. (Macri, Zoratto, & Laviola, 2011), summarizes evidence from laboratory rodent studies and suggests that the link between neonatal stress exposures and adult phenotypic reactivity follows a U-shaped, curvilinear relation. The conclusions of these three papers support, at the very least, further consideration of curvilinear associations between early life stress and HPA axis regulation.

Recent work from our laboratory provides some additional evidence. Using an ethnically diverse longitudinal sample of 338 kindergarten children, we examined the effects of cumulative contextual stressors on children's developing HPA axis regulation (Bush, Obradovic, et al., 2011). Chronic HPA axis regulation was assessed using cumulative, multiday measures of cortisol in both the fall and spring seasons of the kindergarten year. Hierarchical linear regression analyses revealed that contextual stressors related to ethnic minority status, SES, and family adversity each uniquely predicted children's daily HPA activity and that some of those associations were curvilinear in conformation. Results showed that the quadratic, U-shaped influences of family SES and family adversity operate in different directions to predict children's HPA axis regulation such that children from both the low- and high-SES families demonstrated higher levels of daily cortisol than their peers from middle-SES families and children from families with moderate adversity demonstrated higher daily cortisol than did those at either ends of the adversity continuum. Results further suggested that these associations differed for white and ethnic minority children, with the opposing patterns of findings potentially reflecting different biological responses to environmental adversity by subgroup and/or different ranges of exposure to the stressors within subgroups. In total, this study revealed that early childhood experiences contribute to shifts in one of the principal neurobiological systems thought to contribute to allostatic load, and findings suggested that analyses of allostatic load and developmental theories accounting for its accrual would benefit from an inclusion of curvilinear associations in tested predictive models.

Evidence of BSC Within "Positive" Environments

As a result of the field's focus on contextual risk for pathology over contexts that promote optimal development, the majority of studies reviewed above emphasize the negative impacts of adverse exposures or deprivation on children's neurobiology. These studies tell us little about whether enriched environments produce optimized neurobiological development of the same magnitude as that negatively affected by adverse environments. Moreover, we cannot yet be certain whether extremely enriched contexts might counteract detrimental effects of adversity or themselves contribute to such effects, as shown in a recently reported mouse experiment (Christakis, Ramirez, & Ramirez, 2012). Examination of intervention efforts with children exposed to early adversity and possessing stress reactivity phenotypes will broaden evidence for how contextual experience can shape the development of children's physiology.

The Bucharest Early Intervention Project is a novel study where institutionally reared Romanian children who had been abandoned in the first few years of life were randomized to either remain under institutional care or be placed in (relatively) enriched environments via in-home foster care placements (Nelson et al., 2007). It has provided compelling evidence for differential susceptibility to adversity and intervention effects (i.e., both negative and positive environments) (Drury, Gleason, et al., 2012). Specifically, children with either of the "more sensitive" genotypes (in this study, the 5HTTLPR s/s or BDNF Val66Met met carriers) demonstrated the *lowest* levels of indiscriminate behavior in the enriched foster care environment and the *highest* levels in the continued institutionalization context. Children with either of the "less sensitive" alleles (in this study, 5HTTLPR l-carriers or of BDNF val/val) demonstrated little difference in levels of indiscriminate behaviors over time and no group x genotype interaction. Strikingly, this pattern was amplified when GxGxE tests were conducted, revealing that the BSC effect was largest for children with both

sensitive genotypes relative to those with just one; children with no plasticity alleles demonstrated no intervention effect on levels of indiscriminate behavior over time. These findings add to the growing body of literature supporting a differential susceptibility model of gene × environment interactions in developmental psychopathology, but it remains to be seen whether the differential effects on behavior are mediated by individual's neurobiological changes.

Thus far, the limited empirical investigation of intensive interventions suggests that some effects of biological embedding are not entirely reversible but can be overcome. For example, animal models demonstrate that rat pups deprived of maternal care have reduced hippocampal volume and poorer hippocampal-dependent learning compared to pups with enriched maternal care. Creating peripubertal "enriched care" environments for the deprived pups, however, led to learning and memory aptitude similar to high-care pups (Bredy, Humpartzoomian, Cain, & Meaney, 2003). Importantly, these improvements in function occurred without accompanying changes in hippocampal volume, suggesting that malleable early life mechanisms allow for compensatory pathways to provide for typical behavior despite enduring structural deficits.

Additional promise for recovery through intervention can be found in the recent results of Suomi's primate rearing experiment, described above. Although peer-reared monkeys exhibited higher cortisol levels in infancy and in response to stress, 16 months after monkeys were relocated to a large social environment consisting of infants from all three experimental rearing conditions, all rearing groups were indistinguishable from one another physiologically and behaviorally (Dettmer et al., 2012), suggesting transition to more normative environments can allow for recalibration of systems.

The Bucharest Early Intervention Project has also shown that early intervention to correct a deeply impoverished early environment can improve brain structure and function as well as cognitive and emotional capabilities. Examination of brain structure and function using MRI and EEG techniques revealed that children randomized to the intervention exhibited increased cortical white matter, relative to children remaining in institutions (Sheridan, Fox, Zeanah, McLaughlin, & Nelson, 2012). This finding suggests the potential for "catch up" brain growth in human children, even following extreme deprivation. Further results point to behavioral improvements as well, indicating that children in the foster care intervention demonstrated higher levels of positive affect and attention at both 30 and 42 months of age and improved cognitive outcomes at age 42 and 54 months, compared to children who remained institutionalized (Ghera et al., 2009; Nelson et al., 2007). Children who were transitioned to foster care at earlier ages demonstrated the most marked improvements, suggesting possible sensitive periods for cognitive development. Studies of foster care children living in the United States have similarly provided evidence that psychosocial interventions may indeed modify children's disrupted biological systems, such as cortisol diurnal rhythms (Dozier et al., 2006; Fisher, Stoolmiller, Gunnar, & Burraston, 2007). Together, these observed associations suggest some negative effects on neurobiology can be reversed or compensated for with early childhood interventions, emphasizing the importance of both enrichment and adversity-reduction interventions in creating good developmental environments for all children.

Is Reactivity or Sensitivity "Maladaptive"?

The identification of factors contributing to the activation and dysregulation of physiological systems designed to maintain the allostatic balance has been thought of as essential for the design of prevention/intervention efforts (Lupien et al., 2006). However, in recent years, scholars have begun to consider that the alterations in individual biological systems in response to environmental adversity, although sometimes seen as "harmful" or "maladaptive," may actually be an appropriate physiologic coping response to the organism's physical or social context. Thus, rather than being interpreted as pathogenic, high reactivity would index heightened biological

sensitivity to the quality of the environment, a characteristic with demonstrable adaptive features in certain rearing environments. Studies in rats and monkeys, for example, have revealed that "negative" neurobiological effects of "low-quality" maternal care can actually contribute to adaptive physiologic and behavioral responses under future stressful conditions (Lyons, Parker, & Schatzberg, 2010; Oomen et al., 2010). Human children exhibiting muted or hyperreactivity in adverse contexts might be responding adaptively to chronic stressors, and although such physiological system modifications may do harm in the long run (e.g., allostatic load effects on pathology), they likely allow for improved functioning over the short term. Also, modifications such as enhanced amygdala reactivity to neutral stimuli (Tottenham & Sheridan, 2010) may be a favorable response for children living in a high-crime neighborhood, protecting one from physical harm albeit increasing risk for affective dysregulation. As such, variation in physiological outcomes sometimes found for minorities (e.g., Bush, Obradovic, et al., 2011), relative to majority population levels, may be legitimately adaptive to contextual demands and might also reflect unique population characteristics that have other value for those populations (Garcia-Coll, Akerman, & Cicchetti, 2000).

Biological Pathways Linking Early Life Experience to Later Psychopathology

Throughout this chapter, we have focused on highlighting the accumulating evidence for biological embedding of early experience and the manner in which biological sensitivity can moderate the effects of stress on developing physiology and behavior. Far less empirical evidence exists for explicit examination of these processes linking early adversity with subsequent psychopathology (Pollak, 2005). In rat and nonhuman primate studies, adverse early life exposures, such as maternal separation or low-quality maternal care, have been shown to result in subsequent HPA axis, autonomic and immune system changes in response to stress, as well as marked behavioral changes in adulthood such as anxiety-like behavior, anhedonia, social dysfunction, predisposition to alcohol abuse, decreased appetite, and sleep disruptions (Dettmer et al., 2012; Liu et al., 1997; Plotsky & Meaney, 1993; Provencal et al., 2012; Sanchez, Ladd, & Plotsky, 2001). Although animal research lends itself to the rigorous study of environmental effects on biology, it has limitations in its ability to model human experiences of early life stress or developmental psychopathology. On the other hand, researchers studying children with mental health problems find it challenging to incorporate biological assessment into their studies and to follow individuals for the long periods of time required to assess these life course processes. Burghy and colleagues provide a particularly useful study that bridges several of the concepts reviewed above (Burghy et al., 2012). Their findings suggest that stress exposure during infancy increases adolescent depression and anxiety and decreases amygdala-vmPFC resting-state connectivity via cortisol elevations in childhood. They also reveal important gender differences for this vulnerability to dysregulated affect, as well as a developmental sensitive period for these effects. The sample size of 66 youth merits caution for generalization of the findings, but the rich breadth of longitudinal data, strong theory-driven hypotheses, and sophisticated statistical modeling in this study make it an exemplar of the advances being made in this area.

One impediment to uncovering the relations between adversity and psychopathology is that the majority of behavioral and emotional pathologies are likely to result from constellations of aberrant biological systems. Considerable recent attention has been given to early adverse experience effects on the complex and varied neurobiology of depression (Bogdan & Hariri, 2012; Heim, Plotsky, & Nemeroff, 2004). For example, progressive effects on developing stress physiology might explain findings supporting the "kindling hypothesis," in which an increase in spontaneous dysregulation or a lowering of the threshold for experiencing life stressors leads to easier triggering of depressive episodes (Monroe

& Harkness, 2005). As precise, biologically plausible models of psychopathology that consider multiple stress-response systems are developed (Pollak, 2005), our ability to seek and understand the manner in which early experience manifests as health and pathology will be greatly improved as well.

Future Directions

The body of work reviewed in this chapter is advancing, and the opportunities for new research are vast. Although the developmental sequelae of early adversity are well documented, current understanding of the manner in which those experiences "get under the skin" to specifically affect psychopathology is quite limited. Going forward, the most important advances will derive from analyses of prospective, longitudinal datasets that allow for improved inference regarding causal effects of early experience on biological development and subsequent mental health. Understanding the developmental etiology of physiologic function across systems is important in its own right, but these physiologic systems are also mechanisms for the effects of environment on psychopathology and also moderators of the effects of concurrent and later-occurring experiences. Future inquiry should investigate specific pathways through which biological stress responses, shaped by early life adversity, contribute to the development of psychopathology. Building upon informative animal models, various pathways have been proposed, yet few are tested longitudinally in humans as was done by Burghy et al. (2012) described above. When investigating depression, for example, ANS and HPA axis dysregulation are likely to impact cognitive appraisals, emotional and reward processing, and behavior in a manner that heightens risk for prodromes of depression such as anhedonia, social withdrawal, and emotional dysregulation. Early life adversity, such as peer victimization, may lead to ineffective coping behaviors such as rumination, particularly for stress-sensitive children, which eventually may lead to depression, as suggested by Rudolph and colleagues (2011).

Explicit tests of these types of pathways will provide crucial information for the prevention of psychopathology. Additionally, with advances in neuroscience and human molecular genetics, next steps include identifying common variation in the genes and their expression that influence the functioning or availability of components in these stress-disease pathways.

Future work must also advance theory. For example, there is the need for research to determine whether these behavioral, physiologic, and genetic markers of susceptibility to contextual factors constitute the same phenomena expressed at different levels of assessment or represent different types of susceptibility (Obradović & Boyce, 2009). Along these lines, Belsky and Pluess (2013) propose that there are "plasticity phenotypes" such that, rather than just having plasticity in specific systems or genes, individuals as a whole can be seen as differentially susceptible or not to environment. Additionally, the burgeoning field of cultural neuroscience suggests that cultural factors are important contexts that shape neurobiology and require further consideration than has been given previously (Chiao, 2009). All of these endeavors should take account of the breadth of positive buffering factors that operate across the life span, which will take us a step further in understanding healthy behavioral and emotional development.

Such apparent malleability of biological processes by contextual influences points to the value of integrating biological measures into the design and evaluation of preventive interventions (Cicchetti & Gunnar, 2008). In particular, given its ease of collection and low cost for assay, daily cortisol arousal or cortisol reactivity is beginning to prove useful for detecting effects of interventions (Fisher et al., 2007). As costs go down for other neurobiological assessments, feasibility of using sophisticated biomarkers to advance our interventions for psychopathology will improve, such as demonstrating improvements in neural development (Sheridan, Fox, et al., 2012).

In reviewing this literature, we hope to stimulate a new generation of research that will illuminate the manner in which early life contexts interact with children's biology to predict health

and pathology as well as shape children's developing biology. We hope this work supports powerful insights into both typical and atypical development of children and will highlight clear opportunities for the prevention of the development of psychopathology. For the millions of children around the world who begin their lives in adverse circumstances, we should heed the evidence for sensitive periods of development and biological embedding of experience and act to improve their lives before neurobiological processes become well established and place them at risk for psychopathology.

References

Adler, N. E., Boyce, W. T., Chesney, M. A., Cohen, S., Folkman, S., Kahn, R. L., et al. (1994). Socioeconomic status and health: The challenge of the gradient. *American Psychologist, 49*(1), 15–24.

Adler, N. E., Bush, N. R., & Pantell, M. S. (2012). Rigor, vigor, and the study of health disparities. *Proceedings of the National Academy of Sciences of the United States of America, 109*, 17154–17159. doi:10.1073/pnas.1121399109.

Adler, N. E., & Stewart, J. (2010). Preface to the biology of disadvantage: Socioeconomic status and health. *Annals of the New York Academy of Sciences, 1186*, 1–4. NYAS5385 [pii]10.1111/j.1749-6632.2009.05385.x.

Alkon, A., Lippert, S., Vujan, N., Rodriquez, M. E., Boyce, W. T., & Eskenazi, B. (2006). The ontogeny of autonomic measures in 6- and 12-month-old infants. *Developmental Psychobiology, 48*(3), 197–208. doi:10.1002/dev.20129.

American Psychological Association, T. F. o. S. S. (2007). *Report of the APA task force on socioeconomic status*. Washington, DC: American Psychological Association.

Andersen, S. L., & Teicher, M. H. (2008). Stress, sensitive periods and maturational events in adolescent depression. *Trends in Neurosciences, 31*(4), 183–191. http://dx.doi.org/10.1016/j.tins.2008.01.004.

Anisman, H., Zaharia, M. D., Meaney, M. J., & Merali, Z. (1998). Do early-life events permanently alter behavioral and hormonal responses to stressors? *International Journal of Developmental Neuroscience, 16*(3–4), 149–164.

Bakermans-Kranenburg, M. J., Van, I. M. H., Pijlman, F. T., Mesman, J., & Juffer, F. (2008). Experimental evidence for differential susceptibility: Dopamine D4 receptor polymorphism (DRD4 VNTR) moderates intervention effects on toddlers' externalizing behavior in a randomized controlled trial. *Developmental Psychology, 44*(1), 293–300. doi:10.1037/0012-1649.44.1.293. 2007-19851-030 [pii].

Barr, C. S., Dvoskin, R. L., Gupte, M., Sommer, W., Sun, H., Schwandt, M. L., et al. (2009). Functional CRH variation increases stress-induced alcohol consumption in primates. *Proceedings of the National Academy of Sciences of the United States of America, 106*(34), 14593–14598. doi:10.1073/pnas.0902863106.

Belsky, J. (1997). Variation in susceptibility to environmental influence: An evolutionary argument. *Psychological Inquiry, 8*(3), 182–186.

Belsky, J. (2005). Differential susceptibility to rearing influence: An evolutionary hypothesis and some evidence. In B. Ellis & D. Bjorklund (Eds.), *Origins of the social mind: Evolutionary psychology and child development* (pp. 139–163). New York: Guilford Press.

Belsky, J., Bakermans-Kranenburg, M. J., & Van IJzendoorn, M. H. (2007). For better and for worse: Differential susceptibility to environmental influences. *Current Directions in Psychological Science, 16*(6), 300–304.

Belsky, J., & Pluess, M. (2009). Beyond diathesis stress: Differential susceptibility to environmental influences. *Psychological Bulletin, 135*(6), 885–908. 2009-19763-005 [pii]10.1037/a0017376.

Belsky, J., & Pluess, M. (2013). Beyond risk, resilience and dysregulation: Phenotypic plasticity and human development. *Development & Psychopathology, 25,* 1243–1261.

Berntson, G. G., Cacioppo, J. T., & Quigley, K. S. (1993). Cardiac psychophysiology and autonomic space in humans: Empirical perspectives and conceptual implications. *Psychological Bulletin, 114*(2), 296–322.

Bogdan, R., & Hariri, A. R. (2012). Neural embedding of stress reactivity. [10.1038/nn.3270]. *Nature Neuroscience, 15*(12), 1605–1607.

Borghol, N., Suderman, M., McArdle, W., Racine, A., Hallett, M., Pembrey, M., et al. (2012). Associations with early-life socio-economic position in adult DNA methylation. *International Journal of Epidemiology, 41*(1), 62–74. doi:10.1093/ije/dyr147.

Boyce, W. T. (1996). Biobehavioral reactivity and injuries in children and adolescents. In M. H. Bornstein & J. Genevro (Eds.), *Child development and behavioral pediatrics: Toward understanding children and health.* Mahwah, NJ: Erlbaum.

Boyce, W. T. (2004). Social stratification, health and violence in the very young. *Annals of the New York Academy of Sciences, 1036,* 47–68.

Boyce, W. T. (2007). A biology of misfortune: Stress reactivity, social context, and the ontogeny of psychopathology in early life. In A. Masten (Ed.), *Multilevel dynamics in developmental psychopathology: Pathways to the future* (34th ed., pp. 45–82). Minneapolis, MN: University of Minnesota.

Boyce, W. T., Chesney, M., Alkon–Leonard, A., Tschann, J., Adams, S., Chesterman, B., et al. (1995). Psychobiologic reactivity to stress and childhood respiratory illnesses: Results of two prospective studies. *Psychosomatic Medicine, 57,* 411–422.

Boyce, W. T., & Ellis, B. J. (2005). Biological sensitivity to context: I. An evolutionary–developmental theory of the origins and functions of stress reactivity. *Development and Psychopathology, 17*(2), 271–301.

Boyce, W. T., Obradović, J., Bush, N. R., Stamperdahl, J., Kim, Y. S., & Adler, N. E. (2012). Social stratification, classroom climate, and the behavioral adaptation of kindergarten children. Proceedings of the National Academy of Sciences. doi: 10.1073/pnas.1201730109.

Braveman, P., & Egerter, S. (2008). *Overcoming obstacles to health: Report to the Robert Wood Johnson Foundation Commission to build a healthier America.* Princeton, NJ: Robert Wood Johnson Foundation. Retrieved from http://www.commissiononhealth.org

Bredy, T. W., Humpartzoomian, R. A., Cain, D. P., & Meaney, M. J. (2003). Partial reversal of the effect of maternal care on cognitive function through environmental enrichment. *Neuroscience, 118*(2), 571–576. doi:10.1016/s0306-4522(02)00918-1.

Bredy, T. W., Sun, Y. E., & Kobor, M. S. (2010). How the epigenome contributes to the development of psychiatric disorders. [Research Support, N.I.H., Extramural Research Support, Non-U.S. Gov't Review]. *Developmental Psychobiology, 52*(4), 331–342.

Burghy, C. A., Stodola, D. E., Ruttle, P. L., Molloy, E. K., Armstrong, J. M., Oler, J. A., et al. (2012). Developmental pathways to amygdala-prefrontal function and internalizing symptoms in adolescence. [10.1038/nn.3257]. *Nature Neuroscience, 15*(12), 1736–1741. doi: http://www.nature.com/neuro/journal/v15/n12/abs/nn.3257.html#supplementary-information

Bush, N. R., Adler, N., & Boyce, W. T. (2013). *Mechanisms for socioeconomic health disparities: SES predicts longitudinal change in children's ANS reactivity.* Unpublished work.

Bush, N. R., Alkon, A., Stamperdahl, J., Obradović, J., & Boyce, W. T. (2011). Differentiating challenge reactivity from psychomotor activity in studies of children's psychophysiology: Considerations for theory and measurement. *Journal of Experimental Child Psychology, 110*(1), 62–79.

Bush, N. R., Guendelman, M., Adler, N. E., & Boyce, W. T. (2013a). *BDNF allelic variants moderate social disparities in children's chronic cortisol expression.* Manuscript submitted for publication.

Bush, N. R., Guendelman, M., Adler, N. E., & Boyce, W. T. (2013b). *Serotonin transporter allelic variants moderate social disparities in children's chronic cortisol expression.* Unpublished manuscript.

Bush, N. R., Obradovic, J., Adler, N., & Boyce, W. T. (2011). Kindergarten stressors and cumulative adrenocortical activation: The "first straws" of allostatic load? *Development and Psychopathology, 23*(4), 1089–1106. doi:10.1017/s0954579411000514.

Carlson, M., & Earls, F. (1997). Psychological and neuroendocrinological sequelae of early social deprivation in institutionalized children in Romania. *Annals of the New York Academy of Sciences, 807,* 419–428.

Chen, E., Cohen, S., & Miller, G. E. (2010). How low socioeconomic status affects 2-year hormonal trajectories in children. *Psychological Science, 21*(1), 31–37. doi:10.1177/0956797609355566.

Chen, E., Langer, D. A., Raphaelson, Y. E., & Matthews, K. A. (2004). Socioeconomic status and health in adolescents: The role of stress interpretations. *Child Development, 75*(4), 1039–1052.

Chen, E., Matthews, K. A., & Boyce, W. T. (2002). Socioeconomic differences in children's health: How and why do these relationships change with age? *Psychological Bulletin, 128*(2), 295–329.

Chiao, J. Y. (2009). Cultural neuroscience: A once and future discipline. In Y. C. Joan (Ed.), *Progress in brain research* (Vol. 178, pp. 287–304). Amsterdam: Elsevier.

Christakis, D. A., Ramirez, J. S. B., & Ramirez, J. M. (2012). Overstimulation of newborn mice leads to behavioral differences and deficits in cognitive performance. *Scientific Reports, 2*. doi: 10.1038/srep00546

Cicchetti, D., & Gunnar, M. (2008). Integrating biological measures into the design and evaluation of preventative interventions. *Development and Psychopathology, 20*, 737–743.

Cicchetti, D., & Rogosch, F. A. (2001). The impact of child maltreatment and psychopathology on neuroendocrine functioning. *Development and Psychopathology, 13*(4), 783–804.

Cohen, S., Janicki-Deverts, D., Chen, E., & Matthews, K. A. (2010). Childhood socioeconomic status and adult health. *Annals of the New York Academy of Sciences, 1186*(1), 37–55. doi:10.1111/j.1749-6632.2009.05334.x.

Cohen, S., Kesler, R., & Underwood, L. (1995). Strategies for measuring stress in studies of psychiatric and physical disorders. In R. Cohen, R. C. Kessler, & L. G. Underwood (Eds.), *Measuring stress: A guide for health and social scientists* (pp. 3–28). New York: Oxford University Press.

Conti, G., Hansman, C., Heckman, J. J., Novak, M. F. X., Ruggiero, A., & Suomi, S. J. (2012). Primate evidence on the late health effects of early-life adversity. *Proceedings of the National Academy of Sciences of the United States of America, 109*(23), 8866–8871. doi:10.1073/pnas.1205340109.

Cummings, E. M., El-Sheikh, M., Kouros, C. D., & Keller, P. S. (2007). Children's skin conductance reactivity as a mechanism of risk in the context of parental depressive symptoms. *Journal of Child Psychology and Psychiatry, 48*(5), 436–445. JCPP1713 [pii] 10.1111/j.1469-7610.2006.01713.x.

D'Angiulli, A., Van Roon, P. M., Weinberg, J., Oberlander, T. F., Grunau, R. E., Hertzman, C., et al. (2012). Frontal EEG/ERP correlates of attentional processes, cortisol and motivational states in adolescents from lower and higher socioeconomic status. *Frontiers in Human Neuroscience, 6*. doi: 10.3389/fnhum.2012.00306.

de Kloet, E. R., Sibug, R. M., Helmerhorst, F. M., & Schmidt, M. (2005). Stress, genes and the mechanism of programming the brain for later life. *Neuroscience and Biobehavioral Reviews, 29*(2), 271–281. doi:10.1016/j.neubiorev.2004.10.008.

De Meyer, T. (2011). Telomere length integrates psychological factors in the successful aging story, but what about the biology? *Psychosomatic Medicine, 73*(7), 524–527. doi:10.1097/PSY.0b013e31822ed876.

Del Giudice, M., Ellis, B. J., & Shirtcliff, E. A. (2011). The adaptive calibration model of stress responsivity [Research Support, N.I.H., Extramural Research Support, Non-U.S. Gov't Review]. *Neuroscience and Biobehavioral Reviews, 35*(7), 1562–1592.

DeSantis, A. S., Adam, E. K., Doane, L. D., Mineka, S., Zinbarg, R. E., & Craske, M. G. (2007). Racial/ethnic differences in cortisol diurnal rhythms in a community sample of adolescents. *The Journal of Adolescent Health, 41*(1), 3–13. doi:10.1016/j.jadohealth.2007.03.006.

Dettling, A. C., Parker, S. W., Lane, S., Sebanc, A., & Gunnar, M. R. (2000). Quality of care and temperament determine changes in cortisol concentrations over the day for young children in childcare. *Psychoneuroendocrinology, 25*(8), 819–836.

Dettmer, A. M., Novak, M. A., Suomi, S. J., & Meyer, J. S. (2012). Physiological and behavioral adaptation to relocation stress in differentially reared rhesus monkeys: Hair cortisol as a biomarker for anxiety-related responses. *Psychoneuroendocrinology, 37*(2), 191–199. doi:10.1016/j.psyneuen.2011.06.003.

Dienstbier, R. A. (1989). Arousal and physiological toughness – Implications for mental and physical health. *Psychological Review, 96*(1), 84–100.

Dozier, M., Manni, M., Gordon, M. K., Peloso, E., Gunnar, M. R., Stovall-McClough, K. C., et al. (2006). Foster children's diurnal production of cortisol: An exploratory study. *Child Maltreatment, 11*(2), 189–197. doi:10.1177/1077559505285779.

Drury, S. S., Gleason, M. M., Theall, K. P., Smyke, A. T., Nelson, C. A., Fox, N. A., et al. (2012). Genetic sensitivity to the caregiving context: The influence of 5httlpr and BDNF val66met on indiscriminate social behavior. *Physiology & Behavior, 106*(5), 728–735. doi:10.1016/j.physbeh.2011.11.014.

Drury, S. S., Theall, K., Gleason, M. M., Smyke, A. T., De Vivo, I., Wong, J. Y. Y., et al. (2012). Telomere length and early severe social deprivation: Linking early adversity and cellular aging. *Molecular Psychiatry, 17*(7), 719–727. doi:10.1038/mp.2011.53.

Ellis, B. J., & Boyce, W. T. (2011). Differential susceptibility to the environment: Toward an understanding of sensitivity to developmental experiences and context. *Development and Psychopathology, 23*(1), 1–5. doi:10.1017/s095457941000060x.

Ellis, B. J., Boyce, W. T., Belsky, J., Bakermans-Kranenburg, M. J., & van Ijzendoorn, M. H. (2011). Differential susceptibility to the environment: An evolutionary-neurodevelopmental theory. *Development and Psychopathology, 23*(1), 7–28. doi:10.1017/s0954579410000611.

Ellis, B. J., Essex, M. J., & Boyce, W. T. (2005). Biological sensitivity to context: II. Empirical explorations of an evolutionary-developmental theory. *Development and Psychopathology, 17*(2), 303–328.

Ellis, B. J., McFadyen-Ketchum, S., Dodge, K. A., Pettit, G. S., & Bates, J. E. (1999). Quality of early family relationships and individual differences in the timing of pubertal maturation in girls: A longitudinal test of an evolutionary model. *Journal of Personality & Social Psychology, 77*(2), 387–401.

El-Sheikh, M. (2005). The role of emotional responses and physiological reactivity in the marital conflict-child functioning link. *Journal of Child Psychology and Psychiatry, 46*(11), 1191–1199. PP418 [pii] 10.1111/j.1469-7610.2005.00418.x.

El-Sheikh, M., Keller, P. S., & Erath, S. A. (2007). Marital conflict and risk for child maladjustment over time: Skin conductance level reactivity as a vulnerability factor. *Journal of Abnormal Child Psychology, 35*(5), 715–727. doi:10.1007/s10802-007-9127-2.

Engert, V., Efanov, S. I., Dedovic, K., Duchesne, A., Dagher, A., & Pruessner, J. C. (2010). Perceived early-life maternal care and the cortisol response to repeated psychosocial stress. *Journal of Psychiatry & Neuroscience, 35*(6), 370–377. doi:10.1503/jpn.100022.

Entringer, S., Epel, E. S., Kumsta, R., Lin, J., Hellhammer, D. H., Blackburn, E. H., et al. (2011). Stress exposure in intrauterine life is associated with shorter telomere length in young adulthood. *Proceedings of the National Academy of Sciences, 108*(33), E513–E518. doi:10.1073/pnas.1107759108.

Entringer, S., Epel, E., LIn, J., Buss, C., Shahbaba, B., Blackburn, E. H., et al. (2013). Maternal psychosocial stress during pregnancy is associated with newborn leukocyte telomere length. *American Journal of Obstetrics and Gynecology, 208*, 134.e131–134.e137.

Epel, E. S., Blackburn, E. H., Lin, J., Dhabhar, F. S., Adler, N. E., Morrow, J. D., et al. (2004). Accelerated telomere shortening in response to life stress. *Proceedings of the National Academy of Sciences of the United States of America, 101*(49), 17312–17315.

Essex, M. J., Boyce, W. T., Hertzman, C., Lam, L. L., Armstrong, J. M., Neumann, S. M. A., et al. (2013). Epigenetic vestiges of early developmental adversity: Childhood stress exposure and DNA methylation in adolescence. *Child Development, 84*(1), 58–75. doi:10.1111/j.1467-8624.2011.01641.x.

Essex, M. J., Klein, M. H., Cho, E., & Kalin, N. H. (2002). Maternal stress beginning in infancy may sensitize children to later stress exposure: Effects on cortisol and behavior. *Biological Psychiatry, 52*(8), 776–784.

Evans, G. W., Chen, E., Miller, G., & Seeman, T. (2012). How poverty gets under the skin. In V. Maholmes & R. B. King (Eds.), *The Oxford handbook of poverty and child development* (pp. 13–26). Oxford: Oxford University Press.

Evans, G. W., & Kim, P. (2007). Childhood poverty and health: Cumulative risk exposure and stress dysregulation. *Psychological Science, 18*(11), 953–957. PSCI2008 [pii] 10.1111/j.1467-9280.2007.02008.x.

Evans, G. W., Kim, P., Ting, A. H., Tesher, H. B., & Shannis, D. (2007). Cumulative risk, maternal responsiveness, and allostatic load among young adolescents. *Developmental Psychology, 43*(2), 341–351. 2007-02739-006 [pii] 10.1037/0012-1649.43.2.341.

Fernald, L. C., Burke, H. M., & Gunnar, M. R. (2008). Salivary cortisol levels in children of low-income women with high depressive symptomatology. *Development and Psychopathology, 20*, 423–436.

Fisher, P. A., Stoolmiller, M., Gunnar, M. R., & Burraston, B. O. (2007). Effects of a therapeutic intervention for foster preschoolers on diurnal cortisol activity. *Psychoneuroendocrinology, 32*(8–10), 892–905. doi:10.1016/j.psyneuen.2007.06.008.

Fox, S. E., Levitt, P., & Nelson, C. A. (2010). How the timing and quality of early experiences influence the development of brain architecture [Review]. *Child Development, 81*(1), 28–40.

Ganzel, B. L., Morris, P. A., & Wethington, E. (2010). Allostasis and the human brain: Integrating models of stress from the social and life sciences. *Psychological Review, 117*(1), 134–174. doi:10.1037/a0017773.

Garcia-Coll, C., Akerman, A., & Cicchetti, D. (2000). Cultural influences on developmental processes and outcomes: Implications for the study of development and psychopathology. *Development and Psychopathology, 12*, 333–356.

Ghera, M. M., Marshall, P. J., Fox, N. A., Zeanah, C. H., Nelson, C. A., Smyke, A. T., et al. (2009). The effects of foster care intervention on socially deprived institutionalized children's attention and positive affect: Results from the BEIP study. *Journal of Child Psychology and Psychiatry, 50*(3), 246–253. doi:10.1111/j.1469-7610.2008.01954.x.

Giedd, J. N., Vaituzis, A. C., Hamburger, S. D., Lange, N., Rajapakse, J. C., Kaysen, D., Vauss, Y. C., & Rapoport, J. L. (1996). Quantitative MRI of the temporal lobe, amygdala, and hippocampus in normal human development: Ages 4-18 years. *Journal of Comparative Neurology, 366*, 223–230.

Goldstein, L. H., Trancik, A., Bensadoun, J., Boyce, W. T., & Adler, N. E. (1999). Social dominance and cardiovascular reactivity in preschoolers: Associations with SES and health. *Annals of the New York Academy of Sciences, 896*, 363–366.

Green, J., McLaughlin, K. A., Berglund, P. A., Gruber, M., Sampson, N., Zaslavsky, A., et al. (2010). Childhood adversities and adult psychiatric disorders in the national comorbidity survey replication i: Associations with first onset of dsm-iv disorders. *Archives of General Psychiatry, 67*(2), 113–123. doi:10.1001/archgenpsychiatry.2009.186.

Gunnar, M. R., Frenn, K., Wewerka, S. S., & Van Ryzin, M. J. (2009). Moderate versus severe early life stress: Associations with stress reactivity and regulation in 10-12-year-old children. *Psychoneuroendocrinology, 34*(1), 62–75. S0306-4530(08)00217-5 [pii] 10.1016/j.psyneuen.2008.08.013.

Gunnar, M. R., Sebanc, A. M., Tout, K., Donzella, B., & van Dulmen, M. H. (2003). Peer rejection, temperament, and cortisol activity in preschoolers. *Developmental Psychobiology, 43*(4), 346–358.

Gunnar, M. R., Tout, K., de Haan, M., Pierce, S., & Stansbury, K. (1997). Temperament, social competence, and adrenocortical activity in preschoolers. *Developmental Psychobiology, 31*, 65–85.

Gunnar, M. R., & Vazquez, D. M. (2001). Low cortisol and a flattening of expected daytime rhythm: Potential indices of risk in human development. *Development and Psychopathology, 13*(3), 515–538.

Gunnar, M. R., & Vazquez, D. (2006). Stress neurobiology and developmental psychopathology. In D. Cicchetti &

D. J. Cohen (Eds.), *Developmental psychopathology* (Vol. 2, pp. 533–577). Hoboken, NJ: Wiley.

Hackman, D. A., & Farah, M. J. (2009). Socioeconomic status and the developing brain. *Trends in Cognitive Science, 13*(2), 65–73. S1364-6613(08)00263-5 [pii] 10.1016/j.tics.2008.11.003.

Hammock, E. A. D., & Levitt, P. (2006). The discipline of neurobehavioral development: The emerging interface of processes that build circuits and skills. *Human Development, 49*(5), 294–309.

Heim, C., Plotsky, P. M., & Nemeroff, C. B. (2004). Importance of studying the contributions of early adverse experience to neurobiological findings in depression. *Neuropsychopharmacology, 29*(4), 641–648. doi: http://www.nature.com/npp/journal/v29/n4/suppinfo/1300397s1.html

Hertzman, C. (1999). The biological embedding of early experience and its effects on health in adulthood. *Annals of the New York Academy of Sciences, 896*, 85–95.

Hertzman, C. (2012). Putting the concept of biological embedding in historical perspective. *Proceedings of the National Academy of Sciences of the United States of America, 109*, 17160–17167. doi:10.1073/pnas.1202203109.

Hertzman, C., & Boyce, W. T. (2010). How experience gets under the skin to create gradients in developmental health. *Annual Review of Public Health, 31*, 329–347. doi:10.1146/annurev.publhealth.012809.103538.

Hertzman, C., & Wiens, M. (1996). Child development and long-term outcomes: A population health perspective and summary of successful interventions. *Social Science and Medicine, 43*(7), 1083–1095.

Keating, D. P., & Hertzman, C. (1999). *Developmental health and the wealth of nations: Social, biological, and educational dynamics*. New York: Guilford Press.

King, J. A., Barkley, R. A., & Barrett, S. (1998). Attention-deficit hyperactivity disorder and the stress response. *Biological Psychiatry, 44*(1), 72–74.

Kishiyama, M. M., Boyce, W. T., Jimenez, A. M., Perry, L. M., & Knight, R. T. (2009). Socioeconomic disparities affect prefrontal function in children. *Journal of Cognitive Neuroscience, 21*(6), 1106–1115. doi:10.1162/jocn.2009.21101.

Klimes-Dougan, B., Hastings, P. D., Granger, D. A., Usher, B. A., & Zahn-Waxler, C. (2001). Adrenocortical activity in at-risk and normally developing adolescents: Individual differences in salivary cortisol basal levels, diurnal variation, and responses to social challenges. *Development and Psychopathology, 13*, 695–719.

Knafo, A., Israel, S., & Ebstein, R. P. (2011). Heritability of children's prosocial behavior and differential susceptibility to parenting by variation in the dopamine receptor D4 gene. *Development and Psychopathology, 23*(01), 53–67. doi:10.1017/S0954579410000647.

Kroenke, C. H., Epel, E., Adler, N., Bush, N. R., Obradovic, J., Lin, J., et al. (2011). Autonomic and adrenocortical reactivity and buccal cell telomere length in kindergarten children. *Psychosomatic Medicine, 73*(7), 533–540. doi:10.1097/PSY.0b013e318229acfc.

Levine, S. (2005). Developmental determinants of sensitivity and resistance to stress. *Psychoneuroendocrinology,* 30(10), 939–946. S0306-4530(05)00090-9 [pii] 10.1016/j.psyneuen.2005.03.013.

Liu, D., Diorio, J., Tannenbaum, B., Caldji, C., Francis, D., Freedman, A., et al. (1997). Maternal care, hippocampal glucocorticoid receptors, and hypothalamic-pituitary-adrenal responses to stress. *Science, 277*, 1659–1662.

Loman, M. M., & Gunnar, M. R. (2009). Early experience and the development of stress reactivity and regulation in children. *Neuroscience and Biobehavioral Reviews.* doi: S0149-7634(09)00075-X[pii].10.1016/j.neubiorev.2009.05.007

Lupien, S. J., King, S., Meaney, M. J., & McEwen, B. S. (2000). Child's stress hormone levels correlate with mother's socioeconomic status and depressive state. *Biological Psychiatry, 48*(10), 976–980. S0006-3223(00)00965-3 [pii].

Lupien, S. J., Ouellet-Morin, I., Hupbach, A., Tu, M. T., Buss, C., Walker, D., et al. (2006). Beyond the stress concept: Allostatic load–a developmental biological and cognitive perspective. In D. Cicchetti & D. J. Cohen (Eds.), *Developmental psychopathology, Vol 2: Developmental neuroscience* (Vol. 2, pp. 578–628). Hoboken, NJ: Wiley.

Luthar, S. S., Lyman, E. L., & Crossman, E. J. (2014). Resilience and positive psychology. In M. Lewis & K. Rudolph (Eds.), *Handbook of developmental psychopathology*. New York: Springer.

Lyons, D. M., Parker, K. J., & Schatzberg, A. F. (2010). Animal models of early life stress: Implications for understanding resilience. *Developmental Psychobiology, 52*(5), 402–410. doi:10.1002/dev.20429.

Macri, S., Zoratto, F., & Laviola, G. (2011). Early-stress regulates resilience, vulnerability and experimental validity in laboratory rodents through mother-offspring hormonal transfer. *Neuroscience and Biobehavioral Reviews, 35*(7), 1534–1543. doi:10.1016/j.neubiorev.2010.12.014.

Makinodan, M., Rosen, K. M., Ito, S., & Corfas, G. (2012). A critical period for social experience–dependent oligodendrocyte maturation and myelination. *Science, 337*(6100), 1357–1360. doi:10.1126/science.1220845.

Masten, A. (2012). Risk and resilience in development. In P. D. Zelazo (Ed.), *Oxford handbook of developmental psychology*. Oxford: Oxford Press.

McEwen, B. S. (1998). Protective and damaging effects of stress mediators. *New England Journal of Medicine, 338*, 171–179.

McEwen, B. S. (2000). Effects of adverse experiences for brain structure and function. *Biological Psychiatry, 48*(8), 721–731.

McEwen, B. S. (2007). Physiology and neurobiology of stress and adaptation: Central role of the brain. *Physiological Reviews, 87*(3), 873–904. 87/3/873 [pii] 10.1152/physrev.00041.2006.

McEwen, B. S., & Stellar, E. (1993). Stress and the individual. Mechanisms leading to disease. *Archives of Internal Medicine, 153*(18), 2093–2101.

McGrath, J. J., Matthews, K. A., & Brady, S. S. (2006). Individual versus neighborhood socioeconomic status and race as predictors of adolescent ambulatory blood pressure and heart rate. *Social Science & Medicine, 63*(6), 1442–1453. S0277-9536(06)00152-3 [pii] 10.1016/j.socscimed.2006.03.019.

McLoyd, V. C. (1998). Socioeconomic disadvantage and child development. *American Psychologist, 53*(2), 185–204.

Meaney, M. J. (2010). Epigenetics and the biological definition of gene x environment interactions. *Child Development, 81*(1), 41–79.

Meaney, M. J., Aitken, D. H., Van Berkel, C., Bhatnagar, S., & Sapolsky, R. M. (1988). Effect of neonatal handling on age-related impairments associated with the hippocampus. *Science, 239*, 766–768.

Miller, G. E., Chen, E., & Zhou, E. S. (2007). If it goes up, must it come down? Chronic stress and the hypothalamic-pituitary-adrenocortical axis in humans. *Psychological Bulletin, 133*(1), 25–45. doi:10.1037/0033-2909.133.1.25.

Monroe, S. M., & Harkness, K. L. (2005). Life stress, the "Kindling" hypothesis, and the recurrence of depression: Considerations from a life stress perspective. *Psychological Review, 112*(2), 417–445. doi:10.1192/bjp.168.1.68 10.1016/s0165-0327(02)00112-x.

Nelson, C. A., Zeanah, C. H., Fox, N. A., Marshall, P. J., Smyke, A. T., & Guthrie, D. (2007). Cognitive recovery in socially deprived young children: The Bucharest early intervention project. *Science, 318*(5858), 1937–1940. doi:10.1126/science.1143921.

O'Donovan, A., Tomiyama, A. J., Lin, J., Puterman, E., Adler, N. E., Kemeny, M., et al. (2012). Stress appraisals and cellular aging: A key role for anticipatory threat in the relationship between psychological stress and telomere length. *Brain, Behavior, and Immunity, 26*(4), 573–579. http://dx.doi.org/10.1016/j.bbi.2012.01.007.

Oberlander, T. F., Weinberg, J., Papsdorf, M., Grunau, R., Misri, S., & Devlin, A. M. (2008). Prenatal exposure to maternal depression, neonatal methylation of human glucocorticoid receptor gene (NR3C1) and infant cortisol stress response. *Epigenetics, 3*(2), 97–106.

Obradović, J., & Boyce, W. T. (2009). Individual differences in behavioral, physiological, and genetic sensitivities to contexts: Implications for development and adaptation. *Developmental Neuroscience, 31*(4), 300–308.

Obradović, J., Bush, N. R., Stamperdahl, J., Adler, N. E., & Boyce, W. T. (2010). Biological sensitivity to context: The interactive effects of stress reactivity and family adversity on socioemotional behavior and school readiness. [Review]. *Child Development, 81*(1), 270–289.

Oomen, C. A., Soeters, H., Audureau, N., Vermunt, L., van Hasselt, F. N., Manders, E. M. M., et al. (2010). Severe early life stress hampers spatial learning and neurogenesis, but improves hippocampal synaptic plasticity and emotional learning under high-stress conditions in adulthood. *Journal of Neuroscience, 30*(19), 6635–6645. doi:10.1523/jneurosci.0247-10.2010.

Oosterlaan, J., Geurts, H. M., Knol, D. L., & Sergeant, J. A. (2005). Low basal salivary cortisol is associated with teacher-reported symptoms of conduct disorder. *Psychiatry Research, 134*(1), 1–10. doi:10.1016/j.psychres.2004.12.005.

Oosterman, M., De Schipper, J. C., Fisher, P., Dozier, M., & Schuengel, C. (2010). Autonomic reactivity in relation to attachment and early adversity among foster children. *Development and Psychopathology, 22*(01), 109–118. doi:10.1017/S0954579409990290.

Piatti, V. C., Davies-Sala, M. G., Esposito, M. S., Mongiat, L. A., Trinchero, M. F., & Schinder, A. F. (2011). The timing for neuronal maturation in the adult hippocampus is modulated by local network activity. *Journal of Neuroscience, 31*(21), 7715–7728. doi:10.1523/jneurosci.1380-11.2011.

Plotsky, P. M., & Meaney, M. J. (1993). Early, postnatal experience alters hypothalamic corticotropin-releasing factor (CRF) mRNA, median eminence CRF content and stress-induced release in adult rats. *Brain Research. Molecular Brain Research, 18*(3), 195–200.

Pollak, S. D. (2005). Early adversity and mechanisms of plasticity: Integrating affective neuroscience with developmental approaches to psychopathology. *Development and Psychopathology, 17*(3), 735–752. doi:10.1017/s0954579405050352.

Provencal, N., Suderman, M. J., Guillemin, C., Massart, R., Ruggiero, A., Wang, D. S., et al. (2012). The Signature of maternal rearing in the methylome in rhesus macaque prefrontal cortex and T cells. *Journal of Neuroscience, 32*(44), 15626–15642. doi:10.1523/jneurosci.1470-12.2012.

Puterman, E., & Epel, E. (2012). An intricate dance: Life experience, multisystem resiliency, and rate of telomere decline throughout the lifespan. *Social and Personality Psychology Compass, 6*(11), 807–825.

Rudolph, K. D., Troop-Gordon, W., & Granger, D. A. (2010). Peer victimization and aggression: Moderation by individual differences in salivary cortiol and alpha-amylase. *Journal of Abnormal Child Psychology, 38*(6), 843–856. doi:10.1007/s10802-010-9412-3.

Rudolph, K. D., Troop-Gordon, W., & Granger, D. A. (2011). Individual differences in biological stress responses moderate the contribution of early peer victimization to subsequent depressive symptoms. *Psychopharmacology, 214*(1), 209–219. doi:10.1007/s00213-010-1879-7.

Rutter, M. (2012). Resilience as a dynamic concept. *Development and Psychopathology, 24*(2), 335–344. doi:10.1017/s0954579412000028.

Saffery, R., Morley, R., Carlin, J. B., Joo, J.-H. E., Ollikainen, M., Novakovic, B., et al. (2012). Cohort profile: The peri/post-natal epigenetic twins study. *International Journal of Epidemiology, 41*(1), 55–61. doi:10.1093/ije/dyr140.

Sahin, E., Colla, S., Liesa, M., Moslehi, J., Muller, F. L., Guo, M, et al. (2011). Telomere dysfunction induces metabolic and mitochondrial compromise (vol 470, pg 359, 2011). *Nature, 475*(7355). doi: 10.1038/nature10223

Sanchez, M. M., Ladd, C. O., & Plotsky, P. M. (2001). Early adverse experience as a developmental risk factor for later psychopathology: Evidence from rodent and primate models. *Development and Psychopathology, 13*(3), 419–449.

Sapolsky, R. M. (1994). The physiological relevance of glucocorticoid endangerment of the hippocampus. *Brain Corticosteroid Receptors, 746,* 294–307.

Sapolsky, R. M., Romero, L. M., & Munck, A. U. (2000). How do glucocorticoids influence stress responses? Integrating permissive, suppressive, stimulatory, and preparative actions. *Endocrine Reviews, 21,* 55–89.

Seeman, T., Epel, E., Gruenewald, T., Karlamangla, A., & McEwen, B. S. (2010). Socio-economic differentials in peripheral biology: Cumulative allostatic load. *Annals of the New York Academy of Sciences, 1186,* 223–239.

Seeman, T., Gruenewald, T., Karlamangla, A., Sidney, S., Liu, K. A., McEwen, B., et al. (2010). Modeling multisystem biological risk in young adults: The coronary artery risk development in young adults study. *American Journal of Human Biology, 22*(4), 463–472. doi:10.1002/ajhb.21018.

Seeman, T., McEwen, B. S., Rowe, J. W., & Singer, B. H. (2001). Allostatic load as a marker of cumulative biological risk: MacArthur studies of successful aging. *Proceedings of the National Academy of Sciences of the United States of America, 98*(8), 4770–4775. doi:10.1073/pnas.081072698 081072698 [pii].

Selye, H. (1950). *Stress: The physiology and pathology of exposure to stress.* Montreal, QC: Acta Medical Publishers.

Selye, H. (1956). Stress and psychiatry. *American Journal of Psychiatry, 113*(5), 423–427.

Shalev, I. (2012). Early life stress and telomere length: Investigating the connection and possible mechanisms. A critical survey of the evidence base, research methodology and basic biology. *Bioessays, 34*(11), 943–952. doi:10.1002/bies.201200084.

Shannon, K. E., Beauchaine, T. P., Brenner, S. L., Neuhaus, E., & Gatzke-Kopp, L. (2007). Familial and temperamental predictors of resilience in children at risk for conduct disorder and depression. *Development and Psychopathology, 19*(3), 701–727. S0954579407000351 [pii] 10.1017/S0954579407000351.

Sheridan, M. A., Fox, N. A., Zeanah, C. H., McLaughlin, K. A., & Nelson, C. A. (2012). Variation in neural development as a result of exposure to institutionalization early in childhood. *The Proceedings of the National Academy of Sciences of the United States of America, 109*(32), 12927–12932. doi:10.1073/pnas.1200041109.

Sheridan, M. A., Sarsour, K., Jutte, D., D'Esposito, M., & Boyce, W. T. (2012). The Impact of Social Disparity on Prefrontal Function in Childhood. *PLoS ONE, 7*(4). doi: 10.1371/journal.pone.0035744

Shirtcliff, E. A., Granger, D. A., Booth, A., & Johnson, D. (2005). Low salivary cortisol levels and externalizing behavior problems in youth. *Development and Psychopathology, 17,* 167–184.

Simon, N. M., Smoller, J. W., McNamara, K. L., Maser, R. S., Zalta, A. K., Pollack, M. H., et al. (2006). Telomere shortening and mood disorders: preliminary support for a chronic stress model of accelerated aging [Comparative Study Research Support, N.I.H., Extramural Research Support, Non-U.S. Gov't]. *Biological Psychiatry, 60*(5), 432–435.

Smider, N. A., Essex, M. J., Kalin, N. H., Buss, K. A., Klein, M. H., Davidson, R. J., et al. (2002). Salivary cortisol as a predictor of socioemotional adjustment during kindergarten: A prospective study. *Child Development, 73,* 75–92.

Staff, R. T., Murray, A. D., Ahearn, T. S., Mustafa, N., Fox, H. C., & Whalley, L. J. (2012). Childhood socioeconomic status and adult brain size: Childhood socioeconomic status influences adult hippocampal size. *Annals of Neurology, 71*(5), 653–660. doi:10.1002/ana.22631.

Sterling, P., & Eyer, J. (1989). Allostasis: A new paradigm to explain arousal pathology. In S. Fisher & J. Reason (Eds.), *Handbook of life stress, cognition and health* (pp. 629–649). Oxford: Wiley.

Sumner, M. M., Bernard, K., & Dozier, M. (2010). Young children's full-day patterns of cortisol production on child care days. *Archives of Pediatrics & Adolescent Medicine, 164*(6), 567–571.

Swain, J. E., Lorberbaum, J. P., Kose, S., & Strathearn, L. (2007). Brain basis of early parent-infant interactions: Psychology, physiology, and in vivo functional neuroimaging studies. *Journal of Child Psychology and Psychiatry, 48*(3–4), 262–287. JCPP1731 [pii] 10.1111/j.1469-7610.2007.01731.x.

Talge, N. M., Neal, C., & Glover, V. (2007). Antenatal maternal stress and long-term effects on child neurodevelopment: How and why? *Journal of Child Psychology and Psychiatry, 48*(3–4), 245–261.

Tarullo, A. R., & Gunnar, M. R. (2006). Child maltreatment and the developing HPA axis. *Hormones and Behavior, 50*(4), 632–639. doi:10.1016/j.yhbeh.2006.06.010.

Taylor, Z. E., Spinrad, T. L., Vanschyndel, S. K., Eisenberg, N., Huynh, J., Sulik, M. J., et al. (2013). Sociodemographic risk, parenting, and effortful control: Relations to salivary alpha-amylase and cortisol in early childhood. *Developmental Psychobiology, 55*(8), 869–80.

Theall, K. P., Drury, S. S., & Shirtcliff, E. A. (2012). Cumulative neighborhood risk of psychosocial stress and allostatic load in adolescents. *American Journal of Epidemiology, 176,* S164–S174. doi:10.1093/aje/kws185.

Tomiyama, A. J., O'Donovan, A., Lin, J., Puterman, E., Lazaro, A., Chan, J., et al. (2012). Does cellular aging relate to patterns of allostasis? An examination of basal and stress reactive HPA axis activity and telomere length. *Physiology & Behavior, 106*(1), 40–45. doi:10.1016/j.physbeh.2011.11.016.

Tottenham, N., & Sheridan, M. A. (2010). A review of adversity, the amygdala and the hippocampus: a consideration of developmental timing. *Frontiers in Human Neuroscience, 3.* doi: 10.3389/neuro.09.068.2009

Werner, E. E. (2012). Children and war: Risk, resilience, and recovery. *Development and Psychopathology, 24*(2), 553–558. doi:10.1017/s0954579412000156.

Whittle, S., Yap, M. B. H., Sheeber, L., Dudgeon, P., Yücel, M., Pantelis, C., et al. (2011). Hippocampal volume and sensitivity to maternal aggressive behavior: A prospective study of adolescent depressive symptoms. *Development and Psychopathology, 23*(01), 115–129. doi:10.1017/S0954579410000684.

Wolkowitz, O. M., Epel, E. S., Reus, V. I., & Mellon, S. H. (2010). Depression gets old fast: Do stress and depression accelerate cell aging? *Depression and Anxiety, 27*(4), 327–338. doi:10.1002/da.20686.

Zalewski, M., Lengua, L. J., Kiff, C. J., & Fisher, P. A. (2012). Understanding the relation of low income to HPA-axis functioning in preschool children: Cumulative family risk and parenting as pathways to disruptions in cortisol. *Child Psychiatry & Human Development, 43*(6), 924–942. doi:10.1007/s10578-012-0304-3.

Temperament Concepts in Developmental Psychopathology

16

John E. Bates, Alice C. Schermerhorn, and Isaac T. Petersen

The concept of temperament is useful for distinguishing between one child and another and between the child and the social environment. Temperament traits have been regarded as the core of personality and have been shown by research to have important associations with developmental psychopathology. For decades, developmental psychopathology research using temperament has been growing vigorously. We found 1,441 peer-reviewed articles on temperament published between 2009 and June of 2012. Seventy percent of these considered temperament in relation to concepts representing the broader domain of developmental psychopathology, such as behavior problems, externalizing, internalizing, and psychiatric diagnoses.[1] Consistent with the vigor of this area of research, numerous major reviews, edited volumes, and monographs on temperament's relations with developmental psychopathology have appeared in recent years, including Seifer (2000) in the previous edition of this handbook; Caspi and Shiner (2006), Degnan, Almas, and Fox (2010), De Pauw and Mervielde (2010), Kiff, Lengua, and Zalewski (2011), Rothbart (2011), Zentner and Shiner (2012), and Klein, Dyson, Kujawa, and Kotov (2012), just to cite a few of the more recent reviews. We have also contributed reviews (e.g., Bates & Pettit, 2007; Bates, Schermerhorn, & Goodnight, 2010; Bates, Schermerhorn, & Petersen, 2012; Rothbart & Bates, 2006; Wachs & Bates, 2010). This chapter explains our conceptual definition of temperament and how it contributes to the development of psychopathology. This chapter also considers a few measurement issues and some key findings about temperament's role in developmental psychopathology.

This chapter concerns the intersection of temperament, environment, and adjustment. Temperament and environment are overlapping but relatively distinct conceptual domains. The domain of adjustment is wholly embedded in the much larger domain of environment (i.e., only has meaning in relation to social relationships); and a substantial part of the overlap between temperament and environment includes the domain of adjustment.

Temperament concepts are as old as ancient Greek philosophy and as new as the current research on genetic and neural bases of human behavior (Rothbart, 2011). Temperament came into active use in developmental science only in the 1960s, dating especially to the New York Longitudinal Study (Thomas, Chess, & Birch, 1968). The surge in interest in temperament can

---

[1] The complete list of search terms entered into the search tool, PsycInfo: psychopathology, adaptation, adjustment, competence, externalizing, internalizing, antisocial, depression, anxiety, aggression, disorder, and of course, temperament. This may have missed studies of variables we would consider temperament that were given other names.

J.E. Bates, Ph.D. (✉) • I.T. Petersen
Department of Psychological and Brain Sciences,
Indiana University, Bloomington, IN 47405, USA
e-mail: batesj@indiana.edu

A.C. Schermerhorn, Ph.D.
Department of Psychology, University of Vermont,
Burlington, VT 05405, USA

M. Lewis and K.D. Rudolph (eds.), *Handbook of Developmental Psychopathology*,
DOI 10.1007/978-1-4614-9608-3_16, © Springer Science+Business Media New York 2014

be related to the field's shift toward more complex systems models of the development of psychopathology, which resulted partly from arguments such as Bell's (1968) landmark assertion that children influence their own socialization by affecting the parenting they receive. The surge can also be related to the growth of developmental research in general and technological advances, e.g., in multivariate statistical analysis. Temperament concepts came with references to biological processes in the child. They therefore added a dimension to the dominant mid-twentieth-century models of psychopathology, which tended to focus almost exclusively on social environment causes, especially the domain of parent effects (Bates, 1989b). In the first decades after temperament's scientific introduction, several different perspectives on how to define temperament were evident, and there was fairly vigorous discussion of the strengths and weaknesses of the perspectives (see Seifer, 2000, for a review of the definitional perspectives past and present). Definitions do make a difference and there is continued discussion about how best to define temperament concepts (e.g., Aron, Aron, & Jagiellowicz, 2012); however, conceptual differences between the perspectives at the present are relatively modest (Lemery, Goldsmith, Klinnert, & Mrazek, 1999; Rothbart & Bates, 2006). We find scientific questions about specific measures of temperament and their usefulness in describing development of the most interest and will focus on dimensions included in three- and five-factor models of temperament and personality.

We perceive a general convergence on a basic definition first promoted by Rothbart and her colleagues (e.g., Rothbart, 2011; Rothbart & Bates, 2006). Our operating definition is that temperament is a rubric covering traits in negative and positive emotional reactivity and cognitively higher order self-regulation. These reactivity and regulation dimensions can summarize a wide swath of individual differences in human (and animal) behavior. For example, Big 3 and Big 5 models of temperament and personality typically involve high vs. low positive emotionality, high vs. low negative emotionality (often subdivided as

fearful vs. angry emotion), and impulsivity vs. self-regulation and constraint. These models have provided a relatively simple but comprehensive dimensional structure for basic behavioral differences, traits that appear relatively early and are relatively stable across development (Rothbart & Bates, 2006). Temperament traits are based in individual differences in biological structures and processes, such as genes for dopamine, and neural functions, such as amygdala response to threat stimuli and greater right vs. left EEG activation as a marker of negative vs. positive emotionality. However, it is apparent that the phenotypes of temperament behavior patterns are far from simply mapped onto biological markers. We think of the reactivity and self-regulation differences as based in neural systems that are intricately balanced. For example, effortful self-regulation allows management and redirection of both approach- and avoidance-producing emotions, while emotional responses inscribe learning events with meaning and ultimately shape cognitive regulation habits (Barkley, 2012; Lewis & Todd, 2007).

Processes involving child characteristics could influence both the child's environment, such as good self-regulation producing increased parental acceptance (Lengua, 2006), and how the child responds to experiences, such as how genes for serotonin interact with family stress and developmental stages in forecasting anxiety and depression (Petersen et al., 2012). Conversely, processes involving environmental influences could influence child biological functioning, such as when chaotic and threatening environments are associated with abnormal brain processing of social stimuli (Pollak, Klorman, Thatcher, & Cicchetti, 2001), abnormal diurnal patterns of cortisol (Dettling, Parker, Lane, Sebanc, & Gunnar, 2000), or even epigenetic methylation of genes controlling cortisol responses (Champagne et al., 2004). The focus of this chapter is, of course, on the effects of children's biologically based traits rather than on how environment shapes biology. However, the latter findings remind us that any phenotypical measure of temperament could reflect a developmental product of both relatively inborn and experientially developed biological traits. The measurement of temperament is not as simple as the concept of temperament. Measurement issues will be considered after consideration of developmental psychopathology questions.

Concepts of developmental psychopathology or adjustment provide an essential context for the study of temperamental differences between children. We can see evidence of interest in the origins of children's behavioral adjustment growing with the fields of psychology and psychiatry and the areas of clinical and developmental psychology across the nineteenth and twentieth centuries, but the earliest instance we have seen of use of the term *developmental psychopathology* as a comprehensive summary of previous research and a clear, developmental systems vision of future directions was Achenbach's classic 1974 text. By now, the term developmental psychopathology has come to represent a dominant perspective (Cicchetti, 2006; Sroufe & Rutter, 1984). Developmental psychopathology is a field of immense breadth and complexity. It is an approach to research that embraces cross-disciplinary, multilevel, and dynamic concepts, from the fundamental biological processes to the psychological and sociological systems. It is concerned with elucidating processes in both adaptive and maladaptive development. In the service of achieving a dynamic and systemic understanding of development, it integrates the emerging findings and methods of so many basic and applied areas of research that it is nearly impossible to draw boundaries around the field (Cicchetti, 2006). Developmental psychopathology models, even ones most creatively and authoritatively focused on parenting and other environmental variables (e.g., Patterson, Reid, & Dishion, 1992), almost invariably touch on biological levels of child differences.

Developmental psychopathology, just like temperament, contains some differences of perspective, and just as a temperament construct coming from one perspective can have somewhat different meanings than one coming from another perspective, so can developmental psychopathology constructs. Our interest is primarily in developmental psychopathology constructs coming from a dimensional perspective, in which distinc-

tions between individuals are relatively continuous and ordered, as in a spectrum. Categorical, more molar, and configural concepts of psychopathology, such as conduct disorder vs. depression, are quite relevant to questions about temperamental roots (Loeber & Burke, 2011), but we have focused on the more general dimensions of externalizing and internalizing behavior problems. These dimensions have provided convenient summaries of complex growth patterns of the individual children's adjustment in samples representing a broad range of risks and adaptations. Externalizing and internalizing problems tend to be correlated, but they can be analytically separated in their growth parameters and in their temperament antecedents (Keiley, Lofthouse, Bates, Dodge, & Pettit, 2003). The externalizing and internalizing dimensions, despite not being fully independent, can be used to summarize the largest portion of cases of psychopathology at all ages of development. There may be a need, however, for a third dimension, as foreseen in Eysenck's (1992) personality inventory. Eysenck's three dimensions were extraversion-introversion, neuroticism, and psychoticism. Perhaps the hypothetical third dimension involves exceptionally disordered thought processes, such as what happens in autism spectrum disorders, in psychotic disorders, and to perhaps a lesser degree in extreme hostility and cruelty. Autism spectrum and psychotic disorders have externalizing and internalizing elements but appear at this point to be less well accounted for by externalizing and internalizing and less well accounted for by temperament variables than the disruptive behavior disorders and anxiety and mood disorders.[2]

To summarize our points so far about temperament and developmental psychopathology, in the domain of temperament, the key trait dimensions found so far include (1) positive emotionality, which covers variability in approach motivation, activity, and joy; (2) negative

---

[2] Because developmental exploration of a third dimension of psychopathology in relation to temperament is not highly developed, it is not a focus of this chapter. For similar reasons, the chapter also does not focus on temperament origins of positive adjustment dimensions that might be independent of the pathology dimensions.

emotionality, which appears to begin as one dimension and with development becomes two—fearfulness and frustration/anger; and (3) self-regulation, a complex dimension we see as centered on effortful attention, which allows situation-appropriate modification of emotional/motivational responses and inhibition of both approach and avoidance actions (Rothbart & Bates, 2006). And in the domain of developmental psychopathology, the key trait dimensions found so far include (1) externalizing behavior problems, which involve overassertive, aggressive, oppositional, and attention-demanding behaviors as well as rule-breaking, stealing, and everyday cruel behaviors, and (2) internalizing behavior problems, which involve fearful, tense, anxious, and depressed behaviors. We do not consider here, because they have been of little interest in temperament studies so far, thought disorders, which might include psychotic problems and extreme cruelty.

A Social Process Model of Temperament in Developmental Psychopathology

As important as specifying particular dimensions of behavioral adjustment is specifying social-development processes in the emergence, continuity, and change of adjustment. We tend to think of psychopathology vs. competent adjustment of children as arising from a combination of initial child traits (assuming strong biological roots even if child behaviors are responsive to the environment from the beginning), initial parent traits (which reflect the parent's personality and also respond to the child from the beginning), and broader social context as it influences the child's experience, such as deviant peers or marital and economic stress (which reflect the parents' personalities and may in some part respond to the child's needs and personality). From this rough framework, we aim to identify particular interfaces or correspondences between traits and environments and ineffectually resolved conflicts between children and their environments.

Temperament traits are inherently defined in relation to particular incentive situations (Bates, 1989b; Rothbart & Bates, 1998), and so are psychopathology traits. For example, the trait of fearfulness, based in Gray's (1991) conceptual brain network, the Behavioral Inhibition System, is described not only in terms of frequency and extent of an individual's fearful affect and inhibition and withdrawal but also in terms of the environmental situation's degree of threat of punishment (or non-reward). If a situation, for example, is highly threatening, almost all children would seek protection, so temperament differences in fearfulness would be hard to see. However, if it is only mildly or moderately threatening, temperamental differences in fearfulness would be more apparent (Buss, 2011). Correspondingly, psychopathology dimensions are also framed by situations. Anxiety disorders, for example, are noted in relation to actual level of threat.

We find it most useful to think of temperament as a component in what becomes a dynamic process of transactions between the child and environment, gradually producing adjustment outcomes. Temperament only probabilistically influences a child's response to a situation, just as situations only probabilistically influence a child's response, but over many encounters, hour by hour, day by day, the child-environment system organizes itself. Outcomes follow patterns but are the products of dynamic, interactive processes, so they are not completely determined (Thelen & Smith, 1998). The causal processes can involve dramatically transformative events but most often involve myriad, subtle transactions (Sameroff, 2010) between the child and the social environment. Equilibria are attained in the child-environment relationship, with attractors in a state space (Granic & Patterson, 2006; Thelen & Smith, 1998), but habitual child–parent interaction patterns do sometimes change. Changes over time in maladaptive patterns of behavior appear more likely than changes in adaptive ones—the bias is toward amelioration, according to a relatively old literature (Kohlberg, LaCrosse, & Ricks, 1972), and the essence of psychopathology is not simply the experience of conflict with the environment in development but also failure of the developmental system to right itself. Most young children have moments of heightened distress, tantrums, and aggression, but most of them learn, with the help of parents, teachers, siblings, and friends, effective ways to solve the problems and minimize the distress, tantrums, and aggression. Even in the middle-childhood era, parents often mount successful campaigns to solve problems with their children (Goodnight, Bates, Pettit, & Dodge, 2008), and both informal observations and emerging research suggest that children themselves often contribute to their families' resolution of issues and reductions of conflict (Eisenberg et al., 1999; Schermerhorn, Chow, & Cummings, 2010).

Social environment settings can be described in terms of prevalence of particular kinds of situations (Wachs, 2000). How prevalent a given incentive is may have implications for the emergence of particular qualities of the child. For example, twin research suggests that emotionally positive child behavior is significantly influenced by the environment (Goldsmith, Buss, & Lemery, 1997), which seems likely to be due to the prevalence of parental warmth. In the other direction, an emotionally positive child disposition may evoke increases in parents' warmth (Lengua & Kovacs, 2005). Social environment and child temperament tendencies can also relate in a more interactive way. The implications of the environment for child adjustment may depend on child temperament, and the reverse. As will be discussed in more detail later, parenting that works for one kind of child may not for another, and under some regimes of parenting, a child with a temperamental risk for psychopathology may avoid significant levels of pathology.

Situations start out fairly simple for a very young child—feeding, affection, soothing, stimulation, and small shares of autonomy—but gradually become more complex. In the complexity of human adaptation, there are multiple, often conflicting needs and ambiguous cues for action. For example, common situations include both reward and punishment cues and children learn how to detect the cues and balance their responses (Newman & Wallace, 1993). Situations also have cognitive meanings with complex norms for emotional and behavioral responses (Dodge, Coie, & Lynam, 2006; Lewis & Todd, 2007). In children's pursuit of the social and material events that meet their needs, there sometimes are conflicts with the environment. How these are resolved determines qualities of child adjustment. Poor resolutions with chronic distortions and inefficiencies in people meeting their social and psychological needs are the essence of psychopathology. The most salient needs are for protection, the feeling of security and belonging, and the needs for effective action, learning, and feelings of efficacy. The core developmental tasks (Sroufe & Rutter, 1984) involve meeting these needs. The initial, characteristic biases in a child involving needs for protection can be characterized in terms of temperamental fearfulness and irritability. The feeling of security and belonging appear to come from a sense of generally dependable response and support from caregivers, especially at times of distress (Ainsworth, Blehar, Waters, & Wall, 1979), and in general, as measured so far, these traits do not appear to have strong roots in temperament, although some aspects of attachment behavior, such as crying in the Strange Situation, may have such roots (Vaughn & Shin, 2011). Effective action, learning, and self-efficacy grow in importance with the child's physical and cognitive capacities, and ideal environments are supportive of growth in these areas—providing developmentally appropriate affordances for the child's practice of effective and smoothly regulated actions upon the world.

Accompanying the child's growth in competencies, perhaps even shaping some aspects of it, are child temperament and parent–child relationship variables. As mentioned, initial temperament biases involve positive and negative emotionality and early-appearing self-regulatory traits. Approach motivations and actions create many opportunities for basic learning and more advanced social learning. Tendencies in the environment relative to children's needs have been extensively described, especially in terms of parenting—one of the longest and most vigorous research traditions in developmental science. Parenting traits have often been statistically summarized on two or three broad dimensions, including warmth and control, both supportive and negative, with sensitive responsiveness to the child's lead often linked to warmth but sometimes regarded as separate (Bugental & Grusec, 2006). Environmental differences in warmth and responsiveness would pertain to the child's needs for affection, soothing, protection, belonging, learning, and efficacy. Environmental positive and negative control would pertain to how children's needs for autonomy and self-regulation are negotiated.

Child temperament can be seen as reflecting differences between children in some of their psychological needs. These include not only the fear, distress, approach, joy, and frustration that we have already mentioned but also needs for loving, empathy, and caring. Also relevant is self-consciousness. Self-consciousness is viewed by Barkley (2012) as the most central of the executive functions, and individual differences in it relate to effortful self-regulation. Deriving from self-consciousness and effortful control, secondary needs with a more indirect connection to temperament include needs such as shame resolution and identity (Schore, 1994). Environmental qualities in the child's life—especially parenting—involve complementary and clashing emotions and behaviors. In response to fearfulness and distress, parents may feel and act protectively and provide confident soothing. In response to approach and joy, parents may feel love and joy and behave in affectionate, synchronously responsive ways, and when the situation is right (which they can partly engineer), they may encourage autonomous exploration. In response to tokens of the child's needs for connection, parents may feel responsible and act in conscientious (predictable, dependable) and attached ways. In response to the child's needs for self-regulation, parents may withhold protection when it is not really needed, and they may explicitly model and shape cognitive skills, e.g., by

facilitating the internalization of language to guide behavior (Kopp, 1982).

In summary, in using a social process model of temperament in psychopathology, we aim to identify parallel correspondences between temperament and parenting, temperament and adjustment, and parenting and adjustment dimensions. The model would suggest that temperamental dispositions toward high levels of approach, reward-seeking, excessive efforts to control others, and frustrated emotion would be associated with externalizing problems; temperamental dispositions toward fearful emotion, safety-seeking, and behavioral inhibition would be associated with internalizing problems; and temperamental dispositions toward low levels of effortful self-regulation would be associated with both externalizing and internalizing problems. Low effortful control—perhaps expressed as low ability to direct attention away from a positive goal or a minor threat—would lead to conflicts between the child and environment, perhaps developmentally earlier in the case of failure to self-regulate impulsive action (an aggressive child would likely cause early difficulties for the family) and perhaps later in the case of failure to regulate fearfulness (parents can avoid conflict in the short term by overprotecting an over-fearful child but put the child at risk in later developmental tasks). However, these suggested processes assume an average environment. We recognize that the combination of the dimensions is not likely to be modeled in simple terms. Additive combinations have not been sufficient to explain outcomes to a satisfying degree, even allowing for our difficulties in operationalizing the dimensions of temperament, parenting, and adjustment. Some children experience severe environmental challenges and lack of support yet develop as well as others with better environments, and some children begin with difficult temperament traits and end up with no more problems than easier children. And even where there are additive combinations of the variables, there are likely complex cascades of influence across eras of development (Cox, Mills-Koonce, Propper, & Gariépy, 2010; Dodge et al., 2009) rather than simple influences. In this social process model of temperament in developmental psychopathology, mechanisms involving both temperament and environment help explain the relative balance of poorly resolved conflict and positive support across development and ultimately, the growth of psychopathology.

A Note on Measurement

Temperament measures are not the same as the temperament concepts, as much as we might strive for them to closely correspond. Methods for assessing temperament are crucial to their empirical meanings. Concepts of temperament refer to enduring dispositions, based in neurobiological systems, in responses to relevant situations. Measures, however, may reflect relatively momentary rather than enduring tendencies or tendencies that correspond to a specific situation more than to a general type of situation. For example, a young child's response to a novel stimulus in a laboratory task may reflect not only the hypothetical level of fearfulness of the child but also the child's general sense of being protected by their parent (Nachmias, Gunnar, Mangelsdorf, Parritz, & Buss, 1996) or being unable to cope on a particular day (e.g., due to an unresolved conflict with the parent or to deficient sleep). It may also reflect a trait that is associated with but not the same as fearfulness—sensitivity to the environment or tendency to deeply process new stimuli (Aron et al., 2012). Established measures are often interpreted in terms of a single dimension of temperament, such as negative emotionality, but any given behavior or set of behaviors in similar situations can actually represent multiple concepts of temperament. For example, the child's angry/frustrated emotionality can mark not only the tendency toward distress but also tendencies toward approach and mastery, as well as lagging growth in effortful self-regulation. In addition, a psychophysiological measure might map only approximately onto a behavioral dimension of temperament (Rothbart & Bates, 2006). Therefore, because we think of temperament variables as conceptual tools for describing

natural phenomena rather than the phenomena themselves, our interpretations of measures are always provisional.

Each kind of measure has its own strengths and weaknesses—its own construct validational network of meanings. Caregiver ratings of child behavior across multiple modes of response in multiple incentive conditions are the most commonly used operationalization of temperament. Barkley (2012) has made a strong argument that caregiver ratings of child self-regulatory traits can have much greater validity than structured laboratory tasks, mainly because of the lack of ecological validity of the "cold cognitive" measures. Caregiver ratings are convenient, inexpensive, and psychometrically well understood. They do include components of subjectivity in the rater, but these are not greater than the components of objectivity, e.g., convergence with observer ratings (Bates et al., 2010; Bates & Bayles, 1984). So, especially concerning their advantages in the degree of ecological validity, caregiver ratings are useful in studies of development. Observational measures are often used, too, despite their greater expense. The most frequent observational approach is to measure child response to experimentally controlled situations, e.g., a room filled with a specified set of strange and noisy toys. Increasingly, there have also been biological measures of temperament-like constructs, such as sympathetic and parasympathetic responses, and cortisol reactions. Such measures are presumably more endophenotypical than overt behavior measures. There are even some reports of findings of genetic markers. A recent study (Raby et al., 2012), not explicitly about temperament, but nevertheless relevant, shows that serotonin transporter genotypes associated with lower transcriptional efficiency were associated with the infants' expressions of distress in the Strange Situation. Studies have sometimes found that distress in the Strange Situation is predicted by temperamental negative emotionality (Vaughn & Shin, 2011), so by analogy, serotonin transporter gene transcriptional efficiency could influence how an individual responds to other stressors and thus may explain why some individuals are particularly susceptible to experience anxiety and depression in stressful environments (Petersen et al., 2012). No measure is unambiguous, not even the serotonin transporter gene, but a number of points of convergence have been found between different parent report scales, reports and observation, and bio-measures. The basic point here is that the concepts of temperament serve to organize a complex array of measures. Cross-measure generalizations can be drawn but should be viewed as provisional. Progress has been made, but construct development and validation (Cronbach & Meehl, 1955) are always ongoing.

Associations Between Temperament and Developmental Psychopathology

This section considers two basic ways temperament could be developmentally related to adjustment—direct, linear connections and indirect and nonlinear ones. The most direct connections involve simple, linear processes, such as a psychopathology trait, e.g., social anxiety, representing a version of a similar temperament trait, such as distress in novel situations. Also linear, but more indirect, are influences that temperament might have upon the environment that then shape the development of child adjustment. Nonlinear processes involve interactions between different dimensions of temperament or between temperament and environmental variables in producing outcomes.

Processes to Account for Linkage

Accounts of temperament's role would ideally include developmental processes through which temperament contributes to psychopathology. At least ten possible processes have been envisioned (Rothbart & Bates, 2006), including multiple subtypes of *direct effects*, such as fearful temperament increasing odds of the conditioning that produces an anxiety disorder; of complexly *mediated effects*, such as early irritability shaping conflictual, coercive relationships with parents and others, which then shape disordered emotion and behavior; and

of mechanisms involving *moderated effects*, such as early irritability predicting behavior problems mainly among children who also are low in temperamental effortful control or children who have parents low in effective discipline. The following section summarizes emerging findings on predictive linkages and where possible and on mechanisms by which temperament relates to adjustment outcomes. First, the section on differential linkage shows support for relatively direct models of transmission from temperament to psychopathology. Next, some findings with mediation models are highlighted, in which temperament influences social transactional patterns that, in turn, help create (or fail to suppress) emotional and behavioral problems. Mediated mechanisms are demanded by theory, but empirical demonstrations of them are relatively sparse. And finally, some of the relatively extensive research on moderator mechanisms is summarized.

Linear Connections

Differential Linkage Model

There appears to be continuity of styles of temperamental reactivity and self-regulation that eventually support homologous styles of social adjustment. Based on the accumulation of temperament-adjustment links emerging through the 1980s, including a number of longitudinal studies, we proposed what we have called the differential linkage model, in which the various temperament traits predict conceptually related dimensions of psychopathology (Bates, 1989a; Bates & Bayles, 1984). This model is not fully differentiated yet, but it is more constrained than the most general models in which a multiplicity of temperament traits predicts adjustment as a unitary variable. The general pattern is for the fearful dimensions of temperament, especially discomfort in novelty, to predict later internalizing problems better than they predict externalizing problems, for the self-regulation dimensions of temperament to inversely predict later externalizing problems better than they predict internalizing problems (even though, theoretically, aspects of self-regulation should also predict internalizing problems), and for dimensions of negative emotionality and "difficult" temperament to predict both internalizing and externalizing problems more or less equally. Although much further work is needed, e.g., for clarifying the aspects of temperamental self-regulation that might be more strongly related to internalizing problems than externalizing, the general outlines and some variants of the pattern have been noted by a number of reviewers (e.g., Bates et al., 2012; De Pauw & Mervielde, 2010; Saudino, 2005). The linkages cannot be simply attributed to having similar item contents in temperament and pathology measures, because several studies have shown that removal of content that is most clearly overlapping does not appreciably reduce the association between temperament and adjustment measures. The links are also beginning to show up in associations between laboratory measures of temperament and similar dimensions of adjustment, e.g., novelty fear predicting anxiety symptoms (Kagan & Fox, 2006). Similar patterns of differential association have been emerging in biomarkers of temperament-relevant traits, such as high sympathetic nervous system arousal predicting anxiety (Manassis & Bradley, 1994) and low resting sympathetic nervous system arousal and low vagal reactivity predicting externalizing problems (El-Sheikh et al., 2009).

The differential linkage of temperament and adjustment is paralleled by the general findings of differential linkages between adjustment variables across time—i.e., early internalizing predicting later internalizing better than later externalizing and vice versa (Keiley et al., 2003). It is reassuring that the different dimensions of adjustment have at least somewhat separable roots in temperament. Not all elements of the model are clearly differentiated yet. The main overlap is the fact that difficultness and negative emotionality dimensions of temperament predict both internalizing and externalizing problems. This overlap, however, is consistent with the substantial co-occurrence of internalizing and externalizing problems epidemiologically and the fact that both dimensions involve negative emotion expressions (Achenbach, 1991; Mikolajewski, Allan, Hart, Lonigan, & Taylor, 2013). Another possible overlap is that low levels of effortful control might be involved in both internalizing and externalizing problems. This possibility is based on theory—effortful control ability would allow children to avoid anxiety problems by redirecting attention and inhibiting dominant fear responses and performing nondominant, but counterphobic responses—and also based on a few findings (Gartstein, Putnam, & Rothbart, 2012), including fMRI findings of less activation of brain regions involved in attention and cognitive control in inhibited adults than in uninhibited adults (Clauss, Cowan, & Blackford, 2011). And, assuming the centrality of these abilities, they would also be useful for avoiding impulsive approach (Newman & Wallace, 1993) and aggression and performing socially appropriate forms of assertion. Finally, another partial overlap involves temperamental fearfulness, which is sometimes found to predict lower levels of subsequent externalizing behavior (Kochanska, Aksan, & Joy, 2007), and not just high levels of internalizing behavior.

Further studies are needed to put some detail into the picture of temperament roots of psychopathology. One recent example of findings generally consistent with the differential linkage pattern is the study of mothers' perceptions by Gartstein et al. (2012), relating infancy and toddlerhood temperament to preschool age internalizing and externalizing problems. This study's findings support the model and point to possible refinements. The study used a differentiated negative affectivity (NA) construct, with separate measures for six different kinds of NA. Four of the six kinds, including low soothing, fearfulness, and sadness (as would be expected) and also frustration (as might not have been expected), predicted internalizing problems at preschool age. A slightly different four, including frustration, motor activation, as well as sadness and low levels of soothing, predicted externalizing problems. Fear and discomfort did *not* predict externalizing (confirming our original model). From another perspective, the comparison of the size of correlations showed that frustration was more strongly predictive of externalizing than internalizing behavior. The surgency dimension, including activity level, impulsivity, and several positive affectivity scales, did not predict internalizing problems, but by toddlerhood, it did predict externalizing problems. However, only one of the six scales, activity level, predicted as an individual scale. The self-regulation dimension's effortful control factor from toddlerhood predicted externalizing to a stronger degree than internalizing problems. Of the six orienting and self-regulation scales, attentional focusing and inhibitory control were inverse predictors of later preschool externalizing problems and the others—low pleasure in low-intensity events or affiliativeness, soothability by caregivers, or ability to shift attention were not. The basic conclusion, in summary, is that early temperament dimensions predict later adjustment problems, at least internalizing and externalizing problems, to a substantial degree and in a logical pattern. The differential linkage pattern of findings suggests something about the temperament core of adjustment, but this is only the beginning of an account of the temperament's role in developmental psychopathology. There may turn out to be meaningful sub-threads of the temperament-psychopathology linkage.

Mediator Models

Theoretically, as mentioned, early temperament could have its effect on the development of adjustment via impact on environmental factors. One example of a mediational model is the study of Kiel and Buss (2011), in which toddlers' fearful temperament predicted age-5 social withdrawal partly via mothers' protective behavior in toddlerhood. This mediated effect of maternal protectiveness was moderated by mothers' accuracy in predicting their toddlers' distress when exposed to standard novelty experiences. If mothers were accurate, their protectiveness explained a portion of the temperament-to-outcome linkage, but not if they were inaccurate. A second example is one in which low positive affectivity predicted low social support, which accounted for some of the linkage between low positive affectivity and depressive symptoms (Wetter & Hankin, 2009). Another example is provided by Zalewski, Lengua, Wilson, Trancik,

and Bazinet (2011), who found that child self-regulation of frustration mediated between early temperamental effortful control and later depression and conduct problems. A pattern of low behavioral display of frustration in response to an experimenter repeatedly interrupting and changing a token sort task but normal levels of psychophysiological reactivity and subjective report of frustration predicted later symptoms of depression; and a more or less opposite pattern—high behavioral display of frustration and normal physiological and subjective frustration—predicted, to a trend degree, conduct problems. Finally, we mention a study by Zhou, Main, and Wang (2010), which suggests that child effortful control was associated with low levels of later externalizing problems via high academic achievement. Of the four studies mentioned, only one provided the classical 3-wave demonstration of mediation (predictor at the first measurement occasion, mediator at the second, and outcome at the third; Zalewski et al., 2011). We have seen very few other such studies, which is consistent with the relatively small numbers of such findings mentioned in previous reviews. Perhaps this is related to the methodological challenges in demonstrating mediation in longitudinal studies, as discussed by Cole and Maxwell (2003).

Nonlinear Connections

Another kind of model of how temperament is related to later psychopathology is a moderator model—the implications of temperament for adjustment may depend on environmental differences or vice versa, or the implications of one temperament dimension may depend on an individual's level of a second temperament dimension. Despite studies on moderator effects having their own methodological challenges (McClelland & Judd, 1993), they have been published at a much faster rate than studies on mediation effects. Some patterns have been at least roughly replicated. Studies have considered how all three major dimensions of temperament, negative emotionality/inhibition, positive emotionality/

approach, and effortful control, interact with the major dimensions of parenting environment, warmth and control (both effective and harsh), as well as with a number of other qualities of children's environments (Bates et al., 2012; Bates & Pettit, 2007; Bush, Lengua, & Colder, 2010). This increasingly rich literature is not detailed here, but we do offer some theoretical remarks, some general summaries, and a few recent examples. There are almost no full replications across studies in the area, but there are beginning to be some converging findings, and the fact that similar patterns are found despite differences in measurement suggests some meaningful phenomena have been discovered.[3] We think of the different dimensions of temperament as reflecting particular sensitivities, e.g., fearful/inhibited temperament as sensitivity to threats or positive emotionality/approaching temperament as sensitivity to rewards (and perhaps comparative insensitivity to threats). The emerging literature suggests that the developmental implication of a temperament trait depends on the functionality of the trait in the child's environment. Specific generalizations are limited by the differences in measures and designs—e.g., comparisons across studies are often challenged by the key temperament measures representing relatively unique and complex mixtures of more basic temperament dimensions. However, some broad generalizations are still fair.

Negative Emotionality X Environment

First, to consider interactions involving temperamental negative emotionality, children who are negatively emotional—especially if the emotion responds to novel people and places—are more likely than other children to develop adjustment

problems if they are in either an overly supportive (Arcus, 2001; Kiff, Lengua, & Bush, 2011) or denigrating (Rubin, Burgess, & Hastings, 2002) environment. Subsequent studies have shown both kinds of moderated linkage between behavioral inhibition X challenging vs. harsh parenting and later anxiety problems, but the literature has not yet established the conditions under which the patterns do and do not hold (Kiff, Lengua, & Zalewski, 2011).

Another example of negative emotionality's prediction of later adjustment being moderated by environmental characteristics is the widely cited finding of Pluess and Belsky (2010): Children who were high on a composite of adverse temperament traits including negative emotionality showed a stronger predictive relation between the quality of parenting they received (sensitive, positively involved) and their social and academic adjustment than did the temperamentally easy children. That is, quality of the parent–child relationship mattered more for temperamentally difficult children than it did for easy ones. Difficult children with high-quality parenting even had slightly better outcomes than easy children with high-quality parenting. Mesman et al. (2009) provide a similar pattern of findings, in which children's linear slopes of externalizing problems were an interactive function of the child's adverse temperament and maternal sensitivity. In addition, the study by Kim and Kochanska (2012) is also relevant. In this study, self-regulation was not viewed as an antecedent for development, but rather as an outcome. Higher levels of mother–child "mutually responsive orientation," or harmonious, well-synchronized, positive involvement at 15 months predicted observed self-regulation (i.e., success in inhibitory control and compliance on "do" and "don't" tasks) at age 25 months, but only for children who were high in negative emotionality (anger in a frustrating situation and with parents) at age 7 months. Adding to the growing collection of crossover interactions involving negative emotionality, this study found that children who were high in negative emotionality and in high mutuality relationships with their mothers turned out to be more self-regulated at 25 months than

---

[3] Nevertheless, we keep in mind that the phenotypes we call temperament, whether caregiver ratings, observations of behavior, or observations of psychophysiological process, necessarily reflect a history of transactions with the social environment as well as inborn tendencies. At the same time, the phenotypes we call environment also reflect a history of transactions with the child as well as inborn tendencies (of the parents and children).

children who were low in negativity, whereas in low mutuality relationships, highly negative children turned out to have lower self-regulation than the low negative children. In a similar but not crossover interaction, Kochanska, Philibert, and Barry (2009) reported that children with the risk allele of the serotonin transporter gene, which we interpret as related to temperamental negative emotionality, showed low levels of self-regulation across early childhood if they had been insecurely attached to their mother, but showed levels of self-regulation that were as high as the children without the risk allele if they had been securely attached.

To summarize, although the studies suggest that all children benefit from good quality care, more negatively reactive children appear to need and respond to good-quality care (or its absence or unpredictability) to a somewhat stronger degree than children lower on negative emotionality. There is some thinking that such findings imply that more is involved than simply the amount of negativity the child shows, suggesting an evolutionarily based alertness to the affordances of the social environment (e.g., Ellis, Boyce, Belsky, Bakermans-Kranenburg, & Van Ijzendoorn, 2011). Alertness is an interesting possible frame, but evidence for this interpretation is limited at this point. At the moment, there appears to be more support for an interpretation centered on the implications of temperamental negative emotionality. Studies have not provided a precise delineation of the core, endophenotypical temperament, or environmental features in such interactions. The pattern may or may not apply to all of the theoretical dimensions of temperament that could be represented in the negativity composites (e.g., high approach-related frustration, high sensitivity, high distress from novelty or sensory stimuli, low self-soothing). Already, a different pattern has emerged for more particularly fearful negative emotionality—in which temperamentally fearful children develop fewer anxiety problems when their parents are neither too undercutting nor too protective from social and other consequences.

Positive Emotionality X environment

A second domain of temperament X environment interactions in the development of behavioral adjustment involves children's positive emotionality or extraversion (Rothbart & Bates, 2006). What parenting environment would be especially relevant for children high or low on positive emotionality in the development of behavioral adjustment? The important parent–child conflicts for children high on positive emotionality would pertain to the child's need for upper-limit control (Bell, 1968), involving excessive, poorly modulated actions (Newman & Wallace, 1993), as well as self-centered and dysregulated bids for control of others' attention and action (Spivack, Marcus, & Swift, 1986). An earlier study of ours considered the role of a temperament dimension of resistance to control (of approach behaviors), which we assume to pertain, in part, to children's strength of approach tendencies. Early resistant temperament predicted later externalizing adjustment, but more so if the early mother behavior pattern involved relatively low levels of control of the child (Bates, Pettit, Dodge, & Ridge, 1998). Of course, an alternative interpretation of the behaviors marked as resistance to control is a lack of effortful self-regulation, which itself could be a temperamental variation, especially in early childhood. Indeed, we think that as individual differences in effortful control emerge in year 2 and beyond, more and more of the phenotypes of positive and negative emotionality also reflect the child's regulatory dispositions and skills. A second, more recent example has used a dopamine gene (*DRD4*) measure, regarded as a possible root of temperament. This interpretation of *DRD4* is supported by the demonstrated approach and approach-regulation functions of dopamine (Bakermans-Kranenburg & van Ijzendoorn, 2007) (also see Ellis et al., 2011). Children with the risk allele for this gene show a stronger linkage between sensitive parenting and child non-aggressiveness than do children without the risk allele, who show little aggressiveness whether they get low or high sensitivity from their parents.

Effortful Control X Environment

A third domain involves relatively early-appearing differences in child effortful self-regulation. This, like all temperament concepts, is not simple; it can be defined in terms of neuro-cognitive development, but it must also include neuroaffective development, because motivation is an important part of regulation (Barkley, 2012; Rothbart & Bates, 2006). There may be related but distinct endophenotypes within the domain of effortful control, including an ability to direct attention away from distressing stimuli, an ability to direct attention in response to abstract task demands, a working memory to keep goals and procedures in mind, a sense of self (Barkley, 2012), an ability to respond to another person's request or command (a major facet of our ICQ scale of resistance to control or unmanageability of approach behaviors; Bates et al., 1998), and eventually to be able to inhibit behaviors on the basis of internal representations (Barkley, 2012). It would be convenient if these all turned out to be part of an organized developmental sequence, but it is possible that they are not so tightly linked. The abilities may have separate threads of development, starting with their constellations of genes and psychophysiological signatures. However, despite many unresolved conceptual and methodological issues, we are especially encouraged by the literature on how early self-regulation interacts with environmental variables in forecasting later adjustment. It provides the promise of improved focus of prevention programs. Young children who are lagging in their ability to inhibit approach responses are at risk for developing externalizing behavior problems, but especially so if they experience below-average levels of parental management (Bates et al., 1998). A similar pattern, from another perspective, involves peer influences. Peer influences—whether toward deviant or nondeviant behavior—were the largest for youths who were low in ability to inhibit their own reward-seeking actions in a game with a mixture of rewarded and punished stimuli, according to findings of a study by Goodnight, Bates, Newman, Dodge, and Pettit (2006). Similarly, peer deviance was less associated with the delinquent behavior of youths who were temperamentally more regulated, responsive, and positive (Mrug, Madan, & Windle, 2012).

Other Temperament Interactions

Temperament X temperament interactions are also of interest. Just as the meaning of a temperament trait should depend on its social-environmental context, so should the meaning of a temperament trait be framed by the individual's other temperament traits. So far, a solid handful of studies have emerged showing that negative emotionality matters more for the development of behavior problems when it is accompanied by low effortful control, for externalizing (Eisenberg et al., 2000), internalizing (Lonigan, Vasey, Phillips, & Hazen, 2004), and both internalizing and externalizing outcomes (Muris, Meesters, & Blijlevens, 2007).

Other temperament variables might also interact. A few examples of expanded interaction models are starting to emerge, too. One is the finding by Buss, Davis, and Kiel (2011) of a 3-way interaction between fearful temperament, a physiological stress composite (summing indexes of cortisol, sleep deficit, low birth weight, and cardiac vagal tone), and also a more purely environmental composite of parent personality and social class in predicting child anxiety problems at age 3 years. Children who had high temperamental fear and had a high-stress environment showed the strongest association between the physiological stress index and later levels of anxiety problems. Physiological stress was not much associated with later anxiety in a low-stress environment. And non-fearful children showed few anxiety problems whether they were high in physiological stress responses or in a high-stress environment or not. The Buss et al. (2011) study provides an example of a temperament X temperament X environment interaction effect. A second example is the finding of Schermerhorn et al. (2013) that children high in novelty distress who were also high on resistance to control (unmanageability) were especially likely to develop later externalizing problems if they were in a high-stress environment. This was as predicted because it was assumed that chronic arousal due to family stress would amplify dysregulated, aggressive tendencies especially for the more fearful children.

Summary

The studies described are just a sampling of the many noteworthy descriptions of temperament X environment interactions in the literature. Findings of temperament X environment interactions in the development of adjustment were expected theoretically, in a general sense, many years before advances in methods allowed the first converging findings on particular patterns of interaction (Bates et al., 1998). Close replications are much needed in this area (as well as other areas of developmental research—Duncan, Engel, Claessens, & Dowsett, 2012). However, there are enough converging patterns that we can hypothesize some specific temperament X environment interactions in shaping development. First, young children who are high on one aspect of general negative emotionality component, irritability, which might reflect, in part, sensitive awareness of environment, will be especially sensitive to family deficits in warmth and effective parental control and excesses in harsh control and therefore in such families be more likely to develop behavior problems. And they may also be especially advantaged when their family has the opposite parenting qualities. Second, children who are high on a particular kind of negative emotionality, fearfulness, would be especially sensitive to the environments' affordances of security and protection, and those with too little support or too few growth challenges are especially likely to develop anxiety problems. Third, young children whose effortful self-regulation abilities are slow in developing will be especially sensitive to properties of effective control. It appears likely that the higher the early self-regulation, the fewer the conflicts the child has

with the environment and the fewer the chances to perfect skills of coercive control and the more chances the child is given to pursue rewarding prosocial and autonomous skills. However, with caregivers who effectively scaffold the slowly developing self-control of the child, even the child who is low in self-regulation can end up with a socially successful adjustment. Several other temperament X environment contours are emerging (Bates, 2012), but the three listed represent the three of most interest to us at this time. The patterns described are quite complex. However, none of the interaction effects described so far accounts for large amounts of variance. It will be interesting to see the extent to which models with multiple temperament and multiple environmental dimensions, extending beyond Buss et al. (2011) and Schermerhorn et al. (2013), ultimately provide more precise descriptions of adjustment outcomes.

Conclusion

The evidence suggests that temperament traits are implicated in the development of psychopathology, at least the most common, internalizing and externalizing dimensions of adjustment. It is likely that the measured phenotypes of child temperament reflect some degree of experience, but it also appears likely that behavioral phenotypes are systematically associated with biological processes, including genes, neurotransmitters, and psychophysiological responses, and that these have comparable associations with behavioral adjustment. Biological processes are not, in theory, free of environmental influences, but they are regarded as more based in constitution than behavioral phenotypes. We have summarized evidence suggesting that particular temperament dimensions are differentially predictive of particular adjustment dimensions in ways that fit the concepts. For example, children's early fearful temperament predicts later anxiety problems better than it predicts later lack of aggression, and early impulsivity traits predict later aggressive problems better than anxious problems. Although such predictions are quite robust, they do not predict so much of the variance or provide such a precise theoretical account that they can be considered of high practical value. Toward this, research has recently been testing models of how temperament might influence environment qualities that then account for the development of adjustment differences. A number of such mediational findings have been offered but too few for confident cross-study generalizations. The relative lack of such mediational findings may be due to methodological challenges (such as having the relevant measures at the right times across development), but it may also pertain to a more substantive possibility—that temperament does not have a consistent impact on parent–child relationships. Although there are a number of findings of associations between child temperament and parental behavior in aggregate, the effects are quite limited (Bates et al., 2012). This relative lack of findings could reflect a failure to include measures at the right level of individual or social processes. However, it is also possible that some of this relative lack of findings might mean that parents are adaptable—they can respond to children's temperament traits in more and less functional ways, thus influencing the likelihood of behavior problems developing out of the child's early personality. This possibility has recently acquired a relatively large number of empirical examples, with some converging findings on how child temperament traits matter more for future adjustment in some environments than others. Environments that compensate for child temperament risks—e.g., sensitive management for a negatively reactive child or effective control for an impulsive child or low stress for a child with both high unmanageability and high novelty distress—reduce the association between a temperament risk and later adjustment. In addition, with development, children are increasingly able to self-regulate, another way that adverse temperaments can be prevented from causing social conflicts and emotional and behavioral problems, as shown by the findings of interactions between negative emotionality or fearfulness X effortful control in predicting adjustment. Patterns such as these and others we have mentioned are particularly interesting to us because they raise testable

intervention questions (Bates, 2012). For example, in parent behavioral therapy for children with early anxiety and negative emotionality problems, would it be helpful to emphasize, relative to the other elements of the intervention, the parents' finding ways to increase their power to withhold attention from anxious coercion and to promote child mastery efforts? Would it lead to more effective problem solving and ultimately better reductions of child anxious coercion?

The current directions of research are quite exciting. Studies are using more precisely described biological endophenotypes and genotypes that both map onto and extend concepts of temperament and developmental psychopathology. And studies are using more precisely described and theoretically grounded environment dimensions that are also advancing understanding of how transactional processes between child and environment shape development. Rich longitudinal studies, more frequent in recent years, are highly useful for evaluating the mediator, moderator, and mediated moderation processes that are theoretically involved in linking temperament and later adjustment. Finally, another trend, just gathering momentum (e.g., Scott & O'Connor, 2012) is for experimental—usually intervention—studies to evaluate treatment X temperament interactions. Such studies will not establish developmental process, but they will be an important complement to longitudinal studies. As the area of research proceeds, findings will begin to show practical usefulness for designing prevention and early intervention programs. Many behavior problems have a temperament core, but the reverse does not have to be true—temperament traits do not have to become behavior problems.

References

Achenbach, T. M. (1991). *Manual for the child behavior checklist and 1991 profile*. Burlington, VT: Department of Psychiatry, University of Vermont.

Ainsworth, M. D. S., Blehar, M. C., Waters, E., & Wall, S. (1979). *Patterns of attachment: A psychological study of the strange situation*. Oxford, England: Lawrence Erlbaum.

Arcus, D. (2001). Inhibited and uninhibited children: Biology in the social context. In T. D. Wachs & G. A. Kohnstamm (Eds.), *Temperament in context* (pp. 43–60).

Mahwah, NJ: Lawrence Erlbaum Associates Publishers.

Aron, E. N., Aron, A., & Jagiellowicz, J. (2012). Sensory processing sensitivity: A review in the light of the evolution of biological responsivity. *Personality and Social Psychology Review*. doi:10.1177/1088868311434213.

Bakermans-Kranenburg, M. J., & van Ijzendoorn, M. H. (2007). Research review: Genetic vulnerability or differential susceptibility in child development: The case of attachment. *Journal of Child Psychology and Psychiatry, 48*(12), 1160–1173.

Barkley, R. A. (2012). *Executive functions: What they are, how they work, and why they evolved*. New York, NY: The Guilford.

Bates, J. E. (1989a). Applications of temperament concepts. In G. A. Kohnstamm, J. E. Bates, & M. K. Rothbart (Eds.), *Temperament in childhood* (pp. 322–355). Oxford, England: Wiley.

Bates, J. E. (1989b). Concepts and measures of temperament. In G. A. Kohnstamm, J. E. Bates, & M. K. Rothbart (Eds.), *Temperament in childhood* (pp. 3–26). Oxford, England: Wiley.

Bates, J. E. (2012). Temperament as a tool in promoting early childhood development. In S. L. Odum, E. P. Pungello, & N. Gardner-Neblett (Eds.), *Infants, toddlers, and families in poverty: Research implications for early child care* (pp. 153–177). New York: The Guilford.

Bates, J. E., & Bayles, K. (1984). Objective and subjective components in mothers' perceptions of their children from age 6 months to 3 years. *Merrill-Palmer Quarterly, 30*(2), 111–130.

Bates, J. E., & Pettit, G. S. (2007). Temperament, parenting, and socialization. In J. E. Grusec & P. D. Hastings (Eds.), *Handbook of socialization: Theory and research* (pp. 153–177). New York: The Guilford.

Bates, J. E., Pettit, G. S., Dodge, K. A., & Ridge, B. (1998). Interaction of temperamental resistance to control and restrictive parenting in the development of externalizing behavior. *Developmental Psychology, 34*(5), 982–995.

Bates, J. E., Schermerhorn, A. C., & Goodnight, J. A. (2010). Temperament and personality through the lifespan. In M. E. Lamb & A. Freund (Eds.), *Handbook of lifespan development* (pp. 208–253). Hoboken, NJ: Wiley.

Bates, J. E., Schermerhorn, A. C., & Petersen, I. T. (2012). Temperament and family processes. In M. Zentner & R. Shiner (Eds.), *The handbook of temperament*. New York: The Guilford.

Bell, R. Q. (1968). A reinterpretation of the direction of effects in studies of socialization. *Psychological Review, 75*(2), 81–95.

Bugental, D. B., & Grusec, J. E. (2006). *Socialization processes*. Hoboken, NJ: Wiley.

Bush, N. R., Lengua, L. J., & Colder, C. R. (2010). Temperament as a moderator of the relation between neighborhood and children's adjustment. *Journal of Applied Developmental Psychology, 31*(5), 351–361.

Buss, K. A. (2011). Which fearful toddlers should we worry about? Context, fear regulation, and anxiety risk. *Developmental Psychology, 47*, 804–819.

Buss, K. A., Davis, E. L., & Kiel, E. J. (2011). Allostatic and environmental load in toddlers predicts anxiety in preschool and kindergarten. *Development and Psychopathology, 23*(4), 1069–1087.

Caspi, A., & Shiner, R. L. (2006). *Personality development*. Hoboken, NJ: Wiley.

Champagne, F. A., Chretien, P., Stevenson, C. W., Zhang, T. Y., Gratton, A., & Meaney, M. J. (2004). Variations in nucleus accumbens dopamine associated with individual differences in maternal behavior in the rat. *The Journal of Neuroscience, 24*(17), 4113–4123.

Cicchetti, D. (2006). *Development and psychopathology* (2nd ed., Vol. 1). Hoboken, NJ: Wiley.

Clauss, J. A., Cowan, R. L., & Blackford, J. U. (2011). Expectation and temperament moderate amygdala and dorsal anterior cingulate cortex responses to fear faces. *Cognitive, Affective, & Behavioral Neuroscience, 11*(1), 13–21.

Cole, D. A., & Maxwell, S. E. (2003). Testing mediational models with longitudinal data: Questions and tips in the use of structural equation modeling. *Journal of Abnormal Psychology, 112*(4), 558–577.

Cox, M. J., Mills-Koonce, R., Propper, C., & Gariépy, J.-L. (2010). Systems theory and cascades in developmental psychopathology. *Development and Psychopathology, 22*(3), 497–506.

Cronbach, L. J., & Meehl, P. E. (1955). Construct validity in psychological tests. *Psychological Bulletin, 52*(4), 281–302.

De Pauw, S. S. W., & Mervielde, I. (2010). Temperament, personality and developmental psychopathology: A review based on the conceptual dimensions underlying childhood traits. *Child Psychiatry and Human Development, 41*(3), 313–329.

Degnan, K. A., Almas, A. N., & Fox, N. A. (2010). Temperament and the environment in the etiology of childhood anxiety. *Journal of Child Psychology and Psychiatry, 51*(4), 497–517.

Dettling, A. C., Parker, S. W., Lane, S., Sebanc, A., & Gunnar, M. R. (2000). Quality of care and temperament determine changes in cortisol concentrations over the day for young children in childcare. *Psychoneuroendocrinology, 25*(8), 819–836. doi:10.1016/S0306-4530(00)00028-7.

Dodge, K. A., Coie, J. D., & Lynam, D. (2006). Aggression and antisocial behavior in youth. In N. Eisenberg, W. Damon, & R. M. Lerner (Eds.), *Handbook of child psychology* (Social, emotional, and personality development 6th ed., Vol. 3, pp. 719–788). Hoboken, NJ: Wiley.

Dodge, K. A., Malone, P. S., Lansford, J. E., Miller, S., Pettit, G. S., & Bates, J. E. (2009). A dynamic cascade model of the development of substance-use onset: I. Introduction. *Monographs of the Society for Research in Child Development, 74*(3), 1–31.

Duncan, G., Engel, M., Claessens, A., & Dowsett, C. (2012). *The value of replication in developmental research*. Unpublished manuscript. School of Education, UC, Irvine.

Eisenberg, N., Fabes, R. A., Shepard, S. A., Guthrie, I. K., Murphy, B. C., & Reiser, M. (1999). Parental reactions to children's negative emotions: Longitudinal relations to quality of children's social functioning. *Child Development, 70*(2), 513–534.

Eisenberg, N., Guthrie, I. K., Fabes, R. A., Shepard, S., Losoya, S., Murphy, B. C., et al. (2000). Prediction of elementary school children's externalizing problem behaviors from attention and behavioral regulation and negative emotionality. *Child Development, 71*(5), 1367–1382.

Ellis, B. J., Boyce, W. T., Belsky, J., Bakermans-Kranenburg, M. J., & Van Ijzendoorn, M. H. (2011). Differential susceptibility to the environment: An evolutionary-neurodevelopmental theory. *Development and Psychopathology, 23,* 7–28.

El-Sheikh, M., Kouros, C. D., Erath, S., Cummings, E. M., Keller, P., & Staton, L. (2009). Marital conflict and children's externalizing behavior: Pathways involving interactions between parasympathetic and sympathetic nervous system activity. *Monographs of the Society for Research in Child Development, 74,* vii–79.

Eysenck, H. J. (1992). The definition and measurement of psychoticism. *Personality and Individual Differences, 13*(7), 757–785. doi:10.1016/0191-8869(92)90050-Y.

Gartstein, M. A., Putnam, S. P., & Rothbart, M. K. (2012). Etiology of preschool behavior problems: Contributions of temperament attributes in early childhood. *Infant Mental Health Journal, 33,* 197–211.

Goldsmith, H. H., Buss, K. A., & Lemery, K. S. (1997). Toddler and childhood temperament: Expanded content, stronger genetic evidence, new evidence for the importance of environment. *Developmental Psychology, 33*(6), 891–905.

Goodnight, J. A., Bates, J. E., Newman, J. P., Dodge, K. A., & Pettit, G. S. (2006). The interactive influences of friend deviance and reward dominance on the development of externalizing behavior during middle adolescence. *Journal of Abnormal Child Psychology, 34*(5), 573–583. An official publication of the International Society for Research in Child and Adolescent Psychopathology.

Goodnight, J. A., Bates, J. E., Pettit, G. S., & Dodge, K. A. (2008). Parents' campaigns to reduce their children's conduct problems: Interactions with temperamental resistance to control. *European Journal of Developmental Science, 2,* 100–119.

Granic, I., & Patterson, G. R. (2006). Toward a comprehensive model of antisocial development: A dynamic systems approach. *Psychological Review, 113*(1), 101–131.

Gray, J. A. (1991). The neuropsychology of temperament. In J. Strelau & A. Angleitner (Eds.), *Explorations in temperament: International perspectives on theory and measurement. Perspectives on individual differences* (pp. 105–128). New York, NY: Plenum.

Kagan, J., & Fox, N. A. (2006). Biology, culture, and temperamental biases. In N. Eisenberg, W. Damon, & R. M. Lerner (Eds.), *Handbook of child psychology* (Social, emotional, and personality development 6th ed., Vol. 3, pp. 167–225). Hoboken, NJ: Wiley.

Keiley, M. K., Lofthouse, N., Bates, J. E., Dodge, K. A., & Pettit, G. S. (2003). Differential risks of covarying and pure components in mother and teacher reports of externalizing and internalizing behavior across ages 5 to 14. *Journal of Abnormal Child Psychology, 31*(3), 267–283.

Kiel, E. J., & Buss, K. A. (2011). Prospective relations among fearful temperament, protective parenting, and social withdrawal: The role of maternal accuracy in a moderated mediation framework. *Journal of Abnormal Child Psychology, 39*(7), 953–966.

Kiff, C. J., Lengua, L., & Bush, N. (2011). Temperament variation in sensitivity to parenting: Predicting changes in depression and anxiety. *Journal of Abnormal Child Psychology, 39*(8), 1199–1212. doi:10.1007/s10802-011-9539-x.

Kiff, C. J., Lengua, L. J., & Zalewski, M. (2011). Nature and nurturing: Parenting in the context of child temperament [Article]. *Clinical Child and Family Psychology Review, 14*(3), 251–301. doi:10.1007/s10567-011-0093-4.

Kim, S., & Kochanska, G. (2012). Child temperament moderates effects of parent–child mutuality on self-regulation: A relationship-based path for emotionally negative infants. *Child Development, 83*(4), 1275–1289.

Klein, D. L., Dyson, M. W., Kujawa, A. J., & Kotov, R. (2012). Temperament and internalizing disorders. In M. Zentner & R. L. Shiner (Eds.), *The handbook of temperament* (pp. 541–561). New York: The Guilford.

Kochanska, G., Aksan, N., & Joy, M. E. (2007). Children's fearfulness as a moderator of parenting in early socialization: Two longitudinal studies. *Developmental Psychology, 43*(1), 222–237.

Kochanska, G., Philibert, R. A., & Barry, R. A. (2009). Interplay of genes and early mother-child relationship in the development of self-regulation from toddler to preschool age. *Journal of Child Psychology and Psychiatry, 50*(11), 1331–1338.

Kohlberg, L., LaCrosse, J., & Ricks, D. (1972). The predictability of adult mental health from childhood behavior. In B. Wolman (Ed.), *Manual of child psychopathology* (pp. 1217–1284). New York: McGraw-Hill.

Kopp, C. B. (1982). Antecedents of self-regulation: A developmental perspective [Peer Reviewed]. *Developmental Psychology, 18*(2), 199–214. doi:10.1037/0012-1649.18.2.199.

Lemery, K. S., Goldsmith, H. H., Klinnert, M. D., & Mrazek, D. A. (1999). Developmental models of infant and childhood temperament. *Developmental Psychology, 35*(1), 189–204.

Lengua, L. J. (2006). Growth in temperament and parenting as predictors of adjustment during children's transition to adolescence. *Developmental Psychology, 42*(5), 819–832.

Lengua, L. J., & Kovacs, E. A. (2005). Bidirectional associations between temperament and parenting and the prediction of adjustment problems in middle childhood. *Journal of Applied Developmental Psychology, 26*(1), 21–38.

Lewis, M. D., & Todd, R. M. (2007). The self-regulating brain: Cortical-subcortical feedback and the development of intelligent action. *Cognitive Development, 22*(4), 406–430.

Loeber, R., & Burke, J. D. (2011). Developmental pathways in juvenile externalizing and internalizing problems. *Journal of Research on Adolescence, 21*(1), 34–46.

Lonigan, C. J., Vasey, M. W., Phillips, B. M., & Hazen, R. A. (2004). Temperament, anxiety, and the processing of threat-relevant stimuli. *Journal of Clinical Child and Adolescent Psychology, 33*(1), 8–20.

Manassis, K., & Bradley, S. J. (1994). The development of childhood anxiety disorders: Toward an integrated model. *Journal of Applied Developmental Psychology, 15*(3), 345–366. doi:10.1016/0193-3973(94)90037-X.

McClelland, G. H., & Judd, C. M. (1993). Statistical difficulties of detecting interactions and moderator effects. *Psychological Bulletin, 114*(2), 376–390.

Mesman, J., Stoel, R., Bakermans-Kranenburg, M. J., van Ijzendoorn, M. H., Juffer, F., Koot, H. M., et al. (2009). Predicting growth curves of early childhood externalizing problems: Differential susceptibility of children with difficult temperament. *Journal of Abnormal Child Psychology, 37*(5), 625–636.

Mikolajewski, A., Allan, N., Hart, S., Lonigan, C., & Taylor, J. (2013). Negative affect shares genetic and environmental influences with symptoms of childhood internalizing and externalizing disorders. *Journal of Abnormal Child Psychology, 41*, 411–423. doi:10.1007/s10802-012-9681-0.

Mrug, S., Madan, A., & Windle, M. (2012). Temperament alters susceptibility to negative peer influence in early adolescence. *Journal of Abnormal Child Psychology, 40*(2), 201–209.

Muris, P., Meesters, C., & Blijlevens, P. (2007). Self-reported reactive and regulative temperament in early adolescence: Relations to internalizing and externalizing problem behavior and "Big Three" personality factors. *Journal of Adolescence, 30*(6), 1035–1049.

Nachmias, M., Gunnar, M., Mangelsdorf, S., Parritz, R. H., & Buss, K. (1996). Behavioral inhibition and stress reactivity: The moderating role of attachment security. *Child Development, 67*(2), 508–522. doi:10.1111/j.1467-8624.1996.tb01748.x.

Newman, J. P., & Wallace, J. F. (1993). Diverse pathways to deficient self-regulation: Implications for disinhibitory psychopathology in children. *Clinical Psychology Review. Special Issue: Disinhibition disorders in childhood, 13*(8), 699–720.

Patterson, G. R., Reid, J. B., & Dishion, T. J. (1992). *Antisocial boys*. Eugene, OR: Castalia.

Petersen, I. T., Bates, J. E., Goodnight, J. A., Dodge, K. A., Lansford, J. E., Pettit, G. S., et al. (2012). Interaction between serotonin transporter polymorphism (5-HTTLPR) and stressful life events in adolescents'

trajectories of anxious/depressed symptoms. *Developmental Psychology, 48*(5), 1463–1475.

Pluess, M., & Belsky, J. (2010). Differential susceptibility to parenting and quality child care. *Developmental Psychology, 46*, 379–390.

Pollak, S. D., Klorman, R., Thatcher, J. E., & Cicchetti, D. (2001). P3b reflects maltreated children's reactions to facial displays of emotion. *Psychophysiology, 38*, 267–274.

Raby, K. L., Cicchetti, D., Carlson, E. A., Cutuli, J. J., Englund, M. M., & Egeland, B. (2012). Genetic and caregiving-based contributions to infant attachment. *Psychological Science, 23*(9), 1016–1023. doi:10.1177/0956797612438265.

Rothbart, M. K. (2011). *Becoming who we are: Temperament and personality in development*. New York, NY: The Guilford.

Rothbart, M. K., & Bates, J. E. (1998). *Temperament*. Hoboken, NJ: Wiley.

Rothbart, M. K., & Bates, J. E. (2006). Temperament. In N. Eisenberg, W. Damon, & R. M. Lerner (Eds.), *Handbook of child psychology* (Social, emotional, and personality development 6th ed., Vol. 3, pp. 99–166). Hoboken, NJ: Wiley.

Rubin, K. H., Burgess, K. B., & Hastings, P. D. (2002). Stability and social-behavioral consequences of toddlers' inhibited temperament and parenting behaviors. *Child Development, 73*(2), 483–495.

Sameroff, A. J. (2010). A unified theory of development: A dialectic integration of nature and nurture. *Child Development, 81*(1), 6–22.

Saudino, K. J. (2005). Behavioral genetics and child temperament. *Developmental & Behavioral Pediatrics, 26*, 214–223.

Schermerhorn, A. C., Bates, J. E., Goodnight, J. A., Lansford, J. E., Dodge, K. A., & Pettit, G. S. (2013). Temperament moderates associations between exposure to stress and children's externalizing problems. *Child Development, 84*, 1579–1593.

Schermerhorn, A. C., Chow, S.-M., & Cummings, E. M. (2010). Developmental family processes and interparental conflict: Patterns of microlevel influences. *Developmental Psychology, 46*(4), 869–885.

Scott, S., & O'Connor, T. G. (2012). An experimental test of differential susceptibility to parenting among emotionally-dysregulated children in a randomized controlled trial for oppositional behavior. *Journal of Child Psychology and Psychiatry, 53*, 1184–1193. doi:10.1111/j.1469-7610.2012.02586.x.

Schore, A. N. (1994). *Affect regulation and the origin of the self*. Mahwah, NJ: Erlbaum.

Seifer, R. (2000). Temperament and goodness of fit: Implications for developmental psychopathology. In A. J. Sameroff, M. Lewis, & S. M. Miller (Eds.), *Handbook of developmental psychopathology* (2nd ed., pp. 257–276). Dordrecht, Netherlands: Kluwer.

Spivack, G., Marcus, J., & Swift, M. (1986). Early classroom behaviors and later misconduct. *Developmental Psychology, 22*(1), 124–131. doi:10.1037/0012-1649.22.1.124.

Sroufe, L. A., & Rutter, M. (1984). The domain of developmental psychopathology. *Child Development, 55*(1), 17–29.

Thelen, E., & Smith, L. B. (1998). Dynamic systems theories. In R. M. Lerner (Series Ed.) & W. Damon (Vol. Ed.), *Handbook of child psychology: Vol. 1. Theoretical models of human development* (5th ed., pp. 563–634). New York: Wiley.

Thomas, A., Chess, S., & Birch, H. G. (1968). *Temperament and behavior disorders in children.* Oxford, England: New York University Press.

Vaughn, B. E., & Shin, N. (2011). Attachment, temperament, and adaptation: One long argument. In D. Cicchetti & G. I. Roisman (Eds.), *Minnesota symposia on child psychology: The origins and organization of adaptation and maladaptation* (Vol. 36, pp. 55–107). Hoboken, NJ: Wiley.

Wachs, T. D. (2000). *Necessary but not sufficient: The respective roles of single and multiple influences on individual development.* Washington, DC: American Psychological Association.

Wachs, T. D., & Bates, J. E. (2010). Temperament. In J. G. Bremner & T. D. Wachs (Eds.), *Wiley-Blackwell handbook of infant development* (pp. 592–622). Malden, MA: Wiley-Blackwell.

Wetter, E. K., & Hankin, B. L. (2009). Mediational pathways through which positive and negative emotionality contribute to anhedonic symptoms of depression: A prospective study of adolescents. *Journal of Abnormal Child Psychology, 37*(4), 507–520.

Zalewski, M., Lengua, L. J., Wilson, A. C., Trancik, A., & Bazinet, A. (2011). Emotion regulation profiles, temperament, and adjustment problems in preadolescents. *Child Development, 82*(3), 951–966.

Zentner, M., & Shiner, R. (Eds.). (2012). *Handbook of temperament.* New York: The Guilford.

Zhou, Q., Main, A., & Wang, Y. (2010). The relations of temperamental effortful control and anger/frustration to Chinese children's academic achievement and social adjustment: A longitudinal study. *Journal of Educational Psychology, 102*(1), 180–196.

Puberty as a Developmental Context of Risk for Psychopathology

Karen D. Rudolph

Puberty is a formative transition, marked by a confluence of biological, psychological, and social challenges. During this stage, youth experience dramatic physical transformations that signal their passage into adulthood. Moreover, this period is typified by extensive brain remodeling and alterations in hormonal systems involved in sexual maturation (Susman & Dorn, 2009) and stress reactivity (Gunnar, Wewerka, Frenn, Long, & Griggs, 2009). Beyond these physical and biological changes, youth undergo psychological and social reorganization reflected in changing self-perception and self-regulation (Hyde, Mezulis, & Abramson, 2008), shifts in the dynamics of interpersonal relationships (Rudolph, 2009), and contextual changes such as school transitions (Eccles, Lord, Roeser, Barber, & Hernandez Jozefowicz, 1997). Although this period of rapid development provides an opportunity for positive growth, unfortunately it also represents a backdrop for the development of psychopathology (Gunnar et al., 2009). In particular, research documents striking increases in multiple forms of psychopathology, including anxiety (Hayward et al., 1997), depression (Rudolph, Hammen, & Daley, 2006), antisocial behavior (Lahey et al., 2006), and substance use (Patton et al., 2004) across the pubertal transition.

Despite significant advances in the field's understanding of puberty as a context of risk for psychopathology, many questions still remain about how, why, and under what conditions this transition can derail youth development. To synthesize contemporary theory and research as well as suggest directions for further inquiry, this chapter proposes a multi-faceted framework illustrating how the complex linkages between youth and their environments contribute to trajectories of mental health across this sensitive period (see Fig. 17.1). This developmentally informed framework emphasizes how the biological and physical changes of puberty (including *status, timing, perceived timing, and tempo*) interact and transact with its psychological context (*personal risks*) and social context (*contextual risks*) to explain individual differences in the consequences of puberty as well as the processes through which puberty contributes to *psychopathology*. Reflecting emerging *sex differences* in trajectories of psychopathology (Lahey et al., 2006; Rudolph et al., 2006), significant attention is devoted to understanding specific risk in girls and boys. Moreover, this model considers how *genes and gene expression* combined with *early experience* jointly influence puberty itself as well as associated personal and contextual risks in ways that either exacerbate or even confound the effects of puberty.

Nature and Course of Puberty

Consistent with a developmental psychopathology framework (Cicchetti & Cohen, 2006; Sameroff & MacKenzie, 2003), which emphasizes

K.D. Rudolph, Ph.D. (✉)
Department of Psychology, University of Illinois,
Urbana-Champaign, Champaign, IL 61820, USA
e-mail: krudolph@illinois.edu

M. Lewis and K.D. Rudolph (eds.), *Handbook of Developmental Psychopathology*,
DOI 10.1007/978-1-4614-9608-3_17, © Springer Science+Business Media New York 2014

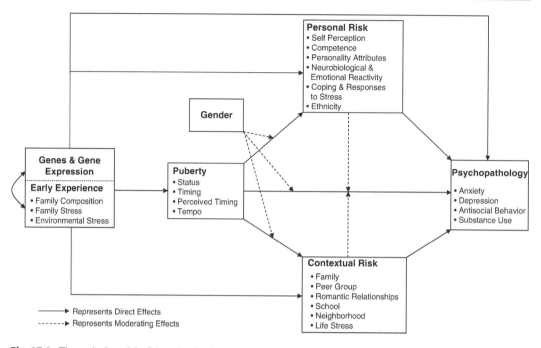

Fig. 17.1 Theoretical model of the role of puberty as a developmental context of risk for psychopathology

the synergistic interactions and dynamic transactions among multiple systems (biological, cognitive, emotional, and behavioral) and levels (personal, interpersonal, societal) of development, the pubertal transition must be situated within a developmental context (Negriff & Susman, 2011). Within this context, the passage through puberty represents not just a physical but also a psychological and social process (Graber, Nichols, & Brooks-Gunn, 2010; Mendle, Turkheimer, & Emery, 2007; Negriff & Susman, 2011; Rudolph, 2009). Specifically, the physical changes of puberty carry a strong "social stimulus value" (Brooks-Gunn & Warren, 1989, p. 41) in that they serve as an explicit signal to both youth and significant others of entrance into a new life stage. Thus, pubertal changes convey personal and social meaning about new roles, expectations, and status (Graber, 2003; Graber et al., 2010).

Puberty involves a network of connected yet distinct biological and physical changes [for reviews, see Styne and Grumbach (2007) and Susman and Dorn (2009)]. Development begins with activation of the adrenal glands, resulting in rising levels of adrenal steroid (dehydroepiandrosterone [DHEA], androstenedione) and gonadal (estrogen, testosterone) hormones. These hormonal changes eventuate in a series of morphological and other physical transformations, including the emergence of secondary sex characteristics (pubic hair growth, breast, and penis development); growth spurt; changes in body shape, size, and composition; and menarche in girls/spermarche in boys. Puberty unfolds over the course of several years, with the onset of hormonal changes preceding observable physical changes.

On average, the onset and time course of puberty differs across sex, with girls undergoing changes earlier than boys; however, there is significant intra- and interindividual variation in the timing, duration, and rate of change across various dimensions of development (Susman & Dorn, 2009). Capturing this variability, developmental scientists have studied several related, yet distinct, indexes of maturation [see Fig. 17.1; for reviews, see Dorn and Biro (2011) and Shirtcliff, Dahl, and Pollak (2009)]. Pubertal status refers to youths' absolute level of maturation, as reflected in either biological (hormonal) or physical (morphological/somatic) indicators. Status is assessed using physical exams (considered the "gold standard") or parent and/or youth report of observed physical changes. Pubertal timing, or youths' level of maturation relative to peers, has been measured as youths' pubertal status residualized on their chronological age or, within girls, as age at menarche (in single-age samples, measures of status essentially reflect timing). Perceived pubertal timing refers to youths' subjective judgments of their stage of maturation relative to peers, as reflected in direct report of whether they perceive their development to be earlier, later, or the same as their peers. A small body of research examines pubertal tempo or the rate at which puberty unfolds. Although these indexes of puberty share some common variance, each represents a unique aspect of the transition that may have specific implications for the development of psychopathology (Conley & Rudolph, 2009; Dorn & Biro, 2011; Dubas, Graber, & Petersen, 1991; Marceau, Ram, Houts, Grimm, & Susman, 2011; Shirtcliff et al., 2009).

Models of Puberty and Psychopathology

Developmental scientists have proposed diverse models to explain the emergence of psychopathology and sex differences therein across the pubertal transition. Some theories highlight the biological and physical context whereas others highlight the psychological and social context. Reflecting these varying emphases, models of puberty-psychopathology linkages include (a) direct effects [biological and physical changes directly trigger psychopathology (Angold, Costello, Erkanli, & Worthman, 1999; Angold, Worthman, & Costello, 2003)]; (b) indirect effects [biological and physical changes stimulate psychological and social disruption, which heighten risk for psychopathology (Conley, Rudolph, & Bryant, 2012; Graber, Brooks-Gunn, & Archibald, 2005; Graber, Brooks-Gunn, & Warren, 2006)]; and (c) interactive effects [biological and physical changes interact with psychological and social

challenges to trigger psychopathology (Conley & Rudolph, 2009; Graber, 2003; Magnusson, 1988; Rudolph & Troop-Gordon, 2010)]. In this section, we review empirical research on biological, psychological, and social changes associated with different indexes of puberty and we present various models that implicate puberty in risk for psychopathology.

Biological Changes

Biological changes at puberty can influence psychopathology through (a) proximal modulatory effects of gonadotropins/gonadal steroids (e.g., luteinizing hormone [LH], follicle-stimulating hormone [FSH], testosterone, estradiol) and adrenal steroids (e.g., DHEA and its sulfate [DHEAS], androstenedione) as well as interactions with other neurotransmitter and hormonal systems involved in central nervous system reactivity and stress regulation and (b) long-lasting organizational effects of hormones on neural development (Angold et al., 1999; Buchanan, Eccles, & Becker, 1992; Hayward & Sanborn, 2002; Susman & Dorn, 2009). Despite evidence for direct hormone-affect and hormone-behavior links (discussed later), these effects are small and inconsistent.

Changes in brain structure and function at puberty also can contribute to risk for psychopathology [for reviews, see Dahl (2004) and Ladouceur (2012)]. Contemporary cognitive and affective neuroscience perspectives focus on a growing disjuncture between brain systems involved in the regulation of arousal, motivation, and emotion and those involved in cognitive modulation of behavior (e.g., executive functions that guide judgment and decision making). Specifically, these theories propose an emerging imbalance during puberty reflected in increasing reactivity of sublimbic regions involved in emotion processing (e.g., amygdala, ventral striatum) accompanied by a lag in the maturation of the prefrontal cortex and associated cognitive control processes; this maturational gap is thought to contribute to emotion dysregulation and subsequent risk for psychopathology (Dahl & Gunnar, 2009; Ladouceur, 2012).

Preliminary research supports this temporal mismatch perspective. Evidence from both animal and human studies suggests that puberty-linked sex steroids influence the connectivity between prefrontal cortical and subcortical limbic regions [for a review, see Ladouceur (2012)]. At a structural level, puberty and associated sex hormones are associated with changes in grey and white matter, with accompanying implications for cognitive-affective integration [for a review, see Ladouceur (2012)]. At a physiological level, advancing puberty is associated with heightened physiological reactivity to emotions (Silk et al., 2009). Moreover, increasing neurobiological sensitivity to stress across adolescence is reflected in elevated hypothalamic–pituitary–adrenal (HPA) axis and sympathetic nervous system reactivity (Gunnar et al., 2009; Stroud et al., 2009). Significant changes also occur in neural (e.g., dopaminergic) systems underlying sensation seeking and sensitivity to reward and punishment (Quevedo, Benning, Gunnar, & Dahl, 2009; Steinberg, 2008). Research using both behavioral and neuroimaging approaches suggests that cognitive control is more easily compromised by emotionally salient information or reward incentives in adolescents compared to adults (Ladouceur, 2012). These structural, functional, and behavioral changes may, in turn, contribute to a variety of problems (e.g., risk-taking behavior, emotion dysregulation, avoidance) that heighten risk for psychopathology.

In sum, early research provides promising leads regarding increasing biological risk for psychopathology at adolescence as well as some specific evidence that these changes are driven by advancing pubertal maturation. However, longitudinal investigations using various indexes of puberty and explicit tests of mediation are needed to carefully elucidate how puberty-specific changes in biological modulation and reactivity contribute to emerging psychopathology and the sex differences therein over the course of adolescence.

Psychological and Social Changes

Beyond the effects of hormonal changes and brain reorganization, a number of theoretical perspectives consider puberty within a psychological and social context (Graber, 2003; Mendle et al., 2007; Negriff & Susman, 2011; Paikoff & Brooks-Gunn, 1991), highlighting the role of indirect pathways wherein physical changes create psychological instability and social disruption, which in turn heighten risk for psychopathology. Indirect-effect models underscore how these processes differ across sex, such that pubertal changes often confer a disadvantage for girls but an advantage for boys. Yet, contemporary perspectives suggest a more complex and nuanced outlook on sex differences, acknowledging both costs and benefits of puberty in girls and boys (Huddleston & Ge, 2003; Mendle & Ferrero, 2012; Mendle et al., 2007), as detailed below.

Pubertal Status

Pubertal changes may induce some positive expectations and even a sense of excitement given their symbolic value of encroaching adulthood (Brooks-Gunn, 1984). At the same time, these changes confront youth with the ambiguity and challenges of entering a new life stage, including the consolidation of self-identity and the negotiation of more complex and emotionally charged relationships (Caspi & Moffitt, 1991; Paikoff & Brooks-Gunn, 1991; Rudolph, 2009; Simmons & Blyth, 1987). Within the family, tension may arise as youth and parents attribute different meaning to advancing maturation, with parents focusing on increasing responsibility and risk and youth focusing on increasing privilege and autonomy (Paikoff & Brooks-Gunn, 1991; Rudolph, 2009; Steinberg, 1987). Within the peer group, physical changes signal readiness to participate in more mature sexual and romantic relationships; this development again may trigger conflicting feelings of positive anticipation and trepidation. More broadly, youth experience these signs of increasing physical maturity before Western societies typically grant social maturity (e.g., autonomy), resulting in asynchrony between different levels of development (Haynie, 2003; Moffitt, 1993).

Beyond these universal implications, girls and boys have some unique experiences. In girls, physical changes (e.g., increases in body fat and weight gain, breast development, onset of menarche) can foster psychological discomfort and social stress, particularly within Western cultures where they represent a move away from cultural ideals of thinness and attractiveness. These changes may undermine girls' sense of self and heighten their sensitivity to social scrutiny. In boys, physical changes (e.g., increases in height and musculature, a deepening voice and growth of body hair, genital development) represent a move toward cultural ideals of masculinity, strength, and athleticism; because these changes are personally and socially valued, they may boost self-esteem and confer prestige, which can protect boys against harassment and social stress. Thus, pubertal changes historically have been viewed as undesirable for girls but desirable for boys, prompting the belief that advancing maturity serves as a risk factor for psychopathology in females but a protective factor in males.

Pubertal Timing

Beyond the social stimulus value of pubertal changes, the timing of the transition may be a key determinant of psychopathology (Graber et al., 2006; Negriff & Susman, 2011; Weichold, Silbereisen, & Schmitt-Rodermund, 2003). The *maturational-deviance* hypothesis (Petersen & Taylor, 1980) implicates off-time development—both earlier and later than peers—as a risk factor. When youth mature off-time, they stand out as different at a time when social comparison processes are particularly salient and peer group conformity is of paramount importance. This discrepancy may trigger a sense of alienation from peers, with accompanying self-doubt and social stress. Also of interest is youths' subjective sense of being off-time relative to peers, which may accentuate feelings of deviance and insecurity (Tobin-Richards, Boxer, & Petersen, 1983).

Although off-time development, in general, may exert adverse effects, some perspectives highlight the particular risk associated with maturing earlier than peers. According to the *stage-termination* or *developmental readiness* perspective, early-maturing youth face the transition without sufficient developmental preparation or contextual support (Petersen & Taylor, 1980). Thus, early-maturing youth are thought to enter this transition at a distinct disadvantage relative to their peers (Caspi & Moffitt, 1991). According to the *risky social context* perspective, early-maturing youth are more likely than their on-time- and late-maturing peers to enter complex and potentially risky social relationships through affiliations with older and norm-breaking peers (Magnusson, 1988; Weichold et al., 2003). Together, the stage-termination and risky social context perspectives imply that developing earlier than one's peers propels youth into especially challenging social contexts when they are psychologically and cognitively ill-prepared to navigate their complexity.

Neither the stage-termination nor the risky social context hypotheses inherently implicates sex-differentiated effects of puberty—that is, both early-maturing girls and boys may suffer from being ill-prepared to cope with puberty as well as from having insufficient social support or affiliating with risky peer groups. However, it is important to keep in mind the differing psychological significance of off-time development in girls and boys. First, in light of sex differences in the time course of puberty, early-maturing girls experience the earliest timing whereas late-maturing boys experience the latest timing. Thus, these two groups are the most deviant from the overall peer network, suggesting that they may be at highest risk. Moreover, early-maturing girls not only confront changes prior to their peers but also show lasting differences in their body size and shape [heavier weight and higher body mass index; BMI (Lee et al., 2007)]. Second, given that girls and boys have different subjective and objective experiences of the pubertal transition, early-maturing girls may suffer more adverse psychological (e.g., threats to self-perception) and social (e.g., heightened stress) costs, whereas early-maturing boys may reap some benefits from being the first to attain the socially desirable male attributes of puberty and associated prestige. Yet, boys potentially still incur some risks due to their participation in risky social contexts. These sex differences must be taken into account when considering the implications of off-time maturation for the development of psychopathology.

Pubertal Tempo

Recently, developmental scientists have considered an often-neglected aspect of maturation—pubertal tempo—or the rate at which maturation occurs within an individual. According to the *maturation compression* perspective, youth who experience a rapid progression through puberty undergo changes faster than they or their environment can acclimate [Mendle, Harden, Brooks-Gunn, and Graber (2010); see also Marceau et al. (2011)]. In some ways, pubertal tempo is distinct from timing in that risk associated with a rapid tempo can emerge regardless of age of pubertal onset. However, it is possible that when youth undergo rapid maturation at a later age, assimilation to these changes is easier given that youth are approaching the status of their already-developed peers and are more prepared to cope with (and perhaps anxiously awaiting) the changes.

Psychological Effects of Puberty

Research generally suggests that more advanced pubertal status, and particularly early maturation, provide psychological challenges for girls but advantages for boys. Girls with more advanced pubertal status and early actual and perceived timing experience lower self-esteem, poorer body image, and more weight concerns (Benjet & Hernández-Guzmán, 2002; Tobin-Richards et al., 1983; Williams & Currie, 2000). Of note, a small amount of research suggests possible curvilinear associations, such that girls who are in mid-development (or who perceive themselves on time) report a better body image (Tobin-Richards et al., 1983) and more positive feelings about puberty (Dubas et al., 1991) than those who are less and more advanced; however, girls with more advanced status (or who perceive themselves as early) still show a disadvantage compared to those with less advanced status [or who perceive themselves as late (Tobin-Richards et al., 1983)]. In boys, early theory and research suggested that early maturation conferred a variety of psychological benefits that persisted through adulthood

(Jones, 1957; Mussen & Jones, 1957). Moreover, boys who are more advanced in their physical maturation (or who perceive themselves as early developing) report higher self-perceived attractiveness and a more positive body image (Alsaker, 1992; Tobin-Richards et al., 1983; Wichstrom, 1999) compared to late-maturing boys, who show more self-derogation and a more negative body image (Alsaker, 1992; Benjet & Hernández-Guzmán, 2002; Silbereisen & Kracke, 1997). Thus, research on the psychological effects of puberty generally is consistent with the conventional idea that this transition serves as a risky period for the emergence of psychopathology in girls but not boys.

Social Effects of Puberty

In girls, maturation has some perceived social advantages, as reflected in self-perceptions of popularity within opposite-sex relationships (Simmons, Blyth, & McKinney, 1983) as well as more self-rated peer support, liking, and attractiveness [for breast development, Brooks-Gunn and Warren (1988) and Tobin-Richards et al. (1983)] and higher levels of peer- and teacher-rated popularity (Reynolds & Juvonen, 2011). At the same time, these social benefits are intertwined with costs, such as being exposed to teasing, rumors, sexual harassment, and relational victimization from same- and other-sex peers (Brooks-Gunn, 1984; Craig, Pepler, Connolly, & Henderson, 2001; McMaster, Connolly, Pepler, & Craig, 2002; Reynolds & Juvonen, 2011), more physical (violent) victimization (Haynie & Piquero, 2006), and more general peer stress [e.g., poor friendship quality, peer isolation, or conflict (Conley et al., 2012)]. Perhaps explaining some of this stress, early-maturing girls befriend older peers and peers who approve of, or engage in, norm-breaking behavior (Magnusson, Stattin, & Allen, 1985; Stattin & Magnusson, 1990; Weichold et al., 2003). Moreover, romantic attractions, dating, and sexual activity emerge at younger ages in early-maturing girls (Compian & Hayward, 2003; Silbereisen & Kracke, 1997). The frequent instability and associated risks of early romantic relationships may lead early-maturing girls to face more stress within other-sex relationships (Llewellyn, Rudolph, & Roisman, 2012). Finally, puberty stimulates challenges as parents and daughters adapt to changing family dynamics (Paikoff & Brooks-Gunn, 1991), including more emotional distance and conflict [for advancing maturity, Steinberg, 1987] and less parental acceptance [for early maturation, Hill, Holmbeck, Marlow, Green, and Lynch (1985)]. These many social changes and challenges may set the stage for heightened psychopathology.

In boys, more advanced puberty reduces stress within the peer group (Conley et al., 2012). More advanced and early-maturing boys also experience less stressful (Llewellyn et al., 2012) and better quality other-sex relationships in the short term (Rodriguez-Tomé et al., 1993) and long term (Taga, Markey, & Friedman, 2006). However, early-maturing boys may still experience stress associated with inadequate support networks, earlier exposure to romantic and sexual relationships, and engagement in risky peer contexts (Weichold et al., 2003). Indeed, more advanced and early-maturing boys more often are targets of same-sex and other-sex sexual harassment and relational victimization (Craig et al., 2001; McMaster et al., 2002) as well as physical (violent) victimization (Haynie & Piquero, 2006). Reflecting heightened family disruption, puberty is associated with more emotional distance (for advancing maturity) and conflict [for early maturation, Steinberg (1987)]. Thus, puberty appears to present boys with social opportunities as well as challenges, thereby implicating puberty in both heightened and dampened risk for psychopathology across this transition.

Summary of Biological, Psychological, and Social Effects of Puberty

Theory and research implicate the progression through puberty as a pivotal developmental context of risk. Hormonal changes as well as brain reorganization heighten youths' emotionality and

stress reactivity as well as their inclination toward both reward seeking and avoidance. Moreover, advancing maturation, particularly when experienced off-time (and especially early) relative to peers, predicts adverse changes in self-image and heightened stress within peer, other-sex, and family relationships. These changes may, in turn, contribute to well-documented rises in psychopathology across adolescence. Despite some relatively greater costs of puberty in girls and some relatively greater benefits of puberty in boys, there are reasons to believe that this transition may heighten risk for certain forms of psychopathology in both sexes.

Empirical Research on Puberty and Psychopathology

There are several excellent reviews of research on puberty and psychopathology (Mendle & Ferrero, 2012; Mendle et al., 2007; Negriff & Susman, 2011; Weichold et al., 2003). Rather than providing a comprehensive review of this research, we highlight key findings with representative citations. We focus in particular on two domains of risk that have received significant theoretical and empirical attention: internalizing psychopathology (anxiety and depression) and externalizing psychopathology (aggression, antisocial and norm-breaking behavior, and substance use).

Internalizing Psychopathology

Research generally supports the idea that puberty contributes to internalizing psychopathology in girls and to the emerging sex difference at adolescence (Angold, Costello, & Worthman, 1998; Conley & Rudolph, 2009; Ge, Conger, & Elder, 2001; Hayward & Sanborn, 2002). However, research also implicates advancing and early pubertal maturation as a contributor to internalizing psychopathology in boys [for reviews, see Huddleston and Ge (2003) and Mendle and Ferrero (2012)], suggesting a more complex picture than originally thought.

Establishing a direct connection between hormonal changes and depression, findings from the Great Smoky Mountains Study linked higher levels of androgen and estradiol with depression in girls (Angold et al., 1999). Moreover, the Angold et al. study revealed a threshold effect, such that when sex steroid levels (combined testosterone and estradiol) reached the upper 30th percentile, girls were five times as likely to be depressed as those with lower levels; when they reached the upper 10 %, there was an additional quadrupling in the rates of depression (Angold et al., 2003). This study also showed that pubertal status, as reflected in hormone levels, served as a stronger predictor of depression and the sex difference therein than did chronological age (Angold et al., 1998). The link between estradiol and depressive affect in girls may be most salient during the period of rapid rise in hormone levels (Brooks-Gunn & Warren, 1989). Of interest, in the National Institute of Mental Health study of puberty and psychopathology, links emerged between high-for-age hormones (reflecting earlier maturation) and depressive symptoms. In girls, high-for-age FSH was associated with sad affect. In boys, high-for-age adrenal androgens but low-for-age estradiol and testosterone/estradiol ratio were associated with sad affect (Susman et al., 1985).

Studies that measure physical maturation and somatic changes, as reflected in clinician, parent, and/or youth reports on the Pubertal Development Scale (Petersen, Crockett, Richards, & Boxer, 1988) and the Tanner Stages (Morris & Udry, 1980) or menarcheal status, also implicate puberty as a contributor to rising rates of depression and associated distress during adolescence. In girls, a consistent picture emerges in which *more* advanced status is associated with higher levels of anxiety (Carter, Silverman, & Jaccard, 2011) and depression (Benjet & Hernández-Guzmán, 2002; Ge, Elder, Regnerus, & Cox, 2001; Hayward, Gotlib, Schraedley, & Litt, 1999; Siegel, Aneshensel, Taub, Cantwell, & Driscoll, 1998; Wichstrom, 1999). In boys, some studies link *less* advanced pubertal status to higher levels of depression (Conley & Rudolph, 2009) and internalizing symptoms (Laitinen-Krispijn, van

der Ende, & Verhulst, 1999). Moreover, some research provides direct evidence that pubertal status accounts for the sex difference in depression (Ge, Conger, et al., 2001). Studies examining the timing of this difference suggest that the preponderance of depression in females compared to males emerges at mid-puberty (Angold et al., 1998; Conley & Rudolph, 2009).

Research also supports the contribution of timing and perceived timing of puberty to internalizing symptoms and the sex difference therein. Consistent with the stage-termination or risky social context perspectives, a consistent corpus of research suggests that early-maturing girls (based on actual and perceived timing) experience heightened depressive mood, symptoms, and disorders (Conley & Rudolph, 2009; Ge, Conger et al., 2001; Graber, Lewinsohn, Seeley, & Brooks-Gunn, 1997; Graber, Seeley, Brooks-Gunn, & Lewinsohn, 2004; Kaltiala-Heino, Kosunen, & Rimpela, 2003; Stice, Presnell, & Bearman, 2001; Wichstrom, 1999; cf. Angold et al., 1998), feelings of anxiety (Silbereisen & Kracke, 1997), panic attacks (Hayward et al., 1997), internalizing symptoms (Caspi & Moffitt, 1991; Hayward et al., 1997), and general psychological distress (Ge, Conger, & Elder, 1996) compared to their on-time- or late-maturing peers [for reviews, see Mendle et al. (2007) and Negriff and Susman (2011)]. However, consistent with a maturational-deviance perspective, a small amount of research also links late maturation in girls with poorer psychological adjustment (Dorn, Susman, & Ponirakis, 2003; Graber et al., 1997). Accelerated pubertal tempo predicted girls' internalizing symptoms in one study (Marceau et al., 2011) but not in others (Ge et al., 2003; Mendle et al., 2010).

Among boys, findings are mixed [for reviews, see Huddleston and Ge (2003), Mendle and Ferrero (2012), and Negriff and Susman (2011)]. Whereas some research links late actual or perceived maturation with elevated depression and internalizing symptoms (Conley & Rudolph, 2009; Dorn et al., 2003; Siegel et al., 1998; cf. Angold et al., 1998), other research implicates early maturation (Natsuaki, Biehl, & Ge, 2009; Silbereisen & Kracke, 1997; Susman et al., 1985) or both (Alsaker, 1992; Graber et al., 1997; Kaltiala-Heino, Kosunen, & Rimpela, 2003) with elevated depression, anxiety, and internalizing symptoms. Research also reveals contradictory findings regarding pubertal tempo in boys: Accelerated tempo predicted the highest risk for depressive or internalizing symptoms in two studies (Ge et al., 2003; Mendle et al., 2010), the lowest risk for depression in another study (Laitinen-Krispijn et al., 1999), and was not predictive in a fourth study (Marceau et al., 2011).

In sum, with a few exceptions, research consistently supports the contribution of puberty to internalizing symptoms. These consequences have been documented for hormonal and morphological changes as well as objective and subjective indicators of timing and tempo of maturation. Across studies, research supports the stage-termination or risky social context perspectives, which implicate especially adverse effects of early timing, and to a lesser extent the maturational-deviance perspective, which implicates adverse effects of both early and late timing. Although some studies suggest that pubertal maturation contributes to observed sex differences in internalizing symptoms during adolescence (a preponderance in girls), both early and late timing predict risk among boys.

Externalizing Psychopathology

Research paints a consistent picture regarding the contribution of puberty to externalizing psychopathology. With regard to hormones, elevated levels of androgens (e.g., testosterone, androstenedione) are linked with low frustration tolerance and aggression, with stronger associations emerging in boys than in girls (Olweus, Mattsson, Schalling, & Low, 1988; Susman et al., 1987; for a review, see Buchanan et al., 1992). Rapid changes in estradiol and DHEAS are linked with aggression in girls (Graber et al., 2006). In the Great Smoky Mountain Study, more advanced Tanner Stage was associated with greater substance use in both girls and boys (Costello, Sung, Worthman, & Angold, 2007), whereas another study reported a stronger link between pubertal

status and delinquency in girls than boys (Flannery, Rowe, & Gulley, 1993).

Across various indexes of actual and perceived pubertal timing, risk for externalizing psychopathology is similar for girls and boys. Compared to their on-time- and late-maturing peers, early-maturing girls and boys show elevated levels of aggression and antisocial behavior, such as oppositional defiant and conduct disorder symptoms, truancy, theft, vandalism, and bullying (Caspi & Moffitt, 1991; Felson & Haynie, 2002; Flannery et al., 1993; Ge, Brody, Conger, Simons, & Murry, 2002; Graber et al., 1997; Kaltiala-Heino, Marttunen, Rantanen & Rimpela, 2003; Lynne, Graber, Nichols, Brooks-Gunn & Botvin, 2007; Magnusson et al., 1985; Storvall & Wichstrom, 2002; Susman et al., 2007) as well as risky and norm-breaking behavior, including smoking and earlier and more frequent sexual activity (Flannery et al., 1993; Magnusson et al., 1985). Both early-maturing boys and girls also engage in earlier and higher rates of alcohol and substance use/abuse (Kaltiala-Heino, Koivisto, Marttunen, & Sari, 2011; Schelleman-Offermans, Knibbe, Engels, & Burk, 2011; Stice et al., 2001), whereas late-maturing boys engage in lower rates of substance use (Graber et al., 1997). In one study, faster pubertal tempo predicted more externalizing symptoms in girls but only inconsistently predicted externalizing symptoms in boys (Marceau et al., 2011).

Despite this general consensus that early timing represents a risk factor for externalizing psychopathology, a few studies have yielded discrepant results. For example, higher rates of delinquency and disruptive behavior (Graber et al., 2004; Williams & Dunlop, 1999) and substance use (Dorn et al., 2003; Graber et al., 2004) have been found in late-maturing boys or in both early- and late-maturing boys (Andersson & Magnusson, 1990).

In sum, research on the contribution of puberty to externalizing psychopathology is quite consistent and generally reveals similar patterns for girls and boys. Most of the evidence supports the stage-termination or risky social context perspectives, in that early puberty has a particularly deleterious effect; however, a small amount of research suggests a possible maturational-deviance effect in boys. Of note, studies supporting this effect either had small sample sizes (e.g., Dorn et al., 2003) or showed inconsistent results across types of delinquency (Williams & Dunlop, 1999) or across time (Andersson & Magnusson, 1990; Graber et al., 1997, 2004). Discrepancies also may result from different approaches to measuring puberty (e.g., clinician vs. youth/parent reports of physical changes vs. subjective assessments of perceived timing). Thus, additional inquiry is needed to determine the robustness of the maturational-deviance effect.

Integrative Models of Puberty and Psychopathology

Despite a substantial body of evidence linking puberty and psychopathology, much of this research focuses on rather simplistic main effects. Drawing from developmental perspectives on psychopathology (Cicchetti & Cohen, 2006; Sameroff & MacKenzie, 2003), Fig. 17.1 illustrates how puberty interacts and transacts with characteristics of youth (*personal risks*) and their contexts (*contextual risks*) to shape trajectories of mental health. Taking this developmental approach (a) helps to clarify the reasons for individual variation in the consequences of puberty (Caspi & Moffitt, 1991; Conley & Rudolph, 2009; Ge & Natsuaki, 2009; Graber, 2003; Rudolph & Troop-Gordon, 2010) and (b) elucidates *how* and *why* puberty contributes to subsequent psychopathology (Ge & Natsuaki, 2009; Graber et al., 2005; Rudolph, 2009). The following two sections describe models accounting for such interactions and pathways.

Individual Differences: Interactive Models of Puberty-Psychopathology Linkages

Although puberty is a universal experience, there are significant individual differences in its connotation, significance, and consequences. Indeed,

the many changes that mark this transition have the potential to confer either advantages or risks (Gunnar et al., 2009). Reflecting this individual variation, personal-accentuation and contextual-amplification models of puberty (described below) propose that characteristics of youth and their contexts magnify or temper the contribution of puberty to psychopathology. An emerging body of research supports the idea that risk associated with puberty is intensified in youth with personal or contextual risks and dampened in youth without these risks.

Personal-Accentuation Effects

According to a personal-accentuation model (Caspi & Moffitt, 1991; Ge et al., 1996; Rudolph & Troop-Gordon, 2010), early maturation accentuates preexisting individual differences in vulnerability. More specifically, this model proposes that individual differences are magnified across periods of social change, such as the pubertal transition. During these times, strong internal resources buffer youth whereas inadequate internal resources accentuate vulnerability, making youth particularly ill-equipped to deal effectively with the demands of puberty. A few studies support this model. For example, early maturation interacts with prior emotional distress (internalizing symptoms and depression) to predict subsequent psychopathology (Ge et al., 1996; Rudolph & Troop-Gordon, 2010). Similarly, early menarche magnifies aggression and delinquent behavior in girls who show prior externalizing symptoms (Caspi & Moffitt, 1991). Personality attributes (depressive personality traits and a negative self-focus) and maladaptive responses to stress also accentuate the contribution of early maturation to psychopathology. Specifically, early maturation predicts subsequent depression in youth who show high levels of depressive personality traits and a tendency toward negative self-focus (for girls) as well as fewer effortful engagement and more disengagement and involuntary (i.e., uncontrolled) responses to stress (Rudolph & Klein, 2009; Rudolph & Troop-Gordon, 2010). Moreover, early menarche predicts aggression in youth who show maladaptive responses to stress (Sontag, Graber, Brooks-Gunn & Warren, 2008). Directly assessing biological stress responses, Susman and colleagues (2010) found that late maturation was associated with delinquent behavior in boys with high cortisol reactivity whereas early maturation was associated with delinquent behavior in boys with low cortisol reactivity; no interactive effects were found in girls. Of importance, several studies suggest a moderating effect of ethnicity [for a review, see Negriff and Susman (2011)] although other research indicates comparable effects across ethnic groups (Ge, Brody, Conger, & Simons, 2006; Lynne et al., 2007), suggesting the need for further inquiry.

Contextual-Amplification Effects

According to a contextual-amplification model (Caspi, Lynam, Moffitt, & Silva, 1993; Ge & Natsuaki, 2009; Graber, 2003; Rudolph, 2009; Rudolph & Troop-Gordon, 2010), exposure to challenging social contexts magnifies the contribution of puberty to psychopathology. This perspective assumes that youth who encounter the pubertal transition with compromised social networks or who gravitate toward riskier contexts (e.g., affiliating with older peers) during the transition face the synergistic effects of multiple social challenges; puberty also may interact with the normative social-developmental stressors of adolescence (e.g., increasing complexity of peer relationships, entrance into romantic relationships, school transitions) to heighten risk (Magnusson, 1988). These amplification effects may be particularly salient in early-maturing youth, perhaps due to their heightened biological reactivity to stress (Natsuaki, Klimes-Dougan et al., 2009) or insufficient cognitive and emotional resources (Ge & Natsuaki, 2009).

Several studies support contextual-amplification effects for internalizing psychopathology. Specifically, more advanced pubertal status and early maturation interact with various aspects of girls' social contexts to predict anxiety, depression, and associated distress. Amplification effects have been found for the sex composition of peer groups (Ge et al., 1996), the quality of peer relationships (Blumenthal, Leen-Feldner, Trainor, Babson, & Bunaciu, 2009; Conley & Rudolph, 2009), engagement in romantic relationships (Hayward & Sanborn, 2002; Natsuaki, Biehl, et al., 2009), and exposure to life stress (Ge, Conger, et al., 2001; Silberg et al., 1999). Early maturation also predicts subsequent depression and psychological distress in youth exposed to recent family adversity and maternal depression (Rudolph & Troop-Gordon, 2010) as well as paternal hostility (Ge et al., 1996). Of interest, there are some sex-differentiated effects: In one study, exposure to peer stress exacerbated the depressogenic effect of *early* maturation in girls and *late* maturation in boys (Conley & Rudolph, 2009). In another study, the sex difference in depression was accounted for by the main and interactive effects of early maturation and life stress (Ge, Conger et al., 2001). Finally, a recent study using a genetically informed design found sex differences in the *timing* of pubertal amplification; specifically, more advanced pubertal status moderated environmental influences on depressive symptoms in both girls and boys, but the effect emerged earlier in girls than in boys, paralleling the delay in pubertal development in boys relative to girls (Edwards, Rose, Kaprio, & Dick, 2011).

Research also supports contextual-amplification effects for risk-taking behavior and externalizing psychopathology. Early maturation predicts norm-breaking behavior, violence, and delinquency in girls who associate with older peers (Magnusson et al., 1985), attend a mixed-sex school (Caspi et al., 1993), are exposed to neighborhood disadvantage (Obeidallah, Brennan, Brooks-Gunn, & Earls, 2004), and are heavily involved in peer or heterosexual relationships and settings that expose them to older and delinquent peers (Stattin, Kerr, & Skoog, 2011). Early maturation also interacts with heightened peer stress to predict overt and relational aggression in girls (Sontag, Graber, & Clemans, 2011). In boys, having delinquent friends exacerbates the contribution of more advanced maturation to delinquency and precocious sexuality (Felson & Haynie, 2002). In mixed-sex samples, early maturation predicts more externalizing psycho-pathology (Ge et al., 2002) and substance use (Lynne-Landsman, Graber, & Andrews, 2010) in the context of poor parenting and high household risk (e.g., low socioeconomic status, poor family relationships, parental substance use). Of inter-est, one study using a behavior genetic design found that early maturation increases girls' sensi-tivity to nonshared environmental influences on delinquency, whereas genetic factors may be more predictive of delinquency in late-maturing girls (Harden & Mendle, 2012).

Summary

Mounting evidence indicates that individual dif-ferences in youth and their contexts potentiate or temper the mental health consequences of puberty. Future research will need to determine the precise role of early vulnerability and risk. For example, the adverse effects of early maturation may, in part, reflect exacerbation of prior disorder (Caspi & Moffitt, 1991). However, because a history of psychopathology accentuates the effect of puberty on subsequent disorder even after adjusting for recent symptoms (Rudolph & Troop-Gordon, 2010), it seems that prior psychopathology also may foster core competence deficits that heighten risk during the pubertal transition. Prior vulnera-bility also may alter the context of puberty such that the pubertal transition poses a greater chal-lenge. For example, early-maturing depressed youth generate more stress in their relationships (Rudolph, 2008) and show more affiliation with deviant peers (Ge et al., 1996) than on-time- and late-maturing depressed youth. Thus, youth with prior vulnerabilities actually may face more chal-lenging contexts and experience less positive social support during puberty, thereby exacerbat-ing their risk. It also will be important to determine whether the amplifying effects of stress within peer and family relationships are driven merely by the synergistic effect of simultaneous stressors or whether this stress reflects others' differential responses to puberty (Paikoff & Brooks-Gunn, 1991). Finally, youth with a history of psychopa-thology and other vulnerabilities or those who enter into risky social contexts may have a genetic

predisposition to psychopathology that is expressed during adolescence. Clearly, integrative models of puberty and psychopathology must con-sider many complicated interactions among youth, social contexts, and developmental change.

Developmental Cascades: Process Models of Puberty-Psychopathology Linkages

Theories of development (Masten & Cicchetti, 2010) and psychopathology (Cicchetti & Cohen, 2006; Sameroff & MacKenzie, 2003) also high-light the early emerging and recursive transac-tions between youth and their environments over time. Puberty may serve as a catalyst for a cascade of changes in adolescents and their social contexts that continuously reinforce each other, eventually instilling risk for psychopathology. Understanding how these cycles unfold over time requires eluci-dating specific pathways that underlie puberty-psychopathology linkages—that is, processes through which the physical changes of puberty are translated into psychological and social dis-ruption and consequent psychopathology (Graber et al., 2005, 2010; Mendle et al., 2007; Rudolph, 2009; Rudolph, Troop-Gordon, Lambert, & Natsuaki, in press). As reflected in earlier sec-tions of this chapter, such pathways may involve intrapersonal (*personal risk*) and interpersonal (*contextual risk*) processes (see Fig. 17.1).

Intrapersonal Risk Pathways

Although research documents diverse intraper-sonal correlates of puberty (e.g., changes in self-perception, emotionality, stress reactivity, and risk taking) that could contribute to subsequent psychopathology, few studies directly examine whether these factors account for puberty-psychopathology linkages. In girls, one study found low social and academic competence mediated the concurrent association between menarcheal status and internalizing and external-izing symptoms (Negriff, Hillman, & Dorn, 2011), and another found that poor body image accounted for the concurrent association between early menarche and depression (Stice et al., 2001). Heightened emotional arousal also accounts for the concurrent association between early maturation and depressive symptoms in girls (Graber et al., 2006). In a study by Sontag and colleagues (Sontag et al., 2008), maladaptive responses to social stress mediated the concurrent association between early menarche and aggression in girls. Shedding light on emerging sex differences at adolescence, a recent study revealed that heightened cortisol reactivity to social stress partially accounted for higher concurrent levels of internalizing symptoms in early-maturing girls but not in boys (Natsuaki, Klimes-Dougan et al., 2009). Some intriguing recent results also reveal that more advanced pubertal maturation is associated with heightened ventrolateral prefrontal cortex reactivity to threat (i.e., angry relative to neutral faces), which is correlated with depressive symptoms (Forbes, Phillips, Silk, Ryan, & Dahl, 2011). In a recent longitudinal study examining multiple types of personal risk (Rudolph et al., in press), heightened negative self-focus, anxious arousal, social problems, and maladaptive responses to stress accounted for an enduring effect of early maturation on girls' depression across several years. Increasing negative self-focus, anxious arousal, and social problems accounted for a progressive effect of early maturation on boys' depression. Collectively, these studies implicate multiple possible intrapersonal pathways from puberty to psychopathology.

Interpersonal Risk Pathways

As discussed earlier, puberty, particularly when experienced early relative to peers, sparks a host of social challenges within the peer group (teasing and victimization, affiliation with older and norm-breaking peers), romantic relationships (early involvement in sexual and romantic relationships, heightened stress), and family relationships (more emotional distancing and conflict). Such contextual changes may reflect homophily or selection effects [e.g., associating with similar—more mature—peers, engaging in risky social contexts (Stattin et al., 2011; Weichold et al., 2003)]; evoc-

ative effects [e.g., eliciting adverse interpersonal reactions (Conley et al., 2012; Ge & Natsuaki, 2009; Paikoff & Brooks-Gunn, 1991)]; or stress-generation effects [e.g., creating conflict within relationships, Rudolph (2008)]. Regardless of their origin, these pernicious contexts can then contribute to psychopathology.

Several studies support interpersonal pathways linking puberty and psychopathology and illustrate differential risk in girls and boys. In one study, exposure to peer stress partially mediated the contribution of both more advanced pubertal status and early maturation to subsequent depression in girls but not in boys (Conley et al., 2012). In another study, being the victim of rumor spreading among peers partially mediated the contribution of early maturation to depressive symptoms in girls (Reynolds & Juvonen, 2011). Exposure to stress within other-sex relationships also partially mediates the early menarche-depression association in girls (Llewellyn et al., 2012). Although there is less evidence in boys, one study did find that increases in peer stressors over time mediated the contribution of early pubertal maturation and rapid pubertal tempo to changes in boys' depressive symptoms (Mendle, Harden, Brooks-Gunn, & Graber, 2012). A recent study revealed sex differences in the timing of interpersonal risk effects (Rudolph et al., in press). In girls, deviant peer affiliation and interpersonal stress accounted for an enduring effect of early maturation on depression. In boys, increasing interpersonal stress over time accounted for a progressive effect of early maturation on depression. With regard to externalizing psychopathology, mediating effects have been found for deviant peer affiliation (Haynie, 2003; Lynne et al., 2007; Negriff, Ji, & Trickett, 2011; Stattin & Magnusson, 1990) as well as involvement in romantic relationships (Haynie, 2003) and sexual activity (Negriff, Susman, & Trickett, 2011). Moreover, exposure to negative life events mediates between rising levels of estradiol and DHEAS and aggression in girls (Graber et al., 2006). Overall, research supports the idea that the transition through puberty, particularly when it is encountered early relative to one's peers, contributes to challenges and disruption in youths' social contexts, which in turn heighten risk for psychopathology.

Summary

Although research clearly establishes the passage through puberty, particularly its timing, as a risk factor for psychopathology, considerably less is known about the explanatory processes. Direct tests of mediation are beginning to elucidate possible mechanisms, but much work remains to fully understand how biological and physical transformations prompt psychological and social changes that heighten risk. Unfortunately, much of this process-oriented research relies on concurrent designs (for exceptions, see Mendle et al., 2012; Rudolph et al., in press), thus undermining our ability to determine how processes evolve over time. Moreover, most research on indirect pathways examines the contribution of early maturation to psychopathology in girls, with less work examining processes in boys and almost no attention to the processes through which late maturation creates risk. It may be that different pathways explain risk across sex, with girls' heightened risk accounted for by both psychological and social disruption and boys' heightened risk accounted for by deviant peer affiliation, exposure to victimization, and family disturbances. Future investigations also need to broaden the scope of mediators and consider integrated intrapersonal and interpersonal pathways. For instance, early maturation may foster insecurity or alienation from the peer group that causes youth to engage in maladaptive social behaviors (e.g., high reassurance seeking, withdrawal), which then elicit adverse social responses and consequent psychopathology (Rudolph, 2009). Research will therefore need to incorporate long-term prospective designs that track puberty, intrapersonal and interpersonal changes, and psychopathology in both girls and boys across the adolescent years.

Summary and Future Directions

The field has witnessed noteworthy advances in theory and research aimed at elucidating how, why, and for whom puberty contributes to the emergence of psychopathology across adolescence. This work clearly implicates puberty as a catalyst for biological, psychological, emotional, and social disequilibrium that has the potential to set youth on a trajectory of increasing risk. Yet, research also clearly documents significant individual differences in how youth traverse this stage and their consequent health and development. Moreover, although there is a strong consensus that puberty serves as an impetus for the well-documented escalating risk for psychopathology across adolescence, some research supports sex-specific risk, whereas other research supports risk for multiple types of psychopathology in both girls and boys. Progress in the field undoubtedly will require continued elaboration of integrative models embedded within a multilevel conceptualization of development and tested with sophisticated longitudinal designs that consider the complex interactions and dynamic transactions between youth and their environments over time. Moreover, with some exceptions, much of the supportive evidence relies on continuous assessments of symptoms rather than diagnoses of disorders. It will therefore be important to determine whether puberty-associated risk is expressed only as transient subclinical symptoms or is translated into clinically significant disorders characterized by enduring symptoms and associated impairment. The final sections of this chapter discuss several specific areas in need of development.

Considering the Relative Contribution of Different Indexes of Puberty

Despite the robust evidence for links between puberty and psychopathology across various indexes of maturation, there are some inconsistencies. It will be important for future studies to include different indexes to unpack their relative contributions. To be sure, there is significant overlap among the various indexes of maturation, including hormone levels, morphological/physical status, actual timing (calculated as status residualized on age or age at menarche), perceived timing (reflected in subjective assessments of one's timing relative to peers), and tempo; however, each of these indexes may carry unique meaning and thus have varying implications for development (Dorn & Biro, 2011; Shirtcliff et al., 2009).

Hormone levels provide a window into the physiological processes of puberty and thus may be especially well suited for efforts to understand puberty-induced changes in brain structure and function and their sequelae (e.g., biological reactivity to stress and regulatory processes involved in the modulation of cognition, emotion, and behavior); however, wide within- and between-individual fluctuations in hormonal levels make them an imprecise indicator of pubertal stage (Susman & Dorn, 2009). Indexes of physical status vary in salience, with some more observable (e.g., breast development), personally and culturally meaningful (e.g., onset of menarche), or socially relevant (e.g., heightened muscularity and athleticism) than others (e.g., skin changes). Those with greater social stimulus value may exert a stronger influence on self and other perceptions and relationships (Brooks-Gunn, 1984; Paikoff & Brooks-Gunn, 1991). Particular somatic manifestations also may be viewed as more or less desirable, perhaps accounting for the mixed findings regarding social advantages versus disadvantages. As discussed, the timing of maturation may be important when considering the psychological and social context of puberty. Moreover, perceived timing likely has strong implications for social comparison and peer relationships. Indeed, in studies comparing actual and perceived timing, subjective perceptions often have stronger predictive value (Alsaker, 1992; Conley & Rudolph, 2009; Siegel et al., 1998; cf. Silbereisen & Kracke, 1997, for some outcomes). Finally, given recent findings suggesting the value of assessing intraindividual change in maturation [i.e., tempo, Marceau et al. (2011) and Mendle et al. (2010, 2012)], research will need to use more dynamic analytic frameworks that account for changes in puberty over time.

Also on the agenda should be efforts to examine nonlinear associations between puberty and psychopathology. As discussed earlier, there are contrasting findings regarding the contribution of early versus late timing to psychopathology, particularly in boys. These discrepancies may result in part from the presence of curvilinear associations. If the maturational-deviance hypothesis holds—that is, both early and late timing carry costs relative to on-time development—studies examine linear associations or categorizing youth as early maturing versus on-time/late maturing may yield misleading findings. Moreover, tests of puberty-psychopathology linkages are dependent upon the age and maturational range within a sample. It is possible that studies revealing effects of early timing overlook the full range of late-developing youth and studies revealing effects of late timing overlook the full range of early-developing youth. Consequently, studies may capture only part of the curvilinear association between puberty and psychopathology.

A few studies do indeed support curvilinear associations. In two studies, both early- and late-maturing girls and boys showed higher levels of depressed mood or symptoms than those with on-time maturation [for actual timing, Natsuaki, Biehl et al. (2009), for perceived timing, Wichstrom (1999)]. In another study, a curvilinear association between perceived timing and depression was found across sex although the precise nature of this pattern differed: In girls, perceived early timing and to a lesser extent late timing were associated with more depression relative to on-time development (resulting in a positive linear association); in boys, perceived late timing and to a lesser extent early timing were associated with more depression relative to on-time development (resulting in a negative linear association). If only linear patterns had been examined, incomplete conclusions would have been drawn (Conley & Rudolph, 2009). Research using categorical analyses similarly reveals that both early and late maturation pose risk for depression in girls [for perceived timing, Graber et al. (1997), for perceived timing, Siegel et al. (1998)], and in boys [for perceived timing, Alsaker (1992), for perceived timing, Graber et al. (1997), for actual timing, Kaltiala-Heino, Kosunen, et al. (2003)], and for externalizing psychopathology in boys [for actual timing, Williams and Dunlop (1999)]. It is clear that an exclusive focus on linear effects will obscure some key findings.

Distinguishing Short Versus Long-Term Pathways

Inconsistent findings also may result from a failure to distinguish short- versus long-term effects of puberty. Most early studies supporting puberty-psychopathology linkages relied on cross-sectional designs. Although more recent research integrates longitudinal analysis, much of this work is relatively short term with far less investigation of lasting effects across adolescence or adulthood. Yet, it is possible, and indeed likely, that the influence of puberty on psychopathology varies over time and across developmental stages. Moreover, it is critical to understand whether the effects of puberty reflect temporary stage-specific disruptions or enduring changes over the life course.

On the one hand, puberty may exert short-term effects—for better or worse—that dissipate over time. Conceivably, the challenges faced by off-time youth may resolve as peers catch up in status (for early-maturing youth) or as they themselves progress through puberty (for late-maturing youth). Moreover, some of the advantages afforded to early-maturing boys, such as athleticism and social prestige, may become less salient as other boys gain similar characteristics. Indeed, risks associated with early maturation may gain traction over time as early-maturing boys begin to suffer the harmful consequences of engaging in risky social contexts. If this *temporary effects* model holds, discrepancies across studies could stem in part from differences in the timing of assessments (earlier vs. later in development, concurrent vs. longitudinal effects). Alternatively, it is possible that once off-time youth are set upon a trajectory of risk, internal and external forces continue to channel them along this path, thereby perpetuating or even exacerbating early risk. If this *enduring effects* model holds, one would expect a similar pattern of findings over time.

For internalizing psychopathology, research generally supports an enduring effects model, particularly for early-maturing girls. Studies examining effects across several years of adolescence suggest that early maturation in girls predicts stable high (Rudolph et al., in press) or increasing (Ge, Conger, et al., 2001) trajectories of depression; similar effects were found in 3rd–6th grade girls (Mendle et al., 2010). Two studies that followed girls from 1st to 9th grade (DeRose, Shiyko, Foster, & Brooks-Gunn, 2011) and age 12–23 (Natsuaki, Biehl, et al., 2009) found curvilinear trajectories, such that early puberty predicted increasing internalizing symptoms across early to mid-adolescence and slight declines through later adolescence and early adulthood. Two follow-up studies in adulthood revealed mixed findings: Whereas one found that perceived early timing predicted higher rates of lifetime depression at age 24 (Graber et al., 2004), another found that early menarche did not predict depressive symptoms at age 21 after accounting for a number of other contributors (Foster, Hagan, & Brooks-Gunn, 2008). Although most research focuses on the long-term effects of early maturation, one study found that girls with perceived late maturation had higher rates of depressive disorders during adolescence (Graber et al., 1997) but not adulthood (Graber et al., 2004).

In boys, studies supporting adverse effects of late maturation often use cross-sectional designs (Dorn et al., 2003; Kaltiala-Heino, Kosunen, & Rimpela, 2003) and measures of perceived timing (Graber et al., 1997; Siegel et al., 1998), whereas studies supporting adverse effects of early maturation (Ge, Elder, et al., 2001; Mendle et al., 2010, 2012; Natsuaki, Biehl et al., 2009) or accelerated tempo (Ge, et al., 2003; Mendle et al., 2010, 2012) often use longitudinal designs (cf. Ge et al., 1996, 2006) and measures of actual timing. Consistent with this pattern, one study found that late maturation predicted higher initial levels of depression that declined over time, whereas early maturation predicted lower initial levels of depression that increased over time (Rudolph et al., in press). Findings for boys may therefore conform more to a temporary effects model, wherein late maturation and early maturation have short-lived consequences at different times or during different developmental stages. However, even when early maturation predicts depression over time in boys, early-maturing girls typically still show the highest absolute risk (Natsuaki, Biehl, et al., 2009).

For externalizing psychopathology, several investigations support an enduring effects model through adolescence, with mixed findings for adult outcomes. In boys, Ge, Elder et al. (2001) found that early maturation in 7th grade predicted more externalizing symptoms in 8th, 9th, and 10th grades; perceived early timing also predicted delinquency in boys and girls across several grades (Lynne et al., 2007). One study found enduring effects of early puberty on substance use across two years in boys but only temporary effects in girls (Kaltiala-Heino et al., 2011), whereas another found only temporary effects of early and late maturation in boys (Andersson & Magnusson, 1990). The few long-term follow-up studies document weak to no lasting effects of early maturation on externalizing psychopathology in adulthood (Magnusson et al., 1985; Stattin & Magnusson, 1990) although one study found that perceived late maturation in boys predicted lifetime disruptive behavior and current substance use disorders in early adulthood (Graber et al., 2004).

Overall, research generally supports enduring effects of early maturation on internalizing psychopathology across adolescence, particularly in girls; in boys, a preliminary synthesis of the literature suggests possible early adverse effects of late maturation but longitudinal adverse effects of early maturation but more research is needed to determine the pattern of long-term effects in boys. For externalizing psychopathology, there is mixed support for temporary versus enduring effects of early maturation across adolescence in girls and boys. Although there is some support for small lasting effects through adulthood, risk generally seems to temper over time. Given evidence for personal-accentuation and contextual-amplification effects, it is likely that the strength of long-term effects depends in part on early or intervening risks. Thus, considerably more research is needed to identify for whom trajectories of psychopathology progress toward stable or increasing psychopathology and for whom the early effects of puberty dissipate over time. Moreover, efforts must be directed toward identifying the processes that maintain long-term effects.

Disentangling the Predictors Versus Consequences of Pubertal Timing

Now that the field has amassed robust evidence for the predictive contribution of puberty, especially early maturation, to psychopathology, it is critical to disentangle the putative mental health effects of pubertal timing per se from its predictors and correlates (Harden & Mendle, 2012; Mendle & Ferrero, 2012). Figure 17.1 summarizes several predictors of puberty, particularly with regard to its timing. Notably, genes account for a large proportion of the variance in pubertal timing (from 40 to 50 % in some studies to over 80 % in others), with greater heritability in girls than in boys (Eaves et al., 2004; Ge, Natsuaki, Neiderhiser, & Reiss, 2007). Thus, early-maturing youth may have genetic predispositions that also heighten risk for personal risks, exposure to/construction of risky social contexts (through passive, evocative, or active gene-environment correlations), and/or psychopathology (Ellis, 2004; Harden & Mendle, 2012; Mendle & Ferrero, 2012). Genes that contribute to pubertal timing also may drive heightened sensitivity to social context in off-time youth (through gene × environment interactions), as reflected in observed contextual-amplification effects. Yet behavior genetic analyses also reveal small (often nonsignificant) shared and moderate nonshared environmental effects on pubertal timing (Eaves et al., 2004; Ge et al., 2007).

Summarizing research on environmental contributors to pubertal timing, Ellis (2004) concluded that these effects are multi-determined, reflecting "developmental plasticity in response to particular ecological conditions" (p. 948). Consistent with psychosocial acceleration and paternal investment theories (e.g., Belsky, Steinberg, & Draper, 1991), exposure to early family adversity (e.g., abuse, more coercive and less positive relationships, father absence) forecasts earlier maturation in girls—presumably as an evolutionary adaptation designed to accelerate reproductive maturity and lower levels of parental investment—whereas better marital quality and more supportive relationships forecast later maturation in girls. There is less support for a stress-suppression theory (i.e., elevated levels of stress-linked adrenal hormones, such as cortisol, suppress activity of the HPG axis); however, animal research does show a suppressive effect of stress on HPG, and some research in humans suggests that severe environmental stress may predict later maturation in girls, presumably as an evolutionary adaptation designed to delay puberty until better times [for reviews, see Ellis (2004) and Susman and Dorn (2009)]. It is therefore feasible that psychosocial stress can accelerate or inhibit puberty as reflected in a curvilinear association (Ellis, 2004). Of importance, the same forms of environmental adversity that predict off-time maturation may contribute to the types of intrapersonal risks (e.g., poor self-image, heightened biological stress reactivity) and interpersonal risks (e.g., poor-quality peer and romantic relationships, precocious sexuality, affiliation with norm-breaking peers, stress generation) and psychopathology believed to stem from individual differences in pubertal timing (Graber, 2003; Mendle & Ferrero, 2012; Natsuaki, Klimes-Dougan et al., 2009).

Beyond genetic and environmental contributions to the timing of puberty, off-time development could be associated with different hormonal profiles or with different susceptibility of the brain to pubertal changes. Research has not yet directly investigated whether there are hormonal differences across individuals as a function of maturational timing. Even if the hormonal profiles of on-time and off-time maturers are relatively similar, the brain may be more susceptible to the effects of hormonal changes when puberty is experienced earlier in development, perhaps due to immaturity of neural systems underlying cognitive regulatory skills, suggesting possible biologically driven effects of early maturation (Harden & Mendle, 2012;

Mendle & Ferrero, 2012; Susman & Dorn, 2009). Other potential contributors to pubertal timing (e.g., obesity, endocrine disruptors; for a review, see Susman & Dorn, 2009) also may directly influence the emergence of psychopathology, thereby creating spurious or complex associations with off-time development.

In sum, it is essential for future research to directly examine the question of whether pubertal timing per se makes a unique contribution to psychopathology beyond the effects of prior genetic and environmental liability and other factors linked to timing. To complicate this issue, the types of environmental adversity contributing to off-time development (e.g., family adversity) may be genetically determined (Harden & Mendle, 2012), further confounding efforts to disentangle the predictors versus consequences of pubertal timing. Genetically informed and longitudinal designs will be required to elucidate potential transactional and/or interactional effects of genes and gene expression, environmental adversity, pubertal timing, and psychopathology.

Puberty as a Stage of Resilience

Although prevailing theory and research target puberty as a developmental context of risk for psychopathology, developmental scientists increasingly are considering the notion that puberty also can serve as a period of resilience during which at-risk youth are redirected toward healthier developmental trajectories. Exposure to early adversity (e.g., family disruption, maltreatment, deprivation) is thought to calibrate stress-response systems early in life, thereby lowering youths' threshold for developing psychopathology in response to subsequent stress (Boyce & Ellis, 2005). This idea is supported by evidence of increasing psychopathology during adolescence in youth exposed to early adversity (Esposito & Gunnar, 2014). Moreover, one study revealed that this process of stress sensitization is particularly salient in girls progressing through puberty (Rudolph & Flynn, 2007). Yet, puberty represents a second period of developmental plasticity during which considerable reprogramming occurs in stress-response systems (Dahl, 2004). The *pubertal stress recalibration hypothesis* argues that puberty provides a window of opportunity during which stress-response systems can be recalibrated based on current demands, such that youth who were exposed to early adversity but then experience supportive, low stress conditions during adolescence may rebound, allowing for protection against psychopathology (DelGiudice, Ellis, & Shirtcliff, 2011; Esposito & Gunnar, 2014). Validation of this hypothesis awaits support from rigorous prospective longitudinal research, but it provides tantalizing possibilities for taking advantage of the opportunities afforded by this complex developmental stage.

Conclusion

The transition through adolescence, as embodied in the biological, physical, psychological, and social changes of puberty, can operate as a turning point in development—an opportunity for positive growth or a presage to intrapersonal and interpersonal disruptions and emerging risk for psychopathology. The next generation of theory and research should involve rigorous prospective designs directed toward identifying how puberty intersects with other risks and competencies to determine long-term trajectories of mental health, with an eye toward identifying resources that can protect vulnerable youth. In this way, future research can help inform efforts to redirect youths' trajectories such that puberty serves as a stepping stone rather than a stumbling block for successful adolescent and adult development.

References

Alsaker, F. D. (1992). Pubertal timing, overweight, and psychological adjustment. *The Journal of Early Adolescence, 12*, 396–419.

Andersson, T., & Magnusson, D. (1990). Biological maturation in adolescence and the development of drinking habits and alcohol abuse among young males: A prospective longitudinal study. *Journal of Youth and Adolescence, 19*, 33–41.

Angold, A., Costello, E. J., Erkanli, A., & Worthman, C. M. (1999). Pubertal changes in hormone levels and depression in girls. *Psychological Medicine, 29*, 1043–1053.

Angold, A., Costello, E. J., & Worthman, C. M. (1998). Puberty and depression: The roles of age, pubertal status and pubertal timing. *Psychological Medicine, 28*, 51–61.

Angold, A., Worthman, C., & Costello, E. J. (2003). Puberty and depression. In C. Hayward (Ed.), *Gender differences at puberty* (pp. 137–164). New York, NY: Cambridge University Press.

Belsky, J., Steinberg, L., & Draper, P. (1991). Childhood experience, interpersonal development, and reproductive strategy: An evolutionary theory of socialization. *Child Development, 62*, 647–670.

Benjet, C., & Hernández-Guzmán, L. (2002). A short-term longitudinal study of pubertal change, gender, and psychological well-being of Mexican early adolescents. *Journal of Youth and Adolescence, 31*, 429–442.

Blumenthal, H., Leen-Feldner, E. W., Trainor, C. D., Babson, K. A., & Bunaciu, L. (2009). Interactive roles of pubertal timing and peer relations in predicting social anxiety symptoms among youth. *Journal of Adolescent Health, 44*, 401–403.

Boyce, W. T., & Ellis, B. J. (2005). Biological sensitivity to context: I. An evolutionary-developmental theory of the origins and functions of stress reactivity. *Development and Psychopathology, 17*, 271–301.

Brooks-Gunn, J. (1984). The psychological significance of different pubertal events to young girls. *The Journal of Early Adolescence, 4*, 315–327.

Brooks-Gunn, J., & Warren, M. P. (1988). The psychological significance of secondary sexual characteristics in nine- to eleven-year-old girls. *Child Development, 59*, 1061–1069.

Brooks-Gunn, J., & Warren, M. P. (1989). Biological and social contributions to negative affect in young adolescent girls. *Child Development, 60*, 40–55.

Buchanan, C. M., Eccles, J. S., & Becker, J. B. (1992). Are adolescents the victims of raging hormones: Evidence for activation effects of hormones on moods and behavior at adolescence. *Psychological Bulletin, 111*, 62–107.

Carter, R., Silverman, W. K., & Jaccard, J. (2011). Sex variations in youth anxiety symptoms: Effects of pubertal development and gender role orientation. *Journal of Clinical Child and Adolescent Psychology, 40*, 730–41.

Caspi, A., Lynam, D., Moffitt, T. E., & Silva, P. A. (1993). Unraveling girls' delinquency: Biological, dispositional, and contextual contributions to adolescent misbehavior. *Developmental Psychology, 29*, 19–30.

Caspi, A., & Moffitt, T. E. (1991). Individual differences are accentuated during periods of social change: The sample case of girls at puberty. *Journal of Personality and Social Psychology, 61*, 157–168.

Cicchetti, D., & Cohen, D. J. (Eds.). (2006). *Developmental psychopathology* (2nd ed.). Hoboken, NJ: Wiley.

Compian, L., & Hayward, C. (2003). Gender differences in opposite sex relationships: Interactions with puberty. In C. Hayward (Ed.), *Gender differences at puberty* (pp. 77–92). New York, NY: Cambridge University Press.

Conley, C. S., & Rudolph, K. D. (2009). The emerging sex difference in adolescent depression: Interacting contributions of puberty and peer stress. *Development and Psychopathology, 21*, 593–620.

Conley, C. S., Rudolph, K. D., & Bryant, F. B. (2012). Explaining the longitudinal association between puberty and depression: Sex differences in the mediating effects of peer stress. *Development and Psychopathology, 24*, 691–701.

Costello, E. J., Sung, M., Worthman, C., & Angold, A. (2007). Pubertal maturation and the development of alcohol use and abuse. *Drug and Alcohol Dependence, 88*(Suppl 1), S50–S59.

Craig, W. M., Pepler, D., Connolly, J., & Henderson, K. (2001). Developmental context of peer harassment in early adolescence: The role of puberty and the peer group. In J. Juvonen & S. Graham (Eds.), *Peer harassment in school: The plight of the vulnerable and victimized* (pp. 242–262). Los Angeles, CA: Guilford Press.

Dahl, R. E. (2004). *Adolescent brain development: A period of vulnerabilities and opportunities Annals of the New York Academy of Sciences, 1021*, 1–22.

Dahl, R. E., & Gunnar, M. R. (2009). Heightened stress responsiveness and emotional reactivity during pubertal maturation: Implications for psychopathology. *Development and Psychopathology, 21*, 1–6.

DelGiudice, M., Ellis, B. J., & Shirtcliff, E. A. (2011). The adaptive calibration model of stress responsivity. *Neuroscience and Biobehaval Reviews, 35*, 1562–1592.

DeRose, L. M., Shiyko, M. P., Foster, H., & Brooks-Gunn, J. (2011). Associations between menarcheal timing and behavioral developmental trajectories for girls from age 6 to age 15. *Journal of Youth and Adolescence, 40*, 1329–1342.

Dorn, L. D., & Biro, F. M. (2011). Puberty and its measurement: A decade in review. *Journal of Research on Adolescence, 21*, 180–195.

Dorn, L. D., Susman, E. J., & Ponirakis, A. (2003). Pubertal timing and adolescent adjustment and behavior: Conclusions vary by rater. *Journal of Youth and Adolescence, 32*, 157–167.

Dubas, J. S., Graber, J. A., & Petersen, A. C. (1991). A longitudinal investigation of adolescents' changing perceptions of pubertal timing. *Developmental Psychology, 27*, 580–586.

Eaves, L., Silberg, J., Foley, D., Bulik, C., Maes, H., Erkanli, A., et al. (2004). Genetic and environmental influences on the relative timing of pubertal change. *Twin Research, 5*, 471–481.

Eccles, J. S., Lord, S. E., Roeser, R. W., Barber, B. L., & Hernandez Jozefowicz, D. M. (1997). The association of school transitions in early adolescence with developmental trajectories through high school. In J. Schulenberg, J. L. Maggs, & K. Hurrelmann (Eds.), *Health risks and developmental transitions during adolescence* (pp. 283–320). Cambridge: Cambridge University Press.

Edwards, A. C., Rose, R. J., Kaprio, J., & Dick, D. M. (2011). Pubertal development moderates the importance of environmental influences on depressive symptoms in adolescent girls and boys. *Journal of Youth and Adolescence, 40*, 1383–93.

Ellis, B. J. (2004). Timing of pubertal maturation in girls: An integrated life history approach. *Psychological Bulletin, 130*, 920–958.

Esposito, E., & Gunnar, M. R. (2014). Early deprivation and developmental psychopathology. In M. Lewis & K. D. Rudolph (Eds.), *Handbook of developmental psychopathology* (3rd ed., pp. 371–388). New York, NY: Plenum Press.

Felson, R. B., & Haynie, D. L. (2002). Pubertal development, social factors, and delinquency among adolescent boys. *Criminology, 40*, 967–988.

Flannery, D. J., Rowe, D. C., & Gulley, B. L. (1993). Impact of pubertal status, timing, and age on adolescent sexual experience and delinquency. *Journal of Adolescent Research, 8*, 21–40.

Forbes, E. E., Phillips, M. L., Silk, J. S., Ryan, N. D., & Dahl, R. E. (2011). Neural systems of threat processing in adolescents: Role of pubertal maturation and relation to measures of negative affect. *Developmental Neuropsychology, 36*, 429–452.

Foster, H., Hagan, J., & Brooks-Gunn, J. (2008). Growing up fast: Stress exposure and subjective "weathering" in emerging adulthood. *Journal of Health and Social Behavior, 49*, 162–177.

Ge, X., Brody, G. H., Conger, R. D., & Simons, R. L. (2006). Pubertal maturation and African American children's internalizing and externalizing symptoms. *Journal of Youth and Adolescence, 35*, 531–540.

Ge, X., Brody, G. H., Conger, R. D., Simons, R. L., & Murry, V. M. (2002). Contextual amplification of pubertal transition effects on deviant peer affiliation and externalizing behavior among African American children. *Developmental Psychology, 38*, 42–54.

Ge, X., Conger, R. D., & Elder, G. H. (1996). Coming of age too early: Pubertal influences on girls' vulnerability to psychological distress. *Child Development, 67*, 3386–3400.

Ge, X., Conger, R. D., & Elder, G. H. (2001). Pubertal transition, stressful life events, and the emergence of gender differences in adolescent depressive symptoms. *Developmental Psychology, 37*, 404–417.

Ge, X., Elder, G. H., Regnerus, M., & Cox, C. (2001). Pubertal transitions, perception of being overweight, and adolescents' psychological maladjustment: Gender and ethnic differences. *Social Psychology Quarterly, 64*, 363–375.

Ge, X., Kim, I. J., Brody, G. H., Conger, R. D., Simons, R. L., Gibbons, F. X., et al. (2003). It's about timing and change: Pubertal transition effects on symptoms of major depression among African American youths. *Developmental Psychology, 39*, 430–439.

Ge, X., & Natsuaki, M. (2009). In search of explanations for early pubertal timing effects on developmental psychopathology. *Current Directions in Psychological Science, 18,* 327–331.

Ge, X., Natsuaki, M. N., Neiderhiser, J. M., & Reiss, D. (2007). Genetic and environmental influences on pubertal timing: Results from two national sibling studies. *Journal of Research on Adolescence, 17,* 767–788.

Graber, J. A. (2003). Puberty in context. In C. Hayward (Ed.), *Gender differences at puberty* (pp. 307–325). New York, NY: Cambridge University Press.

Graber, J. A., Brooks-Gunn, J., & Archibald, A. B. (2005). Links between girls' puberty and externalizing and internalizing behaviors: Moving from demonstrating effects to identifying pathways. In D. M. Stoff & E. J. Susman (Eds.), *Developmental psychobiology of aggression* (pp. 87–113). New York, NY: Cambridge University Press.

Graber, J. A., Brooks-Gunn, J., & Warren, M. P. (2006). Pubertal effects on adjustment in girls: Moving from demonstrating effects to identifying pathways. *Journal of Youth and Adolescence, 35,* 413–423.

Graber, J. A., Lewinsohn, P. M., Seeley, J. R., & Brooks-Gunn, J. (1997). Is psychopathology associated with the timing of pubertal development? *Journal of the American Academy of Child and Adolescent Psychiatry, 36,* 1768–1776.

Graber, J. A., Nichols, T. R., & Brooks-Gunn, J. (2010). Putting pubertal timing in developmental context: Implications for prevention. *Developmental Psychobiology, 52,* 254–262.

Graber, J. A., Seeley, J. R., Brooks-Gunn, J., & Lewinsohn, P. M. (2004). Is pubertal timing associated with psychopathology in young adulthood? *Journal of the American Academy of Child and Adolescent Psychiatry, 43,* 718–726.

Gunnar, M. R., Wewerka, S., Frenn, K., Long, J. D., & Griggs, C. (2009). Developmental changes in HPA activity over the transition to adolescence: Normative changes and associations with puberty. *Development and Psychopathology, 21,* 69–85.

Harden, K. P., & Mendle, J. (2012). Gene environment interplay in the association between pubertal timing and delinquency in adolescent girls. *Journal of Abnormal Psychology, 121,* 73–87.

Haynie, D. L. (2003). Contexts of risk? Explaining the link between girls' pubertal development and their delinquency involvement. *Social Forces, 82,* 355–397.

Haynie, D. L., & Piquero, A. R. (2006). Pubertal development and physical victimization in adolescence. *Journal of Research in Crime and Delinquency, 43,* 3–35.

Hayward, C., Gotlib, I. J., Schraedley, P. K., & Litt, I. F. (1999). Ethnic differences in the association between pubertal status and symptoms of depression in adolescent girls. *Journal of Adolescent Health, 25,* 143–149.

Hayward, C., Killen, J. D., Wilson, D. M., Hammer, L. D., Litt, I. F., Kraemer, H. C., et al. (1997). Psychiatric risk associated with early puberty in adolescent girls. *Journal of the American Academy for Child and Adolescent Psychiatry, 36,* 255–262.

Hayward, C., & Sanborn, K. (2002). Puberty and the emergence of gender differences in psychopathology. *Journal of Adolescent Health, 30,* 49–58.

Hill, J. P., Holmbeck, G. N., Marlow, L., Green, T. M., & Lynch, M. E. (1985). Menarcheal status and parent–child relations in families of seventh-grade girls. *Journal of Youth and Adolescence, 14,* 301–316.

Huddleston, J., & Ge, X. (2003). Boys at puberty: Psychosocial implications. In C. Hayward (Ed.), *Gender differences at puberty* (pp. 113–134). New York, NY: Cambridge University Press.

Hyde, J. S., Mezulis, A. H., & Abramson, L. Y. (2008). The ABCs of depression: Integrating affective, biological, and cognitive models to explain the emergence of the gender difference in depression. *Psychological Review, 115,* 291–313.

Jones, M. C. (1957). The later careers of boys who were early- or late-maturing. *Child Development, 28,* 113–128.

Kaltiala-Heino, R., Koivisto, A., Marttunen, M., & Sari, F. (2011). Pubertal timing and substance use in middle adolescence: A 2-year follow-up study. *Journal of Youth and Adolescence, 40,* 1288–1301.

Kaltiala-Heino, R., Kosunen, E., & Rimpela, M. (2003). Pubertal timing, sexual behaviour and self-reported depression in middle adolescence. *Journal of Adolescence, 26,* 531–545.

Kaltiala-Heino, R., Marttunen, M., Rantanen, P., & Rimpela, M. (2003). Early puberty is associated with mental health problems in middle adolescence. *Social Science and Medicine, 57,* 1055–1064.

Ladouceur, C. D. (2012). Neural systems supporting cognitive-affective interactions in adolescence: The role of puberty and implications for affective disorders. *Frontiers in Integrative Neuroscience, 6,* 65. doi:10.3389/fnint.2012.00065.

Lahey, B. B., Van Hulle, C. A., Waldman, I. D., Rodgers, J. L., D'Onofrio, B. M., Pedlow, S., et al. (2006). Testing descriptive hypotheses regarding sex differences in the development of conduct problems and delinquency. *Journal of Abnormal Child Psychology, 34,* 737–755.

Laitinen-Krispijn, S., van der Ende, J., & Verhulst, F. C. (1999). The role of pubertal progress in the development of depression in early adolescence. *Journal of Affective Disorders, 54,* 211–215.

Lee, J. M., Appugliese, D., Kaciroti, N., Corwyn, R. F., Bradley, R. H., & Lumeng, J. C. (2007). Weight status in young girls and the onset of puberty. *Pediatrics, 119,* e624–e630.

Llewellyn, N., Rudolph, K. D., & Roisman, G. I. (2012). Other-sex relationship stress and sex differences in the contribution of puberty to depression. *Journal of Early Adolescence, 32,* 824–850.

Lynne, S. D., Graber, J. A., Nichols, T. R., Brooks-Gunn, J., & Botvin, G. J. (2007). Links between pubertal timing, peer influences, and externalizing behaviors among urban students followed through middle school. *Journal of Adolescent Health, 40,* 181e.7–181e.13.

Lynne-Landsman, S. D., Graber, J. A., & Andrews, J. A. (2010). Do trajectories of household risk in childhood moderate pubertal timing effects on substance initiation in middle school? *Developmental Psychology, 46,* 853–868.

Magnusson, D. (1988). *Individual development from an interactional perspective: A longitudinal study.* Hillsdale, NJ: Lawrence Erlbaum.

Magnusson, D., Stattin, H., & Allen, V. L. (1985). Biological maturation and social development: A longitudinal study of some adjustment processes from mid-adolescence to adulthood. *Journal of Youth and Adolescence, 14,* 267–283.

Marceau, K., Ram, N., Houts, R., Grimm, K., & Susman, E. J. (2011). Individual differences in boys' and girls' timing and tempo of puberty: Modeling development with nonlinear growth models. *Developmental Psychology, 47,* 1389–1409.

Masten, A. S., & Cicchetti, D. (2010). Developmental cascades. *Development and Psychopathology, 22,* 491–495.

McMaster, L. E., Connolly, J., Pepler, D., & Craig, W. M. (2002). Peer to peer sexual harassment in early adolescence: A developmental perspective. *Development and Psychopathology, 14,* 91–105.

Mendle, J., & Ferrero, J. (2012). Detrimental psychological outcomes associated with pubertal timing in adolescent boys. *Developmental Review, 32,* 49–66.

Mendle, J., Harden, K. P., Brooks-Gunn, J., & Graber, J. A. (2010). Development's tortoise and hare: Pubertal timing, pubertal tempo, and depressive symptoms in boys and girls. *Developmental Psychology, 46,* 1341–1353.

Mendle, J., Harden, K. P., Brooks-Gunn, J., & Graber, J. A. (2012). Peer relationships and depressive symptomatology in boys at puberty. *Developmental Psychology, 48,* 429–435.

Mendle, J., Turkheimer, E., & Emery, R. E. (2007). Detrimental psychological outcomes associated with early pubertal timing in adolescent girls. *Developmental Review, 27,* 151–171.

Moffitt, T. (1993). Adolescence-limited and life-course-persistent antisocial behavior: A developmental taxonomy. *Psychological Review, 100,* 674–701.

Morris, N. M., & Udry, J. R. (1980). Validation of a self-administered instrument to assess stage of adolescent development. *Journal of Youth and Adolescence, 9,* 271–280.

Mussen, P. H., & Jones, M. C. (1957). Self-conceptions, motivations and interpersonal attitudes of late- and early maturing boys. *Child Development, 28,* 243–256.

Natsuaki, M. N., Biehl, M. C., & Ge, X. (2009). Trajectories of depressed mood from early adolescence to young adulthood: The effects of pubertal timing and adolescent dating. *Journal of Research on Adolescence, 19,* 47–74.

Natsuaki, M. N., Klimes-Dougan, B., Ge, X., Shirtcliff, E. A., Hastings, P. D., & Zahn-Waxler, C. (2009). Early pubertal maturation and internalizing problems in adolescence: Sex differences in the role of cortisol reactivity to interpersonal stress. *Journal of Clinical Child and Adolescent Psychology, 38,* 513–524.

Negriff, S., Hillman, J. B., & Dorn, L. D. (2011). Does competence mediate the associations between puberty and internalizing or externalizing problems in adolescent girls? *Journal of Adolescent Health, 49,* 350–356.

Negriff, S., Ji, J., & Trickett, P. K. (2011). Exposure to peer delinquency as a mediator between self-report pubertal timing and delinquency: A longitudinal study of mediation. *Development and Psychopathology, 23,* 293–304.

Negriff, S., & Susman, E. J. (2011). Pubertal timing, depression, and externalizing problems: A framework, review, and examination of gender differences. *Journal of Research on Adolescence, 21,* 717–746.

Negriff, S., Susman, E. J., & Trickett, P. K. (2011). The developmental pathway from pubertal timing to delinquency and sexual activity from early to late adolescence. *Journal of Youth and Adolescence, 40,* 1343–56.

Obeidallah, D., Brennan, R. T., Brooks-Gunn, J., & Earls, F. (2004). Links between pubertal timing and neighborhood contexts: Implications for girls' violent behavior. *Journal of the American Academy of Child and Adolescent Psychiatry, 43,* 1460–1468.

Olweus, D., Mattsson, A., Schalling, D., & Low, H. (1988). Circulating testosterone levels and aggression in adolescent males: A causal analysis. *Psychosomatic Medicine, 50,* 261–272.

Paikoff, R. L., & Brooks-Gunn, J. (1991). Do parent–child relationships change during puberty? *Psychological Bulletin, 110,* 47–66.

Patton, G. C., McMorris, B. J., Toumbourou, J. W., Hemphill, S. A., Donath, S., & Catlano, R. F. (2004). Puberty and the onset of substance use and abuse. *Pediatrics, 114,* 300–306.

Petersen, A. C., Crockett, L., Richards, M., & Boxer, A. (1988). A self-report measure of pubertal status: Reliability, validity, and initial norms. *Journal of Youth and Adolescence, 17,* 117–133.

Petersen, A. C., & Taylor, B. (1980). The biological approach to adolescence: Biological change and psychological adaptation. In J. Adelson (Ed.), *Handbook of adolescent psychology* (pp. 117–155). New York, NY: Wiley.

Quevedo, K. M., Benning, S. D., Gunnar, M. G., & Dahl, R. E. (2009). The onset of puberty: Effects on the psychophysiology of defensive and appetitive motivation. *Development and Psychopathology, 21,* 27–45.

Reynolds, B. M., & Juvonen, J. (2011). The role of early maturation, perceived popularity, and rumors in the emergence of internalizing symptoms among adolescent girls. *Journal of Youth and Adolescence,, 40,* 1407–22.

Rodriguez-Tomé, H., Bariaud, F., Cohen Zardi, M. F., Delmas, C., Jeanvoine, B., & Szylagyi, P. (1993). The effects of pubertal changes on body image and relations with peers of the opposite sex in adolescence. *Journal of Adolescence, 16,* 421–438.

Rudolph, K. D. (2008). Developmental influences on interpersonal stress generation in depressed youth. *Journal of Abnormal Psychology, 117,* 673–679.

Rudolph, K. D. (2009). The interpersonal context of adolescent depression. In S. Nolen-Hoeksema & L. M. Hilt (Eds.), *Handbook of depression in adolescents* (pp. 377–418). New York, NY: Routledge.

Rudolph, K. D., & Flynn, M. (2007). Childhood adversity and youth depression: The role of gender and pubertal status. *Development and Psychopathology, 19*, 497–521.

Rudolph, K. D., Hammen, C., & Daley, S. E. (2006). Mood disorders. In D. A. Wolfe & E. J. Mash (Eds.), *Behavioral and emotional disorders in adolescents: Nature, assessment, and treatment* (pp. 300–342). New York, NY: Guilford Press.

Rudolph, K. D., & Klein, D. N. (2009). Exploring depressive personality traits in youth: Origins, correlates, and developmental consequences. *Development and Psychopathology, 21*, 1155–1180.

Rudolph, K. D., & Troop-Gordon, W. (2010). Personal-accentuation and contextual-amplification models of pubertal timing: Predicting youth depression. *Development and Psychopathology, 22*, 433–451.

Rudolph, K. D., Troop-Gordon, W., Lambert, S. F., & Natsuaki, M. N. (in press). Long-term consequences of pubertal timing for youth depression: Identifying personal and contextual pathways of risk. *Development and Psychopathology*.

Sameroff, A. J., & MacKenzie, M. J. (2003). Research strategies for capturing transactional models of development: The limits of the possible. *Development and Psychopathology, 15*, 613–640.

Schelleman-Offermans, K., Knibbe, R. A., Engels, R. C. M. E., & Burk, W. J. (2011). The effect of pubertal and psychosocial timing on adolescents' alcohol use: What role does alcohol-specific parenting play? *Journal of Youth and Adolescence, 40*, 1302–1314.

Shirtcliff, E. A., Dahl, R. A., & Pollak, S. D. (2009). Pubertal development: Correspondence between hormonal and physical development. *Child Development, 8*, 327–337.

Siegel, J. M., Aneshensel, C. S., Taub, B., Cantwell, D. P., & Driscoll, A. K. (1998). Adolescent depressed mood in a multiethnic sample. *Journal of Youth and Adolescence, 27*, 413–427.

Silbereisen, R. K., & Kracke, B. (1997). Self-reported maturational timing and adaptation in adolescence. In J. Schulenberg, J. L. Maggs, & K. Hurrelman (Eds.), *Health risks and developmental transitions during adolescence* (pp. 85–109). Cambridge: Cambridge University Press.

Silberg, J., Pickles, A., Rutter, M., Hewitt, J., Simonoff, E., Maes, H., et al. (1999). The influence of genetic factors and life stress on depression among adolescent girls. *Archives of General Psychiatry, 56*, 225–232.

Silk, J. S., Siegle, G. J., Whalen, D. J., Ostapenko, L. J., Ladouceur, C. D., & Dahl, R. E. (2009). Pubertal changes in emotional information processing: Pupillary, behavioral, and subjective evidence during emotional word identification. *Development and Psychopathology, 21*, 7–26.

Simmons, R. G., & Blyth, D. A. (1987). *Moving into adolescence: The impact of pubertal change and school context*. New York, NY: Aldine de Gruyter.

Simmons, R. G., Blyth, D. A., & McKinney, K. L. (1983). The social and psychological effects of puberty on white females. In J. Brooks-Gunn & A. C. Petersen (Eds.), *Girls at puberty: Biological and psychosocial perspectives* (pp. 229–272). New York, NY: Plenum Press.

Sontag, L. M., Graber, J. A., Brooks-Gunn, J., & Warren, M. P. (2008). Coping with social stress: Implications for psychopathology in young adolescent girls. *Journal of Abnormal Child Psychology, 36*, 1159–1174.

Sontag, L. M., Graber, J. A., & Clemans, K. H. (2011). The role of peer stress and pubertal timing on symptoms of psychopathology during early adolescence. *Journal of Youth and Adolescence, 40*, 1371–1382.

Stattin, H., Kerr, M., & Skoog, T. (2011). Early pubertal timing and girls' problem behavior: Integrating two hypotheses. *Journal of Youth and Adolescence, 40*, 1271–1287.

Stattin, H., & Magnusson, D. (1990). *Pubertal maturation in female development*. Hillsdale, NJ: Erlbaum.

Steinberg, L. (1987). Impact of puberty on family relations: Effects of pubertal status and pubertal timing. *Developmental Psychology, 23*, 451–460.

Steinberg, L. (2008). A social neuroscience perspective on adolescent risk-taking. *Developmental Review, 28*, 78–106.

Stice, E., Presnell, K., & Bearman, S. K. (2001). Relation of early menarche to depression, eating disorders, substance abuse, and comorbid psychopathology among adolescent girls. *Developmental Psychology, 37*, 608–619.

Storvall, E. E., & Wichstrom, L. (2002). Do the risk factors associated with conduct problems in adolescents vary according to gender? *Journal of Adolescence, 25*, 183–202.

Stroud, L. R., Foster, E., Papandonatos, G., Handwerger, K., Granger, D. A., Kivlighan, K. T., et al. (2009). Stress response and the adolescent transition: Performance versus social rejection stress. *Development and Psychopathology, 21*, 47–68.

Styne, D. M., & Grumbach, M. M. (2007). Control of puberty in humans. In O. H. Pescovitz & E. C. Walvoord (Eds.), *When puberty is precocious* (pp. 51–82). Totowa, NJ: Humana Press.

Susman, E. J., Dockray, S., Granger, D. A., Blades, K. T., Randazzo, W., Heaton, J. A., et al. (2010). Cortisol and alpha amylase reactivity and timing of puberty: Vulnerabilities for antisocial behaviour in young adolescents. *Psychoneuroendocrinology, 35*, 557–569.

Susman, E. J., Dockray, S., Schiefelbein, V. L., Herwehe, S., Heaton, J. A., & Dorn, L. D. (2007). Morningness/eveningness, morning-to-afternoon cortisol ratio, and antisocial behavior problems during puberty. *Developmental Psychology, 43*, 811–822.

Susman, E. J., & Dorn, L. D. (2009). Puberty: Its role in development. In R. M. Lerner & L. Steinberg (Eds.), *Handbook of adolescent psychology, Volume 1, Individual bases of adolescent development* (3rd ed., pp. 115–151). Hoboken, NJ: Wiley.

Susman, E. J., Inoff-Germain, G., Nottelmann, E. D., Loriaux, D. L., Cutler, G. B., Jr., & Chrousos, G. P. (1987). Hormones, emotional dispositions, and aggressive attributes in young adolescents. *Child Development, 58*, 1114–1134.

Susman, E. J., Nottelmann, E. D., Inoff-Germain, G. E., Dorn, L. D., Cutler, G. B., Loriaux, D. L., et al. (1985). The relation of relative hormonal levels and physical development and social-emotional behavior in young adolescents. *Journal of Youth and Adolescence, 14*, 245–264.

Taga, K., Markey, C., & Friedman, H. (2006). A longitudinal investigation of associations between boys' pubertal timing and adult behavioral health and well-being. *Journal of Youth and Adolescence, 35*, 401–411.

Tobin-Richards, M. H., Boxer, A. M., & Petersen, A. C. (1983). The psychological significance of pubertal change: Sex differences in perceptions of self during early adolescence. In J. Brooks-Gunn & A. C. Petersen (Eds.), *Girls at puberty: Biological and psychosocial perspectives* (pp. 127–154). New York, NY: Plenum Press.

Weichold, K., Silbereisen, R. K., & Schmitt-Rodermund, E. (2003). Short-term and long-term consequences of early versus late physical maturation in adolescents. In C. Hayward (Ed.), *Gender differences at puberty* (pp. 241–276). New York, NY: Cambridge University Press.

Wichstrom, L. (1999). The emergence of gender difference in depressed mood during adolescence: The role of intensified gender socialization. *Developmental Psychology, 35*, 232–245.

Williams, J. M., & Currie, C. (2000). Self-esteem and physical development in early adolescence: Pubertal timing and body image. *The Journal of Early Adolescence. Special Issue: Self-Esteem in Early Adolescence: Part II, 20*, 129–149.

Williams, J. M., & Dunlop, L. C. (1999). Pubertal timing and self-reported delinquency among male adolescents. *Journal of Adolescence, 22*, 157–171.

Part IV

Early Childhood Disorders

Attachment Disorders: Theory, Research, and Treatment Considerations

18

Howard Steele and Miriam Steele

Over the last decade, there have been considerable advances in the scientific understanding of the origins and developmental course of attachment disorders conceived of both in the narrow diagnostic psychiatric sense, with respect to reactive attachment disorder (DSM 1980, 1994, 1999) and in the more general sense with respect to diverse forms of attachment-related disorders across the lifespan. This chapter is organized into three sections. The first section concerns familiar ground to many, i.e., infant–parent patterns of attachment, which serves as a background to the spectrum of attachment patterns including secure, insecure, disorganized, and nonattached. The second section elaborates on a model for understanding attachment disorders by way of summarizing recent research on a typical problem in childhood, i.e., the emergence, maintenance, and/or prevention of impulse-control difficulties that have to do with aggression. Attachment insecurities play a role in all range of childhood and adult psychological disorders as many have demonstrated via clinical work (e.g., Brisch, 2012), longitudinal developmental research (e.g., Grossmann, Grossmann, & Watters, 2005), and meta-analytic reports (e.g., Fearon, Bakermans-Kranenburg, van IJzendoorn, Lapsly, & Roisman, 2010). Direct effects of early attachment upon long-term mental health are difficult to establish, often involving a mediating or moderating role for attachment rather than a direct causal role per se. This has become evident from studies of the onset and course of children's externalizing disorders, and so the second section of this chapter devotes itself to summarizing this recent work that may help refine our thinking about the influence of attachment upon mental health outcomes in general and reactive attachment disorder in particular. Finally, the third section focuses in some detail on the phenomenon of reactive attachment disorder, a diagnosis first identified in 1980, yet the syndrome of RAD fits with observations of institutionalized infants from previous decades (e.g., Provence & Lipton, 1962; Spitz, 1945) and would serve as a fitting account for many of the children adopted out of institutions since the 1980s. The development of these adoptees has been studied longitudinally, detailed in three recent monographs from the Society for Research in Child Development (McCall, van IJzendoorn, Juffer, Groark & Groza 2011; Rutter, Sonuga-Burke, Beckett, Castle, Kreppner et al., 2010; The St. Petersburgh-USA Orphanage Research Team, 2008).

Infant–Parent Patterns of Attachment

Attachment is a term with multiple meanings including biological, social, and psychological processes present in the human and other animals

H. Steele, Ph.D. (✉) • M. Steele, Ph.D.
Department of Psychology, New School for
Social Research, New York, NY, USA
e-mail: SteeleH@newschool.edu

M. Lewis and K.D. Rudolph (eds.), *Handbook of Developmental Psychopathology*,
DOI 10.1007/978-1-4614-9608-3_18, © Springer Science+Business Media New York 2014

from birth if not before (Bowlby, 1969). The term "attachment" is applied both to observable behavior and to unseen internal mental and affective processes. The "internal working model" of self and attachment figures is assumed to become consolidated, organized, and stable in the final quarter of the first year. In the 1-year old child, there is robust evidence that individual differences in attachment patterns are observable in the context of a filmed 20-min sequence involving child and parent in a playroom-like setting, including a stranger, and typically two separations from, followed by two reunions with, the parent (Ainsworth, Blehar, Waters, & Wall, 1978). This observational paradigm is the gold standard measure of attachment in early childhood (with 13, 169 citations to it in print as of March 2014, with over 150 new citations appearing in the literature with each passing month). Results based on careful reviews by reliable raters of infant–caregiver interactions in the Strange Situation with a special focus on reunion behavior represent a reliable and valid indication of the extent to which a 1-year-old child has experienced sensitive and responsive care over the first year of life with a given caregiver. And, looking forward, there are significant links from observed behavior in the Strange Situation at 1 year with mother (or father) to emotion-regulation, social competence, and mental health throughout the childhood and adolescent years (e.g., Fearon et al., 2010; Lewis, Feiring, & Rosenthal, 2000; Sroufe, 2005).

The normal developmental trajectory of attachment from birth onwards includes an initial period, up to about 6 months, where an infant's bids for contact/comfort are nonselective insofar as she/he will typically accept sensitive ministrations from an unfamiliar person (Bowlby, 1969). But by 8–9 months of age, the healthy infant shows stranger anxiety (Bowlby, 1960; Spitz, 1950). And, by 1 year in the Strange Situation, signs of typical selective secure or insecure (avoidant or resistant) attachments are reliably observed (Ainsworth et al., 1978).

The Three Main Patterns of Infant–Parent Attachment and Infant Temperament

The securely attached infant shows signs of a clear preference of being with the parent, protests separation, and settles quickly upon reunion showing pleasure and a return to play. The infant with an insecure-avoidant attachment shows a lack of preference regarding mother or stranger, is nonchalant regarding separation, and avoids the parent upon reunion, looking away or moving away. The infant with an insecure-resistant attachment markedly prefers the mother to the stranger, protests separation loudly, and is inconsolable upon reunion in an angry or passive manner. Interestingly, temperament, once hotly debated as a possible cause of these differences, is now widely seen as a possibly influential factor upon the type of security or the type of insecurity shown, *not whether a child will be securely or insecurely attached* (see Belsky & Rovine, 1987; van IJzendoorn & Bakermans-Kranenburg, 2012, for a thorough account of this issue). By "type" of security or "type" of insecurity, the focus is upon how inhibited or lacking in inhibition a child will be when displaying his or her pattern of attachment. Importantly, securely attached children include a widely varying range of temperaments including those lacking inhibition and so are oriented toward exploration and play who therefore show reserve in displaying proximity seeking upon reunion. Whether this reserve looks like avoidance (A) or security (B) hinges on a comparison between how the infant behaves with the parent upon reunion and how he behaved with the stranger. If there is a clear preference for the parent, security (B1 or B2) is the valid conclusion. If the reserve shown toward the parent is matched to or greater than the reserve shown the stranger, an avoidant (A1 or A2) attachment is the valid conclusion. Though children with avoidant attachments tend not to cry at all during separation, salivary cortisol assays (obtained prior to, 15 min after and 30 min after the Strange Situation observation) have confirmed that they are nonetheless distressed (Spangler & Grossmann, 1993), belying the reserve shown, which should be seen as a defensive (avoidant) posture.

At the other end of the temperamental spectrum, there are some infants who are highly inhibited, easily overwhelmed, and show excessive crying upon reunion, yet some settle within the 3-min reunions of the Strange Situation, while others remain upset after 3 min. The latter group of infants are said to have an insecure-resistant (C1 or C2) attachment, while the former group who eventually settle within the 3 min are said to have a secure (B3 or B4) attachment. So while temperament does not determine a secure versus insecure attachment, it may play a role in influencing how a child shows his or her security (in the range from B1 to B4) or insecurity (in the range from A1–A2 to C1–C2).

With respect to the highly inhibited or easily distressed child, individual differences in parental sensitivity are likely to determine whether the highly reactive child develops a resistant or secure attachment. This has potentially long-term implications for these high reactive infants because should they develop insecure-resistant attachments to mother, they are at significantly increased risk of later developing anxiety disorders of the internalizing variety (Warren, Huston, Egeland, & Sroufe, 1997).

Infant–Parent Attachments, Prevalence Rates, Caregiving, and Cultural Influences

Secure attachments arise from optimally sensitive and responsive care, consistently seen in 55 % of community samples (van IJzendoorn & Kroonenberg, 1988). Notably, a central feature of this optimal care is prompt responsiveness on the part of the caregiver to infant distress, where the infant has had the common experience of repair following rupture, recovery following distress. The insecure patterns, avoidance and resistance, consistently found in approximately 30 % of community samples where familiarity with

disappointment in response to unduly neglectful or intrusive care seem to be the normative childhood experience (van IJzendoorn & Kroonenberg, 1988). In the avoidant case, the child opts for *flight* in the face of distress—a strategy adopted to deny or isolate distressing feelings, more common in cultures that emphasize independence over dependence, e.g., Northern Germany. In the resistant case, the child opts for *fight* in the face of distress, protesting loudly either with anger or passivity—more often seen in cultures that emphasize dependence of children and downplay independence, e.g., Japan and Israel. Thus, while proportions of security (55–65 %) are stable across cultures, insecurity (avoidance versus resistance) tends to vary somewhat across cultures with avoidance being more prevalent in northern Europe and America and resistance being more prevalent in Japan and Israel (van IJzendoorn & Sagi-Schwartz, 2008).

The Collapse of Attachment Strategies: Disorganization

Importantly the Ainsworth Strange Situation has also yielded reliable indications of the extent to which disorganized-disoriented behavioral responses, what Bowlby (1980) regarded as the normal response to loss, prevail among some infants as a likely consequence of overwhelming fear felt in the primary attachment relationship (Main & Solomon, 1990) and the still more extreme and disturbing phenomenon of attachment-disordered behavior (DSM 1980, 1994, 1999; Zeanah, Smyke, Koga, Carlson, & The BEIP Core Group, 2005). Disorganization appears to reflect a temporary breakdown of an organized strategy (shown through freezing, crying uncontrollably, and hiding from the parent).

Disorganized-disoriented attachments were first identified by Main and Solomon (1990) and have been extensively studied in the years since, e.g., in 2006 a meta-analysis reported on the causes of infant–mother attachment disorganization in 851 families (Madigan et al., 2006). Infant–mother disorganization is typically linked to frightened or frightening caregiving and/or abusive behavior (Hesse & Main, 2006) and unresolved states of mind concerning past loss or trauma (Madigan et al., 2006). The anomalous disorganized-disoriented infant response to the Strange Situation is seen in 15 % of community samples, but in 40–80 % of clinical samples, such as depressed mothers or infants where maltreatment is suspected (Lyons-Ruth & Jacobvitz, 2008). Disorganized attachments to mother at 1 year have been linked longitudinally to dissociative symptoms during adolescence, assessed via self-, peer, and teacher report (Carlson, 1998). This indicates that fear in one's earliest and most important relationship can leave one vulnerable to a persisting ease for entering trance-like states that take one away from typical perceptions of reality. A core emotional experience that would appear to become overwhelming for the toddler developing disorganized behavior would appear to be profound shame. This suggestion is based in part on the classic description of toddlerhood in terms of the psychosocial dilemma between shame/doubt on the one hand and autonomy on the other (Erikson, 1951) and is also informed by the description of shame discussed by Lewis (1992). For Lewis, shame is that negative self-evaluative emotion that "encompasses *the whole of ourselves*; it generates a wish to hide, to disappear, or even to die" (Lewis, 1992, p. 2). When the experience is pervasive and feels inescapable, self-harm and dissociative problems become inevitable. We take up this point in the final section of this chapter where multiple models of attachment, within the same individual, are discussed with respect to reactive attachment disorder.

Interestingly, for toddlers who show disorganized-disoriented behavior with a caregiver in the Strange Situation, it has been possible to readily assign a best-fitting alternate attachment strategy, avoidant, resistant, or secure. However, making the assumption of a selective attachment to the observed caregiver, easily arrived at with community and clinical samples, is often not a valid assumption with infants living in institutional settings. In this latter case, serious questions have been raised about the extent of attachment formation on account of many infants observed in institutional settings who show a curious absence of attachment behaviors that would otherwise be expected. This was initially identified by Elizabeth Carlson in her work scoring Strange Situation responses among infants living in Romanian orphanages (Zeanah et al., 2005). In other words, early maltreatment and neglect appear capable of disrupting the normal biological, social, and psychological processes involved in typical development from a nonselective to a selective attachment, keeping a child "stuck" in the nonselective phase prevailing in—and typically limited to—the first 6 months of age (see Roy, Rutter, & Pickles, 2004).

Attachment Experiences and Risk of (or Protection Against) Psychopathology

This section provides an update to one of the central claims of attachment theory, namely, that there are near- and long-term adverse or beneficial effects of early infant–parent attachment on mental health outcomes (Bowlby (1969/1982). For purely illustrative reasons, the focus of this section is upon externalizing disorders that affect 1–10 % of typically developing children.

The Case of Externalizing Disorders

Antisocial, aggressive behavior was the focus of Bowlby's initial (1944) report on how deficits in early caregiving may lead to an absence of normative moral restraints and a corresponding reliance on aggressive or delinquent actions. The prevalence of such difficulties, and the social angst and economic costs they engender, has led to extensive research on externalizing problems, many that included assessments of the early child–mother relationship. A recent meta-analysis explored the extent to which insecure and/or disorganized attachment may be linked to children's externalizing problems (Fearon et al., 2010). Fearon et al. reviewed 69 samples ($N = 5,947$) which showed that insecure and disorganized child–mother attachments significantly increase the risk for externalizing problems, $d = 0.31$ (94 % CI: 0.23–0.40). More pronounced effects were found for boys ($d = 0.35$), clinical samples ($d = 0.49$), and from observation-based outcome assessments ($d = 0.58$). Robust as these effects are, Fearon et al. point out that their meta-analytic results cannot speak to issues of causality, do not address the possible influence of child–father attachments owing to too few studies included with fathers, and the effects are "uncorrected for the influence of relevant third variables….that could amplify or attenuate the association between attachment and externalizing problems" (Fearon et al., 2010, pp. 448–449).

As to the relevance of fathers, and a third variable that may moderate or mediate the effect of early attachment on later antisocial behaviors, the role of heavy-handed and power-assertive behavior by mothers or fathers has been implicated in the longitudinal work of Kochanska, Barry, Stellern, and O'Bleness (2009). Kochanksa et al. found evidence for moderated meditational effects such that in the context of insecure child–parent attachments, parental power assertion predicted children's resentful opposition, which then predicted antisocial conduct. Models of effect looked similar for mothers and fathers. This mechanism of influence was absent when secure child–parent relationships had been observed in infancy. The effects appeared most marked in the context of early disorganized attachments and support the Fearon et al. view that other variables such as parental power assertion are likely to interact with insecurity/disorganization to produce externalizing problems. Overall, early insecurity served as a catalyst igniting a developmental journey toward adversarial interactions with parents and childhood externalizing behavior problems. In contrast, early security was observed to defuse or moderate this maladaptive trajectory. It may also have been the case that parental insensitivity during infancy and later parental power assertions were responsible for the early insecurity and the later externalizing problems—insofar as the context that led to insecurity did not change and so the aggressive correlates of early insecurity were unaltered. In other words, as Lewis (1997) noted, if the context remains the same, the child's behavior is likely to remain the same.

Two other studies of externalizing behavior have implications for how we think about attachment disorders since they looked at both attachment and genetics (Bakermans-Kranenburg & van IJzendoorn, 2006; Bakermans-Kranenburg, van IJzendoorn, Pijlman, Mesman, & Juffer, 2008). This work speaks to the differential susceptibility children have to the caregiving environment, carried by one or other genetic polymorphism (e.g., DRD4). For example, Bakermans-Kranenburg and van IJzendoorn (2006) found that maternal insensitivity was linked to oppositional and aggressive behavior, but only in the presence of the DRD4 7-repeat allele. There was a sixfold increase in externalizing behavior in children with the 7-repeat allele who were exposed to insensitive care, in comparison to children with neither insensitive care nor the 7-repeat allele. The differential susceptibility hypothesis is that the very same long allele which may lead to heightened risk in the context of insensitive care will also hasten developmental advances and resilience in the context of sensitive care. To test this hypothesis, Bakermans-Kranenburg and colleagues (2008) explored whether children with the 7-repeat allele were more sensitive to a systematic intervention by manipulation of the caregiving environment than children without the 7-repeat allele. They found that children with the DRD4 7-repeat allele were indeed more susceptible than similarly aggressive children without the long repeat allele to an intervention aimed at enhancing maternal sensitivity and positive discipline strategies. In other words, a heightened sensitivity to the caregiving environment will be a "risk" factor when in the context of insensitive care and a "resilience" factor in the context of sensitive care or other favorable experiences, including a supportive sibling, friend, teacher, or therapist. This chapter next considers the example of sustained pathogenic care that may lead to children developing reactive attachment disorder (RAD), a rare but perplexing difficulty.

Reactive Attachment Disorder

What Is RAD? Current Diagnostic Nosology

RAD refers to a distinct class of adjustment problems, namely, challenging behavior underpinned by core deficits in self and social development, seemingly specific to children growing up in contexts of impersonal institutional rearing or chronically maltreating environments. Thus, the constellation of disturbed behavior known as RAD is assumed to be a response to an extreme variation from the average expectable environment.

Most of the research on RAD summarized in this chapter, conducted over the last 20 years, was based on versions of DSM prior to the introduction of DSM V in late 2013. According to DSM IV-R, reactive attachment disorder was thought of as having two types, inhibited and disinhibited:

- Inhibited type: hypervigilant, excessively inhibited, highly ambivalent, and contradictory responses
- Disinhibited type: diffuse attachments, marked by indiscriminate sociability and inability to exhibit appropriate selective attachments

Both stipulate that RAD should have the following features:

- Be differentiated from pervasive developmental disorders
- Is likely to occur in relation to abusive or impoverish child care
- Onset age before 5 years
- Markedly disturbed and developmentally inappropriate social relatedness

Zeanah and Gleason (2010) proposed changes to RAD diagnoses for DSM V that have been implemented into DSM V. Zeanah and Gleason's suggestions incorporated into DSM V amount to retaining only the previously considered inhibited form of RAD as RAD, and assigning a new diagnostic label to the indiscriminately friendly form, i.e. Social Engagement Disorder. These separate syndromes are called for on account of their distinctive phenotypic characteristics, correlates, course, and response to intervention, despite their close connection as deriving from pathogenic care. The disinhibited type, often referred to as showing indiscriminately friendliness or IF, has become disinhibited social engagement disorder while the inhibited type has become the only form of reactive attachment disorder. The latter label is thought to best merit the RAD label as once the provision of a reliable and sensitive caregiver is made available, inhibition typically changes into responsiveness and a selective attachment. Disinhibited social engagement disorder occurs in children with and without selective attachments, even among children with secure attachments, and is far more persistent over time, likely to follow a path akin to Attention Deficit Hyperactivity Disorder, less amenable to intervention, and so distinguishable from (inhibited) reactive attachment disorder syndrome. The research and clinical value of restricting use of the term RAD to the inhibited, as opposed to disinhibited, response to pathogenic care will be a question for DSM VI to take up.

RAD formally entered the psychiatric literature with the 3rd edition of the Diagnostic and Statistical Manual of the American Psychiatric Association and became further reified over successive iterations of DSM (1980, 1994, 1999). RAD has been applied, sometimes too loosely, in respect of waves of children who were adopted in large numbers to Western Europe and North America throughout the 1980s and 1990s from child care institutions or orphanages in the former Soviet Union, Eastern Europe, China, and parts of Africa (McCall et al. 2011; Rutter et al. 2010; Steele, Steele, Archer, Jin, & Herreros, 2009; The St. Petersburgh-USA Orphanage Research Team, 2008). Observations and clinical studies of these children confirmed that two overarching types of troubled behavior occurred, both the inhibited and a more common and disinhibited type (Zeanah & Gleason, 2010). Both of these forms of RAD are relatively rare in the population at large, but are very common among abandoned, previously institutionalized children (O'Connor & Zeanah, 2003). Although the overall prevalence of RAD is extremely low with rates less than 1 % in the overall population (Richters & Volkmar, 1994), this number soars to 40 % or more when institutionalized children, radically deprived of consistent and sensitive care, are later studied (O'Connor & Zeanah, 2003).

In addition to being reified in the psychiatric classifications of disorder (DSM and ICD), the phenomenon of RAD is also detailed in the Diagnostic Classification of Mental Health and Developmental Disorders in Infancy and Early Childhood (Zero to Three, 2005). In this infant/child psychiatry publication, the terms "deprivation/maltreatment disorder" and "reactive attachment disorder" are linked as twin diagnostic concepts, underlining the close connection between gross deviations from the average expectable environment and consequent disturbances in the domain of social relations with accompanying disturbances in emotion-regulation and attention (Zeanah & Gleason, 2010).

This represents progress toward a nuanced understanding of RAD that was not available to the authors of DSM III in the late 1970s as this was a time when they were deliberately moving away from the perceived conflation of explanation and description that typified DSM I and II, pursuing instead the task of reliable description as an end in itself. Thus, when RAD was introduced into DSM III in 1980, it was irrevocably limited to descriptions of behavior, yet also included a firm reference to causation. To this day, it is only post-traumatic stress disorder and RAD where the diagnostic criteria include the requirement that a significant trauma rest in the individual's past. RAD should only be diagnosed *in the context of a history of highly pathogenic care*.

Reactive Attachment Disorder and the Surge in International Adoptions from Institutional Settings

Institutional rearing due to its regimented nature, high child-to-caregiver ratios, multiple shifts, and frequent changes of caregivers almost inevitably deprives children of reciprocal interactions with stable caregivers. In this respect, institutional care implies structural neglect. A considerable number of studies have shown that children growing up in orphanages are at risk in various domains of functioning, including their physical, socio-emotional, and cognitive development.

Catch-up rates following adoption into a typical family arrangement, following early institutional rearing, have been studied extensively in recent years and meta-analytic reviews have been published (Juffer & van IJzendoon, 2009; van IJzendoorn & Juffer, 2006). The findings illustrate remarkable evidence of plasticity and catch-up following early institutional rearing. Catch-up is observed first in the domain of physical development, with children assuming a place on normal growth curves within 6 months of receiving appropriate nutrition and stimulation. Development catch-up typically takes longer in the domain of cognition, with some persisting language and cognitive delays being evident for years in a substantial group of children adopted out of institutions. Finally, the slowest catch-up occurs in the social domain, which may be seen as testament to the relevance of the diagnostic term RAD. As many as 10 years post-adoption, fully one-third of adoptees show signs of RAD. This means, of course, that the majority of adoptees do *not* present with RAD. And these consequences of early institutional rearing are most marked in those children who remained longer during infancy and beyond in some cases, living in the institution from which they were adopted. In other words, there is a dose-response relationship between length of time in early institutional living and later post-adoption developmental delays. Rutter and Sonuga-Barke (2010) summarized results from their 15-year follow-up of children adopted in the UK out of Romanian orphanages at the end of the communist regime compared to a group of English adoptees and their adoptive parents. This well-controlled study found a range of specific long-term developmental deficits persisting for the adoptees from Romania who spent more than their first 6 months in the institution. Among the many lessons to draw from this longitudinal research, then, is to make every effort possible to place a child without parents in an adoptive home or long-term foster caregiving relationship as soon as possible. This notion receives support from a meta-analysis reviewing age at time of adoption and a child's attachment security in the adoptive family (Van den Dries, Juffer, van IJzendoorn, & Bakermans-Kranenburg,

2009). Children who were adopted before 12 months of age were similarly securely attached as their non-adopted peers, whereas children adopted after their first birthday showed less attachment security than non-adopted children.

Attachment difficulties were seen in many tens of thousands of adopted children among 200,000 brought to US homes between 1995 and 2005 (Merz & McCall, 2010). Yet most adoptees do not meet diagnostic criteria for RAD, indicative of robust evidence of catch-up after the provision of adequate care by adoptive parents (Bakersman-Kranenburg et al., 2011), illustrating the possibility of altering fate (Lewis, 1997). For those adoptees who do show RAD, a sizable number of their adoptive parents have, for understandable reasons, been strident in seeking quick fixes for their children's "affectless psychopathy," as Bowlby (1944) predicted. The extraordinary and urgent needs of these adoptive parents for support were met occasionally by mental health workers applying well-meaning but untested treatments. Most infamously, among these untested interventions is holding therapy, the forced holding of a child against his or her will in order to provide contact/comfort that the child was deprived of in infancy and so begin the process of establishing a secure attachment. No matter that the child was 5, 10, or 15 years of age, holding therapy was applied against the will of the youth being forcibly held. This nondevelopmental and intrusive intervention is *not* based on attachment theory and research (Steele, 2003). Since holding therapy led to the tragic deaths (by suffocation) of a number of a children, caution has been sounded by responsible mental health providers about the vital lessons to be learned from the "holding therapy" debacle (Chaffin et al., 2006) and the need for reliable and valid interventions to be made available to adoptive parents seeking help.

Charles Zeanah and his colleagues cautioned against overuse of the term RAD, recommending a distinction between children where the primary and exclusive difficulty is one of attachment disorder versus the children with primary difficulties of ADHD or conduct disorder, with a secondary difficulty concerning pathogenic care and attachment difficulties (Gleason et al.,

2011). This classification holds much promise in terms of delineating the specificity and sensitivity of the RAD diagnosis and is supported by the Bucharest Early Intervention Project (BEIP) where evidence-derived criteria for these two types were derived. This work involved Gleason et al.'s observation of 120 children, beginning in the 2nd year of life, four times during an intervention, and was aimed at showing that foster care could bring about change for children with RAD. Initially, 40 (32 %) of the children met criteria for indiscriminately social/disinhibited RAD, but this number diminished by half by 30 months and remained stable through 54 months. These children with the disinhibited form of RAD had some ADHD symptoms but did *not* on the whole meet the diagnostic criteria for ADHD. This work demonstrated that RAD appears to be a distinctive disorder, separate from ADHD, and also showed that two forms of RAD, the inhibited and lacking inhibition forms, could be identified, with some stability over time. But this work by Gleason and colleagues highlights a conceptual challenge: how do we understand the phenomena whereby a child can exhibit behaviors consistent with both RAD, inhibited or uninhibited forms, and also be securely attached to the caregiver? This speaks to the research and clinical question of what in the individual child's current functioning reflects earliest experiences? And what in the individual's functioning reflects current experiences? RAD may reflect what is earliest and persisting in a child's inner world, while that inner world may also hold in a segregated or fragile fashion representations of current more secure interactions with the adoptive or foster parent. Put differently, but consistent with this picture, RAD is thought to reside within the child whose early experiences of neglect and maltreatment constitute profound deprivation, and the consequences of this adversity are fairly pervasive and yet the very same child may still be open to responding to positive security-promoting qualities of the present parent–child relationship and, when distressed, will be able to turn to the new caregiver for protection, inhibiting or setting aside the concerns that lead him/her to show RAD-like symptoms at other times.

Multiple Models of Attachment Arising from Radically Differing Experiences

It could also be that for some of these children, they may suffer from having multiple models of two different sources. Multiple models may, for example, arise as Bowlby (1980) postulated from experiences of a caregiver who behaves in markedly contradictory ways, i.e., at times nurturing and at times abusive. Yet another possible source of multiple models may be seen to arise within the internal world of the child who either had many different caregivers, most of whom did not make their mark as especially connected to the child as would be the case in institutional care or for the cases that arise from children in foster care, those that may have had the experience of being perpetually in transition. Their representational worlds may contain elements including a range of diverse and possibly conflicting representations from many and often abrupt changes of caregivers, understandably giving rise to feelings of confusion and fear that persist in the mind and become active at times, even when newer more positive experiences have engendered some sense of trust in the child. It could well be that in such cases we are witnessing the child who demonstrates elements of both RAD and secure attachment.

This latter suggestion may draw some support from recent empirical findings from the BEIP study (McGoron et al., 2012). This report includes a regression analysis showing that security of attachment in the Strange Situation at 42 months mediates the link between 30-month caregiving quality based on 1.5 h "home" observations and 54-month measures of indiscriminately social/disinhibited reactive attachment disorder (RAD) derived from the previously validated disturbances of attachment interview (DAI) developed by Smyke, Dumitrescu, and Zeanah (2002). In other words, the significance of the link between early caregiving quality and later RAD (disinhibited form) held, but only for those children who were insecurely attached at 42 months. The inhibited form of RAD in the BEIP sample was too small a number (six) for the meditational regression analysis to be meaningful, and most of the children (five) in this small group were actually securely attached.

Until recently, the only validated measure of RAD was the DAI (Smyke et al., 2002), i.e., reliance on caregiver report, but a recent paper based on 74 Portuguese toddlers living in an institution provided validating evidence for an observational measure of RAD embedded in the classic Strange Situation (Oliveira et al. (2012). Olivera et al. demonstrated significant correlations between DAI reports of indiscriminate behavior (IB) and independent observations of actual IB with the stranger in the Strange Situation. Preadmission experiences of the institutionalized children in their biological families—namely, prenatal risk and extent of maternal emotional neglect were shown to be predictors of IB, with emotional neglect mediating the influence of prenatal risk on IB (Oliveira et al., 2012). The observational measure, known as the Rating of Infant and Stranger Engagement (Rise), was developed by Lyons-Ruth and colleagues (Riley, Atlas-Corbett, & Lyons-Ruth, 2005) and was initially validated in their study of home-reared at-risk children, but the Oliveira, Soares, Marins, Silva, Marques, et al. (2012) report showed its relevance to children living in institutions. In future use with adopted children or children in foster care, the RISE may prove a useful tool for further exploring how RAD, and IB or Social Engagement Disorder, in particular, are distinct from, or overlapping with, the classic typical patterns of child–parent attachment.

Improving the Lives of Abandoned or Orphaned Children Within the Institutional Setting in Their Home Countries

In our own research on the circumstances that can improve the lives of abandoned children living in child care institutions, we visited two of the 3,000 child care institutions in China (Steele, Steele, Archer, Jin, & Herreros, 2009). Our mission was to set up a research study that might demonstrate the effectiveness of a granny program which would increase the quantity and quality of caregivers available to look after toddlers living in a child care institution. We collected Strange Situation observations of toddlers with their favorite caregiver in one of two types of institutions with (N = 50+) and without (N = 50+) the granny program. We showed that improving the quality of care served to significantly lessen evidence of attachment disorganization and increase evidence of attachment security.

With a marked decline in international adoptions over recent years, as countries such as China and Russia, previously open to sending their abandoned children abroad, are now taking steps within their borders to provide foster care, adoption, or improvements to the quality of institutional care. This should lead international rates of RAD to decline. In the effort to improve institutional care, tools for rating and teaching social and emotional skills to caregivers may find wide applications (e.g., McCall, Groark, & Fish, 2010). McCall et al. present results from a Nicaraguan orphanage showing that their 18-item rating scale can be reliably applied, with minimal training, even using observational periods as short as 5 min. The scales are flexible to accommodate to individual differences in caregivers attending to children from birth to 4 and from 4 to 8 years of age.

The work of clinicians aiming to shift the fractured internal worlds of individuals with attachment disorders should continue to be informed by state-of-the-art research that combines many facets of development including physical, social, emotional, psychophysiological, and genetic. Some exemplar efforts of research in this context with implications for adoption and foster care have appeared recently (e.g., De Schipper, Oosterman, & Scheungel, 2012). Specifically, De Schipper et al. found that shy children who had more sensitive foster parents were more likely to be securely attached, while for non-shy children differing levels of parental sensitivity had no noticeable effects on attachment security.

Discussion and Conclusions

While the early observations and studies of infants in institutions together with the early reviews of pioneering work from the last century (Bowlby,

1951; Spitz, 1945) evocatively described the pernicious impact on children's development that comes about as a result of "experiments in nature" (Cicchetti, 2002) that are apparent in institutions or maltreating environments, we have extended observations into empirically based measures of these children's initial developmental deficits and their ability to "catch up" if given the opportunity to do so (Bakersman-Kranenburg et al. 2011). Research documents how the move from deprived environments to ones of more benign or positive caregiving contexts can be achieved and maintained across a range of socio-emotional, cognitive, and physical developmental indices. Studies of institutionalized infants (e.g., Zeanah et al., 2005), those abandoned children who move into foster care (Dozier, Stovall, Albus, & Bates, 2001) or placements with adoptive parents (Steele et al., 2008), point to characteristics of parents that facilitate radical changes toward organization and security for children. This literature will be an ongoing source of influence upon future research and clinical work (e.g., Steele, Murphy, & Steele, 2010) that has the potential to radically and positively impact the lives of parents with adverse trauma histories and their children at risk of maltreatment.

Yet much current research also points to characteristics of individual children that influence their susceptibility to the caregiving they receive (e.g., Bakermans-Kranenburg & van IJzendoorn, 2006; Bakermans-Kranenburg et al. (2008). Belsky and Puess (2009) place the differential susceptibility findings in an evolutionary perspective, arguing that in any given family, it makes survival sense to equip some children with extreme sensitivity to the environment, as it may change, and other children with much less sensitivity to small variations in the environment as these may be misleading given the overall stability of the environment. In respect of differential susceptibility, which may affect parents as much as children, we are only at the beginning of understanding how to identify those most, and those least, at risk. And what if we could reliably distinguish membership in these groups? Would we leave in the orphanage the child who is LESS impacted by his/her environment and favor for "early release" the child who is MORE impacted? These questions arise from the limited resources available to address the problem of pathogenic care endemic to institutional settings. The problem must be worked on from multiple angles. First, the quality of care within child care institutions needs to be improved and consistently monitored. Second, movement of children to high quality foster care or adoptive care should be sought. Third, training, support, and monitoring of foster care workers are called for just as treatment trials are needed of interventions aimed to achieve and maintain secure attachments between adoptees and their adoptive parents.

With respect to adoptive parents who are frequently the ones to experience the immediate impact of RAD when a child is adopted, typically from another country, there is considerable advice available from those who have worked with RAD problems and adoptive parents (e.g., Leiberman, 2003). Lieberman points to four phenomena that she has repeatedly noticed in work with young adopted children with RAD and their adoptive parents (1) the adoptive parents are distressed and often overwhelmed with feelings of guilt, shame, or anger; (2) the adoptive parents tended to overlook or downplay the child's anxiety and need for care; (3) the parents often fail to read the child's attachment cues, responding with authority and discipline, rather than a mix of limit setting and reassurance or warmth; and (4) the adoptive parents were insufficiently prepared by the adoptive agency. One piece of preparatory advice needs to point out the extreme sensitivity to rejection and shame-proneness the adopted child will have. Thus, ordinary discipline tactics, e.g., time-out, will amplify the child's shame and pain without producing agreeable behavior. A more appropriate strategy in these circumstances is time-in, i.e., stay close with me at my side as "I need your help." A learning experience can then follow that will help alter fate for the child with RAD, away from his or her history of deep shaming experiences toward a future with a firmly rooted sense of acceptance by others and a corresponding strong sense of self-worth linked to self-efficacy.

It is 50 years since Provence and Lipton (1962) assembled the compelling evidence of the time regarding the serious debilitating effects of institutional care upon infants. And while institutional care of children in the developed Western world has been more or less eliminated, the quality of care available to children in Western countries is by no means void of the conditions known to lead to attachment disorders. And in many countries throughout the world, institutional care of young children remains the norm for abandoned children. Children and caregivers in orphanages around the world deserve to benefit from training, research, and clinical tools known to diminish the likelihood of attachment disorders in the narrow sense of RAD. And for attachment disorders in the broad sense to be minimized, a renewed effort toward preventing child maltreatment, and child psychopathology in all its variants, is urgently called for. To paraphrase John Bowlby, a society that values its children must cherish, monitor, and support those who provide care to its children: birth parents, foster parents, adoptive parents, stepparents, child care workers, religious figures, sports coaches and managers, teachers, and all others involved in caregiving to children.

Acknowledgment The authors are grateful to the NIH HRSA R40 funding mechanism (R40MC23629-01-00) for support during the time of preparing this chapter.

References

Ainsworth, M. D., Blehar, M. C., Waters, E., & Wall, S. (1978). *Patterns of attachment: A psychological study of the Strange Situation*. Hillsdale, NJ: Lawrence Erlbaum.

American Psychiatric Association. (1980). *Diagnostic and statistical manual of mental disorders* (3rd ed.). Washington, DC: Author.

American Psychiatric Association. (1994). *Diagnostic and statistical manual of mental disorders* (4th ed.). Washington, DC: Author.

American Psychiatric Association. (1999). *Diagnostic and statistical manual of mental disorders* (4, Text rev. th ed.). Washington, DC: Author.

Bakersman-Kranenburg, M. J, Steele, H., Zeanah, C. H., Muhamedrahimov, R. J., Vorria, P, Dobrovo-Krol, N. A., Steele, M., van IJzendoorn, M. H., Juffer, F., &

Gunnar, M. R. (2011). Attachment and emotional development in institutional care: Characteristics and catch-up. In R. B. McCall, M. H. van IJzendoorn, F. Juffer, C. J. Groark, & V. K. Groza (Eds.), Children without permanent parents: Research, practice, and policy (pp. 62–91). *Monographs of the Society for Research in Child Development, 76*, Serial No. 301.

Bakermans-Kranenburg, M., & van IJzendoorn, M. H. (2006). Gene-environment interaction of the dopamine d4 receptor (DRD4) and observed maternal insensitivity predicting externalizing behavior in preschoolers. *Developmental Psychobiology, 48*, 406–409.

Bakermans-Kranenburg, M. J., van IJzendoorn, M. H., Pijlman, F. T. A., Mesman, J., & Juffer, F. (2008). Differential susceptibility to intervention: Dopamine D4 receptor polymorphism (DRD4 VNTR) moderates effects on toddlers' externalizing behaviour in a randomized control trial. *Developmental Psychology, 44*, 293–300.

Belsky, J., & Puess, M. (2009). Beyond diathesis stress: Differential susceptibility to environmental influences. *Psychological Bulletin, 135*, 885–908.

Belsky, J., & Rovine, M. (1987). Temperament and attachment security in the strange situation: An empirical rapprochement. *Child Development, 58*, 787–795.

Bowlby, J. (1944). Forty-four juvenile thieves: Their characters and home-life. *International Journal of Psychoanalysis, 25*, 19–53.

Bowlby, J. (1951). *Maternal care and mental health*. Geneva: World Health Organization.

Bowlby, J. (1960). Separation anxiety. *International Journal of Psychoanalysis, 41*, 89–113.

Bowlby, J. (1969/1982). *Attachment and loss: Vol. 1. Attachment*. London: Hogarth Press and the Institute of Psychoanalysis.

Bowlby, J. (1980). *Attachment and loss: Vol. 2: Separation*. London: Hogarth Press and the Institute of Psychoanalysis.

Brisch, K. (2012). *Treating attachment disorders: From theory to therapy* (2nd ed.). New York: Guilford Press.

Carlson, E. A. (1998). A prospective longitudinal study of attachment disorganization/disorientation. *Child Development, 69*, 1107–1128.

Chaffin, M., Hanson, R., Saunders, B. E., Nichols, T., Barnett, D., Zeanah, C. H., et al. (2006). Report of the APSAC task force on attachment therapy, reactive attachment disorder, and attachment problems. *Child Maltreatment, 11*, 76–89.

Cicchetti, D. (2002). Editorial: Experiments of Nature: Contributions to developmental theory. *Development and Psychopathology, 15*, 833–835.

De Schipper, J. C., Oosterman, M., & Scheungel, C. (2012). Temperament, disordered attachment and parental sensitivity in foster care: Differential findings on attachment security for shy children. *Attachment and Human Development, 14*, 349–365.

Dozier, M., Stovall, K. C., Albus, K., & Bates, B. (2001). Attachment for infants in foster care: The role of cargiver state of mind. *Child Development, 72*, 1467–1477.

Erikson, E. (1951). *Childhood and society*. New York: WW Norton.

Fearon, R. P., Bakermans-Kranenburg, M. J., van IJzendoorn, M. H., Lapsly, A.-M., & Roisman, G. I. (2010). The significance of insecure attachment and disorganization in the development of children's externalizing behavior: A meta-analytic study. *Child Development, 81*, 435–456.

Gleason, M. M., Fox, N. A., Dury, S., Smyke, A., Egger, H. L., Nelson, C. A., III, et al. (2011). Validity of evidence-derived criteria for reactive attachment disorder: Indiscriminately social/disinhibited and emotionally withdrawn/inhibited subtypes. *Journal of the American Academy of Child and Adolescent Psychiatry, 50*, 216–231.

Grossmann, K. E., Grossmann, K., & Watters, E. (2005). *Attachment from infancy to adulthood: The major longitudinal studies*. New York: Guilford Press.

Hesse, E., & Main, M. (2006). Frightening, threatening and dissociative (FR) parental behavior as related to infant D attachment in low-risk samples: Description, discussion, and interpretations. *Development and Psychopathology, 18*, 309–343.

Juffer, F., & van IJzendoon, M. H. (2009). International adoption comes of age: Development of international adoptees from a longitudinal and meta-analytic perspective. In G. M. Wrobel & E. Neil (Eds.), *International advances in adoption research for practice* (pp. 169–192). Chichester, UK: Wiley-Blackwell.

Kochanska, G., Barry, R. A., Stellern, S. A., & O'Bleness, J. J. (2009). Early attachment organization moderates the parent-child mutually coercive pathway to children's anti-social conduct. *Child Development, 80*, 1297–1309.

Leiberman, A. (2003). The treatment of attachment disorder in infancy and early childhood: Reflections from clinical intervention with later-adopted foster care children. *Attachment and Human Development, 5*, 279–282.

Lewis, M. (1992). *Shame: The exposed self*. New York: The Free Press.

Lewis, M. (1997). *Altering fare: Why the past does not predict the future*. New York: Guilford Press.

Lewis, M., Feiring, C., & Rosenthal, S. (2000). Attachment over time. *Child Development, 71*(3), 707–720.

Lyons-Ruth, K., & Jacobvitz, D. (2008). Attachment disorganization: Genetic factors, parenting contexts, and developmental transformations from infancy to adulthood. In J. Cassidy & P. R. Shaver (Eds.), *Handbook of attachment theory, research and clinical applications* (2nd ed., pp. 666–697). New York: Guilford Press.

Madigan, S., Bakermans-Kranenburg, M. J., van IJzendoorn, M. H., Moran, G., Pederson, D. R., & Benoit, D. (2006). Unresolved states of mind, anomalous parental behavior, and disorganized attachment:

A review and meta-analysis of a transmission gap. *Attachment and Human Development, 8*, 89–111.

Main, M., & Solomon, J. (1990). Procedures for identifying infants as disorganized/disoriented during the Ainsworth Strange Situation. In M. T. Greenberg, D. Cicchetti, & E. M. Cummings (Eds.), *Attachment during the preschool years: Theory, research and intervention* (pp. 121–160). Chicago: University of Chicago Press.

McCall, R. B., van IJzendoorn, M. H., Juffer, F., Groark, C. J., & Groza, V. K. (Eds.). (2011). Children without permanent parents: Research, practice, and policy. *Monographs of the Society for Research in Child Development, 76*, Serial No. 301.

McCall, R. B., Groark, C. J., & Fish, L. (2010). A caregiver-child social/emotional and relationship rating scale (CCSERRS). *Infant Mental Health Journal, 31*, 201–219.

McGoron, L., Gleason, M. M., Smyke, A. T., Drury, S. S., Nelson, C. A., III, Gregas, M. C., et al. (2012). Recovering from early deprivation: Attachment mediates effects of caregiving on psychopathology. *Journal of the American Academy of Child and Adolescent Psychiatry, 51*, 683–693.

Merz, E. C., & McCall, R. B. (2010). Behavior problems in children adopted from psychosocially depriving institutions. *Journal of Abnormal Child Psychology, 38*, 459–470.

O'Connor, T., & Zeanah, C. H. (2003). Attachment disorders: Assessment strategies and treatment approaches. *Attachment and Human Development, 5*, 223–244.

Oliveira, P. S., Soares, I., Martins, C., Silva, J. R., Marques, S., Baptista, J., et al. (2012). Indiscriminate attachment behavior observed in the Strange Situation among institutionalized toddlers: Relations to caregiver report and early family risk. *Infant Mental Health Journal, 33*, 187–196.

Provence, S., & Lipton, R. (1962). *Infants in institutions: A comparison of their development with family-reared infants during the first year of life.* New York: International Universities Press.

Richters, M., & Volkmar, F. (1994). Reactive attachment disorder of infancy or early childhood. *Journal of the American Academy of Child and Adolescent Psychiatry, 33*, 328–332.

Riley, C., Atlas-Corbett, A., & Lyons-Ruth, K. (2005). Rating of Infant-Stranger Engagement (RISE) coding system. Unpublished manual, Harvard Medical School at the Cambridge Hospital, Department of Psychiatry, Cambridge, MA.

Roy, P., Rutter, M., & Pickles, A. (2004). Institutional care: Associations between overactivity, and lack of selectivity in social relationships. *Journal of the Child Psychology and Psychiatry, 45*, 866–873.

Rutter, M., Sonuga-Barke, E. J., Beckett, C., Castle, J., Kreppner, R., et al. (Eds.). (2010). Deprivation-specific psychological patterns: Effects of institutional deprivation. *Monographs of the Society for Research in Child Development, 75*, Serial No. 295.

Rutter, M., & Sonuga-Barke, E. J. (2010). Conclusions: Overview of findings from the ERA study, inferences, and research implications. In M. Rutter, E. J. Sonuga-Barke, C. Beckett, J. Castle, J. Kreppner, R. Kumsta, et al. (Eds.), *Deprivation-specific psychological patterns: Effects of institutional deprivation* (pp. 232–247). Monographs of the Society for Research in Child Development, 75, Serial No. 295.

Smyke, A. T., Dumitrescu, A., & Zeanah, C. H. (2002). Attachment disturbances in young children: I: the continuum of caretaking causality. *Journal of the American Academy of Child and Adolescent Psychiatry, 41*, 972–982.

Spangler, G., & Grossmann, K. E. (1993). Biobehavioral organization in securely and insecurely attached infants. *Child Development, 64*, 1439–1450.

Spitz, R. (1945). Hospitalism: An inquiry into the genesis of psychiatric conditions in early childhood. *Psychoanalytic Study of the Child, 1*, 53–73.

Spitz, R. (1950). Anxiety in infancy: A study of its manifestations in the first year of life. *Internation Journal of Psychoanalysis, 31*, 138.

Sroufe, A. L. (2005). Attachment and development: A prospective longitudinal study from birth to adulthood. *Attachment and Human Development, 7*, 349–367.

Steele, H. (2003). Holding therapy is not attachment therapy. *Attachment and Human Development, 5*, 219.

Steele, M., Hodges, J., Kaniuk, J., Steele, H., Asquith, K., & Hillman, S. (2009). Attachment Representations and Adoption Outcome: On the use of narrative assessments to track the adaptation of previously maltreated children in their new families. In B. Neil & G. Wrobel (Eds.), *International advances in adoption research for practice* (pp. 193–216). New York: Wiley.

Steele, M., Hodges, J., Kaniuk, J., Steele, H., Hillman, S., & Asquith, K. (2008). Forecasting outcomes in previously maltreated children: The use of the AAI in a longitudinal attachment study. In H. Steele & M. Steele (Eds.), *Clinical applications of the Adult Attachment Interview* (pp. 427–451). New York: Guilford Press.

Steele, M., Murphy, A., & Steele, H. (2010). Identifying therapeutic action in an attachment-based intervention with high-risk families. *Clinical Social Work Journal, 38*, 61–72.

Steele, M., Steele, H., Archer, M., Jin, X., & Herreros, F. (2009). Enhancing security and diminishing disorganization among Chinese orphans: Beneficial effects of a granny program. Symposium presentation at SRCD, Denver, April 2, 2009.

The St. Petersburgh-USA Orphanage Research Team (2008). The effects of early social-emotional and relationship experience on the development of young orphanage children. *Monographs of the Society for Research in Child Development, 73*, Serial No. 291.

Van den Dries, L., Juffer, F., van IJzendoorn, M. H., & Bakermans-Kranenburg, M. J. (2009). Fostering

Security? A meta-analysis of attachment in adopted children. *Children and Youth Services Review, 31,* 410–421.

van IJzendoorn, M. H., & Bakermans-Kranenburg, M. J. (2012). Integrating temperament and attachment: The differntial susceptibility paradigm. In M. Zentner & R. L. Shiner (Eds.), *Handbook of temperament* (pp. 403–424). New York: Guilford Press.

van IJzendoorn, M. H., & Juffer, F. (2006). The Emanuel Miller Memorial Lecture 2006: Adoption as intervention. Meta-analtyic evidence of massive catch-up and plasticity in physical, socio-emotional, and cognitive development. *Journal of Child Psychology and Psychiatry, 47,* 1228–1245.

van IJzendoorn, M. H., & Kroonenberg, P. M. (1988). Cross-cultural patterns of attachment: A meta-analysis of the strange situation. *Child Development, 59,* 147–156.

van IJzendoorn, M. H., & Sagi-Schwartz, A. (2008). Cross-cultural patterns of attachment: Universal and contextual dimensions. In J. Cassidy & P. R. Shaver (Eds.), *Handbook of attachment theory, research and clinical applications* (2nd ed.). New York: Guilford Press.

Warren, S., Huston, L., Egeland, B., & Sroufe, L. A. (1997). Child and adolescent anxiety disorders and early attachment. *Journal of the American Academy of Child and Adolescent Psychiatry, 36,* 637–644.

Zeanah, C. H., & Gleason, M. M. (2010). *Reactive attachment disorder: A review for DSM V.* Washington, DC: American Psychiatric Association.

Zeanah, C. H., Smyke, A. T., Koga, S., Carlson, E., & The BEIP Core Group. (2005). Attachment in institutionalized and community children in Romania. *Child Development, 76,* 1015–1028.

Zero to Three. (2005). *Diagnostic classification of mental health and developmental disorders of infancy and early childhood: Revised edition (DC:0-3R).* Washington, DC: Zero to Three Press.

Early Deprivation and Developmental Psychopathology

Elisa A. Esposito and Megan R. Gunnar

Psychology has long been fascinated by the development of children who suffer extreme deprivation early in life. From questions about whether language will develop in the absence of linguistic input to the lore surrounding presumed feral children (for a review, see Rutter, 1981), we ponder the limits of human resilience and the importance of critical periods in the life stories of these children. Initiated by geopolitical events, the early 1990s saw a sudden surge in the number of children who experienced severe early deprivation being adopted by highly resourced families in the USA and other industrialized countries. At first the children came primarily from Eastern Europe and Russia; later China became a major sending country. At its peak in the mid-2000s, around 27,000 children were being adopted each year by US families, with the majority coming from countries that used institutions to care for wards of the state. This number has fallen drastically in the last few years due to changing rules in birth countries and the economic recession. Nonetheless, we now have thousands of children available for study who are recovering from significantly adverse early life conditions whose lives provide testimony to both the impact of early experiences on neurobehavioral development and the resilience and plasticity of the human nervous system.

E.A. Esposito, M.A. (✉) • M.R. Gunnar, Ph.D.
Institute of Child Development, University
of Minnesota, Minneapolis, MN 55455, USA
e-mail: espos016@umn.edu

Prevalence of Psychopathology

"How are the children?" is not only a Masai greeting but also the question we often ask about children adopted from institutions or other deprived circumstances. The answer, particularly with regard to psychopathology, depends on which outcomes are examined. Much of the initial work focused on the problems typically seen in other groups of maltreated children, notably attention, externalizing, and internalizing problems. With the exception of attention problems, which are highly prevalent in these children, internalizing and externalizing problems are not observed at high frequencies, especially in childhood. This is the conclusion of a large meta-analysis conducted by Juffer and van Ijzendoorn (2005). They included multiple studies that had reported on Child Behavior Checklist (CBCL) total, internalizing, and externalizing scale scores in domestic and international adoptees. They concluded that domestic adoptees had more behavior problems than international adoptees, but on the whole, most adoptees were problem-free despite being taken more often to mental health clinics. Following a large group of children adopted into the UK from Romania, Rutter and colleagues drew somewhat similar conclusions with regard to internalizing and externalizing problems during childhood (Rutter, Kreppner, & O'Connor, 2001). The researchers noted a wide range of outcomes for the children, despite severe and global deprivation early in life. When children had problems, they were not ones of conduct, anxiety, or depression. Rather, the authors argued that there were specific problems associated with severe, early deprivation: attention-deficit/hyperactivity, quasi-autism, severe mental delay, and disinhibited attachment disorder. As the researchers followed these Romanian children into adolescence, however, conduct and affective pathology emerged in a significant number of cases. Reviewing these cases, the English and Romanian Adoption (ERA) study team concluded that psychopathology emerged predominantly in those youth who suffered one or more of the deprivation-specific disorders listed earlier and thus was a phenomenon secondary to the primary deficits produced by early deprivation (Kreppner et al., 2010). Said differently, the pathology emerging in adolescence for these children reflected a developmental cascade such that failure to succeed on earlier salient developmental tasks undermined later developing capacities.

In the years since the Juffer and van Ijzendoorn meta-analysis and Rutter and colleagues' argument for deprivation-specific problems, the nature of the problems suffered by children residing in and adopted from conditions of deprivation has been examined more thoroughly. Quasi-autism has been examined in fewer samples of children, while more general issues of delays/deficits in intersubjectivity/theory of mind have been examined more widely. Attention problems have received considerable attention. The possibility that attention problems may reflect deficits in reward systems functioning (e.g., Sonuga-Barke & Fairchild, 2012) has stimulated the study of sensitivity to reward among youth with early life histories of deprivation. The argument that indiscriminately friendly behavior reflects a form of reactive attachment disorder has given way to the argument that this odd and intrusive social behavior is its own phenomenon. More recent work has also questioned the absence of internalizing problems for these children. Although perhaps not meeting clinical criteria in childhood, the evidence is mounting that early experiences amplify the reactivity of the distributed neural systems involved in fear, thus increasing the risk of internalizing pathologies.

Chapter Overview

There have been many advances in the study of early deprivation and later emotional and behavioral problems. What is only beginning, however, is examination of how the impact of deprivation on cognitive and affective systems mediates the development of affective and behavioral pathologies. This chapter will cover the following issues. First, we will outline several, not mutually exclusive, theoretical perspectives on the effects of early deprivation. Second, we will briefly outline effects of early deprivation on physical health and physical growth. Often overlooked or only dealt with to rule out malnutrition as a source of influence, we argue that health and physical growth effects need to be studied in concert with neurobiological impacts if we are to understand how early deprivation influences brain and behavioral development. Next, we will outline what we know about key domains affected by early deprivation: attention problems, executive functions, intersubjectivity/theory of mind, attachment, indiscriminately friendly behavior, emotion understanding, and anxiety. We follow this with a section on neurobiological studies of early deprivation, noting where the findings may help explain some of the behavioral effects and where we need more information. Finally, we will consider how altered functioning in the domains we have discussed in combination with puberty and the changing demands and social contexts of adolescence may contribute to the rise in psychopathology during adolescence in youth exposed to deprivation early in life.

Perspectives on Early Deprivation

Adverse early experiences can be sorted into stimulation that should not be there (e.g., physical abuse) and the absence of stimulation that should be there (e.g., changing visual input). Deprivation would seem to imply that we are only dealing with the latter; however, the distinction is not that clear. In some instances lack of input produces conditions that confront the organism with stimuli that should not be there (e.g., lack of medical care with increased exposure to pathogens). Nonetheless, when viewed cautiously, the idea that deprivation involves the absence of expectable stimulation can be helpful. From this perspective, Greenough's argument about experience-expectant and experience-dependent neural development has been evoked as an organizing framework (see Zeanah et al., 2003). Experience-expectant neural systems are those whose development *requires* the presence of stimulation that is available under nearly all conditions and thus supports species-typical development (e.g., exposure to patterned light is necessary for the development of the visual cortex). Experience-dependent neural development involves systems that adapt to local conditions of stimulation and thus supports behaviors that may be culturally, family, or individually specific (e.g., early, prolonged exposure to a particular language eventually makes it impossible to discriminate phonemes from unfamiliar languages). Under conditions of stimulus deprivation, we would predict that experience-expectant neural development would be delayed or undermined, leading to delays/deficits in the development of typical developmental milestones in cognitive, emotion, and motor development. Because the neural systems underlying these competencies may have sensitive periods for development, we might expect that if children are older at removal from deprivation, full recovery may not be possible.

Indeed, when institutional settings lack developmentally appropriate visual, auditory, proprioceptive, motor, and linguistic stimulation, children fall behind in all developmental milestones and their ability to catch up to age norms reflects the age of removal and placement in a more enriched context, as evidenced by data on both IQ (e.g., Nelson et al., 2007) and language development (e.g., Windsor, Moraru, Nelson, Fox, & Zeanah, 2012). Note that the papers just cited come from the Bucharest Early Intervention Project (BEIP), a study that involved random assignment to care as usual or to removal from the institution for placement in study-supported foster care. The BEIP results mirror all the studies that have not had the advantage of random

assignment, and lend support to the argument that effects are due, at least in part, to early deprivation rather than to potential associated factors (e.g., parental IQ, prenatal experiences).

An alternative or additional model of early deprivation invokes the idea that regulatory systems of the human infant and young child evolved to function in relationships with a few consistent caregivers (Bowlby, 1969). Certainly, close contact with another adult human being during infancy is part of the expectable environment of our species. The absence of that expectable environment activates counter-regulatory systems, including systems mediating the mammalian stress response. Based on animal models of maternal deprivation, chronic deprivation in early life can be viewed as a form of chronic stress which alters future behavior via activity of the hypothalamic-pituitary-adrenocortical (HPA) axis, stress-related neuropeptides (e.g., corticotropin-releasing hormone produced at extrahypothalamic sites), and neurotransmitters (e.g., serotonin, NE) (Faturi et al., 2010). Early adverse care may also alter the functioning of stress-mediating systems and other systems needed to manage challenge and threat via epigenetic mechanisms resulting in potentially long-lasting effects of stress-stimulating experiences of early deprivation (McClelland, Korosi, Cope, Ivy, & Baram, 2011).

Thus, we have two models: (1) stimulation is needed for brain development; absent or deficient stimulation during sensitive periods will produce long-term deficits; and (2) lack of consistent adults serving their regulatory functions stimulates the neurobiology of stress resulting in epigenetic changes in the adaptive systems that manage threat and challenge. At first glance, both models might apply, but to different facets of early deprivation effects. To some extent that seems true, as the stimulation-rich institutions that lack consistent caregivers result in children who struggle with some of the deprivation-specific effects noted earlier (e.g., indiscriminate friendliness, attention problems) but not others (e.g., general intelligence/language development; Tizard & Hodges, 1978). On the other hand, low levels of expectable stimulation have been shown in rodents to produce epigenetic changes in a gene critical for regulating the stress neuraxis, even though this effect is not mediated by activation of stress-mediating systems, but rather seems to be a reflection simply of reduced stimulation (Meaney & Szyf, 2005). Making matters more complicated, this effect occurs within the normal range of maternal care and thus is not the result of deprivation of expectable input. It is probably more in the realm of Greenough's experience-dependent neural development. Nonetheless, this epigenetic alteration results in heightened fearfulness, stress reactivity, and vulnerability to the disorders of aging.

Although more intense deprivation produces more dramatic effects in animal models (McClelland et al., 2011), it is not obvious where one would draw the line between effects due simply to low levels of expectable stimulation and effects due to lack of regulatory input triggering the activation of counter-regulatory systems. Likewise, this example points to the fluidity in boundaries between experience-expectant and experience-dependent processes. It is likely that we are simply going to need to understand much more about the molecular mechanisms through which early deprivation impacts different developing systems and the developmental cascades that early alterations can then play into before we can sort out these different perspectives on early deprivation.

Physical Health and Growth

Children adopted from institutional care often arrive in their new families with existing medical conditions, such as infectious diseases (e.g., Hepatitis B), the presence of intestinal parasites, and/or nutrient deficiency (Johnson, 2001). The extent of medical conditions varies with both the degree of preadoption deprivation and the health problems endemic in the children's birth countries. Health problems range in severity but commonly include infectious diseases, parasites, and other treatable medical conditions. Increasingly, problems requiring surgical intervention (e.g., cleft palate) and physical deformities (e.g., lack of an arm)

are being seen as children without such needs find adoption homes in their birth countries. Fisher, Ames, Chisholm and Savoie (1997) reported that 85 % of children in their sample had at least one medical problem at adoption. We and other researchers note similar percentages (e.g., Loman, Wiik, Frenn, Pollak, & Gunnar, 2009). The frequency of different medical conditions seen at adoption varies by country of origin, reflecting an incredibly broad spectrum of preadoption experience: Children adopted from China are more likely to present with lead exposure (Miller & Hendrie, 2000), whereas diagnoses of fetal alcohol syndrome (FAS) are more common among children adopted from institutions in Eastern Europe (Johnson & Gunnar, 2011). The latter provides a critical challenge for understanding the independent effects of institutional deprivation on neurobiological and cognitive development, because similar cognitive sequelae are observed for both prenatal alcohol exposure and early deprivation. The need for medical treatment typically decreases over time (Johnson, 2001); however, some families are burdened with frequent medical visits and procedures during their first months and years as a family. Sadly, the effect of the child's initial health on parenting stress and children's psychosocial development has not been considered in studies of post-institutionalized children.

In addition to the presence of medical conditions, children adopted from institutions are often smaller than their non-adopted age-mates. Children currently residing in institutions are much more likely to meet criteria for stunted growth (Johnson et al., 2010). Again, the duration of early deprivation predicts the degree of growth failure: Estimates of growth deceleration are as high as 1 month of linear growth lost per 3 months spent in institutional care (Miller & Hendrie, 2000). Van Ijzendoorn, Bakermans-Kranenburg, and Juffer (2007) conducted a meta-analysis of 33 studies and found that the duration of institutionalization not only predicted greater growth delays but also was related to less complete catch-up in height and weight following removal from the institutional setting. Post-adoptive caregiving experiences have also been demonstrated to significantly impact the rate of catch-up growth. Johnson et al. (2010) found that high positive regard for the child and sensitivity uniquely predicted increases in catch-up in height and weight, whereas caregiver detachment was negatively correlated with gains in height.

There is considerable discussion over whether growth delays index malnutrition or reflect the impact of chronic stress on the growth hormone-insulin-like growth factor axis (GH-IGF-1) system. Generally speaking, weight-for-age scores cannot be used to index malnutrition; weight-for-height or BMI indices is what is needed. In some institutions, as many as 30 % of infants have extremely low BMIs, suggesting marked levels of malnutrition. On the other hand, there are many instances of normal BMI but strikingly small height-for-age (Sonuga-Barke, Schlotz, & Rutter, 2010). Linear growth may reflect the GH-IGF-1 system, particularly beyond infancy. This system can be downregulated in the presence of increased HPA axis activity (Johnson & Gunnar, 2011).

Allostasis is the process of maintaining stability through change and it has been used to describe the way that stress-mediating systems operate to preserve viability (McEwen, 2000). Allostatic load reflects the physiological alterations induced by chronic or repeated activation of allostatic mediating systems. In adults, biological markers such as high blood pressure, larger waist-hip ratios, and serum cholesterol have been used as indices of allostatic load. Because of the role that stress may play in linear growth, we have recently argued that growth delay is an allostatic load index (Johnson, Bruce, Tarullo, & Gunnar, 2011). Furthermore, we have demonstrated that the more linearly growth delayed children are at adoption, the more dysregulated the HPA axis is years after adoption and the more evidence of deprivation-specific neurobehavioral problems the children exhibit (i.e., attention problems and indiscriminate friendliness; Johnson et al., 2011).

Early deprivation not only impacts linear growth, but it may also affect the timing of puberty. Puberty, in turn, may have powerful impacts on the neurodevelopment of children adopted from conditions of deprivation. We will briefly review the evidence for early puberty here. Puberty is delayed for children who continue to live under highly depriving circumstances throughout childhood and adolescence. The shift to earlier onset puberty is observed when children who were deprived early in life move into well-resourced, nutritionally rich environments (for a review, see Johnson & Gunnar, 2011). With that move comes rapid linear growth and it is not clear whether it is the early delay or the rapid post-adoption growth that is critical in affecting the biological clocks regulating pubertal timing. What does seem to be clear is that for girls, but not necessarily for boys, there is an increased risk of early-onset puberty, sometimes as early as 6–7 years of age. Even for girls who do not enter puberty that early, a shift of 6–12 months earlier than age-mates has been reported. There is, of course, good evidence that earlier puberty can be a risk factor for internalizing and externalizing in girls (Graber, Nichols, & Brooks-Gunn, 2010). As earlier puberty may be co-occurring with other deprivation-induced social-cognitive deficits, it may be of particular concern.

Finally, there is emerging evidence that early deprivation and neglect may have long-term impacts on health through effects on the immune system and mechanisms of cellular growth and repair. Although not yet described for institutionalized and post-institutionalized children, there is evidence that maltreatment during development is associated with increased production of proinflammatory immune factors and epigenetic changes in macrophages that make them resistant to regulation by glucocorticoids (for a review, see Miller, Chen, & Parker, 2011). Along with unhealthy lifestyle choices, these "under the skin" effects of early adversity heighten the risk for metabolic syndrome and a host of diseases of aging. There is also increasing evidence that inflammatory processes may play a role in the development and/or expression of depression (Miller et al., 2011). Adding to the advances to the aging clock, early adversity may also impact the length of telomere. Telomeres are regions of repetitive nucleotide sequences at the ends of chromosomes which, like aglets (the plastic ends of shoe laces), protect the chromosome from deterioration or fusion with neighboring chromosomes. Cell division and stress shorten telomeres, explaining why both aging and stress are associated with disease and death. The BEIP group recently reported that duration of institutional care was inversely associated with telomere length (Drury et al., 2011). Thus, although the health issues induced by early deprivation are largely reversible once children are placed in supportive homes, there is increasing evidence that these early experiences do get under the skin and affect systems that can influence physical and emotional health throughout life.

Cognitive Sequelae

General Intelligence

The most common means for assessing the impact of early deprivation on cognitive development has been measures of general intelligence. Early reports made strong claims that damage to children's IQ following early institutionalization was irreparable, but later research demonstrated that the quality of caregiving in the institution and the duration of deprivation experienced directly predict IQ (Hodges & Tizard, 1989a; Nelson et al., 2007). Although IQ is negatively impacted by the experience of early institutional care, children who are subsequently placed into supportive family settings experience substantial catch-up. Findings from the ERA and BEIP studies demonstrate that the majority of children perform within the normal range on tests of general intelligence within the first year or so of removal from the institution. Even those children who exhibited the most severe delays continue to improve across childhood and into adolescence (e.g., Beckett, Castle, Rutter, & Sonuga-Barke, 2010). Although measures of general intelligence are useful for providing an initial index of the impact of early deprivation on global cognitive functioning, they severely limit our ability to understand which underlying cognitive—and neural—systems are affected and the extent to which they recover following placement into a supportive family context. This limitation has

prompted recent efforts to uncover the effects of early deprivation on specific domains of cognitive functioning.

Attention Problems and Hyperactivity

Converging evidence from multiple groups of researchers has shown that children who experience early deprivation are at heightened risk for developing attention problems, with some samples showing ADHD rates of over 40 % (Miller, Chan, Tirella, & Perrin, 2009). The pattern of attention and hyperactivity problems presents a sufficient burden that the ERA team has classified it as one of their deprivation-specific problems (Kreppner, O'Connor, Rutter, & The English Romanian Adoptees Study, 2001). There is evidence to suggest that the heightened risk for attention problems is not merely the result of poor nutrition or inadequate cognitive stimulation: Children who were reared in high-quality institutions also demonstrated patterns of overactivity and inattentive behavior compared to children reared in foster families. Of greatest interest here is that these difficulties are related to indiscriminately friendly behavior, the core behavior used in diagnosing the disinhibited form of reactive attachment disorder (Bruce, Tarullo, & Gunnar, 2009; Roy, Rutter, & Pickles, 2004). Attention problems appear to ameliorate somewhat over time, though the catch-up in this domain appears to follow a particularly protracted course, and may not become obvious for years after removal from the institution (Stevens et al., 2008). Despite their prevalence in this population, hyperactivity and inattention are not universal consequences of institutional rearing. Similar to other outcomes reviewed here, longer duration of deprivation independently predicts the severity of these problems (Kreppner et al., 2001), and the impact of deprivation on this system appears to be moderated by the dopamine transporter polymorphism (Stevens et al., 2008).

The persistence of attention deficits into late childhood and adolescence despite years of more normative stimulation makes it plausible that these deficits reflect the impact of depriving conditions on early neural maturation. Children exposed to institutional rearing have shown decreased levels of high-frequency power and increased levels of low-frequency power in EEG (Tarullo, Garvin, & Gunnar, 2011), a pattern associated with ADHD (Barry, Clarke, & Johnstone, 2003) and which may indicate delayed neural maturation. Indeed, this atypical power distribution has been shown to partially mediate the relationship between institutional rearing and symptoms of ADHD in early childhood (McLaughlin et al., 2010).

Researchers are still not certain that deprivation-induced attention problems and ADHD arising in the absence of early deprivation and adversity are comparable. Sonuga-Barke and Rubia (2008) found that although the profiles of attention problems in post-institutionalized children (specifically males) were highly similar to comparison cases of typical ADHD, post-institutionalized children appeared to have greater deficits in inhibitory control, but lower levels of conduct problems. This investigation is promising, but limited by a small sample size—future studies are needed to clarify whether the clinically relevant attention problems experienced by children with and without a history of institutional rearing are comparable.

Executive Functions

The protracted course of prefrontal cortex development may allow for fine-tuning of the neural systems that underlie specific cognitive processes such as executive functions, attention, and theory of mind. Nonetheless, there is increasing evidence that early experiences can have profound impacts on later developing systems. Recent evidence suggests that executive functions may be particularly affected by early deprivation. Pollak et al. (2010) used a battery of cognitive tasks to assess post-institutionalized children's working memory, attention, executive control, and learning abilities. Two comparison groups were employed: children adopted from foster care overseas as an adoption control and children reared in birth fami-

lies of the same high education and income as the adopting families. Even though they had been in their adoptive homes for 6 years or more, the early deprived children performed more poorly on tests of inhibitory control, visual and auditory attention, and working memory. Surprisingly, they performed comparably to controls on tasks that required planning and sequencing (i.e., Stockings of Cambridge) and rule learning and manipulation. The Bucharest group repeated this analysis with comparable findings (Bos, Fox, Zeanah, & Nelson, 2009). In both of these studies, executive deficits were more severe among children who had spent more time in institutional care. Consistent with duration of deprivation associations with greater impairment, in a small sample of youth who nearly all were adopted from Russia and Eastern European countries later than the two previous samples, impairments were more severe and even the Stockings of Cambridge task was affected (Bauer, Hanson, Pierson, Davidson, & Pollak, 2009).

Impairments in executive functioning have been noted in a number of pathological conditions, including but not restricted to ADHD. Problems with these functions likely also contribute to academic difficulties, which in developmental cascades may lead children and youth to associate with groups of children whose behavior problems increase the risk of conduct disorder. In families of high achievers, as is often the case for the families who adopt internationally, academic difficulties may create stress for the adopted children, thereby increasing the risk of anxiety and depression. Such cascades have not yet been examined in research on post-institutionalized children, but would be a potentially fruitful direction for research.

Theory of Mind

Theory of mind (ToM), or the ability to think about others' mental states, develops rapidly over the first 5 years of life, and research suggests that early adversity may compromise the child's ability to successfully coordinate social attention and communication (e.g., Rogosch, Cicchetti,

Shields, & Toth, 1995). In an initial study, preschool-aged children who were currently in an institutional care setting performed more poorly on tests of ToM compared to comparison children after controlling for age, language skills, and nonverbal intelligence (Yagmurlu, Berument, & Celimli, 2005). A history of early institutionalization uniquely predicts ToM performance over and above verbal ability, suggesting a disruption of the developmental precursors necessary for social cognition (Tarullo, Bruce, & Gunnar, 2007). As mentioned earlier, the early development of inhibitory control and set shifting, which allow children to take the perspective of others, is negatively impacted by the experience of early deprivation. Deficits in ToM may underlie the type of quasi-autistic features (e.g., deficits in communication and the ability to form reciprocal social relationship; stereotypic behaviors) exhibited by some post-institutionalized children. Indeed, statistical mediation has been shown, although because the ToM measures were given long after the autistic behavior was noted, this study could not establish ToM difficulties as a temporal precursor to the development of quasi-autism (Colvert et al., 2008). Taken together, it becomes clear that the experience of severe, global, early deprivation is sufficient to disrupt the neural and cognitive foundations of complex social cognition so that these difficulties persist over time and may play a role in the subsequent development of more pervasive social problems.

Emotion Perception

In light of evidence that post-institutionalized children are at heightened risk for experiencing social difficulties (e.g., Fisher et al., 1997), researchers have also investigated the extent to which early deprivation affects children's ability to understand others' emotional displays. While still living in the institutional setting, children performed significantly worse on an emotion understanding task compared to their community-raised peers (Sloutsky, 1997). A more recent study on preschool-aged children adopted from Eastern European institutions found that they had more difficulty accurately identifying facial expressions of emotion as well as matching emotional displays to an appropriate emotional context. As expected, a longer duration of institutionalization predicted poorer performance on these tasks, but children who had spent more time in their adoptive homes had relatively better performance (Wismer Fries & Pollak, 2004). Subsequent research on a group of older post-institutionalized children found no differences in emotion understanding compared to non-adopted controls (Tarullo et al., 2007), suggesting that the previously noted differences may more accurately represent delays in development of emotion understanding, rather than lasting deficits. The role that the post-adoption environment plays in catch-up in this area is highlighted by findings that suggest more supportive parenting shortly after adoption predicts greater emotion understanding (Garvin, Tarullo, Van Ryzin, & Gunnar, 2012).

In contrast to the findings presented here, longitudinal research by the BEIP suggests that a history of institutional rearing does not impact children's ability to discriminate emotional expression. Despite group differences in the amplitude of ERP components in infancy (Parker, Nelson, & Bucharest Early Intervention Project, 2005), behavioral assessments failed to yield significant differences at baseline, 13–30-month and 42-month follow-ups. However, it should be noted that the stimuli used in these studies consisted of static photos of prototypical peak facial expressions, so it remains to be seen whether a history of early institutional deprivation affects children's ability to interpret mixed or more subtle emotional displays (Jeon, Moulson, Fox, Zeanah, & Nelson, 2010).

Social and Affective Sequelae

It has been suggested that although cognitive functions improve following removal from institutional care, social functions and problems both may be more intransigent and may increase with age. Given the impairments/delays just discussed with regard to executive functions and ToM, the idea that cognitive problems desist while social ones persist is not wholly accurate. It probably reflects an overreliance on IQ as the index of cognitive functioning. Nonetheless, there is evidence that socioemotional problems may increase with age and thus with time in the family, which if true, is the opposite of what one would expect if a supportive family serves to ameliorate the impact of early deprivation. This pattern would suggest the presence of sleeper effects, whereby early deprivation induces impairments in socioemotional abilities that emerge long after birth (Maurer, Mondloch, & Lewis, 2007). Alternatively, early deprivation may limit the child's ability to develop the same ultimate level of expertise that a child who was not deprived early in life is able to achieve. Or finally, delays or impairments in socioemotional abilities may become more debilitating with age as the nature and demands of the peer group become more sophisticated. Regardless of whether any of these patterns hold, it does appear that social and emotional challenges are persistent for some post-institutionalized children and youth.

Attachment

While in the institutional setting many children have no discriminating attachment to any caregiver, a high proportion of organized attachment relationships that are formed in these settings are atypical (see review, Bakermans-Kranenburg et al., 2011). Reactive attachment disorder (RAD) is characterized by emotional withdrawal and a lack of attachment behaviors (i.e., failure to use a caregiver as a source of comfort), whereas indiscriminate use of attachment behaviors with non-caregivers characterizes disinhibited social engagement disorder, which was formerly considered a disinhibited subtype of RAD (American Psychiactric Association, 2013). Both of these disorders are noted in children currently residing in institutions. Although the earliest research on post-institutionalized children's ability to form secure attachment relationships with their adoptive families painted a grim picture, decades of research in this area has provided firm evidence that children with a history of institutional

rearing are able to form attachment relationships with caregivers and that a substantial minority of these relationships are classified as secure. The BEIP study provides the best evidence for the course of RAD subtypes following adoption. Smyke et al. (2012) found that within approximately 1 year of placement, children randomized to high-quality foster care resembled never-institutionalized controls on a measure of signs of inhibited RAD. Children randomized to foster care also displayed fewer signs of disinhibited RAD compared to those who remained in the institution, but they continued to show more signs of the disorder compared to the never-institutionalized group up to 8 years of age. This study also found that children removed from the institution earlier (before 24 months of age) displayed fewer signs of disinhibited RAD at 30 and 54 months of age compared to their later-adopted peers. The data on age at adoption parallels previous findings suggesting that a longer duration of institutionalization predicts lower rates of secure attachment to adoptive caregivers.

Two major issues should be considered when interpreting the evidence on attachment quality among post-institutionalized youth. First, measuring attachment security beyond infancy presents a major challenge. Second, the core feature in disinhibited RAD is a marked lack of wariness and social approach, often referred to as indiscriminate friendliness. These behaviors and diagnoses of the disinhibited form of RAD have been shown to co-occur with behaviors reflecting a secure attachment. Though some would argue that these findings represent a failure to accurately assess children's attachment security, recent revisions to diagnostic criteria reflect a growing consensus that the disinhibited subtype is not an attachment disorder, but rather reflects a disorder of disinhibited social engagement (Zeanah & Gleason, 2010).

Indiscriminate Friendliness or Disinhibited Social Engagement

At its core, indiscriminate friendliness represents a lack of developmentally appropriate social reticence around unfamiliar adults. It also includes behaviors such as frequent attempts to approach and engage strangers, a willingness to go away with strangers, failure to check back with the caregiver in unfamiliar situations, and asking strangers intrusive or personal questions. It is of note that these behaviors are truly neither indiscriminate nor friendly. Post-institutionalized children may show a strong initial approach to strangers compared to typically developing children, but are in fact more likely to approach familiar persons than strangers. Further, these interactions are described as non-reciprocal, impersonal, and superficial (O'Connor, Bredenkamp, & Rutter, 1999). Both parent report and laboratory observation have demonstrated significantly higher frequencies of indiscriminately friendly behaviors among post-institutionalized children compared to those adopted from foster care or raised in birth families (Bruce et al., 2009; Chisholm, Carter, Ames, & Morison, 1995; O'Connor et al., 1999; O'Connor & Rutter, 2000). These behaviors also appear to persist for years following the transition into the adoptive family (Chisholm, 1998), through middle childhood (Smyke et al., 2012) and adolescence (The English and Romanian Adoptees (ERA) Study Team, 2010; Kreppner et al., 2010).

The etiology of these behaviors remains unclear. Indiscriminate friendliness is predicted by duration of institutional care, but may not be a function of global deprivation per se (Bruce et al., 2009; O'Connor & Rutter, 2000). These behavioral patterns may emerge as a function of the persistent disruption of early caregiving relationships, as evidenced by the prevalence of indiscriminate friendliness among children from high-quality institutions with high caregiver turnover (Hodges & Tizard, 1989b). Children in foster care also exhibit these behaviors. Notably, a recent analysis showed that indiscriminate friendliness in foster care children was not predicted by the severity of physical or sexual abuse, but instead by the severity of neglect and the frequency of changes in caregivers in the first few years of life (Pears, Bruce, Fisher, & Kim, 2010). Taken together, these findings do suggest that the

lack of conditions necessary for forming stable attachments also results in indiscriminate behavior, although the two phenomena may not be isomorphic.

Although this analysis suggests that lack of experience with stable attachment figures underlies the behavior, others have argued that it is learned through reinforcement. Specifically, they argue that indiscriminate behavior gets the child social rewards and so becomes part of the child's repertoire (Chisholm, 1998). Others have suggested that indiscriminate friendliness reflects social obtuseness and thus is related to problems in perspective taking and theory of mind discussed earlier (O'Connor et al., 1999).

More consistently, indiscriminate friendliness has been associated with problems of attention and behavior regulation (Bruce et al., 2009; Chisholm, 1998; O'Connor et al., 1999; O'Connor, Marvin, Rutter, Olrick, & Britner, 2003; Roy et al., 2004). Further support for the underlying role of attention problems or more general disinhibition comes from an EEG study demonstrating that the atypical power distribution associated with ADHD symptomatology in institutionalized children also predicts indiscriminate friendliness in children after adoption (Tarullo et al., 2011). These deficits in inhibitory control may mediate the relationship between early caregiving disruptions and indiscriminate friendliness (Pears et al., 2010). Taken together, the evidence to date suggests that indiscriminately friendly behavior reflects changes in neural circuitry underlying regulatory processes that typically develop in the context of stable and supportive early caregiver-child relationships.

Anxiety

In animal models of early maternal deprivation, anxiety is one of the more consistent outcomes. Increased fearfulness and heightened reactivity of the HPA axis are interpreted as evidence that early life stress enhances the risk of anxiety and depression (Sanchez, Ladd, & Plotsky, 2001). Neither the ERA study (Rutter et al., 2001), our earlier work (Gunnar, van Dulmen, & The International Adoption Project Team, 2007), nor the meta-analysis by Juffer and van Ijzendoorn (2005) found evidence for increased anxiety symptoms among post-institutionalized children. However, the reason may be that parental report was used and parents of adopted children both under- and overreport anxiety symptoms. In a recent study, we asked parents and children to report on their anxiety symptoms using the MacArthur Health and Behavioral Questionnaire (Wiik et al., 2011). The children were 8 through 11 years old. Parents of both post-institutionalized children and children adopted from foster care overseas described their children as more anxious than did parents of children born and raised in their birth families. Note that both the ERA study and Gunnar and van Dulmen (2007) used other adopted children as the comparison group, so these data are consistent in evidence that anxiety is not a sequela of early deprivation. However, the children did not agree. The children's data clearly indicated that the children adopted from foster care overseas were no more anxious than non-adopted children, whereas the post-institutionalized children were more anxious and their reported anxiety symptoms increased with duration of institutional care. As discussed below, the children's data are consistent with evidence from imaging studies of increased amygdala volume (Mehta et al., 2009; Tottenham et al., 2010) and amygdala reactivity to threat stimuli (Maheu et al., 2010; Tottenham et al., 2011) among children who are deprived and neglected early in life. Furthermore, as noted earlier, adolescence ushers in a marked rise in anxiety and depressive disorders among early deprived as compared to other adopted children (Kreppner et al., 2010), and thus we may expect that the substrate for anxiety and depression is primed by the impact of their early experiences. A better understanding of the processes through which early experiences heighten risk for anxiety and depression, as well as all of the other behaviors just discussed, will be achieved through improving our understanding of the impact of these experiences on neurodevelopment.

Neurobiological Correlates of Early Deprivation

Studies using a variety of neuroimaging techniques have begun to elucidate the extent to which early deprivation impacts the development of brain structure and function (see review, Nelson, Bos, Gunnar, & Sonuga-Barke, 2011). Over the course of development, neural circuitry involved in processing lower-level information develops earlier, and higher-level processes build on lower-level ones (Fox, Levitt, & Nelson, 2010). By examining neural development in the context of early institutional rearing, researchers can explore issues related to sensitive periods for optimal development as well as long-term plasticity within various systems.

The first indication that early deprivation had an adverse impact on neural development in humans came from measurements of head circumference, which is highly correlated with brain size during infancy. Growth delays in this domain among post-institutionalized children are marked, catch-up following adoption lags far behind gains made in height and weight (Van Ijzendoorn et al., 2007), and measurements of head circumference in Romanian adoptees were found to partially mediate the relationship between the duration of early deprivation and the later presence of deprivation-specific problems (Sonuga-Barke, Schlotz, & Rutter 2010). Recent MRI studies have found that children who experienced early deprivation had significantly smaller head circumference as well as lower total brain, gray matter, and white matter volume (Mehta et al., 2009; Sheridan, Fox, Zeanah, McLaughlin, & Nelson, 2012), suggesting that early deprivation presents a global insult to neural development.

Beyond global impacts, more nuanced effects are also being documented. Chugani et al. (2001) used positron emission tomography (PET) with children who spent more than 1 year in Romanian institutions. Compared to non-adopted children and healthy adults, post-institutionalized children demonstrated deficits in impulsivity and attention and showed significantly decreased metabolism in several brain areas involved in attention and behavior regulation, including the orbitofrontal cortex, infralimbic prefrontal cortex, amygdala, and hippocampus (e.g., Elliott, Dolan, & Frith, 2000; Kerr & Zelazo, 2004).

Cerebellar volume was examined in a recent study of predominantly Russian/Eastern European youth who experienced extremely long durations (in some cases more than 6 years) of institutional care prior to adoption (Bauer et al., 2009). Reduced volume of one lobe (left and right superior-posterior) was noted which was shown to statistically mediate performance on a memory (delayed match to sample) and planning (Stockings of Cambridge) task.

Early deprivation has also been noted to produce lasting changes in amygdala structure and function. As noted earlier, in several studies longer periods of early deprivation have been associated with greater amygdala volumes (Mehta et al., 2009; Tottenham et al., 2010). In animal models, chronic stress has been shown to increase dendritic branching in the amygdala (e.g., Vyas, Pillai, & Chattarji, 2004), which presumably corresponds to heightened sensitivity and reactivity to threat. Functional studies tend to support the heightened reactivity view, as several now demonstrate a greater increase in BOLD signal in response to threat stimuli (Maheu et al., 2010; Tottenham et al., 2011). Furthermore, Tottenham et al. (2011) found that post-institutionalized children showed greater amygdala activation to distractor faces in an emotional Go-No-Go task, indicating that they were less able to suppress responses to irrelevant but emotionally salient stimuli.

One view is that early life stress shifts neural processing towards sensitivity to threat, facilitating the kind of rapid response that may support survival in a hostile environment, but might impair the type of thinking and reflection needed in an information society. Notably, however, although chronic stress has been shown to reduce hippocampal volume and impair declarative memory, studies of post-institutionalized youth have not reported smaller hippocampi (Mehta et al., 2009; Tottenham et al., 2010).

This, however, is consistent with other studies of prepubertal children exposed to neglect and maltreatment early in life (e.g., De Bellis et al., 1999) and is a finding that may change when children are studied following puberty.

In addition to structural and functional imaging, researchers have begun to use diffusion tensor imaging to examine the integrity of white matter tracts. Two studies have reported decreased fractional anisotropy in the uncinate fasciculus, a limbic pathway connecting structures in the medial temporal lobe (e.g., amygdala) to the orbitofrontal cortex (Eluvathingal et al., 2006; Govindan, Behen, Helder, Makki, & Chugani, 2010). However, only one of these studies demonstrated that the degree of white matter disorganization was related to the duration of early deprivation (Govindan et al., 2010). Fractional anisotropy is associated with age-related maturation; decreases in this measure may indicate a lack or loss of myelination. Another study indicated that children exposed to early institutional care have a more diffuse cortical fiber distribution of axons originating in the caudate and terminating in the frontal cortex (Behen et al., 2009). Although evidence remains sparse, these changes in connectivity may be the result of insufficient synaptic pruning or a lack of experience-expected stimulation (Govindan et al., 2010) during the time spent in the institution.

Most important to consider is the potential effect of inefficient or disrupted structural connectivity on the functioning of broad neural networks that underlie complex behaviors. In the domain of social functioning, where multiple brain regions are recruited as part of larger networks to attend to and simultaneously process verbal and nonverbal information, the inability of the network to function appropriately may explain part of the discrepancy between what appears to be normal emotion understanding capabilities in the laboratory (Jeon et al., 2010) and reported social difficulties (Gunnar et al., 2007).

Thus far, all of the structural and functional imaging studies of post-institutionalized children and youth have been cross-sectional. They thus highlight the differences noted between children exposed to deprivation early in life and those exposed to less or no deprivation. They do not allow examination of changes in brain structure and function when children are removed from institutional deprivation and placed in families. The glass, thus, seems half empty when in fact it is very likely that much recovery and rebound occurs.

The closest we can get to demonstration of rebound and resilience in neural measures are in data provided by the BEIP study. As noted earlier, the BEIP group reported that children in institutional care showed a pattern of EEG activity that suggested delayed neural maturation. Specifically, over the first few years of life, the power or activity in resting brain wave activity shifts from slower waves (e.g., theta) to faster oscillations (e.g., alpha, beta, and gamma). Compared to children reared in their families, during the infancy and toddler periods, children living in institutions were delayed in the maturation of EEG patterns and showed more relative power in the lower-frequency theta band and less in the higher-frequency alpha band (for a review, see Vanderwert, Marshall, Nelson, Zeanah, & Fox, 2010). However, once some of the children were placed in foster care homes run by the BEIP group, things began to change. At 42 months, children placed before 2 years of age exhibited more of the expected ratio of alpha to theta power, although those placed later did not (see Vanderwert et al., 2010). Similar findings were reported at 8 years of age (Vanderwert et al., 2010). Specifically, EEG data from children who entered foster care before age two were comparable to that obtained from children who had never been institutionalized. Meanwhile, power in the alpha band of children who entered foster care after their second birthday was comparable to that of children in the "care as usual" comparison group, some of whom were still living in institutions.

Most recently, researchers in the BEIP group employed structural MRI when the children were approximately 9 years of age. Children who experienced institutional care (regardless of intervention status) had smaller total cortical gray matter compared to controls. Although this domain does not seem to show recovery at this age, researchers did see effects of intervention on total cortical white matter volume. Children in the care as usual group had significantly smaller white matter volumes compared to never-institutionalized children. Children randomized to the foster care intervention had larger white matter volumes than the care as usual group, but did not significantly differ from the other two groups. Of greatest interest, the researchers found that white matter volume not only significantly predicted alpha power but significantly *mediated* the relationship between institutional experience and alpha power (Sheridan et al., 2012). These findings are relevant to our understanding of the role of early deprivation and early intervention in the development of psychopathology because, as noted earlier, EEG power-mediated effects of early deprivation on ADHD in the BEIP study (McLaughlin et al., 2010), and in work in our lab, are also associated with indiscriminately friendly behavior (Tarullo et al., 2011). Thus, at least two of what Rutter and colleagues termed "deprivation-specific problems" may reflect processes related to reduced/delayed myelination, which may in turn be amenable to some degree of recovery with supportive care. However, consistent with the behavioral data, these EEG data indicate that duration of exposure and time of removal from deprivation are critical variables in predicting neural recovery. In addition, age at assessment may also be important, a possibility that becomes more obvious as we turn to the next section on adolescence and puberty.

Adolescence: Period of Risk and Opportunity

Adolescence is a period of both risk and opportunity. Although this is true for all young people, it may be especially true for those who begin their lives under conditions of deprivation and neglect. The challenge of adolescence has long been noted to be greater for adopted children than those raised in their biological families, presumably because of the additional issues adoption creates for identity formation (Nickman et al., 2005). However, there also may be critical opportunities in this period.

Specifically, increased neural plasticity as a function of pubertal changes may facilitate recalibration of neural systems adapted initially to deprived conditions and this recalibration may enhance or reduce risk for psychopathology depending on what the young person experiences during adolescence (Romeo, 2010).

There is now significant evidence that puberty is associated with an increase in activity of the hypothalamic-pituitary-adrenocortical (HPA) axis, which is believed to increase risk for depression in youth who are at genetic and/or experiential risk (e.g., Gunnar, Wewerka, Frenn, Long, & Griggs, 2009). Early life stress has significant impacts on the developing stress system (Tarullo & Gunnar, 2006). Nonetheless, there is emerging evidence that with puberty the HPA axis of children who were deprived early in life may normalize to that of non-stressed children if their pubertal conditions are benign. This was demonstrated in a study of 12- and 13-year-old children who ranged widely in pubertal status (Quevedo, Johnson, Loman, LaFavor, & Gunnar, 2012). The study examined the cortisol awakening response (CAR), a measure of HPA axis activity that tends to be blunted under conditions of chronic stress. A blunted pattern was observed for youth who had been adopted from institutions early in life and were early in pubertal development, but among those at more advanced stages of pubertal development, the CAR was similar to that seen among low-risk youth born and raised in their biological families. Although longitudinal work is needed, it appeared that the CAR normalized with puberty. Notably, this was a psychiatrically healthy sample of post-institutionalized youth who were doing well at home and in school. The pubertal stress recalibration hypothesis would predict that with puberty stress and threat systems recalibrate in light of current threat and stress. Thus, for youth with early adverse histories and significant current life stressors, recalibration may heighten reactivity of stress and threat systems further, increasing risk of psychopathology.

Indeed, as noted earlier, there is evidence that adolescence is associated with clinical depression and conduct problems emerging in post-institutionalized youth who did not show these problems earlier in development (Sonuga-Barke, Schlotz, & Kreppner, 2010). Other researchers have also noted that adolescence and young adulthood are periods of heightened psychopathology for youth who experienced prolonged periods of early life adversity (Tieman, van der Ende, & Verhulst, 2005). Consistent with the stress recalibration hypothesis, Rutter and colleagues have argued that in the ERA study the adolescent increase in depression and conduct problems was primarily observed among the youth who earlier had exhibited one or more deprivation-specific problems (i.e., ADHD, quasi-autism, disinhibited attachment, or severe cognitive delay; Sonuga-Barke, Schlotz, & Kreppner 2010). These would be the youth who should struggle the most with the complexity of the adolescent years as their deprivation-induced issues would be expected to complicate peer relations and academic success. Peer rejections and academic struggles, in turn, should create significant psychosocial stress as the context for recalibration of threat and stress systems. However, as yet there is no evidence that stress is the mediator of the adolescent rise in either depression or conduct issues. It is equally possible that other developmental cascades may explain why adolescence is a particularly problematic time for many, but not all, youth who begin their lives under conditions of deprivation and neglect. What is needed are studies examining alternative biologically plausible pathways from childhood into adolescence to understand the role of puberty and the psychosocial challenges of adolescence in fostering both greater risk and opportunities for youth with adverse histories.

Summary and Conclusions

A straightforward story of recovery from early life adversity would tell us that the effects of early deprivation ameliorate over time with adoption into a supportive and well-resourced environment. However, years of research have demonstrated that the story is not so simple: Although many children who have been exposed to early deprivation do not suffer any long-term negative consequences, others continue to experience a host of cognitive, emotional, and physical health difficulties that place them at increased risk for developing psychopathology across the lifespan. Alterations in early neural development, which may reflect delays or deficits, underlie behavioral issues (e.g., problems of inattention; McLaughlin et al., 2010) and potentially affect the degree to which children perceive their environments as adverse and threatening (e.g., Tottenham et al., 2011). As these children develop across childhood, they are expected to meet higher expectations for academic success—and tend to fall behind their non-adopted peers (Beckett et al., 2010)—in addition to negotiating increasingly complex social environments, which require more sophisticated theory of mind and emotion understanding skills. Individuals with early difficulties in these domains and/or who are more likely to perceive their social environment as threatening may experience greater stress as a result of a reduced ability to meet the demands of their developmental level. Further, as mentioned earlier in the chapter, girls who experience early puberty in the context of deficits in social cognition and peer difficulties may be at particular risk for the development of internalizing and externalizing disorders during the transition to adolescence. As the ERA study reported, adolescents who display deprivation-induced deficits in childhood are more likely to develop psychopathology in adolescence (Kreppner et al., 2010). In line with the pubertal recalibration hypothesis, early deficits (or failure to completely catch up) in the cognitive or socioemotional domains or failure to create a secure attachment with a primary caregiver may create an environment that does not allow stress systems to fully recalibrate to adolescents' resource-rich environments. A better understanding of the neurobiological impact of early deprivation, as well as the mechanisms by which early adversity affects developing competencies, will allow researchers to better identify factors that predict or facilitate rebound, so that potential interventions can be more effectively tailored. Although the number of children being adopted from institutions into the USA and other industrialized countries has fallen sharply since the beginning of the economic recession, the number of children who experience severe deprivation and neglect has not declined. Thus, continuing to increase our understanding of how early deprivation and neglect impacts the developing child is still a critical imperative.

References

American Psychiactric Association. (2000). *Diagnostic and statistical manual of mental disorders (text rev)* (4th ed.). Washington, DC: Author.

Bakermans-Kranenburg, M. J., Steele, H., Zeanah, C. H., Muhamedrahimov, R. J., Vorria, P., Dobrova-Krol, N. A., et al. (2011). Attachment and emotional development in institutional care: Characteristics and catch-up. In R. B. McCall, M. H. van IJzendoorn, F. Juffer, C. J. Groark, and V. K. Groza (Eds.), Children without permanent parents: Research, practice, and policy. *Monographs of the Society for Research in Child Development, 76*(4), 62–91.

Barry, R. J., Clarke, A. R., & Johnstone, S. J. (2003). A review of electrophysiology in attention-deficit/hyperactivity disorder: I. Qualitative and quantitative electroencephalography. *Clinical Neurophysiology, 114*, 171–183.

Bauer, P. M., Hanson, J. L., Pierson, R. K., Davidson, R. J., & Pollak, S. D. (2009). Cerebellar volume and cognitive functioning in children who experienced early deprivation. *Biological Psychiatry, 66*(12), 1100–1106.

Beckett, C., Castle, J., Rutter, M., & Sonuga-Barke, E. J. (2010). VI. Institutional deprivation, specific cognitive functions, and scholastic achievement: English and Romanian Adoptee (ERA) study findings. *Monographs of the Society for Research in Child Development, 75*(1), 125–142.

Behen, M. E., Muzik, O., Saporta, A. S. D., Wilson, B. J., Pai, D., Hua, J., et al. (2009). Abnormal fronto-striatal connectivity in children with histories of early deprivation: A diffusion tensor imaging study. *Brain Imaging and Behavior, 3*(3), 292–297.

Bos, K. J., Fox, N., Zeanah, C. H., & Nelson, C. A. (2009). Effects of early psychosocial deprivation on the development of memory and executive function. *Frontiers in Behavioral Neuroscience, 3*, 16.

Bowlby, J. (1969). *Attachment and loss: Volume 1. Attachment.* New York, NY: Basic Books.

Bruce, J., Tarullo, A. R., & Gunnar, M. R. (2009). Disinhibited social behavior among internationally adopted children. *Development and Psychopathology, 21*(1), 157–171.

Chisholm, K., Carter, M. C., Ames, E. W., & Morison, S. J. (1995). Attachment security and indiscriminately friendly behavior in children adopted from Romanian orphanages. *Development and Psychopathology, 7,* 283–294.

Chisholm, K. (1998). A three year follow-up of attachment and indiscriminate friendliness in children adopted from Romanian orphanages. *Child Development, 69,* 1092–1106.

Chugani, H. T., Behen, M. E., Muzik, O., Juhasz, C., Nagy, F., & Chugani, D. C. (2001). Local brain functional activity following early deprivation: A study of postinstitutionalized Romanian orphans. *NeuroImage, 14*(6), 1290–1301.

Colvert, E., Rutter, M., Kreppner, J., Beckett, C., Castle, J., Groothues, C., et al. (2008). Do theory of mind and executive function deficits underlie the adverse outcomes associated with profound early deprivation? Findings from the English and Romanian adoptees study. *Journal of Abnormal Child Psychology, 36*(7), 1057–1068.

De Bellis, M., Keshavan, M. S., Clark, D. B., Casey, B. J., Giedd, J. N., Boring, A. M., et al. (1999). Developmental traumatology. Part II: Brain development. *Biological Psychiatry, 45,* 1271–1284.

Drury, S. S., Theall, K., Gleason, M. M., Smyke, A. T., DeVivo, I., Wong, J. Y., et al. (2011). Telomere length and early severe social deprivation: Linking early adversity and cellular aging. *Molecular Psychiatry, 17,* 719–727.

Elliott, R., Dolan, R. J., & Frith, C. D. (2000). Dissociable functions in the medial and lateral orbitofrontal cortex: Evidence from human neuroimaging studies. *Cerebral Cortex, 10*(3), 308–317.

Eluvathingal, T. J., Chugani, H. T., Behen, M. E., Juhasz, C., Muzik, O., Maqbool, M., et al. (2006). Abnormal brain connectivity in children after early severe socioemotional deprivation: A diffusion tensor imaging study. *Pediatrics, 117*(6), 2093–2100.

Faturi, C. B., Tiba, P. A., Kawakami, S. E., Catallani, B., Kerstens, M., & Sucheki, D. (2010). Disruptions of the mother-infant relationship and stress-related behaviours: Altered corticosterone secretion does not explain everything. *Neuroscience and Biobehaval Reviews, 34,* 821–834.

Fisher, L., Ames, E. W., Chisholm, K., & Savoie, L. (1997). Problems reported by parents of Romanian orphans adopted to British Columbia. *International Journal of Behavioral Development, 20*(1), 67–82.

Fox, S. E., Levitt, P., & Nelson, C. A. (2010). How the timing and quality of early experiences influence the development of brain architecture. *Child Development, 81*(1), 28–40.

Garvin, M. C., Tarullo, A. R., Van Ryzin, M., & Gunnar, M. R. (2012). Postadoption parenting and socioemotional development in postinstitutionalized children. *Development and Psychopathology, 24*(1), 35–48.

Govindan, R. M., Behen, M. E., Helder, E., Makki, M. I., & Chugani, H. T. (2010). Altered water diffusivity in cortical association tracts in children with early deprivation identified with tract-based spatial statistics (TBSS). *Cerebral Cortex, 20*(3), 561–569.

Graber, J. A., Nichols, T. R., & Brooks-Gunn, J. (2010). Putting pubertal timing in developmental context: Implications for prevention. *Developmental Psychobiology, 52,* 254–262.

Gunnar, M. R., van Dulmen, M. H., & The International Adoption Project Team. (2007). Behavior problems in post-institutionalized internationally-adopted children. *Development & Psychopathology, 19,* 129–148.

Gunnar, M. R., Wewerka, S., Frenn, K., Long, J. D., & Griggs, C. (2009). Developmental changes in HPA activity over the transition to adolescence: Normative changes and associations with puberty. *Development & Psychopathology, 21,* 69–85.

Hodges, J., & Tizard, B. (1989a). IQ and behavioural adjustment of ex-institutional adolescents. *Journal of Child Psychology and Psychiatry, and Allied Disciplines, 30,* 53–75.

Hodges, J., & Tizard, B. (1989b). Social and family relationships of ex-institutional adolescents. *Journal of Child Psychology and Psychiatry, and Allied Disciplines, 30,* 77–97.

Jeon, H., Moulson, M. C., Fox, N., Zeanah, C., & Nelson, C. A. (2010). The effects of early institutionalization on the discrimination of facial expressions of emotion in young children. *Infancy, 15*(2), 209–221.

Johnson, D. E. (2001). Medical and developmental sequelae of early childhood institutionalization in Romania. In C. A. Nelson (Ed.), *The Minnesota symposia on child psychology* (Effects of early adversity on neurobehavioral development, Vol. 31, pp. 113–162). Mahwah, NJ: Erlbaum.

Johnson, A. E., Bruce, J., Tarullo, A. R., & Gunnar, M. R. (2011). Growth delay as an index of allostatic load in young children: Predictions to disinhibited social approach and diurnal cortisol activity. *Development and Psychopathology, 23*(3), 859–871.

Johnson, D. E., & Gunnar, M. R. (2011). Growth failure in institutionalized children. *Monographs of the Society for Research in Child Development, 76*(4), 92–126.

Johnson, D. E., Guthrie, D., Smyke, A. T., Koga, S. F., Fox, N. A., Zeanah, C. H., et al. (2010). Growth and associations between auxology, caregiving environment, and cognition in socially deprived Romanian children randomized to foster vs ongoing institutional care. *Archives of Pediatrics & Adolescent Medicine, 164*(6), 507–516.

Juffer, F., & van Ijzendoorn, M. H. (2005). Behavior problems and mental health referrals of international adoptees: A meta-analysis. *JAMA, 293*(20), 2501–2515.

Kerr, A., & Zelazo, P. D. (2004). Development of "hot" executive function: The children's gambling task. *Brain and Cognition, 55,* 148–157.

Kreppner, J., Kumsta, R., Rutter, M., Beckett, C., Castle, J., Stevens, S., et al. (2010). IV. Developmental course of deprivation-specific psychological patterns: Early manifestations, persistence to age 15, and clinical features. *Monographs of the Society for Research in Child Development, 75*(1), 79–101.

Kreppner, J. M., O'Connor, T. G., Rutter, M., & The English Romanian Adoptees Study. (2001). Can inattention/overactivity be an institutional deprivation syndrome? *Journal of Abnormal Child Psychology, 29*(6), 513–528.

Loman, M. M., Wiik, K. L., Frenn, K. A., Pollak, S. D., & Gunnar, M. R. (2009). Postinstitutionalized children's development: Growth, cognitive, and language outcomes. *Journal of Developmental and Behavioral Pediatrics, 30*(5), 426–434.

Maheu, F. S., Dozier, M., Guyer, A. E., Mandell, D., Peloso, E., Poeth, K., et al. (2010). A preliminary study of medial temporal lobe function in youths with a history of caregiver deprivation and emotional neglect. *Cognition, Affect, and Behavioral Neuroscience, 19*, 34–49.

Maurer, D., Mondloch, C. J., & Lewis, T. L. (2007). Sleeper effects. *Developmental Science, 10*, 40–47.

McClelland, S., Korosi, A., Cope, J., Ivy, A., & Baram, T. Z. (2011). Emerging roles of epigenetic mechanisms in the enduring effects of early-life stress and experience on learning and memory. *Neurobiology of Learning and Memory, 96*, 79–88.

McEwen, B. (2000). Allostasis and allostatic load: Implications for neuropsychopharmacology. *Neuropsychopharmacology, 22*, 108–124.

McLaughlin, K. A., Fox, N. A., Zeanah, C. H., Sheridan, M. A., Marshall, P., & Nelson, C. A. (2010). Delayed maturation in brain electrical activity partially explains the association between early environmental deprivation and symptoms of attention-deficit/hyperactivity disorder. *Biological Psychiatry, 68*(4), 329–336.

Meaney, M. J., & Szyf, M. (2005). Environmental programming of stress responses through DNA methylation: Life at the interface between a dynamic environment and a fixed genome. *Dialogues in Clinical Neuroscience, 7*, 103–123.

Mehta, M. A., Golembo, N. I., Nosarti, C., Colvert, E., Mota, A., Williams, S. C. R., et al. (2009). Amygdala, hippocampal and corpus callosum size following severe early institutional deprivation: The English and Romanian Adoptees Study Pilot. *Journal of Child Psychology and Psychiatry, 50*(8), 943–951.

Miller, L. C., Chan, W., Tirella, L., & Perrin, E. (2009). Outcomes of children adopted from Eastern Europe. *International Journal of Behavioral Development, 33*(4), 289–298.

Miller, G. E., Chen, E., & Parker, K. J. (2011). Psychological stress in childhood and susceptibility to the chronic diseases of aging: Moving towards a model of behavioral and biological mechanisms. *Psychological Bulletin, 137*, 959–997.

Miller, L. C., & Hendrie, N. W. (2000). Health of children adopted from China. *Pediatrics, 105*(6), E76.

Nelson, C. A., Bos, K., Gunnar, M. R., & Sonuga-Barke, E. J. S. (2011). The neurobiological toll of early human deprivation. *Monographs of the Society for Research in Child Development, 76*(4), 127–146.

Nelson, C. A., Zeanah, C. H., Fox, N. A., Marshall, P. J., Smyke, A. T., & Guthrie, D. (2007). Cognitive recovery in socially deprived young children: The Bucharest Early Intervention Project. *Science, 318*(5858), 1937–1940.

Nickman, S. L., Rosenfeld, A. A., Fine, P., Macintyre, J. C., Pilowsky, D. J., Howe, R. A., et al. (2005). Children in adoptive families: Overview and update. *Journal of the American Academy of Child and Adolescent Psychiatry, 44*(10), 987–995.

O'Connor, T. G., Bredenkamp, D., & Rutter, M. (1999). Attachment disturbances and disorders in children exposed to early severe deprivation. *Infant Mental Health Journal, 20*(1), 10–29.

O'Connor, T. G., Marvin, R. S., Rutter, M., Olrick, J. T., & Britner, P. A. (2003). Child–parent attachment following early institutional deprivation. *Development and Psychopathology, 15*(1), 19–38.

O'Connor, T. G., & Rutter, M. (2000). Attachment disorder behavior following early severe deprivation: Extension and longitudinal follow-up. English and Romanian Adoptees Study Team. *Journal of the American Academy of Child and Adolescent Psychiatry, 39*(6), 703–712.

Parker, S. W., Nelson, C. A., & Bucharest Early Intervention Project. (2005). The impact of early institutional rearing on the ability to discriminate facial expressions of emotion: An event-related potential study. *Child Development, 76*(1), 54–72.

Pears, K. C., Bruce, J., Fisher, P. A., & Kim, H. K. (2010). Indiscriminate friendliness in maltreated foster children. *Child Maltreatment, 15*, 64–75.

Pollak, S. D., Nelson, C. A., Schlaak, M. F., Roeber, B. J., Wewerka, S. S., Wiik, K. L., et al. (2010). Neurodevelopmental effects of early deprivation in postinstitutionalized children. *Child Development, 81*(1), 224–236.

Quevedo, K., Johnson, A. E., Loman, M. L., LaFavor, T. L., & Gunnar, M. (2012). The confluence of adverse early experience and puberty on the cortisol awakening response. *International Journal of Behavioral Development, 36*(1), 19–28.

Rogosch, F. A., Cicchetti, D., Shields, A., & Toth, S. L. (1995). Parenting dysfunction in child maltreatment. In M. Bornstein (Ed.), *Handbook of parenting* (Vol. 4, pp. 127–159). Hillsdale, NJ: Erlbaum.

Romeo, R. D. (2010). Pubertal maturation and programming of hypothalamic-pituitary-adrenal reactivity. *Frontiers of Neuroendocrinology, 31*, 232–240.

Roy, P., Rutter, M., & Pickles, A. (2004). Institutional care: Associations between overactivity and lack of selectivity in social relationships. *Journal of Psychology and Psychiatry, 45*(4), 866–873.

Rutter, M. (1981). *Maternal deprivation reassessed*. New York: Penguin.

Rutter, M., Kreppner, J., & O'Connor, T. G. (2001). Specificity and heterogeneity in children's responses to profound institutional privation. *British Journal of Psychiatry, 179*, 97–103.

Sanchez, M. M., Ladd, C. O., & Plotsky, P. (2001). Early adverse experience as a developmental risk factor for later psychopathology: Evidence from rodent and primate models. *Development & Psychopathology, 13*, 419–450.

Sheridan, M. A., Fox, N. A., Zeanah, C. H., McLaughlin, K. A., & Nelson, C. A. (2012). Variation in neural development as a result of exposure to institutionalization early in childhood. *Proceedings of the National Academy of Sciences, 109*, 12927–12932.

Sloutsky, V. M. (1997). Institutional care and developmental outcomes of 6- and 7-year-old children: A contextual perspective. *International Journal of Behavioral Development, 20*, 131–151.

Smyke, A. T., Zeanah, C. H., Gleason, M. M., Drury, S. S., Fox, N. A., Nelson, C. A., et al. (2012). A randomized controlled trial comparing foster care and institutional care for children with signs of reactive attachment disorder. *American Journal of Psychiatry, 169*, 508–514.

Sonuga-Barke, E. J., & Fairchild, G. (2012). Neuroeconomics of attention-deficit/hyperactivity disorder: Differential influences of medial, dorsal, and ventral prefrontal brain networks on suboptimal decision making? *Biological Psychiatry, 72*, 126–133.

Sonuga-Barke, E. J. S., & Rubia, K. (2008). Inattentive/overactive children with histories of profound institutional deprivation compared with standard ADHD cases: A brief report. *Child: Care, Health and Development, 34*(5), 596–602.

Sonuga-Barke, E. J., Schlotz, W., & Kreppner, J. (2010). V. Differentiating developmental trajectories for conduct, emotion, and peer problems following early deprivation. *Monographs of the Society for Research in Child Development, 75*(1), 102–124.

Sonuga-Barke, E. J., Schlotz, W., & Rutter, M. (2010). VII. Physical growth and maturation following early severe institutional deprivation: Do they mediate specific psychopathological effects? *Monographs of the Society for Research in Child Development, 75*(1), 143–166.

Stevens, S. E., Sonuga-Barke, E. J. S., Kreppner, J. M., Beckett, C., Castle, J., Colvert, E., et al. (2008). Inattention/overactivity following early severe institutional deprivation: Presentation and associations in early adolescence. *Journal of Abnormal Child Psychology, 36*(3), 385–398.

Tarullo, A. R., Bruce, J., & Gunnar, M. R. (2007). False belief and emotion understanding in post-institutionalized children. *Social Development, 16*(1), 57–78.

Tarullo, A. R., Garvin, M. C., & Gunnar, M. R. (2011). Atypical EEG power correlates with indiscriminately friendly behavior in internationally adopted children. *Developmental Psychology, 47*(2), 417–431.

Tarullo, A. R., & Gunnar, M. R. (2006). Child maltreatment and the developing HPA axis. *Hormones and Behavior, 50*, 632–639.

The English and Romanian Adoptees (ERA) Study Team. (2010). II. Methods and measures used for follow-up at 15 years of the English and Romanian Adoptee (ERA) study. *Monographs of the Society for Research in Child Development, 75*(1), 21–47.

Tieman, W., van der Ende, J., & Verhulst, F. C. (2005). Psychiatric disorders in young adult intercountry adoptees: An epidemiological study. *American Journal of Psychiatry, 162*, 592–598.

Tizard, B., & Hodges, J. (1978). The effect of early institutional rearing on the development of eight-year-old children. *Journal of Child Psychology and Psychiatry and Allied Disciplines, 19*, 99–118.

Tottenham, N., Hare, T. A., Millner, A., Gilhooly, T., Zevin, J. D., & Casey, B. J. (2011). Elevated amygdala response to faces following early deprivation. *Developmental Science, 14*(2), 190–204.

Tottenham, N., Hare, T. A., Quinn, B. T., McCarry, T. W., Nurse, M., Gilhooly, T., et al. (2010). Prolonged institutional rearing is associated with atypically large amygdala volume and difficulties in emotion regulation. *Developmental Science, 13*(1), 46–61.

Van Ijzendoorn, M. H., Bakermans-Kranenburg, M. J., & Juffer, F. (2007). Plasticity of growth in height, weight, and head circumference: Meta-analytic evidence of massive catch-up after international adoption. *Journal of Developmental and Behavioral Pediatrics, 28*(4), 334–343.

Vanderwert, R. E., Marshall, P. J., Nelson, C. A., Zeanah, C. H., & Fox, N. A. (2010). Timing of intervention affects brain electrical activity in children exposed to severe psychosocial neglect. *PLoS ONE, 5*, e11415.

Vyas, A., Pillai, A. G., & Chattarji, S. (2004). Recovery after chronic stress fails to reverse amygdaloid neuronal hypertrophy and enhanced anxiety-like behavior. *Neuroscience, 128*(4), 667–673.

Wiik, K. L., Loman, M. M., Van Ryzin, M. J., Armstrong, J. M., Essex, M. J., Pollak, S. D., et al. (2011). Behavioral and emotional symptoms of post-institutionalized children in middle childhood. *Journal of Child Psychology & Psychiatry, 52*(1), 56–63.

Windsor, J., Moraru, A., Nelson, C. A., Fox, N. A., & Zeanah, C. H. (2012). Effect of foster care on language learning at eight years: Findings from the Bucharest Early Intervention Project. *Journal of Child Language, 14*, 1–23.

Wismer Fries, A. B., & Pollak, S. D. (2004). Emotion understanding in postinstitutionalized Eastern European children. *Development and Psychopathology, 16*(2), 355–369.

Yagmurlu, B., Berument, S. K., & Celimli, S. (2005). The role of institution and home contexts in theory of mind development. *Journal of Applied Developmental Psychology, 26*(5), 521–537.

Zeanah, C. H., & Gleason, M. M. (2010). Reactive attachment disorder: A review for DSM-V. Retrieved from http://www.dsm5.org/ProposedRevisions/Pages/proposedrevision.

Zeanah, C. H., Nelson, C. A., Fox, N. A., Smyke, A. T., Marshall, P., Parker, S. W., et al. (2003). Designing research to study the effects of institutionalization on brain and behavioral development: The Bucharest Early Intervention Project. *Development and Psychopathology, 15*, 885–907.

Prematurity and Failure to Thrive: The Interplay of Medical Conditions and Development

Stephanie Blenner, L. Kari Hironaka,
Douglas L. Vanderbilt, and Deborah A. Frank

Introduction

Prematurity and failure to thrive are two classic biopsychosocial conditions which present short- and long-term challenges to families and to the physical health and neuropsychological and socio-emotional development of children. Prematurity is a common perinatal condition, while failure to thrive typically affects children in infancy and early childhood. Each occurs disproportionately but not exclusively in the context of poverty with associated stressors. Both conditions have the potential to profoundly impact the developing brain at vulnerable periods during neurogenesis. Fortunately, adverse consequences from both may be mitigated to varying degrees by appropriate interventions with child and family. Understanding the pathophysiology and need for multidisciplinary intervention is predicated on appreciating the developmental underpinnings of each condition. Effective treatment requires collaboration between clinicians skilled in medical differential diagnosis and treatment, developmental specialists, nutritionists, social workers, and mental health professionals.

S. Blenner, M.D. (✉) • L.K. Hironaka, M.D., M.P.H.
D.A. Frank, M.D.
Boston University School of Medicine,
Boston, MA 02118, USA
e-mail: Stephanie.Blenner@bmc.org

D.L. Vanderbilt, M.D.
Keck School of Medicine, University of Southern
California, Los Angeles, CA 90089, USA

Prematurity

Epidemiology

Prematurity, being born at less than 37 weeks gestation, impacts a child's subsequent developmental trajectory, as well as their neuropsychologic and mental health outcomes. While rates of prematurity are highest in developing countries, rate of preterm births in the USA remains at 12 % and increased annually in the USA prior to stabilizing in 2007 (Martin, Osterman, & Sutton, 2010). Improvements in medical and technological support have resulted in improved survival rates for preterm infants over the past 3 decades; however, there continues to be significant morbidity associated with prematurity, particularly among those born at earlier gestation (Stoll et al., 2010). Sequelae include increased rates of physical, cognitive, developmental, learning, and social-emotional difficulties. Some of these challenges are a direct result of an infant's early birth and associated medical and sensorineural complications. Many also reflect the co-occurring impact of known individual, family, and community factors that are associated a priori with higher risk of a child being born prematurely.

Premature birth occurs for a range of reasons, both maternal and fetal. The decision to deliver an infant prior to term can be made when severe medical complications, like placental abruption, eclampsia, infection, or fetal conditions requiring delivery, threaten the survival of the mother or infant. The majority of early births, though, occur spontaneously. Understanding of the reasons and mechanism why early delivery occurs is evolving (Behrman & Butler, 2007). There may be physical factors, such as cervical incompetence or multiple gestation, that result in a mother delivering before term. Inadequate maternal nutrition, poor prenatal care, substance exposure, demographic factors like age and race ethnicity, and psychosocial stressors are associated with and may be etiologic contributors to premature birth. The role of prenatal stress, inflammation, and the hormonal and cytokine milieu is increasingly recognized as potential pathophysiologic mediators of early delivery (Coussons-Read et al., 2012).

Classification of Prematurity

As understanding and research around prematurity has increased, the classification system used to define the degree of prematurity has evolved. Until relatively recently, prematurity was often classified in the literature based on birth weight using the designations of low birth weight (LBW, <2,500 g), very low birth weight (VLBW, <1,500 g), and extremely low birth weight (ELBW, <1,000 g). Despite having been commonly used, this classification system is not ideal, particularly in outcomes research, because infants who are "small for gestational age" or SGA are included in a low birth weight sample together with premature infants. Small for gestational age infants have birth weights lower than the 10th percentile for their gestational age but have had a longer gestation than the premature infants whose birth weights fall within the same range and are appropriate for gestational age (AGA). SGA infants experience developmental trajectories and unique risk that differ from those of similar weight preterm infants (Garite, Clark, & Thorp, 2004).

Instead of relying on birth weight, the current classification system uses the weeks of gestation to divide premature infants into risk groups. Preterm infants are born at less than 37 weeks gestation, very preterm infants are born less than 32 weeks gestation, and extremely preterm infants are born less than 28 weeks gestation. "Late preterm" refers to infants born between 34 and 36 weeks gestation, who are increasingly recognized as being at greater risk for poorer health and neurodevelopment compared to infants born at term (Quigley, et al. 2012).

Medical Complications That May Impact Development

While the degree of prematurity is an important predictor of neurodevelopmental and psychological functioning, medical complications occurring during preterm birth and perinatally influence a child's ultimate outcome. Many of the complications that affect premature infants reflect the immaturity of key body systems like the lungs, gastrointestinal tract, immune system, and brain. Respiratory distress syndrome, infection, feeding and nutritional issues, patent ductus arteriosus, and conditions like necrotizing enterocolitis can decrease odds of survival and increase risk of adverse sequelae in survivors.

One common neurologic complication of prematurity, intraventricular hemorrhage involves the germinal matrix, a highly vascular periventricular area unique to the preterm brain and vulnerable to bleeding in the period immediately after birth. Bleeding occurs due to a combination of fragility of the germinal matrix structure, perturbations in cerebral blood flow accompanying birth and medical procedures, and coagulation abnormalities (Ballabh, 2010). IVH is diagnosed by cranial ultrasound and graded using a severity scale of 1 through 4. Infants who experience IVH associated with white matter or parenchymal damage have increased risk of adverse developmental outcomes including cerebral palsy (O'Shea et al., 2012).

Neonatal Intensive Care

To address the preterm infant's immaturity following interruption of normal intrauterine development, the neonatal field has evolved increasingly specialized approaches to care over the past 50 years (Aylward, 2005). Medical intervention in a tertiary level neonatal intensive care unit (NICU), while technical, involves increasing integration of developmental care and family support. After discharge from the NICU, neonatal follow-up programs track the development of former preterm infants as part of most pediatric hospital programs.

There have been many challenges in meeting the developmental and social-emotional needs of preterm infants and their families. This partly reflects the early history of the field which focused on technological intervention. The emergence of the initial components of specialized care for preterm infants dates to the turn of the twentieth century with development of the incubator in France in the late 1800s (Weil & Tang, 2011). This technology was then introduced in the USA through "incubator baby shows," exhibits featuring preterm infants at expos and fairs around the country (Baker, 1996). Subsequently, care transitioned to hospital-based nurseries and, in the 1960s, neonatal intensive care units began to be established in major hospitals. Despite many technological advances after the advent of NICUs, including adaptation of the ventilator for infants and ability to deliver intravenous nutrition, there was little recognition for the developmental or social-emotional needs of these infants. Through the mid-1970s, due to concerns about maintaining sterile conditions, parents were often excluded from the NICU and had highly limited, if any, contact with their newborns during the weeks or months of hospitalization (Davis, Mohay, & Edwards, 2003).

Subsequent to this period, studies showed no increase in infant infection rates with parental contact. Additional studies demonstrated the transactional nature of infant development and importance of early attachment and the parent–child relationship justifying increased parental involvement in neonatal care from birth when medically possible. As a greater number of younger gestational age infants are surviving and being cared for in the NICU, there has been an increasing shift from considering not just technologic intervention and survival but also how to provide developmentally supportive care to minimize long-term neurodevelopmental and social-emotional morbidity.

There are now a range of interventions that have been implemented in modern NICUs to optimize a child's development. Currently, breastfeeding when possible is recognized to confer not only medical benefits but also neurodevelopmental advantage for preterm infants (Quigley, Hockley, Carson, et al., 2012; Vohr et al., 2006). Breast milk provides immunologic factors and contains essential long-chain polyunsaturated fatty acids which are important in early brain development. Use of expressed or banked breast milk for feeding when breastfeeding is not possible has been advocated for these reasons, though one recent study found lower than optimal DHA levels in pooled donor banked milk than in expressed maternal breast milk (Baack, Norris, Yao, & Colaizy, 2012). Breastfeeding also provides additional close contact and social stimulation for the infant.

Kangaroo mother care (KMC) is an approach to preterm care that originated in Colombia but used around the world. The primary component of kangaroo care, along with breastfeeding and close monitoring, is direct skin-to-skin contact between infant and the mother but also with the father and other family members. In a Cochrane analysis, this has been associated with improved medical outcomes including decreased morbidity and shorter hospital stay (Conde-Agudelo, Belizán, & Diaz-Rossello, 2011). The impact on development has been less clear and limited by few studies and short follow-up periods. Griffith Quotients for Psychomotor Development at 6 and 12 months corrected age were not different for infants who had been randomized to KMC versus traditional care (Charpak, Ruiz-Pelaez, de Figueroa, & Charpak, 2001). However, a more stimulating home environment was found in the Kangaroo care group (Tessier et al., 2003) on follow-up at one year corrected age.

The Newborn Individualized Developmental Care and Assessment Program (NIDCAP) is an example of a comprehensive program that incorporates individualized care and environmental modification based on an infant's neurosensory maturation. The program aims to improve state regulation to impact child outcome. Implementation of NIDCAP requires extensive training and programmatic commitment. Some studies have found improved outcomes in several domains for infants who participated in NIDCAP (Baron & Rey-Casserly, 2010), but findings vary across studies and are limited by methodologic issues, small samples, and brief follow-up periods (Wallin & Eriksson, 2009). The key components of any intervention program are those that enhance parental sensitive responsiveness to the infant's signals in a developmental systems conceptual approach (Guralnick, 2012).

Effect of Prematurity on Parental Functioning

Though strides have been made to make the NICU experience more supportive of families and infants, preterm birth is still often experienced by parents as a traumatic event that precipitates a range of reactions, including posttraumatic stress and depressive symptoms. Loss of the healthy idealized child, separation from the infant, and exposure to an intensely medical environment combine in ways that may generate an initial traumatic reaction (Alcorn, O'Donovan, Patrick, Creedy, & Devilly, 2010). Parental symptoms can include anxiety, sleep problems, dissociation, hypervigilance, numbing, and avoidance of medical visits. These symptoms can persist in the caregiving of a medically ill child (Peebles-Kleiger, 2000). On parent response scales and interviews, the classic posttraumatic stress disorder (PTSD) symptomatology of increased arousal, re-experiencing, and avoidance is seen in mothers acutely in the days after the birth (Vanderbilt, Bushley, Young, & Frank, 2009) and up to 14 months postpartum in both mothers and fathers (DeMier, Hynan, Harris et al., 1996; Kersting et al., 2004; Shaw, Bernard, Deblois et al., 2009). Mothers of VLBW newborns who have been in the NICU report more symptoms of anxiety and depression acutely and ongoing psychological distress and parenting

stress compared to mothers of healthy term newborns (Doering, Moser, & Dracup, 2000; Carter, Mulder, Bartram, & Darlow, 2005). Poverty exacerbates the vulnerability for PTSD symptoms related to preterm births and ongoing poorer child outcomes (Breslau et al., 2009).

Depressive symptoms in parents are also common. While the baseline prevalence of postpartum depression (PPD) among women is 10–15 % (CDC, 2008), preterm birth raises the rate to 40 % in the early postpartum period (Vigod, Villegas, Dennis, & Ross, 2010). Clinically relevant PPD symptoms following VLBW infant birth can be seen in the range of 12–60 % (Davis, et. al., 2003; Singer, Salvator, Guo, et al., 1999). Prenatal depression is a strong predictor of PPD and long-term child effects (Field, 2011). The hormonal changes after childbirth and the traumatic experience of unanticipated delivery, separation from the infant, and the NICU milieu make mothers of preterm infants especially vulnerable to PPD. Parental distress increases with the severity of child illness in the NICU (Klebanov, Brooks-Gunn, & McCormick, 1994). Depressive symptoms are highest at the infant's discharge from the hospital, decrease in most studies by 6 months of age, but may be more severe and sustained in lower socioeconomic minority populations (Poehlmann, Schwichtenberg, Bolt et al., 2009).

Parental Response and Impact on Child

Emotional distress among parents in the NICU can have intergenerational consequences to the developing infant. Parents' PTSD symptoms affect their own physical and emotional health, which can have implications for the health, developmental, and behavioral outcomes of their high-risk infants (Schnurr & Jankowski, 1999). Quinnell found almost 6 % of the variance in cognitive performance at 30 months among high-risk infants explained by maternal posttraumatic stress related to infants' prematurity (Quinnell, 2001). Higher levels of maternal anxiety assessed during the infant's NICU hospitalization were associated with lower cognitive development and more internalizing behavior problems when children were 24 months corrected age (Zelkowitz, Na, Wang, Bardin, & Papageorgiou, 2011). Sleep and eating problems are more prevalent among premature toddlers of parents experiencing PTSD symptoms (Pierrehumbert, Nicole, Muller-Nix et al., 2003). A potential mechanism to these behavioral problems was seen in a study that showed increased maternal emotional stress contributing to more negative parenting behaviors and increased behavioral problems in their preterm children at age 4 years (Assel et al., 2002).

Maternal depression in general postpartum populations has been shown to affect risk of poorer child cognitive development, behavioral functioning, feeding and growth, and less appropriate use of health care services (Field, Sandberg, Garcia et al., 1985, Mounts, 2009). Chronicity, timing, and severity of maternal postnatal depression may account for variations seen among studies (NICHD, 1999; Grace, Evindar, & Stewart, 2003). Among mothers with preterm births, persistent postnatal depression at 9 months predicted lower cognitive functioning in the toddlers at 16 months (McManus & Poehlmann, 2012). The challenges of parenting a preterm child, depression, and traumatic stress can lead to negative maternal recollections of the birth experience which predict greater report of internalizing and total problems at 5 years of age for preterm but not full-term children (Latva, Korja, Salmelin et al., 2008). Mothers of low birth weight children were more likely to rate their child as having a behavioral problem compared to teachers. The strongest predictors were caregiving quality and maternal depression but not child biological factors (Spiker, Kraemer, Constantine et al., 1992).

Influence on Attachment

An extensive literature highlights the importance of early parent–child relationships as providing the foundation for later development. Positive parent–child relationship can offer some buffer against biological and environmental risk factors including prematurity and other associated risks. Maladaptive attachment relationships contribute to lower scores on cognitive, behavior, and adaptive assessment (Belsky & Fearon, 2002) and can contribute to health problems such as obesity (Anderson, Gooze, Lemeshow, & Whitaker, 2012).

Parents develop an internal representation of the child even before the child is born which can have an ongoing effect on the quality of the relationship (Benoit, Parker, & Zeanah, 1997). Parental internal representations of their infant impact parent–child interaction with preterm infants being especially sensitive to the protective or risk aspects in the relationship. Stern observed less positive interactions and appraisals among mothers playing with infants randomly labeled "preterm" as compared to "full term" (Stern, Karraker, Sopko, & Norman, 2000). Prematurity moderates the association between depression and attachment at 12 months and affects the security of the attachment relationship (Poehlmann & Fiese, 2001; Mangelsdorf et al., 1996).

Preterm infants are also active participants in the interactions with their parents, although their social development may differ from term infants. In a controlled study, preterm infants showed equal positive affect as their full-term counterparts in a parent–child interaction procedure, but they showed more negative affect, had a smaller latency to negative affect, and were less facially responsive than full-term infants (Hsu & Jeng, 2008). Prematurity dyads in general show lower rates of "sensitive maternal style and cooperative infant interaction style" at 6 months, and infants were at higher risk for problems with sleeping, eating, and behavioral problems at 18 months (Forcada-Guex, Pierrehumbert, Borghini, Moessinger, & Muller-Nix, 2006).

The additional effects of PTSD and maternal depression associated with preterm birth can lead to poorer synchrony in the parent–child relationship. As noted, parental symptoms of PTSD, such as dissociation, hypervigilance, and numbing, may decrease parental ability to respond sensitively to infant cues (Bosquet Enlow et al., 2011). For example, sleep dysregulation was related to poor parent–infant bonding among mothers with

PTSD symptoms (Hairston et al., 2011). Maternal PTSD symptoms arising from premature birth are associated with less sensitive and more controlling maternal behaviors (Muller-Nix, Forcada-Guex, Pierrehumbert et al., 2004; Feeley et al., 2011). Even after controlling for medical risks, maternal anxiety showed a moderate association with infant facial responsivity, again suggesting an important a complex interaction between maternal internal experiences and infant behaviors.

Many studies of maternal postnatal depression support a relationship between depression and attachment (Wan & Green, 2009). Though one recent large cohort study in the Netherlands found pre- and postnatal depression did not have an effect on infant–maternal attachment at 14 months (Tharner et al., 2012), other studies have found maternal postnatal depressive symptoms lower the quality of the infant–maternal interaction in preterm dyads, result in greater rates of insecure attachment in the child, and raise the risk of distorted attachment representations in the mother (Korja, Savonlahti, Ahlqvist-Bjorkroth et al., 2008). One study identified insecure attachment relationships as occurring more frequently with parental subclinical depressive symptoms in preterm infants but not in term infants (Poehlmann & Fiese, 2001). Attachment disruption due to parent depression and anxiety also leads to lower infant social engagement, unregulated fear regulation, and increased stress reactivity (Feldman, Granat, Pariente et al., 2009). Maternal unresolved grief also has been associated with insecure attachment at 16 months among infants born preterm (Shah, Clements, & Poehlmann, 2011).

Vulnerable Child Syndrome

Vulnerable child syndrome is a constellation of parental perception and behaviors involving perceived increased child vulnerability after resolution of medical difficulties and can be seen in families who have experienced preterm birth (Perrin, West, & Culley, 1989). This influences parent behavior. For example, if parents perceive their child to be unusually vulnerable, they are more likely to use emergency services (Chambers, Mahabee-Gittens, & Leonard, 2011).

The "vulnerable child syndrome" also impacts the child's development and behavior. Controlling for medical severity among premature infants, parental perception of vulnerability correlated with maternal anxiety at neonatal discharge and developmental outcomes in 1-year-olds (Allen et al., 2004). NICU graduates deemed vulnerable by their parents on the Childhood Vulnerability Scale are found to have increased total behavioral problems on the Child Behavioral Checklist (De Ocampo, Macias, Saylor, & Katikaneni, 2003). This dynamic can continue throughout childhood into young adulthood, with parents of adults born preterm assessing their parenting styles as more protective and VLBW women retrospectively reporting their mothers as more protective and authoritarian (Pyhala et al., 2011).

Child Outcomes in Prematurity

In considering the burgeoning body of literature on outcomes related to prematurity, it is important to note that there have been changes in the sample characteristics of infants studied over time. Many of the longer term and adult outcome studies reflect the premature population of the 1980s or earlier which typically consisted of VLBW or very preterm infants. More recent study samples typically include the increasing numbers of ELBW or extremely preterm infants surviving after birth at less than 28 weeks. Changes in medical care and family support as neonatology has evolved have differentially impacted these changing samples and their neurodevelopmental and social-emotional outcomes across time. Additionally, outcome measures have changed as newer versions of tests and scales are used to study cognitive or behavioral outcomes and can impact outcome comparisons across studies from different time periods (Vohr et al., 2012).

Prematurity and Social-Emotional Development

Prematurity's impact can extend into the realm of social-emotional development. Several studies have not found overall differences in baseline temperament between preterm and term groups (Gray, Edwards, O'Callaghan, & Cuskelly, 2012; Olafsen et al., 2008; Larroque et al., 2005). Infants born at less than 29 weeks in one study did not show significant differences in temperament from term infants at 9 months of age unless they had abnormalities on neonatal cerebral ultrasound or developmental delays (Larroque et al., 2005). However, preterm infants rated by their mothers as having a more difficult temperament were more susceptible to early negative parenting (Poehlmann et al., 2011). Studies of young adults born prematurely have shown differences in psychosocial functioning into adulthood even in samples that do not have psychiatric diagnoses or major disabilities related to their prematurity. One study found that ELBW adults in their 20s without diagnosed psychiatric or neurosensory impairment reported higher rates of shyness, inhibition, and lower emotional well-being than peers born at normal weight (Schmidt, Miskovic, Boyle, & Saigal, 2008).

Low birth weight premature cohorts also have shown higher rates of positive screens on the Modified Checklist for Autism in Toddlers (M-CHAT) (Limperopoulos et al., 2008). The Extremely Low Gestational Age Newborns (ELGAN) Study found increased risk of scoring positive on the M-CHAT at 10 % even after controlling for medical severity (Kuban et al., 2009). Later analysis found global impairments in motor, cognitive, vision, and hearing contributed to many of the false positives (Luyster et al., 2011). Epidemiological studies have noted that pre- and perinatal factors such as prematurity, low Apgar scores, and growth restriction increase the risk of autism in Scandinavian cohorts (Buchmayer et al., 2009; Haglund & Källén, 2011). A recent study of children born at less than 2,000 g and assessed periodically through age 21 found an estimated autism spectrum disorder (ASD) prevalence rate of 5 % in the cohort studied which was higher than Centers for Disease Control estimates at the time among the general population (Pinto-Martin et al., 2011).

Children born preterm also have higher reported rates of emotional and behavioral disorders at preschool and school age (Vanderbilt &

Gleason, 2011). This association is strongest in extremely preterm infants (Johnson et al., 2010), but has been identified to some degree even in preschoolers born between 32 and 35 weeks gestation (Potijk, de Winter, Bos, Kerstjens, & Reijneveld, 2012). The most common difficulties seen in former preterms are attentional problems followed by internalizing or anxiety symptoms (Lund, Vik, Skranes, Brubakk, & Indredavik, 2011). A national cohort study from Sweden found higher rates of ADHD medication usage at school age as the degree of gestational immaturity increased, with children born between 23 and 28 weeks having an adjusted risk double that of children born at term (Lindström, Lindblad, & Hjern, 2011). As with cognitive outcomes, increased medical risk impacts emotional, behavioral, and psychiatric outcomes. In a recent large cohort assessed at age 16, history of intraventricular hemorrhage increased the risk for depressive disorder and obsessive–compulsive disorder, while parenchymal lesions increased the risk for attention-deficit/hyperactivity disorder-inattentive type and obsessive–compulsive disorder (Whitaker et al., 2011).

In contrast to higher rates of attentional difficulties and internalizing behavior, meta-analysis did not identify increased rates of externalizing behaviors or risk-taking in former preterm school-aged children (Aarnoudse-Moens et al., 2009). Into adolescence, young adults born extremely preterm self-report fewer problems with externalizing behavior and decreased rates of alcohol use (Hallin & Stjernqvist, 2011) and other risk behaviors (Strang-Karlsson et al., 2008).

Failure to Thrive

Failure to thrive (FTT) is a term used to describe an infant or toddler with inadequate or less than expected weight gain. Rather than a distinct disorder, it is often the final common pathway for a host of medical, social-emotional, nutritional, and environmental factors that result in inadequate weight gain (Gahagan, 2006). Although there is no clear consensus on the definition of failure to thrive, it is often defined by crossing two major percentile lines on a standard growth chart: weight-for-age less than the third or fifth percentile over a period of time or weight-for-height less than the tenth percentile. Typically, consideration of both growth velocity and absolute anthropomorphic measurements helps to distinguish FTT from normal fluctuations in the rate of growth that may occur in early infancy or children who are small but growing normally (Wright, 2000). Unfortunately, there is no single anthropomorphic measurement that adequately identifies all children with clinically important growth delays (Olsen et al., 2007). However, the appropriate diagnosis and management of FTT is of key importance as children with failure to thrive are at risk for long-lasting negative effects on their physical, cognitive, and behavioral development.

In the 1940s, Spitz described institutionalized infants with significant growth retardation and developmental delay using the terms "hospitalism" or "anaclitic depression" (Spitz, 1945). For children with similar symptoms who were living at home with their mothers, this concept was extended and thought to be secondary to "maternal deprivation" (Coleman & Provence, 1957; Patton & Gardner, 1962). Historically, failure to thrive had been attributed to maternal inadequacy whose "treatment" was through maternal therapy or foster care placement. This conceptualization has been replaced by a more complex multifactorial model, that informs our current approach to FTT.

Failure to thrive is more accurately referred to as "growth faltering" (Wright, 2000) or "malnutrition" in its more severe form. Typically, there are three basic mechanisms that can result in growth faltering or failure to thrive: (1) loss of calories through malabsorption, (2) increased caloric expenditure (i.e., congenital heart disease, hyperthyroidism, asthma), and (3) inadequate caloric intake (i.e., severe neurologic dysfunction, oral-motor aversion, interactive feeding disorder, unusual dietary beliefs, inadequate economic resources for a healthful diet, etc.). Certain genetic and dysmorphic conditions (i.e., trisomy 21, fetal alcohol syndrome) manifest with deficits in height poorly responsive to nutritional interventions, but do not explain under-weight for height. However, regardless of the mechanism, failure to thrive has been associated with clinically important growth, developmental, and behavioral outcomes as well as alterations in the ability to resist infection.

Based upon data collected from the 2010 United Nations' surveys, it has been estimated that 16 % of children less than 5 years of age were underweight and 27 % were stunted worldwide (Lutter et al., 2011). Undernutrition was more prevalent in Africa and Asia but also commonly seen in Latin America (Lutter et al., 2011). In the developed world, data from birth cohorts suggest the prevalence of FTT to be between 4 and 10 % over the first 9–12 months of life (Blair, Drewett, Emmett, Ness, & Emond, 2004; Wright et al., 2006a, 2006b). In the USA, approximately 80 % of children present before 18 months of age (Cole & Lanham, 2011). Although there are differences in the presentation and diagnostic evaluation of FTT in developing and developed countries, failure to thrive continues to be a common condition of young children throughout the world.

The evaluation of a child with FTT is influenced by the child's clinical presentation and growth parameters. Wasting is described as a deficit in weight for height and is a sign of acute malnutrition. Stunting is defined as decreased height for age and reflects more chronic malnutrition. Underweight is defined as decreased weight for age and can reflect acute or chronic malnutrition. Typically, weight decreases first, followed by height, and then head circumference (Kistin & Bauchner, 2008). A comprehensive assessment begins with a thorough history including a dietary and feeding history, review of systems, pregnancy and past medical history, developmental history, social history, and review of social-emotional and material resources. The child requires a complete physical exam looking for signs of illness, dysmorphic features, and other abnormalities. The laboratory assessment of a child with failure to thrive depends upon the history obtained, symptoms described, and physical exam. A "shotgun approach" to the evaluation has been shown to be neither cost effective nor likely to provide much diagnostic yield (Berwick, Levy, & Kleinerman, 1982). Instead, the history and physical exam must be used to thoughtfully guide the medical management and therapeutic approach to the child with FTT.

Traditionally, the etiology of a child's inadequate weight gain was often dichotomized into "organic" versus "nonorganic" origins. "Organic FTT" was used to describe a medical condition or organ system dysfunction that results in FTT; "nonorganic FTT" was used to describe inadequacies in the home or social environment that impact a child's ability to maintain adequate growth. However, with an increasing recognition of the complex interplay between the multiple factors contributing to a child's growth, the dichotomy of "organic FTT" and "nonorganic FTT" as discrete entities is no longer regarded as clinically useful. Instead, considering the "transactional model" of child, caregiver, and environmental factors that interact to create a condition of poor growth offers greater insight into the complex processes that result in FTT (Blenner, Wilbur, & Frank, 2008; Frank & Zeisel, 1988; Sameroff & Mackenzie, 2003).

Parent Characteristics/Risk Factors

Parental characteristics such as education have previously been viewed as risk factors for FTT. The Avon Longitudinal Study of Parents and Children (ALSPAC), a UK birth cohort of over 11,000 infants, identified low parental height and higher parity as associated with slower infant weight gain, but did not find associations between FTT and other parental factors such as parental education (Blair et al., 2004). Results from the Gateshead Millennium Baby Study, another UK cohort with data on over 700 infants, also failed to demonstrate a significant relationship between maternal education and FTT (Wright et al., 2006a, 2006b). However, the relationship between maternal education and FTT may differ between the developed and developing world. Analyses of data from India demonstrated continued disparities in rates of undernutrition associated with maternal education (Subramanyam, Kawachi, Berkman, & Subramanian, 2010). Results of these large cohort studies emphasize the importance of assessing the

broader social environment, including the national and cultural context, when evaluating the relevancy of various risk factors.

Studies assessing the relationship between maternal depression and failure to thrive in young children have demonstrated mixed results, conveying a complex interaction between these two conditions depending on the social context. A review of the evidence suggests that the strength of the relationship depends upon other socioeconomic factors (Stewart, 2007). Surkan and colleagues performed a meta-analysis of maternal depression and early childhood growth in the developing world, including both adjusted and unadjusted analyses. Based on their results, the odds ratio for the association between maternal depression and child underweight was 1.5 (CI: 1.2–1.8); and the odds ratio between maternal depression and child stunting was 1.4 (CI: 1.2–1.7) (Surkan, Kennedy, Hurley, & Black, 2011). However, two large cohort studies from the developed world have failed to demonstrate a significant sustained association (Grote et al., 2010; Wright et al., 2006a, 2006b). Evaluation of a birth cohort by Santos and colleagues in Brazil also failed to demonstrate a positive association between maternal depressive symptoms and child underweight (Santos, Matijasevich, Rodrigues Domingues, Barros, & Barros, 2010). This suggests that the relationship between maternal depressive symptomatology and child underweight may vary depending on the broader socioeconomic and cultural context.

Although previous small studies have posited an association between failure to thrive and maternal eating habits (McCann, Stein, Fairburn, & Dunger, 1994; Altemeier, O'Connor, Sherrod, & Vietze, 1985), an evaluation of data from the Avon Longitudinal Study of Parents and Children (ALPSAC) failed to demonstrate a relationship between infant undernutrition and maternal dieting or history of a maternal eating disorder (Blair et al., 2004). Results from this large birth cohort and more recent case–control studies suggest a lack of a significant association between maternal eating attitudes and infant FTT (Blair et al., 2004; Chatoor, Ganiban, Hirsch, Borman-Spurrell, & Mrazek, 2000).

Other studies suggest that children with failure to thrive are more likely to demonstrate patterns of insecure attachment than typically growing peers. In a study by Chatoor and colleagues, when compared to picky or healthy eating controls, infants with FTT had higher rates of insecure attachment, although the majority of children with FTT demonstrated secure attachment patterns (Chatoor, Ganiban, Colin, Plummer, & Harmon, 1998). The authors concluded that insecure attachment may intensify feeding difficulties and increase the risk for more severe malnutrition. Mothers of children with FTT are more likely to describe insecure attachment representations based upon the Adult Attachment Interview than mothers of healthy eaters (Chatoor et al., 2000). It was hypothesized that parents with insecure attachment representations may demonstrate decreased sensitivity to their infants, resulting in an increased risk of maladaptive feeding and FTT (Chatoor et al., 2000). Results of these studies emphasize the importance of considering the qualities of the maternal–child relationship when assessing a child who presents with FTT but acknowledge that the majority of infants with FTT have secure attachment relationships.

Parental perception of a toddler's temperamental traits may also contribute to the risk for failure to thrive. In a small study by Chatoor and colleagues, when compared to healthy eaters, mothers of children with FTT tended to report higher rates of difficult, negatively adaptive, dependent, irregular, sober, and unstoppable temperamental characteristics (Chatoor et al., 2000). Whether or not the parental perceptions of a toddler's temperament correlated with objective descriptions of the toddler was not ascertained. Some of the reported child characteristics may themselves be sequelae of macro- or micronutrient deficiencies. For example, Lozoff and colleagues described decreased activity, poor soothability, and negative mood along with increased clinginess and wariness seen in children with iron-deficiency anemia (Lozoff et al., 1998, 2008).

In a minority of cases, failure to thrive can be the result of child neglect. Although the risk of failure to thrive as a manifestation of child neglect

was highlighted in a clinical report by the American Academy of Pediatrics' Committee on Child Abuse and Neglect (Block, Krebs, The Committee on Child Abuse and Neglect, & The Committee on Nutrition, 2005), a highly regarded group of researchers in the field have countered that the prevalence of child neglect among cases of FTT is not common (Black et al., 2006). Although child neglect is clearly within the complex multifactorial differential of failure to thrive, serious consideration of neglect as an important etiology should be reserved for cases in which there are clearly concerning signs. Black and colleagues argued that abuse and neglect should be most strongly considered in cases where there is the "intentional withholding of food from the child; strong beliefs in health and/or nutritional regimens that jeopardize a child's well-being; and/or a family that is resistant to recommended interventions despite a multidisciplinary team approach" (Black et al., 2006). They argue that child neglect should not be considered a diagnosis of exclusion when no other etiology can be determined, but should be considered when specific case-based factors suggest it (Black et al., 2006).

Child Characteristics

A child with failure to thrive may demonstrate a range of physical and psychosocial characteristics that contribute to inadequate weight gain. Children with low birth weight (LBW: <2,500 g) are at an increased risk of developing postnatal failure to thrive (Dusick, Poindexter, Ehrenkranz, & Lemons, 2003; De Curtis & Rigo, 2004). Data from the Neonatal Research Network suggest that 89 % of extremely low birth weight babies (ELBW: <1,000 g) have growth failure at 36 weeks corrected age. By 18–22 months corrected age, 40 % still had anthropomorphic measurements below the tenth percentile (Dusick et al., 2003). In a similar study, 22 % of very low birth weight babies (VLBW: <1,500 g) were small for gestational age (SGA) at birth, but 97 % showed growth failure by hospital discharge (Lemons et al., 2001). The authors of these studies emphasize the critical importance of providing aggressive nutritional support to low birth weight babies in the newborn period, both before and after discharge. In addition, these studies highlight the importance of early and appropriate prenatal care to help prevent outcomes of prematurity and low birth weight.

Late preterm children, infants born between 34 and 36 weeks gestational age, are also at a higher risk for developing failure to thrive. Using data from a 2004 Brazilian birth cohort, Santos and colleagues found that late preterm children were 1.87 (0.50; 7.01) times more likely to be wasted, 2.30 (1.40; 3.77) times more likely to be stunted, and 3.36 (1.56; 7.23) times more likely to be underweight at 24 months of age (Santos et al., 2009).

Children with failure to thrive may have a medical condition that is associated with their poor weight gain. As part of the evaluation of a child who presents with FTT, it is important to carefully look for the presence of an acute or chronic medical condition that contributes to the inadequate weight gain. The participation of an experienced pediatric health provider, ideally one working with a multidisciplinary team that includes nutritionists and social workers, is essential. The list of conditions associated with FTT is extensive and beyond the scope of this review. Commonly occurring conditions include genetic or nongenetic syndromes, developmental disorders such as autism or cerebral palsy, cleft lip or palate, adenoidal-tonsillar hypertrophy/obstructive sleep apnea, dental caries, gastroesophageal reflux, food allergies, celiac disease, asthma, cystic fibrosis, congenital heart disease, hepatitis, HIV, and enteric pathogens (Blenner et al., 2008). These conditions may be associated with one or more of the three basic mechanisms that result in failure to thrive: (1) loss of calories through malabsorption, (2) increased caloric expenditure, and (3) inadequate caloric intake. However, the identification of one or more of these conditions must be viewed in the context of other parental, child, and social factors which contribute to the presentation of failure to thrive. As previously discussed, the larger social context is often of critical importance whether or not other physiologic derangements are identified.

Social Context

Poverty has long been thought to be the most important social risk factor associated with failure to thrive; however, some recent longitudinal British cohort studies suggest that this relationship may not be as robust as previously envisioned in some developed countries. The Avon Longitudinal Study of Parents and Children (ALPSAC) failed to demonstrate a relationship between social class and failure to thrive (Blair et al., 2004). Similarly, Wright and colleagues analyzed data from the Gateshead Millennium Baby Study and found no association between FTT and socioeconomic status (Wright et al., 2006a, 2006b). Interestingly, there were about twice the number of infants with FTT in the highest and lowest quintiles of affluence (Wright et al., 2006a, 2006b). The researchers argue that the lack of a clear association with poverty may be secondary to the protective effects of the UK welfare food scheme, similar to the US Women Infants and Children program (WIC). In addition, it has been postulated that children with socioeconomic risk factors are more likely to be referred to a subspecialty clinic for further evaluation and management (Wright et al., 2006a, 2006b; Sullivan, 2004). In the USA, cross-sectional data from large national datasets also failed to demonstrate a clear association between low-income levels and child undernutrition (Wang, Monteiro, & Popkin, 2002; Casey, Szeto, Lensing, Bogle, & Weber, 2001). However, in a study utilizing data from the National Longitudinal Study of Youth (1979–1988), Miller and colleagues suggest that persistent poverty is positively associated with increased stunting and wasting (Miller & Korenman, 1994). This raises questions as to whether long-term poverty is a better measurement than short-term income as a risk factor for undernutrition in the developed world. Studies from the developing world continue to find an association with childhood undernutrition and household wealth, suggesting the potential for a differential association between poverty and FTT in the developed and developing world (Subramanyam et al., 2010; Wang et al., 2002).

Frank and colleagues described a phenomenon they termed "heat or eat," where children of families who were participating in the Low-Income Home Energy Assistance Program (LIHEAP) were at decreased risk for anthropomorphic measurements suggestive of undernutrition (Frank et al., 2006). This relationship held in adjusted analysis when controlled for a number of socioeconomic risk factors including participation in other assistance program benefits (i.e., WIC, SNAP, TANF, etc.) (Frank et al., 2006). This highlights the tightrope upon which many low-income families walk when a cold winter can mean the difference between a healthy or an underweight infant and the importance of maintaining programs that provide nutritional and economic support to underserved, at-risk, families.

Feeding Characteristics

In 1994, the DSM-IV introduced Feeding Disorders of Infancy and Early Childhood as one of its diagnostic disorders. It included the following characteristics: "(1) The persistent failure to eat adequately, as reflected by significant failure to gain weight or significant weight loss over at least 1 month; (2) There is no gastrointestinal or other general medical condition severe enough to account for the feeding disturbance; (3) The feeding disturbance is also not better accounted for by another mental disorder or lack of available food; and (4) The onset of the disorder must be before age 6 years" (APA, 1994). The DSM-5 no longer includes Feeding Disorders of Infancy and Early Childhood as a diagnosis and introduces the diagnosis of Avoidant/Restrictive Food Intake Disorder. Chatoor and colleagues, in conjunction with one of the infant and preschool working groups of the American Academy of Child and Adolescent Psychiatry, also created a more detailed diagnostic classification scheme for feeding disorders in young children. It is described as follows (Chatoor, 2002):

1. Feeding disorder of state regulation (onset newborn period)
   This categorization is used to describe an infant who cannot reach or maintain a state of calm alertness that is necessary for effective feeding. The infant may be too sleepy or too agitated to feed appropriately. Infants with this type of feeding disorder tend to present in the newborn period and require the use of calming techniques to promote feeding (i.e., feeding in a darkened room, massaging, etc.). Until a baby can adequately regulate his or her state, he or she may require supplemented feeding through an NG tube.

2. Feeding disorder of reciprocity (onset 2–6 months of age)
   Feeding disorder of reciprocity is used to describe feeding difficulties resulting from a lack of appropriate social responsiveness (i.e., smiling, babbling, etc.) during feeding with the primary caregiver. This type of feeding disorder may be associated with decreased maternal–child reciprocity or maternal psychosocial issues. Treatment often requires intensive work with both the child and parent to improve the mutual responsiveness of the dyad.

3. Infantile anorexia (onset 6 months–3 years)
   Infantile anorexia is often characterized by frequent food refusal. The onset may occur as a child transitions from spoon-feeding to self-feeding. Typically, the child does not know how to effectively communicate hunger and seems to lack interest in food. Parents often respond by trying to regulate their child's intake. Temperamentally, children with infantile anorexia are described as being difficult, intense, curious, and irregular. An escalation of the mother–infant conflict during feeding is often associated with poorer weight gain. A study by Wright and colleagues suggests that the degree to which the caregiver responds to food refusal may be associated with poorer weight gain (Wright et al., 2006a, 2006b). The helpful treatment of infantile anorexia often requires addressing the child's temperament and the parent–infant relationship.

4. Sensory food aversions (onset during the introduction of baby or table foods)
   Sensory food aversions can present during the introduction of baby or table foods. This feeding disorder is characterized by food refusal based upon "specific tastes, textures, smells, or appearances of foods." Sensory food aversions differ from "pickiness" in that they must

be associated with specific nutritional deficiencies or oral-motor delays (i.e., resistance to eating food that requires chewing). Treatment includes emphasizing the importance of encouraging, but not forcing, a child to eat a broader array of foods. Tying the consumption of certain foods to contingencies (i.e., TV time or dessert) tends to backfire as children often shift their interest away from these contingency-dependent foods (Birch, Birch, Marlin, & Kramer, 1982). Feeding therapy with an occupational therapist or speech-language pathologist may help to gradually expand a child's range of foods. In addition, the use of a nutritional supplement and/or vitamin may also support a child's nutritional needs while decreasing parental pressure to expand his range of foods.

5. Feeding disorder associated with current medical conditions (onset all ages)

There are certain medical conditions that may be associated with increased distress with feeding and whose primary symptom may be that of food refusal. Food allergies and silent reflux are two examples of the type of condition that may be difficult to diagnose and may present with food refusal. Typically, children with this type of feeding disorder are interested in initiating a feed, but show distress or refusal over the course of the meal. Medical management of the underlying condition may improve symptoms, but does not always completely alleviate the feeding issue. Treatment may require ongoing feeding therapy, use of supplementation, and in more extreme cases, tube feedings.

6. Posttraumatic feeding disorder (onset all ages)

Children who experience a posttraumatic feeding disorder experience food refusal following a traumatic event or repeated insults such as "choking, severe vomiting, or insertion of an endotracheal tube." The child may be triggered by reminders of the traumatic event such as the sight of a bib or bottle and show intense resistance when approached by food or refuse to swallow when food is placed in his mouth. Posttraumatic feeding disorder can be a severe problem requiring the use of a gastric tube and intense feeding therapy to overcome the oral aversion. There are various approaches to supporting a child with this type of feeding disorder through feeding therapy or a desensitization program that can take months to years.

Olsen and colleagues also reviewed the association between failure to thrive and age of onset (Olsen, Skovgaard, Weile, Petersen, & Jørgensen, 2010), with findings that roughly corresponded with the classification scheme outlined by Chatoor and colleagues. Using the Copenhagen Child Cohort, a birth cohort of 6,090 children born in the year 2000, they described risk factors associated with FTT among three different age groups. The study included data collected from home-visitation public health nurses who assessed the health and development of the child as well as the quality of the mother–child interaction. FTT that began in children aged birth to 2 weeks was associated with low birth weight and gestational age, single parenthood, and maternal tobacco use. Onset of FTT between 2 weeks and 4 months was associated with congenital disorders, significant medical conditions, and mother–child relationship issues. Finally, onset between 4 and 8 months was associated with feeding problems that arose de novo in otherwise healthy children.

Interventions

A multidisciplinary team approach is the mainstay of effective management for the child with failure to thrive. Typically, the multidisciplinary team includes a pediatrician, dietitian, social worker, mental health clinician, and an occupational or speech-language therapist (Showers, Mandelkron, Coury, & McCleery, 1986; Bithoney et al., 1989). In general, goals in management include the following: (1) provision of adequate calories, protein, and micronutrients; (2) nutritional counseling of the family; (3) supportive economic assistance; (4) treatment of medical conditions associated with FTT; (5) psychosocial support for families; and (6) addressing developmental needs through EI or school-based services (Shah, 2002; Blenner et al., 2008). Multidisciplinary teams provide the breadth of resources to help address the multiple parental, child, and social environmental factors that often contribute to a child who is failing to gain adequate weight.

Given the complexities of the management of FTT, many have felt that the optimal treatment of FTT is conducive to a home-visitation model. Black and colleagues conducted a randomized controlled trial of home visitation of young children with nonorganic failure to thrive and longitudinal follow-up until 8 years of age. Participants included low-income urban families of children with failure to thrive and no significant medical complications. Children were randomized into clinical care through a multidisciplinary growth and nutrition clinic versus multidisciplinary clinical care with weekly home intervention for 1 year. At the 12-month follow-up, children made improvements in anthropomorphic measurements regardless of study arm. However, children in the home-intervention group demonstrated better receptive language skills and more child-oriented home environments as measured by the Home Observation Measure of the Environment (HOME) than the clinic-only group (Black, Dubowitz, Hutcheson, Berenson-Howard, & Starr, 1995). This cohort of children was reassessed at 8 years of age with 74 % and 78 % retention. Although there were no differences between the two groups in terms of IQ, reading, or mother-reported behavior problems, children in the home-intervention group had fewer teacher-reported internalizing problems and improved work habits (Black, Dubowitz, Krishnakumar, & Starr, 2007).

In a similar study, Raynor and colleagues sought to determine whether home visitation by a specialist health visitor would affect the outcome of children with FTT (Raynor, Rudolf, Cooper, Marchant, & Cottrell, 1999). Children were randomized to receive standard care in an outpatient failure to thrive clinic versus receiving an additional specialist health visitor intervention for 12 months. Both groups demonstrated good weight gain and improvement in their developmental scores and energy intake. However, the control group demonstrated more referrals for dietary services, social service involvement, hospital admissions, and missed clinical appointments. The more coordinated approach of the trained specialist health visitor resulted in an overall decrease in health service utilization (Raynor et al., 1999).

Conclusion

Prematurity and failure to thrive are both important and common biopsychosocial conditions affecting infants and young children which have long-lasting implications for the physical, neuropsychological, and socioemotional development of children. These are complex conditions that benefit from a multidisciplinary team approach to assess the interwoven medical, social-emotional, nutritional, and environmental factors that influence both short- and long-term outcomes. Fortunately, by focusing interventions on addressing the mutable risk factors affecting both premature and underweight children, we can help to decrease negative outcomes associated with these conditions and promote healthy development for these children.

References

Aarnoudse-Moens, C. S., Weisglas-Kuperus, N., van Goudoever, J. B., & Oosterlaan J. (2009) Meta-analysis of neurobehavioral outcomes in very preterm and/or very low birth weight children. *Pediatrics 124*(2), 717–28.

Alaimo, K., Olson, C. M., & Frongillo, E. A. (2001). Low family income and food insufficiency in relation to overweight in US children – is there a paradox? *Archives of Pediatrics & Adolescent Medicine, 155*, 1161–1167.

Alcorn, K. L., O'Donovan, A., Patrick, J. C., Creedy, D., & Devilly, G. J. (2010). A prospective longitudinal study of the prevalence of post-traumatic stress disorder resulting from childbirth events. *Psychological Medicine, 40*(11), 1849–59.

Allen, E. C., Manuel, J. C., Legault, C., Naughton, M. J., Pivor, C., & O'Shea, T. M. (2004). Perception of child vulnerability among mothers of former premature infants. *Pediatrics, 113*(2), 267–73.

Altemeier, W. A., O'Connor, S. M., Sherrod, K. B., & Vietze, P. M. (1985). Prospective study of antecedents for nonorganic failure to thrive. *Journal of Pediatrics, 106*, 360–65.

American Psychiatric Association. (1994). *Diagnostic and statistical manual of mental disorders* (4th ed.).

Washington, DC: American Psychiatric Association.

Anderson, S. E., Gooze, R. A., Lemeshow, S., & Whitaker, R. C. (2012). Quality of early maternal–child relationship and risk of adolescent obesity. *Pediatrics, 129*(1), 132–40.

Assel, M. A., Landry, S. H., Swank, P. R., Steelman, L., Miller-Loncar, C., & Smith, K. E. (2002). How do mothers' childrearing histories, stress and parenting affect children's behavioural outcomes? *Child: Care, Health and Development, 28*(5), 359–68.

Aylward, G. P. (2005). Neurodevelopmental outcomes of infants born prematurely. *Journal of Developmental and Behavioral Pediatrics, 26*(6), 427–40.

Baack, M. L., Norris, A. W., Yao, J., & Colaizy, T. (2012). Long-chain polyunsaturated fatty acid levels in US donor human milk: Meeting the needs of premature infants? *Journal of Perinatology, 32*(8), 598–603.

Baker, J. P. (1996). *The machine in the nursery: Incubator technology and the origins of newborn intensive care.* Baltimore, London: Johns Hopkins University Press.

Ballabh, P. (2010). Intraventricular hemorrhage in premature infants: Mechanism of disease. *Pediatric Research, 67*(1), 1–8.

Baron, I. S., & Rey-Casserly, C. (2010). Extremely preterm birth outcome: A review of four decades of cognitive research. *Neuropsychology Review, 20*(4), 430–52.

Behrman, R. E., & Butler, A. S. (2007). *Preterm birth: Causes, consequences, and prevention.* Washington, DC: National Academies Press.

Belsky, J., & Fearon, R. M. (2002). Infant-mother attachment security, contextual risk, and early development: A moderational analysis. *Development and Psychopathology, 14*(2), 293–310.

Benoit, D., Parker, K. C. H., & Zeanah, C. H. (1997). Mothers' representations of their infants assessed prenatally: Stability and association with infants' attachment classifications. *Journal of Child Psychology and Psychiatry, 38*(3), 307–13.

Berwick, D. M., Levy, J. C., & Kleinerman, R. (1982). Failure to thrive: Diagnostic yield of hospitalisation. *Archives of Disease in Childhood, 57*, 347–351.

Birch, L. L., Birch, D., Marlin, D., & Kramer, L. (1982). Effects of instrumental eating on children's food preferences. *Appetite, 3*, 125–134.

Bithoney, W. G., McJunkin, J., Michalek, J., Egan, H., Snyder, J., & Munier, A. (1989). Prospective evaluation of weight gain in both nonorganic and organic failure-to-thrive children: An outpatient trial of multidisciplinary team intervention strategy. *Journal of Developmental & Behavioral Pediatrics, 10*, 27–31.

Black, M. M., Dubowitz, H., Casey, P. H., Cutts, D., Drewett, R. F., Drotar, D., et al. (2006). Failure to thrive as distinct from child neglect. *Pediatrics, 117*, 1456–1458.

Black, M. M., Dubowitz, H., Hutcheson, J., Berenson-Howard, J., & Starr, R. H. (1995). A randomized clinical trial of home intervention for children with failure to thrive. *Pediatrics, 95*, 807–814.

Black, M. M., Dubowitz, H., Krishnakumar, A., & Starr, R. H. (2007). Early intervention and recovery among children with failure to thrive: Follow-up at age 8. *Pediatrics, 120*, 59–69.

Blair, P. S., Drewett, R. F., Emmett, P. M., Ness, A., & Emond, A. M. (2004). Family, socioeconomic and prenatal factors associated with failure to thrive in the Avon Longitudinal Study of Parents and Children (ALSPAC). *International Journal of Epidemiology, 33*, 839–847.

Blenner, S., Wilbur, M. B., & Frank, D. A. (2008). Food insecurity and failure to thrive. In M. L. Wolraich, P. H. Dworkin, D. D. Drotar, & E. C. Perrin (Eds.), *Developmental-behavioral pediatrics: Evidence and practice* (pp. 768–779). Philadelphia, PA: Mosby Elsevier.

Block, R. W., Krebs, N. F., The Committee on Child Abuse and Neglect, & The Committee on Nutrition. (2005). Failure to thrive as a manifestation of child neglect. *Pediatrics, 116*, 1234–1237.

Boddy, J., Skuse, D., & Andrews, B. (2000). The developmental sequelae of nonorganic failure to thrive. *Journal of Child Psychology and Psychiatry, 41*(8), 1003–1014.

Bosquet Enlow, M., Kitts, R. L., Blood, E., Bizarro, A., Hofmeister, M., & Wright, R. J. (2011). Maternal posttraumatic stress symptoms and infant emotional reactivity and emotion regulation. *Infant Behavior & Development, 34*(4), 487–503.

Brennan, P. A., Hammen, C., Andersen, M. J., Bor, W., Najman, J. M., & Williams, G. M. (2000). Chronicity, severity, and timing of maternal depressive symptoms: Relationships with child outcomes at age 5. *Developmental Psychology, 36*(6), 759–66.

Breslau, J., Miller, E., Breslau, N., Bohnert, K., Lucia, V., & Schweitzer, J. (2009). The impact of early behavior disturbances on academic achievement in high school. *Pediatrics, 123*(6), 1472–6.

Buchmayer, S., Johansson, S., Johansson, A., Hultman, C. M., Sparén, P., & Cnattingius, S. (2009). Can association between preterm birth and autism be explained by maternal or neonatal morbidity? *Pediatrics, 124*(5), e817–25.

Burkhardt, M. C., Beck, A. F., Kahn, R. S., & Klein, M. D. (2012). Are our babies hungry? Food insecurity among infants in urban clinics. *Clinical Pediatrics, 51*(3), 238–243.

Carter, J. D., Mulder, R. T., Bartram, A. F., & Darlow, B. A. (2005). Infants in a neonatal intensive care unit: Parental response. *Archives of Disease in Childhood. Fetal and Neonatal Edition, 90*(2), F109–13.

Casey, P. H., Szeto, K., Lensing, S., Bogle, M., & Weber, J. (2001). Children in food-insufficient, low-income families – prevalence, health, and nutritional status. *Archives of Pediatrics & Adolescent Medicine, 155*, 508–514.

Centers for Disease Control and Prevention (CDC). (2008). Prevalence of self-reported postpartum depressive symptoms–17 states, 2004–2005. *MMWR. Morbidity and Mortality Weekly Report, 57*(14), 361–6.

Chambers, P. L., Mahabee-Gittens, E. M., & Leonard, A. C. (2011). Vulnerable child syndrome, parental perception of child vulnerability, and emergency department usage. *Pediatric Emergency Care, 27*(11), 1009–13.

Charpak, N., Ruiz-Pelaez, J. G., de Figueroa, C. Z., & Charpak, Y. (2001). A randomized, controlled trial of kangaroo mother care: Results of follow-up at 1 year of corrected age. *Pediatrics, 108*(5), 1072–9.

Chatoor, I. (2002). Feeding disorders in infants and toddlers: Diagnosis and treatment. *Child and Adolescent Psychiatric Clinics of North America, 11*, 163–83.

Chatoor, I., Ganiban, J., Colin, V., Plummer, N., & Harmon, R. J. (1998). Attachment and feeding problems: A reexamination of nonorganic failure to thrive and attachment insecurity. *Journal of the American Academy of Child and Adolescent Psychiatry, 37*(11), 1217–1224.

Chatoor, I., Ganiban, J., Hirsch, R., Borman-Spurrell, E., & Mrazek, D. A. (2000). Maternal characteristics in toddler temperament in infantile anorexia. *Journal of the American Academy of Child and Adolescent Psychiatry, 39*(6), 743–751.

Chee, C. Y., Chong, Y. S., Ng, T. P., et al. (2008). The association between maternal depression and frequent non-routine visits to the infant's doctor—a cohort study. *Journal of Affective Disorders, 107*(1–3), 247–53.

Cole, S. Z., & Lanham, J. S. (2011). Failure to thrive: An update. *American Family Physician, 83*(7), 829–834.

Coleman, R. W., & Provence, S. (1957). Environmental retardation (hospitalism) in infants living in families. *Pediatrics, 15*, 285–92.

Conde-Agudelo, A., Belizán, J. M., & Diaz-Rossello, J. (2011). Kangaroo mother care to reduce morbidity and mortality in low birthweight infants. *Cochrane Database of Systematic Reviews, 16*(3), CD002771.

Cook, J. T., & Frank, D. A. (2008). Food security, poverty, and human development in the United States. *Annals of the New York Academy of Sciences, 1136*, 193–209.

Corbett, S. S., Drewett, R. F., & Wright, C. M. (1996). Does a fall down a centile chart matter? The growth and developmental sequelae of mild failure to thrive. *Acta Paediatrica, 85*(11), 1278–83.

Coussons-Read, M. E., Lobel, M., Carey, J. C., Kreither, M. O., D'Anna, K., Argys, L., et al. (2012). The occurrence of preterm delivery is linked to pregnancy-specific distress and elevated inflammatory markers across gestation. *Brain, Behavior, and Immunity, 26*(4), 650–9.

Davis, L., Edwards, H., Mohay, H., & Wollin, J. (2003). The impact of very premature birth on the psychological health of mothers. *Early Human Development, 73*(1–2), 61–70.

Davis, L., Mohay, H., & Edwards, H. (2003). Mothers' involvement in caring for their premature infants: An historical overview. *Journal of Advanced Nursing, 42*(6), 578–586.

DeMier, R. L., Hynan, M. T., Harris, H. B., et al. (1996). Perinatal stressors as predictors of symptoms of post-traumatic stress in mothers of infants at high risk. *Journal of Perinatology, 16*(4), 276–80.

Dennis, C. L. (2004). Influence of depressive symptomatology on maternal health service utilization and general health. *Archives of Women's Mental Health, 7*(3), 183–92.

De Curtis, M., & Rigo, J. (2004). Extrauterine growth restriction in very low birthweight infants. *Acta Paediatrica, 93*(12), 1563–1568.

De Ocampo, A. C., Macias, M. M., Saylor, C. F., & Katikaneni, L. D. (2003). Caretaker perception of child vulnerability predicts behavior problems in NICU graduates. *Child Psychiatry and Human Development, 34*(2), 83–96.

Doering, L. V., Moser, D. K., & Dracup, K. (2000). Correlates of anxiety, hostility, depression, and psychosocial adjustment in parents of NICU infants. *Neonatal Network, 19*(5), 15–23.

Drotar, D., & Strum, L. (1992). Personality development, problem solving, and behavior problems among preschool children with early histories of non-organic failure to thrive: A controlled study. *Journal of Developmental and Behavioral Pediatrics, 13*(4), 266–273.

Dusick, A. M., Poindexter, B. B., Ehrenkranz, R. A., & Lemons, J. A. (2003). Growth failure in the preterm infant: Can we catch up? *Seminars in Perinatology, 27*(4), 302–310.

Feeley, N., Zelkowitz, P., Cormier, C., Charbonneau, L., Lacroix, A., & Papageorgiou, A. (2011). Posttraumatic stress among mothers of very low birthweight infants at 6 months after discharge from the neonatal intensive care unit. *Applied Nursing Research, 24*(2), 114–7.

Feldman, R., Granat, A., Pariente, C., et al. (2009). Maternal depression and anxiety across the postpartum year and infant social engagement, fear regulation, and stress reactivity. *Journal of the American Academy of Child and Adolescent Psychiatry, 48*(9), 919–27.

Field, T. (2011). Prenatal depression effects on early development: A review. *Infant Behavior & Development, 34*(1), 1–14.

Field, T. A., Sandberg, D., Garcia, R., et al. (1985). Pregnancy problems, postpartum depression, and early mother–infant interactions. *Developmental Psychology, 21*, 1152–6.

Flynn, H. A., Davis, M., Marcus, S. M., et al. (2004). Rates of maternal depression in pediatric emergency department and relationship to child service utilization. *General Hospital Psychiatry, 26*(4), 316–22.

Forcada-Guex, M., Pierrehumbert, B., Borghini, A., Moessinger, A., & Muller-Nix, C. (2006). Early dyadic patterns of mother-infant interactions and outcomes of prematurity at 18 months. *Pediatrics, 118*(1), e107–14.

Frank, D. A., Neault, N. B., Skalicky, A., Cook, J. T., Wilson, J. D., Levenson, S., et al. (2006). Heat or eat: The Low Income Home energy Assistance Program and nutritional and health risks among children less than 3 years of age. *Pediatrics, 118*(5), e1293–e1302.

Frank, D. A., & Zeisel, S. H. (1988). Failure to thrive. *Pediatric Clinics of North America, 35*, 1187–1206.

Gahagan, S. (2006). Failure to thrive: A consequence of undernutrition. *Pediatrics in Review, 27*(1), e1–11.

Garite, T. J., Clark, R., & Thorp, J. A. (2004). Intrauterine growth restriction increases morbidity and mortality among premature neonates. *American Journal of Obstetrics and Gynecology, 191*(2), 481–7.

Grace, S. L., Evindar, A., & Stewart, D. E. (2003). The effect of postpartum depression on child cognitive development and behavior: A review and critical analysis of the literature. *Archives of Women's Mental Health, 6*(4), 263–74.

Gray, P. H., Edwards, D. M., O'Callaghan, M. J., & Cuskelly, M. (2012). Parenting stress in mothers of preterm infants during early infancy. *Early Human Development, 88*(1), 45–9.

Gress-Smith, J. L., Luecken, L. J., Lemery-Chalfant, K., & Howe, R. (2012). Postpartum depression prevalence and impact on infant health, weight, and sleep in low-income and ethnic minority women and infants. *Maternal and Child Health Journal, 16*(4), 887–93.

Grote, V., Vik, T., von Kries, R., Luque, V., Socha, J., Verduci, E., et al. (2010). Maternal postnatal depression and child growth: a European cohort study. *BMC Pediatrics, 10*, 14.

Guralnick, M. J. (2012). Preventive interventions for preterm children: Effectiveness and developmental mechanisms. *Journal of Developmental and Behavioral Pediatrics, 33*(4), 352–64.

Haglund, N. G., & Källén, K. B. (2011). Risk factors for autism and Asperger syndrome. Perinatal factors and migration. *Autism, 15*(2), 163–83.

Hairston, I. S., Waxler, E., Seng, J. S., Fezzey, A. G., Rosenblum, K. L., & Muzik, M. (2011). The role of infant sleep in intergenerational transmission of trauma. *Sleep, 34*(10), 1373–83.

Hallin, A. L., & Stjernqvist, K. (2011). Adolescents born extremely preterm: Behavioral outcomes and quality of life. *Scandinavian Journal of Psychology, 52*(3), 251–6.

Hay, D. F., Pawlby, S., Sharp, D., et al. (2001). Intellectual problems shown by 11-year-old children whose mothers had postnatal depression. *Journal of Child Psychology and Psychiatry, 42*(7), 871–89.

Holditch-Davis, D., Bartlett, T. R., Blickman, A. L., & Miles, M. S. (2003). Posttraumatic stress symptoms in mothers of premature infants. *Journal of Obstetric, Gynecologic, & Neonatal Nursing, 32*(2), 161–71.

Hsu, H. C., & Jeng, S. F. (2008). Two-month-olds' attention and affective response to maternal still face: A comparison between term and preterm infants in Taiwan. *Infant Behavior & Development, 31*(2), 194–206.

Johnson, S., Hollis, C., Kochhar, P., Hennessy, E., Wolke, D., & Marlow, N. (2010). Psychiatric disorders in extremely preterm children: Longitudinal finding at age 11 years in the EPICure study. *Journal of the American Academy of Child & Adolescent Psychiatry, 49*(5), 453–63.e1.

Jyoti, D. F., Frogillo, E. A., & Jones, S. J. (2005). Food insecurity affects school children's academic performance, weight gain, and social skills. *Journal of Nutrition, 135*, 2831–2839.

Kelleher, K. J., Casey, P. H., Bradley, R. H., Pope, S. K., Whiteside, L., Barrett, K. W., et al. (1993). Risk factors and outcomes for failure to thrive in low birth weight preterm infants. *Pediatrics, 91*(5), 941–948.

Kersting, A., Dorsch, M., Wesselmann, U., Lüdorff, K., Witthaut, J., Ohrmann, P., et al. (2004). Maternal posttraumatic stress response after the birth of a very low-birth-weight infant. *Journal of Psychosomatic Research, 57*(5), 473–6.

Kistin, C. J., & Bauchner, H. (2008). A picture is worth a thousand words. *Archives of Disease in Childhood. Education and Practice Edition, 93*, 177–189.

Klebanov, P. K., Brooks-Gunn, J., & McCormick, M. C. (1994). Classroom behavior of very low birth weight elementary school children. *Pediatrics, 94*(5), 700–8.

Korja, R., Savonlahti, E., Ahlqvist-Bjorkroth, S., et al. (2008). Maternal depression is associated with mother–infant interaction in preterm infants. *Acta Paediatrica, 97*(6), 724–30.

Kuban, K. C., O'Shea, T. M., Allred, E. N., Tager-Flusberg, H., Goldstein, D. J., & Leviton, A. (2009). Positive screening on the Modified Checklist for Autism in Toddlers (M-CHAT) in extremely low gestational age newborns. *The Journal of Pediatrics, 154*(4), 535–540.e1.

Kurstjens, S., & Wolke, D. (2001). Effects of maternal depression on cognitive development of children over the first 7 years of life. *Journal of Child Psychology and Psychiatry, 42*(5), 623–36.

Larroque, B., N'guyen The Tich, S., Guédeney, A., Marchand, L., Burguet, A., & Epipage Study Group. (2005). Temperament at 9 months of very preterm infants born at less than 29 weeks' gestation: The Epipage study. *Journal of Developmental and Behavioral Pediatrics, 26*(1), 48–55.

Latva, R., Korja, R., Salmelin, R. K., et al. (2008). How is maternal recollection of the birth experience related to the behavioral and emotional outcome of preterm infants? *Early Human Development, 84*(9), 587–94.

Lemons, J. A., Bauer, C. R., Oh, W., Korones, S. B., Papile, L. A., Stoll, B. J., et al. (2001). Very low birth weight outcomes of the National Institute of Child Health and human development neonatal research network, January 1995 through December 1996. NICHD Neonatal Research Network. *Pediatrics, 107*(1), E1.

Limperopoulos, C., Bassan, H., Sullivan, N. R., Soul, J. S., Robertson, R. L., Jr., Moore, M., et al. (2008). Positive screening for autism in ex-preterm infants: Prevalence and risk factors. *Pediatrics, 121*(4), 758–65.

Lindström, K., Lindblad, F., & Hjern, A. (2011). Preterm birth and attention-deficit/hyperactivity disorder in schoolchildren. *Pediatrics, 127*(5), 858–65.

Lozoff, B., Clark, K. M., Jing, Y., Armony-Sivan, R., Angelilli, M. L., & Jacobson, S. W. (2008). Dose–response relationships between iron-deficiency with or without anemia and infant social-emotional behavior. *Journal of Pediatrics, 152*(5), 696–702.

Lozoff, B., Klein, N. K., Nelson, E. C., McClish, D. K., Manuel, M., & Chacon, M. E. (1998). Behavior of infants with Iron deficiency anemia. *Child Development, 69*(1), 24–36.

Lund, L. K., Vik, T., Skranes, J., Brubakk, A. M., & Indredavik, M. S. (2011). Psychiatric morbidity in two low birth weight groups assessed by diagnostic interview in young adulthood. *Acta Paediatrica, 100*(4), 598–604.

Lutter, C. K., Daelmans, B. M. E. G., deOnis, M., Kothari, M. T., Ruel, M. T., Arimond, M., et al. (2011). Undernutrition, poor feeding practices, and low coverage of key nutrition interventions. *Pediatrics, 128*, e1418–e1427.

Luyster, R. J., Kuban, K. C., O'Shea, T. M., Paneth, N., Allred, E. N., Leviton, A., et al. (2011). The Modified Checklist for Autism in Toddlers in extremely low gestational age newborns: Individual items associated with motor, cognitive, vision and hearing limitations. *Paediatric and Perinatal Epidemiology, 25*(4), 366–76.

Makrides, M., Gibson, R. A., McPhee, A. J., Yelland, L., Quinlivan, J., & Ryan, P. (2010). Effect of DHA supplementation during pregnancy on maternal depression and neurodevelopment of young children: A randomized controlled trial. *JAMA, 304*(15), 1675–83.

Mandl, K. D., Tronick, E. Z., Brennan, T. A., et al. (1999). Infant health care use and maternal depression. *Archives of Pediatrics & Adolescent Medicine, 153*(8), 808–13.

Mangelsdorf, S. C., Plunkett, J. W., Dedrick, C. F., Berlin, M., Meisels, S. J., McHale, J. L., et al. (1996). Attachment security in very low birth weight infants. *Developmental Psychology, 32*(5), 914–920.

Martin, J. A., Osterman, M. J., & Sutton, P. D. (2010). Are preterm births on the decline in the United States? Recent data from the National Vital Statistics System. *NCHS Data Brief, 39*, 1–8.

McCann, J. B., Stein, A., Fairburn, C. G., & Dunger, D. B. (1994). Eating habits and attitudes of mothers of children with non-organic failure to thrive. *Archives of Disease in Childhood, 70*, 234–36.

McManus, B. M., & Poehlmann, J. (2012). Maternal depression and perceived social support as predictors of cognitive function trajectories during the first 3 years of life for preterm infants in Wisconsin. *Child: Care, Health and Development, 38*(3), 425–34.

Miller, J. E., & Korenman, S. (1994). Poverty and children's nutritional status in the United States. *American Journal of Epidemiology, 140*, 233–243.

Minkovitz, C. S., Strobino, D., Scharfstein, D., et al. (2005). Maternal depressive symptoms and children's receipt of health care in the first 3 years of life. *Pediatrics, 115*(2), 306–14.

Mounts, K. O. (2009). Screening for maternal depression in the neonatal ICU. *Clinics in Perinatology, 36*, 137–152.

Muller-Nix, C., Forcada-Guex, M., Pierrehumbert, B., et al. (2004). Prematurity, maternal stress and mother–child interactions. *Early Human Development, 79*(2), 145–58.

Murray, L., Hipwell, A., Hooper, R., et al. (1996). The cognitive development of 5-year-old children of postnatally depressed mothers. *Journal of Child Psychology and Psychiatry, 37*(8), 927–35.

Murray, L., Arteche, A., Fearon, P., Halligan, S., Croudace, T., & Cooper, P. (2010). The effects of maternal postnatal depression and child sex on academic performance at age 16 years: A developmental approach. *Journal of Child Psychology and Psychiatry, 51*(10), 1150–9.

National Institutes of Child Health and Human Development Early Child Care Research Network Bethesda MD US. (1999). Chronicity of maternal depressive symptoms, maternal sensitivity, and child functioning at 36 months. *Developmental Psychology, 35*(5), 1297–1310.

Olafsen, K. S., Kaaresen, P. I., Handegård, B. H., Ulvund, S. E., Dahl, L. B., & Rønning, J. A. (2008). Maternal ratings of infant regulatory competence from 6 to 12 months: influence of perceived stress, birth-weight, and intervention: A randomized controlled trial. *Infant Behavior & Development, 31*(3), 408–21.

Olsen, E. M., Petersen, J., Skovgaard, A. M., Weile, B., Jørgensen, T., & Wright, C. M. (2007). Failure to thrive: The prevalence and concurrence of anthropometric criteria in a general infant population. *Archives of Disease in Childhood, 92*, 109–114.

Olsen, E. M., Skovgaard, A. M., Weile, B., Petersen, J., & Jørgensen, T. (2010). Risk factors for weight faltering in infancy according to age of onset. *Paediatric and Perinatal Epidemiology, 24*, 370–382.

O'Shea, T. M., et al. (2012). Intraventricular hemorrhage and developmental outcomes at 24 months of age in extremely preterm infants. *Journal of Child Neurology, 27*(1), 22–29.

Patel, V., DeSouza, N., & Rodrigues, M. (2003). Postnatal depression and infant growth and development in low income countries: A cohort study from Goa, India. *Archives of Disease in Childhood, 88*, 34–7.

Patel, V., Rahman, A., Jacob, K. S., & Hughes, M. (2004). Effect of maternal mental health on infant growth in low income countries: New evidence from South Asia. *BMJ, 328*, 820–3.

Patton, R. G., & Gardner, L. I. (1962). Influence of family environment on growth: The syndrome of "maternal deprivation". *Pediatrics, 957–962*.

Peebles-Kleiger, M. J. (2000). Pediatric and neonatal intensive care hospitalization as traumatic stressor: Implications for intervention. *Bulletin of the Menninger Clinic, 64*(2), 257–80.

Perrin, E. C., West, P. D., & Culley, B. S. (1989). Is my child normal yet? Correlates of vulnerability. *Pediatrics, 83*(3), 355–63.

Petrou, S., & Kupek, E. (2010). Poverty and childhood undernutrition in developing countries: A multinational cohort study. *Social Science & Medicine, 71*(7), 1366–1373.

Pierrehumbert, B., Nicole, A., Muller-Nix, C., et al. (2003). Parental post-traumatic reactions after premature birth: Implications for sleeping and eating problems in the infant. *Archives of Disease in Childhood. Fetal and Neonatal Edition, 88*(5), F400–4.

Pinto-Martin, J. A., Levy, S. E., Feldman, J. F., Lorenz, J. M., Paneth, N., & Whitaker, A. H. (2011). Prevalence of autism spectrum disorder in adolescents born weighing <2000 grams. *Pediatrics, 128*(5), 883–91.

Poehlmann, J., & Fiese, B. H. (2001). The interaction of maternal and infant vulnerabilities on developing attachment relationships. *Development and Psychopathology, 13*(1), 1–11.

Poehlmann, J., Schwichtenberg, M. A. J., Bolt, D., et al. (2009). Predictors of depressive symptom trajectories in mothers of infants born preterm or low birthweight. *Journal of Family Psychology, 23*(5), 690–704.

Poehlmann, J., Schwichtenberg, A. J., Shlafer, R. J., Hahn, E., Bianchi, J. P., & Warner, R. (2011). Emerging self-regulation in toddlers born preterm or low birth weight: Differential susceptibility to parenting? *Development and Psychopathology, 23*(1), 177–93.

Potijk, M. R., de Winter, A. F., Bos, A. F., Kerstjens, J. M., & Reijneveld, S. A. (2012). Higher rates of behavioural and emotional problems at preschool age in children born moderately preterm. *Archives of Disease in Childhood, 97*(2), 112–7.

Pyhala, R., et al. (2011). Parental bonding after preterm birth: Child and parent perspectives in the Helsinki study of very low birth weight adults. *The Journal of Pediatrics, 158*(2), 251–256.

Quigley, M. A., Hockley, C., Carson, C., Kelly, Y., Renfrew, M. J., & Sacker, A. (2012). Breastfeeding is associated with improved child cognitive development: A population-based cohort study. *Journal of Pediatrics, 160*(1), 25–32.

Quigley, M. A., et al. (2012). Early term and late preterm birth are associated with poorer school performance at age 5 years: a cohort study. *Archives of Disease in Childhood. Fetal and Neonatal Edition, 97*(3): F167–73.

Quinnell FA (2001) Postpartum posttraumatic stress as a risk factor for atypical cognitive development in high-risk infants. Doctoral dissertation. University of Wisconsin. Milwaukee, Wisconsin.

Rahman, A., Iqbal, Z., Bunn, J., et al. (2004). Impact of maternal depression on infant nutritional status and illness. *Archives of General Psychiatry, 61*(9), 946–52.

Ravn, I. H., Smith, L., Smeby, N. A., Kynoe, N. M., Sandvik, L., Bunch, E. H., et al. (2012). Effects of early mother-infant intervention on outcomes in mothers and moderately and late preterm infants at age 1 year: A randomized control trial. *Infant Behavior & Development, 35*, 36–47.

Raynor, P., Rudolf, M. C., Cooper, K., Marchant, P., & Cottrell, D. (1999). A randomized controlled trial of specialist health visitor intervention for failure to thrive. *Archives of Disease in Childhood, 80*, 500–506.

Rudolf, M. C. J., & Logan, S. (2005). What is the long term outcome for children who fail to thrive? A systematic review. *Archives of Disease in Childhood, 90*, 925–931.

Sameroff, A. J., & Mackenzie, M. J. (2003). Research Strategies for capturing transactional models of development: The limits of the possible. *Development and Psychopathology, 15*(3), 613–40.

Sannino, P., Plevani, L., Bezze, E., & Cornalba, C. (2011). The 'broken' attachment between parents and preterm infant: How and when to intervene. *Early Human Development, 87*(Suppl 1), S81–2.

Santos, I. S., Matijasevich, A., Domingues, M. R., Barros, A. J., Victora, C. G., & Barros, F. C. (2009). Late preterm birth is a risk factor for growth faltering in early childhood: A cohort study. *BMC Pediatrics, 9*, 71.

Santos, I. S., Matijasevich, A., Rodrigues Domingues, M., Barros, A. J. D., & Barros, F. C. F. (2010). Long-lasting maternal depression and child growth at 4 years of age: A cohort study. *The Journal of Pediatrics, 157*, 401–6.

Saxe, G., Vanderbilt, D., & Zuckerman, B. (2003). Traumatic stress in injured and ill children. *PTSD Research Quarterly, 14*(2), 1–7.

Schmidt, L. A., Miskovic, V., Boyle, M. H., & Saigal, S. (2008). Shyness and timidity in young adults who were born at extremely low birth weight. *Pediatrics, 122*(1), e181–7.

Schnurr, P. P., & Jankowski, M. K. (1999). Physical health and post-traumatic stress disorder: Review and synthesis. *Seminars in Clinical Neuropsychiatry, 4*(4), 295–304.

Seng, J. S., Low, L. K., Sperlich, M., Ronis, D. L., & Liberzon, I. (2011). Post-traumatic stress disorder, child abuse history, birthweight and gestational age: A prospective cohort study. *BJOG, 118*(11), 1329–39.

Shah, M. D. (2002). Failure to thrive in children. *Journal of Clinical Gastroenterology, 35*(5), 371–374.

Shah, P. E., Clements, M., & Poehlmann, J. (2011). Maternal resolution of grief after preterm birth: Implications for infant attachment security. *Pediatrics, 127*(2), 284–92.

Shaw, R. J., Bernard, R. S., Deblois, T., et al. (2009). The relationship between acute stress disorder and posttraumatic stress disorder in the neonatal intensive care unit. *Psychosomatics, 50*(2), 131–7.

Showers, J., Mandelkron, R., Coury, D. L., & McCleery, J. (1986). Non-organic failure to thrive: Identification and intervention. *Journal of Pediatric Nursing, 1*, 240–246.

Singer, L. T., Salvator, A., Guo, S., et al. (1999). Maternal psychological distress and parenting stress after the birth of a very-low-birth-weight infant. *JAMA, 281*(9), 799–805.

Spiker, D., Kraemer, H. C., Constantine, N. A., et al. (1992). Reliability and validity of behavior problem checklists as measures of stable traits in low birth weight, premature preschoolers. *Child Development, 63*(6), 1481–96.

Spitz, R. (1945). Hospitalism. *Psychoanalytic Study of the Child, 1*, 53.

Stern, M., Karraker, K. H., Sopko, A. M., & Norman, S. (2000). The prematurity stereotype revisited: Impact on mothers' interactions with premature and full-term infants. *Infant Mental Health Journal, 21*(6), 495–509.

Stewart, R. C. (2007). Maternal depression and infant growth: A review of recent evidence. *Maternal and Child Nutrition, 3*(2), 94–107.

Stoll, B. J., Hansen, N. I., Bell, E. F., Shankaran, S., Laptook, A. R., Walsh, M. C., et al. (2010). Neonatal outcomes of extremely preterm infants from the NICHD Neonatal Research Network. *Pediatrics, 126*(3), 443–456.

Strang-Karlsson, S., Räikkönen, K., Pesonen, A. K., Kajantie, E., Paavonen, E. J., Lahti, J., et al. (2008). Very low birth weight and behavioral symptoms of attention deficit hyperactivity disorder in young adulthood: The Helsinki study of very-low-birth-weight adults. *The American Journal of Psychiatry, 165*(10), 1345–53.

Subramanyam, M. A., Kawachi, I., Berkman, L. F., & Subramanian, S. V. (2010). Socioeconomic inequalities in childhood undernutrition in India: Analyzing trends between 1992 and 2005. *PLoS One, 5*(6), e11392.

Sullivan, P. B. (2004). Commentary: The epidemiology of failure-to-thrive in infants. *International Journal of Epidemiology, 33*, 847–848.

Surkan, P. J., Kennedy, C. E., Hurley, K. M., & Black, M. M. (2011). Maternal depression and early childhood growth in developing countries: Systematic review and meta-analysis. *Bulletin of the World Health Organization, 89*(8), 608–15.

Tessier, R., Cristo, M. B., Velez, S., Giron, M., Nadeau, L., Figueroa, Z., et al. (2003). Kangaroo mother care: A method for protecting high-risk low birth weight and premature infants against developmental delay. *Infant Behavior & Development, 26*(3), 384–97.

Tharner, A., Luijk, M. P., van Ijzendoorn, M. H., Bakermans-Kranenburg, M. J., Jaddoe, V. W., Hofman, A., et al. (2012). Maternal lifetime history of depression and depressive symptoms in the prenatal and early postnatal period do not predict infant–mother attachment quality in a large, population-based Dutch cohort study. *Attachment & Human Development, 14*(1), 63–81.

Trapolini, T., McMahon, C. A., & Ungerer, J. A. (2007). The effect of maternal depression and marital adjustment on young children's internalizing and externalizing behaviour problems. *Child: Care, Health and Development, 33*(6), 794–803.

Treyvaud, K., Doyle, L. W., Lee, K. J., Roberts, G., Cheong, J. L., Inder, T. E., et al. (2011). Family functioning, burden and parenting stress 2 years after very preterm birth. *Early Human Development, 87*(6), 427–31.

Vanderbilt, D., Bushley, T., Young, R., & Frank, D. A. (2009). Acute posttraumatic stress symptoms among urban mothers with newborns in the neonatal intensive care unit: A preliminary study. *Journal of Developmental and Behavioral Pediatrics, 30*(1), 50–6.

Vanderbilt, D., & Gleason, M. M. (2011). Mental health concerns of the premature infant through the lifespan. *Pediatric Clinics of North America, 58*(4), 815–32. ix.

Vigod, S. N., Villegas, L., Dennis, C. L., & Ross, L. E. (2010). Prevalence and risk factors for postpartum depression among women with preterm and low-birth-weight infants: A systematic review. *BJOG, 117*(5), 540–50.

Vohr, B. R., Stephens, B. E., Higgins, R. D., Bann, C. M., Hintz, S. R., Das, A., et al. (2012). Are outcomes of extremely preterm infants improving? Impact of Bayley Assessment on outcomes. *The Journal of Pediatrics, 161*(2), 222–8.

Vohr, B. R., Poindexter, B. B., Dusick, A. M., McKinley, L. T., Wright, L. L., Langer, J. C., et al. (2006). Beneficial effects of breast milk in the neonatal intensive care unit on the developmental outcome of extremely low birth weight infants at 18 months of age. *Pediatrics, 118*(1), e115–23.

Wallin, L., & Eriksson, M. (2009). Newborn Individual Development Care and Assessment Program (NIDCAP): A systematic review of the literature. *Worldviews on Evidence-based Nursing, 6*(2), 54–69.

Wan, M. W., & Green, J. (2009). The impact of maternal psychopathology on child–mother attachment. *Archives of Women's Mental Health, 12*(3), 123–34.

Wang, Y., Monteiro, C., & Popkin, B. M. (2002). Trends of obesity and underweight in older children and adolescents in the United States, Brazil, China, and Russia. *American Journal of Clinical Nutrition, 75*, 971–977.

Weil, M. H., & Tang, W. (2011). From intensive care to critical care medicine: A historical perspective. *American Journal of Respiratory and Critical Care Medicine, 183*(11), 1451–3.

Whitaker, A. H., Feldman, J. F., Lorenz, J. M., McNicholas, F., Fisher, P. W., Shen, S., et al. (2011). Neonatal head ultrasound abnormalities in preterm infants and adolescent psychiatric disorders. *Archives of General Psychiatry, 68*(7), 742–52.

Wright, C. M. (2000). Identification and management of failure to thrive: A community perspective. *Archives of Disease in Childhood, 82*, 5–9.

Wright, C. M., Parkinson, K. N., & Drewett, R. F. (2006a). How does maternal and child feeding behavior relate to weight gain and failure to thrive? Data from a prospective birth cohort. *Pediatrics, 117*, 1262–1269.

Wright, C. M., Parkinson, K. N., & Drewett, R. F. (2006b). The influence of maternal socioeconomic and emotional factors on infant weight gain and weight faltering (failure to thrive): data from a prospective birth cohort. *Archives of Disease in Childhood, 91*, 312–317.

Zelkowitz, P., Na, S., Wang, T., Bardin, C., & Papageorgiou, A. (2011). Early maternal anxiety predicts cognitive and behavioural outcomes of VLBW children at 24 months corrected age. *Acta Paediatrica, 100*(5), 700–4.

Eleanor L. McGlinchey and Allison G. Harvey

Sleep and Sleep Disturbance

Sleep is fundamental for multiple domains of health and functioning across development. There is a 60–80 % increase in the odds of being a short sleeper among children who are obese (Cappuccio et al., 2008), there is robust evidence that sleep deprivation undermines emotion regulation among youth (McGlinchey et al., 2011; Talbot, McGlinchey, Kaplan, Dahl, & Harvey, 2010), and inadequate sleep compromises learning (Dewald et al., 2010; Sadeh, Gruber, & Raviv, 2003). Clearly, inadequate or disturbed sleep in childhood and adolescence may have immediate adverse effects in domains important for optimal development, with potential long-term consequences of great concern.

For the clinician wanting to provide effective prevention, diagnosis, and treatment of sleep problems or appropriate referral for the evalua-tion of more serious disorders, knowledge and clinical skills are needed in two major areas. First, it is important to understand normal sleep physiology and the normal development of sleep patterns in children and adolescents. Second, it is important to have knowledge of common sleep disorders in children and teens. In addition to knowledge of these common disorders, it is important to develop clinical skills relevant to assessing sleep habits, diagnosing sleep disorders, and understanding treatment principles, particularly behavioral interventions that can have several advantages relative to pharmacologic interventions.

Sleep Across Development

Beginning in infancy, the brain cycles through stages of neural activity/behavioral states which correspond to periods of wakefulness and different stages of sleep. "Mature" sleep is divided into two major categories: rapid eye movement (REM) sleep and non-REM (NREM) sleep. NREM sleep is subdivided into 4 stages: Stage 1 occurs at transitions of sleep and wakefulness; Stage 2 is characterized by frequent bursts of rhythmic electroencephalography (EEG) activity, called sleep spindles, and high-voltage slow spikes, called K-complexes; Stages 3 and 4 (also called slow wave sleep or delta sleep) represent the deepest stages of sleep and are comprised largely of high-voltage EEG activity in the

E.L. McGlinchey, Ph.D.
Division of Child and Adolescent Psychiatry,
Columbia University Medical Center,
New York State Psychiatric Institute, New York,
NY 10032, USA

A.G. Harvey, Ph.D. (✉)
Department of Psychology,
The Golden Bear Sleep and Mood Research Clinic,
Clinical Science Program and Psychology Clinic,
University of California, Berkeley,
CA 94720-1650, USA
e-mail: aharvey@berkeley.edu

slowest (delta) frequency range. In newborn infants, each sleep cycle is around 60 min, with 50 % in "active sleep" and 50 % in "quiet sleep." Active sleep is similar to REM sleep in adults and involves head movements, rapid eye movements, fast and irregular respiration, and increased heart rate. Quiet sleep is similar to NREM sleep in adults and involves few movements. By about 2 years of age, active sleep declines to 20–25 %. By 6–11 years of age, clearer cycles of sleep, each about 90 min, emerge such that the amount of Stages 3 and 4 sleep and REM reduces and Stage 2 sleep increases (Hoban, 2004). By around 11 years of age, slow wave sleep is at 40 % and continues to decline across adolescence. REM sleep is retained across childhood, adolescence, adulthood, and older adults, whereas slow wave sleep decreases across the age range.

Two independent regulatory processes interact to regulate the timing, intensity, and duration of sleep: a homeostatic sleep process and a circadian sleep process (Borbély, 1982; Borbély & Achermann, 2005). The first, often called "Process S," represents a sleep–wake-dependent homeostatic component of sleep that increases as a function of previous wakefulness and gradually decreases over the course of a sleep period. The second process, often called "Process C," is the circadian component, which arises from the endogenous pacemaker in the suprachiasmatic nuclei (SCN) (Reppert & Weaver, 2002). At the molecular level, intrinsically rhythmic cells within the SCN generate rhythmicity via an autoregulatory transcription–translation feedback loop regulating expression of circadian genes. The process by which the pacemaker is set to a 24-h period and kept in appropriate phase with seasonally shifting day length is called entrainment, which occurs via zeitgebers. The primary zeitgeber is the daily alteration of light and dark (Roennebert & Foster, 1997). The SCN is also responsive to non-photic cues such as arousal/locomotor activity, social cues, feeding, sleep deprivation, and temperature (Mistlberger, Antle, Glass, & Miller, 2000).

The Nature of Sleep Disturbance in Children

Sleep disruption is the most common parental concern addressed with pediatricians (Ferber, 1985). Problems at bedtime and frequent overnight wakings are highly prevalent in young children and teens. Recent estimates indicate that as many as 20–30 % of infants, toddlers, and young children experience sleep problems (Lozoff, Wolf, & Davis, 1985; Mindell, 1996, 1999). Unfortunately, untreated sleep problems first presenting in infancy are known to persist during school-aged years and often become chronic (Pollock, 1994; Zuckerman, Stevenson, & Bailey, 1987). The hypothesis has been that there are neurodevelopmental, biological, and circadian factors, influenced by environmental and behavioral factors, all working together to support the sometimes elusive milestone of "sleeping through the night." In other words, although sleep consolidation and sleep regulation develop primarily through the process of maturation of the neural and circadian systems, the environment and context in which this maturation takes place also have an influence on sleep and disorders of sleep (Mirmiran, Maas, & Ariagno, 2003; Sadeh & Anders, 1993).

There are many potential factors that constitute vulnerability toward sleep problems. Additionally, there are factors that appear to maintain night wakings, making them more difficult to reverse. The most common vulnerability factor has been associated with child temperament; namely, children who are known to be difficult to calm are least likely to fall asleep or stay asleep without the assistance of a caregiver (Carey, 1974; Owens-Stively et al., 1997). There is also a relationship between current medical issues or history of serious medical problems and sleep difficulties in young children. It can be particularly difficult for caregivers of children with medical problems to tease apart when a child should be comforted at bedtime as opposed to setting a limit.

Additional factors that may perpetuate sleep problems in young children include caregiver attributes including symptoms of depression (Gress-Smith, Luecken, Lemery-Chalfant, & Howe, 2012) and parental work schedule (Sinai & Tikotzky, 2012). Recent research also suggests that when the parental expectations for sleep behavior do not match the typical development of childhood sleep habits, poor sleep among young children is common (Tikotzky & Sadeh, 2009). Research also suggests that these caregiver factors reduce the ability for the parent to set clear limits and structure appropriate bedtime routines.

Finally, there are environmental factors that may exacerbate problems that the child has with falling asleep or also with parental difficulties in setting clear limits for bedtime (Mindell, Kuhn, Lewin, Meltzer, & Sadeh, 2006). Some examples are housing arrangements where family members sleep in the same room as the child. However, as is the case with parental attributes, the influence of the family of origin's culture and socioeconomic status should be considered when interpreting the potential causes or maintaining factors in childhood sleep problems.

Common Sleep Disorders in Children and Teens: Description, Assessment, and Treatment

Given the potential perpetuating and maintaining factors in childhood sleep problems presented above, there are opportunities to use behavioral modification strategies to treat the maladaptive behaviors. Knowledge about assessment, diagnosis, and treatment of sleep difficulties across development is critical. Moreover, this knowledge provides a critical foundation of expertise relevant to understanding (and effectively intervening in) a broad range of common emotional and health problems in children and adolescents.

Problems Going to Sleep and Staying Asleep in Young Children

Bedtime struggles and middle of the night wakings are not only a source of sleep disruption for children and their parents but also can be a source of conflict and negative emotion among family members, contributing to negative parent–child interactions and marital discord. One aspect of the difficulty is that young children often show a "paradoxical" reaction when obtaining insufficient or inadequate sleep. That is, sleep-deprived young children (whether from insufficient or disrupted sleep) often look irritable, impulsive, with some symptoms of distractibility and emotional lability, and may seem overly active.

Interventions for bedtime problems and night wakings are founded on principles of learning and behavior (e.g., reinforcement, extinction, shaping). Treatments involve training parents with a therapist guiding interventions on how to change their child's problematic sleep habits or sleep-related behaviors. The different behavioral interventions for early childhood sleep difficulties and the level of empirical support for each has been reviewed in a recent practice parameters paper commissioned by the American Association for Sleep Medicine (Mindell et al., 2006). The first of these interventions is unmodified extinction and involves having the parents put the child to bed at a designated bedtime and then ignoring any crying, tantruming, or calling out by the child until a set time the next morning (although parents monitor for illness, injury, etc.). The effective use of extinction requires parental consistency. No matter how long the crying lasts, parents must ignore this every night. Otherwise, the child will only learn to cry longer the next time. One difficulty with this approach is that postextinction response bursts may occur. That is, often at some later date, there is a return of the original bedtime resistance or overnight waking. Parents must again avoid inadvertently reinforcing the inappropriate behavior following such a postextinction burst. The common term used in the media and self-help books to describe unmodified extinction techniques is the "cry it out" approach (Ferber, 1985). The difficulty with the use of unmodified extinction procedures is that it is often perceived as stressful by parents and many are not able to ignore the crying long enough for the procedure to be effective. An alternative to unmodified extinction is extinction with parental presence. In this variant, the parent stays in the child's room at bedtime but ignores the child and his/her problematic behavior. For some parents this procedure helps them to be more consistent and is more acceptable to them.

Another intervention based on extinction principals is "Graduated Extinction." Parents are instructed to ignore bedtime crying and tantrums on a specified schedule of check-ins. The period between check-ins is often tailored with the guidance of a therapist with considerations for the child's age, temperament, and the parents' judgment of how long they can tolerate the child's crying. Parents can also choose to check on their child on a fixed schedule (e.g., every 5 min) or with incrementally longer intervals (e.g., 5 min, 10 min, then 15 min). When using incrementally longer intervals, increases across successive checks within the same night or across successive nights can gradually reduce to no check-ins. Parents should only comfort their child for a brief period and no longer than a minute. Through the use of Graduated Extinction, the child will develop "self-soothing" skills so that he/she falls asleep independently without the parent. In self-help books, this type of intervention is often referred to as "sleep training" (Mindell, 2005).

Behavioral interventions can also include powerful methods for increasing homeostatic drive to sleep, such as developmental adaptations of stimulus control and sleep restriction which involve a small amount of sleep restriction that builds the homeostatic process.

Positive Routines are an intervention that involves the parents developing a routine at bedtime that is characterized by quiet and enjoyable activities for the child. Faded bedtime is often used with Positive Routines and involves taking the child out of bed for predetermined periods of time when the child does not fall asleep. Bedtime is also delayed so that sleep onset occurs quickly and so that the cues for sleep are paired with the enjoyable activities from the Positive Routines procedure. Once the behavioral chain of events is well established and the child falls asleep more quickly, bedtime is moved earlier by 15–30 min over successive nights until an age-appropriate bedtime goal is achieved. In addition, when overnight wakings are the primary problem, scheduled

awakenings can be used. This procedure involves the parent awakening and comforting their child approximately 15–30 min before a typical awakening. Prior to using this strategy, a baseline of the number and timing of the nighttime awakenings must be established. Preemptive awakenings are then scheduled and can involve rocking or nursing the child back to sleep. Over consecutive nights, scheduled awakenings are faded out, by gradually increasing the time span between awakenings. Scheduled awakenings have been shown to increase the duration of consolidated sleep (Rickert & Johnson, 1988).

Another approach to treatment of sleep disturbances is to *prevent* their occurrence. A number of behavioral interventions have been incorporated into new parent education programs. These programs typically focus on early establishment of positive sleep habits. Education in these programs targets bedtime routines, development of a consistent schedule, parental soothing techniques during sleep initiation, and parent response to nighttime awakenings. Additionally, almost all programs recommend that parents should put babies to bed "drowsy but awake" so that they can develop independent sleep initiation skills. Moreover, this can help babies return to sleep without parental intervention following naturally occurring nighttime arousals. Among the forms of behavioral health services for children, no other treatment has been more thoroughly researched or broadly applied as parent education training (Kazdin, 2005).

In a recent review of behavioral interventions, the average percentage of infants and young children who improved was 82 % (range 10–100 %) (Mindell et al., 2006). Overall, the weight of the evidence from controlled group studies supports unmodified extinction and parent education/prevention. Graduated Extinction, bedtime fading/positive routines, and scheduled awakenings are also well supported in empirical literature. Standardized bedtime routines and positive reinforcement techniques have often been incorporated as part of a multicomponent treatment package; however, there is limited empirical support for their effectiveness as stand-alone interventions.

Problems Going to Sleep and Staying Asleep in Older Children and Adolescents

Insomnia

Insomnia is a common complaint among older children and adolescents, particularly sleep-onset insomnia. Cognitive behavioral treatments for insomnia (CBT-I) include a range of powerful behavioral adjustments to sleep. The evidence that CBT-I produces reliable and durable changes in sleep *in adults* has been summarized in multiple meta-analyses (Morin, Culbert, & Schwartz, 1994; Murtagh & Greenwood, 1995; Smith et al., 2002) and two practice parameters papers commissioned by the American Academy of Sleep Medicine (Morin et al., 1999, 2006). Among youth, there is less evidence for the use of CBT-I; however, this is a growing area of research. For example, Bootzin and Stevens (2005) conducted an uncontrolled trial of CBT-I for adolescents with insomnia and substance use problems ($n=55$). Self-reported drug problems declined for completers at follow-up evaluations while continuing to increase for non-completers. Improved sleep was also associated with decreased aggression (Bootzin & Stevens, 2005).

In our experience, there are a range of important components of a behavioral intervention for insomnia. A brief description of each follows:

(a) *Functional analysis/case formulation and goal setting*. The frequency, intensity, and duration as well as the antecedents, behaviors, and consequences will be assessed across four time points: before bed (e.g., use of technology), during the night (e.g., cell phone left on), on waking (e.g., severe sleepiness, lethargy), and during the day (e.g., caffeine use). Goals are identified and operationalized.

(b) *Motivational enhancement (ME)*. This component is critical given that eveningness is associated with poor self-regulation (Digdon & Howell, 2008). A recent meta-analysis (Hettema, Steele, & Miller, 2005) found that ME significantly increases youth motivation. ME involves a straightforward review of perceived pros and cons of change (Miller & Rollnick, 2002) recognizing that many sleep-incompatible/interfering behaviors used by youth are rewarding (e.g., text messaging with friends).

(c) *Sleep and circadian education* (Kaplan & Harvey, 2009). Guided by the teens' interest, this may include the association with weight gain (Cappuccio et al., 2008), eating poorly (Spiegel, Tasali, Penev, & Van Cauter, 2004), and/or attractiveness (Seidel et al., 1984). Second, we provide education on the circadian system, the environmental influences acting on it (particularly light), and the tendency if left unchecked to move toward a delayed phase. Third, sleep inertia is defined and normalized. Sleep inertia is the 5–20-min period on waking that is the normal transitional state between sleep and wakefulness (Tassi & Muzet, 2000). We acknowledge that these feelings are not pleasant but do not necessarily indicate having had a poor night of sleep.

(d) *Shifting and regularizing the sleep–wake window*. Stimulus control (Bootzin, 1972) is an important component for regularizing the sleep–wake cycle and strengthening the association between the bed and sleeping (Bootzin, 1972; Bootzin & Stevens, 2005). Building the motivation for the teen to wake at the same time [including on weekends (Crowley & Carskadon, 2010)] is a key focus. The routine wake-up time promotes sleepiness in the evening, particularly when naps are avoided, which enables the teen to progressively move their bedtime forward by 20–30 min per week (small enough that the circadian system can adapt).

(e) *Wind down*. Typically youth need assistance to devise a "wind-down" period of 30–60 min prior to sleep in which relaxing, sleep-enhancing activities are introduced, *in dim light conditions*. The latter is important for helping the circadian phase advance, as well as for the maintenance of entrainment on a less owl-like schedule (Wyatt, Stepanski, & Kirkby, 2006). A central issue is the use of electronic media (Internet, cell phones, MP3 players). ME and behavioral experiments are used to facilitate individuals voluntarily *choosing* an electronic curfew. It is crucial to acknowledge that contact with peers is a vital aspect of adolescents' social environment and to work with teens on alternatives to pre-bed social interaction. We introduce behavioral strategies to limit pre-bedtime technology use (e.g., keeping phone chargers in the kitchen).

(f) *Wake up.* This is individualized but typically includes not hitting snooze on the alarm, opening the curtains to let sunlight in, spending the first 30–60 min after waking outside or in a room with bright lights, and making the bed so the incentive to get back in is reduced.

(g) *Unhelpful beliefs about sleep.* Altering beliefs about sleep is important (Edinger, Wohlgemuth, Radtke, Marsh, & Quillian, 2001). Typical unhelpful beliefs about sleep held by youth include "there is no point going to bed earlier because I won't be able to fall asleep," "sleep is a waste of time," and "I can train myself to get less sleep." Guided discovery and individualized experiments test the validity and utility of the beliefs (Harvey, Sharpley, Ree, Stinson, & Clark, 2007; Ree & Harvey, 2004).

(h) *Bedtime worry, rumination, and vigilance.* Many youth attribute difficulty getting to sleep to negative (worry/rumination) and positive thoughts (Harvey, Schmidt, Scarna, Semler, & Goodwin, 2005). As anxiety (Espie, 2002) and negative or positive worry/ rumination (Harvey, 2005) are antithetical to sleep onset, it is important to manage bedtime worry, rumination, and anxiety. This is individualized but can include savoring (McMakin, Siegle, & Shirk, 2011), cognitive therapy to evaluate worry and rumination, diary writing or scheduling a "worry period" to process worry prior to bedtime, and creating a "to-do" list.

(i) *Daytime coping.* Teens typically believe that the only way they can feel less tired in the daytime is to sleep more. Hence, behavioral experiments are devised to allow the teen to *experience* the energy-generating effects of activity (Ree & Harvey, 2004). This is also an opportunity to develop a list of "energy-generating" and "energy-sapping" activities which can be used to manage daytime tiredness, the "post-lunch" circadian dip in alertness, and build resilience toward inevitable bouts of sleep deprivation that occasionally occur.

(j) *Relapse prevention.* The goal is to consolidate gains and prepare for setbacks. A critical element is to stress the need for regularizing the sleep schedule after treatment which is critical for maintaining the more adaptive relationship between entrained circadian phase and the earlier sleep–wake schedule. It is guided by an individualized summary of learning and achievements. Areas needing further intervention are addressed by setting specific goals and creating plans for achieving each goal.

Delayed Sleep Phase Syndrome

There is evidence that the onset of puberty triggers a change toward a distinct evening preference among approximately 40 % of teens (Carskadon, Acebo, Richardson, Tate, & Seifer, 1997; Gianotti & Cortesi, 2002; Lee, Hummer, Jechura, & Mahoney, 2004; Roenneberg et al., 2004; Tonetti, Fabbri, & Natale, 2008), which is then exacerbated by various social (e.g., importance of peers, parents less involved in decisions regarding bed and waketimes), psychological (e.g., increased pressure at school), and behavioral factors (e.g., use of social media in bed and during the night). Together these factors can contribute to a tendency toward eveningness or, in the extreme, delayed sleep phase syndrome (DSPS) (Okawa, Uchiyama, Ozaki, Shibui, & Ichikawa, 1998; Regestein & Monk, 1995). Problems with delayed sleep in children and adolescents can be further compounded by large differences between weekday and weekend schedules. For example, an adolescent who has been going to bed at 3 AM and getting up at noon during a vacation tries to go bed at 10 PM the Sunday night before the first day back at school finds that his/her physiology is quite resistant to sleep. For a few days, he/she manages to get up for school by overriding the system (despite inadequate sleep) but then takes a long nap after school. Despite numerous nights of trying to go to bed at 10 PM, he/she is unable to shift his/her circadian system back to an earlier phase.

There is a small treatment literature on DSPS in teens (Okawa et al., 1998; Regestein & Monk, 1995) (Gradisar et al., 2011), including the use of timed light with teens (Crowley, Acebo, & Carskadon, 2007), as well as practice parameters (Sack et al., 2007) that indicate evidence for timed light exposure (with a light box) and planned and regular sleep schedules (chronotherapy) *in adults*. Two developmental adaptations may be appropriate although note that these require future research. First, teens tend not to be motivated to use a light box; hence, we suggest the use of natural morning light and evening dim light with youth-selected electronic curfews. Second, traditional chronotherapy involving progressively delaying bedtimes and waketimes until reaching the desired alignment tend to be highly disruptive to family and work schedules (Czeisler et al., 1981; Thorpy, Korman, Spielman, & Glovinsky, 1988; Weitzman et al., 1981), so we suggest adopting a planned sleep modification protocol derived from circadian principles involving moving bedtimes earlier by 20–30 min per week.

There is a subgroup of adolescents who appear to have trouble following an early schedule but are not particularly troubled by their late schedule. These adolescents are not motivated to correct the problem, are not particularly troubled by their recurrent experiences of being late for or missing school, and do not show great motivation to change their late-night habits. These adolescents are essentially choosing a late-night schedule. Unless the clinician is able to alter the larger realm of priorities and motivators, these adolescents are very unlikely to respond to any treatment of a sleep/schedule problem.

Daytime Sleepiness/Difficulty Waking up for School

After the onset of puberty and throughout the adolescent period, the most prevalent sleep complaints tend to center on difficulty waking up for school in the morning and the associated difficulties with daytime sleepiness, tiredness, and irritability. It is important to emphasize that there is a broad continuum of severity. This ranges from normative/mild difficulties that appear to affect up to half of all high school students in the USA and result in at least some symptoms (National Sleep Foundation, 2006) to a much smaller subset of adolescents with severe difficulties with sleep and schedules that result in significant impairments (such as failures in school) and often meet full criteria for DSPS. At the current time, there is an absence of empirical data to help delineate precisely when to diagnose adolescents as having DSPS disorder from the much larger set of youth with mild to moderate problems with erratic and late sleep schedules. One pragmatic approach is that clinicians understand both the physiological and social influences that contribute to these problems and apply sound behavioral principles aimed at improving and increasing sleep in any adolescent who shows evidence of suboptimal sleep as a result of late-night and erratic schedules, as already described. In the adolescents with true sleepiness (not simply complaints of fatigue) two main categories of problems should be considered: (1) inadequate amounts of sleep and (2) circadian and scheduling disorders. Circadian disorders were discussed above (DSPS). In terms of inadequate amounts of sleep, the most common cause of mild to moderate sleepiness in adolescents is an inadequate number of hours in bed. A combination of social schedules leading to late nights with early morning school requirements can significantly compress the number of hours of sleep. Part-time jobs, sports activities, hobbies, and active social lives can exacerbate this problem. The catch-up sleep of naps, weekends, and holidays can also contribute to the problem by leading to erratic schedules and even later nights. In taking a sleep history, it is important to ask specific questions about bedtime schedules. Many families will say the adolescent "usually" goes to bed at a certain time, but when asked for an exact time covering the previous few nights, a much later hour is reported. When assessing the amount of sleep an adolescent is getting, it is important to obtain details of bedtime (such as when the child gets into bed as well as lights-out time), estimates of sleep latency, nighttime arousals, time of getting up in the morning, difficulty getting up, and the frequency, timing, and duration of daytime naps. It is also essential to get details of sleep–wake schedules on weekends, as well as during the school week. When this type of specific information is obtained either by interview or by having the family maintain a sleep diary, evidence of inadequate sleep is often evident. A prospective detailed sleep diary provides the most reliable information.

When inadequate sleep is identified, simply recommending that the adolescent go to bed earlier is not likely to be effective. Often, the primary role of the clinician is to help the entire family understand and acknowledge the consequences resulting from the inadequate sleep. Sleep deprivation frequently contributes to many factors that the family identifies as problems, including falling asleep in school, oversleeping in the morning, fatigue, and irritability. In cases in which the adolescent's school or social functioning is significantly impaired by sleep problems, a strict behavioral contract that is agreed upon by the family can be essential. The contract should specify hours in bed (with only *small* deviations on the weekends) and should target the specific behaviors contributing to bad sleep habits, such as specific late-night activities, erratic napping, or oversleeping for school. The choice of rewards for successes and negative consequences for failures, as well as an accurate method of assessing compliance, are essential components of the contract.

Other behavioral components include education about sleep inertia, which is defined and normalized. Sleep inertia is the 5–20-min period on waking that is the normal transitional state between sleep and wakefulness (Tassi & Muzet, 2000). We acknowledge that these feelings are not pleasant but do not necessarily indicate having had a poor night of sleep. This is individualized but typically includes not hitting snooze on the alarm, opening the curtains to let sunlight in, spending the first 30–60 min after waking outside or in a room with bright lights, and making the

bed so the incentive to get back in is reduced. Teens typically believe that the only way they can feel less tired in the daytime is to sleep more. Hence, behavioral experiments are devised to allow the teen to *experience* the energy-generating effects of activity (Ree & Harvey, 2004). This is also an opportunity to develop a list of "energy-generating" and "energy-sapping" activities which can be used to manage daytime tiredness, the "post-lunch" circadian dip in alertness, and build resilience toward inevitable bouts of sleep deprivation that occasionally occur.

Note on Use of Medications for Treating Sleep Difficulties in Children and Adolescents

One contentious issue in the domain of treating sleep problems in children and adolescents with difficulty going to sleep is the use of medications to promote sleep onset (Owens, Rosen, & Mindell, 2003). Indeed, there are large numbers of medications prescribed for children of all ages in attempt to hasten sleep onset. Adult sleep pharmacology has seen numerous advances, including new generation agents with a much better specificity for sleep, duration of action, and relatively low risk and side effects *in adults*. Therefore, one might logically argue that some of these medications might represent treatment options for insomnia in children and adolescents. However, until we have empirical data and controlled trials using these medications in youth (including dosing, side effects, and efficacy), we are reluctant to advocate any specific medication at this time. We note that while there have been trials of melatonin for teens (Jan et al., 2000; Szeinberg, Borodkin, & Dagan, 2000), there are safety concerns about the impact on the reproductive endocrine system (Arendt, 1997; Malpaux, Thiéry, & Chemineau, 1999; Wyatt, 2007). Also, there are questions about whether the sleep obtained confers the full benefit of "natural" sleep or sleep in the absence of medications (Seibt et al., 2008). For example, Seibt and colleagues (2008) investigated the impact of zolpidem (Ambien) on the development of the visual system in kittens 28–41 days old. As expected, zolpidem *increased* NREM sleep by 27 % and *increased* total sleep over the 8-h period. However, rather alarmingly, zolpidem *reduced* cortical plasticity by 50 %. The authors concluded that *hypnotics that produce more "physiological" sleep based on EEG may actually impair critical sleep-dependent brain processes during development*. This finding should stimulate new research into the safety of certain pharmacologic agents, particularly regarding impacts on the developing bodies and brains of children and adolescents. There may also be implications for adults who continue to need sleep for growth, repair, learning, plasticity, and optimal emotional functioning.

The Child with Parasomnias

Parasomnias occur commonly in children as sudden, partial awakenings from deep, non-REM sleep into a mixed state which has some aspects of being awake and some aspects of being in a deep sleep. There appear to be at least two routes to this mixed state: (1) difficulty leaving deep sleep (Stage 3 and 4) at the end of the first sleep cycle or (2) a sudden disturbance or disruption during the middle of deep sleep. The events include sleepwalking, night terrors, and confused partial arousals (some enuretic events can also occur as partial arousals). Although the specific types of arousal (sleepwalking versus night terror) are sometimes considered separate entities. These behaviors represent a spectrum of related phenomena with respect to sleep physiology. The *intense* events (with screaming, agitated flailing, and running) represent the extreme *end* of a spectrum of partial arousal behaviors that occur in mild forms (such as calm mumbling or a few awkward movements) in many children. The events can last from a few seconds to 20 min, with an average duration of about 3 min. The termination is usually as sudden as the initiation, with a rapid return to deep sleep. During the events, the children may seem confused, often not recognizing their parents, being inconsolable, and often appearing incoherent.

Overtiredness from any source (whether sleep deprivation, sleep disruption, or erratic schedule) can increase or precipitate partial arousals. Any time a child is adjusting to getting less sleep, or has disturbed nighttime sleep, the physiological compensation is to get deeper sleep (especially in the first 1 to 2 h after sleep onset). This deep "recovery" sleep appears to be fertile ground for partial arousal events. A second theme of associated features is in the realm of psychological/emotional factors. Particularly with respect to night terrors, much has been written about the association with particular psychological states, such as anxiety, trauma, stressful events, and repressed aggression (Ferber, 1989; Klackenberg, 1982). These psychological factors may contribute to sleep loss. For example, emotional and behavioral problems are also associated with difficulty falling asleep, as occurs with depression and anxiety in children (Ryan et al., 1987). Likewise, externalizing disorders, such as attention-deficit disorder and conduct disorder, can be accompanied by oppositional behaviors around bedtime, which may delay sleep onset, as well as occasional difficulties falling asleep (Ryan et al., 1987).

When a parasomnia is suspected, the clinical interview should include obtaining a careful history of all sleep-related habits, as well as the characteristics, pattern, and frequency of the events. The pattern of events should also be assessed. Occurrence in the first third of the night and an increased frequency corresponding to periods of being overly tired are strongly suggestive of typical partial arousal events.

Given the wide range of intensity and clinical significance of these nocturnal partial arousals, the key to therapy is matching the appropriate intervention to the degree of problem. That is, mild sleepwalking or an occasional night terror in a young child requires only some parental reassurance with general suggesstions regarding improved sleep habits and the likelihood that the events will decrease over time. First, educate the family about the events (and what to do during the actual partial arousal event). For mild to moderate events, the parents should try to direct the child to go back to bed and back to sleep. Physically taking the child by the hand and leading him/her back to bed during a mild event can also be effective. Usually, however, the event needs to take its course and will end spontaneously. During more agitated arousals, interventions trying to direct the child back to bed can result in increased arousal and can inadvertently prolong the event. In general, if mild directing of the child does not work, the parents should let the episode run its course. One very important caveat to this advice is with respect to the *need to prevent self-injury*. Eliminating factors such as sleeping on the top bunk bed, having a bedroom near the top of the stairs, or having windows or dangerous objects in the room are major considerations.

Second, encourage a regular sleep–wake schedule with good sleep habits. The parents should consider an earlier bedtime if there is any evidence that the child is getting inadequate sleep. Specific causes of delayed bedtime or difficulty falling asleep should also be directly addressed. It is important to try to improve the overall quantity and/or quality of sleep of the child when applicable.

Third, help the child feel safe, secure, and relaxed at bedtime and to identify and express sources of stress, anxiety, and fear in a supportive environment. If there is evidence that anxiety and unexpressed anger may contribute to the frequency of these partial arousal events, the family should be encouraged to facilitate their child expressing sources of anxieties, fears, anger, and conflicts in healthy ways while awake. Age-appropriate suggestions of positive family interactions within this realm can be very helpful. Also, helping children focus on positive images and positive relaxation exercises can help to foster feelings of safety and security at bedtime.

Finally, for the more frequent, repetitive, intense, and agitated sleep terrors, these can be treated effectively through the use of scheduled awakenings (Durand, 2002; Durand & Mindell, 1990). Similar to the scheduled awakenings described previously, the child is lightly awakened and allowed to fall back to sleep 15–30 min prior to the usual time of the episodes (Durand, 2008). After about a week of this intervention, the sleep terrors typically are reduced or eliminated.

Sleep-Disordered Breathing

Sleep apnea and a related set of problems called sleep-disordered breathing can contribute to fragmented sleep (and possibly intermittent hypoxia; Gozal & Kheirandish, 2006; Kheirandish & Gozal, 2006) that can contribute to daytime difficulties with cognitive and affective functioning. In particular, difficulties with irritability, attentional difficulties, and emotional lability can be created and/or exacerbated by sleep-disordered breathing in children. Although the actual number of minutes of arousal during the night may be small, the repeated, chronic, but brief disruptions in sleep can lead to significant daytime symptoms in children. It is important to note that the child is usually unaware of waking up, and the parent often describes very restless sleep but usually does not describe the child's waking up completely. The most frequent symptoms reported by families include loud chronic snoring (or noisy breathing); restless sleep with unusual sleeping positions (attempts by the child to move and open the airway); a history of problems with tonsils, adenoids, and/or ear infections; and signs of inadequate nighttime sleep.

In medical centers with pediatric sleep facilities consultation with a child sleep specialist can be extremely helpful in sorting out decisions in these cases. A few recent references provide excellent reviews of the complex issues (Ferber, 1996; Marcus, 1997). In 2011, the first of three papers was published on the respiratory indications for polysomnography (PSG) in children (Aurora et al., 2011). Standard recommendations for PSG use in children with suspected sleep-related breathing disorders include PSG as a necessary assessment tool for the diagnosis of obstructive sleep apnea (OSAS), and PSG is indicated pre- and postoperatively for adenotonsillectomies. Moreover, PSG is indicated for positive airway pressure (PAP) titration in children diagnosed with OSAS.

Restless Leg Syndrome and Periodic Limb Movement Disorder

Similar to the situation with OSAS (and even more controversial) is the situation regarding restless leg syndrome (RLS) and periodic limb movement disorder (PLMD) in children. Periodic limb movement in sleep (PLMS) is characterized by periodic episodes of repetitive and highly stereotypic limb movements during sleep (American Academy of Sleep Medicine, 2005). PLMD is defined by the presence of periodic limb movement during sleep associated with symptoms of insomnia or excessive daytime sleepiness (Chesson et al., 1999). RLS is a clinical diagnosis characterized by disagreeable leg sensations that usually occur prior to sleep onset. PLMD and RLS are distinct entity but can coexist. Most patients with PLMD do not manifest RLS symptoms; however, approximately 80 % of patients with RLS have PLMS (Montplaisir et al., 1997).

PLMD has been described in children with somewhat different clinical presentation. Children with PLMD may present with nonspecific symptoms such as growing pains, restless sleep, and hyperactivity (Picchietti & Walters, 1999). These symptoms are most often unnoticed by their parents, although a family history of RLS and PLMD is common. In a series of studies, Picchietti and colleagues suggested an increased prevalence of PLMD among children with attention-deficit/hyperactivity disorder (ADHD) (Picchietti, England, Walters, Willis, & Verrico, 1998). Other studies have suggested that the sleep fragmentation secondary to these disorders are an important contribution to ADHD and that particularly in the context of symptoms and/or a positive family history of RLS/PLMS that sleep studies should be performed if there is any question that sleep fragmentation is contributing to daytime impairments with attentional control (Corteses et al., 2005; Hoban & Chervin, 2005).

In terms of treatment, the guideline from the Standard of Practice Committee of the American Academy of Sleep Medicine states that no specific recommendation can be made regarding treatment of children with RLS or PLMD (Littner et al., 2004). There is limited information on the dopaminergic medications in children, and other medications have not been adequately studied in children. There is some evidence that children with PLMD may have low iron storage as evidenced by low serum ferritin and iron. Children with low serum ferritin (<50 µg/L) have been reported to respond favorably to iron therapy (Simakajornboon et al., 2003). However, currently, there are no long-term data on the use of iron treatment. These children also appear to benefit from avoiding caffeine and behavioral interventions to improve sleep habits.

Narcolepsy

Narcolepsy is a chronic neurological disorder characterized by excessive daytime sleepiness. The classic tetrad of symptoms in narcolepsy includes (1) sleep attacks, (2) cataplexy (the sudden loss of muscle tone without change of consciousness), (3) sleep paralysis (inability to move after waking up), and (4) hypnagogic hallucinations (dreamlike imagery before falling asleep). These symptoms do not all occur together or consistently in many cases of narcolepsy. Particularly in younger patients, signs of sleepiness may be the only initial symptom. Cataplexy is typically provoked by laughter, anger, or sudden emotional changes. It may be as subtle as a slight weakness in the legs or as dramatic as a patient's falling to the floor limp and unable to move. If cataplectic attacks last long enough, full sleep can occur.

Narcolepsy affects approximately 1 in 10,000 people in the USA. Narcolepsy is a neurologic disorder that appears to be caused by an abnormality in the hypocretin/orexin system—often by a loss of hypocretin neurons in the lateral hypothalamus and usually low CSF levels of hypocretin. About 10 % of narcoleptics are members of familial clusters; however, genetic factors alone are apparently insufficient to cause the disease. Hence, obtaining a family history of narcolepsy and/or excessive sleepiness can be helpful, though it is negative in many cases. Although traditionally the onset of narcolepsy is thought to be late adolescence and adulthood, there are well-documented cases that begin in early childhood.

The diagnosis of narcolepsy requires evaluation in a sleep laboratory. Patients with narcolepsy show early REM periods near sleep onset, fragmented nighttime sleep, excessive daytime sleepiness in objective nap studies during the day, and sleep-onset REM periods in naps. In prepubertal children, this diagnosis can be very difficult to establish (Kotagal, Hartse, & Walsh, 1990). Repeat studies may be necessary before reaching a final diagnosis.

Treatment of narcolepsy is generally focused on (1) education and counseling of the patient and family, (2) adherence to a regular schedule to obtain optimal sleep with good sleep habits (often including scheduled naps), (3) use of short-acting stimulant medication for treatment of daytime sleepiness (with drug holidays to avoid buildup of tolerance), and (4) use of REM-suppressant medications (such as protriptyline) when symptoms of cataplexy are problematic.

The differential diagnosis of narcolepsy includes consideration of *idiopathic hypersomnia*. Some patients have significantly increased sleep needs without evidence of the REM abnormalities seen in narcolepsy. There is often a familial history of excessive sleep needs, and these individuals show clear objective sleepiness in nap studies despite having obtained what appears to be adequate amounts of nighttime sleep. Hypersomnia disorders may be managed behaviorally (Harvey & Li, 2009; Kaplan & Harvey, 2009).

Conclusions

In this chapter we have reviewed several important principles relevant to the assessment, diagnosis, and treatment of sleep problems in children and adolescents. We have underscored the evidence for interactions between sleep and the regulation of behavior, emotion, and learning and the importance of sleep disturbance to many aspects of child psychiatry (and behavioral pediatrics). We have consistently emphasized behavioral principles and behavioral approaches to these problems because we believe that there is great pragmatic value in understanding and implementing these in many domains of clinical practice. There are few risks—and potentially many benefits—from increasing and enhancing sleep in children and adolescents through cognitive and behavioral interventions.

Although behavioral interventions for sleep disturbances in childhood and adolescence are clearly effective, there are areas requiring future research. Importantly, individual treatment components (e.g., extinction, stimulus control) and delivery of treatment including the format, duration, and mechanism of delivery (e.g., group, Internet based, etc.) need to be systematically examined with regard to efficacy, adherence, and cost-effectiveness. Furthermore, the impact of potential moderating variables (e.g., child temperament, household socioeconomic status, etc.) on treatment outcomes needs to be researched. Moreover, follow-up studies on the potential long-term impact that behavioral interventions may have on the persistence of sleep problems in adulthood need to be evaluated. Perhaps most important, the use of behavioral treatments in other populations including children ages 6–11 years old and children with special needs (e.g., children with autism spectrum disorders, mental retardation, neurodevelopmental disabilities) and children with chronic medical and psychiatric conditions needs to be investigated.

References

American Academy of Sleep Medicine. (2005). *International classification of sleep disorders (ICSD): Diagnostic and coding manual* (2nd ed.). Westchester, IL: Author.

Arendt, J. (1997). Safety of melatonin in long-term use (?). *Journal of Biological Rhythms, 12*, 673–681.

Aurora, R. N., Zak, R. S., Karippot, A., Lamm, C. I., Morgenthaler, T. I., Auerbach, S. H., et al. (2011). Practice parameters for the respiratory indications for polysomnography in children. *Sleep, 34*, 379–388.

Bootzin, R. R. (1972). Stimulus control treatment for insomnia. *Proceedings of the American Psychological Association, 7*, 395–396.

Bootzin, R. R., & Stevens, S. J. (2005). Adolescents, substance abuse, and the treatment of insomnia and daytime sleepiness. *Clinical Psychology Review, 25*, 629–644.

Borbély, A. A. (1982). A two process model of sleep regulation. *Human Neurobiology, 1*(3), 195–204.

Borbély, A. A., & Achermann, P. (2005). Sleep homeostasis and models of sleep regulation. In M. H. Kryger, T. Roth, & W. C. Dement (Eds.), *Principles and practice of sleep medicine* (3rd ed., pp. 405–417). Philadelphia, PA: Elsevier Saunders.

Cappuccio, F. P., Taggart, F. M., Kandala, N. B., Currie, A., Peile, E., Stranges, S., et al. (2008). Meta-analysis of short sleep duration and obesity in children and adults. *Sleep, 31*, 619–626.

Carey, W. B. (1974). Night waking and temperament in infancy. *Journal of Pediatrics, 84*, 756–758.

Carskadon, M. A., Acebo, C., Richardson, G. S., Tate, B. A., & Seifer, R. (1997). An approach to studying circadian rhythms of adolescent humans. *Journal of Biological Rhythms, 12*, 278–289.

Chesson, A. L., Jr., Wise, M., Davila, D., Johnson, S., Littner, M., Anderson, W. M., et al. (1999). Practice parameters for the treatment of restless legs syndrome and periodic limb movement disorder. An American Academy of Sleep Medicine Report. Standards of Practice Committee of the American Academy of Sleep Medicine. *Sleep, 22*(7), 961–968.

Corteses, S., Konofal, E., Lecendreus, M., Arnulf, I., Mouren, M. C., & Darra, F. (2005). Restless legs syndrome and attention-deficit/hyperactivity disorders: A review of the literature. *Sleep, 28*, 1007–1013.

Crowley, S. J., Acebo, C., & Carskadon, M. A. (2007). Sleep, circadian rhythms, and delayed phase in adolescence. *Sleep Medicine, 8*, 602–612.

Crowley, S. J., & Carskadon, M. A. (2010). Modifications to weekend recovery sleep delay circadian phase in older adolescents. *Chronobiology International, 27*, 1469–1492.

Czeisler, C. A., Richardson, G. S., Coleman, R. M., Zimmerman, J. C., Moore-Ede, M. C., Dement, W. C., et al. (1981). Chronotherapy: Resetting the circadian clocks of patients with delayed sleep phase insomnia. *Sleep, 4*, 1–21.

Dewald, J. F., Meijer, A. M., Oort, F. J., Gerard, A., Kerkhof, G. A., & Bogels, S. M. (2010). The influence of sleep quality, sleep duration and sleepiness on school performance in children and adolescents: A meta-analytic review. *Sleep Medicine Reviews, 14*, 179–189.

Digdon, N. L., & Howell, A. J. (2008). College students who have an eveningness preference report lower self-control and greater procrastination. *Chronobiology International, 26*, 1029–1046.

Durand, V. M. (2002). Treating sleep terrors in children with autism. *Journal of Positive Behavior Interventions, 4*(66–72).

Durand, V. M. (2008). *When children don't sleep well: Interventions for pediatric sleep disorders, therapist guide*. New York: Oxford University Press.

Durand, V. M., & Mindell, J. A. (1990). Behavioral treatment of multiple childhood sleep disorders. *Effects on child and family. Behavior Modification, 14*(1), 37–49.

Edinger, J. D., Wohlgemuth, W. K., Radtke, R. A., Marsh, G. R., & Quillian, R. E. (2001). Does cognitive-behavioral insomnia therapy alter dysfunctional beliefs about sleep? *Sleep, 24*, 591–599.

Espie, C. A. (2002). Insomnia: Conceptual issues in the development, persistence, and treatment of sleep disorder in adults. *Annual Review of Psychology, 53*, 215–243.

Ferber, R. (1985). *Solve your child's sleep problems*. New York: Simon & Schuster.

Ferber, R. (1989). Sleeplessness in the child. In M. H. Kryger, T. Roth, & W. C. Dement (Eds.), *Principles and practice of sleep medicine* (pp. 633–639). Philadelphia, PA: WB Saunders.

Ferber, R. (1996). Clinical assessment of child and adolescent sleep disorders. In R. E. Dahl (Ed.), *Child and Adolescent Psychiatric Clinics of North America* (pp. 569–580). Philadelphia, PA: W.B. Saunders.

Gianotti, F., & Cortesi, F. (2002). Sleep patterns and daytime function in adolescence: An epidemiological survey of an Italian high school student sample. In M. A. Carskadon (Ed.), *Adolescent sleep patterns: Biological, social, and psychological influences* (pp. 132–147). Cambridge: Cambridge University Press.

Gozal, D., & Kheirandish, L. (2006). Oxidant stress and inflammation in the snoring child: Confluent pathways to upper airway pathogenesis and end-organ morbidity. *Sleep Medicine Reviews, 10*, 83–96.

Gradisar, M., Dohnt, H., Gardner, G., Paine, S., Starkey, K., Menne, A., et al. (2011). A randomized controlled trial of cognitive-behavior therapy plus bright light therapy for adolescent delayed sleep phase disorder. *Sleep, 34*.

Gress-Smith, J. L., Luecken, L. J., Lemery-Chalfant, K., & Howe, R. (2012). Postpartum depression prevalence and impact on infant health, weight, and sleep in low-income and ethnic minority women and infants. *Maternal and Child Health Journal, 16*(4), 887–893.

Harvey, A. G. (2005). Unwanted intrusive thoughts in insomnia. In D. A. Clark (Ed.), *Intrusive thoughts in clinical disorders: Theory, research, and treatment* (pp. 86–118). New York: Guilford Press.

Harvey, A. G., & Li, D. (2009). Managing sleep disturbance in bipolar disorder. *Current Psychiatry Reviews, 5*, 194–201.

Harvey, A. G., Schmidt, D. A., Scarna, A., Semler, C. N., & Goodwin, G. M. (2005). Sleep-related functioning in euthymic patients with bipolar disorder, patients with insomnia, and subjects without sleep problems. *American Journal of Psychiatry, 162*, 50–57.

Harvey, A. G., Sharpley, A. L., Ree, M. J., Stinson, K., & Clark, D. M. (2007). An open trial of cognitive therapy for chronic insomnia. *Behaviour Research and Therapy, 45*, 2491–2501.

Hettema, J., Steele, J., & Miller, W. R. (2005). A meta-analysis of research on motivational interviewing treatment effectiveness. *Annual Review of Clinical Psychology, 1*, 91–111.

Hoban, T. F. (2004). Sleep and its disorders in children. *Seminars in Neurology, 24*, 327–340.

Hoban, T. F., & Chervin, R. D. (2005). Pediatric sleep-related breathing disorders and restless legs syndrome: How children are different. *The Neurologist, 11*, 325–337.

Jan, J. E., Hamilton, D., Seward, N., Fast, D. K., Freeman, R. D., & Laudon, M. (2000). Clinical trials of controlled-release melatonin in children with sleep-wake cycle disorders. *Journal of Pineal Research, 29*, 34–39.

Kaplan, K. A., & Harvey, A. G. (2009). Hypersomnia across mood disorders: A review and synthesis. *Sleep Medicine Reviews, 13*, 275–285.

Kazdin, A. E. (2005). *Parent management training: Treatment for oppositional, aggressive, and antisocial behavior in children and adolescents.* New York: Oxford University Press.

Kheirandish, L., & Gozal, D. (2006). Neurocognitive dysfunction in children with sleep disorders. *Developmental Science, 9*, 388–399.

Klackenberg, G. (1982). Somnambulism in childhood–prevalence, course and behavioral correlations. A prospective longitudinal study (6–16 years). *Acta Paediatrica Scandinavica, 71*(3), 495–499.

Kotagal, S., Hartse, K. M., & Walsh, J. K. (1990). Characteristics of narcolepsy in preteenaged children. *Pediatrics, 85*(2), 205–209.

Lee, T. M., Hummer, D. L., Jechura, T. J., & Mahoney, M. M. (2004). Pubertal development of sex differences in circadian function: An animal model. *Annals of the New York Academy of Science, 1021*, 262–275.

Littner, M. R., Kushida, C., Anderson, W. M., Bailey, D., Berry, R. B., Hirshkowitz, M., et al. (2004). Practice parameters for the dopaminergic treatment of restless legs syndrome and periodic limb movement disorder. *Sleep, 27*(3), 557–559.

Lozoff, B., Wolf, A. W., & Davis, N. S. (1985). Sleep problems seen in pediatric practice. *Pediatrics, 75*(3), 477–483.

Malpaux, B., Thiéry, J. C., & Chemineau, P. (1999). Melatonin and the seasonal control of reproduction. *Reproduction, Nutrition, Development, 39*, 355–366.

Marcus, C. L. (1997). Management of obstructive sleep apnea in childhood. *Current Opinion in Pulmonary Medicine, 3*, 464–469.

McGlinchey, E. L., Talbot, L. S., Chang, K. H., Kaplan, K. A., Dahl, R. E., & Harvey, A. G. (2011). The effect of sleep deprivation on vocal expression of emotion in adolescents and adults. *Sleep, 34*, 1233–1241.

McMakin, D. L., Siegle, G. J., & Shirk, S. R. (2011). Positive Affect Stimulation and Sustainment (PASS) module for depressed mood: A preliminary investigation of treatment-related effects. *Cognitive Therapy and Research, 35*, 217–226.

Miller, W. R., & Rollnick, S. (2002). *Motivational interviewing: Preparing people for change.* New York: Guilford Press.

Mindell, J. A. (1996). Treatment of child and adolescent sleep disorders. In R. Dahl (Ed.), *Child and adolescent Psychiatric Clinics of North America: Sleep disorder* (pp. 741–752). Philadelphia, PA: W. B. Saunders.

Mindell, J. A. (1999). Empirically supported treatments in pediatric psychology: Bedtime refusal and night wakings in young children. *Journal of Pediatric Psychology, 24*, 465–481.

Mindell, J. A. (2005). *Sleeping through the night* (2nd ed.). New York: Harper Collins.

Mindell, J. A., Kuhn, B., Lewin, D. S., Meltzer, L. J., & Sadeh, A. (2006). Behavioral treatment of bedtime problems and night wakings in infants and young children. *Sleep, 29*, 1263–1276.

Mirmiran, M., Maas, Y. G. H., & Ariagno, R. L. (2003). Development of fetal and neonatal sleep and circadian rhythms. *Sleep Medicine Reviews, 7*(4), 321–334.

Mistlberger, R. E., Antle, M. C., Glass, J. D., & Miller, J. D. (2000). Behavioral and serotonergic regulation of circadian rhythms. *Biological Rhythm Research, 31*, 240–283.

Montplaisir, J., Boucher, S., Poirier, G., Lavigne, G., Lapierre, O., & Lesperance, P. (1997). Clinical, polysomnographic, and genetic characteristics of restless legs syndrome: A study of 133 patients diagnosed with new standard criteria. *Movement Disorders, 12*(1), 61–65.

Morin, C. M., Bootzin, R. R., Buysse, D. J., Edinger, J. D., Espie, C. A., & Lichstein, K. L. (2006). Psychological and behavioral treatment of insomnia: An update of recent evidence (1998–2004). *Sleep, 29*, 1396–1406.

Morin, C. M., Culbert, J. P., & Schwartz, S. M. (1994). Nonpharmacological interventions for insomnia: A meta-analysis of treatment efficacy. *American Journal of Psychiatry, 151*, 1172–1180.

Morin, C. M., Hauri, P. J., Espie, C. A., Spielman, A. J., Buysse, D. J., & Bootzin, R. R. (1999). Nonpharmacologic treatment of chronic insomnia. An American Academy of Sleep Medicine review. *Sleep, 22*, 1134–1156.

Murtagh, D. R., & Greenwood, K. M. (1995). Identifying effective psychological treatments for insomnia: A meta-analysis. *Journal of Consulting and Clinical Psychology, 63*, 79–89.

National Sleep Foundation. (2006). *Adolescent sleep needs and patterns: Research report and resource guide.* Washington, DC: National Sleep Foundation.

Okawa, M., Uchiyama, M., Ozaki, S., Shibui, K., & Ichikawa, H. (1998). Circadian rhythm sleep disorders in adolescents: Clinical trials of combined treatments based on chronobiology. *Psychiatry and Clinical Neurosciences, 52*, 483–490.

Owens, J. A., Rosen, C. L., & Mindell, J. A. (2003). Medication use in the treatment of pediatric insomnia: Results of a survey of community-based pediatricians. *Pediatrics, 111*(5 Pt 1), 628–635.

Owens-Stively, J., Frank, N., Smith, A., Hagino, O., Spirito, A., Arrigan, M., et al. (1997). Child temperament, parenting discipline style, and daytime behavior in childhood sleep disorders. *Journal of Developmental and Behavioral Pediatrics, 18*, 314–321.

Picchietti, D. L., England, S. J., Walters, A. S., Willis, K., & Verrico, T. (1998). Periodic limb movement disorder and restless legs syndrome in children with attention-deficit hyperactivity disorder. *Journal of Child Neurology, 13*(12), 588–594.

Picchietti, D. L., & Walters, A. S. (1999). Moderate to severe periodic limb movement disorder in childhood and adolescence. *Sleep, 22*(3), 297–300.

Pollock, J. I. (1994). Night-waking at five years of age: Predictors and prognosis. *Journal of Child Psychology & Psychiatry & Allied Disciplines, 35*(4), 699–708.

Ree, M., & Harvey, A. G. (2004). Insomnia. In J. Bennett-Levy, G. Butler, M. Fennell, A. Hackman, M. Mueller, & D. Westbrook (Eds.), *Oxford guide to behavioural experiments in cognitive therapy* (pp. 287–305). Oxford: Oxford University Press.

Regestein, Q. R., & Monk, T. H. (1995). Delayed sleep phase syndrome: A review of its clinical aspects. *American Journal of Psychiatry, 152*, 602–608.

Reppert, S. M., & Weaver, D. R. (2002). Coordination of circadian timing in mammals. *Nature, 418*, 935–941.

Rickert, V. I., & Johnson, C. M. (1988). Reducing nocturnal awakening and crying episodes in infants and young children: A comparison between scheduled awakenings and systematic ignoring. *Pediatrics, 81*(2), 203–212.

Roenneberg, T., Kuehnle, T., Pramstaller, P. P., Ricken, J., Havel, M., Guth, A., et al. (2004). A marker for the end of adolescence. *Current Biology, 14*, R1038.

Roennebert, T., & Foster, R. G. (1997). Twilight times: Light and the circadian system. *Photochemistry and Photobiology, 66*, 549–561.

Ryan, N. D., Puig-Antich, J., Ambrosini, P., Rabinovich, H., Robinson, D., Nelson, B., et al. (1987). The clinical picture of major depression in children and adolescents. *Archives of General Psychiatry, 44*(10), 854–861.

Sack, R. L., Auckley, D., Carskadon, M. A., Wright, K. P. J., Vitiello, M. V., & Zhdanova, I. V. (2007). Circadian rhythm sleep disorders: Part II, advanced sleep phase disorder, delayed sleep phase disorder, free-running disorder, and irregular sleep-wake rhythm: An American academy of sleep medicine review. *Sleep: Journal of Sleep and Sleep Disorders Research, 30*, 1484–1501.

Sadeh, A., & Anders, T. F. (1993). Infant sleep problems: Origins, assessment, interventions. *Infant Mental Health Journal, 14*(1), 17–34.

Sadeh, A., Gruber, R., & Raviv, A. (2003). The effects of sleep restriction and extension on school-age children: What a difference an hour makes. *Child Development, 74*, 444–455.

Seibt, J., Aton, S. J., Jha, S. K., Coleman, T., Dumoulin, M. C., & Frank, M. G. (2008). The non-benzodiazepine hypnotic zolpidem impairs sleep-dependent cortical plasticity. *Sleep, 31*, 1381–1391.

Seidel, W. F., Ball, S., Cohen, S., Patterson, Y., Yost, D., & Dement, W. C. (1984). Daytime alertness in relation to mood, performance, and nocturnal sleep in chronic insomniacs and noncomplaining sleepers. *Sleep, 7*, 230–238.

Simakajornboon, N., Gozal, D., Vlasic, V., Mack, C., Sharon, D., & McGinley, B. M. (2003). Periodic limb movements in sleep and iron status in children. *Sleep, 26*(6), 735–738.

Sinai, D., & Tikotzky, L. (2012). Infant sleep, parental sleep and parenting stress in families of mothers on maternity leave and in families of working mothers. *Infant Behavior and Development, 35*(2), 179–186.

Smith, M. T., Perlis, M. L., Park, A., Smith, M. S., Pennington, J., Giles, D. E., et al. (2002). Comparative meta-analysis of pharmacotherapy and behavior therapy for persistent insomnia. *American Journal of Psychiatry, 159*, 5–11.

Spiegel, K., Tasali, E., Penev, P., & Van Cauter, E. (2004). Brief communication: Sleep curtailment in healthy young men is associated with decreased leptin levels, elevated ghrelin levels, and increased hunger and appetite. *Annals of Internal Medicine, 141*, 846–850.

Szeinberg, A., Borodkin, K., & Dagan, Y. (2000). Melatonin treatment in adolescents with delayed sleep phase syndrome. *Clinical Pediatrics, 45*, 809–818.

Talbot, L. S., McGlinchey, E. L., Kaplan, K. A., Dahl, R. E., & Harvey, A. G. (2010). Sleep deprivation in adolescents and adults: Changes in affect. *Emotion, 10*(6), 831–841.

Tassi, P., & Muzet, A. (2000). Sleep inertia. *Sleep Medicine Reviews, 4*, 341–353.

Thorpy, M. J., Korman, E., Spielman, A. J., & Glovinsky, P. B. (1988). Delayed sleep phase syndrome in adolescents. *Journal of Adolescent Health Care, 9*, 22–27.

Tikotzky, L., & Sadeh, A. (2009). Maternal sleep-related cognitions and infant sleep: A longitudinal study from pregnancy through the 1st year. *Child Development, 80*(3), 860–874.

Tonetti, L., Fabbri, M., & Natale, V. (2008). Sex difference in sleep-time preference and sleep need: A cross-sectional survey among Italian pre-adolescents, adolescents, and adults. *Chronobiology International, 25*, 745–759.

Weitzman, E. D., Czeisler, C. A., Coleman, R. M., Spielman, A. J., Zimmerman, J. C., Dement, W., et al. (1981). Delayed sleep phase syndrome: A chronobiological disorder with sleep-onset insomnia. *Archives of General Psychiatry, 38*, 737–746.

Wyatt, J. K. (2007). Circadian rhythm sleep disorders in children and adolescents. *Sleep Medicine Clinics, 2*, 387–395.

Wyatt, J. K., Stepanski, E. J., & Kirkby, J. (2006). Circadian phase in delayed sleep phase syndrome: Predictors and temporal stability across multiple assessments. *Sleep, 29*, 1075–1080.

Zuckerman, B., Stevenson, J., & Bailey, V. (1987). Sleep problems in early childhood: Continuities, predictive factors, and behavioral correlates. *Pediatrics, 80*(5), 664–671.

Part V

Disruptive Behavior Disorders

A Developmental Perspective on Attention-Deficit/Hyperactivity Disorder (ADHD)

22

Susan B. Campbell, Jeffrey M. Halperin, and Edmund J.S. Sonuga-Barke

Attention-deficit/hyperactivity disorder (ADHD), among the most common psychiatric disorders of childhood, has been the subject of research for over a century (Barkley, 1997, 2006). The intense interest in ADHD has produced a huge corpus of empirical data on putative etiological factors, the complex genetic and neurobiological mechanisms that appear to underlie ADHD, profiles of behavioral and cognitive functioning that characterize the disorder, the developmental course of ADHD from early childhood to adulthood, and treatments that are effective for some children with a diagnosis of ADHD. At the same time, specific causal mechanisms remain elusive, and the general consensus is that there are multiple causal pathways to ADHD, with environmental factors primarily serving to exacerbate or ameliorate symptom expression in children who are at some degree of biological risk for the disorder (Nigg, Willcutt, Doyle, & Sonuga-Barke, 2005; Sonuga-Barke, Auerbach, Campbell, Daley, & Thompson, 2005).

In this chapter, we will first discuss diagnostic criteria for ADHD and its clinical presentation across the age range from early childhood to early adulthood. We will also examine the current diagnostic nomenclature as described in DSM-IV-TR (2000) and the proposed changes that are being considered for DSM-V (Coghill & Seth, 2011; http://www.dsm5.org). We will briefly review recent epidemiological studies of ADHD. Etiological considerations, with an emphasis on recent genetic and neurobiological findings, will be discussed, followed by an examination of other factors that may be important in understanding the etiological heterogeneity of ADHD. When the research on ADHD is considered from a developmental psychopathology perspective (Cummings, Davies, & Campbell, 2000; Sonuga-Barke & Halperin, 2010), the etiological heterogeneity, high level of comorbidity, and biological and psychosocial/family correlates of ADHD underscore the need to posit multiple developmental pathways to the disorder (Sonuga-Barke et al., 2005; Sonuga-Barke & Halperin, 2010). Furthermore, these initial pathways are likely to be mediated and moderated by a variety of within child and family contextual factors that are associated with either the diminution of symptoms over time or their exacerbation. These issues will be addressed, as will their implications for the treatment of ADHD (Sonuga-Barke & Halperin, 2010), especially in early childhood (Halperin, Bédard, & Curchack-Lichtin, 2012; Halperin & Healey, 2011). Throughout, directions for future research will be noted.

S.B. Campbell, Ph.D. (✉)
Department of Psychology, University of Pittsburgh,
Pittsburgh, PA 15260, USA
e-mail: sbcamp@pitt.edu

J.M. Halperin, Ph.D.
Department of Psychology, Queens College
and the Graduate Center, City University
of New York, Flushing, NY 11367, USA

E.J.S. Sonuga-Barke, Ph.D.
Department of Psychology, University of
Southampton, Southampton, SO17 1B5, UK
and
Ghent University, Ghent, Belgium

M. Lewis and K.D. Rudolph (eds.), *Handbook of Developmental Psychopathology*,
DOI 10.1007/978-1-4614-9608-3_22, © Springer Science+Business Media New York 2014

Diagnostic Issues

Over the last 60 years, various terms have been used to describe the disorder that we now call ADHD, including hyperkinetic impulse disorder, minimal brain dysfunction, hyperactivity, attention deficit disorder, and most recently, ADHD (Barkley, 2006). These differences in terminology reflect different conceptions of the primary symptoms and putative underlying pathophysiology of the disorder, despite general agreement that the core features are inattention, impulsivity, and hyperactivity. The DSM-IV (American Psychiatric Association, 2000) includes three distinct subtypes of ADHD: the combined type requiring at least six symptoms of inattention (out of a possible nine) and six symptoms of hyperactivity-impulsivity (out of a possible nine); the inattentive type requiring at least six symptoms of inattention, but fewer than six symptoms of hyperactivity-impulsivity; and the hyperactive-impulsive type requiring at least six hyperactivity-impulsivity symptoms, but fewer than six symptoms of inattention (see Table 22.1). In addition, symptoms must be present for at least 6 months, be inappropriate for the child's age and developmental level, be evident by age 7, be of concern across settings (e.g., home and school), interfere with social and/or academic functioning, and not be due to another disorder such as autism. Research on ADHD over the last 20 years or so has primarily utilized these diagnostic criteria or focused on the symptoms listed in the DSM-IV, although some longitudinal studies that have followed children from the 1980s to adulthood (e.g., Barkley, Fischer, Smallish, & Fletcher, 2006; Mannuzza, Klein, Bessler, Malloy, & Hynes, 1997) began when earlier criteria were in use.

Debates about the diagnostic criteria, both for ADHD and for childhood disorders more generally (e.g., Coghill & Sonuga-Barke, 2012; Pickles & Angold, 2003), have emphasized the pros and cons of using a categorical in contrast to a dimensional approach, a topic that is beyond the scope of this chapter. In regard to ADHD, this debate has been intertwined with arguments about the validity and diagnostic utility of the subtypes.

Table 22.1 Symptoms of ADHD in the DSM-IV and proposed for the *DSM-V*

Inattention	Hyperactivity	Impulsivity
Fails to attend to details, careless	Often fidgets or squirms	Blurts out answers
Difficulty sustaining attention	Is often restless	Difficulty awaiting turn
Does not listen	Often runs about or climbs	Interrupts or intrudes on others
Does not follow instructions	Excessively loud or noisy	*Tends to act without thinking*
Difficulty organizing tasks	Often "on the go"	*Is often impatient*
Avoids tasks requiring mental effort	Talks excessively	*Is uncomfortable doing things slowly*
Often loses things		*Finds it difficult to resist temptations*
Easily distracted		
Often forgetful		

Note: Symptoms added to the DSM-V are in italics

For example, Milich, Balentine, and Lynam (2001) have contended that the inattentive type of ADHD should be considered a separate categorical disorder. In contrast, Lahey and Willcutt (2010) have argued for inclusion of a dimensional characterization of inattention and hyperactivity-impulsivity rather than nominal or categorical subtypes. This is because a longitudinal study showed that the subtypes are inherently unstable (Lahey, Pelham, Loney, Lee, & Willcutt, 2005). On reflection, it is hardly surprising that when children are followed from early to middle childhood, they shift from one subtype to another. These shifts across subtypes illustrate a number of problems with the diagnostic criteria including the arbitrariness of symptom thresholds that may lead to artifactual classifications (e.g., a child with six inattention and six hyperactivity-impulsivity symptoms will get a different subtype diagnosis than a child with six inattention and five hyperactivity-impulsivity symptoms), developmental changes in symptom expression as a function of both maturation and changing social and cognitive demands (e.g., Hart, Lahey, Loeber, Applegate, & Frick, 1995), and the likelihood that different symptoms will be emphasized by different reporters as a function of situational demands and expectations (e.g., parents may be especially aware of impulsivity, but teachers may be more aware than parents of inattention).

It is noteworthy, however, that different patterns of deficits and comorbidities are associated with the combined in contrast to the inattentive type in some studies, with children with combined symptoms more likely to evidence comorbid oppositional and conduct problems (e.g., Beauchaine, Hinshaw, & Pang, 2010) and children with the inattentive type more likely to show comorbid anxiety and learning problems (e.g., Milich et al., 2001; Willcutt & Pennington, 2000). Furthermore, severity and subtype designation are somewhat confounded (Lahey & Willcutt, 2010). Although all children with an ADHD diagnosis looked worse than controls over an 8-year follow-up, children with the combined-type diagnosis at intake looked worse on a range of measures of academic and social functioning at follow-up than children with an initial diagnosis of either inattentive or hyperactive-impulsive type; indeed, whereas 82 % of children with a combined designation met criteria for ADHD (regardless of type) 8–9 years later, only about half (53.8 %) of those with either of the other subtype designations did. These results underscore the complexity of trying to describe the heterogeneity of ADHD across the inattention and hyperactivity-impulsivity dimensions, while adhering to a categorical diagnostic system and taking severity and variability in symptom expression over time into account.

Another problem with the DSM-IV is the generally vague and nonspecific description of symptoms. Although the DSM-IV states that symptoms must be "inappropriate for age and developmental level," there are no guidelines delineating what to expect of children of different ages from preschool age to adolescence when the clinical presentation and associated symptoms vary widely. More recent research on adult ADHD has added another level of complexity to the diagnostic picture, both in terms of symptom thresholds and clinical presentation (Barkley, Murphy, & Fischer, 2007; Faraone et al., 2006). Finally, as already noted, ADHD is almost always comorbid with another disorder, including oppositional defiant and conduct disorders, anxiety disorders, and learning difficulties (Angold, Costello, & Erklani, 1999; Willcutt & Pennington, 2000). These co-occurring problems complicate clinical management of the disorder, as well as research on clinical presentation, cognitive and social profiles, developmental course, and family correlates.

The revisions to the diagnostic criteria for ADHD, proposed in the DSM-V (see Coghill & Seth, 2011; http://www.dsm5.org) and currently being tested in field trials, may or may not solve some of these problems. Four new impulsivity symptoms are proposed (see Table 22.1), meant to better capture the poor self-regulation that is a hallmark of the disorder. In addition, the descriptions of some symptoms have been enhanced to clarify the clinical presentation in late adolescence and early adulthood. The age of onset criterion has been changed to require only that several symptoms were evident by age 12; in contrast, in the DSM-IV more impairing symptoms had to be evident by age 7. This change is likely to result in an increase in the prevalence of the inattentive presentation and allow for the diagnosis of more late-onset cases, but it is unlikely to enhance our understanding of the emergence, developmental course, or etiology of ADHD. In addition, the criteria for a diagnosis in late adolescence or early adulthood require only four symptoms of either inattention or hyperactivity-impulsivity, further widening the net of individuals likely to receive the diagnosis.

The biggest change proposed in the DSM-V involves the subtype designations. In an attempt to recognize the instability of ADHD subtypes, the fact that clinical presentation is likely to change with age, and the heterogeneity of symptoms across the dimensions of inattention and hyperactivity-impulsivity, subtypes will now be specified as "current presentation," based on the symptom picture in the last 6 months. This allows for developmental changes and tries to avoid reifying subtypes. Further, the inattentive presentation is divided into two: *predominately inattentive* allows for three to five symptoms of hyperactivity-impulsivity, whereas the *restrictive inattentive* presentation allows for no more than two symptoms of hyperactivity-impulsivity. This may result in even more confusion about the inattentive type than currently exists, but the ongoing field trials, meant to test the appropriateness of these new criteria, may lead to further modifications. Although the proposed revisions include elaborations of the clinical presentation of ADHD in older adolescents and adults, they still do a poor job of describing symptoms in younger children or discussing potential early developmental markers, despite attempts to diagnose this disorder in younger and younger children (Egger & Angold, 2006; Zito et al., 2000). An emphasis on impairment and social context is especially important when assessing ADHD and related problems in young children (Campbell, 2002; Egger & Angold, 2006; Healey, Miller, Castelli, Marks, & Halperin, 2008). Perhaps further refinement will lead to a clearer distinction between emerging ADHD symptoms in preschool-age children and age-related and transient behaviors reflecting high energy, exuberance, and/or uneven development.

Developmental Course and Clinical Presentation

Despite variations in both the conceptualization of and diagnostic criteria for ADHD over the last several decades, the clinical picture remains essentially unchanged. Children with ADHD are most often referred for assessment between the of ages 5 and 8 when their high energy level, fidgetiness and difficulty sitting still, disorganization, lack of persistence on cognitive tasks, poor concentration, difficulty regulating behavior in social situations, and lack of social judgment lead to a myriad of social and academic problems. Difficulties are evident at home where children with ADHD often have problems following rules and routines; may create disturbances at mealtime, bedtime, or family outings; are in frequent conflict with siblings; and rarely complete homework without parental supervision. In the classroom, children with ADHD often stand out because of their lack of attention to ongoing lessons, failure to follow classroom rules and routines, activity level, inappropriate and disruptive behavior, and difficulty working either independently or collaboratively with classmates on group projects. In the peer group, children with ADHD are often avoided or actively rejected because of their insensitive or overbearing behavior; they may provoke fights, disrupt the activities of others, barge into a game and try to change the rules, or have difficulty taking turns and recognizing the needs of others.

Although ADHD is often not identified until children enter school, a developmental psychopathology perspective mandates a focus on the early emergence of ADHD. Most theoretical conceptualizations of early signs or precursors of ADHD (e.g., Campbell, 2002; Nigg, Goldsmith, & Sachek, 2004; Sonuga-Barke et al., 2005) focus partly on infant temperament, especially high levels of reactivity (approach, negative emotionality, activity level) and low levels of regulation (impulsivity, attentional control) (Nigg et al., 2004; Rothbart & Bates, 1998) as potential risk factors for later ADHD. Based on the consensus that temperamental characteristics are highly heritable, moderately stable within developmental periods, and form the building blocks for later personality (Nigg et al., 2004; Rothbart & Bates, 1998), it is likely that active, irritable, easily aroused, difficult to soothe infants will be more likely than their more quiet and manageable counterparts to develop ADHD (see Sonuga-Barke et al., 2005). In one prospective study of children at risk for ADHD because of elevated symptoms in their fathers, Auerbach et al. (2008) found that both mothers and fathers of high-risk infants reported higher levels of activity and negative affect and lower levels of attentional and inhibitory control than did parents of control infants. By 24 months, group differences in effortful control were also apparent. Early dysregulation of affect, attention, activity level, and impulse control may cascade into more serious problems, especially in the context of cognitive delays and/or harsh and inconsistent parenting (Campbell, 2002; Graziano, Calkins, & Keane, 2011; Sonuga-Barke et al., 2005). Given the heritability of these behaviors, it is also likely that some children showing these problems early will be raised in families where at least one parent is also impulsive and dysregulated (Mokrova, O'Brien, Calkins, & Keane, 2010).

By toddlerhood and the preschool period, children with signs of emerging ADHD are likely to be extremely overactive, difficult to calm down, rambunctious, noncompliant, and prone to temper tantrums in the face of parental prohibitions (Campbell, 2002). Cognitive and language delays may also be evident, along with difficulties on measures of executive functioning and school readiness (Campbell & von Stauffenberg, 2009; DuPaul & Kern, 2011). Furthermore, these children are likely to have problems in the peer group, given their difficulties taking turns, sharing toys, following rules, and playing quietly. Moreover, their poor ability to regulate behavior in response to others may result in high levels of reactive aggression that in turn leads to peer rejection. For example, Campbell, Pierce, March, Ewing, and Szumowski (1994) studied preschool boys with elevated ratings of hyperactivity and impulsivity on observational measures of activity, regulation, and compliance in the laboratory and their preschool classrooms. Compared to control boys, boys at risk for ADHD were more active during free play and structured tasks, less focused on specific toys during play, less able to resist touching a tempting but forbidden toy, and less compliant with their mother during a toy cleanup. In their preschool classrooms, at-risk boys were observed to be more disruptive with peers and less compliant with teachers. More recent studies of preschoolers at risk for ADHD and associated behavior problems have likewise reported that poorer regulation of emotion and attention predicted chronic problems across ages 2–5 (Hill, Degnan, Calkins, & Keane, 2006), including specific links between observed effortful control and cross-informant ratings of inattention and impulsivity at age 3 (Olson, Sameroff, Kerr, Lopez, & Wellman, 2005). Other studies have indicated that preschoolers with ADHD show more difficulties on measures of executive functioning (Berwid et al., 2005; Sonuga-Barke, Dalen, Daley, & Remington, 2002). These difficulties even result in some children being asked to leave their child care or preschool setting. In one study, 16 % of preschoolers with a diagnosis of ADHD had been expelled from preschool or child care (Egger & Angold, 2006). Moreover, longitudinal studies indicate that ADHD identified in early childhood often persists through middle childhood and into adolescence (Lee, Lahey, Owens, & Hinshaw, 2008; Pierce, Ewing, & Campbell, 1999).

School entry brings its own set of challenges as children need to follow stricter rules for self-regulation of behavior, follow classroom routines, attend to lessons and assignments, and cooperate in a larger peer group setting (Campbell & von Stauffenberg, 2008). Teachers routinely note that children with ADHD do more poorly on academic tasks and have more peer problems (e.g., Lahey & Willcutt, 2010; Lee & Hinshaw, 2006). Laboratory assessments reveal more difficulties on a range of executive function tests including those assessing verbal and nonverbal working memory, response inhibition, vigilance, and planning (Willcutt, Doyle, Nigg, Faraone, & Pennington, 2005) in comparison to children without any diagnosis, but the degree to which these deficits are specific to ADHD remains in question (Frazier, Demaree, & Youngstrom, 2004; Halperin & Schulz, 2006). Furthermore, follow-up studies from school age to adolescence indicate that problems persist in most children with a diagnosis and especially in those with comorbid disorders (e.g., Barkley, Fischer, Edelbrock, & Smallish, 1990; Biederman et al., 1996). Children with ADHD are at heightened risk for adolescent psychopathology (Mannuzza et al., 1991; Miller et al., 2008), including higher rates of antisocial behavior (Barkley et al., 1990; Mannuzza et al., 1991), substance use disorders (Mannuzza et al., 1991; Molina & Pelham, 2003), personality disorders (Miller et al., 2008), and persistent ADHD symptoms (Mannuzza et al., 1991; Mick et al., 2011). They also have poorer academic and employment histories, more automobile accidents and driving impairments, and more difficulties with friendships and intimate relationships (Barkley, 2006; Barkley, Guevremont, Anastopoulos, DuPaul, & Shelton, 1993). These follow-up studies have focused almost exclusively on boys, but studies following girls with ADHD through adolescence also indicate that problems in academic and social functioning persist, as do ADHD symptoms (Hinshaw, Owens, Sami, & Fargeon, 2006; Mick et al., 2011).

Studies of children with ADHD followed into adulthood also indicate high levels of persistent problems. For example, Barkley, Fischer, Smallish, and Fletcher (2004) followed a sample of children with and without ADHD into early adulthood (mean age 20–21); the ADHD group reported a range of negative outcomes including more arrests, thefts, assaults, and drug use. However, when the ADHD group was divided into those with and without co-occurring CD, only the comorbid group differed from controls; young adults with a history of both ADHD and CD not only were more likely to engage in substance use, but they used a greater variety of substances including alcohol, cocaine, and hallucinogens, and they used these more often than either control subjects or young adults with a history of ADHD alone. A growing body of research has shown that ADHD, but especially ADHD and CD, acts as a risk factor for drug use and smoking (Harty, Ivanov, Newcorn, & Halperin, 2011; Molina, Bukstein, & Lynch, 2002). In addition, data from Barkley et al. (2006) and others (Mannuzza et al., 1997; Weiss & Hechtman, 1993) indicate poorer academic and educational achievement, lower job satisfaction and employment stability, and less stable friendships and marital relationships in adults with a childhood history of ADHD. Although comorbid antisocial behavior accounts for some of these poor outcomes, academic and occupational difficulties are also associated with ADHD alone (Barkley et al., 2006).

Follow-up studies to adulthood indicate that although problems are not outgrown, the nature of symptoms may change, with gross motor activity less salient, but internal feelings of restlessness evident (Weiss & Hechtman, 1993). A recent increase in the number of college students with ADHD has also been reported (Weyant & DuPaul, 2006); they are more likely than comparison students to seek help with academic and social problems in college counseling centers; they also, not surprisingly, have lower grade point averages, are more likely to be on academic probation, and are more likely to drop out than students without ADHD. This is consistent with the long-term follow-up studies of Barkley et al. (2006) and Mannuzza et al. (1997) cited above, who likewise reported that their ADHD subjects had lower academic achievement and occupational success than controls, even with cognitive ability controlled.

Epidemiology

In studies assessing representative samples of preschool children, rates of ADHD range from 2 % to 5.7 % depending on whether impairment criteria must be met and clinical consensus is required (Egger & Angold, 2006). In general, rates are lower than in school-age children, presumably because expectations for self-control, activity, and inattention are lower. However, follow-up studies indicate (e.g., Lahey et al., 2005; Lee et al., 2008) that when rigorous diagnostic criteria are utilized to diagnose 4- and 5-year-olds with ADHD, problems are likely to persist to school entry and beyond. At the same time, Egger and Angold (2006) report that certain defining symptoms, especially those on the hyperactivity-impulsivity dimension, are very frequent in young children including difficulty sitting still, talking excessively, and often interrupting others. This highlights the importance of not overpathologizing typical behavior (Campbell, 2002), despite the importance of accurately identifying children and families in need of intervention (Egger & Angold, 2006; Halperin et al., 2012).

In school-age children and adolescents, the prevalence of ADHD varies widely based on whether impairment criteria are employed and whether data are obtained from both parents and teachers. The DSM-IV (American Psychiatric Association, 2000) estimates the prevalence of ADHD to range from 3 % to 7 % of school-age children. Using data from the 1,420 9- to 13-year-olds participating in the Great Smoky Mountain Study, Costello, Mustillo, Erklani, Keeler, and Angold (2003) estimated cumulative prevalence at 4.1 % by age 16, but with a marked sex difference

(1.1 % in girls and 7.0 % in boys). According to the Centers for Disease Control website (http://www.CDC.gov), parents report that approximately 9.5 % of children between the ages of 4 and 17 have ever been diagnosed with ADHD, with 13.2 % of boys and 5.6 % of girls receiving a diagnosis. The CDC also reports that the prevalence of ADHD increased systematically between 1997 and 2007, primarily reflected in higher rates of ADHD diagnoses among adolescents. This is presumably at least partly a reflection of the recent emphasis on identifying and treating ADHD in high school and college students (Weyant & DuPaul, 2006) as well as in adults more generally (Barkley et al., 2007).

Etiological Models

Etiological models focus on genetic and environmental influences, their correlations and interactions, and their effects on brain structure and function, which presumably mediate symptom expression. Yet research has not adequately integrated findings across these multiple levels of analysis or been informed by a developmental perspective (e.g., Coghill, Nigg, Rothenberger, Sonuga-Barke, & Tannock, 2005; Sonuga-Barke & Halperin, 2010). More research is needed to establish clear links between putative underlying genetic and neural processes and the behavioral manifestations of ADHD.

Genetic and Environmental Influences and Gene–Environment Interplay

Genetic factors shape ADHD developmental pathways, although ADHD is not a genetic disorder in any simple sense (Thapar, O'Donovan, & Owen, 2005). Genetic explanations of ADHD have been driven by data from family and twin studies showing that the condition is familial and highly heritable, with heritability estimates averaging around 76 % (Faraone et al., 2005). Attempts to identify the source of these genetic effects using a candidate gene approach to detect common genetic variants associated with ADHD have had limited success (Neale et al., 2010). A meta-analysis indicated small but significant effects for a number of putative functional variants in genes regulating brain neurochemistry especially in the dopamine system (e.g., D4 and the dopamine transporter (DAT1); Faraone et al., 2005). Common variants in genes in other neuromodulator systems (i.e., serotonin and norepinephrine; Oades et al., 2008) have also been implicated along with genes regulating more general brain function and growth (e.g., Brophy, Hawi, Kirley, Fitzgerald, & Gill, 2002). Despite these isolated findings, candidate gene associations account for little variation in ADHD expression (Faraone et al., 2005; Neale et al., 2010). Linkage studies have not found replicable disease susceptibility loci for ADHD. Hypothesis-free genome-wide association studies which tag a very large number of markers of common genetic variants in very large samples, while confirming the overall genetic contribution to ADHD, have failed to identify genome-wide significant effects for individual markers (Neale et al., 2010).

Several factors might account for the gap between the high heritability estimates and very small effects of common genetic variants. First, if genetic effects on ADHD are solely due to common genetic variants, a large number of markers of diminishingly small effect will be implicated (Faraone et al., 2005), and much larger samples will be required to detect genetic variants of smaller and smaller effects (Neale et al., 2010). Second, if one assumes genetic heterogeneity—with ADHD in different individuals determined by different genetic variants—then the goal is to create more uniform subgroups by identifying biologically meaningful networks of genetic variants (Poelmans, Pauls, Buitelaar, & Franke, 2011) or partitioning genetic heterogeneity on the basis of intermediate, potentially genetically more simple, pathophysiological or behavioral phenotypes. Third, genetic effects in ADHD may not result from common variants but rather from rare variants with larger effects (Gibson, 2012). Recent findings of an increased rate of de novo and inherited chromosomal deletions and/or duplications (so-called copy number variants—CNVs) in ADHD (Lionel et al., 2011) have spurred interest, despite inconsistencies in the gene system affected and the lack of specificity to ADHD. Fourth, and most relevant from a developmental perspective, virtually all genetic studies are cross sectional, and many combine participants with wide age ranges, potentially obfuscating developmental variation in genetic effects and related behaviors. By combining children and adolescents in the same sample, developmentally sensitive relations between genes, brain, and behavior are likely to remain undetected.

Another reason why genetic main effects are difficult to isolate may be that gene–environment associations rather than genetic main effects drive high heritability estimates; these effects are not captured in genetic studies that do not take environmental factors into account. Such a view is at the heart of a developmental psychopathology framework and consistent with the argument that the study of genes cannot be isolated from the study of environments (Rutter, 2000, 2006). ADHD has been associated with increased levels of pre-, peri-, and postnatal environmental risk, although the effects are small and their causal status difficult to discern due to the observational nature of most studies (Taylor & Rogers, 2005). The dominant focus has been on *prenatal factors.* Both maternal smoking (Thapar et al., 2003) and alcohol consumption (Vaurio, Riley, & Mattson, 2008) during pregnancy have been suggested as environmental risk factors. Maternal use of drugs of abuse (Linares et al., 2006) and drugs prescribed for therapeutic reasons may also be implicated, although it is difficult to disentangle these effects from variations in maternal psychological disorder during pregnancy. Furthermore, maternal stress, perhaps via dysregulation of the HPA axis, may play a role (O'Connor, Heron, Golding, & Glover, 2003). Prematurity (Bhutta, Cleves, Casey, Craddock, & Anand, 2002) and pregnancy complications (Ben Amor et al., 2005) are also associated with ADHD, although these risks are not specific to ADHD and the direction of causality is often unclear (Taylor & Rogers, 2005).

In addition to these pre- and perinatal risk factors, parenting and family stress may be implicated in ADHD and also represent examples of gene–environment correlation or interaction. ADHD symptoms elicit negative, intrusive, and harsh responses from parents (Campbell, Pierce, Moore, Marakovitz, & Newby, 1996; Seipp & Johnston, 2005) which are thought to set up negative cycles of parent–child interaction that perpetuate and exacerbate patterns of impairment in ADHD. Links between harsh parenting and the aggravation of symptoms may reflect the reciprocal relations between impulsive parents and impulsive children. The extent to which this can induce ADHD itself or alter its long-term trajectory, rather than potentiate the emergence of comorbid social and emotional problems remains to be determined. Parent training interventions, in as much as they reduce core ADHD symptoms, provide support for the therapeutic value of positive parenting, clear and proactive limit-setting, and family structure (see below), regardless of how these problems initially began.

In addition to the social–emotional aspects of the family environment, the degree of intellectual and physical stimulation that a child receives may affect brain development and in turn behavior in children with ADHD (Halperin & Healey, 2011). Animal research has clearly documented the positive impact of environmental enrichment, cognitive stimulation, and physical exercise on neural and behavioral development. To the extent that children with ADHD show delays in brain development (Shaw et al., 2007), the degree to which the child's environment provides adequate stimulation may alter risk and affect the trajectory of the disorder. Interventions such as working memory training (Klingberg et al., 2005) or more broadly based cognitive enhancement programs (Halperin et al., 2013; Tamm, Nakonezny, & Hughes, 2012) highlight the potential of the postnatal environment to change the brain and the behavior of children with ADHD, although findings are largely preliminary and further research is clearly needed.

Nevertheless, the high level of covariation among genetic and environmental risks, nested within patterns of lifestyle and economic adversity, makes it difficult to separate genetic from environmental effects (Taylor & Rogers, 2005).

For instance, recent studies using adoption and artificial conception designs have suggested that many of the reported effects of maternal smoking may be due to genetic effects shared by mothers who smoke during pregnancy and their ADHD offspring (Nomura, Marks, & Halperin, 2010; Thapar et al., 2009).

Most importantly, we need to consider gene by environment interactions (G×E). For example, genes may moderate the effects of environmental exposures—as in the classic study whereby carrying a risk or susceptibility genotype of the serotonin transporter determined the long-term effects on mood of adverse social environments (Caspi et al., 2003). ADHD G×E studies to date have focused on dopamine genes, with evidence that genotypes moderate the effects of prenatal exposure to nicotine and alcohol (e.g., Becker, El-Faddagh, Schmidt, Esser, & Laucht, 2008; Brookes et al., 2006). Postnatal social influences may also be moderated by genetic factors. Serotonin and/or dopamine genes may moderate the effects of social adversity increasing risk for externalizing problems in general, as well as ADHD in particular (Lahey et al., 2011; Sonuga-Barke et al., 2009). Notably, children with the DRD4 7-repeat allele, as compared to those without that allele, were found to be more sensitive to the quality of parenting received (Sheese, Voelker, Rothbart, & Posner, 2007) and to respond better to parenting interventions (Bakermans-Kranenburg, Van Ijzendoorn, Mesman, Alink, & Juffer, 2008), again, suggesting genetic differences in the degree to which environmental factors influence developmental trajectories in children with ADHD. Most recently variations in DAT1 were found to moderate the responses of children with ADHD to behavioral parent training (van den Hoofdakker et al., 2012).

A second possibility is that environmental exposures moderate genetic effects through epigenetic modifications of the genome. In brief the epigenetic hypothesis is that environmental exposure can modify the expression of ADHD risk genes altering the likelihood of the condition. While such effects are well established in animal models, human epigenetics is in its infancy (see Meaney, 2010 for a discussion). Exploring the role of epigenetic mechanisms in ADHD represents a major research priority.

This framework highlights the potential significance of the developmental timing of putative risk and protective processes by raising the possibility that these processes operate both early and later in development. Although genetic factors are typically thought of as operating in a fixed way across the life span, that is unlikely to be the case. In contrast our model of ADHD pathogenesis makes a distinction between early and late operating genetic effects—this begs the question of whether genetic factors are implicated in determining continuity, discontinuity, and progression of the disorder. Greven, Asherson, Rijsdijk, and Plomin (2011) demonstrated, using longitudinal twin data, that patterns of stability and change in ADHD symptoms were the result of relatively stable genetic influences but also newly appearing influences emerging at different points across the life span. With regard to environmental influences, key questions relate to the primacy of early experience and sensitive periods (Do adverse environments have to be experienced during specific time windows? Can early adversity be overcome by later environmental enrichment?). There are currently very few studies that have the relevant combination of genetic/high-risk designs and longitudinal data to address these issues.

Neurobiological Mediators

According to our framework, genetic and environmental risk set the context for the development of ADHD via structural and functional alterations in key brain networks. Testing such a mediational model requires answers to three questions (1) In what way are ADHD developmental pathways related to altered developmental trajectories of brain structure and function? (2) Are such alterations associated with genetic and environmental factors shown to be linked to ADHD? (3) Do these ADHD-related neurodevelopmental alterations differentially operate early or late in development? Because so few studies of brain function have been longitudinal, our capacity to address these questions is limited.

ADHD and Brain Structure

Structural alterations in multiple brain systems have been implicated in ADHD (Sonuga-Barke & Fairchild, 2012). As compared to typically developing peers, studies have reported significantly smaller brains in children and adolescents with ADHD in contrast to non-ADHD controls (Castellanos et al., 2002) with the cerebellum, corpus callosum, and striatal (i.e., caudate nucleus, putamen and globus pallidus; Ellison-Wright, Ellison-Wright, & Bullmore, 2008) and frontal regions (e.g., dorsolateral prefrontal cortex) (DLPFC; Valera, Faraone, Murray, & Seidman, 2007) especially affected. Others have reported that children with ADHD evidence reduced cortical thickness, especially in the DLPFC (Batty et al., 2010). There is also evidence of altered patterns of cortical folding—effects often related to early environmental factors (Wolosin, Richardson, Hennessey, Denckla, & Mostofsky, 2009). Diffusion tensor imaging suggests alterations in white matter integrity in a range of fiber pathways thought to subserve cognitive functions implicated in ADHD (van Ewijk, Heslenfeld, Zwiers, Buitelaar, & Oosterlaan, 2012). Key regions in reward and emotion processing networks such as the ventral striatum and the amygdala may also be implicated (Carmona et al., 2009; Plessen et al., 2006).

The few studies that have examined developmental changes in brain structure related to ADHD have demonstrated some continuity in group differences over time, although several differences between those with and without ADHD in childhood were no longer evident by adolescence (Castellanos et al., 2002). More recent analyses of cortical thickness have supported the notion of a delayed developmental pattern in ADHD rather than a fixed deficit such that children with ADHD follow a trajectory of cortical development that is similar to but delayed by 2–3 years relative to their typically developing peers (Shaw et al., 2007). Emerging evidence from this longitudinal study of cortical thickness suggests that remission of symptoms may be associated with relative normalization of brain structure (Shaw et al., 2007). Consistent with this, neuroimaging (Schulz, Newcorn, Fan, Tang, & Halperin, 2005) and neuropsychological (Halperin, Trampush, Miller, Marks, & Newcorn, 2008) prospective studies of children with ADHD suggest parallels between clinical improvement and structural and functional normalization of the brain, although these latter studies also show evidence for enduring neural anomalies irrespective of clinical improvement.

ADHD and Brain Chemistry

The hypothesis that ADHD is a dopamine (DA) dysregulation disorder is partially supported by genetic, imaging, and pharmacological studies (Oades et al., 2005; Pliszka, 2005). PET studies have produced mixed results with some suggesting that ADHD is a hypo-dopaminergic and others a hyper-dopaminergic syndrome. This is supported by the fact that DA agonists (e.g., methylphenidate) reduce ADHD symptoms, probably through the increase of extracellular DA (Pliszka, 2005). DA neurons innervate brain networks (see below) implicated in ADHD. Methylphenidate improves functioning across some neuropsychological domains deficient in ADHD (e.g., Bush et al., 2008). The DA hypothesis is further supported by genetic studies implicating DA genes (see above) and by studies using animal models with pharmacological lesions and gene knockouts of catecholamine systems (Madras, Miller, & Fischman, 2005). Clearly other neurochemicals, such as norepinephrine (Arnsten, Steere, & Hunt, 1996) and serotonin (Oades et al., 2008), are also implicated in ADHD. Because the interactions among neurotransmitters are complex, it is difficult to isolate the effects of one (e.g., DA) from the others (e.g., serotonin or acetylcholine).

ADHD and Brain Function

Simple models of ADHD as a disorder of executive function have been replaced by models of pathophysiological heterogeneity (Durston, van Belle, & de Zeeuw, 2011; Halperin et al., 2008; Nigg, 2006; Sonuga-Barke, Bitsakou, & Thompson, 2010). At the neuropsychological level, ADHD is associated with deficits in a range of executive functions (Willcutt et al., 2005), especially in inhibitory control (Barkley, 1997), working memory (Rapport et al., 2008), planning, and attentional flexibility (Willcutt et al., 2005). Functional neuroimaging data suggest that inhibitory-based deficits are linked to hypoactivation in the prefrontal cortex (Rubia, Smith, Brammer, Toone, & Taylor, 2005) and the dorsal striatum (Vaidya, Bunge, Dudukovic, & Zalecki, 2005), while working memory deficits implicate a network linking posterior regions of the prefrontal and anterior regions of the parietal cortex (Dickstein, Bannon, Castellanos, & Milham, 2006). Altered patterns of functional connectivity between key executive brain regions have also been identified.

Altered motivational and reward-related processes are also implicated in ADHD. Functional MRI studies suggest hypoactivation in the ventral striatum/nucleus accumbens and the orbitofrontal cortex in response to anticipated rewards (Scheres, Milham, Knutson, & Castellanos, 2006). Findings are less clear at the behavioral level with some studies suggesting that ADHD children are less sensitive to reinforcement, while others suggest oversensitivity. A consistent finding is that ADHD individuals respond differently to delayed reward (e.g., Marco et al., 2009). Alternatively, data suggest that ADHD is associated with delay aversion (a negative affective state induced by delay cues) and that escape from delay is a primary motivator for ADHD (Sonuga-Barke et al., 2010). Consistent with this view, brain regions involved in processing negative emotional stimuli (amygdala and anterior insula) are hyperactivated to cues of impending delay.

The default mode network (Broyd et al., 2009) is also attracting increased attention. This "resting state network" is active during rest and deactivates during task performance (Sonuga-Barke & Castellanos, 2007). During task performance activity in this network is associated with intermittent errors thought to reflect attentional lapses. In individuals with ADHD, this network shows reduced connectivity during rest (Fair et al., 2011) and not the typical decline in activity during rest-to-task transitions (e.g., Peterson et al., 2009), both effects that can be normalized with stimulant medication (e.g., Liddle et al., 2011).

Research on reward and delay highlights the context dependent nature of ADHD deficits. An alternative perspective on this issue is provided by the state regulation model, which posits that children with ADHD have particular difficulties regulating their psychophysiological state during periods of under- or overactivation (Wiersema, Van der Meere, Antrop, & Roeyers, 2006). ADHD children may be less capable of effectively allocating effort to regulate suboptimal states (Sergeant, 2005). Although the biological basis of this model is not well studied, supporting evidence comes from the repeated finding that performance in children with ADHD deteriorates under fast and slow event rate conditions, which should reduce activation/arousal (Metin, Roeyers, Wiersema, van der Meere, & Sonuga-Barke, 2012).

Integration from a Developmental Psychopathology Perspective

Children with ADHD are heterogeneous with respect to symptom picture, patterns of comorbidity, types of impairment, and family dysfunction. Developmentally, such heterogeneity is reflected in diverse trajectories of ADHD marked by differential patterns of continuity, discontinuity, and progression in clinical presentation (Lahey et al., 2005; Willoughby, Pek, Greenberg, & The Family Life Project Investigators, 2012). This clinical diversity is almost certainly mirrored in underlying pathogenesis—with ADHD risk associated with an array of interacting genetic and environmental factors—and mediated by multiple brain networks, with different individuals affected in different ways and to varying degrees. The field, however, is hampered by a dependence on simplistic disease models of etiology, built on the notion that ADHD is the result of a fixed and stable pattern of core dysfunction. A developmental psychopathology perspective offers an alternative formulation which provides a dynamic and flexible account of the pathogenesis of complex and heterogeneous conditions, such as ADHD (e.g., Halperin et al., 2013; Sonuga-Barke & Halperin, 2010). This approach moves beyond a merely *descriptive developmental approach* (characterizing patterns of change across the life span) to an *explanatory developmental approach*, that considers the processes underpinning diverse developmental patterns and focuses on the dynamic interplay among different causal factors and pathogenic processes.

We posit that the clinical syndrome is a manifestation of neurodevelopmental liability, mediated by alterations in brain structure and function in response to multiple interacting early- (genetic and prenatal) and later-operating genetic and environmental risk and resilience factors, and later environmental protective processes (Rutter, 2000, 2006). Furthermore, building on a recent review that provides compelling evidence against discrete (or unique) causal factors or pathophysiological conditions marking diagnostic boundaries across the ADHD continuum of severity (Coghill & Sonuga-Barke, 2012), our model assumes a spectrum of liability for ADHD that is related to clinical severity in a dose-like manner.

Consistent with this view, we argue that multiple, rather than single, deficit models of ADHD reflect the heterogeneity in both the clinical picture and the underlying genetic and neurobiological patterns discussed above. ADHD is almost certainly not a single neurobiological entity but rather an umbrella term covering a range of different phenotypes, each with a specific pathophysiological profile. The notion of multiple deficits that may be distinct in some children and overlap in others is most clearly illustrated by data on cognitive and motivational functioning in children with ADHD. Indeed evidence indicates that each deficit (e.g., executive, reward/delay, state regulation) affects only a minority of cases (Sonuga-Barke et al., 2010). Distinct groups of ADHD children affected exclusively by either executive function problems or delay aversion and timing problems have been identified (Sonuga-Barke et al., 2010). On the basis of this and other data, multiple pathway models have been proposed (Coghill et al., 2005; Durston et al., 2011; Nigg, 2006; Sonuga-Barke et al., 2005), building on the functionally segregated nature of reward and cognitive anterior brain systems (Winstanley, Eagle, & Robbins, 2006).

Furthermore, as noted by Coghill et al. (2005), cognitive and executive dysfunctions appear to be more closely associated with the inattention dimension and poor academic achievement. Motivational deficits and delay aversion, on the other hand, appear to be associated with hyperactivity and impulsivity. Presumably some children have deficits in all of these areas. Considering these deficits in the broader context of family, school, and peer functioning, one can posit that the academic and regulatory difficulties that emerge from delayed development of executive functions in school-age children may cascade into more serious learning and interpersonal problems, possibly associated with school failure, poor decision-making, and peer rejection. Similarly, the high activity level and impulsivity associated with difficulties in reward processing may be reflected not only in symptoms of ADHD but also in higher levels of noncompliance at home, reactive aggression with peers, and disruptive behavior in the classroom. A stressful family context may also exacerbate problems via harsh parenting, inadequate support for self-regulation, and poor role models. It is well-documented that more severe family adversity, including marital conflict, parental psychopathology, and stressful life events, is associated with persistent ADHD over and above co-occurring ODD and CD (Biederman, Faraone, & Monuteaux, 2002; Counts, Nigg, Stawicki, Rappeley, & Von Eye, 2005). In contrast, supportive parenting paired with clear limit-setting may be reflected in a decline in symptoms and better social and academic functioning. Treatment outcome data (see below) suggest the importance of parent management and the parent–child relationship for children with ADHD.

Although follow-up studies indicate that problems persist in many children with ADHD, especially those with the combined presentation and comorbid conduct problems, little is known about developmental continuities and age-related changes in the psycho-pathophysiological underpinnings of ADHD or about brain structure and function in ADHD at different developmental periods. However, it is clear that individuals with ADHD are affected by cognitive problems across the life span (Seidman, 2006) with motivational and energetic factors also playing a role in preschool, childhood, adolescence, and adulthood (e.g., Marco et al., 2009; Wiersema et al., 2006). A few recent studies suggest that developmental change may be evident in underlying cognitive and neural processes, related to continuity and discontinuity in the clinical manifestations of ADHD. Halperin and colleagues (2008) found that individuals who showed a persistent pattern of disorder from childhood through adolescence could be distinguished from those who remitted on the basis of the integrity of their executive or effortful control processes, a finding which the authors argue is consistent with the idea that recovery from ADHD is associated with emergence of well-functioning executive control. However, the so-called ADHD remitters continued to show impairments on less consciously controlled cognitive processes, despite improvements in executive control. These findings are consistent with preliminary fMRI data indicating that the magnitude of prefrontal activation in response to inhibition in adolescents with childhood ADHD corresponds to the persistence of symptoms; those who were less symptomatic appeared more like never-ADHD controls (Schulz et al., 2005).

In studies of the transition from preschool to school, earlier delays in executive functions seem to predict the onset or persistence of disorder or symptoms (Campbell & von Stauffenberg, 2009; Wahlstedt, Thorell, & Bohlin, 2008). Imaging studies of brain function have not been designed or powered to identify systematic differences in brain structure or function in different age groups, but consistencies in alterations have been seen for school-age, adolescent, and adult samples. Structural effects seem to show a degree of continuity although the one longitudinal morphometric study found that early childhood differences in striatal volume are reduced by adolescence and cerebellar differences become more prominent (Castellanos et al., 2002). However, two interesting studies of brain structure and function may challenge this view by demonstrating that the brains of ADHD children share characteristics of developmentally younger children. Shaw et al. (2007) reported that ADHD children were delayed, rather than deficient in cortical growth, especially in areas linked to executive control. Clarke, Barry, McCarthy, Selikowitz, and Brown (2002) identified a subgroup of ADHD children who they designated as having patterns of brain activity that were typical of developmentally younger children on the basis of their EEGs. Taken together, these studies suggest that developmental delays and individual differences in brain function and structure as well as associated cognitive processes are reflected in the clinical heterogeneity and variations in the developmental course of ADHD. Longitudinal studies are needed that examine neural and cognitive processes in the same children with ADHD and link changes in brain function to changing cognitive and symptom patterns across development, while also taking family context, including parenting style, into account.

Treatment

Evidence-based treatments for children with ADHD include an array of pharmacological and psychosocial approaches. FDA-approved medications include psychostimulants (i.e., methylphenidate and amphetamines) and more recently approved non-stimulant medications (i.e., atomoxetine and guanfacine). Behavioral interventions in the forms of parent management training (PMT) and contingency management in the classroom have been studied extensively. While these interventions generally provide symptom relief, at least in the short term, they also have limitations (see below). As such, efforts have been ongoing to develop novel non-pharmacological interventions for ADHD, several of which incorporate a developmental psychopathology perspective. Below, we briefly review current evidence-based medication and psychosocial treatments for ADHD and then discuss emerging interventions that show promise.

Medication

Psychostimulants are the most commonly prescribed medications for treating children with

ADHD. There are numerous preparations of both methylphenidate and amphetamine. Perhaps the biggest change in stimulant medication treatment over the past decade has been the shift from short-term preparations to those with effects lasting throughout most of the day. In addition, the approval of non-stimulant medications provides an alternative for those who do not respond well to stimulants or whose parents are concerned about their misuse. While the available non-stimulants may not be as effective as long-acting psychostimulants (Hanwella, Senanayake, & de Silva, 2011), they are helpful for many children who do not respond well to stimulants or as a supplement to stimulant treatment, and they do not raise the social concerns associated with treating children with a drug of potential abuse.

The precise mechanisms by which these medications exert their impact on ADHD symptoms are not known. Most theories posit that stimulant medications work by enhancing dopamine in the striatum (Volkow et al., 2012), although others have focused on their effect on noradrenergic alpha-2 receptors in the prefrontal cortex (Arnsten et al., 1996). Both non-stimulant medications have direct actions only on the noradrenergic system; atomoxetine selectively blocks the norepinephrine transporter (primarily in the prefrontal cortex) which has secondary effects on dopamine as well, whereas guanfacine is a highly specific alpha-2a receptor agonist.

For most children with ADHD, these medications are highly effective for reducing the core symptoms of ADHD as well as enhancing compliance and academic success and decreasing aggression (Conners, 2000; Greenhill, Halperin, & Abikoff, 1999). Stimulants are well tolerated by most children with ADHD, although a substantial number experience side effects (Swanson et al., 2007; Wigal et al., 2006). Further, many parents and teachers, especially of young children, feel uncomfortable using medication as a treatment for children with ADHD (Pisecco, Huzinec, & Curtis, 2001; Power, Hess, & Bennett, 1995) and questions about long-term medication effects remain Therefore, there is a renewed focus on psychosocial interventions for children with ADHD.

Evidence-Based Psychosocial Interventions

Many parents of children with ADHD prefer psychosocial interventions prior to or instead of medication. This is particularly the case in preschool children, where the American Academy of Pediatrics (Wolraich et al., 2011) recommends such interventions prior to the initiation of medication. Evidence-based psychosocial interventions typically employ a behavior modification model implemented through PMT and/or school-based contingency management programs. Studies of PMT have shown improvements in ADHD symptoms (Anastopoulos, Shelton, DuPaul, & Guevremont, 1993; Sonuga-Barke, Daley, Thompson, Laver-Bradbury, & Weeks, 2001), oppositional problems and impairment (Erhardt & Baker, 1990; Pisterman et al., 1992), and parent functioning (Anastopoulos et al., 1993; Pisterman et al., 1992; Sonuga-Barke et al., 2001). However, PMT is generally more effective for decreasing oppositional and defiant behaviors than core ADHD symptoms. Contingency management in the classroom has been shown to improve classroom behavior and academic productivity as reflected in teacher reports, classroom observations, and academic tests (Fabiano et al., 2007; Pelham, Wheeler, & Chronis, 1998). While behavioral interventions are effective, benefits often do not generalize to other settings, they are difficult to implement, and they may be less effective than stimulant medications (MTA Cooperative Group, 1999).

Limitations of Current Treatments

Although currently employed pharmacological and psychosocial treatments can be effective in reducing symptoms of ADHD and comorbid conditions, a substantial proportion of treated children continue to exhibit clinically significant levels of ADHD symptoms and associated impairment (Swanson et al., 2001). ADHD children usually function better following treatment, yet they remain deviant relative to peers in social and academic functioning. Furthermore, treatment-related gains are rarely maintained beyond the termination of active treatment, and both psychopharmacological (Molina et al., 2007, 2009) and behavioral interventions (Molina et al., 2007; Pelham & Fabiano, 2008) have minimal impact on long-term outcomes of children with ADHD. While it could be argued that ADHD is a chronic condition that requires long-term treatment, perhaps throughout much of the life span, long-term adherence to both medication and behavioral interventions is generally poor (MTA Cooperative Group, 2004). For behavioral interventions to provide lasting benefits, parents and teachers need to implement highly intensive interventions over long periods of time, but this is extremely challenging. Thus, despite short-term benefits of these evidence-based treatments, the lack of "normalization" for many children, the limited generalization of treatment effects, poor long-term adherence, and the lack of evidence for improved long-term outcomes are problematic.

Developmental Psychopathology Perspectives on Treatment for ADHD

Unlike static or fixed deficit models, the developmental psychopathology perspective views ADHD as a manifestation of neurodevelopmental liability, mediated by changes in brain structure and function in response to multiple genetic and environmental risk and resilience factors (Rutter, 2000, 2006). As such, the goal of treatment is to reduce environmental risk and enhance resilience and protective processes. While there may be several potential treatment targets for accomplishing these goals, ongoing research has largely focused on two: the improvement of parent–child relationships and the facilitation of neural development. These approaches often target younger children, when brains and behavioral patterns may be more "plastic" or amenable to change and because, theoretically, relatively modest effects early on can have substantial cascading effects on the long-term trajectory (Halperin et al., 2012).

Several developmentally sensitive early interventions include a more traditional PMT component which provides guidance in the provision of structure and rule-based reinforcement. Incorporated into the intervention are strategies for promoting parental warmth and improving the quality of the parent–child relationship (Bor, Sanders, & Markie-Dadds, 2002; Sonuga-Barke et al., 2001; Thompson et al., 2009). In contrast to PMT with older children, these interventions with preschoolers yield evidence of persisting benefits beyond the termination of active treatment.

In addition, as the trajectory of ADHD is likely mediated by brain structure and function, several novel interventions focus on promoting neural development through the employment of computer-based training (Klingberg et al., 2005; Shalev, Tsal, & Mevorach, 2007), targeted cognitive skill development (Thompson et al., 2009), physical exercise (Berwid & Halperin, 2012), and play (Halperin et al., 2013; Tamm et al., 2012). Play-based interventions are noteworthy in that they aim to facilitate neurodevelopment within a context that promotes improved parent–child relationships (Halperin & Healey, 2011). While the impact of these approaches on brain development has not been systematically evaluated, preliminary data suggest that behavioral improvements last at least several months beyond the termination of active treatment.

Summary and Conclusions

Much progress has been made in describing the developmental course of ADHD from preschool age to early adulthood and recognizing that the clinical picture is likely to emerge from a heterogeneous set of correlated and interacting genetic and environmental risk factors. In addition, there is growing evidence that subgroups of children with ADHD show different patterns of cognitive and motivational deficits, some of which appear to be linked to delays in brain maturation. Specific comorbidities also vary widely, although the majority of children with ADHD have some comorbid condition. Thus, ADHD is best conceptualized as a final common manifestation of multiple neurobiological risks that may be exacerbated or ameliorated by experiences in the family and school setting. Symptom patterns and severity of impairment are strongly associated with family adversity and parenting competence and are likely to reflect both general risks for disorder (e.g., parental psychopathology, family conflict, harsh parenting) and risks specific to ADHD (e.g., paternal ADHD). Treatment programs that begin early and are aimed at modifying the parent–child relationship and children's cognitive and attentional processing appear promising.

References

American Psychiatric Association. (2000). *Diagnostic and statistical manual of mental disorders* (Text revision). Washington, DC: Author.

Anastopoulos, A. D., Shelton, T. L., DuPaul, G. J., & Guevremont, D. C. (1993). Parent training for attention-deficit hyperactivity disorder: Its impact on parent functioning. *Journal of Abnormal Child Psychology, 21*, 581–596.

Angold, A., Costello, J., & Erklani, A. (1999). Comorbidity. *Journal of Child Psychology and Psychiatry, 40*, 57–87.

Arnsten, A. F., Steere, J. C., & Hunt, R. D. (1996). The contribution of alpha 2-noradrenergic mechanisms to prefrontal cortical cognitive function. Potential significance for attention-deficit hyperactivity disorder. *Archives of General Psychiatry, 53*, 448–455.

Auerbach, J. G., Berger, A., Atzaba-Poria, N., Arbelle, S., Cypin, N., Friedman, A., et al. (2008). Temperament at 7, 12, and 25 months in children at familial risk for ADHD. *Infant and Child Development, 17*, 321–338.

Bakermans-Kranenburg, M. J., Van Ijzendoorn, M. H., Mesman, J., Alink, L. R., & Juffer, F. (2008). Effects of an attachment-based intervention on daily cortisol moderated by dopamine receptor D4: A randomized control trial on 1-to 3-year-olds screened for externalizing behavior. *Development and Psychopathology, 20*, 805–820.

Barkley, R. A. (1997). Behavioral inhibition, sustained attention, and executive functions: Constructing a unifying theory of ADHD. *Psychological Bulletin, 121*, 65–94.

Barkley, R. A. (2006). *Attention deficit/hyperactivity disorder: A handbook for diagnosis and treatment* (3rd ed.). New York: Guilford.

Barkley, R. A., Fischer, M., Edelbrock, C., & Smallish, L. (1990). Adolescent outcome of hyperactive children diagnosed by research criteria: I. An 8-year prospective follow-up study. *Journal of the American Academy of Child and Adolescent Psychiatry, 29*, 546–557.

Barkley, R. A., Fischer, M., Smallish, L., & Fletcher, K. (2004). Young adult follow-up of hyperactive children: Antisocial activities and drug use. *Journal of Child Psychology and Psychiatry, 45*, 195–211.

Barkley, R. A., Fischer, M., Smallish, L., & Fletcher, K. (2006). Young adult outcome of hyperactive children: Adaptive functioning in major life activities. *Journal of the American Academy of Child and Adolescent Psychiatry, 45*, 192–202.

Barkley, R. A., Guevremont, D. C., Anastopoulos, A. D., DuPaul, G. J., & Shelton, T. L. (1993). Driving-related risks and outcomes of attention-deficit hyperactivity disorder in adolescents and young-adults – A 3-year to 5-year follow-up survey. *Pediatrics, 92*, 212–218.

Barkley, R. A., Murphy, K., & Fischer, M. (2007). *ADHD in adults: What the science says*. New York: Guilford.

Batty, M. J., Liddle, E. B., Pitiot, A., Toro, R., Groom, M. J., Scerif, G., et al. (2010). Cortical gray matter in attention-deficit hyperactivity disorder: A structural magnetic resonance imaging study. *Journal of the American Academy of Child and Adolescent Psychiatry, 49*, 229–238.

Beauchaine, T. P., Hinshaw, S. P., & Pang, K. L. (2010). Comorbidity of attention-deficit/hyperactivity disorder and early onset conduct disorder: Biological, environmental, and developmental mechanisms. *Clinical Psychology: Science and Practice, 17*, 327–336.

Ben Amor, L., Grizenko, N., Schwartz, G., Lageix, P., Baron, C., Ter-Stepanian, M., et al. (2005). Perinatal complications in children with attention-deficit hyperactivity disorder and their unaffected siblings. *Journal of Psychiatry and Neuroscience, 30*, 120–126.

Becker, K., El-Faddagh, M., Schmidt, M. H., Esser, G., & Laucht, M. (2008). Interaction of dopamine transporter genotype with prenatal smoke exposure on ADHD symptoms. *Journal of Pediatrics, 152*, 263–269.

Berwid, O. G., Curko Kera, E. A., Marks, D. J., Santra, A., Bender, H. A., & Halperin, J. M. (2005). Sustained attention and response inhibition in young children at risk for attention deficit hyperactivity disorder. *Journal of Child Psychology and Psychiatry, 46*, 1219–1229.

Berwid, O. G., & Halperin, J. M. (2012). Emerging support for a role of exercise in attention-deficit/hyperactivity disorder intervention planning. *Current Psychiatry Reports, 14*(5), 543–551.

Bhutta, A. T., Cleves, M. A., Casey, P. H., Craddock, M. M., & Anand, K. J. (2002). Cognitive and behavioral outcomes of school-aged children who were born preterm: A meta-analysis. *Journal of the American Medical Association, 288*, 728–737.

Biederman, J., Faraone, S., Milberger, S., Curtis, S., Chen, L., Marrs, A., et al. (1996). Predictors of persistence and remission of ADHD into adolescence: Results from a four-year prospective follow-up. *Journal of the American Academy of Child and Adolescent Psychiatry, 35*, 343–351.

Biederman, J., Faraone, S., & Monuteaux, B. (2002). Differential effect of environmental adversity by gender: Rutter's index of adversity in a group of boys and girls with and without ADHD. *American Journal of Psychiatry, 159*, 1556–1562.

Bor, W., Sanders, M. R., & Markie-Dadds, C. (2002). The effects of the Triple P-Positive Parenting Program on preschool children with co-occurring disruptive behavior and attentional/hyperactive difficulties. *Journal of Abnormal Child Psychology, 30*, 571–587.

Brookes, K. J., Mill, J., Guindalini, C., Curran, S., Xu, X. H., Knight, J., et al. (2006). A common haplotype of the dopamine transporter gene associated with attention-deficit/hyperactivity disorder and interacting with maternal use of alcohol during pregnancy. *Archives of General Psychiatry, 63*, 74–81.

Brophy, K., Hawi, Z., Kirley, A., Fitzgerald, M., & Gill, M. (2002). Synaptosomal-associated protein 25 (SNAP-25) and attention deficit hyperactivity disorder (ADHD): Evidence of linkage and association in the Irish population. *Molecular Psychiatry, 7*, 913–917.

Broyd, S. J., Demanuele, C., Debener, S., Helps, S. K., James, C. J., & Sonuga-Barke, E. J. S. (2009). Default-mode brain dysfunction in mental disorders: A systematic review. *Neuroscience and Biobehavioral Reviews, 33*, 279–296.

Bush, G., Spencer, T. J., Holmes, J., Shin, L. M., Valera, E. M., Seidman, L. J., et al. (2008). Functional magnetic resonance imaging of methylphenidate and placebo in attention-deficit/hyperactivity disorder during the multi-source interference task. *Archives of General Psychiatry, 65*, 102–114.

Campbell, S. B. (2002). *Behavior problems in preschool children: Clinical and developmental issues* (2nd ed.). New York: Guilford.

Campbell, S. B., Pierce, E. W., Moore, G., Marakovitz, S., & Newby, K. (1996). Boys' externalizing problems at elementary school: Pathways from early behavior problems, maternal control, and family stress. *Development and Psychopathology, 8*, 701–720.

Campbell, S. B., Pierce, E. W., March, C. L., Ewing, L. J., & Szumowski, E. K. (1994). Hard-to-manage preschool boys: Symptomatic behavior across contexts and time. *Child Development, 65*, 836–851.

Campbell, S. B., & von Stauffenberg, C. (2008). Child characteristics and family processes that predict behavioral readiness for school. In A. Booth & A. C. Crouter (Eds.), *Early disparities in school readiness: How do families contribute to successful and unsuccessful transitions into school?* (pp. 225–258). Mahwah, NJ: Erlbaum.

Campbell, S. B., & von Stauffenberg, C. (2009). Delay and inhibition as early predictors of ADHD symptoms in third grade. *Journal of Abnormal Child Psychology, 37*, 1–15.

Carmona, S., Proal, E., Hoekzema, E. A., Gispert, J. D., Picado, M., Moreno, I., et al. (2009). Ventro-striatal reductions underpin symptoms of hyperactivity and impulsivity in attention-deficit/hyperactivity disorder. *Biological Psychiatry, 66*, 972–977.

Caspi, A., Sugden, K., Moffitt, T. E., Taylor, A., Craig, I. W., Harrington, H., et al. (2003). Influence of life stress on depression modified by a polymorphism in the 5-HTT gene. *Science, 301*, 386–389.

Castellanos, F. X., Lee, P. P., Sharp, W., Jeffries, N. O., Greenstein, D. K., Clasen, L. S., et al. (2002). Developmental trajectories of brain volume abnormalities in children and adolescents with attention-deficit/hyperactivity disorder. *Journal of the American Medical Association, 288*, 1740–1748.

Clarke, A. R., Barry, R. J., McCarthy, R., Selikowitz, M., & Brown, C. R. (2002). EEG evidence for a new conceptualisation of attention deficit hyperactivity disorder. *Clinical Neurophysiology, 113*, 1036–1044.

Coghill, D., Nigg, J., Rothenberger, A., Sonuga-Barke, E., & Tannock, R. (2005). Wither causal models in the neuroscience of ADHD? *Developmental Science, 8*, 105–114.

Coghill, D., & Seth, S. (2011). Do the diagnostic criteria for ADHD need to change? *European Child and Adolescent Psychiatry, 20*, 75–81.

Coghill, D., & Sonuga-Barke, E. J. S. (2012). Categories versus dimensions in the classification and conceptualization of child and adolescent mental disorders – implications of recent empirical study. *Journal of Child Psychology and Psychiatry, 53*, 469–489.

Conners, C. K. (2000). Forty years of methylphenidate treatment in attention-deficit/hyperactivity disorder. *Journal of Attention Disorders, 6*(Suppl. 1), S17–S30.

Costello, E. J., Mustillo, S., Erkanli, A., Keeler, G., & Angold, A. (2003). Prevalence and development of psychiatric disorders in childhood and adolescence. *Archives of General Psychiatry, 60*, 837–844.

Counts, C. A., Nigg, J. T., Stawicki, J. A., Rappeley, M. D., & Von Eye, A. (2005). Family adversity in DSM-IV ADHD combined and inattentive subtypes and associated disruptive behavior problems. *Journal of the American Academy of Child and Adolescent Psychiatry, 44*, 690–698.

Cummings, E. M., Davies, P., & Campbell, S. B. (2000). *Developmental psychopathology and family process: Research, theory, and clinical implications*. New York: Guilford.

Dickstein, S. G., Bannon, K., Castellanos, F. X., & Milham, M. P. (2006). The neural correlates of attention deficit hyperactivity disorder: An ALE meta-analysis. *Journal of Child Psychology and Psychiatry, 47*, 1051–1062.

DuPaul, G. J., & Kern, L. (2011). *Young children with ADHD: Early identification and intervention*. Washington, DC: American Psychological Association.

Durston, S., van Belle, J., & de Zeeuw, P. (2011). Differentiating frontostriatal and fronto-cerebellar circuits in attention-deficit/hyperactivity disorder. *Biological Psychiatry, 69*, 1178–1184.

Egger, H. L., & Angold, A. (2006). Common emotional and behavioral disorders in preschool children: Presentation, nosology, and epidemiology. *Journal of Child Psychology and Psychiatry, 47*, 313–337.

Ellison-Wright, I., Ellison-Wright, Z., & Bullmore, E. (2008). Structural brain change in attention deficit hyperactivity disorder identified by meta-analysis. *BMC Psychiatry, 8*, 51.

Erhardt, D., & Baker, B. L. (1990). The effects of behavioral parent training on families with young hyperactive children. *Journal of Behavior Therapy and Experimental Psychiatry, 21*, 121–132.

Fabiano, G. A., Pelham, W. E., Gnagy, E. M., Burrows-MacLean, L., Coles, E. K., Chacko, A., et al. (2007). The single and combined effects of multiple intensities of behavior modification and methylphenidate for children with ADHD in a classroom setting. *School Psychology Review, 36*, 195–216.

Fair, D. A., Posner, J., Nagel, B. J., Bathula, D., Dias, T. G., Mills, K. L., et al. (2011). Atypical default network connectivity in youth with attention-deficit/hyperactivity disorder. *Biological Psychiatry, 68*, 1084–1091.

Faraone, S. V., Biederman, J., Spencer, T., Mick, E., Murray, K., Petty, C., et al. (2006). Diagnosing adult attention deficit hyperactivity disorder: Are late onset and subthreshold diagnoses valid? *American Journal of Psychiatry, 163*, 1720–1729.

Faraone, S. V., Perlis, R. H., Doyle, A. E., Smoller, J. W., Goralnick, J. J., Holmgren, M. A., et al. (2005). Molecular genetics of attention-deficit/hyperactivity disorder. *Biological Psychiatry, 57*, 1313–1323.

Frazier, T. W., Demaree, H. A., & Youngstrom, E. A. (2004). Meta-analysis of intellectual and neuropsychological test performance in attention-deficit/hyperactivity disorder. *Neuropsychology, 18*, 543–555.

Gibson, S. (2012). Rare and common variants: Twenty arguments. *Nature Reviews Genetics, 13*, 135–145.

Graziano, P. A., Calkins, S. D., & Keane, S. P. (2011). Sustained attention development during toddlerhood to preschool period: Associations with toddlers' emotion regulation strategies and maternal behavior. *Infant and Child Development, 20*, 389–408.

Greenhill, L. L., Halperin, J. M., & Abikoff, H. (1999). Stimulant medications. *Journal of the American Academy of Child and Adolescent Psychiatry, 38*, 503–512.

Greven, C. U., Asherson, P., Rijsdijk, F. V., & Plomin, R. (2011). A longitudinal twin study on the association between inattentive and hyperactive-impulsive ADHD symptoms. *Journal of Abnormal Child Psychology, 39*, 623–632.

Halperin, J. M., Bédard, A. C. V., & Curchack-Lichtin, J. T. (2012). Preventive interventions for ADHD: A neurodevelopmental perspective. *Neurotherapeutics, 9*(3), 531–541.

Halperin, J. M., & Healey, D. M. (2011). The influences of environmental enrichment, cognitive enhancement, and physical exercise on brain development: Can we alter the developmental trajectory of ADHD? *Neuroscience and Biobehavioral Reviews, 35*, 621–634.

Halperin, J. M., Marks, D. J., Bédard, A. C. V., Chacko, A., Curchack, J. T., Yoon, C. A., et al. (2013). Training executive, attention and motor skills (TEAMS): A proof-of-concept study in preschool children with ADHD. *Journal of Attention Disorders, 17*(8), 711–721.

Halperin, J. M., & Schulz, K. P. (2006). Revisiting the role of the prefrontal cortex in the pathophysiology of attention-deficit/hyperactivity disorder. *Psychological Bulletin, 132*, 560–581.

Halperin, J. M., Trampush, J. W., Miller, C. J., Marks, D. J., & Newcorn, J. H. (2008). Neuropsychological outcome in adolescents/young adults with childhood ADHD: Profiles of persisters, remitters, and controls. *Journal of Child Psychology and Psychiatry, 49*, 958–966.

Hanwella, R., Senanayake, M., & de Silva, V. (2011). Comparative efficacy and acceptability of methylphenidate and atomoxetine in treatment of attention deficit hyperactivity disorder in children and adolescents: A meta-analysis. *BMC Psychiatry, 11*, 176.

Hart, E. L., Lahey, B. B., Loeber, R., Applegate, B., & Frick, P. J. (1995). Developmental change in attention-deficit hyperactivity disorder in boys: A four-year longitudinal study. *Journal of Abnormal Child Psychology, 23*, 729–749.

Harty, S. C., Ivanov, I., Newcorn, J. H., & Halperin, J. M. (2011). The impact of conduct disorder and stimulant medication on later substance use in an ethnically diverse sample of individuals diagnosed with ADHD in childhood. *Journal of Child and Adolescent Psychopharmacology, 21*, 331–339.

Healey, D. M., Miller, C. J., Castelli, K. L., Marks, D. J., & Halperin, J. M. (2008). The impact of impairment criteria on the rates of ADHD diagnoses in preschoolers. *Journal of Abnormal Child Psychology, 36*, 771–778.

Hill, A. L., Degnan, K. A., Calkins, S. D., & Keane, S. P. (2006). Profiles of externalizing behavior problems for boys and girls across preschool: The roles of emotion regulation and inattention. *Developmental Psychology, 42*, 913–928.

Hinshaw, S. P., Owens, E. B., Sami, N., & Fargeon, S. (2006). Prospective follow-up of girls with attention-deficit/hyperactivity disorder into adolescence: Evidence for continuing cross-domain impairment. *Journal of Consulting and Clinical Psychology, 74*, 489–499.

Klingberg, T., Fernell, E., Olesen, P. J., Johnson, M., Gustafsson, P., Dahlström, K., et al. (2005). Computerized training of working memory in children with ADHD–a randomized, controlled trial. *Journal of the American Academy of Child and Adolescent Psychiatry, 44*, 177–186.

Lahey, B. B., Pelham, W. E., Loney, J., Lee, S., & Willcutt, E. (2005). Instability of DSM-IV subtypes of ADHD from preschool through elementary school. *Archives of General Psychiatry, 62*, 896–902.

Lahey, B. B., Rathouz, P. J., Lee, S. S., Chronis-Tuscano, A., Pelham, W. E., Waldman, I. D., et al. (2011). Interactions between early parenting and a polymorphism of the child's dopamine transporter gene in predicting future child conduct disorder symptoms. *Journal of Abnormal Psychology, 120*, 33–45.

Lahey, B. B., & Willcutt, E. G. (2010). Predictive validity of a continuous alternative to nominal subtypes of attention-deficit/hyperactivity disorder for DSM-V. *Journal of Clinical Child and Adolescent Psychology, 39*, 761–775.

Lee, S. S., & Hinshaw, S. P. (2006). Predictors of adolescent functioning in girls with attention deficit hyperactivity disorder (ADHD): The role of childhood ADHD, conduct problems, and peer status. *Journal of Clinical Child and Adolescent Psychology, 35*, 356–368.

Lee, S. S., Lahey, B. B., Owens, E. B., & Hinshaw, S. P. (2008). Few preschool boys and girls with ADHD are well-adjusted during adolescence. *Journal of Abnormal Child Psychology, 36*, 373–383.

Liddle, E. B., Hollis, C., Batty, M. J., Groom, M. J., Totman, J. J., Liotti, M., et al. (2011). Task-related default mode network modulation and inhibitory control in ADHD: Effects of motivation and methylphenidate. *Journal of Child Psychology and Psychiatry, 52*, 761–771.

Linares, T. J., Singer, L. T., Kirchner, H. L., Short, E. J., Min, M. O., Hussey, P., et al. (2006). Mental health outcomes of cocaine-exposed children at 6 years of age. *Journal of Pediatric Psychology, 31*, 85–97.

Lionel, A. C., Crosbie, J., Barbosa, N., Goodale, T., Thiruvahindrapuram, B., Rickaby, J., et al. (2011). Rare copy number variation discovery and cross-disorder comparisons identify risk genes for ADHD. *Science Translational Medicine, 3*.

Madras, B. K., Miller, G. M., & Fischman, A. I. (2005). The dopamine transporter and attention-deficit/hyperactivity disorder. *Biological Psychiatry, 57*, 1397–1409.

Mannuzza, S., Klein, R. G., Bessler, A., Malloy, P., & Hynes, M. E. (1997). Educational and occupational outcome of hyperactive boys grown up. *Journal of the American Academy of Child and Adolescent Psychiatry, 36*, 1122–1127.

Mannuzza, S., Klein, R. G., Bonagura, N., Malloy, P., Giampino, T. L., & Addalli, K. A. (1991). Hyperactive boys almost grown up. V. Replication of psychiatric status. *Archives of General Psychiatry, 48*, 77–83.

Marco, R., Miranda, A., Schlotz, W., Melia, A., Mulligan, A., Muller, U., et al. (2009). Delay and reward choice in ADHD: An experimental test of the role of delay aversion. *Neuropsychology, 23*, 367–380.

Meaney, M. J. (2010). Epigenetics and the biological definition of gene × environment interaction. *Child Development, 81*, 41–79.

Metin, B., Roeyers, H., Wiersema, R., van der Meere, J., & Sonuga-Barke, E. (2012). A meta-analytic study of event rate effects on go/no-go performance in attention-deficit hyperactivity disorder. *Biological Psychiatry, 72*(12), 990–996.

Mick, E., Byrne, D., Fried, R., Monuteaux, M., Faraone, S. V., & Biederman, J. (2011). Predictors of ADHD persistence in girls at 5-year follow-up. *Journal of Attention Disorders, 15*, 183–192.

Milich, R., Balentine, A., & Lynam, D. (2001). ADHD combined type and ADHD predominantly inattentive type are distinct and unrelated disorders. *Clinical Psychology: Science and Practice, 8*, 463–488.

Miller, C. J., Flory, J. D., Miller, S. R., Harty, S. C., Newcorn, J. H., & Halperin, J. M. (2008). Childhood ADHD and the emergence of personality disorders in adolescence: A prospective follow-up study. *Journal of Clinical Psychiatry, 69*, 1476–1483.

Mokrova, I., O'Brien, M., Calkins, S., & Keane, S. (2010). Parental ADHD symptomatology and ineffective parenting: The connecting link of home chaos. *Parenting: Science and Practice, 10*, 119–135.

Molina, B. S., Bukstein, O. G., & Lynch, K. G. (2002). Attention-deficit/hyperactivity disorder and conduct disorder symptomatology in adolescents with alcohol use disorder. *Psychology of Addictive Behavior, 16*, 161–164.

Molina, B. S., Flory, K., Hinshaw, S. P., Greiner, A. R., Arnold, L. E., Swanson, J. M., et al. (2007). Delinquent behavior and emerging substance use in the MTA at 36 months: Prevalence, course, and treatment effects. *Journal of the American Academy of Child and Adolescent Psychiatry, 46*, 1028–1040.

Molina, B. S., Hinshaw, S. P., Swanson, J. M., Arnold, L. E., Vitiello, B., Jensen, P. S., et al. (2009). The MTA at 8 years: Prospective follow-up of children treated for combined-type ADHD in a multisite study. *Journal of the American Academy of Child and Adolescent Psychiatry, 48*, 484–500.

Molina, B. S., & Pelham, W. E., Jr. (2003). Childhood predictors of adolescent substance use in a longitudinal study of children with ADHD. *Journal of Abnormal Psychology, 112*, 497–507.

MTA Cooperative Group. (1999). 14-Month randomized clinical trial of treatment strategies for attention deficit hyperactivity disorder. *Archives of General Psychiatry, 56*, 1073–1086.

MTA Cooperative Group. (2004). National Institute of Mental Health Multimodal Treatment Study of ADHD follow-up: 24-Month outcomes of treatment strategies for attention-deficit/hyperactivity disorder. *Pediatrics, 113*, 754–761.

Neale, B. M., Medland, S. E., Ripke, S., Asherson, P., Franke, B., Lesch, K. P., et al. (2010). Meta-analysis of genome-wide association studies of attention-deficit/hyperactivity disorder. *Journal of the American Academy of Child and Adolescent Psychiatry, 49*, 884–897.

Nigg, J. (2006). *What causes ADHD?* New York: Guilford.

Nigg, J. T., Goldsmith, H. H., & Sachek, J. (2004). Temperament and attention-deficit/hyperactivity disorder: The development of a multiple pathway model. *Journal of Clinical Child and Adolescent Psychology, 33*, 42–53.

Nigg, J. T., Willcutt, E. G., Doyle, A. E., & Sonuga-Barke, E. J. S. (2005). Causal heterogeneity in attention-deficit/hyperactivity disorder: Do we need neuropsychologically impaired subtypes? *Biological Psychiatry, 57*, 1224–1230.

Nomura, Y., Marks, D. J., & Halperin, J. M. (2010). Prenatal exposure to maternal and paternal smoking on attention deficit hyperactivity disorder symptoms and diagnosis in offspring. *Journal of Nervous and Mental Disease, 198*, 672–678.

Oades, R. D., Lasky-Su, J., Christiansen, H., Faraone, S. V., Sonuga-Barke, E. J., Banaschewski, T., et al. (2008). The influence of serotonin- and other genes on impulsive behavioral aggression and cognitive impulsivity in children with attention-deficit/hyperactivity disorder (ADHD): Findings from a family-based association test (FBAT) analysis. *Behavioral and Brain Functions, 4*, 4–48.

Oades, R. D., Sadile, A. G., Sagvolden, T., Viggiano, D., Zuddas, A., Devoto, P., et al. (2005). The control of responsiveness in ADHD by catecholamines: Evidence for dopaminergic, noradrenergic and interactive roles. *Developmental Science, 8*, 122–131.

O'Connor, T. G., Heron, J., Golding, J., & Glover, V. (2003). Maternal antenatal anxiety and behavioural/emotional problems in children: A test of a programming hypothesis. *Journal of Child Psychology and Psychiatry, 44*, 1025–1036.

Olson, S. L., Sameroff, A. J., Kerr, D., Lopez, N. L., & Wellman, H. M. (2005). Developmental foundations of externalizing problems in young children: The role of effortful control. *Development and Psychopathology, 17*, 25–45.

Pelham, W. E., Jr., & Fabiano, G. A. (2008). Evidence-based psychosocial treatments for attention-deficit/hyperactivity disorder. *Journal of Clinical Child and Adolescent Psychology, 37*, 184–214.

Pelham, W. E., Jr., Wheeler, T., & Chronis, A. (1998). Empirically supported psychosocial treatments for attention deficit hyperactivity disorder. *Journal of Clinical Child Psychology, 27*, 190–205.

Peterson, B. S., Potenza, M. N., Wang, Z. S., Zhu, H., Martin, A., Marsh, R., et al. (2009). An fMRI study of the effects of psychostimulants on default-mode processing during Stroop task performance in youths with ADHD. *American Journal of Psychiatry, 166*, 1286–1294.

Pickles, A., & Angold, A. (2003). Natural categories or fundamental dimensions: On carving nature at the joints and the re-articulation of psychopathology. *Development and Psychopathology, 15*, 613–640.

Pierce, E. W., Ewing, L. J., & Campbell, S. B. (1999). Diagnostic status and symptomatic behavior of hard-to-manage preschool children in middle childhood and early adolescence. *Journal of Clinical Child Psychology, 28*, 44–57.

Pisecco, S., Huzinec, C., & Curtis, D. (2001). The effect of child characteristics on teachers' acceptability of classroom-based behavioral strategies and psychostimulant medication for the treatment of ADHD. *Journal of Clinical Child Psychology, 30*, 413–421.

Pisterman, S., Firestone, P., McGrath, P., Goodman, J. T., Webster, I., Mallory, R., et al. (1992). The role of parent training in treatment of preschoolers with ADDH. *American Journal of Orthopsychiatry, 62*, 397–408.

Plessen, K. J., Bansal, R., Zhu, H. T., Whiteman, R., Amat, J., Quackenbush, J. A., et al. (2006). Hippocampus and amygdala morphology in attention-deficit/hyperactivity disorder. *Archives of General Psychiatry, 63*, 795–807.

Pliszka, S. R. (2005). The neuropsychopharmacology of attention-deficit/hyperactivity disorder. *Biological Psychiatry, 57*, 1385–1390.

Poelmans, G., Pauls, D. L., Buitelaar, J. K., & Franke, B. (2011). Integrated genome-wide association study findings: Identification of a neurodevelopmental network for attention deficit hyperactivity disorder. *American Journal of Psychiatry, 168*, 365–377.

Power, T. J., Hess, L. E., & Bennett, D. S. (1995). The acceptability of interventions for attention-deficit hyperactivity disorder among elementary and middle school teachers. *Journal of Developmental and Behavioral Pediatrics, 16*, 238–243.

Rapport, M. D., Alderson, R. M., Kofler, M. J., Sarver, D. E., Bolden, J., & Sims, V. (2008). Working memory deficits in boys with attention-deficit/hyperactivity disorder (ADHD): The contribution of central executive and subsystem processes. *Journal of Abnormal Child Psychology, 36*, 825–837.

Rothbart, M., & Bates, J. E. (1998). Temperament. In W. Damon (Series Ed) & N. Eisenberg (Vol. Ed.), *Handbook of child psychology* (Vol. 3. Social, emotional, and personality development, 5th ed., pp. 105–176). New York: Wiley.

Rubia, K., Smith, A. B., Brammer, M. J., Toone, B., & Taylor, E. (2005). Abnormal brain activation during inhibition and error detection in medication-naive adolescents with ADHD. *American Journal of Psychiatry, 162*, 1067–1075.

Rutter, M. (2000). Psychosocial influences: Critiques, findings, and research needs. *Development and Psychopathology, 12*, 375–405.

Rutter, M. (2006). *Genes and behavior: Nature-nurture interplay explained*. Malden, MA: Blackwell.

Scheres, A., Milham, M. P., Knutson, B., & Castellanos, F. X. (2006). Ventral striatal hyporesponsiveness during reward anticipation in attention-deficit/hyperactivity disorder. *Biological Psychiatry, 61*, 720–724.

Schulz, K. P., Newcorn, J. H., Fan, J., Tang, C. Y., & Halperin, J. M. (2005). Brain activation gradients in ventrolateral prefrontal cortex related to persistence of ADHD in adolescent boys. *Journal of the American Academy of Child and Adolescent Psychiatry, 44*, 47–54.

Seidman, L. J. (2006). Neuropsychological functioning in people with ADHD across the lifespan. *Clinical Psychology Review, 26*, 466–485.

Seipp, C. M., & Johnston, C. (2005). Mother-son interactions in families of boys with attention deficit/hyperactivity disorder with and without oppositional behavior. *Journal of Abnormal Child Psychology, 33*, 87–98.

Sergeant, J. A. (2005). Modeling attention-deficit/hyperactivity disorder: A critical appraisal of the cognitive-energetic model. *Biological Psychiatry, 57*, 1248–1255.

Shalev, L., Tsal, Y., & Mevorach, C. (2007). Computerized progressive attentional training (CPAT) program: Effective direct intervention for children with ADHD. *Child Neuropsychology, 13*, 382–388.

Shaw, P., Eckstrand, K., Sharp, W., Blumenthal, J., Lerch, J. P., Greenstein, D., et al. (2007). Attention deficit/hyperactivity disorder is characterized by a delay in cortical maturation. *Proceedings of the National Academy of Science, 104*, 199649–199654.

Sheese, B. E., Voelker, P. M., Rothbart, M. K., & Posner, M. I. (2007). Parenting quality interacts with genetic variation in dopamine receptor D4 to influence temperament in early childhood. *Development and Psychopathology, 19*, 1039–1046.

Sonuga-Barke, E. J., Auerbach, J., Campbell, S. B., Daley, D., & Thompson, M. (2005). Preschool varieties of hyperactive and dysregulated behaviour: Multiple pathways between risk and disorder. *Developmental Science, 8*, 141–150.

Sonuga-Barke, E. J., Bitsakou, P., & Thompson, M. (2010). Beyond the dual pathway model: Evidence for the dissociation of timing, inhibitory, and delay-related impairments in attention-deficit/hyperactivity disorder. *Journal of the American Academy of Child and Adolescent Psychiatry, 49*, 345–355.

Sonuga-Barke, E. J., & Castellanos, F. X. (2007). Spontaneous attentional fluctuations in impaired states and pathological conditions: A neurobiological hypothesis. *Neuroscience and Biobehavioral Reviews, 31*, 977–986.

Sonuga-Barke, E. J., Dalen, L., Daley, D., & Remington, B. (2002). Are planning, working memory, and inhibition associated with individual differences in preschool ADHD symptoms? *Developmental Neuropsychology, 21*, 255–272.

Sonuga-Barke, E. J., Daley, D., Thompson, M., Laver-Bradbury, C., & Weeks, A. (2001). Parent-based therapies for preschool attention-deficit/hyperactivity disorder: A randomized, controlled trial with a community sample. *Journal of the American Academy of Child and Adolescent Psychiatry, 40*, 402–408.

Sonuga-Barke, E. J., & Fairchild, G. (2012). Neuroeconomics of attention-deficit/hyperactivity disorder: Differential influences of medial, dorsal, and ventral prefrontal brain networks on suboptimal decision making? *Biological Psychiatry, 72*, 126–133.

Sonuga-Barke, E. J., & Halperin, J. (2010). Developmental phenotypes and causal pathways in attention deficit/hyperactivity disorder: Potential targets for early intervention? *Journal of Child Psychology and Psychiatry, 51*, 368–398.

Sonuga-Barke, E. J., Oades, R. D., Psychogiou, L., Chen, W., Franke, B., Buitelaar, J., et al. (2009). Dopamine and serotonin transporter genotypes moderate sensitivity to maternal expressed emotion: The case of conduct and emotional problems in attention-deficit/hyperactivity disorder. *Journal of Child Psychology and Psychiatry, 50*, 1052–1063.

Swanson, J. M., Elliott, G. R., Greenhill, L. L., Wigal, T., Arnold, L. E., Vitiello, B., et al. (2007). Effects of stimulant medication on growth rates across three years in the MTA follow-up. *Journal of the American Academy of Child and Adolescent Psychiatry, 46*, 1015–1027.

Swanson, J. M., Kraemer, H. C., Hinshaw, S. P., Arnold, L. E., Conners, C. K., Abikoff, H. B., et al. (2001). Clinical relevance of the primary findings of the MTA: Success rates based on severity of symptoms at the end of treatment. *Journal of the American Academy of Child and Adolescent Psychiatry, 40*, 168–179.

Tamm, L., Nakonezny, P. A., & Hughes, C. W. (2012). An open trial of a metacognitive executive function training for young children with ADHD. *Journal of Attention Disorders*. doi:10.1177/1087054712.

Taylor, E., & Rogers, J. W. (2005). Early adversity and developmental disorders. *Journal of Child Psychology and Psychiatry, 46*, 451–467.

Thapar, A., Fowler, T., Rice, F., Scourfield, J., van den Bree, M., Thomas, H., et al. (2003). Maternal smoking during pregnancy and attention deficit hyperactivity disorder symptoms in offspring. *American Journal of Psychiatry, 160*, 1985–1989.

Thapar, A., O'Donovan, M., & Owen, M. J. (2005). The genetics of attention deficit hyperactivity disorder. *Human Molecular Genetics, 14*, 272–275.

Thapar, A., Rice, F., Hay, D., Boivin, J., Langley, K., van den Bree, M., et al. (2009). Prenatal smoking might not cause attention-deficit/hyperactivity disorder: Evidence from a novel design. *Biological Psychiatry, 66*, 722–727.

Thompson, M. J., Laver-Bradbury, C., Ayres, M., Le Poidevin, E., Mead, S., Dodds, C., et al. (2009). A small-scale randomized controlled trial of the revised new forest parenting programme for preschoolers with attention deficit hyperactivity disorder. *European Child and Adolescent Psychiatry, 18*, 605–616.

Vaidya, C. J., Bunge, S. A., Dudukovic, N. M., & Zalecki, C. A. (2005). Altered neural substrates of cognitive control in childhood ADHD: Evidence from functional magnetic resonance imaging. *American Journal of Psychiatry, 162*, 1605–1613.

Valera, E. M., Faraone, S. V., Murray, K. E., & Seidman, L. J. (2007). Meta-analysis of structural imaging findings in attention-deficit/hyperactivity disorder. *Biological Psychiatry, 61*, 1361–1369.

van den Hoofdakker, B. J., Nauta, M. H., Dijck-Brouwer, D. A. J., van der Veen-Mulders, L., Sytema, S., Emmelkamp, P. M., et al. (2012). Dopamine transporter gene moderates response to behavioral parent training in children with ADHD: A pilot study. *Developmental Psychology, 48*, 567–574.

van Ewijk, H., Heslenfeld, D. J., Zwiers, M. P., Buitelaar, J. K., & Oosterlaan, J. (2012). Diffusion tensor imaging in attention deficit/hyperactivity disorder: A systematic review and meta-analysis. *Neuroscience and Biobehavioral Reviews, 36*, 1093–1106.

Vaurio, L., Riley, E. R., & Mattson, S. N. (2008). Differences in executive functioning in children with heavy prenatal alcohol exposure or attention-deficit/hyperactivity disorder. *Journal of the International Neuropsychological Society, 14*, 119–129.

Volkow, N. D., Wang, G. J., Tomasi, D., Kollins, S. H., Wigal, T. L., Newcorn, J. H., et al. (2012). Methylphenidate-elicited dopamine increases in ventral striatum are associated with long-term symptom improvement in adults with attention deficit hyperactivity disorder. *Journal of Neuroscience, 32*, 841–849.

Wahlstedt, C., Thorell, L. B., & Bohlin, G. (2008). ADHD symptoms and executive function impairment: Early predictors of later behavioral problems. *Developmental Neuropsychology, 33,* 160–178.

Weiss, G., & Hechtman, L. (1993). *Hyperactive children grown up* (2nd ed.). New York: Guilford.

Weyant, L. L., & DuPaul, G. (2006). ADHD in college students. *Journal of Attention Disorders, 10,* 9–19.

Wiersema, R., Van der Meere, J., Antrop, I., & Roeyers, H. (2006). State regulation in adult ADHD: An event-related potential study. *Journal of Clinical and Experimental Neuro-psychology, 28,* 1113–1126.

Wigal, T., Greenhill, L., Chuang, S., McGough, J., Vitiello, B., Skrobala, A., et al. (2006). Safety and tolerability of methylphenidate in preschool children with ADHD. *Journal of the American Academy of Child and Adolescent Psychiatry, 45,* 1294–1303.

Willcutt, E. G., Doyle, A. E., Nigg, J. T., Faraone, S. V., & Pennington, B. F. (2005). Validity of the executive function theory of attention-deficit/hyperactivity disorder: A meta-analytic review. *Biological Psychiatry, 57,* 1336–1346.

Willcutt, E. G., & Pennington, B. F. (2000). Comorbidity between reading disability and attention- deficit/hyperactivity disorder: Differences by gender and subtype. *Journal of Learning Disorders, 33,* 179–191.

Willoughby, M., Pek, J., Greenberg, M. T., & The Family Life Project Investigators. (2012). Parent-reported attention deficit/hyperactivity symptomatology in preschool-aged children: Factor structure, developmental change, and early risk factors. *Journal of Abnormal Child Psychology, 40*(8), 1301–1312.

Winstanley, C. A., Eagle, D. M., & Robbins, T. W. (2006). Behavioral models of impulsivity in relation to ADHD: Translation between clinical and preclinical studies. *Clinical Psychology Review, 26,* 379–395.

Wolraich, M., Brown, L., Brown, R. T., DuPaul, G., Earls, M., Feldman, H. M., et al. (2011). ADHD: Clinical practice guideline for the diagnosis, evaluation, and treatment of attention-deficit/hyperactivity disorder in children and adolescents. *Pediatrics, 128,* 1007–1022.

Wolosin, S. M., Richardson, M. E., Hennessey, J. G., Denckla, M. B., & Mostofsky, S. H. (2009). Abnormal cerebral cortex structure in children with ADHD. *Human Brain mapping, 30,* 175–184.

Zito, J. M., Daniel, J. S., dosReis, S., Gardner, J. F., Boles, M., & Lynch, F. (2000). Trends in the prescribing of psychotropic medications to preschoolers. *Journal of the American Medical Association, 283,* 1025–1030.

A Developmental Model of Aggression and Violence: Microsocial and Macrosocial Dynamics Within an Ecological Framework

23

Thomas J. Dishion

Overview

In this chapter an ecological framework is proposed for understanding the development of individual differences in aggression and violence from childhood to adulthood. The model is based on three organizing hypotheses. The first hypothesis is that aversive social behaviors and threats can function to "coerce" the immediate social environment (i.e., microdynamics) such that aggressive behavior is strengthened over time (Patterson, 1982). The second hypothesis is that some aggressive individuals join within social networks; as such, aggression amplifies in lethality and frequency through social contagion dynamics (i.e., macrodynamics) and then culminates in violence (Dishion & Tipsord, 2011). The third hypothesis is that aggression and violence are predictable and preventable and that interventions that target the key micro- and macrodynamics social processes relevant to each developmental period can reduce individual levels of aggression and prevalence of aggression and violence in the community (Biglan, 2003). In this chapter, each hypothesis is discussed in the context of developmental patterns of aggression and violence.

T.J. Dishion, Ph.D. (✉)
Department of Psychology & Prevention
Research Center, Arizona State University,
Tempe, AZ 85287, USA
e-mail: Dishion@asu.edu

It is increasingly clear that one must consider both biological and environmental factors to understand the emergence of aggression and violence that develop by adulthood. Caspi and colleagues, for example, tested a model with a gene by environment interaction that accounted for adult violence in males. In this model, boys with the MAO-A single-nucleotide polymorphism who also had been exposed to parental maltreatment in early childhood were the most likely to be violent adult offenders (Caspi et al., 2002). There is compelling evidence that factors such as impulsivity and poor self-regulation render children more vulnerable to harsh and pathogenic environments (Dishion & Patterson, 2006). However, in general, genetic vulnerabilities account for very little of the overall variance in aggression and violence. In contrast, environmental experiences, which are often amenable to intervention, account for a relatively large proportion of the variance in individual differences in aggression and violence. Those interventions that target and improve the parenting environment, for example, completely mitigate genetic vulnerability for multiple forms of problem behavior (Brody et al., 2009). Thus, the primary focus of this chapter is the social dynamics underlying the emergence of aggression and the ensuing amplification to violence.

An ecological framework can be a useful organizing structure for thinking about systems of influence on aggression as a child develops over time (Bronfenbrenner, 1979; Hinde, 1974). While examining a child's ecology, one can parse the social environment into specific microsocial and macrosocial influences (Dishion & Patterson, 2006). Microsocial influences involve relatively immediate action and reaction patterns in which aggressive behavior is learned and amplified. In terms of the development of aggression, parent–child, sibling–child, and peer–child interactions are the most frequently studied relationships.

Macrosocial dynamics evolve over longer periods of time, and their functional significance is less apparent in the study of social interaction patterns. For example, engaging with a gang network in a community can confer status, basic resources, and potential sexual partners (see Dishion, Ha, & Véronneau, 2012), which are functional outcomes that are both immediate and deferred over the course of days, weeks, months, and years. This perspective is helpful when studying the development of aggression in children in that one examines the child's movement from the family, to peers and teachers in school, to friendships, and eventually to an intimate partner, adult family relationships, and relationship networks in the community (e.g., military service, gangs, coworkers, extended family).

From an ecological perspective, when aggression evokes gang membership, it has shaped the social context and network of the individual. This sort of macrosocial function is often of interest to evolutionary psychologists (e.g., Belsky, Steinberg, & Draper, 1991; Ellis, Figueredo, Brumbach, & Schlomer, 2009), but in actuality, selection by consequences occurs at all levels of social interaction (Biglan, 2003). Behavior is shaped by the momentary reactions of the audience and by the biologically driven survival function of procreation and group affili-

ation (Dishion et al., 2012; Dishion & Patterson, 2006).

When relationship niches are considered in the context of the life course, attention must be given to the functional dynamics in each relationship and to the dynamics of movement from one relationship to another (i.e., macrosocial). Figure 23.1 summarizes the interlocking microsocial and macrosocial dynamics that define the evolution of socialization experiences that have been found to underlie the development of aggression and violence beginning in early childhood and continuing through early adulthood. From a biosocial perspective, genetic and other biological characteristics (e.g., sex, puberty) of the child motivate developmental progressions and interact with microsocial and macrosocial dynamics to account for individual differences in aggression and violence.

One of the core achievements in developmental psychopathology is the ability to map the transformation from minor problems in self-regulation to development of serious forms of aggression in young adulthood. Several research groups have referred to the unfolding of socialization experiences leading to various forms of adolescent problem behavior as a *developmental cascade* (Dodge, Greenberg, & Malone, 2008; Masten et al., 2005; Moilanen, Shaw, & Maxwell, 2010). Each developmental stage has its adjustment outcomes and collateral effects, which can be seen as products of the outcome that feed into the developmental cascade toward violence.

Following is a more detailed description of how coercion and contagion dynamics at each stage of development account for variation in aggression.

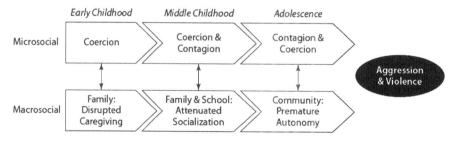

Fig. 23.1 Microsocial and macrosocial dynamics leading to aggression and violence in late adolescence

Coercion and Contagion Dynamics

Coercion is a basic interpersonal dynamic by which individuals use aversive behavior to attain access to rewarding resources and to reduce unpleasant experiences. It can involve being aggressive or unpleasant, or it can play out as emotional manipulation. Although aggression and violence are certainly examples of more extreme forms of coercion, the vast majority of coercive exchanges go unnoticed by the participants. A young child's whining sets the stage for parents to attend to, and potentially reward, the behavior. However, most parents, at some time, reverse the pattern and work to teach the child to use language to make requests rather than rely on whining and crying (Patterson, 1982). The coercion process is inherently bidirectional in that it builds on response tendencies of both the child and the parent. The key to change often lies in parents' ability to regulate their emotional reaction to aversive child behavior rather than yell, withdraw, spoil, or hit and to mindfully manage the child's behavior by using patience and by optimizing opportunities for their child to learn social skills. The link between understanding coercion and promoting family management becomes clear: The latter is the remedy for the former. Positive family management practices reduce the functional utility of coercive dynamics in the family.

Intensive research on the coercion dynamic began in the homes of children referred to outpatient clinics for aggressive behavior (Patterson, 1974). To isolate the underlying patterns that accounted for the coercion dynamic, Patterson and colleagues conducted a series of studies that looked at the conditional probability of a child's aggressive response to a parent's behavior. This series of detailed observational studies revealed the importance of stimulus control in the aggressive exchange (Patterson, 1976; Patterson & Cobb, 1973; Patterson & Moore, 1979). Although work on coercion theory was initially driven by intensive study of clinically aggressive children, the concepts were measured in epidemiologically defined community samples of youths and found

to predict escalations in problem behavior from childhood through adolescence (for a review, see Dishion & Patterson, 2006). When the coercion model was then applied to the design of prevention studies, it was found that targeting coercive parenting practices prevented the escalations in problem behaviors one would expect among high-risk adolescents (Dishion, Patterson, & Kavanagh, 1992) and in families undergoing divorce and remarriage (for a review, see Forgatch & Patterson, 2010). These findings suggested that whatever the origins of coercive dynamics in families, interventions that reduce coercion help reduce antisocial and aggressive behavior in childhood and adolescence.

The peer contagion dynamic is of particular interest with regard to the amplification of children's aggression to other forms of problem behavior. Since the beginning of systematic research on antisocial and delinquent behavior, it was observed that peers are core to the problem, but the influence process was unclear (Dishion & Patterson, 2006). We began to study the microsocial dynamic we called *deviancy training* (Dishion, Capaldi, Spracklen, & Li, 1995; Dishion, Spracklen, Andrews, & Patterson, 1996). We began by carefully observing the adolescent male friendships of a sample of 13- to 14-year-old boys in the Oregon Youth Study (Patterson, Reid, & Dishion, 1992). In these videotaped interactions, we coded the boys' deviant talk and their affective reactions in real time. To study the reinforcement of deviant values in verbal exchanges among peers, one must use an extension of the typical learning approach to studying aggressive behavior. Relational frame theory (Hayes & Hayes, 1992) clarified the mechanisms by which reinforcement of words is equivalent to reinforcement of behavior. A uniquely human capability that comes with language is that rewarding deviant talk is as powerful as rewarding the actual behavior.

We applied the "matching law" to evaluate the extent to which the boys were being selectively reinforced for deviant talk compared with other, more normative topics (i.e., relative rate of reinforcement). In general, we found that the amount of deviant talk in an adolescent friendship was directly proportionate to the friend's relative amount of positive affect in response to deviant versus normative talk (Dishion et al., 1996). Snyder et al. (2008) extended the concept of deviancy training to include young children mocking adult behavior, such as pretending to smoke cigarettes during playtime at school. The studies by Snyder and colleagues also coded positive affect and found that some youths were mutually reinforcing deviant talk and that this dynamic contributed to later increases in antisocial behavior. The idea that peer contagion has a unique influence on future behavior of children and adolescents has been supported by studies of iatrogenic effects, which have indicated that random assignment to group interventions that aggregate high-risk children can potentially increase problem behavior, and that these increases are associated with deviancy training in the sessions (Dishion, McCord, & Poulin, 1999; Dodge, Dishion, & Lansford, 2006).

Coercion and contagion are interpersonal dynamics that often occur outside of the participants' awareness. Coercion is more characteristic of established relationships in which members share a certain level of "fate control," such as parent–child, sibling, and marital relationships. Contagion, on the other hand, is a concept typically applied to understanding how behaviors become disinhibited in the context of age-mates (Dishion & Tipsord, 2011). To study coercion and contagion as real-time behavioral dynamics, it is necessary to code interpersonal events as they unfold over time and to link interpersonal outcomes (ending conflict, mutual laughter) with the coercion and contagion dynamic over time. It is possible, however, to use global ratings of direct observation data to surmise the extent to which a relationship interaction is characterized by either coercion or deviancy training.

Early Childhood

How does a toddler become an oppositional and defiant child? This developmental period is characterized by strong dependence on primary caregivers for nurturance, safety, and socialization (Ainsworth, 1989). This foundation is not to be underestimated; lack of it will set the stage for struggles in other periods of development of self-regulation (Rothbart, Ellis, Rueda, & Posner, 2003) and of correlated problem behaviors, such as oppositional behavior and aggression (Olson, Sameroff, Kerr, Lopez, & Wellman, 2005).

Given the evidence that early-onset antisocial behavior is potentially the most problematic for the child and the community, it stands to reason that considerable work would have been done to examine early-childhood parent–child interactions and interventions. Patterson's theoretical framework of coercive family processes is relevant to understanding how the interaction of child characteristics and parenting practices prompts development of early problem behavior (Patterson, 1982; Patterson et al., 1992). Coercion theory posits that a child's interpersonal style is largely learned within the family and carries over to interactions with others outside the family, such as peers and teachers.

Although numerous studies of parenting in early childhood are conducted, many use measurement shortcuts. For example, parent reports of their own parenting practices are certainly useful, but they may be insufficient when applied to the problem of studying moment-to-moment interaction patterns. A critical impetus to more carefully examine the parent–child dynamic in early childhood was the finding that boys identified by teachers as oppositional had often been on a trajectory of problem behavior since age 2. A tendency for the child to be bold in the face of a fearful stimulus, together with maternal depression at child age 2, has been shown to be the best predictor of the early-onset trajectory (Shaw, Gilliom, Ingoldsby, & Nagin, 2003). A modicum of compassion enables us to appreciate how parenting can be disrupted when isolated mothers care for young children without adequate support (Wahler, 1980). Depression certainly disrupts positive parenting and the critical exchanges between a young child and his or her caregiver (Hops, Sherman, & Biglan, 1990). However, surprisingly little research has identified the effects of caregiver isolation and depression on actual parent–child coercion dynamics.

The study of coercion dynamics presents some difficulty because it requires the measurement of parent–child interaction as it unfolds in real time. With an observed microsocial data stream, one can examine how contingent events lead to escalation of the aversiveness of the interaction. Early on, use of Markov models of social interaction and computation of sequential analyses activated interest among scientists studying microsocial dynamics (Gottman & Roy, 1990), but these models became increasingly suspect, partly because of the base rate problem. Aversive events generally constitute a minority of social events, and the probability of a parent responding aversively contingent on a child's coercive behavior is about .5 of 10 % of the interaction. Given the rarity of aversive exchanges, estimates of coercive interaction patterns were somewhat unreliable (Stoolmiller, 2001).

Snyder and colleagues (Snyder, Edwards, McGraw, Kilgore, & Holton, 1994) were the first to consider intensity and duration as critical parameters of escalating patterns of coercion. In an examination of 10 aggressive and 10 nonaggressive preschool children, parent–child interactions were studied for 10 h. The researchers found that duration of conflict was the key to studying the progression of coercion. Using the Family Process Code, which captures real-time duration of parent–child interactive behavior (Dishion et al., 1983), these researchers determined that parent–child interactions that involved aggressive children were characterized by longer durations of conflict, greater intensity of conflict, and a statistically reliable tendency for the children to be reinforced for their behavior during conflict.

Recently, Smith and colleagues tested the coercion model longitudinally in an ethnically diverse sample of 730 toddlers followed to age 7.5 (Smith, Dishion, Shaw, & Wilson, 2013). Coercive exchanges between parent and child were measured using duration coding and were found to increase from age 2 through age 5, suggesting that coercion dynamics emerge in early childhood and are not in place at age 2. Key to the coercion model is children's noncompliance (Patterson, 1982). Children's noncompliance was rated by coders who

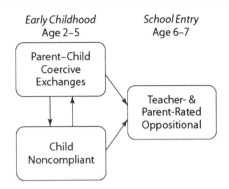

Fig. 23.2 Coercion dynamics in early childhood and oppositional and defiant behavior (adapted from Smith et al., 2013)

watched the videotaped parent–child interaction sessions; mothers rated their child's oppositional behavior at age 2, 3, and 5; and teachers rated the child at age 7.5. Findings from the model are summarized in Fig. 23.2.

The model shown in Fig. 23.2 systematically tested the evocative effects of child noncompliance on parent–child coercion, as well as the reverse. It was hypothesized that these dynamic interaction patterns were prognostic of growth in oppositional behavior in the home from age 2 to 5 and of teachers' rating of oppositional behavior in first or second grade. It is important to note that teacher perceptions of problem behavior in the first two grades of elementary school are highly predictive of more serious problem behavior in adolescence and adulthood (Loeber & Dishion, 1983; Robins & Hill, 1966). As shown in Fig. 23.2, the effects of the unfolding coercion cycle were decidedly bidirectional. It appears that coercion dynamics at age 2 and 3 feed future noncompliance and oppositional behavior problems perceived by parents. However, the reverse is also true: Children's noncompliance and oppositional behavior at age 3 predict later coercive parent–child interactions. It is especially noteworthy that increases in parents' ratings of oppositional child behavior, the average level of noncompliance during the 3-year period, and coercive parent–child interactions predict teacher ratings of oppositional behavior problems. The model fit the data well, and 22 % of the variance in teacher ratings was accounted for by the developmental dynamics underlying family coercion in early childhood.

Data such as these provide some support for the hypothesis that how the parent reacts to their child's behavior can reduce the development of early behavior problems and aggression. Of course, many randomized studies that target parenting practices have revealed consistent effects on reduction in aggression in early childhood; most noteworthy are the findings of Webster-Stratton and colleagues (Webster-Stratton & Reid, 2010). Recent studies have found that randomized assignment to the Family Check-Up (FCU) (Dishion & Stormshak, 2007) resulted in improved child behavior and increased positive parenting (Dishion et al., 2008; Shaw, Dishion, Supplee, Gardner, & Arnds, 2006). In the Dishion et al. (2008), study, changes in parents' use of positive behavior support, observed during videotaped parent–child interactions, mediated the covariation between the intervention and reductions in child problem behavior from ages 2 to 4. Moreover, significant reductions were noted in teachers' ratings of oppositional defiance at age 7.5. The FCU is a brief parenting intervention designed for use in public health or public school settings and emphasizes periodic contact with children and families. In this study, we provided the FCU to families enrolled in the Women, Infants, and Children (WIC) program in three geographically distinct communities (urban, suburban, rural). Results revealed that the number of FCU interventions that a family completed increased the effect sizes on parent ratings of oppositional behavior and teacher ratings of problem behavior at age 7 (Dishion, Brennan, Shaw, McEachern, & Wilson, 2013). Taken together, the findings suggest that parenting is indeed modifiable, and the benefits to children are pronounced and long lasting.

Antisocial Behavior in Childhood

How does oppositional and defiant behavior in early childhood lead to stealing, lying, and fighting in later childhood? In the 1980s the field was concerned with potential specialization in children's antisocial behavior. Patterson's (1982) early work on coercion theory attempted to identify the unique family interaction profiles and treatment needs of children referred for stealing, compared with those of children referred for aggression. This distinction was carried forward in an important review of the literature by Loeber and Schmaling (1985), in which the terms *overt* and *covert* antisocial behavior were coined. Several interesting studies compared the correlates of these two forms of antisocial behavior. It is surprising that overt and covert antisocial behaviors have unique effects on children's lives, despite the fact that the two factors were correlated at about .8 in a community sample (Patterson et al., 1992). Loeber and Stouthamer-Loeber (1998) later clarified that involvement in both covert and overt antisocial behaviors (mixed, early onset) posed the greatest risk for more serious forms of violence and aggression in adolescence. These findings and conclusions were confirmed and extended in a comprehensive approach to longitudinal modeling that combined six data sets (Broidy et al., 2003). All six identified a group characterized by chronic antisocial behavior from childhood to early adolescence. In most youths, as Tremblay would hypothesize, aggression tended to decrease over time (Tremblay, 2000). However, for the chronic group, the level of physical aggression remained stable. Interestingly, only for children in the urban sample, physical aggression actually increased from childhood to early adolescence, suggesting a contextual effect for the communities the youths resided in.

It has become increasingly clear that community-level dynamics have an influence on the peer group, which is readily observable in the context of neighborhoods and playgrounds. Coercion on the playground and deviant peer influence are observable in the first grade in the public school environment (Dishion, Duncan, Eddy, Fagot, & Fetrow, 1994). It is interesting, however, that what is learned on the playground at school is only loosely associated with what the child has learned in the family. Examination of coercive dynamics with parents and those with peers on the playground has indicated a correlation of .19 between the two settings. Thus, it seems that interactions with peers potentially provide a relatively independent influence on the development and growth of antisocial behavior in childhood.

Research by Snyder and colleagues has provided insights about the role of peers in the growth of covert and overt antisocial behavior during childhood. These researchers developed a protocol that enabled the measurement of deviancy training among 5-year-olds in the school context (Snyder et al., 2005).

Snyder's work is seminal with respect to understanding the early development of antisocial behavior. He found that deviancy training and coercion could be identified in peer interactions on the kindergarten playground. Moreover, as would be expected, coercive exchanges were associated with growth in overt forms of antisocial behavior in the ensuing year. That is, children who engaged with peers in a coercive manner were actually seen as more aggressive even by their parents, suggesting for the first time that there may be a carryover from peers to the family early in development. It previously had been assumed that the general direction of influence was from the family to peers (Patterson et al., 1992). Snyder and colleagues also found that deviancy training led to growth in covert antisocial behavior during the ensuing year, as seen by parents and by teachers. Covert and overt antisocial behavior have been associated with a general tendency to engage in antisocial behavior at ages 7 and 8 (Snyder et al., 2008).

Figure 23.3 summarizes findings from the Snyder group (Snyder et al., 2010) regarding the general influence of deviancy training in kindergarten on subsequent development of antisocial behavior by age 9, based on youth report. Note that observed children's deviant talk in kindergarten independently predicted growth of antisocial behavior, controlling for the same behavior at age 5. These findings suggest that organization and structure of informal play settings in public elementary schools are key to learning antisocial behavior patterns that are prognostic of later aggression and violence.

Several prevention trials have indicated that with relative ease, the public school environment can be modified to reduce ambient levels of peer aggression and antisocial behavior. For example, when teachers use the "good behavior game" in classroom settings, levels of aggression drop at a group level; in addition, individual children who experience this intervention are less likely to become antisocial and violent (Kellam, Reid, & Balster, 2008; Petras et al., 2008). It is interesting to note that a relatively brief and focused contextual intervention in the first grade can have such a dramatic effect on growth of serious forms of antisocial and violent behavior in adolescence. As shown in Fig. 23.1, relatively small improvements in microsocial interaction patterns can alter the child's adaptation in school and among peers, which in turn potentiates large reductions in risk over time.

Collateral Effects

In a cascade developmental model, aggressive and antisocial behavior have collateral effects on normative peer relationships and academic

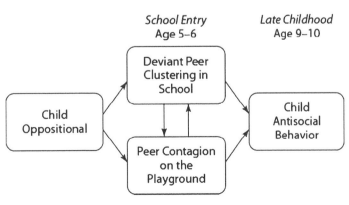

Fig. 23.3 Peer contagion in public elementary school and progressions in antisocial behavior (adapted from Snyder et al., 2010)

achievement. Dodge and Coie's early studies provoked an entire era of research on peer rejection, and the covariation between aggressive behavior and peer rejection is well established. The aggressive child is quickly rejected by normative peers (Coie & Kupersmidt, 1983; Dodge, 1983). In my dissertation work, a general model was developed and tested that revealed that family interaction dynamics were prognostic of antisocial behavior and poor academic achievement, and both of these outcomes were prognostic of peer rejection (Dishion, 1990). Patterson tested the dual failure model, which added a depression overlay to concerns about the antisocial child, in that academic failure and peer rejection were found to be associated with depressed mood (Patterson & Stoolmiller, 1991).

Most relevant to the development of aggression and violence is the tendency to self-organize into deviant peer groups. In longitudinal research on the Oregon Youth Study sample, we found that academic skill deficits, peer rejection, antisocial behavior, and poor parental monitoring combined to predict affiliation with deviant peers in early adolescence (Dishion, Patterson, Stoolmiller, & Skinner, 1991). Stoolmiller's (1990) work with the same sample captured the construct called *wandering*, meaning that antisocial boys actually pulled themselves away from parental supervision and actively shopped for unsupervised settings and activities. It is from this research that we began to think of deviant peer affiliation as fitting the dynamic systems idea of self-organization. The biological and social changes associated with adolescence motivate youths to self-organize into groups, a process often studied intensively by social network researchers.

Given the collateral effects of childhood antisocial behavior on several developmental outcomes, it is important to consider the evidence that it is malleable. Some interventions have been shown to successfully reduce children's antisocial behavior. The first is to motivate and support caregivers' behavior management and supervision. The vast majority of the research on parent management training, which has focused on conduct problems in middle childhood, has shown that supporting parenting practices reduces antisocial behavior (e.g., Kazdin, 2010). Especially noteworthy are Forgatch and Patterson's (2010) findings that effects endure as long as 9 years following intervention. Models of mediation have also revealed that improved parenting practices mediate long-term improvements in children's behavior that endure through adolescence, as documented by reduced court-documented arrest rates. The second promising intervention is to work directly with the child to motivate and support prosocial coping (Kazdin, 2010; Lochman, Boxmeyer, Powell, Barry, & Pardini, 2010). Kazdin and Lochman's work provides empirical support for the idea that building youths' skill in using prosocial strategies for resolving conflict and handling stress can reduce antisocial behavior.

Antisocial Behavior to Violence

How does a troublesome adolescent become a dangerous adult? Puberty is the defining feature of adolescent development, the timing of which transforms the child's motivation to engage and participate in new social contexts. This fundamental change underlies the increasingly rewarding value of peer interaction and enhanced reinforcement for risk-taking (Steinberg et al., 2006). As shown in Fig. 23.1, self-organization into peer groups increases, as does deviant peer clustering for those with a history of school failure and peer rejection. In some contexts with more extreme marginalization, these groups become gangs (Dishion, Nelson, & Yasui, 2005). Research on gangs clearly reveals their strong influence on violent behavior (Thornberry, 1998). Violence is not the only outcome of deviant peer clustering; however, multiple problem behaviors in adolescence are associated with peers, including drug use, high-risk sexual behavior, and other forms of delinquent behavior (see Dishion & Patterson, 2006).

The cascading developmental process is embedded in the evolving family context from early childhood through adolescence. In early childhood, specific parenting practices that scaffold emotion-related self-regulation are at the core of social and emotional development (Eisenberg, Spinrad, & Eggum, 2010). In middle childhood, family management skills that include positive behavior support, limit setting and monitoring, and relationship building are uniquely prognostic of problem behavior and development of social and emotional competence (Patterson et al., 1992). Through adolescence and into young adulthood, these outcomes are determined by how well the caregiver balances the need for autonomy with involved monitoring and guidance (Dishion, Nelson, & Bullock, 2004; Fosco, Caruthers, & Dishion, 2012). Randomized interventions studies clearly indicate that reductions in problem behavior result from targeting family and school risk processes summarized in the developmental cascade process.

The prediction of violence has been one of the more intractable problems of criminology for more than 40 years (Monahan, 1978). For quite some time, the best that could be offered was that the more youths displayed antisocial behavior in childhood, the more likely they were to commit a violent crime in adulthood (Loeber & Farrington, 1998). Advances in developmental theory, longitudinal data analysis, and in measuring interpersonal dynamics, however, have rendered the progression to violence from child antisocial behavior more predictable.

Without question, adolescence and young adulthood are times when youths attend to peer norms and acceptance and establish themselves independently from caregivers. This is not a question of whether autonomy will happen; it is a question of when. For high-risk youths, the shift from family to peers generally occurs earlier, beginning around the onset of puberty and nearly completing by middle, or certainly by late, adolescence. For typically developing youths who are engaged in school, autonomy from caregivers commonly begins in late adolescence and gradually evolves through the twenties, as is indicated by the popularized term *emerging adulthood* (Arnett & Tanner, 2006).

The process of "premature autonomy" among high-risk adolescents has been studied in detail, and interventions have been designed to prevent

it. As suggested by the work of Stoolmiller (1990), the high-risk youth begins to pull away from adult supervision and seek unsupervised time with peers. In response, many parents begin to give up supervision and relinquish the role of caregiving adult. When parenting and friendship interactions were videotaped and systematically coded, longitudinal growth modeling revealed that reduced family management from early to late adolescence and high levels of deviancy training with peers in adolescence predicted continuing antisocial behavior from adolescence through age 24. Most interesting was the interaction term, in that the highest levels of antisocial behavior at age 24 were found with youths whose parents had relinquished monitoring and limit setting and whose friends had engaged in deviancy training (Dishion et al., 2004).

The Broidy et al. (2003) study indicated that aggression is on a downward trend for most youths, except for those who are on a high-risk trajectory, for example, those who live in urban settings. Another approach to longitudinal data is to model trajectories of peer groups and map onto those groups longitudinal changes in antisocial behavior. When Lacourse and colleagues used this strategy, they found that the youths who increased their violent behavior were those who were in the chronically deviant peer group from childhood through adolescence (Lacourse, Nagin, Tremblay, Vitaro, & Claes, 2003). These data suggest that the passage from troublesome to dangerous is by and large not a solitary endeavor and that some peer groups cocreate violence. This finding is consistent with the longitudinal findings by Thornberry (1998) that showed increases in the seriousness of adolescents' problem behavior among urban youths when they became involved in a gang.

Given the consequences of youths self-organizing into deviant clusters, it is essential to know which youths are more vulnerable to gang membership. As one might expect, gangs are more prevalent in specific communities. From a historical perspective, poor and disorganized communities with pockets of marginalized individuals tend to have high rates of crime and gang structures (Sampson & Laub, 1994). For example,

Fig. 23.4 Self-organization into deviant peer clusters, sexual promiscuity, and adolescent problem behavior

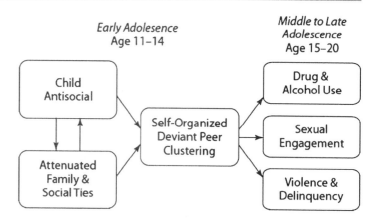

Sampson and Laub (1994) reported that in early nineteenth-century Boston, Irish immigrants were more likely to be involved in crime and gang activity.

As suggested by Fig. 23.1, disrupted parenting in early childhood leads to higher levels of problem behavior in childhood, which immediately translates to early formation of peer networks of like-minded youths. Adolescents with poor academic skills, poor relationships with peers and teachers, and attenuated relationships with parents are more likely to self-organize into deviant peer groups. We propose that this is not an intention-driven process, but that it emerges with changes in puberty and depends on social context. Thus the term *self-organize* is appropriate because rarely is there a leader involved, and selection and influence evolve over time to facilitate increasing levels of problem behavior. Previous research has shown that in careful observation of the microsocial dynamics of adolescents with their friends, youths match their deviant talk to the relative rate of friends' reinforcement of such talk (Dishion et al., 1996). Thus, the youths are influencing each other toward increasingly deviant norms, especially when they self-organize into groups that comprise many antisocial youths.

What is the function of the gang in the life of an adolescent? Interesting work by Pellegrini first linked early-adolescence peer behaviors with sexual selection theory (Pellegrini, 2003). Covariation was found between some problem behaviors and increased dating popularity, but in general the findings did not entirely support sexual

selection theory, perhaps because of the relatively normative nature of the sample.

We hypothesized that deviant peer clustering in early adolescence was an evolutionary-based adaptation to marginalization and stress in families and the school environment. The concept is summarized in Fig. 23.4, in that deviant peer clustering is positioned at the center of progressions to new forms of problem behavior. Consistent with a sexual selection perspective, youths self-organize into deviant peer groups primarily to enhance short-term reproductive potential (see Fig. 23.4). In a two-stage, evolutionary-based analysis of deviant peer clustering in early adolescence, it was predicted that first, socioeconomic status, family attenuation, and peer and school marginalization throughout middle school would predict deviant peer clustering by the end of middle school. Second, it was predicted that deviant peer clustering by ages 13–14 would be prognostic of high levels of sexual activity 2–3 years later (ages 16–17), at a time when 95 % of the youths would have reached puberty. In addition, it was predicted that high levels of sexual activity at ages 16–17 would predict the number of children by ages 23–24 (Dishion et al., 2012). The model fit the data supporting the hypothesis that self-organized deviant peer clustering was an adaptive process that is consistent with a fast life history strategy.

The friendship dynamics that define the deviant peer group determine in part what becomes socialized in the group. When my colleagues and I first intensively studied friendship dynamics, we focused on a sample of boys from a suburban community. We were surprised to find very little negativity or aggression in the friendship interactions (Dishion, Andrews, & Crosby, 1995). Only a handful of the 204 boys participated in coercive exchanges with friends during an observation task. Consequently, we focused primarily on the role of positive reinforcement in deviancy training. However, when we later analyzed friendship interactions among an urban sample of youths, the picture changed. Significantly more than a handful of friendships were characterized by an aggressive posture and overt efforts to exert and maintain dominance over one another. It did not take a rocket scientist to see a connection to gang involvement, in that many of the youths in the friendship interactions were dressed in gang attire and used gang-like mannerisms. We became interested in the idea that specific social interaction patterns presented a coercive stance to the social world that amplified a youth's tendency to become violent in late adolescence to early adulthood. That is, they would become dangerous people.

We came to term the process we had been witnessing *coercive joining* (Van Ryzin & Dishion, 2013); that is, a friendship of two individuals is organized around coercing each other as well as others. When coercion is the organizing theme, the individual who is more likely to escalate or be the most aversive (e.g., physical aggression, assault) has the most influence. Moreover, the dyad is made stronger by joining in coercion; that is, they coerce others and take pride and enjoyment in treating others abusively or with aggression. As is often documented in the literature about gang involvement, the ability to be fearless and highly aggressive is directly linked to status in the group (Raine, 2002). Status is a key outcome of aggression and deviance and is rarely addressed in prevention programs (Ellis et al., 2012).

It is possible that coercive joining in adolescent friendships facilitates the progression from aggression to violence in adolescence (Dishion & Van Ryzin, 2011). In research that included 998 adolescents (Project Alliance 1), 85 % of the sample were observed participating in videotaped interactions with their best friend.

To examine their friendship quality, each youth was asked to report about their satisfaction with the friendship, pleasant activities they shared, and the extent to which they agreed about basic friendship issues. In a model that included antisocial behavior at ages 16–17 and coercive joining and friendship quality that predicted serious violence by ages 22–23, all three predictors were statistically reliable. As one might expect, an interaction effect was found between friendship quality and coercive joining, and youths with the lowest friendship quality and the highest levels of coercive joining were the most violent 5 years later. Coercion in friendships undermines the relationship and socializes youths to become increasingly dangerous.

Figure 23.5 summarizes a longitudinal model of the source of the coercive joining dynamic. One can see that gang involvement at ages 13–14 predicts coercive joining with a friend 3 years later, which in turn uniquely predicts violence by ages 22–23. It is alarming to note that a youth's involvement in gangs uniquely predicts violence nearly 10 years later, even after controlling for their antisocial behavior and coercive joining in friendships. These data provide a clear picture of how youths learn more serious forms of violence in the peer context during adolescence. It is worth noting that in these models, violence was measured comprehensively, including adult arrests for violence, self-reports of carrying weapons, self-reports of violence, and parent reports of adult violence.

In an ecological perspective on development, one must consider the socializing influence of friends and also the contribution of families to adolescent violence. The coercion model suggests that coercive interaction patterns in families provide the basic training for youths to feel comfortable establishing coercive friendships. This hypothesis was tested with a subset of the sample described earlier, who were preselected to also complete family-observation tasks when they were young adolescents (Van Ryzin & Dishion, 2012). Coercive interactions within the family were prognostic of later coercive joining in friendships, which, in turn, predicted violence in young adulthood, controlling for previous levels

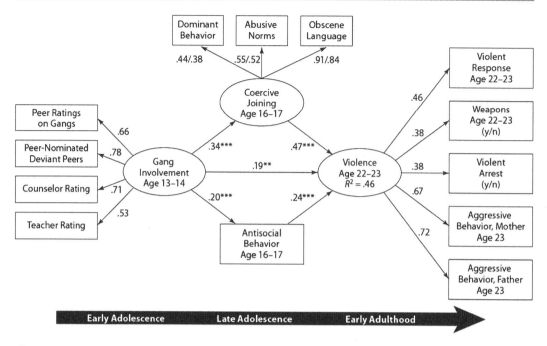

Fig. 23.5 A model for the contribution of coercive joining in friendships and progressions to violence in late adolescence

of antisocial behavior, and even observed deviancy training with friends at ages 16–17. The covariation between observed coercion in the family at ages 12–13 and acting out dangerous behaviors 10 years later was mediated by coercive joining with friends at age 16.

Yet another question regarding the development of violence requires more research: To what extent is violence reinforcing? From systematic research in early childhood, we learned that countering aggression on the playground with more intense aggression reinforced the behavior, leading to more aggression later. Figure 23.6 summarizes the possibility that dangerous threats or acts are reinforcing at an individual and at a group level. For example, in some contexts, an attack on a victim that leads to death or submission can positively impact the status of the offender in a violent community. The person most willing to face potential danger to self in the process of harming others is revered as "dangerous" or "bad." Such a process can be realized only when the ambient level of violence is high, such as in a gang or in the context of war (Patterson, 2012). Ellis and colleagues (2012)

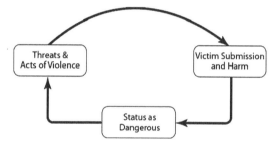

Fig. 23.6 The threat–submission coercion dynamic and dangerousness

make a similar point regarding bullying behavior in early adolescence, that the bully gains status. The entry card is risking one's own safety to inflict harm on others.

If violence is understood to be individually reinforcing with respect to social status, current interventions designed to reduce antisocial behavior at younger ages may have only limited effectiveness. In Project Alliance 1, we individually randomized 999 11-year-olds to either middle school as usual or middle school with the offer of an FCU. Of the families assigned to the intervention group, 25 % agreed to engage in the FCU.

Using intention-to-treat analyses, we found that participation in the FCU was associated with reduced substance use (Dishion, Kavanagh, Schneiger, Nelson, & Kaufman, 2002), and for high-risk youths, changes in substance use were associated with improved parental monitoring practices (Dishion, Nelson, & Kavanagh, 2003). Our research team later found that antisocial behavior by age 18 was reduced for those in the intervention group, an outcome that was partially mediated by long-term reductions in parent–adolescent conflict (Van Ryzin & Dishion, 2012). Using mixture modeling longitudinal data analysis, it was found that randomization to the FCU reduced serious forms of antisocial behavior, including arrests (Connell, Dishion, Yasui, & Kavanagh, 2007). The intervention, on the other hand, did not prevent serious violence.

It is generally the case that randomized intervention studies provide only limited evidence that adolescent violence can be reduced through intensive, family-centered interventions (Henggeler & Schaeffer, 2010). What seems particularly intractable is adolescent involvement in gangs. Malcolm Klein, whose career focused on understanding and intervening with adolescent delinquent gangs, concluded that the best approach is to prevent gangs from forming rather than try to reduce gang influence after they have formed (Klein, 2006).

Summary

Decades of research in development and psychopathology are providing an empirical account of how some children move from minor problems in self-regulation and problem behavior to being dangerous young adults. In many respects, predictors of aggression and violence are similar for males and for females, although less serious violence is apparent among the latter. Clearly, there are deep gender differences with respect to male and female social networks, the role of romantic relationships and sexuality, and need to drop out of the deviance process because of pregnancy and childbirth. Of interest is the finding that academic failure and peer rejection predict

gang membership for boys and for girls. However, ratings of being liked were predictive of gang membership only for boys, suggesting that social status of potential gang members is high among males in early adolescence. This finding and the body of research by Snyder and colleagues reported in this chapter suggest that the developmental time line should be reconsidered with respect to the role of the peer group and the development of aggression. Perhaps by early adolescence, the dominance hierarchies for males in particular are well established, and aggression maintains status and dominance during adolescence, when the introduction of sexual attraction raises the stakes considerably.

Conclusion and Future Directions

At this juncture, two comments and one suggestion for future directions must be made. First, a developmental cascade process seems to account for amplification of deviance over time (Dishion, Véronneau, & Myers, 2010; Dodge et al., 2008). Doubtless, some violent offenders act alone and are not directly supported by a peer group, as described in this chapter. Although many school shootings, for example, have elements of group support and contention as a preamble to violence, many violent and aggressive acts appear to be an outcome of individual rumination that has no clear history in the individual aside from acquisition of a weapon and ammunition.

However, technological advancements in media and communication may alter definitions and forms of peer reinforcement. For example, social media and texting provide a venue for expressing deviant and aggressive values, and peer reactions in these venues may reinforce escalations to more serious and lethal aggressive acts. Sitting in front of a computer and posting violent messages may evoke positive reactions from virtual peers. For youths with poor social skills, positive reactions might be confabulated from ambiguous responses from virtual peers. Thus, many acts of violence that seem solitary may actually evolve from a period of coercion and contagion that is less directly interpersonal, yet powerful in shaping thoughts and behavior nonetheless. Clearly, the salience of media for individuals is likely a function of their own mental health and social isolation, as would be suggested by the matching law formulation. That is, positive responses to violent themes and behavior on social media may be especially influential among isolated individuals with few rewarding, prosocial relationships.

The developmental psychopathology framework has been particularly successful with respect to informing the design of interventions that reduce risk for aggressive and violent behavior. Data suggest that if interventions addressed and reduced the developmental processes described in this chapter, then a significant level of violence in many communities could be curtailed and even prevented. To date, this is a promissory note, and future research should focus more narrowly on the progression from antisocial behavior to violence, to evaluate the optimal timing and focus of violence prevention.

Critical to the success of future prevention is the need to effectively address the peer group dynamics that are seemingly left to run amuck in urban communities immobilized by poverty, joblessness, and marginalization of some of our fellow citizens (Sampson & Laub, 1994). Using historical perspective, we realize that problems of gangs and gang violence are not isolated to a specific group of people defined by culture, religion, or race. Marginalization is an ever-shifting process that changes across eras and geographic boundaries. Self-organization into peer groups that promote violence is an adaptation to inadequate social environments, which are extremely difficult to change ad hoc (Klein, 2006). The process must be addressed earlier, when it unfolds in public schools and neighborhoods characterized by bullying and aggression. Recent efforts to prevent bullying have come down to adults being reminded that it is unacceptable for youths to be unsafe and victimized in schools and public settings (Olweus, 1993). Effective prevention programs mobilize adults to nurture, safeguard, and teach skills to youths to reduce bullying and aggression.

As is clear from the work described in this chapter, researchers' focus to date has been on the dark side of family and peer relationships.

Normative and prosocial family development and peer relationships ordinarily do not get the attention of prevention and intervention researchers. However, all children have the potential to be either kind or violent. Would an effort to promote prosocial behavior, compassion, empathy, and self-regulation add significantly to the impressive array of interventions now available to reduce the dark side of family and peer relationships? It is clear that the kinds of friendships and romantic relationships that emerge from a developmental history of antisocial behavior and violence are not happy and satisfying and, as such, provide very little reinforcement for kindness and compassion. A focus on health promotion may have a unique effect over and above risk reduction strategies for preventing the developmental cascade toward violence and therefore is decidedly worthy of future research.

Acknowledgments The author's work has been supported by National Institutes of Health grants DA07031 and DA16110 to the first author and DA018760 to Anthony Biglan.

References

Ainsworth, M. S. (1989). Attachments beyond infancy. *American Psychologist, 44*(4), 709–716.

Arnett, J. J., & Tanner, J. L. (Eds.). (2006). *Emerging adults in America: Coming of age in the 21st century.* Washington, DC: American Psychological Association.

Belsky, J., Steinberg, L., & Draper, P. (1991). Childhood experience, interpersonal development, and reproductive strategy: An evolutionary theory of socialization. *Child Development, 62*, 647–670.

Biglan, A. (2003). Selection by consequences: One unifying principle for a transdisciplinary science of prevention. *Prevention Science, 4*(44), 213–232.

Brody, G. H., Beach, S. R. H., Philibert, R. A., Chen, Y.-F., Lei, M.-K., Murry, V. M., et al. (2009). Parenting moderates a genetic vulnerability factor in longitudinal increases in youths' substance use. *Journal of Consulting and Clinical Psychology, 77*(1), 1–11.

Broidy, L. M., Tremblay, R. E., Brame, B., Fergusson, D., Horwood, J. L., Laird, R. D., et al. (2003). Developmental trajectories of childhood disruptive behaviors and adolescent delinquency: A six-site, cross-national study. *Developmental Psychology, 39*, 222–245.

Bronfenbrenner, U. (1979). *The ecology of human development* (pp. 3–15). Cambridge, MA: Harvard University Press.

Caspi, A., McClay, J., Moffitt, T., Mill, J., Craig, I. W., Taylor, A., et al. (2002). Role of genotype in the cycle of violence in maltreated children. *Science, 297*, 851–854.

Coie, J. D., & Kupersmidt, J. B. (1983). A behavioral analysis of emerging social status in boys' (possessive) groups. *Child Development, 54*, 1400–1416.

Connell, A., Dishion, T. J., Yasui, M., & Kavanagh, K. (2007). An adaptive approach to family intervention: Linking engagement in family-centered intervention to reductions in adolescent problem behavior. *Journal of Consulting and Clinical Psychology, 75*, 568–579.

Dishion, T. J. (1990). The peer context of troublesome child and adolescent behavior. In P. Leone (Ed.), *Understanding troubled and troublesome youth* (pp. 128–153). Beverly Hills, CA: Sage.

Dishion, T. J., Andrews, D. W., & Crosby, L. (1995). Antisocial boys and their friends in early adolescence: Relationship characteristics, quality, and interactional process. *Child Development, 66*, 139–151.

Dishion, T. J., Brennan, L. M., Shaw, D. S., McEachern, A. D., Wilson, M. N., & Jo. B. (2013). Prevention of problem behavior through annual Family Check-Ups in early childhood: Intervention effects from home to early elementary school. *Journal of Abnormal Child Psychology*, no pagination specified.

Dishion, T. J., Capaldi, D., Spracklen, K. M., & Li, F. (1995). Peer ecology of male adolescent drug use. *Development and Psychopathology, 7*, 803–824.

Dishion, T. J., Duncan, T. E., Eddy, J. M., Fagot, B. I., & Fetrow, R. (1994). The world of parents and peers: Coercive exchanges and children's social adaptation. *Social Development, 3*, 255–268.

Dishion, T. J., Gardner, K., Patterson, G. R., Reid, J. R., Spyrou, S., & Thibodeaux, S. (1983). *The family process code: A multidimensional system for observing family interaction*. Eugene, OR: Child and Family Center.

Dishion, T. J., Ha, T., & Véronneau, M.-H. (2012). An ecological analysis of the effects of deviant peer clustering on sexual promiscuity, problem behavior, and childbearing from early adolescence to adulthood: An enhancement of the life history framework. *Developmental Psychology, 48*, 703–717.

Dishion, T. J., Kavanagh, K., Schneiger, A., Nelson, S., & Kaufman, N. (2002). Preventing early adolescent substance use: A family-centered strategy for public middle school. In R. L. Spoth, K. Kavanagh., & T. J. Dishion (Eds.), Universal family-centered prevention strategies: Current findings and critical issues for public health impact [Special issue]. *Prevention Science, 3*, 191–201.

Dishion, T. J., McCord, J., & Poulin, F. (1999). When interventions harm: Peer groups and problem behavior. *American Psychologist, 54*, 755–764.

Dishion, T. J., Nelson, S. E., & Bullock, B. M. (2004). Premature adolescent autonomy: Parent disengagement and deviant peer process in the amplification of problem behavior [Special issue]. *Journal of Adolescence, 27*, 515–530.

Dishion, T. J., Nelson, S. E., & Kavanagh, K. (2003). The family check-up with high-risk young adolescents: Preventing early-onset substance use by parent monitoring [Special issue]. *Behavior Therapy, 34*, 553–571.

Dishion, T. J., Nelson, S. E., & Yasui, M. (2005). Predicting early adolescent gang involvement from middle school adaptation. *Journal of Clinical Child and Adolescent Psychology, 34*(1), 62–73.

Dishion, T. J., & Patterson, G. R. (2006). The development and ecology of antisocial behavior. In D. Cicchetti & D. J. Cohen (Eds.), *Developmental psychopathology* (Risk, disorder, and adaptation 2nd ed., Vol. 3, pp. 503–541). Hoboken, NJ: Wiley.

Dishion, T. J., Patterson, G. R., & Kavanagh, K. (1992). An experimental test of the coercion model: Linking theory, measurement, and intervention. In J. McCord & R. Trembley (Eds.), *The interaction of theory and practice: Experimental studies of interventions* (pp. 253–282). New York, NY: Guilford.

Dishion, T. J., Patterson, G. R., Stoolmiller, M., & Skinner, M. (1991). Family, school, and behavioral antecedents to early adolescent involvement with antisocial peers. *Developmental Psychology, 27*, 172–180.

Dishion, T. J., Shaw, D. S., Connell, A. M., Gardner, F., Weaver, C. M., & Wilson, M. N. (2008). The family check-up with high-risk indigent families: Preventing problem behavior by increasing parents' positive behavior support in early childhood. *Child Development, 79*(5), 1395–1414.

Dishion, T. J., Spracklen, K. M., Andrews, D. W., & Patterson, G. R. (1996). Deviancy training in male adolescent friendships. *Behavior Therapy, 27*, 373–390.

Dishion, T. J., & Stormshak, E. A. (2007). *Intervening in children's lives: An ecological, family-centered approach to mental health care*. Washington, DC: American Psychological Association.

Dishion, T. J., & Tipsord, J. M. (2011). Peer contagion in child and adolescent social and emotional development. *Annual Review of Psychology, 62*, 189–214.

Dishion, T. J., & Van Ryzin, M. J. (2011). Peer contagion dynamics in problem behavior and violence: Implications for intervention and policy. *ISSBD Bulletin, 60*(2), 6–11.

Dishion, T. J., Véronneau, M.-H., & Myers, M. W. (2010). Cascading peer dynamics underlying the progression from problem behavior to violence in early to late adolescence. *Development and Psychopathology, 22*, 603–619.

Dodge, K. A. (1983). Behavioral antecedents: A peer social status. *Child Development, 54*, 1386–1399.

Dodge, K. A., Dishion, T. J., & Lansford, J. E. (Eds.). (2006). *Deviant peer influences in programs for youth: Problems and solutions*. New York, NY: Guilford.

Dodge, K. A., Greenberg, M. T., & Malone, P. S. (2008). Testing an idealized dynamic cascade model of the development of serious violence in adolescence. *Child Development, 79*, 1907–1921.

Eisenberg, N., Spinrad, T. L., & Eggum, N. D. (2010). Emotion-related self-regulation and its relation to children's maladjustment. *Annual Review of Clinical Psychology, 6*, 495–525.

Ellis, B. J., Del Giudice, M., Dishion, T. J., Figueredo, A. J., Gray, P., Griskevicius, V., et al. (2012). The evolutionary basis of risky adolescent behavior: Implications for science, policy, and practice. *Developmental Psychology, 48*(3), 598–623.

Ellis, B. J., Figueredo, A. J., Brumbach, B. H., & Schlomer, G. L. (2009). Fundamental dimensions of environmental risk: The impact of harsh versus unpredictable environments on the evolution and development of life history strategies. *Human Nature, 20*(2), 204–268.

Forgatch, M. S., & Patterson, G. R. (2010). Parent management training–Oregon model: An intervention for antisocial behavior in children and adolescents. In J. R. Weisz & A. E. Kazdin (Eds.), *Evidence-based psychotherapies for children and adolescents* (pp. 159–178). New York, NY: Guilford.

Fosco, G. M., Caruthers, A. S., & Dishion, T. J. (2012). A six-year predictive test of adolescent family relationship quality and effortful control pathways to emerging adult social and emotional health. *Journal of Family Psychology, 26*(4), 565–575.

Gottman, J. M., & Roy, A. K. (1990). *Sequential analysis: A guide for behavioral researchers*. Cambridge, MA: Cambridge University Press.

Hayes, S. C., & Hayes, L. J. (Eds.). (1992). *Understanding verbal relations*. Reno, NV: Context.

Henggeler, S. W., & Schaeffer, C. (2010). Treating serious antisocial behavior using multisystemic therapy. In J. R. Weisz & A. E. Kazdin (Eds.), *Evidence-based psychotherapies for children and adolescents* (pp. 259–276). New York, NY: Guilford.

Hinde, R. A. (1974). *Biological bases of human social behavior*. New York, NY: McGraw-Hill.

Hops, H., Sherman, L., & Biglan, A. (1990). Maternal depression, marital discord, and children's behavior: A developmental perspective. In G. R. Patterson (Ed.), *Depression and aggression in family interaction* (pp. 18–308). Hillsdale, NJ: Erlbaum.

Kazdin, A. E. (2010). Problem-solving skills training and parent management training for oppositional defiant disorder and conduct disorder. In J. R. Weisz & A. E. Kazdin (Eds.), *Evidence-based psychotherapies for children and adolescents* (pp. 211–226). New York, NY: Guilford.

Kellam, S. G., Reid, J., & Balster, R. L. (2008). Effects of a universal classroom behavior management program in first and second grades on young adult behavioral, psychiatric, and social outcomes. *Drug & Alcohol Dependence, 95*, 5–28.

Klein, M. W. (2006). Peer effects in naturally occurring groups: The case of street gangs. In K. A. Dodge, T. J. Dishion, & J. E. Lansford (Eds.), *Deviant peer influences in programs for youth: Problems and solutions* (pp. 234–250). New York, NY: Guilford.

Lacourse, E., Nagin, D., Tremblay, R. E., Vitaro, F., & Claes, M. (2003). Developmental trajectories of boys' delinquent group membership and facilitation of violent behaviors during adolescence. *Development and Psychopathology, 15*, 183–197.

Lochman, J. E., Boxmeyer, C. L., Powell, N. P., Barry, T. D., & Pardini, D. A. (2010). Anger control training for aggressive youths. In J. R. Weisz & A. E. Kazdin (Eds.), *Evidence-based psychotherapies for children and adolescents* (pp. 227–242). New York: Guilford Press.

Loeber, R., & Dishion, T. J. (1983). Early predictors of male delinquency: A review. *Psychological Bulletin, 94*(1), 68–99.

Loeber, R., & Farrington, D. P. (Eds.). (1998). *Serious & violent juvenile offenders. Risk factors and successful interventions*. Thousand Oaks, CA: Sage.

Loeber, R., & Schmaling, K. B. (1985). Empirical evidence for overt and covert patterns of antisocial conduct problems: A meta-analysis. *Journal of Abnormal Child Psychology, 13*, 337–352.

Loeber, R., & Stouthamer-Loeber, M. (1998). Development of juvenile aggression and violence: Some common misconceptions and controversies. *American Psychologist, 53*, 242–259.

Masten, A. S., Roisman, G. I., Long, J. D., Burt, K. B., Obradović, J., Riley, J. R., et al. (2005). Developmental cascades: Linking academic achievement and externalizing and internalizing symptoms over 20 years. *Developmental Psychology, 41*(5), 733–746.

Moilanen, K. L., Shaw, D. S., & Maxwell, K. L. (2010). Developmental cascades: Externalizing, internalizing, and academic competence from middle childhood to early adolescence. *Development Psychopathology, 22*, 635–653.

Monahan, J. (1978). *The prediction of violent behavior in juveniles: The serious juvenile offender*. Washington, DC: Department of Justice.

Olson, S. L., Sameroff, A. J., Kerr, D. C. R., Lopez, N. L., & Wellman, H. M. (2005). Developmental foundations of externalizing problems in young children: The role of effortful control. *Development & Psychopathology, 17*, 25–45.

Olweus, D. (1993). *Bullying at school: What we know and what we can do*. Oxford, UK: Blackwell.

Patterson, G. R. (1974). Interventions for boys with conduct problems: Multiple settings, treatments, and criteria. *Journal of Consulting and Clinical Psychology, 42*, 471–481.

Patterson, G. R. (1976). The aggressive child: Victim and architect of a coercive system. In E. J. Mash, L. A. Hamerlynck, & L. C. Handy (Eds.), *Behavior modification and families* (pp. 267–316). New York, NY: Brunner/Mazel.

Patterson, G. R. (1982). *A social learning approach: III. Coercive family process*. Eugene, OR: Castalia.

Patterson, G. R. (2012). *Free and moving*. Eugene, OR: Author.

Patterson, G. R., & Cobb, J. A. (1973). Stimulus control for classes of noxious behaviors. In J. F. Knutson (Ed.), *The control of aggression: Implications from basic research* (pp. 144–199). Chicago, IL: Aldine.

Patterson, G. R., & Moore, D. R. (1979). Interactive patterns of units of behavior. In M. E. Lamb, S. J. Suomi, & G. R. Stevenson (Eds.), *Social interaction analysis: Methodological issues.* Madison, WI: University of Wisconsin Press.

Patterson, G. R., Reid, J. B., & Dishion, T. J. (1992). *Antisocial boys.* Eugene, OR: Castalia.

Patterson, G. R., & Stoolmiller, M. (1991). Replications of a dual failure model for boys' depressed mood. *Journal of Consulting and Clinical Psychology, 59,* 491–498.

Pellegrini, A. D. L. (2003). A sexual selection theory: Longitudinal analysis of sexual segregation and integration in early adolescence. *Journal of Experimental Child Psychology, 85,* 257–278.

Petras, H., Kellam, S. G., Brown, C. H., Muthén, B. O., Ialongo, N. S., & Poduska, J. M. (2008). Developmental epidemiological courses leading to antisocial personality disorder and violent and criminal behavior: Effects by young adulthood of a universal preventive intervention in first- and second-grade classrooms. *Drug and Alcohol Dependence, 95*(S1), S45–S59.

Raine, A. (2002). Biosocial studies of antisocial and violent behavior in children and adults: A review. *Journal of Abnormal Child Psychology, 30,* 311–326.

Robins, L. N., & Hill, S. Y. (1966). Assessing the contributions of family structure, class and peer groups to juvenile delinquency. *The Journal of Criminal Law, Criminology and Police Science, 3,* 325–334.

Rothbart, M. K., Ellis, L. K., Rueda, M. R., & Posner, M. I. (2003). Developing mechanisms of temperamental effortful control. *Journal of Personality, 71*(6), 1113–1143.

Sampson, R. J., & Laub, J. H. (1994). Urban poverty and the family context of delinquency: A new look at structure and process in a classic study. *Child Development, 65,* 523–540.

Shaw, D. S., Dishion, T. J., Supplee, L., Gardner, F., & Arnds, K. (2006). Randomized trial of a family-centered approach to the prevention of early conduct problems: Two-year effects of the family check-up in early childhood. *Journal of Consulting and Clinical Psychology, 74*(1), 1–9.

Shaw, D. S., Gilliom, M., Ingoldsby, E. M., & Nagin, D. (2003). Trajectories leading to school-age conduct problems. *Developmental Psychology, 39,* 189–200.

Smith, J. D., Dishion, T. J., Shaw, D. S., & Wilson, M. N. (2013). Indirect effects of fidelity to the Family Check-Up on changes in parenting and early childhood problem behaviors. *Journal of Consulting and Clinical Psychology, 81*(6), 962–974. doi:10.1037/a0033950.

Snyder, J., Edwards, P., McGraw, K., Kilgore, K., & Holton, A. (1994). Escalation and reinforcement in mother–child conflict: Social processes associated with the development of physical aggression. *Development and Psychopathology, 6,* 305–321.

Snyder, J., McEachern, A. D., Schrepferman, L., Just, C., Jenkins, M., Roberts, S., et al. (2010). Contribution of peer deviancy training to the early development of conduct problems: Mediators and moderators. *Behavior Therapy, 27,* 373–390.

Snyder, J., Schrepferman, L., McEachern, A. D., Barner, S., Johnson, K., & Provines, J. (2008). Peer deviancy training and peer coercion: Dual processes associated with early-onset conduct problems. *Child Development, 79*(2), 252–268.

Snyder, J., Schrepferman, L., Oeser, J., Patterson, G., Stoolmiller, M., Johnson, K., et al. (2005). Deviancy training and association with deviant peers in young children: Occurrence and contribution to early-onset conduct problems. *Development & Psychopathology, 17*(2), 397–413.

Steinberg, L., Dahl, R., Keating, D., Kupfer, D. J., Masten, A. S., & Pine, D. S. (2006). The study of developmental psychopathology in adolescence: Integrating affective neuroscience with the study of context. In D. Cicchetti & D. J. Cohen (Eds.), *Developmental psychopathology* (Developmental neuroscience 2nd ed., Vol. 2, pp. 710–741). Hoboken, NJ: Wiley.

Stoolmiller, M. S. (1990). *Parent supervision, child unsupervised wandering, and child antisocial behavior: A latent growth curve analysis* (Unpublished manuscript). University of Oregon, Eugene, OR

Stoolmiller, M. (2001). Synergistic interaction of child manageability problems and parent-discipline tactics in predicting future growth in externalizing behavior for boys. *Developmental Psychology, 37,* 814–825.

Thornberry, T. P. (1998). Membership in youth gangs and involvement in serious and violent offending. In R. Loeber & D. P. Farrington (Eds.), *Serious and violent juvenile offenders: Risk factors and successful interventions* (pp. 147–166). Newbury Park, CA: Sage.

Tremblay, R. E. (2000). The development of aggressive behaviour during childhood: What have we learned in the past century? *International Journal of Behavioral Development, 24,* 129–141.

Van Ryzin, M. J., & Dishion, T. J. (2012). The impact of a family-centered intervention on the ecology of adolescent antisocial behavior: Modeling developmental sequelae and trajectories during adolescence. *Development and Psychopathology, 24,* 1139–1155.

Van Ryzin, M. J., & Dishion, T. J. (2013). From antisocial behavior to violence: A model for the amplifying role of coercive joining in adolescent friendships. *Journal of Child Psychology and Psychiatry, 54*(6), 661–669. doi:10.1111/jcpp.12017.

Wahler, R. G. (1980). The insular mother: Her problems in parent–child treatment. *Journal of Applied Behavior Analysis, 13,* 207–219.

Webster-Stratton, C., & Reid, M. J. (2010). The incredible years parents, teachers, and children training series: A multifaceted treatment approach for children with conduct disorders. In J. R. Weisz & A. E. Kazdin (Eds.), *Evidence-based psychotherapies for children and adolescents* (pp. 194–210). New York, NY: Guilford.

Conduct Disorder

24

Karen L. Bierman and Tyler R. Sasser

Children with conduct disorder (CD) repeatedly violate the rights of others and the basic expectations of society, often exhibiting violent and destructive behaviors that cause great harm to others. Most of these children experience significant adversity in their personal lives, and many show severe deficits in multiple aspects of development and adjustment, including academic underachievement, emotional distress, and troubled interpersonal relationships (Lahey & Waldman, 2012). When CDs persist into adolescence and adulthood, they are extremely costly. Estimates suggest that a severely antisocial youth costs society two to five million dollars, considering the costs of justice system involvement and damages to victims (Cohen & Piquero, 2009), and the yearly cost of youth violence in the USA is estimated at $158 billion (Center for Disease Control and Prevention, 2008). As such, CD represents a serious public health problem, negatively affecting the children and adolescents involved and their families, schools, and communities.

Prevalence estimates suggest that between 4 and 10 % of all children display symptoms severe enough to warrant a diagnosis of CD, with estimates ranging from 6 to 16 % for boys and 2 to 9 % for girls (Offord, Boyle, & Racine, 1991). CDs disproportionately affect socioeconomically disadvantaged families and ethnic minority youth, resulting in serious health disparities (Lahey & Waldman, 2012). Hence, gaining a better understanding of the causes of CD and the nature of its developmental course is critically important, in order to inform effective prevention and intervention efforts.

Definition and Characteristics of Conduct Disorder

Based on the *Diagnostic and Statistical Manual of Mental Disorders*, 5th ed. (DSM-V), CD is diagnosed when youth show a chronic pattern of problem behaviors that involve violations of the basic rights of others and/or of age-appropriate social norms (American Psychiatric Association, 2013). Defining characteristics include aggression (e.g., bullying, threatening, fighting, physical cruelty toward other people or animals), destructive behavior (e.g., vandalism, fire setting), covert antisocial activity (e.g., lying, fraud, theft), and rule breaking (e.g., running away from home, truancy). To warrant a diagnosis of CD, the behaviors must occur for at least a 6-month period and must be severe enough to cause significant impairment in social, academic, or occupational functioning.

K.L. Bierman, Ph.D. (✉)
Department of Psychology, The Pennsylvania State University, University Park, PA 16802, USA
e-mail: kb2@psu.edu

T.R. Sasser, M.S.
Training Interdisciplinary Education Scientists Program, The Pennsylvania State University, University Park, PA 16802, USA

M. Lewis and K.D. Rudolph (eds.), *Handbook of Developmental Psychopathology*, DOI 10.1007/978-1-4614-9608-3_24, © Springer Science+Business Media New York 2014

Developmentally Linked Disorders

In the DSM-V, CD is grouped together with oppositional defiant disorder (ODD) in a category labeled "disruptive, impulse-control, and conduct disorders." ODD are sometimes considered developmental precursors of CD (Lahey, McBurnett, & Loeber, 2000). ODD involves a chronic pattern (at least 6 months) of argumentative, noncompliant, and defiant behavior and includes emotional volatility, irritability, and frequent anger outbursts. Although many of the children diagnosed with CD share the emotional and behavioral characteristics of children diagnosed with ODD (e.g., argumentative, negativistic), CD is distinguished by the additional presence of serious aggressive and/or antisocial behaviors. The risk of a diagnosis of CD is four times higher in children who have a prior diagnosis of ODD, compared with children with no prior diagnosis (Burke, Loeber, & Birmaher, 2002).

CD is also often accompanied by the hyperactive and impulsive behaviors (e.g., acting without thinking, excessive and intrusive behavior) that characterize ADHD, as well as problems with attention control (e.g., difficulty sustaining attention, distractibility, forgetfulness). Epidemiological and clinical samples indicate that 30–50 % of the children diagnosed with ADHD also meet the criteria for CD or ODD, and over 80 % of those diagnosed with CD also meet the criterion for ADHD (Greene et al., 2002).

In turn, these three disorders (CD, ODD, and ADHD) have been implicated as developmental precursors to chronic delinquency, although CD has emerged as the primary unique predictor when all three are included together in predictive analyses (Broidy et al., 2003). For example, studying 503 boys from ages 7 to 25, Byrd, Loeber, and Pardini (2012) found that CD and interpersonal callousness in childhood and adolescence were higher among boys whose delinquency persisted into adulthood relative to those boys whose delinquency desisted across time. ADHD and ODD did not predict delinquency, once CD was taken into account.

In addition, children with CD are at risk for stable psychopathology, and many are diagnosed with antisocial personality disorder in adulthood, a disorder that characterizes approximately 75 % of the prison population (Hare, 1991). In one longitudinal study, 51 % of the children diagnosed with CD attained a diagnosis of antisocial personality disorder in adulthood, whereas only 15 % of the children in the high-risk sample experienced this outcome without childhood CD (Simonoff et al., 2004). Further, the severity of CD behavior during childhood is an important factor predicting adult outcomes. For example, in another longitudinal study, the general rate of adult antisocial personality disorder among children diagnosed with CD in elementary school was approximately 35 %, but the risk rate climbed to 71 % among children who displayed the most severe conduct disorders (eight or more symptoms) (Robins & Price, 1991). These results are similar to those of Broidy et al. (2003) who found that, across six longitudinal data sets, the severity of childhood physical aggression was the primary predictor of the stability of the aggression and the emergence of more violent behavior in adolescence.

In addition, a growing database suggests that the emotional and the behavioral characteristics of youth with disruptive behaviors have predictive value (Pardini, Obradovic, & Loeber, 2006). Although not part of the DSM-IV definitions of ODD or CD, there is a growing evidence suggesting that children who are emotionally insensitive (e.g., callous, unemotional), low in empathy, and lacking in guilt or remorse are at increased risk for more severe and aggressive forms of antisocial behavior, adolescent delinquency, and adult antisocial personality disorder than children without these features (see Pardini & Loeber, 2008). For this reason, in the revised DSM-V, the diagnosis of CD includes a specifier, indicating whether or not the youth also exhibits callous and emotional traits (Moffit et al., 2008; Scheepers, Buitelaar, & Matthys, 2011).

Categorical Versus Dimensional Approaches to Assessment

The DSM (American Psychiatric Association, 2013) diagnostic framework represents a "person-oriented" clinical taxonomy. Children who fall above identified thresholds on key behavioral and emotional indicators are classified together as CD. Although there is heterogeneity among these children in the particular problematic behaviors they display, the assumption is that they have the same core difficulties, as well as commonalities in etiological processes, developmental course, and treatment needs. In the context of studying CD, this clinical approach focuses on children at the extreme end of the aggressive/antisocial behavioral spectrum, in the "disordered" range indicating a need for intervention (Lacourse et al., 2010).

In contrast, in the dimensional approach used in most developmental research on disruptive behavior problems, children are rated along continuous scales, providing a more precise estimate of their relative position on each of the key behavioral, emotional, and cognitive characteristics associated with CD. Studies using dimensional measures of aggression typically focus on the entire distribution, rather than extreme groups. This chapter takes a hybrid approach, including findings from both developmental studies focused on key dimensions of disturbance associated with CD as well as clinical studies of children and adolescents who meet diagnostic criterion for CD.

One advantage of dimensional scales over person-oriented approaches is that they lend themselves to empirical explorations of the structure of conduct problems, particularly the search for dimensions of behavior problems that might characterize distinct subgroups of children with CD (Loeber, Burke, Lahey, Winters, & Zera, 2000). A large number of studies have used factor analyses to characterize the distinct dimensions that represent conduct problems. Looking for general patterns, Lahey and colleagues (1990) applied multidimensional scaling to 64 factor analytic studies that examined the structure of disruptive behaviors. Overall, disruptive behaviors were characterized along two dimensions— overt versus covert and destructive versus nondestructive. Behaviors most characteristic of CD were overt and destructive (e.g., fight, bully, threaten), whereas behaviors most characteristic of ODD were overt but nondestructive (e.g., noncompliant, stubborn, irritable). Covert antisocial

behaviors emerged distinct from overt behaviors; some were destructive (e.g., vandalism, stealing), whereas others were nondestructive (truancy, substance use).

Dimensional measures can also be used in "person-oriented" models, using recently developed latent class and latent profile analyses. For example, using the National Longitudinal Survey of Children and Youth, Lacourse et al. (2010) applied a latent cluster analysis and identified three CD clusters among preteens (ages 12–13): physically aggressive, covert (nonaggressive) antisocial (e.g., stealing, substance use), and mixed-severe aggressive-antisocial. In a follow-up assessment in mid-adolescence, youth in the mixed-severe group had by far the highest level of antisocial and criminal activity. Preteens in the other groups were at higher risk for adolescent criminal activity than preteens without CD behaviors, but at significantly less risk than the mixed-severe group. In this study, the preteens who exhibited the mixed-severe features of aggressive CD were 6 times more likely to sell drugs, 9 times more likely to join a gang, 11 times more likely to carry a weapon, and almost 8 times more likely to be arrested as teenagers than preteens who did not exhibit CD (Lacourse et al., 2010). Severity of aggression, along with the breadth and diversity of involvement in overt and covert antisocial activities, is an important feature of preadolescent CD associated with its long-term course.

In summary, CD is a disorder of behavior and emotion, in which the frequency and severity of an individual's hostile (aggressive, destructive, antisocial) behaviors crosses a threshold indicating significant pathology relative to developmental expectations. CD often coexists with ODD and ADHD, sharing features of impulsivity and emotional volatility, but is differentiated by severe aggressive and antisocial behavior and predicts more negative long-term outcomes. For many children with CD, particularly those who display severe aggression, a diverse array of antisocial behaviors, and a lack of empathy or guilt, antisocial behavior becomes a habitual way of interacting with others and eventually an enduring feature of their personality, wreaking havoc for themselves, their families, and society at large.

Etiology and Developmental Course

Over 50 years of research has focused on uncovering the causes of CDs and understanding the developmental course. It is generally accepted that CDs have multiple causes, emerging and intensifying as a function of escalating developmental processes fueled by both biological (e.g., genes, physiology, temperament) and environmental influences (e.g., parenting, peer socialization, schooling experiences, neighborhood risk) (Lynam et al., 2000). In their review of factors linked empirically with antisocial behavior in childhood, Loeber and Farrington (2000) listed 40 distinct risk factors in five different domains (child, family, school, peers, and neighborhood). Yet, research on these different influences has generally been fragmented, with different investigators studying various biological or environmental influences. The extensive research base provides relatively few integrated models testing transactional processes between multiple biological and environmental influences over time (Burke et al., 2002; Raine, 2002; Tremblay, Hartup, & Archer, 2005). Fortunately, recent advances in the technology of neuropsychological and psychophysiological assessment, combined with methodological advances in modeling complex developmental relations, are creating new opportunities to study dynamic developmental transactions in longitudinal studies of children at risk, offering the opportunity to test more integrative developmental models. In the following section, we first review research describing the developmental course of aggression and conduct problems, and then consider the state of evidence regarding the ways in which biology and environment might transact to affect the developmental course of CD.

Developmental Course

In the DSM-V, CD has two subtypes that are differentiated by age of onset (before or after age 10). This distinction is based upon evidence that CD behaviors that emerge first in childhood differ from those that emerge first in adolescence in terms of their causes, correlates, and consequences (see Moffit et al., 2008). In studies that compare early- and adolescent-onset groups, children in the early-starting group generally show a greater range of social adjustment and learning difficulties and are at greater risk for persisting in violent and criminal behavior and developing antisocial personality disorder than their late-starting counterparts (Moffitt & Caspi, 2001). However, others have argued that many youth with CD do not fall neatly into an early-starting or later-starting category (Simonoff et al., 2004). In part, this is because the process of developing CD unfolds over time with more continuity than a discrete "age of onset" model implies. In addition, factors that affect the developmental course of CD, including the severity of aggression, the existence of concurrent cognitive and learning difficulties, and experiences of peer rejection and victimization may be as (or more) important than age of onset as predictors of the chronicity and severity of CD (Broidy et al., 2003; Tremblay et al., 2005).

In addition, developmental research has shown only mixed evidence for a distinct group of youth with late-starting aggression. Specifically, Broidy et al. (2003) examined developmental trajectories of physical aggression across six longitudinal studies. They found two patterns that emerged with consistency among boys: a small group (4 % on average) of boys with high, stable levels of physical aggression from early elementary school through adolescence (who tended to be the boys with the highest levels of physical aggression in kindergarten) and a large group with stable low levels of aggression across age. A pattern in which aggression increased in early adolescence (consistent with the late-starter model) emerged in some data sets, but not consistently. In general, girls showed similar developmental trajectories as boys, but with lower levels of aggression and a greater likelihood of early desisting (see Broidy et al., 2003). Correspondingly, rather than looking for different developmental determinants for early- and late-starting subtypes of CD, most developmental research has focused on understanding the factors that predict to chronically high levels of aggression, recognizing that different factors may play a role during different phases of development, and account for the widening diversity of antisocial activity that emerges in adolescence (Loeber & Farrington, 2000).

In general, there is a recognition that the developmental course of aggression is dynamic and multifaceted, with stable CD emerging primarily when multiple risk factors cascade to impair adaptive socialization (Beauchaine, Gatzke-Kopp, & Mead, 2007; Dodge, Greenberg, Malone, & CPPRG, 2008). Extensive developmental research has led to the construction of a near-consensual model describing the sequential phases of this negative cascade, which has been validated recently by Dodge and colleagues (2008) using a large longitudinal sample of 754 high-risk children, followed from kindergarten through high school (ages 5–18). In that study, the validated cascade began with contexts of disadvantage (e.g., poverty, single parenthood), frequent parent–child conflict, and harsh, ineffective discipline in early childhood, which predicted child social and cognitive deficits at school entry. At the transition into school, poor learning readiness predicted conduct problem behavior, linked with both peer rejection and academic underachievement. By early adolescence, school disengagement and parent withdrawal led to reduced monitoring and adult limit setting, and affiliation with antisocial peers provided opportunities for substance use and expanded antisocial activity.

Reflecting the multifaceted nature of this negative developmental cascade, children who meet the criterion for CD often have multiple mental health and interpersonal adjustment problems, including depressed mood and suicidal thoughts, conflict-laden interpersonal relationships, early substance use, and precocious sexual activity, with increased risk for sexually transmitted diseases and unwanted pregnancy (Loeber, Farrington, Stouthamer-Loeber, & White, 2008). In adolescence, school disengagement, early substance use, deviant peer affiliation, and the early initiation of sexual activity act as accelerants to the negative developmental cascade, promoting CD (see also Dishion, 2014).

In addition to documenting the general course of early aggression and the emergence of CD, a key focus of developmental research is to uncover the mechanisms of action whereby biological vulnerabilities and socialization experiences transact to accelerate or, alternatively, to deflect trajectories of risk associated with CD. The standard cascade model belies the variation that also occurs in the development of CD, whereby some individuals share similar risk factors in childhood but experience different outcomes (i.e., multifinality) whereas other children experience the same outcome, with differential risk characteristics (i.e., equifinality). Developmental research seeks to understand factors that account for child selection into and continuity within the negative developmental cascade associated with CD, as well as factors that account for variations in development and discontinuities or recovery from the negative cascade. In the next sections, we provide a brief description of the dominant hypotheses regarding the ways in which biological factors and socialization experiences influence CD development, followed by speculative models concerning their interactions.

Physiological Activation of Aggressive Responding

Although a number of different biological factors have been identified as correlates of CD, cohesive developmental models that postulate specific mechanisms of action focus primarily on two different physiological systems underlying (1) the motivation to initiate aggressive behavior and (2) the inclination to react to threat with aggressive behavior. This distinction has its basis in animal models that document distinct neural circuitry underlying predatory versus defensive aggression (Gendreau & Archer, 2005). Animal predatory aggression involves activation in the approach or appetitive motivational system of the brain, and has been viewed as a parallel to human *proactive* aggression—aggression that is instrumental in nature, and goal-oriented, motivated by anticipated rewards (Gregg & Siegel, 2001). Animal defensive aggression involves activation in the more primitive interactive neural circuits associated with the processing of fear and rage, and has been viewed as a parallel to human *reactive* aggression—impulsive aggression that occurs in response to a provocation or frustration, motivated by anger or fear (see also Vitaro & Brendgen, 2005). In turn, empirical evidence suggests that individual differences in the functioning of both of these physiological systems and their corresponding neural circuitry, which often co-occur, may create vulnerability for the development of chronically elevated aggression and CD, as discussed further in the following sections.

The approach or appetitive motivational system involves the lateral hypothalamus and a number of structures that are innervated by neurons releasing dopamine and serotonin and has been a key focus of studies on adults with criminal records or antisocial personality disorder (Raine, 2002). One well-studied model postulates that low levels of physiological arousal [e.g., low resting heart rate and skin conductance levels and long slow-wave electroencephalogram (EEG)] are unpleasant and associated with irritability and hence predispose individuals to seek excitement, initiating risky behaviors to raise their arousal level and stimulate neural pathways associated with reward (e.g., sensation seeking) (Zuckerman, 1994). In addition, psychophysiological underarousal may blunt anxiety and fear of negative consequences (e.g., fearlessness), thereby enhancing the relative salience of rewards and reducing concerns regarding negative consequences or threats or punishment (Beauchaine et al., 2007; Van Goozen, Snoek, Matthys, van Rossum, & van Engeland, 2004). Consistent with this model, a number of studies have documented lower resting heart rates and skin conductance in samples of conduct disordered, aggressive, and delinquent youth compared with nondisruptive youth (Fowles, Kochanska, & Murray, 2000). Further, a few studies suggest that indices of childhood physiological underarousal predict later antisocial behavior. For example, as reported in Raine (2005), low resting heart rate at age 3 predicted aggression at age 11, and low resting heart rate and skin conductance during adolescence

predicted criminal behavior in early adulthood. However, these predictive relations explain relatively small amounts of variance, and there are inconsistencies across studies, with some failing to find the expected relations between child and adolescent aggression and indices of physiological underarousal (Lorber, 2004). Hence, developmental researchers generally postulate that the link between physiological underarousal, child sensation seeking or fearlessness, and chronic aggression is moderated by socialization experiences. Specifically, low levels of physiological arousal may serve as a risk factor that increases the likelihood of developmental processes that, in some cases, cascade in a negative fashion to support aggressive responding. For example, young children with low levels of physiological arousal may initiate frequent impulsive, willful, and risky behaviors, and may be relatively unresponsive to punishment, challenging caregivers to set limits effectively, thus contributing to the initiation of family conflict in early childhood and to ongoing rebellion against teachers and adult authority in later childhood and adolescence, as described in the negative cascade model (Fowles et al., 2000; Joireman, Anderson, & Strathman, 2003). Hypothetically, under alternative conditions of effective limit setting and guidance, individual elevations in sensation seeking and fearlessness are redirected to goal-oriented behavior that is aligned with social norms and expectations and modulated by an awareness and respect for social conventions and the rights of others (e.g., conscience and empathy).

The other physiological system that has attracted considerable attention in developmental research on aggression involves individual differences in children's reactivity to threat or perceived harm (Beauchaine et al., 2007; El-Sheikh, Keller, & Erath, 2007; Gordis, Granger, Susman, & Trickett, 2006). In humans, two linked systems process response to threat (1) a fast-acting system, via the activation of the autonomic nervous system, release of norepinephrine, and parasympathetic reactivity reflected in the elevated heart and respiratory rate that characterize the "fight or flight" response and (2) a slower-acting system, via the activation of the HPA axis and secretion of glucocorticoids (e.g., cortisol) (Gordis et al., 2006).

Beauchaine (2001) has argued that functioning in the first of these systems, the reactivity of the parasympathetic system, affects emotional experiences in ways that can contribute to the onset and developmental course of CD. Specifically, he argues that low respiratory sinus arrhythmia, an aspect of heart rate that reflects parasympathetic system functioning, serves as an index of emotion dysregulation and is associated with emotional outbursts and experiences of extreme anger and aggression (see also Beauchaine et al., 2007). Correspondingly, high levels of vagal reactivity are an indicator of emotional lability and characterize children who react to stress or threat with emotion dysregulation, anger, and reactive aggression. Beauchaine (2001) suggests that it is the interaction of multiple aspects of physiology (e.g., underarousal of the approach-appetitive motivational system combined with deficient vagal modulation of emotion) that contribute to the development of CD. Consistent with this conceptualization, McKay and Halperin (2001) have argued that emotional lability and deficits in the executive functions that regulate emotion are implicated centrally in impulsive aggression and associated with the social dysfunction and chronic externalizing problems associated with CD. They suggest that emotional dysregulation and impulsive aggression are, in part, mediated by the serotonergic (5-HT) system, which moderates vulnerability to environmental adversity and interpersonal threat.

Researchers have also examined cortisol as an indicator of individual differences in stress exposure and stress responding. Much of this research suggests that aggressive youth have low levels of baseline cortisol, which has been interpreted as an index of hyporeactivity and possibly related to callous unemotionality and fearlessness in a manner consistent with physiological underarousal (Pajer, Gardner, Rubin, Perel, & Neal, 2001). However, elevated (rather than suppressed) baseline and reactive cortisol have also been documented in subgroups of antisocial youth. Specifically, McBurnett and colleagues (McBurnett, King, & Scarpa, 2003; McBurnett, Lahey, Rathouz, & Loeber, 2000) found low levels of baseline cortisol characterized only the non-anxious children with CD, whereas higher baseline cortisol levels characterized children with CD and comorbid anxiety. These investigators speculate that only a subset of aggressive youth are hyporeactive and fearless, whereas others are hyperreactive to stress which contributes over time to elevated baseline cortisol levels and concurrent anxious symptoms (McBurnett et al., 2003). Similar findings have been found with reactive cortisol. For example, van Goozen and colleagues (1998) exposed boys with conduct problems to provocation and found elevated reactive cortisol among those who were also highly anxious, but low levels of baseline and reactive cortisol among those who were not anxious.

Consistent with the idea that aggressive children may vary in their reactivity to stress, a related hypothesis is that, whereas proactive aggression is activated by the approach-appetitive motivational system, impulsive-reactive forms of aggression are fueled primarily by hyperreactivity of the stress response system (Stieben et al., 2007). Therefore, youth whose behavior is more intensively characterized by reactive aggression (as opposed to proactive aggression) may show greater parasympathetic system and cortisol reactivity (Vitaro & Brendgen, 2005), whereas youth who display more proactive aggression will instead be characterized by low levels of physiological arousal and hyporeactivity. In support of this model, van Bokhoven et al. (2005) found that boys who were reactively aggressive (based on teacher ratings, with proactive aggression controlled) had significantly higher resting cortisol levels than boys who were less reactively aggressive. Similarly, Hubbard et al. (2002) found that teacher-rated reactive aggression was a correlate of angry nonverbal behaviors and rising skin conductance when second grade children were confronted with a cheating play partner. These findings are also in line with evidence that reactive (but not proactive) aggression is associated with inattention and elevations in temperamental reactivity to unconditioned stimuli such as light or pain (Vitaro, Brendgen, & Tremblay, 2002).

Although heightened stress reactivity has thus been implicated as a risk factor for aggression in some children, individual differences in stress reactivity are heavily affected by socialization experiences, as well as biological tendencies. In general, predictable, consistent, and supportive caregiving fosters well-modulated responses to stress, whereas conditions of environmental threat or deprivation, including harsh punishment, family violence, abuse, or instability amplify stress reactivity (Cicchetti, 2002). Exposure to high levels of stress and threat in the context of low levels of caregiving security and support may trigger dysregulated responding in children with susceptible physiology, thereby instigating angry and reactive aggression (Beauchaine, 2001).

In a landmark study examining the impact of exposure to severe caregiving adversity (e.g., frequent changes in primary caregiver, rejection by the mother, and physical or sexual abuse) in a sample of high-risk youth, Caspi et al. (2002) found that the subset of youth who carried the low-activity allele of MAOA-L appeared most vulnerable to developing violence. Specifically, of the youth who had experienced this severe adversity by age 11, those with the MAOA-L variant (who comprised 12 % of the adversity-exposed sample) accounted for 44 % of the total sample convictions for assault and other violent crimes. The researchers hypothesized that children with the MAOA-L variant are predisposed toward neural hyperreactivity when they are exposed to severe threat, responding with increased serotonin availability which may fuel reactive aggression. Additional research by Meyer-Lindenberg et al. (2006) has demonstrated that, for males, the MAOA-L genotype is associated with amygdala hyperreactivity during emotional arousal. These researchers hypothesize that when this threat hyperreactivity is combined with diminished arousal or activation of the regulatory regions of the prefrontal cortex, the propensity for impulsive aggression is heightened (Meyer-Lindenberg et al., 2006).

In summary, extensive research has explored aspects of physiological and neural responding as possible mechanisms accounting for the increased risk some children face for developing CD. Over the past decade, this research has moved away from single, main effect models and instead sought to understand how individual differences in aggressive and violent tendencies arise as a function of interactions among different physiologic and neural systems. Key contributors may be (1) low levels of physiological arousal that are associated with irritability and motivate willful and sensation-seeking behaviors to stimulate neural pathways associated with reward, (2) blunted sensitivity to negative consequences (e.g., fearlessness) that may reduce the effectiveness of socialization efforts designed to curb or redirect aggressive impulses, and (3) hyperreactivity to threat that is associated with emotion dysregulation and anger, fueling impulsive and reactive aggression. These processes are not mutually exclusive and may work in combination within individuals. That is, youth with or at risk for CD exhibit high rates of both reactive and proactive aggression and, although less often studied together, may also show concurrent elevations in sensation seeking and heightened stress reactivity. Each of these factors is posited to increase vulnerability to CD, but only in the context of socializing experiences that encourage aggressive responding or, alternatively, impede the development of regulatory control, as described in the following sections.

Socialization Experiences Associated with Aggression

There are two prevalent views concerning the mechanisms by which socialization experiences contribute to chronic aggression and emerging CD. One set of models emphasizes the way in which experiences with parents, teachers, and peers promote aggression via processes of instrumental learning (modeling and reinforcement), fostering the development of an aggressive behavioral repertoire that is diversified and well practiced. The other set of models focuses on the impact of socialization on the development of self-regulation, and the ways in which socializing agents foster (or fail to support) the development of inhibitory control, conscience, empathy, and flexible problem-solving, thereby helping children inhibit aggressive impulses and internalize culturally approved standards of behavior.

A prominent set of developmental models postulates that children who learn to display frequent and diverse aggressive and antisocial behaviors receive interpersonal modeling and reinforcement that promote the overlearning and habitual exhibition of these behaviors. In parent–child interactions, caregivers may model aggressive control tactics by yelling, threatening, and hitting their children. They may also inadvertently reinforce child noncompliance and aggression. This occurs when, faced with child misbehavior, parents either give in to child demands (e.g., give a yelling child the toy he/she wants, positive reinforcement) or parents relinquish their attempts at control and leave the child alone (e.g., give up attempts to get a yelling child to go to bed, negative reinforcement) (Granic & Patterson, 2006). In either case, the child successfully uses aggressive tactics to get his or her way, strengthening the habit to behave in similar ways in the future. Over time, children increasingly rely on aggressive and aversive behavior to get what they want, and discouraged (often angry and emotionally distraught) adults abdicate their role, leaving children poorly supervised and vulnerable to risk exposure with siblings and with peers (Granic & Patterson, 2006; Patterson, 1976). Strong empirical evidence supports the hypothesized link between parenting practices and child aggression, with elevated rates of parental criticism, directive control efforts, and punitive punishment each associated with elevated levels of child noncompliant and aggressive behavior (Gershoff, 2002).

Experiences with siblings and with peers can also play a key role in the instrumental training of aggressive and antisocial behavior. Developmental research suggests that highly aggressive children are generally disliked by peers, but nonetheless many develop reciprocated friendships (Miller-Johnson, Coie, Bierman, Maumary-Gremaud, & CPPRG, 2002) and some attain central and influential positions in peer networks (Farmer, Estell, Bishop, O'Neal, & Cairns, 2003).

As early as the preschool years, there is evidence that aggressive children tend to befriend each other and spend time together (Hanish, Martin, Fabes, Leonard, & Herzog, 2005; Snyder, Cramer, Afrank, & Patterson, 2005). By late childhood and early adolescence, peer affiliations become more differentiated into cliques and crowds, and aggressive children tend to affiliate selectively with other aggressive children who have similar positive attitudes toward risk-taking and antisocial activities (Farmer et al., 2003). Increasing evidence suggests that, when aggressive children spend unsupervised time together, these peer relations create niches of social opportunity in which aggressive behavior and rule-breaking talk are modeled and positively reinforced with laughter, interest, and approval. Sometimes termed deviancy training or peer contagion, these experiences amplify aggression over time and provide opportunities and support for antisocial activities (see Dishion, 2014). Peer support for aggressive behavior is particularly likely when students are placed in elementary classrooms that contain many aggressive children, as often happens in poor, urban areas, because in these contexts both deviancy training in friendships and social norm processes in the classroom may support aggressive responding (Powers, Bierman, & CPPRG, 2012).

Complementary to a focus on facets of family and peer socialization that promote a child's learning and use of aggressive behaviors, developmental researchers have called for a focus on family and peer socialization experiences that reduce child aggression, by enhancing children's abilities to inhibit and redirect their aggressive impulses (see Tremblay et al., 2005). Pointing out that aggressive behavior is common in early childhood, but peaks and begins to decline rapidly between the ages of 2 and 4, these developmental researchers argue that the critical developmental capacity is not learning how to express aggression but rather how to inhibit, control, and redirect aggressive impulses.

In the past decade, intensive interest has focused on the development of the executive regulatory skills in the prefrontal cortex as factors that strengthen children's capacities to regulate emotions (e.g., stop and calm down when upset or excited), focus and shift attention, engage in rule-governed behavior, and respond thoughtfully when confronted with social conflicts or frustrations (Hughes, 2011). The executive regulatory system directly influences and is influenced by emotional and autonomic responses to stimulation and plays a central role in the development of empathy, prosocial behavior, conscience, and guilt (Kochanska, Gross, Lin, & Nichols, 2002). These self-regulatory controls each foster desistance from aggression, as they allow the child to inhibit their impulsive reactions to the immediate provocation and engage in more complex and thoughtful analysis of the situation in order to plan an adaptive and socially appropriate responses (Blair, Zelazo, & Greenberg, 2005).

The development of the prefrontal cortex, including language and self-regulatory control skills, is heavily influenced by environmental experiences (Cicchetti, 2002). Under good conditions, caregivers provide sensitive-responsive support, positive guidance, limit setting, and scaffolding to help young children engage in organized and productive exploration of their social and physical environments, thereby promoting sustained attention, emotional understanding, and planning and problem-solving skills (Lengua, Honorado, & Bush, 2007). However, early adversity, including family poverty, maternal depression, low levels of social support, stressful life events, and exposure to violence, can stress children and reduce caregiving availability and support, thereby contributing to delays in the development of executive regulatory control (Lengua et al., 2007). For example, Lengua et al. (2007) found that poverty, contextual risk, family disruptions, and poor-quality parent–child interactions all delayed the pace of development of self-regulatory control in early childhood (before age 8), with the quality of parenting mediating the distal effects of the environment on the children. Similarly, in another study, low levels of maternal responsiveness assessed during the first 2 years of life predicted later disruptive behavior disorders (ODD and CD) in middle childhood (Wakschlag & Hans, 2002). The quality of attachment, reflecting positive parent–child relationships and the degree to which the child is able to derive comfort from the parent's presence, appears to be a particularly important protective (or risk) factor. In a sample of high-risk infants, clinically elevated levels of aggressive behavior at age 5 were found in 44 % of the children who showed disorganized attachments but in only 5 % of the children who were securely attached to their mothers (Lyons-Ruth, Alpern, & Repacholi, 1993); another study found that the majority (60 %) of children with disorganized attachments showed clinically elevated aggressive behavior, as compared with 17 % of their peers with secure attachments (Shaw, Owens, Vondra, Keenan, & Winslow, 1996).

A second set of social influences that can undermine positive self-regulatory and social-emotional development occurs when aggressive children are rejected by their peers. It is well established that aggressive children tend to be disliked by their peers and ostracized from normative peer interactions (Miller-Johnson et al., 2002). In turn, peer rejection predicts future aggressive-disruptive behavior. Peer disliking is thought to amplify aggressive-disruptive behavior in two ways (1) by limiting opportunities for positive peer socialization experiences needed to develop prosocial skills and (2) by exposing children to bullying and victimization by other children (Miller-Johnson et al., 2002; Snyder et al., 2008). Excluded by mainstream peers, disliked children more often play alone or with younger children, providing low levels of exposure to the types of social support and social exchanges that foster social competence and the development of anger management and negotiation skills. Rejection may also make aggressive children more vulnerable to negative peer influence—a social augmentation hypothesis proposed by Dishion, Piehler, & Myers, (2008). Supporting this hypothesis, Snyder et al. (2010) found that the deviancy training processes were more powerful for children who were socially rejected than for children who were well liked by peers.

In addition to their immediate and direct impact on children's aggressive behavior, experiences with parents and peers may also have long-term effects on children, mediated by their influence on children's social information processing. A significant body of research suggests that social experiences influence children's social expectations and reasoning, affecting their selective attention to particular social cues, their attributions regarding the benign versus hostile intentions of others, their goals and values in social interactions, and their decision-making processes regarding behavioral choices (see Fontaine, 2006). Children who have been exposed to repeated conflict in their family and peer interactions may become overly vigilant to social threat and sensitized to the cues of impending conflict, choosing to act aggressively rather than experience vulnerability (Erath, El-Sheikh, & Cummings, 2009).

In summary, it is evident that socialization experiences play a central role in the development and course of CD. Although many children who show elevated aggression in early childhood self-right over time, responding to socialization supports and gaining behavioral control, for others, aggression becomes chronic and develops into the more diverse and serious range of antisocial behaviors that characterize CD. The negative cascade into CD is more likely for children whose families face multiple socioeconomic risks that create child-rearing challenges and increase child exposure to community risks.

In 1976, Patterson aptly characterized the aggressive child as an architect and victim of a coercive system (Patterson, 1976). Children with developing CD are "architects" of a hostile social world for themselves, in the sense that their impulsive, intrusive, and aggressive behaviors evoke high levels of anger, rebuke, rejection, and counteraggression from their parents, siblings, teachers, and peers. They are "victims" in the sense that they are often the recipients of high levels of social mistreatment by adults and other children, who withhold affection and social support from them, and leave them without the nurturant experiences that build empathy, conscience, and self-control.

Transactional Models

Several models describe processes by which multiple risk factors (at biological and environmental levels) propel the negative developmental cascade associated with chronic aggression and CD. In this section, we contrast two types of transactional models (1) models that postulate *parallel developmental processes*, with two distinct pathways to CD, and (2) models that describe *sequential developmental processes*, whereby the differentiated characteristics of youth with CD emerge via paths that open at different times in the sequence of development. Each type of model seeks to explain the presence of severe aggressive and antisocial behavior among the CD youth, as well as the heterogeneity that exists among this group in terms of their psychophysiological responding, emotional characteristics, social adjustment, and cognitive functioning.

Table 24.1 provides a listing of the major areas in which heterogeneity has been documented among subgroups of aggressive youth. As described in the preceding review, these include (1) variations in physiology, including low levels of physiological arousal or heightened stress responding; (2) variations in motivation and postulated neural circuitry characteristic of proactive versus reactive aggression; (3) variations in socialization experiences, including instrumental conditioning (modeling and reinforcement) that supports aggressive behavior, and threat exposure (insufficient support, victimization) that elicits reactive aggression and undermines self-regulatory skill development;

Table 24.1 Areas of documented heterogeneity among conduct problem youth

	Hypothetical parallel process pathways	
Domain of functioning	Dominant/rebellious	Trauma-exposed/angry
Physiology and stress reactivity	Hypo-arousal	Hyperreactivity to threat
Motivation and neural circuitry	Proactive aggression	Reactive aggression
Socialization mechanism	Instrumental learning	High threat/low support caregiving
Emotional characteristics	Callous, unemotional	Anxious, depressed, angry
Cognitive characteristics	Positive aggression beliefs	Low executive regulatory control

(4) variations in emotional characteristics—either unemotional, callous, or emotionally dysregulated—with elevated anxiety, depression, and anger; and (5) variations in cognitive contributions, including positive evaluations of aggression or low executive regulatory control skills.

Developmental theorists have considered the various ways in which these factors may support differentiated and parallel developmental pathways to CD. For example, Hawes, Brennan, and Dadds (2009) hypothesize that one early-onset pathway to CD includes children with low physiological arousal and corresponding emotional insensitivity (low stress reactivity, interpersonal callousness, and lack of empathy) who are resistant to socialization efforts and are at risk for the most severe and chronic antisocial behavior, whereas a second group is comprised of youth who have heightened HPA axis stress reactivity and are exposed to early trauma, triggering elevated hostile-reactive aggression. Along similar lines, Dodge, Lochman, Harnish, Bates, and Pettit (1997) speculated that reactive and proactive aggression have different family correlates, with harsh, unpredictable, and threatening caregiving eliciting impulsive hostility and reactive aggression, and instrumental support (the modeling and reinforcement of aggressive tactics) providing a developmental training ground for proactive aggression.

Although these dual-pathway models are elegant theoretically, they struggle to account for the high levels of co-occurrence among the risk factors in youth with conduct problems. For example, reactive and proactive aggression are highly correlated (average $r = .70$) and typically co-occur, suggesting that although the types of aggression are distinct, they do not distinguish subtypes of human aggressors (see also Bushman & Anderson, 2002). Indeed, in person-centered studies, concurrent profiles reflecting elevations in both reactive and proactive aggression describe the majority of aggressive youth, whereas many fewer are purely reactive and even fewer are purely proactive (Little, Brauner, Jones, Nock, & Hawley, 2003).

Alternatively, *sequential developmental process* models postulate that the heterogeneity observed

in youth who become CD reflects variations in paths taken at several junctures over time that represent important transitions in the development of CD. For example, Vitaro and Brendgen (2005) posit that the aggressive behavior shown in early childhood is primarily reactive, as children with high temperamental reactivity and negative affectivity react to restraint or displeasure. They suggest that proactive aggression does not emerge until later in development, as a function of instrumental learning that occurs when parents are ineffective in managing toddler impulsivity and tantrums, and inadvertently instruct children in the utility of aggression to achieve goals. Hence, this model predicts that the majority of children who show elevated aggression in early childhood will be characterized by reactive aggression, but that by school entry, many will have learned how to use aggressive behavior effectively to gain dominance and autonomy, producing diversified profiles of reactive and proactive aggression. They further hypothesize that, as some of these children develop self-regulatory capacities over the course of early childhood (ages 3–7), the prevalence of their reactive aggression will recede, such that the growth in proactive aggression will dominate in later childhood and adolescence. Consistent with this hypothesis, Lansford, Deater-Deckard, Dodge, Bates, and Pettit (2004) showed that reactive aggression in 1 year predicted subsequent proactive aggression from kindergarten through grade 7, whereas early proactive aggression did not predict subsequent reactive aggression (Fig. 24.1).

A logical corollary of this sequential developmental model is that the elevated levels of callous-unemotional characteristics observed in chronically antisocial youth may not simply reflect constitutional risk (Frick & Sheffield Morris, 2004), but rather result from the interaction between constitution and socialization experiences. For example, a set of studies suggests that children with low skin conductance are more likely than other children to show elevated aggression when they receive harsh punishment (Erath et al., 2009) or are exposed to marital conflict (El-Sheikh et al., 2007). Possibly because they are relatively unfazed by parental hostile

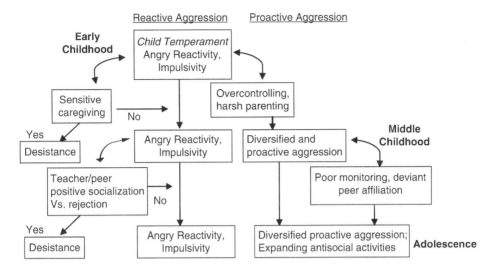

Fig. 24.1 Developmental sequence model

threats, they are more likely to counteraggress in response, making parents' attempts to socialize children with low arousal through harsh punishment especially ineffective and counterproductive (Dadds & Salmon, 2003; Fontaine, McCrory, Boivin, Moffitt, & Viding, 2011).

In summary, research addressing the development of CD is focused increasingly on articulating transactional models and testing dynamic developmental processes. There are concerted efforts to integrate psychophysiological mechanisms with social and psychological processes in developmental research, recognizing that biological factors do not operate in a vacuum, and the interplay between psychophysiological and social risk factors is likely more important than either factor in isolation (Lorber, 2004).

Approaches to Prevention and Intervention

An ongoing hope is that research that expands an understanding of the risk factors and the developmental course of CD will guide continuing improvements in prevention and early intervention design, thereby reducing the prevalence and severity of this costly disorder. A number of evidence-based prevention and intervention approaches have demonstrated efficacy in reducing aggression and antisocial activity (for comprehensive reviews, see Eyberg, Nelson, & Boggs, 2008; Trentacosta & Shaw, 2012). However, substantial work remains to be done to increase intervention efficacy and impact.

Promising approaches to the prevention and treatment of CD include (1) parent management training, designed to reduce overcontrolling and harsh parenting and improve warm support and effective (nonpunitive) limit setting; (2) cognitive-behavioral and social-emotional skill training approaches focused on improving youth problem-solving skills, communication skills, impulse control, and anger management skills; (3) family therapy, focused on making changes within the family system, such as improving communication skills and family interactions, and increasing parental monitoring and limit setting; and (4) multicomponent programs designed to combine parent-focused and youth-focused intervention components.

Parent Management Training

A number of clinic-based parenting programs have demonstrated that parent management training leads to reduced child aggressive and oppositional behavior (McMahon & Forehand, 2005). One of the first of these programs to be developed was the Parent Management Training—Oregon model (Patterson, Chamberlain, & Reid, 1982), which provides weekly parenting sessions focusing on five core parenting skills (1) limit setting, (2) positive parent involvement, (3) monitoring and supervision, (4) encouragement for skill development, and (5) family problem-solving. Additional approaches to parent management training reflect similar principles, but vary in program length, format, or delivery system. For example, the Helping the Noncompliant Child program (McMahon & Forehand, 2005) focuses on younger children (ages 3–8). Parents attend therapy sessions with their young children and practice core parenting skills, including praise and positive feedback for appropriate behavior, ignoring minor problems, giving clear directions, and providing negative consequences for noncompliance. In the Incredible Years parent training program (Webster-Stratton & Reid, 2003), parents meet in groups, and the training process is built around discussions of parenting vignettes. In the Parent–child Interaction Therapy program (Brinkmeyer & Eyberg, 2003), parents practice skills with in vivo coaching and videotaped feedback. Each of these programs has documented positive effects in randomized controlled trials, showing increases in positive parenting practices and decreases in child noncompliant and aggressive behaviors (see Eyberg et al., 2008).

Cognitive-Behavioral and Social-Emotional Skill Training

A second intervention strategy focuses on building youth emotion regulation skills, social interaction skills, and social information processing skills. Research demonstrates that classroom-level interventions that focus on teaching social-emotional skills can promote reductions in aggressive behavior. For example, the PATHS (Promoting Alternative THinking Strategies) Curriculum (Kusche & Greenberg, 1994) includes lessons in areas of self-control, emotional understanding, peer-related social skills, and social

problem-solving. A recent randomized trial involving 2,937 children who either received the program during the early elementary years (grades 1–3) or experienced "usual practice" teaching revealed modest reductions in student aggression and increased prosocial behavior associated with the intervention (according to both teacher and peer report) and improved academic engagement (according to teacher report) (CPPRG, 2010a). Small group social skill training interventions also show promise for reducing aggressive behavior by teaching fair play and conflict management strategies in the early grade school years (for a review, see Bierman & Powers, 2009). Skill training has also shown effectiveness at the older elementary level, particularly when combined with parent training. For example, the Coping Power Program (Lochman & Wells, 2004) consists of 34 structured sessions for aggressive youth focused on topics such as goal setting, organization and planning skills, anger management, social skills, problem-solving skills, and resistance skills. When combined with a parent training program in a randomized trial, Coping Power reduced youth's angry feelings and hostile attributions and improved parent management skills (Lochman & Wells, 2004).

Family Programs for Antisocial Adolescents

Given the negative developmental cascade associated with CD, intervention often becomes more challenging with adolescents. However, some success has been documented. Multisystemic Therapy (MST) (Henggeler & Lee, 2003) is an intensive family treatment program designed for adolescents who have become heavily involved in antisocial activity. The MST model recognizes that adolescent CD is multi-determined and embedded within risk factors operating at the levels of the youth, family, peer group, school, and community context. As such, MST provides intensive, individualized, and home-based services following a set of guiding principles. Goals include improving caregiver discipline practices, enhancing family closeness, decreasing youth association with deviant peers, improving positive peer and school engagement, and developing an indigenous support network to help caregivers achieve and maintain the changes. Supported by a set of randomized trials, MST has proven effective in reducing criminal activity, drug-related arrests, violent offenses, and incarceration (Henggeler, Mihalic, Rone, Thomas, & Timmons-Mitchell, 1998; Sawyer & Borduin, 2011).

Multicomponent Prevention Programs

Prevention of CD is a particularly important goal. Many children at risk for the development of CD can be identified as early as 5–6 years of age, based upon high rates of aggression at the transition into school. Because high-risk children are likely to progress toward more severe and violent problems over time, early intervention may reduce the likelihood that children will become enmeshed in the accumulating risk factors associated with the negative cascade, such as peer rejection, affiliation with deviant peers, and school disengagement.

Based on a developmental model of CD, the Fast Track program was initiated in 1991, using a multicomponent approach to promote positive parenting, strengthen child social and self-regulatory skills, and improve school engagement and peer relationships. The goal of Fast Track was to determine the extent to which a prevention program could prevent serious antisocial outcomes by beginning early, taking a multifaceted approach, and sustaining support from childhood into mid-adolescence. During the elementary years, Fast Track intervention components included parent training groups and home visits to teach parents behavior management skills and improve parent–child relationship quality, classroom-level social-emotional skill training program (the PATHS Curriculum, delivered from first through fifth grade), and additional social skills training groups for highly aggressive children. Individual academic support was also provided, on an as-needed basis. In the middle school years, individualized prevention programs were based on regular assessments of risk and protective factors. Fast Track was evaluated using a randomized, controlled design including 891 high-risk, aggressive children in four locations in the USA. In the early elementary years, when intervention was most intensive, children in the intervention group showed greater gains in child social and academic skills than children in the control group, their parents reduced their use of harsh punishment, and children showed reduced aggression and improved peer relationships. By the end of high school, youth in the intervention group self-reported fewer delinquent behaviors and had fewer juvenile arrests based on court records (CPPRG, 2010b). By age 24, youth in the intervention group were significantly less likely than controls to be diagnosed with an externalizing disorder by either self or peer report, 63 % (intervention group) compared with 74 % (control group) (CPPRG, 2012). These findings speak to the potential of prevention programs to disrupt the maladaptive developmental processes associated with early-starting aggression and to place high-risk children and their parents on a trajectory toward positive adjustment. They also reflect the nature of the challenge, given the high prevalence of externalizing disorder in the high-risk sample, selected based on kindergarten aggression scores.

Summary

Conduct disorder (CD) is one of the most prevalent yet challenging mental health problems in children and adolescents. Often described as intractable, CDs are characterized by a negative developmental cascade, in which early difficulties become compounded over time by failure experiences, victimization, and opportunities for perceived rewards within a deviant lifestyle. A large and expanding research base indicates risk factors that exist at the level of the child's physiology and temperament, the family, the peer group, the school, and the community. Emerging research seeks to clarify divergent developmental processes and mechanisms and hopefully to inform prevention and intervention efforts.

Effective prevention and intervention approaches exist, but they require additional development and research to increase their impact, portability, and cost-effectiveness.

References

American Psychiatric Association. (2013). *Diagnostic and statistical manual of mental disorders* (4th ed.). Washington, DC: Author.

Beauchaine, T. P. (2001). Vagal tone, development, and Gray's motivational theory: Toward an integrated model of autonomic nervous system functioning in psychopathology. *Development and Psychopathology, 13*, 183–214.

Beauchaine, T. P., Gatzke-Kopp, L., & Mead, H. K. (2007). Polyvagal theory and developmental psychopathology: Emotion dysregulation and conduct problems from preschool to adolescence. *Biological Psychology, 74*, 174–184.

Bierman, K. L., & Powers, C. J. (2009). Social skills training to improve peer relations. In K. H. Rubin, W. Bukowski, & B. Laursen (Eds.), *Handbook of peer interactions, relationships, and groups* (pp. 603–621). New York: Guilford.

Blair, C., Zelazo, P. D., & Greenberg, M. T. (2005). The measurement of executive function in early childhood. *Developmental Neuropsychology, 28*, 561–571.

Brinkmeyer, M. Y., & Eyberg, S. M. (2003). Parent–child interaction therapy for oppositional children. In A. E. Kazdein & J. R. Weisz (Eds.), *Evidence-based psychotherapies for children and adolescents* (pp. 204–223). New York: Guilford.

Broidy, L. M., Nagin, D. S., Tremblay, R. E., Bates, J. E., Brame, B., Dodge, K. A., et al. (2003). Developmental trajectories of childhood disruptive behaviors and adolescent delinquency: A six-site, cross-national study. *Developmental Psychology, 39*, 222–245.

Burke, J. D., Loeber, R., & Birmaher, B. (2002). Oppositional defiant disorder and conduct disorder: A review of the past 10 years, part 2. *Journal of the American Academy of Child and Adolescent Psychiatry, 41*, 1275–1293.

Bushman, B. J., & Anderson, C. A. (2002). Human Aggression. *Annual Review of Psychology, 53*, 27–51.

Byrd, A. L., Loeber, R., & Pardini, D. A. (2012). Understanding desisting and persisting forms of delinquency: The unique contributions of disruptive behavior disorders and interpersonal callousness. *Journal of Child Psychology and Psychiatry, 53*, 371–380.

Caspi, A., McClay, J., Moffitt, T. E., Mill, J., Martin, J., Craig, I. W., et al. (2002). Role of genotype in the cycle of violence in maltreated children. *Science, 297*, 851–854.

Center for Disease Control and Prevention. (2008). *Understanding youth violence: Fact sheet*. Retrieved

August 3, 2012, from http://www.cdc.gov/ncipc/pubres/YVFactSheet.pdf

Cicchetti, D. (2002). The impact of social experience on neurobiological systems: Illustration from a constructivist view of child maltreatment. *Cognitive Development, 17*, 1407–1428.

Cohen, M. A., & Piquero, A. R. (2009). New evidence on the monetary value of saving a high-risk youth. *Journal of Quantitative Criminology, 25*, 25–49.

CPPRG. (2010a). The effects of a multiyear universal social-emotional program: The role of student and school characteristics. *Journal of Consulting and Clinical Psychology, 78*, 156–168.

CPPRG. (2010b). Fast Track intervention effects on youth arrests and delinquency. *Journal of Experimental Criminology, 6*, 131–157.

CPPRG. (2012). *Impact of early intervention on externalizing psychopathology at age 24* (Unpublished manuscript).

Dadds, M. R., & Salmon, K. (2003). Punishment insensitivity and parenting: Temperament and learning as interacting risks for antisocial behavior. *Clinical Child and Family Psychology Review, 6*, 69–86.

Dishion, T. J. (2014). A developmental model of aggression and violence: Microsocial and macrosocial dynamics within an ecological framework. In M. Lewis & K. D. Rudolph (Eds.), *Handbook of developmental psychopathology* (3rd ed.). New York: Springer.

Dishion, T. J., Piehler, T. F., & Myers, M. W. (2008). Dynamics and ecology of adolescent peer influences. In M. J. Prinstein & K. A. Dodge (Eds.), *Understanding Peer Influence in Children and Adolescents* (pp. 72–93). New York: Guilford.

Dodge, K. A., Greenberg, M. T., Malone, P. S., & CPPRG. (2008). Testing an idealized dynamic cascade model of the development of serious violence in adolescence. *Child Development, 79*, 1907–1927.

Dodge, K. A., Lochman, J. E., Harnish, J. D., Bates, J. E., & Pettit, G. S. (1997). Reactive and proactive aggression in school children and psychiatrically impaired chronically assaultive youth. *Journal of Abnormal Psychology, 106*, 37–51.

El-Sheikh, M., Keller, P. S., & Erath, S. A. (2007). Marital conflict and risk for child maladjustment over time: Skin conductance level reactivity as a vulnerability factor. *Journal of Abnormal Child Psychology, 35*, 715–727.

Erath, S. A., El-Sheikh, M., & Cummings, E. M. (2009). Harsh parenting and child externalizing behavior: Skin conductance level reactivity as a moderator. *Child Development, 80*, 578–592.

Eyberg, S. M., Nelson, M. M., & Boggs, S. R. (2008). Evidence-based psychosocial treatments for children and adolescents with disruptive behavior. *Journal of Clinical Child and Adolescent Psychology, 37*, 215–237.

Farmer, T. W., Estell, D. B., Bishop, J. L., O'Neal, K. K., & Cairns, B. D. (2003). Rejected bullies or popular leaders? The social relations of aggressive subtypes of rural African American early adolescents. *Developmental Psychology, 39*, 992–1004.

Fontaine, R. G. (2006). Applying systems principles to models of social information processing and aggressive behavior in youth. *Aggression and Violent Behavior, 11*, 64–76.

Fontaine, N. M. G., McCrory, E. J. P., Boivin, M., Moffitt, T. E., & Viding, E. (2011). Predictors and outcomes of joint trajectories of callous-unemotional traits and conduct problems in childhood. *Journal of Abnormal Psychology, 120*, 730–742.

Fowles, D. C., Kochanska, G., & Murray, K. (2000). Electrodermal activity and temperament in preschool children. *Psychophysiology, 37*, 777–787.

Frick, P. J., & Sheffield Morris, A. (2004). Temperament and developmental pathways to conduct problems. *Journal of Clinical Child and Adolescent Psychology, 33*, 54–68.

Gendreau, P. L., & Archer, J. (2005). Subtypes of aggression in humans and animals. In R. E. Tremblay, W. H. Hartup, & J. Archer (Eds.), *Developmental origins of aggression* (pp. 25–46). New York: Guilford.

Gershoff, E. T. (2002). Corporal punishment by parents and associated child behaviors and experiences: A meta-analytic and theoretical review. *Psychological Bulletin, 128*, 539–579.

Gordis, E. B., Granger, D. A., Susman, E. J., & Trickett, P. K. (2006). Asymmetry between salivary cortisol and alpha-amylase reactivity to stress: Relation to aggressivebehaviorinadolescents. *Psychoneuroendocrinology, 31*, 976–987.

Granic, I., & Patterson, G. R. (2006). Toward a comprehensive model of antisocial development: A dynamic systems approach. *Psychological Review, 113*, 101–131.

Greene, R., Biederman, J., Zerwas, S., Monuteaux, M., Goring, J. C., & Faraone, S. (2002). Psychiatric comorbidity, family dysfunction, and social impairment in referred youth with oppositional defiant disorder. *American Journal of Psychiatry, 159*, 1214–1224.

Gregg, T. R., & Siegel, A. (2001). Brain structures and neurotransmitters regulating aggression in cats: Implications for human aggression. *Progress in Neuro-Psychopharmacology & Biological Psychiatry, 25*, 91140.

Hanish, L. D., Martin, C. L., Fabes, R. A., Leonard, S., & Herzog, M. (2005). Exposure to externalizing peers in early childhood: Homophily and peer contagion processes. *Journal of Abnormal Child Psychology, 33*, 267–281.

Hare, R. D. (1991). *The Hare psychopathy checklist—Revised*. Toronto, ON: Multi-Health Systems.

Hawes, D. J., Brennan, J., & Dadds, M. R. (2009). Cortisol, callous-unemotional traits, and pathways to antisocial behavior. *Current Opinions in Psychiatry, 22*, 357–362.

Henggeler, S. W., & Lee, T. (2003). Multisystemic treatment of serious clinical problems. In A. E. Kazdein & J. R. Weisz (Eds.), *Evidence-based psychotherapies for children and adolescents* (pp. 301–322). New York: Guilford.

Henggeler, S. W., Mihalic, S. F., Rone, L., Thomas, C., & Timmons-Mitchell, J. (1998). *Blueprints for violence prevention, book six: Multisystemic therapy*. Boulder, CO: Center for the Study and Prevention of Violence.

Hubbard, J. A., Smithmyer, C. M., Ramsden, S. R., Parker, E. H., Flanagan, K. D., Dearing, K. F., et al. (2002). Observational, physiological, and self-report measures of children's anger: Relations to reactive versus proactive aggression. *Child Development, 73*, 1101–1118.

Hughes, C. (2011). Changes and challenges in 20 years of research into the development of executive functions. *Infant and Child Development, 20*, 251–271.

Joireman, J., Anderson, J., & Strathman, A. (2003). The aggression paradox: Understanding links among aggression, sensation seeking, and the consideration of future consequences. *Journal of Personality and Social Psychology, 84*, 1287–1302.

Kochanska, G., Gross, J. N., Lin, M.-H., & Nichols, K. E. (2002). Guilt in young children: Development, determinants, and relations with a broader system of standards. *Child Development, 73*, 461–482.

Kusche, C. A., & Greenberg, M. T. (1994). *The PATHS curriculum*. Seattle, WA: Developmental Research and Programs.

Lacourse, E., Baillargeon, R., Dupéré, V., Vitaro, F., Romano, E., & Tremblay, R. (2010). Two-year predictive validity of conduct disorder subtypes in early adolescence: A latent class analysis of a Canadian longitudinal sample. *Journal of Child Psychology and Psychiatry, 51*, 1386–1394.

Lahey, B. B., Frick, P. J., Loeber, R., Tannenbaum, B. A., Van Horn, Y., & Christ, M. A. G. (1990). *Oppositional and conduct disorder: I. A meta-analytic review*. Unpublished manuscript, University of Georgia, Athens.

Lahey, B. B., McBurnett, K., & Loeber, R. (2000). Are attention-deficit/hyperactivity disorder and oppositional defiant disorder developmental precursors to conduct disorder? In A. J. Sameroff, M. Lewis, & S. M. Miller (Eds.), *Handbook of developmental psychopathology* (2nd ed., pp. 431–446). New York: Plenum.

Lahey, B. B., & Waldman, I. D. (2012). Annual research review: Phenotypic and causal structure of conduct disorder in the broader context of prevalent forms of psychopathology. *The Journal of Child Psychology and Psychiatry, 53*, 536–557.

Lansford, J. E., Deater-Deckard, K., Dodge, K. A., Bates, J. E., & Pettit, G. S. (2004). Ethnic differences in the link between physical discipline and later adolescent externalizing behaviors. *Journal of Child Psychology and Psychiatry, 45*, 801–812.

Lengua, L. J., Honorado, E., & Bush, N. (2007). Contextual risk and parenting as predictors of effortful control and social competence in preschool children. *Journal of Applied Developmental Psychology, 28*, 40–55.

Little, T. D., Brauner, J., Jones, S. M., Nock, M. K., & Hawley, P. H. (2003). Rethinking aggression: A typological examination of the functions of aggression. *Merrill-Palmer Quarterly, 49*, 343–369.

Lochman, J. E., & Wells, K. C. (2004). The Coping Power Program for preadolescent boys and their parents: Outcome effects at the 1-year follow-up. *Journal of Consulting and Clinical Psychology, 72*, 571–578.

Loeber, R., Burke, J. D., Lahey, B. B., Winters, A., & Zera, M. (2000). Oppositional defiant and conduct disorder: A review of the past 10 years, part 1. *Journal of the American Academy of Child and Adolescent Psychiatry, 12*, 1468–1484.

Loeber, R., & Farrington, D. P. (2000). Young children who commit crime: Epidemiology, developmental origins, risk factors, early interventions, and policy implications. *Development and Psychopathology, 12*, 737–762.

Loeber, R., Farrington, D.P., Stouthamer-Loeber, M., White, H.R. (2008). *Violence and serious theft: Risk and promotive factors from childhood to early adulthood*, Mahwah, NJ: Lawrence Erlbaum.

Lorber, M. F. (2004). Psychophysiology of aggression, psychopathy, and conduct problems: A meta-analysis. *Psychological Bulletin, 130*, 531–552.

Lynam, D. R., Caspi, A., Moffit, T. E., Wikstrom, P., Loeber, R., & Novak, S. (2000). The interaction between impulsivity and neighborhood context on offending: The effects of impulsivity are stronger in poorer neighborhoods. *Journal of Abnormal Psychology, 109*, 563–574.

Lyons-Ruth, K., Alpern, L., & Repacholi, B. (1993). Disorganized infant attachment classification and maternal psychosocial problems as predictors of hostile aggressive behavior in the preschool classroom. *Child Development, 64*, 572–585.

McBurnett, K., King, J., & Scarpa, A. (2003). The hypothalamic-pituitary-adrenal system (HPA) and the development of aggressive, antisocial and substance abuse disorders. In D. Cicchetti & E. Walker (Eds.), *Neurodevelopmental mechanisms in psychopathology* (pp. 324–344). New York, NY: Cambridge University Press.

McBurnett, K., Lahey, B. B., Rathouz, P. J., & Loeber, R. (2000). Low salivary cortisol and persistent aggression in boys referred for disruptive behavior. *Archives of General Psychiatry, 57*, 38–43.

McKay, K. E., & Halperin, J. M. (2001). ADHD, aggression, and antisocial behavior across the lifespan: Interactions with neurochemical and cognitive function. In: Wasserstein, J., Wolf, L. E., & LeFever, F. F. (Eds.), Adult attention deficit disorder: Brain mechanisms and life outcomes. *Annals of the New York Academy of Sciences, 931*, 84–96.

McMahon, R. J., & Forehand, R. L. (2005). *Helping the noncompliant child* (Family-based treatment for oppositional behavior 2nd ed.). New York: Guilford.

Meyer-Lindenberg, A., Buckholtz, J. W., Kolachana, B., Hariri, A. R., Pezawas, L., Blasi, G., et al. (2006). Neural mechanisms of genetic risk for impulsivity and violence in humans. *Proceedings of the National Academy of Sciences of the United States of America, 103*, 6269–6274.

Miller-Johnson, S., Coie, J. D., Bierman, K., Maumary-Gremaud, A., & CPPRG. (2002). Peer rejection and aggression and early starter models of conduct disorder. *Journal of Abnormal Child Psychology, 30*, 217–230.

Moffit, T. E., Arseneault, L., Jaffee, S. R., Kim-Cohen, J., Koenen, K. C., Odgers, C. L., et al. (2008). Research review: DSM-V conduct disorder: Research needs for an evidence base. *Journal of Child Psychology and Psychiatry, 49*, 3–42.

Moffitt, T. E., & Caspi, A. (2001). Childhood predictors differentiate life-course persistent and adolescence-limited antisocial pathways among males and females. *Development and Psychopathology, 13*, 355–375.

Offord, D.R., Boyle, M.H., & Racine, Y.A. (1991). Epidemiology of behavioral and emotional disorders of adolescence. Implications for treatment, research and policy. In R. J. McMahon & P. R. Dev (eds.), *Behavior Disorders of Adolescence: Research, Intervention, and Policy in Clinical and School Settings* (pp. 13–26). Plenum, New York.

Pajer, K., Gardner, W., Rubin, R. T., Perel, J., & Neal, S. (2001). Decreased cortisol levels in adolescent girls with conduct disorder. *Archives of General Psychiatry, 58*, 297–302.

Pardini, D. A., & Loeber, R. (2008). Interpersonal callousness trajectories across adolescence early social influences and adult outcomes. *Criminal Justice and Behavior, 35*, 173–196.

Pardini, D. A., Obradovic, J., & Loeber, R. (2006). Interpersonal callousness, hyperactivity/impulsivity, inattention, and conduct problems as precursors to delinquency persistence in boys: A comparison of three grade-based cohorts. *Journal of Clinical Child and Adolescent Psychology, 35*, 46–59.

Patterson, G. R. (1976). The aggressive child: Victim and architect of a coercive system. In L. A. Hamerlynck, L. C. Handy, & E. J. Mash (Eds.), *Behavior modification and families: 1. Theory and research*. New York: Brunner/Mazel.

Patterson, G. R., Chamberlain, P., & Reid, J. B. (1982). A comparative evaluation of a parent-training program. *Behavior Therapy, 13*, 638–650.

Powers, C. J., Bierman, K. L., & CPPRG. (2012). The multifaceted impact of peer relations on aggressive-disruptive behavior in early elementary school. *Developmental Psychology, 49*(6), 1174–1186.

Raine, A. (2002). Biosocial studies of antisocial and violent behavior in children and adults: A review. *Journal of Abnormal Child Psychology, 30*, 311–326.

Raine, A. (2005). The interaction of biological and social measures in the explanation of antisocial and violent behavior. In D. Stoff & E. Susman (Eds.), *Developmental psychobiology of aggression* (pp. 13–42). New York: Cambridge University Press.

Robins, L. N., & Price, R. K. (1991). Adult disorders predicted by childhood conduct problems: Results from the NIMH Epidemiological Catchment Area project. *Psychiatry, 54*, 116–132.

Sawyer, A. M., & Borduin, C. M. (2011). Effects of multisystemic therapy through midlife: A 21.9-year follow-up to a randomized clinical trial with serious and violent juvenile offenders. *Journal of Consulting and Clinical Psychology, 79*, 643–652.

Scheepers, F. E., Buitelaar, J. K., & Matthys, W. (2011). Conduct disorder and the specifier callous and unemotional traits in the DSM-5. *European Child and Adolescent Psychiatry, 20*, 89–93.

Shaw, D. S., Owens, E. B., Vondra, J. I., Keenan, K., & Winslow, E. B. (1996). Early risk factors and pathways in the development of early disruptive behavior problems. *Development and Psychopathology, 8*, 679–699.

Simonoff, E., Elander, J., Holmshaw, J., Pickles, A., Murray, R., & Rutter, M. (2004). Predictors of antisocial personality. Continuities from childhood to adult life. *The British Journal of Psychiatry, 184*, 118–127.

Snyder, J., Cramer, A., Afrank, J., & Patterson, G. R. (2005). The contributions of ineffective discipline and parental hostile attributions of child misbehavior to the development of conduct problems at home and school. *Developmental Psychology, 41*, 30.

Snyder, J., McEachern, A., Schrepferman, L., Just, C., Jenkins, M., Roberts, S., et al. (2010). Contribution of peer deviancy training to the early development of conduct problems: Mechanisms and moderators. *Behavior Therapy, 41*, 317–328.

Snyder, J., Schrepferman, L., McEachern, A., Barner, S., Johnson, K., & Provines, J. (2008). Peer deviancy training and peer coercion: Dual processes associated with early-onset conduct problems. *Child Development, 79*, 252–268. doi:10.1111/j.1467-8624.2007.01124.x.

Stieben, J., Lewis, M. D., Granic, I., Zelazo, P. D., Segalowitz, S., & Pepler, D. (2007). Neurophysiological mechanisms of emotion regulation for subtypes of externalizing children. *Development and Psychopathology, 19*, 455–480.

Tremblay, R. E., Hartup, W. W., & Archer, J. (2005). *The developmental origins of aggression*. New York: Guilford.

Trentacosta, C. J., & Shaw, D. S. (2012). Preventing early conduct problems and later delinquency. In E.

Grigorenko (Ed.), *Handbook of juvenile forensic psychology and psychiatry* (pp. 311–324). New York: Springer.

van Bokhoven, I., Van Goozen, S. H. M., van Engeland, H. I., Schaal, B., Arseneault, L., Séguin, J. R., et al. (2005). Salivary cortisol and aggression in a population-based longitudinal study of adolescent males. *Journal of Neural Transmission, 112*, 1083–1096.

Van Goozen, S. H., Matthys, W., Cohen-Kettenis, P. T., Gispen-de Wied, C., Wiegant, V. M., & Engeland, H. (1998). Salivary cortisol and cardiovascular activity during stress in oppositional-defiant disorder boys and normal controls. *Biological Psychiatry, 7*, 531–539.

Van Goozen, S. H., Snoek, H., Matthys, W., van Rossum, I., & van Engeland, H. (2004). Evidence of fearlessness in behaviorally disordered children: A study on startle reflex modulation. *Journal of Child Psychology and Psychiatry, 45*, 884–892.

Vitaro, F., & Brendgen, M. (2005). Proactive and reactive aggression: A developmental perspective. In R. E. Tremblay, W. W. Hartup, & J. Archer (Eds.), *The developmental origins of aggression* (pp. 202–222). New York: Guilford.

Vitaro, F., Brendgen, M., & Tremblay, R. E. (2002). Reactively and proactively aggressive children: Antecedent and subsequent characteristics. *Journal of Child Psychology and Psychiatry, 43*, 495–505.

Wakschlag, L. S., & Hans, S. L. (2002). Maternal smoking during pregnancy and conduct problems in high-risk youth: A developmental framework. *Development and Psychopathology, 14*, 351–369.

Webster-Stratton, C., & Reid, M. (2003). The incredible years parents, teachers, and children training series: A multifaceted treatment approach for young children with conduct problems. In A. E. Kazdein & J. R. Weisz (Eds.), *Evidence-based psychotherapies for children and adolescents* (pp. 224–240). New York: Guilford.

Zuckerman, M. (1994). *Behavioral expressions and biosocial bases of sensation seeking*. Cambridge: Cambridge University Press.

Part VI

Emotional Disorders

Depression in Children and Adolescents

Judy Garber and Uma Rao

Depression is one of the most common forms of psychopathology and a leading cause of disability in the world (World Health Organization, 2008). Depressive disorders tend to be recurrent, can be chronic, and are associated with significant impairment (Kessler et al., 2012). Mood disorders are relatively rare during childhood, but the rates increase significantly during adolescence, and many depressed adults recall that their first depression occurred when they were an adolescent. Moreover, some factors associated with risk for depression during adolescence and adulthood have their origin earlier in development. The current chapter describes the diagnostic criteria, continuity and phenomenology, epidemiology, and etiology of depression in children and adolescents from a developmental psychopathology perspective.

The term "depression" has been defined as a symptom (sadness), a syndrome (a constellation of associated symptoms), or a diagnosed disorder (a specific set of symptoms with the same course, prognosis, etiology, and response to treatment). Occasional feelings of sadness in the face of disappointment or loss are natural and expected. When such dysphoria lingers for weeks or months, occurs at the same time as other symptoms (e.g., changes in sleep, appetite, concentration), and affects a person's ability to function, then the individual may be experiencing major depressive disorder (MDD).

Diagnostic Criteria

The criteria for depressive disorders outlined in the fourth edition of the *Diagnostic and Statistical Manual of Mental Disorders-Text Revision* (DSM-IV-TR; American Psychiatric Association, 2000) are essentially the same across development. Two minor variations in DSM-IV are that for children and adolescents (a) irritability is considered a manifestation of dysphoric mood and (b) the duration of dysthymia is one rather than two years. Functional impairment is particularly important for distinguishing depressive disorders from normal mood variability. Thus, according to DSM-IV-TR there are few real developmental differences in the symptoms that comprise the syndromes of major depression or dysthymia.

J. Garber, Ph.D. (✉)
Department of Psychology and Human Development, Vanderbilt University, 0552 Peabody, 230 Appleton Pl., Nashville, TN 37203-5721, USA
e-mail: judy.garber@vanderbilt.edu; jgarber.vanderbilt@gmail.com

U. Rao, M.D.
Kennedy Center, Vanderbilt University, Nashville, TN 37203-5721, USA

Center for Molecular and Behavioral Neuroscience, Meharry Medical College, Nashville, TN, USA

Department of Psychiatry and Behavioral Sciences, Meharry Medical College, Nashville, TN, USA

M. Lewis and K.D. Rudolph (eds.), *Handbook of Developmental Psychopathology*,
DOI 10.1007/978-1-4614-9608-3_25, © Springer Science+Business Media New York 2014

The recently revised DSM-V (American Psychiatric Association, 2013) includes the following changes to mood disorders (Moran, 2013): (a) disruptive mood dysregulation disorder (DMDD) is a new diagnosis intended to identify children who experience extreme irritability without changes in mood that are characteristic of bipolar disorder and to reduce the overdiagnosing of children with bipolar disorder. (b) Premenstrual dysphoric disorder (PMDD) is a new diagnostic entity in *DSM-V* and is no longer in the appendix. Although not unique to adolescents, PMDD can begin after puberty and thus can be diagnosed in adolescent girls. (c) The term "dysthymia" now falls under the diagnosis of "persistent depressive disorder," which includes both chronic MDD and what was previously dysthymic disorder (DD) in DSM-IV-TR. (d) The "grief exclusion" has been eliminated, which now means that patients experiencing severe and persistent major depression related to bereavement can be diagnosed and treated.

Continuity and Phenomenology of Depression

Continuity is central to the study of developmental psychopathology (Rutter & Sroufe, 2000). Three types of continuity are particularly relevant to depression: (a) continuity across symptoms, syndrome, and disorder; (b) continuity in the occurrence of depression from childhood through adulthood; and (c) continuity in symptom manifestation across development.

Continuity Across Depressive Symptoms, Syndrome, and Disorder

How is depressed mood or a combination of depressive symptoms (i.e., syndrome) related to more severe and sustained depressive disorders? Subthreshold levels of depressive symptoms in youth significantly predict the onset of a full MDD in adulthood (Klein, Shankman, Lewinsohn, & Seeley, 2009; Kovacs & Lopez-Duran, 2010), and subthreshold depressive symptoms often are associated with significant functional impairment (Lewinsohn, Solomon, Seeley, & Zeiss, 2000), which then can exacerbate the symptoms further. These patterns indicate evidence of some continuity across levels of severity.

A related issue is whether depression is a continuous dimension versus a categorical entity. Studies using taxometric procedures (Waller & Meehl, 1998) to examine the latent structure of depression in children and adolescents have found evidence for a depression taxon (Richey et al., 2009; Solomon, Ruscio, Seeley, & Lewinsohn, 2006), although others have reported a dimensional solution (Hankin, Fraley, Lahey, & Waldman, 2005). These contrary results are partially due to differences in the measures of depression, informants, sample sizes, and data analytic procedures used. Given the increasing emphasis on dimensional approaches to psychopathology (Insel, 2013), further studies are needed to determine to what extent depression is dimensional, categorical, or some combination of the two. The answer likely will depend upon multiple factors including individuals' ages, personal and family history of depression, methods used to assess depression, data analytic strategies applied, and the underlying processes that explain the dimension versus category of depression.

Continuity of Depression from Childhood to Adulthood

A second type of continuity concerns how stable depression is across development (Avenevoli & Steinberg, 2001). Is there continuity between depressions during childhood and those that occur later in adolescence and adulthood? Are the processes that underlie childhood-onset depression the same as those that produce adolescent- or adult-onset depression?

Depression at the symptom level has been found to be relatively stable in children (e.g., Cole, Martin, Powers, & Truglio, 1996; Hofstra, van der Ende, & Verhulst, 2000). Cole et al. (1996) reported high stability of symptoms assessed by multiple informants over 6 months for children in both grades 3 and 6. In contrast, a prospective study of 3- to 12-year-old children showed a lack of stability in depressive symptoms based on self- and parent report (Pihlakoski et al., 2006). Thus, continuity of depression over time likely depends upon the informant about the symptoms, the amount of time between assessments, and the child's age.

Recurrence, defined as the onset of a new depressive episode, is high in children and adolescents (Kennard, Emslie, Mayes, & Hughes, 2006). Younger age of onset significantly predicts relapse (e.g., Birmaher et al., 1996). MDD has a cumulative probability of recurrence of 40 % by 2 years and 70 % by 5 years (Emslie et al., 1997). A 9-year follow-up study found that 80 % of children with prior dysthymia and 50 % of children with prior MDD had subsequent episodes of depression (Kovacs, 1996a).

Results of investigations of the long-term course of early-onset mood disorders have been inconsistent, however. Some studies have found that prepubertal-onset depression did not show continuity into adulthood, but was sometimes followed by behavioral problems and impaired functioning (e.g., Harrington, Fudge, Rutter, Pickles, & Hill, 1990; Weissman et al., 1999). Other studies (e.g., Dunn & Goodyer, 2006; Fergusson & Woodward, 2002; Kovacs, 1996b) have reported that pediatric-onset depressions recur into adulthood. Copeland, Shanahan, Costello, and Angold (2009), however, showed that depression in adolescence was no longer related to depression in adulthood when they controlled for anxiety and externalizing disorders during adolescence. Finally, other studies (e.g., Geller, Zimerman, Williams, Bolhofner, & Craney, 2001; Weissman et al., 1999) have suggested that some early-onset depressions have a bipolar course that emerges over time.

Differences in the onset, duration, and recurrence of early-onset depression have been linked to demographic (e.g., age, gender), individual (e.g., preexisting diagnosis, negative cognitive style), family (e.g., parental psychopathology), biological (e.g., neurobiological dysregulation), and psychosocial factors (e.g., poor support, stressful life events) (Birmaher et al., 2004;

Garber, 2007; Timbremont & Braet, 200⸱ MDEs might increase vulnerability to sub episodes by creating biological and/or ᵖ logical *scars* that sensitize individuals to later exposure to even low levels of the etiological agent(s). That is, recurrence of depression may result from *kindling*, sensitization, or *scarring* (Lewinsohn, Steinmetz, Larson, & Franklin, 1981; Monroe & Harkness, 2005). The kindling hypothesis asserts that prior episodes of depression "leave behind neurobiological residues that make patients more vulnerable to subsequent episodes" (Post, 1992; p. 1006). Earlier depressions may change individuals in some ways, which then lead to their generating the kinds of stressful situations that are likely to precipitate future episodes (Hammen, 1991). Finally, Teasdale (1983, 1988) proposed a differential activation hypothesis such that vulnerability to subsequent, more severe depressive episodes is influenced by patterns of information processing that occur during earlier, milder depressions. Depressed mood presumably activates negatively biased interpretations of experiences, which then maintain and exacerbate the dysphoria into further clinical depression.

Phenomenology

A third type of continuity concerns whether the manifestation of the symptoms that comprise the syndrome and disorder (i.e., phenomenology) of depression is similar or different across development. That is, do the symptoms that define depressive disorder reflect homotypic versus heterotypic continuity from childhood through adulthood?

Infants have been observed to experience depression-like symptoms such as sadness, irritability, sleep and eating problems, fatigue, withdrawal, apathy, fussiness, and tantrums (Guedeney et al., 2003). Failure to thrive in infants has several similarities to depression such as psychomotor delay, behavioral difficulties, and feeding problems (Raynor & Rudolf, 1996) and may be a manifestation of a mood disorder in babies. In preschool-age children, a specific constellation of depressive symptoms has been identified (Luby et al., 2002). Anhedonia was found to be a specific indicator, and mood symptoms (i.e., sadness and irritability) were found to be sensitive indicators. The most severely impaired preschoolers could be diagnosed using unmodified DSM criteria. The modified criteria, however, identified a larger number of seriously impaired children who would have been missed had only the existing DSM-IV criteria been used (Luby et al., 2003).

The symptoms of depressive disorder might not be isomorphic across the life span (Cicchetti & Toth, 1998; Weiss & Garber, 2003). Therefore, the criteria that define depression in adults may "need to be translated into age-appropriate guidelines for children, sensitive to developmental changes in the children's experience and expression of depression" (Cicchetti & Schneider-Rosen, 1984, p. 7). Although there may be a core set of common depressive symptoms across all ages, other symptoms might be uniquely associated with the syndrome at different developmental levels (Avenevoli & Steinberg, 2001; Kovacs, Obrosky, & Sherrill, 2003).

A meta-analysis of 16 empirical studies comparing the rates of depressive symptoms in different age groups revealed developmental effects for 18 of the 29 (62 %) core and associated depressive symptoms (Weiss & Garber, 2003). Older youth had higher levels of anhedonia, hopelessness, hypersomnia, weight gain, and social withdrawal and lower levels of energy. Adolescents had more vegetative symptoms (i.e., low energy, hypersomnia, weight loss), hopelessness/helplessness, and suicidality than preadolescents (Yorbik, Birmaher, Axelson, Williamson, & Ryan, 2004). Thus, developmental differences exist in the rates of some symptoms in children versus adolescents. Evidence is more mixed regarding age differences in the factor structure of depression (Weiss & Garber, 2003). Overall, although some researchers have argued that there are not developmental differences in depressive symptoms (e.g., Kashani, Rosenberg, & Reid, 1989; Ryan et al., 1987), the evidence does *not* support this conclusion.

Epidemiology: Prevalence of Depression in Childhood and Adolescence

MDD is rarely assessed in infants, uncommon in preschool-age children, relatively infrequent during middle childhood, and increases significantly during adolescence. The overall prevalence estimate of depression in school-age children is 2.8 %, although the rate varies by age, informant, and type of depression (Costello, Foley, & Angold, 2006). Among very young children (i.e., ages 2–5), prevalence rates are 1.4 % for MDD, 0.6 % for DD, and 0.7 % for depression not otherwise specified (NOS)/minor depression (Bufferd, Dougherty, Carlson, & Klein, 2011; Egger & Angold, 2006). In children ages 9, 11, and 13, 3-month prevalence rates are 0.03 % for MDD, .13 % for DD, and 0.45 % for depression NOS (Costello et al., 1996). Overall, the rates of diagnosed depressive disorders in preadolescents are relatively low (Rubio-Stipec, Fitzmaurice, Murphy, & Walker, 2003). When impairment criteria are included, lower rates (3.4 %) are found than when they are not (4.1 %; Canino et al., 2004).

Rates rise significantly through adolescence (Costello, Mustillo, Erkanli, Keeler, & Angold, 2003). In a nationally representative sample of over 3,000 youth, the 12-month prevalence of a mood disorder was 2.5 % in 8- to 11-year-olds and 4.8 % in 12- to 15-year-olds (Merikangas et al., 2010). With impairment criteria, the prevalence was 1.8 % for 8- to 11-year-olds and 3.9 % for 12- to 15-year-olds. Lifetime prevalence rates of MDD in adolescents range from 9 to 24 % (Merikangas & Knight, 2009). The National Comorbidity Survey—Adolescent Supplement, which interviewed over 10,000 adolescents ages 13–18, reported the lifetime prevalence of mood disorders was 14.3 %; when severe impairment or distress was included, prevalence was 11.2 % (Merikangas et al., 2010). Subclinical depression also is quite high, with about 10–20 % of youth experiencing subsyndromal or minor depression (Kessler & Walters, 1998). An even greater percent of youth

(20–50 %) endorse significant levels of depressive symptoms on self-report measures (Kessler, Avenevoli, & Merikangas, 2001).

Sex Differences

Across cultures, epidemiological studies repeatedly find about twice the rate of depression in females compared to males (Weissman & Olfson, 1995). Whereas some researchers have found the rates of MDD to be about equal in preadolescent girls and boys (e.g., Angold & Rutter, 1992; Fleming, Offord, & Boyle, 1989), others have reported higher rates among preadolescent boys than girls (e.g., Angold, Costello, & Worthman, 1998; Steinhausen & Winkler, 2003). Findings of sex differences in minor depression or depressive symptoms have been more mixed (e.g., Gonzalez-Tejera et al., 2005). A meta-analysis of 310 studies using the Children's Depression Inventory found no significant sex differences in self-reported depressive symptoms in children ages 8–12 (Twenge & Nolen-Hoeksema, 2002). By early adolescence, girls begin to show higher levels of depressive symptoms and disorders than boys (Angold, Erkanli, Silberg, Eaves, & Costello, 2002; Costello et al., 2003). Sex differences in the manifestation of depression also have been noted. Young depressed females are more likely than males to experience appetite and weight problems, worthlessness or guilt (Lewinsohn, Rohde, & Seeley, 1998), and suicidality (Yorbik et al., 2004). MDD tends to be more recurrent and insidious in adolescent females than males (Lewinsohn & Essau, 2002).

Explanations of the increasing rates of depression in females during adolescence emphasize the contribution of biological, psychological, interpersonal, and contextual factors and their interactions during the transition to adolescence (Cyranowski, Frank, Young, & Shear, 2000; Hankin & Abramson, 2001; Hyde, Mezulis, & Abramson, 2008; Nolen-Hoeksema & Hilt, 2009; Strauman, Costanzo, & Garber, 2011). Hormonal changes (e.g., levels of androgen and estradiol) during puberty may be one explanation for the emerging sex difference in depression during adolescence (e.g., Angold, Costello, Erkanli, & Worthman, 1999b). Early maturing girls have been found to be at higher risk for depression than their average-maturing peers (Conley & Rudolph, 2009; Copeland et al., 2010), possibly due to psychosocial factors such as increased social expectations and pressures, less peer support, and greater body dissatisfaction (e.g., Stice, Hayward, Cameron, Killen, & Taylor, 2000; Teunissen et al., 2011).

Girls also report higher levels of stress during the transition to adolescence, particularly interpersonal problems, and are more likely than boys to experience depression at the same level of stress (Hankin, Mermelstein, & Roesch, 2007; Shih, Eberhart, Hammen, & Brennan, 2006). Finally, individual differences in temperament, stress responses, rumination, and attention biases to emotional stimuli may produce depression in girls more than boys, particularly under conditions of stress (Else-Quest, Hyed, Goldsmith, & van Hulle, 2006; Kujawa et al., 2011; Nolen-Hoeksema & Hilt, 2009). Thus, sex differences in the rates of depression become increasing evident postpuberty due to biological, psychological, and social factors.

Comorbidity

Comorbidity with depression is very common in children and adolescents, with rates ranging from about 42 % in community samples (e.g., Rohde, Lewinsohn, & Seeley, 1991) to as high as 75 % in clinical samples (e.g., Kovacs, 1996b; Sorensen, Nissen, Mors, & Thomsen, 2005). DD is the most common comorbid disorder with MDD (Kovacs, 1994). Such *double depression* is associated with more severe and longer depressive episodes, a higher rate of other comorbid disorders (e.g., generalized anxiety disorder), more suicidality, and less social competence (Goodman, Schwab-Stone, Lahey, Shaffer, & Jensen, 2000).

The pattern of comorbidity with depression varies across age and sex (Angold, Costello, & Erkanli, 1999a; Wagner, 2003). In younger children, anxiety and depression form a unified, indistinguishable construct, whereas in older children a dual-factor or tripartite model is more common (Cole, Truglio, & Peeke, 1997). In pre-adolescents, depression often co-occurs with separation anxiety, ADHD (Yorbik et al., 2004), and conduct problems (Harrington et al., 2000), whereas in adolescents common comorbid conditions include ODD and substance use disorders, particularly in males, and eating disorders, particularly in females (Lewinsohn, Hops, Roberts, Seeley, & Andrews, 1993). In general, depressions that are comorbid with other disorders have a higher risk of recurrence, longer duration, more suicide attempts, greater functional impairment, less favorable response to treatment, and greater mental health service utilization (Ezpeleta, Domenech, & Angold, 2006; Rudolph & Clark, 2001).

Etiology of Depression in Children and Adolescents

Depression is a heterogeneous condition with a complicated etiology. No single factor is either necessary or sufficient; rather, multiple risk factors and processes interact to produce depression (Cicchetti & Dawson, 2002). We focus here on factors for which there is the most empirical support including genes, neurobiology, temperament, negative cognitions, self-regulation, stressful life events, and interpersonal relationships as well as interactions among these variables. Although some of these variables (e.g., stress) also are associated with other psychiatric conditions (e.g., anxiety), the particular amalgamation of these vulnerability factors with each other is what uniquely results in one condition rather than another (Garber & Hollon, 1991).

Genetic Factors

Behavioral Genetic Studies

Behavioral genetic studies utilizing family, twin, and adoption designs document effects of both genetic and environmental factors for unipolar depression (Lau & Eley, 2008; Rice, 2010; Sullivan, Neale, & Kendler, 2000). Twin studies with children and adolescents reported marked variability in the heritability estimates for depressive symptoms (ranging from 0 to 55 %) as a function of age, sex, and informant (e.g., Bartels et al., 2004; Happonen et al., 2002; Rice, Harold, & Thapar, 2002; Scourfield et al., 2003). The emerging theme from these studies is that the influence of genetic factors on depression is very modest during childhood and increases during adolescence (Rice, 2010). These age-related differences may be partly due to gene–environment correlations, which increase during adolescence as a function of greater independence in selecting and shaping the environment with increasing age (Rice, Harold, & Thapar, 2003). New genetic influences also might emerge during adolescence due to developmental changes (Scourfield et al., 2003) or functional modifications in the genome induced by the changing environment (Bagot & Meaney, 2010).

Heritability estimates for depressive symptoms have indicated negligible differences between males and females (Bartels et al., 2004; Happonen et al., 2002; Scourfield et al., 2003). Some evidence exists of significant interactions between age and sex on heritability estimates in children and adolescents (Eley & Stevenson, 1999; Silberg et al., 1999). In addition, a study of anxiety and depression in 3- to12-year-old children showed that the same genes were expressed in boys and girls (Boomsma, van Beijsterveldt, & Hudziak, 2005). Heritability estimates also have been found to vary by informant (i.e., child, parent, or teacher). For instance, in the Virginia Twin Study, heritability estimates based on children's self-report were lower than those based on parents' reports of children's depression (Eaves et al., 1997).

One twin study that focused on depressive disorders in 12- to 23-year-old (mean = 15 years) females (Glowinski, Madden, Bucholz, Lynskey, & Heath, 2003) found a heritability estimate of 40 % (95 % confidence interval = 24–55), which is consistent with the findings in adults (Sullivan et al., 2000). A comparison of heritability estimates for a broad phenotype comprised of sadness and/or anhedonia lasting 2 weeks versus the diagnosis of MDD indicated that the broad phenotype involved largely shared environmental factors, whereas a diagnosis of MDD was related to both genetic and environmental factors (Glowinski et al., 2003). These findings highlight the importance of precision in diagnostic classification for behavioral and molecular genetic studies (Rice, 2010). The relative contribution of genes and environment across development needs further study with large samples and careful characterization of the phenotypes and epigenetic phenomena (i.e., the shaping of gene expression by the rearing environment without altering the nucleotide sequence) (Bagot & Meaney, 2010).

Molecular Genetics

Molecular genetic studies of child and adolescent depression largely have used a candidate gene approach and have focused particularly on functional polymorphisms in genes involved in emotional regulation and the stress response (Rice, 2010). A few genetic association and pharmacogenetic studies with modest sample sizes have been conducted (Rice, 2010).

Among the candidate genes associated with depressive disorder, the serotonin transporter (5-HTT) gene has been studied in both pediatric and adult samples. Humans exhibit polymorphisms in the 5-HTT gene (SLC6A4), based on the number of variable repeat sequences appearing in the promoter region of the gene, and differ in their transcriptional efficiency. The short (S) variant has reduced serotonin transporter expression compared with the long (L) variant (Lesch et al., 1996). More recently, the long allele was discovered to consist of two variants: L_G, which behaves physiologically like the S allele, and the high-functioning (L_A) variant (Hu et al., 2006).

A small-scale study of children and adolescents using a case–control and family-based association design reported a significant relation between SLC6A4 short variant and depression (Nobile et al., 2004). In a community sample of 200 youth, chronic family stress (but not episodic stress) predicted prospective increases in depressive symptoms over 6 months among individuals with the SLC6A4 short allele (Jenness, Hankin, Abela, Young, & Smolen, 2011). In a study of 346 adolescents at low and high risk for depression, chronic family stress at age 15 predicted higher depression scores at age 20 among individuals with the short allele, but the genetic moderation effects were significant only for females (Hammen, Brennan, Keenan-Miller, Hazel, & Najman, 2010). Kaufman et al. (2004) found that positive social support reduced the effects of SLC6A4 short allele on depressive symptoms in children exposed to maltreatment. In contrast, the Christchurch Health and Development Study that followed a birth cohort of 893 children for up to 30 years did not find that the interaction of SLC6A4 genotypes with life stress predicted depressive symptoms in adult life (Fergusson, Horwood, Miller, & Kennedy, 2011).

Gene-by-gene-by-environment interactions also have been found in association with depression vulnerability. For example, the SLC6A4 short variant interacted with Val66Met polymorphism in the gene encoding brain-derived neurotrophic factor (BDNF) to increase the risk for depressive symptoms in maltreated children, but not in healthy controls (Kaufman et al., 2006). Social support further modified the risk for depression by reducing the severity of depression scores in the high-risk group. Similarly, Hammen and colleagues (Conway, Hammen, Brennan, Lind, & Najman, 2010; Hammen et al., 2010) found that the val158met polymorphism in the catechol-O-methyltransferase (COMT) gene moderated SLC6A4 short variant-by-environment interactions on both depressive symptoms and diagnosis. For val158 homozygotes, the SLC6A4 long allele appeared to be protective at higher stress levels.

Other investigations have demonstrated in high-risk youth who exhibited the SLC6A4 short allele compared to those with the long-allele higher morning cortisol levels (Chen, Joormann, Hallmayer, & Gotlib, 2009; Goodyer, Bacon, Ban, Croudace, & Herbert, 2009) and increased cortisol responses to a laboratory-administered stressor (Gotlib, Joormann, Minor, & Hallmayer, 2008). Moreover, the combination of the short variant and higher morning cortisol levels predicted the onset of depressive disorder over a 12-month follow-up period, controlling for baseline depressive symptoms (Goodyer et al., 2009). In the same study, the combination of Val66Val genotype of the BDNF gene and higher morning cortisol levels increased the risk for a subsequent depressive episode after accounting for the SLC6A4 short variant-by-morning cortisol interactions (Goodyer, Croudace, Dudbridge, Ban, & Herbert, 2010).

With respect to gene-association studies, a genome scan was performed in 146 nuclear families from Hungary consisting of children with either MDD or bipolar disorder and affected siblings (Wigg et al., 2009). No evidence of linkage was found on a genome-wide scan that included 405 microsatellite markers. However, markers on two chromosomes (13q and Xq) showed linkage in regions (D13S779 on 13q and TTTA062 on Xq) previously identified in association with bipolar disorder in adults.

Neurobiology

Sleep Architecture and Electrophysiological Studies

The regulation of sleep is essential to the pathophysiology and treatment of depression. First, there is a significant overlap in the control of sleep and mood regulation (Adrien, 2002; Clarke & Harvey, 2012). Sleep complaints are common in depression and form an essential criterion of the diagnosis (American Psychiatric Association, 2000). Developmental influences on the rates of depression and maturational changes in sleep regulation also imply a close connection between depressive disorders and sleep regulation. Mood disorders are relatively rare prior to puberty but increase dramatically during adolescence (Hankin et al., 1998; Kessler et al., 2001). Sleep regulation at younger ages is relatively "protected" against disruptions. By puberty, however, there is a large drop in slow-wave sleep (Dahl et al., 1990), a decrease in the threshold of arousal to disrupt sleep (Busby, Mercier, & Pivik, 1994), a dramatic increase in daytime sleepiness, and a shift in the circadian pattern, with a preference

for late-night schedules (Carskadon, Orav, & Dement, 1983). Objective sleep changes found in adult MDD are rarely seen in prepubertal depression, gradually emerge after puberty, and are consistent biological findings in later adolescence (Kaufman, Martin, King, & Charney, 2001; Rao, 2011).

In contrast to the consistent findings in adults, sleep architecture measures have shown considerable variability in depressed youth despite significant subjective sleep complaints (e.g., Ivanenko & Johnson, 2008; Rao, 2011). The results vary as a function of age, sex, ethnicity, familial risk, severity of illness, and clinical course (Rao, 2011; Rao, Hammen, & Poland, 2009a, 2009b; Robert et al., 2006). Depressed adolescents have relatively more frequent disturbances in circadian rest-activity rhythms, sleep architecture, and EEG rhythms during sleep than depressed children (e.g., Armitage et al., 2000; Rao, 2011). Robert and colleagues (Armitage, Hoffmann, Emslie, Rintelmann, & Robert, 2006; Robert et al., 2006) found an interaction among age, sex, and depression diagnosis such that depressed adolescent males exhibited most severe sleep problems including the highest proportion of stage 1 sleep, shortest REM latency, and lowest percentage of slow-wave sleep. In contrast, adolescent females had the lowest temporal coherence on sleep microarchitecture analysis.

Changes in sleep architecture and sleep-related EEG rhythms also have been documented in healthy adolescents at high familial risk for depression, and these changes were associated with depression during a prospective follow-up (Morehouse, Kusumakar, Kutcher, LeBlanc, & Armitage, 2002; Rao et al., 2009b). Baseline sleep measures also predicted early recurrence (Armitage et al., 2002; Emslie et al., 2001) and differed between depressed adolescents who had a recurrent unipolar course versus those who developed bipolar disorder (Rao et al., 2002). The observed variability in sleep architecture changes in depressed youth may partly reflect heterogeneity in the longitudinal course of these disorders (Rao, 2011).

Electrophysiological studies have documented reduced left frontal electrical activity in infant and adolescent offspring of depressed mothers (Dawson, Klinger, Panagiotides, Hill, & Spieker, 1992; Tomarken, Dichter, Garber, & Simien, 2004). Evidence of right parietotemporal hypoactivation, but not left frontal hypoactivation, in depressed female adolescents also has been reported (Kentgen et al., 2000). Decreased left frontal EEG activity probably reflects an underactivation of the approach system and reduced positive emotional expression, which also might be a marker of vulnerability to depression (Davidson, Pizzagalli, Nitschke, & Putnam, 2002). Finally, in a sample of adolescent boys, baseline frontal EEG measures predicted the onset of depressive symptoms during a prospective follow-up (Mitchell & Possel, 2012).

Neuroendocrine Studies

Among the neuroendocrine markers of pediatric depression, the hypothalamic–pituitary–adrenal (HPA) system has been a focus of interest, although the findings have been inconsistent (Kaufman et al., 2001; Rao & Chen, 2009). For example, depressed children did not display changes in 24-h cortisol patterns compared to healthy youth. Few differences in basal cortisol secretion have been observed between depressed adolescents and controls; group differences tended to be subtle alterations in normal diurnal patterns. Nonetheless, these subtle differences were relatively robust in predicting the longitudinal clinical course. Higher cortisol secretion in the evening or during sleep, when the HPA axis is relatively quiet, was associated with a longer time to episode recovery (Goodyer, Park, & Herbert, 2001), a propensity for recurrence (Rao et al., 1996; Rao, Hammen, & Poland, 2010), and more suicide attempts (Mathew et al., 2003). Higher cortisol secretion also was detected in at-risk youth who subsequently developed depression (Goodyer, Herbert, Tamplin, & Altham, 2000; Rao et al., 2009b). HPA activity also has been found to vary as a function of exposure to stressful experiences, such that greater HPA activity was observed in youth experiencing particularly high levels of adversity (Kaufman et al., 1997; Rao, Hammen, Ortiz, Chen, & Poland, 2008).

Another neuroendocrine marker possibly related to depression is growth hormone. Although the precise role of growth hormone secretion in depression is not known, it appears to be a marker of central noradrenergic and 5-HT systems (Dinan, 1998). Findings in children and adolescents have been variable (Kaufman et al., 2001; Rao & Chen, 2009). One study reported that depressed children with stressful life events had increased growth hormone secretion compared to youth who had not experienced recent stress, suggesting that environmental factors may have a moderating effect (Williamson, Birmaher, Dahl, al-Shabbout, & Ryan, 1996). In contrast, depressed adolescents who subsequently exhibited suicidal behavior were found to have increased growth hormone secretion during sleep when measured at baseline and manifested blunted growth hormone secretion compared with controls (Coplan et al., 2000). Pharmacological challenge studies have documented blunted growth hormone response to a variety of pharmacological agents in depressed children, as in depressed adults (Dinan, 1998), but less so in depressed adolescents. Pubertal changes and sex might account for some of the variability across children, adolescents, and adults (Kaufman et al., 2001; Zalsman et al., 2006).

Neuroimaging Studies
Structural Neuroimaging Studies

In pediatric samples, structural magnetic resonance imaging (sMRI) studies have revealed reductions in left frontal volume (e.g., in the anterior cingulate and orbitofrontal cortex, and subgenual region of the PFC), particularly in youth with familial depression (Botteron, Raichle, Drevets, Heath, & Todd, 2002; Nolan et al., 2002; Steingard et al., 2002). Additionally, reduced caudate nucleus volume recently was observed in a study of adolescents with depression (Shad, Muddasani, & Rao, 2012).

The hippocampus has been a focal area of research in both animal and human studies because depression is considered to be a stress-sensitive illness and the hippocampus is highly sensitive to stress, particularly early in development (MacQueen & Frodl, 2011; McEwen, 1999; Sapolsky, 2003). The hippocampus also is involved in mood regulation and cognitive function (Campbell & Macqueen, 2004). Studies utilizing both pediatric and adult samples have reported reductions in hippocampal volume in association with depression (MacQueen & Frodl, 2011; McKinnon, Yucel, Nazarov, & MacQueen, 2009). Reduced hippocampal volume has been observed in healthy adolescents at high familial risk for depression, particularly in those who experienced high levels of adversity in child-hood, and this reduced hippocampal volume partly accounted for the increased vulnerability to depression during longitudinal follow-up (Rao et al., 2010). Although morphological changes in the hippocampus have been associated with depression, not all studies have replicated these findings due to variability in methods and sam-ples (Campbell, Marriott, Nahmias, & MacQueen, 2004; McKinnon et al., 2009).

The amygdala also is involved in the stress response as well as in emotional and mood regu-lation. In a pediatric sample of medication-naïve patients with depression, an increased ratio of the amygdala to hippocampal volume was observed compared to age- and gender-matched controls, but this difference was accounted for by the severity of associated anxiety symptoms (MacMillan et al., 2003). Depressed youth also have been found to have significant reductions of left and right amygdala volumes compared with healthy controls (Rosso et al., 2005), but no sig-nificant correlations were found between amyg-dala volumes and depressive symptom severity, age of onset, or episode duration.

Studies utilizing the diffusion tensor imaging (DTI) technique have detected microstructural white matter abnormalities in depressed adoles-cents (Cullen et al., 2010) and in healthy adoles-cents at high familial risk for depression (Huang, Fan, Williamson, & Rao, 2011), suggesting these alterations might be vulnerability markers for depression (Huang, Gundapuneedi, & Rao, 2012). Alterations in glial cells in these networks have been noted in postmortem studies; glial cells protect neurons through the production of myelin and participate in brain metabolism and communication between neurons (Rajkowska & Miguel-Hidalgo, 2007).

Functional Neuroimaging Studies

Functional MRI (fMRI) studies have implicated impaired corticostriatal and corticolimbic circuits (Cusi, Nazarov, Holshausen, Macqueen, & McKinnon, 2012; Mayberg, 2003; Price & Drevets, 2012). Patients with depression show increased neural activity in response to negative cues and diminished neural activity in response to positive stimuli in emotion-related brain cir-cuits (e.g., amygdala and ventral striatum) (Hasler & Northoff, 2011; Leppanen, 2006). Some abnormalities in processing of emotional information were found to persist after symptom remission and also were observed in healthy indi-viduals at high risk for the development of mood disorders. In pediatric samples, similar deficits in these neural networks have been found, although the direction of change (i.e., increased versus decreased response) has not been consistent across studies (e.g., Forbes et al., 2006, Forbes et al., 2009; Gotlib et al., 2010; Hulvershorn, Cullen, & Anand, 2011; Roberson-Nay et al., 2006; Shad, Bidesi, Chen, Ernst, & Rao, 2011; Weir, Zakama, & Rao, 2012).

Studies using magnetic resonance spectros-copy have reported altered biochemical concen-trations in specific regions of the corticostriatal and corticolimbic networks in depressed adults (Ende, Demirakca, & Tost, 2006; Luykx et al., 2012), and changes in the biochemical concentra-tion in response to treatment (Caverzasi et al., 2012). Research in children is consistent with the adult findings, suggesting some developmental continuity (e.g., Hulvershorn et al., 2011; Kondo et al., 2010; Olvera et al., 2010; Yildiz-Yesiloglu & Ankerst, 2006).

Summary of Neurobiological Research

Pediatric depressive disorders may not necessar-ily result from the same etiological processes as in adults, and specific subtypes with familial loading or depression with a recurrent unipolar course may or may not be associated with neuro-biological changes typically observed in adult unipolar depression (Rao & Chen, 2009). Studies of normal volunteers indicate that neurobiological factors change during the course of development and developmentally influenced neurobiological processes may become disrupted during depressive episodes (Rao, 2011; Weir et al., 2012). Prospective studies of high-risk samples indicate that several neurobiological measures are premorbid and may be vulnerability markers for depression (e.g., Goodyer et al., 2009; Huang et al., 2012; Rao et al., 2009b; Rao, Chen et al., 2010). Experiential factors also may influence neurobiological findings (e.g., Kaufman & Charney, 2001; Rao et al., 2008). Longitudinal studies with large samples are needed to examine genetic, developmental, and sociocultural influences on neurobiological factors associated with the onset and course of depression in children and adolescents.

Many important developmental questions regarding the neurobiology of pediatric depression remain. For instance, how do the maturational changes across development relate to the vulnerability and maintenance of depression? Which neurobiological changes are specific to depression and how do family history, severity, symptom patterns, and comorbidity affect the findings? Are the neurobiological changes preexisting vulnerabilities to or consequence of the illness? Are observed neurobiological changes temporary conditions that resolve without any sequelae, but place individuals on a delayed trajectory toward normal development, or are they a permanent disruption to the normal maturational process affecting neurobiological systems? The effect of disease course on the neurobiological substrate also needs to be studied (Frodl et al., 2008). The utility of these neurobiological markers in the diagnosis and prognosis of the disorder should be established as well as neurobiological changes in response to intervention (Caverzasi et al., 2012; Clarke & Harvey, 2012; Gerber & Peterson, 2008).

Temperament

Temperament is a stable and consistent behavioral, emotional, and/or cognitive style (Rothbart & Bates, 2006; Shiner & Masten, 2012) thought to have a genetic or biological basis (e.g., Gray, 1991). Indeed, temperament may serve as an intermediate endophenotype between biology and behavior. Traits that have been particularly linked with depression are negative and positive emotionality and constraint and attentional control (Compas, Connor-Smith, & Jaser, 2004; Klein, Kotov, & Bufferd, 2011; Tackett, 2006).

Negative emotionality (NE) is characterized by sensitivity to negative stimuli, increased wariness, vigilance, physiological arousal, and emotional distress (e.g., anxiety, fear, sadness, anger). *Positive emotionality* (PE) is characterized by sensitivity to reward cues, approach, energy, involvement, sociability, and adventurousness. NE and PE, respectively, are conceptually related to negative (NA) and positive affectivity (PA; Clark & Watson, 1991), neuroticism and extraversion (Eysenck & Eysenck, 1985), the behavioral inhibition and activation systems (Gray, 1991), and difficult temperament and activity/approach (Thomas & Chess, 1977). Although different terms are used, these constructs share much conceptual and empirical overlap (Klein et al., 2011).

According to the tripartite model (Clark & Watson, 1991), high levels of NA are associated with both depression and anxiety, whereas low levels of PA are uniquely related to depression, particularly anhedonia. Evidence consistent with this model has been found in children (e.g., Lonigan, Phillips, & Hooe, 2003; Phillips, Lonigan, Driscoll, & Hooe, 2002). Low PA is a significant risk factor for depression, and low extraversion and low emotional stability predict internalizing problems in both clinical and nonclinical child samples (van Leeuwen, Mervielde, De Clercq, & De Fruyt, 2007). Offspring of depressed parents have lower PA and higher NA than children of nondepressed parents (Olino, Klein, Dyson, Rose, & Durbin, 2010).

Temperament may be a risk for depression (e.g., Caspi, Moffitt, Newman, & Silva, 1996; Goodwin, Fergusson, & Horwood, 2004; Nigg, 2006). For example, children who were inhibited, socially reticent, and easily upset at age 3 had elevated rates of depressive disorders at age 21 (Caspi et al., 1996). Wetter and Hankin (2009) reported that levels of NE and PE significantly predicted changes in anhedonia 5 months later.

Sex differences also have been found in the relation between temperament and mood disorders. Gjerde (1995) reported that shy and withdrawn behavior in girls and higher levels of under-controlled behaviors in boys at ages 3 and 4 predicted chronic depression in adulthood.

The relation between temperament and depression in children has been found to be moderated by parenting behaviors, such as rejection or inconsistent discipline. For example, the link between fearful temperament and depressive symptoms was stronger for girls whose parents were rejecting, whereas parental warmth buffered the relation of child frustration to internalizing problems (Oldehinkel, Veenstra, Ormel, de Winter, & Verhulst, 2006). In families undergoing divorce, low PE predicted higher levels of depression in children experiencing high levels of parental rejection, and impulsivity and depression were significantly associated in children receiving inconsistent parental discipline (Lengua, Wolchik, Sandler, & West, 2000).

Temperament itself can be a *diathesis* that moderates the effect of other risk factors (e.g., stress; rejection) on depression. Under conditions of stress, negative affect leads to emotional arousal, difficulty modulating emotional reactivity, and a greater use of avoidance (Compas et al., 2004). In girls with more reactive temperaments, peer rejection significantly predicted increases in depressed mood (Brendgen, Wanner, Morin, & Vitaro, 2005). Sugimura and Rudolph (2012) reported that in girls with high but not low NE, peer victimization predicted subsequent depressive symptoms. In contrast, boys with high NE had more depressive symptoms regardless of level of victimization, whereas boys with low NE showed more depression only at high levels of victimization. Thus, temperament (e.g., emotionality) may explain individual variation and sex differences in children's depressive reactions to stressors such as parent rejection or peer victimization.

Temperament also may contribute to the development of the cognitive vulnerability to depression (e.g., Garber, 2007; Hankin & Abramson, 2001). Higher levels of withdrawal at ages 1 and 4 interacted with recent life events to predict more negative cognitions at age 11

(Mezulis, Hyde, & Abramson, 2006). Similarly, low PE in early childhood predicted depressive cognitions in middle childhood (Hayden, Klein, & Durbin, 2005). Thus, temperament may be both a direct vulnerability and a diathesis that interacts with other variables (e.g., stress), to predict depression in youth. The link between various temperaments (e.g., frustration, fear, shyness) and depression has tended to vary by age, sex, and family characteristics (Ormel et al., 2005).

Negative Cognitions

Cognitive-stress models of depression (Abramson, Metalsky, & Alloy, 1989; Beck, 1967) assert that negative beliefs and maladaptive information processing are vulnerabilities (i.e., diatheses) that become active in the context of stress. Beck (1967) suggested that negative cognitive schemas (i.e., beliefs about loss, failure, worthlessness) and dysfunctional attitudes bias interpretations of stress; contribute to negative views of the self, world, and future; and thereby result in depression. Hopelessness theory (Abramson et al., 1989) asserts that maladaptive beliefs interact with stressful events to produce negative inferences about the causes, consequences, and self-implications of the events, which then results in hopelessness and depression. Thus, cognitive models of depression posit that various negative cognitions are diatheses that interact with stress to produce depression. Recently, cognitive models have been expanding to incorporate genes and neurobiological processes as more distal diatheses in the causal chain (e.g., Beck, 2008; Hankin, 2012).

Depressed children and adolescents report more hopelessness, cognitive distortions, cognitive errors, negative views of self and future, negative attributional styles, and biases in attention, memory, and information processing as compared to nondepressed children (Abela & Hankin, 2008; Jacobs, Reinecke, Gollan, & Kane, 2008). Prospective studies have shown that these various cognitive vulnerabilities predict increases in depressive symptoms (e.g., Lewinsohn, Joiner, & Rohde, 2001; Rudolph,

Kurlakowsky, & Conley, 2001) and the onset of diagnosed depressive episodes (Bohon, Stice, Burton, Fudell, & Nolen-Hoeksema, 2008; Carter & Garber, 2011; Hankin, Abramson, Miller, & Haeffel, 2004) under conditions of stress. Reviews of over 30 prospective studies (Abela & Hankin, 2008; Lakdawalla, Hankin, & Mermelstein, 2007) indicate that the cognition by stress interaction is a stronger predictor of depression in adolescents than children. This is consistent with the developmental hypothesis that depressive cognitions do not emerge and consolidate until late childhood/ early adolescence and that the association of the cognitive vulnerability with depression becomes stronger with increasing age (e.g., Abela, 2001; Cole et al., 2008; Weisz, Southam-Gerow, & McCarty, 2001).

The relation of cognitive vulnerability to depression also depends on which cognitions are being studied. Abela (2001) suggested that inferential styles about consequences and the self may develop earlier than causal attributions, which require more abstract, higher order thinking. Abela and colleagues (Abela & Payne, 2003; Abela & Sarin, 2002) proposed the *weakest link hypothesis* that individuals are as vulnerable to depression as their most negative inferential style. Indeed, children's most negative inferential style about causes, consequences, or self has been found to interact with stressful events to predict increases in depressive symptoms (Abela & Payne, 2003; Morris, Ciesla, & Garber, 2008). The weakest link approach explains some of the inconsistent findings on cognitive-stress models of depression in children.

Offspring of depressed parents are at increased risk for depression and also have been found to have significantly lower self-worth, a more negative attributional style, and recall fewer positive and more negative self-descriptive words than children of nondepressed parents (e.g., Garber & Robinson, 1997; Taylor & Ingram, 1999). Following a negative mood induction procedure, never-depressed adolescent daughters of depressed mothers showed a clear information-processing bias (Gotlib, Joormann, Minor, & Cooney, 2006). Thus, children who have not yet experienced depression, but who are at risk, show negative cognitions and processing biases that may serve as vulnerabilities to future depression.

Negative cognitions likely develop through modeling parents' negative beliefs, dysfunctional parent–child relationships, exposure to stressful life events, family adversity, negative feedback from others, and emotional abuse (e.g., Garber & Martin, 2002; Gibb, 2002; Hankin, 2005; Rudolph et al., 2001). Early stress exposure and high levels of negative interpersonal events have been found to predict depressive cognitions in children (Garber & Flynn, 2001; Harkness & Lumley, 2008; Mezulis et al., 2006).

The experience of depression itself also predicts negative cognitions (e.g., McCarty, Vander Stoep, & McCauley, 2007; Pomerantz & Rudolph, 2003). Bidirectional relations between depressive symptoms and perceived competence (Cole, Martin, Peeke, Seroczynski, & Hoffman, 1998; Hoffman, Cole, Martin, Tram, & Serocynski, 2000), negative mood and self-criticism (e.g., Park, Goodyer, & Teasdale, 2005; Rudolph, Hammen, & Burge, 1997), and negative cognitions and depressive symptoms (e.g., Hoffman et al., 2000; Lau & Eley, 2008) have been observed in children and adolescents. Hoffman and colleagues reported that children's underestimation of their competence predicted depressive symptoms over time and prior depression predicted a low evaluation of their competence. In a community sample of 515 children in grades 2 through 9, LaGrange et al. (2011) showed that depressive symptoms predicted negative cognitions but not the reverse. Thus, the association between negative cognitions and depression may be reciprocal and may not be directly causal.

Self-Regulation and Coping

Self-regulation is the way individuals stimulate, modify, or manage their thoughts, affect, and behaviors through biological, cognitive, social, and/or behavioral means (Posner & Rothbart, 2007; Thomson, 1994). *Coping* is a subcategory of self-regulation activated in times of stress (Compas, Connor-Smith, Saltzman, Thomsen, & Wadsworth, 2001; Eisenberg, Spinrad, &

Eggum, 2010). Eisenberg et al. (2010) suggested three coping categories: *emotion regulation* refers to direct attempts to manage affect; *problem-focused coping* involves attempts to regulate the situation; and *behavioral regulation* is the management of behaviors resulting from emotional arousal.

Compas et al. (2001) proposed a broader definition of coping that involves intentional regulation of emotions, cognitions, behaviors, physiology, and the environment. That is, coping is the volitional response to stress, whereas involuntary or automatic reactions reflect individual differences in *temperament*. Compas et al. also distinguished between *engagement coping* (i.e., problem solving, cognitive restructuring, positive reappraisal, distraction) and *disengagement coping* (i.e., avoidance, self-blame, emotional discharge, rumination). Whereas engagement coping is associated with lower internalizing symptoms, disengagement coping is associated with higher symptom levels (Compas et al., 2001). In children ages 9 to 12, active coping predicted fewer depressive symptoms, whereas avoidant coping predicted higher levels of depressive symptoms (Lengua, Sandler, West, Wolchik, & Curran, 1999). Flynn and Rudolph (2007) showed that maladaptive responses to stress (i.e., fewer effortful responses and more involuntary, dysregulated responses) accounted for the association between reduced posterior right hemisphere bias (PRHB) and depressive symptoms in adolescents reporting high levels of stress. Flynn and Rudolph suggested that a reduced PRHB heightens stress reactivity by interfering with effective coping and emotion regulation.

Children with good self-regulation skills are better at delaying maladaptive responses and using active coping strategies in response to stressful situations. Poor self-regulation often involves greater use of automatic and reflexive rather than effortful and reflective cognitive, emotional, and behavioral reactions to the environment, and also may trigger disinhibited cognitions, rumination, negative emotions, and depression (e.g., Carver, Johnson, & Joormann, 2008; Compas et al., 2004; Rothbart & Bates, 2006). In a recent study of self-regulation and social motivation, Rudolph, Troop-Gordon, and Llewellyn (2013) found that poor inhibitory control predicted depressive symptoms in girls with high but not low avoidance motivation. Rudolph and colleagues suggested that the combination of poor self-regulation and high avoidance motivation may contribute to difficulties in shifting attention away from concerns about peer disapproval and toward avoidance, social withdrawal, and depressive symptoms. Thus, the inability to purposefully regulate cognitions, emotions, and behaviors can lead to more maladaptive responses to stress (e.g., rumination, emotional arousal, inaction), which then can contribute to and sustain depressive symptoms (Carver et al., 2008; Compas et al., 2001).

Children at risk for depression show greater difficulty inhibiting negative affect, selectively attend to sad facial expressions, use active distraction less, and are less able to generate positive affect in the face of distraction compared to low-risk youth (e.g., Forbes, Fox, Cohn, Galles, & Kovacs, 2006; Joormann, Talbot, & Gotlib, 2007; Silk, Shaw, Forbes, Lane, & Kovacs, 2006). In a sample of 4- to 7-year-old children, Silk et al. (2006) showed that positive reward anticipation in the context of a negative-emotion-inducing task was associated with lower internalizing problems, and this link was stronger for children of depressed as compared to nondepressed mothers. Thus, in children at risk for depression, positive self-regulatory behavior may protect against the negative effects of stress, whereas self-regulation problems may be a marker of vulnerability.

Stressful Life Events and Trauma

Stress has a prominent role in most theories of depression. Depressive symptoms and disorders in children and adolescents are significantly associated with both major and minor undesirable life events, particularly cumulative or chronic stressors (Grant et al., 2006). Depressed youth experience significantly more negative life events compared to nondepressed children (e.g., Goodyer et al., 2000).

The link between stress and depression emerges even before birth. In animals, both antenatal and prepartum stress impact the developing fetus and later physiological and behavioral outcomes in offspring of stressed animals (e.g., Markham & Koenig, 2011; Schneider, Moore, & Kraemer, 2003). In humans, stress in the fetal environment can affect birth weight and the development of the LHPA axis, both of which may be vulnerabilities for depression (Austin, Leader, & Reilly, 2005; Gale & Martyn, 2004). Stress-induced hormonal changes in mothers (e.g., elevated levels of CRH and cortisol) may lead to increased LHPA fetal activity, difficulty habituating to stimuli, temperamental difficulties, reduced birth weight, and slow growth (Kapoor, Dunn, Kostaki, Andrews, & Matthews, 2006; Weinstock, 2005), resulting in increased sensitivity to stress and greater vulnerability to depression as they mature. Infants exposed to high levels of maternal stress (e.g., maternal depression) show elevated cortisol levels when they encounter maternal stress as preschoolers (Essex, Klein, & Kalin, 2002). Moreover, the relation between a family history of mood disorders and depression in preschoolers was found to be mediated by stress (Luby, Belden, & Spitznagel, 2006).

Childhood-onset depression has been linked with more perinatal insults, parental criminal convictions, parental psychopathology, and peer problems (Jaffee et al., 2002). Stressful events increase from childhood through adolescence (Rudolph & Hammen, 1999), with girls reporting greater increases than boys (Garber, 2007), paralleling increases in rates of depression during adolescence (Hankin et al., 1998). This increasing trajectory of stressful events, particularly interpersonal stressors (Hankin et al., 2007; Shih et al., 2006), predicts growth in depressive symptoms for girls but not for boys (Ge, Lorenz, Conger, Elder, & Simons, 1994). Stress also predicts the onset of clinically significant depressive episodes, controlling for prior symptom levels in children and adolescents (Carter & Garber, 2011; Goodyer et al., 2000).

Although no specific stressful event invariably leads to depression, events occurring during childhood and adolescence such as loss, disappointment, separation, interpersonal conflict, relationship breakups, and rejection (Goodyer et al., 2000; Monroe, Rohde, Seeley, & Lewinsohn, 1999; Rueter, Scaramella, Wallace, & Conger, 1999), as well as parents' marital conflict and divorce, family violence, maltreatment, and economic disadvantage, are particularly likely to predict depression in youth (e.g., Gilman, Kawachi, Fitzmaurice, & Buka, 2003; Hankin, 2005; Uhrlass & Gibb, 2007). Physical and sexual abuse are among the most damaging stressors linked with the onset and recurrence of depression (Harkness & Lumley, 2008). The relation between depression and maltreatment is particularly strong in the presence of high familial loading of depression and polymorphisms in SLCGA4 and BNDF genes (Caspi et al., 2003; Kaufman et al., 2004, Kaufman et al., 2006). Moreover, experience of such early adversity may make children more vulnerable or sensitized to depression when exposed to new stressors later in development (Hammen, Henry, & Daley, 2000; Harkness, Bruce, & Lumley, 2006), although this may vary by age and sex (Rudolph & Flynn, 2007).

Social support also may affect the relation between stress and depression. For example, among children with low as compared to high social support, the interaction between genes and childhood maltreatment significantly predicted higher levels of depressive symptoms (Kaufman et al., 2004; Kaufman et al., 2006). Among youth living in highly disordered neighborhoods (i.e., exposure to gangs, harassment, drug dealing), supportive parenting (i.e., use of inductive reasoning) served as a buffer against depressive symptoms (Natsuaki et al., 2007).

The relation between stress and depression likely is bidirectional. In the stress exposure model, stress precedes the onset of depression (Brown, 1993), whereas the stress generation model asserts that depressed individuals' own behaviors create many of the stressors they encounter, which then further exacerbates their depressive symptoms (Hammen, 1991, 2006). Depressed youth (Hankin et al., 2007; Rudolph et al., 2000; Shih et al., 2006) as well as those with maladaptive interpersonal problem-solving styles (Davila, Hammen, Burge, Paley, & Daley, 1995) tend to generate more stress. Several studies (Carter, Garber, Ciesla, & Cole, 2006; Cole, Nolen-Hoeksema, Girgus, & Paul, 2006; Gibb & Alloy, 2006) have found a reciprocal relation between stress and depression, thus highlighting the "vicious cycle" between them.

Interpersonal Relationships

Interpersonal perspectives on depression emphasize the transactions between individuals and their social environment (Hammen, 2006; Joiner & Coyne, 1999). The social context can be both a source of support and a source of stress. Depressed individuals are often the recipient as well as the elicitor of interpersonal difficulties. Depression in children and adolescents is associated with considerable family adversity, peer problems, victimization, and interpersonal rejection (Nolan, Flynn, & Garber, 2003; Rudolph, Flynn, & Abaied, 2008). At the same time, depressed youth may have distorted perceptions of their social world, engage in behaviors that elicit negative responses and conflict with others, and generate additional stressors in their relationships (e.g., Hankin et al., 2007; Rudolph et al., 2008).

Family

Attachment theory (Bowlby, 1980) asserts that children with consistently accessible and supportive caregivers develop cognitive representations, or *working models*, of the self and others as positive and trustworthy. Conversely, children with unresponsive or inconsistent caregivers tend to have insecure attachments and working models of self-criticism, abandonment, and dependency. Insecure attachments increase children's vulnerability to depression when exposed to new interpersonal strains (Brumariu & Kerns, 2010). Securely attached toddlers tend to be more cooperative, persistent, enthusiastic, and higher functioning and show lower levels of depressive symptoms when exposed to stress (Abela et al., 2005; Matas, Arend, & Sroufe, 1978). Insecurely attached children have deficits in social-behavioral and emotion regulation that

can increase their vulnerability to depression (Rudolph et al., 2008).

Maladaptive parenting also is associated with depression. Currently depressed children describe their parents as controlling, rejecting, and unavailable (e.g., Stein et al., 2000). Ratings of parents' psychologically controlling behaviors predict children's depressive symptoms over and above prior depression levels (Barber & Xia, 2013). Hostile child-rearing attitudes predict increases in children's depression (Katainen, Raikkonen, Keskivaara, & Keltikangas-Jarvinen, 1999), whereas positive parent–child relationships (e.g., clear and consistent expectations, good communication, parent supervision, and shared positive activities) are linked with less depression in children (e.g., Borowsky, Ireland, & Resnick, 2001; Resnick et al., 1997).

Observational studies indicate that low warmth, high hostility, harsh discipline, and family conflict predict internalizing symptoms in youth (e.g., Ge, Best, Conger, & Simons, 1996; Sheeber, Hops, Alpert, Davis, & Andrews, 1997), and escalating parent–child conflict predicts increases in adolescents' internalizing symptoms (Rueter et al., 1999). Mothers of depressed children also are less rewarding and more dominant and controlling than mothers of nondepressed children (e.g., Sheeber, Hops, & Davis, 2001). Levels of maternal criticism of children are higher in mothers of depressed children compared to mothers of children with ADHD or healthy controls (Asarnow, Tompson, Woo, & Cantwell, 2001). Thus, convergence across children's, parents', and observers' ratings indicates that depression in children and adolescents is characterized by considerable family dysfunction (Park, Garber, Ciesla, & Ellis, 2008).

Parental depression also is characterized by dysfunctional parenting (e.g., Garber, 2005; Lovejoy, Graczyk, O'Hare, & Neuman, 2000). Such difficulties likely are one important and possibly malleable mechanism of the intergenerational transmission of depression (Goodman, 2007). Hammen and colleagues (Hammen & Brennan, 2001; Hammen, Shih, & Brennan, 2004) showed that depressed mothers had high levels of interpersonal stress that contributed to poor parenting as well as interpersonal deficits, stress, and depression in their children. Bifulco et al. (2002) reported that the relation between maternal and child depression was mediated by child-reported neglect and abuse (see also Hammen et al., 2004; Leinonen, Solantaus, & Punamaki, 2003). Other studies (Jones, Forehand, & Neary, 2001; Kim, Capaldi, & Stoolmiller, 2003), however, have not found that parenting attitudes or behaviors significantly explain the relation between parent and child depression.

One possible mediator of the relation between dysfunctional parenting and offspring depression is children's negative cognitions (Abela, Skitch, Adams, & Hankin, 2006; Garber, Robinson, & Valentiner, 1997; Gibb et al., 2001). For example, negative cognitive style partially mediated the relation between parent abuse and neglect and subsequent depressive symptoms (McGinn, Cukor, & Sanderson, 2005), and between emotional maltreatment in childhood and depressive episodes during young adulthood (Gibb et al., 2001).

Peers

Depressed children and adolescents have both real and perceived peer problems. Depressed youth have actual social skills deficits, poorer quality friendships, and higher teacher-rated peer rejection (e.g., Prinstein, Borelli, Cheah, Simon, & Aikins, 2005; Rudolph et al., 2008; Rudolph & Clark, 2001), and they view themselves to be less socially competent and less accepted, and to have lower quality friendships than their nondepressed peers (Brendgen, Vitaro, Turgeon, & Poulin, 2002; Rudolph et al., 1997). Interestingly, *perceived* rejection, even more than actual peer rejection, predicts increases in depressive symptoms in some children (e.g., Kistner, Balthazor, Risi, & Burton, 1999). Regardless of how much a child is actually liked by peers, those with high levels of rejection sensitivity (Rizzo, Daley, & Gunderson, 2006; Sandstrom, Cillessen, & Eisenhower, 2003) or social-evaluative concerns (Rudolph & Conley, 2005) are especially prone to experiencing depression. Perceiving rejection from others may lead to withdrawal from or hostility toward others, which then may elicit

actual negative reactions from peers, thereby reinforcing the depressed child's negative perceptions. Thus, a self-perpetuating and transactional cycle of cognitive distortions, negative social interactions, peer rejection, and depression may develop (e.g., Rudolph, 2009).

Longitudinal studies have found that persistent interpersonal difficulties such as excessive reassurance seeking (Prinstein et al., 2005), negative feedback seeking (Borelli & Prinstein, 2006), interpersonal rejection (Nolan et al., 2003), and romantic conflicts and breakups (Hankin et al., 2007; Monroe et al., 1999) significantly predict increases in depressive symptoms. Moreover, social-behavioral deficits were found to interact with some of these relationship disturbances to predict depression in youth (Gazelle & Rudolph, 2004; Rizzo et al., 2006). Additionally, low sociometric status and observer ratings of social disengagement in first grade were associated with increases in depressive symptoms in grades 3 and 4 (Schrepferman, Eby, Snyder, & Stropes, 2006).

Interestingly, both bullies and the bullied have high rates of depression (Ivarsson, Broberg, Arvidsson, & Gillberg, 2005; Kaltiala-Heino, Rimpela, Rantanen, & Rimpela, 2000). Children who were friends with highly aggressive peers had high levels of depressive symptoms across two years, controlling for initial depression levels (Mrug, Hoza, & Bukowski, 2004). Spending time with delinquent peers predicted high levels of self-reported depressive symptoms assessed monthly (Connell & Dishion, 2006). Depressed children might select delinquent peers as a way to "fit in" and obtain a sense of belonging not provided by their broader social networks. Deviant peers, however, typically do not give much positive feedback, which then may further exacerbate the youth's depression (Brendgen, Vitaro, & Bukowski, 2000).

Conclusions and Future Directions

Various vulnerability factors have been associated with depression in children and adolescents. Simply examining the independent contribution of these individual risk factors, however, is not sufficient for fully understanding the processes that account for the onset, maintenance, recurrence, and offset of depressive disorders throughout development. Rather, we need multivariate models that explain how the various within-individual, biological, and psychological vulnerabilities synergistically combine with external contextual factors to produce depression across time.

Several integrated models of depression have been formulated that include additive and interactive effects of multiple risk factors (e.g., Beck, 2008; Kendler, Gardner, & Prescott, 2002). The classic paper by Akiskal and McKinney (1975) asserted that most distal causal processes (e.g., stress, low rates of positive reinforcement) go through a common final neuroanatomical pathway to depression. Diathesis-stress models highlight that within-person characteristics, such as genetic or cognitive vulnerability, interact with environmental stressors to produce depression (Abramson et al., 1989; Beck, 2008; Caspi et al., 2003; Kendler et al., 1995; Monroe & Simons, 1991). Interpersonal approaches (e.g., Hammen, 2006; Rudolph et al., 2008) suggest that cognitions about important social relationships may be a risk for depression when stressful interpersonal events occur. Negative cognitive schemas about the self and others may be the result of earlier insecure attachment and interpersonal difficulties. In contrast, Ingram, Miranda and Segal (1998) posited that cognitive processes are the common final pathway through which all social and nonsocial information is processed and linked to depression.

A broad, reciprocal, and dynamic model that describes the transactional relations among biological, psychological, social, and contextual risk processes underlying depression is required to capture the complexity of the disorder. The combination of individual vulnerabilities and contextual factors directly, indirectly (i.e., mediation), and interactively (i.e., moderation) produces depression. Some diatheses are more distal and relatively stable (e.g., temperament), whereas others are potentially malleable (e.g., parenting, coping) and may influence how individuals respond to specific proximal stressors (Compas

et al., 2009). According to this perspective, children who are born with certain biological propensities, such as stress reactivity, an overactive amygdala, or an irritable temperament, will be more vulnerable to the effects of negative life events and less able to effectively self-regulate in the face of stress.

Children learn, in part through interactions with others, about their own ability to cope with stressors and whether others can be counted on for support. Children also learn through social encounters whether they are worthy of others' love and care. Exposure to stressful life events can activate negative affective structures that connect with developing schemas about the self and others (Ingram et al., 1998). A cycle begins in which children develop some symptoms of depression (e.g., irritability, low self-esteem, anhedonia), which then may generate further stressors, such as interpersonal rejection and academic failure. Experience with chronic or severe stressors can produce neurobiological changes (e.g., in the HPA system), which then further maintains or exacerbates the depressive symptoms. Thus, in this *mediated moderation model*, individual diatheses modify the relation between stress and depression and contribute to how the child responds to adverse events. Such responses to stress mediate the effect of individual diatheses on subsequent depression. Individuals with certain biological and/or psychological vulnerabilities who encounter stressful events and respond ineffectively (e.g., involuntary disengagement), so that the stressor is not adequately managed, then likely will develop depression. These escalating stressful circumstances can alter their biochemistry, self-schema, and information processing and lead to further maladaptive behaviors, thereby generating more negative events, particularly within the social domain (Coyne, 1976; Hammen, 2002), and so the cycle continues. This *scarring* (Lewinsohn, Allen, Seeley, & Gotlib, 1999) or *kindling* (Post, 1992) results in dynamic changes in these biopsychosocial systems over time.

The precise genes and neural pathways that produce the endophenotypes (e.g., temperament, negative cognitions) that then interact with specific contextual factors (e.g., exposure to in utero and early, severe, and/or chronic stress) to elicit symptoms of depression remain to be discovered. Future research needs to identify specific genetic risk markers, elucidate the pathophysiology from the genetic polymorphisms to neuroendocrine and neurochemical dysregulation, describe how these biological processes affect persons' appraisals and behaviors in response to environmental events, and determine how the combination of these factors results in the specific symptoms of depression. Are all of these risk factors part of a single causal model, or do different combinations of these mechanisms produce subtypes or explain different manifestations of depression across development?

Theories of depression need to account for differences in the phenomenology of depression in children, adolescents, and adults and increases in the rates of depression from childhood to adolescence, particularly in girls. Are the processes that underlie childhood-onset depression different from those that explain the first onset of depression during adolescence or adulthood? Are causal mechanisms different for first versus recurrent episodes of depression? What accounts for the recurrences of depression across the life span? When and how do depressive vulnerabilities develop, unfold, and change over time? What aspects of growth (e.g., age, pubertal status, cognitive, social, or emotional level) are most related to observed developmental differences in prevalence, phenomenology, and etiology? Finally, are the various risks for depression permanent characteristics of individuals, and through what mechanisms are they turned on and off? What biological and psychosocial processes set off latent vulnerabilities, and, conversely, how does spontaneous remission of depression occur? Do vulnerable individuals no longer have the risk factor(s) or do they develop new skills to compensate for them? If so, can we learn from these naturalistic processes to develop more effective interventions?

Acknowledgements This work was supported, in part, by grants to Judy Garber from the National Institute of Mental Health R01MH64735, and RC1MH088329 and by the Vanderbilt CTSA grant UL1RR024975-01 from NCRR/NIH, and to Uma Rao from the National Institutes of Health (RO1 MH068391, G12 RR003032, UL1 RR024975/ TR000445 and U54 RR026140/ MD007593), and by the Endowed Chair in Brain and Behavior Research at Meharry Medical College.

References

Abela, J. R. Z. (2001). The hopelessness theory of depression: A test of the diathesis-stress and causal mediation components in third and seventh grade children. *Journal of Abnormal Child Psychology, 29*, 241–254.

Abela, J. R. Z., & Hankin, B. L. (2008). Cognitive vulnerability to depression in children and adolescents: A developmental perspective. In J. R. Z. Abela & B. L. Hankin (Eds.), *Handbook of depression in children and adolescents* (pp. 35–78). New York: Guilford.

Abela, J. R. Z., Hankin, B. L., Haigh, E. A. P., Adams, P., Vinokuroff, T., & Trayhern, L. (2005). Interpersonal vulnerability to depression in high-risk children: The role of insecure attachment and reassurance seeking. *Journal of Clinical Child and Adolescent Psychology, 34*, 182–192.

Abela, J. R. Z., & Payne, A. V. L. (2003). A test of the integration of the hopelessness and self-esteem theories of depression in school children. *Cognitive Therapy and Research, 27*, 519–535.

Abela, J. R. Z., & Sarin, S. (2002). Cognitive vulnerability to hopelessness depression: A chain is only as strong as its weakest link. *Cognitive Therapy and Research, 26*, 811–829.

Abela, J. R. Z., Skitch, S. A., Adams, P., & Hankin, B. L. (2006). The timing of parent and child depression: A hopelessness theory perspective. *Journal of Clinical Child and Adolescent Psychology, 35*, 253–263.

Abramson, L. Y., Metalsky, G. I., & Alloy, L. B. (1989). Hopelessness depression: A theory-based subtype of depression. *Psychological Review, 96*, 358–372.

Adrien, J. (2002). Neurobiological bases for the relation between sleep and depression. *Sleep Medicine Reviews, 6*(5), 341–351.

Akiskal, H. S., & McKinney, W. T. (1975). Overview of recent research in depression: Integration of ten conceptual models into a comprehensive clinical framework. *Archives of General Psychiatry, 32*, 285–305.

American Psychiatric Association. (2000). *Diagnostic and statistical manual of mental disorders: DSM-IV-TR*. Washington, DC: American Psychiatric Association.

American Psychiatric Association. (2013). *Diagnostic and statistical manual of mental disorders* (5th ed.). Washington, DC: Author.

Angold, A., Costello, E. J., & Erkanli, A. (1999a). Comorbidity. *Journal of Child Psychology and Psychiatry, and Allied Disciplines, 40*, 57–87.

Angold, A., Costello, E. J., Erkanli, A., & Worthman, C. M. (1999b). Pubertal changes in hormone levels and depression in girls. *Psychological Medicine, 29*, 1043–1053.

Angold, A., Costello, E. J., & Worthman, C. M. (1998). Puberty and depression: The roles of age, pubertal status, and pubertal timing. *Psychological Medicine, 28*, 51–61.

Angold, A., Erkanli, A., Silberg, J., Eaves, L., & Costello, E. J. (2002). Depression scale scores in 8–17-year-olds: Effects of age and gender. *Journal of Child Psychology and Psychiatry, 43*, 1052–1063.

Angold, A., & Rutter, M. (1992). Effects of age and pubertal status on depression in a large clinical sample. *Development and Psychopathology, 4*, 5–28.

Armitage, R., Emslie, G. J., Hoffmann, R. F., Weinberg, W. A., Kowatch, R. A., Rintelmann, J., et al. (2000). Ultradian rhythms and temporal coherence in sleep EEG in depressed children and adolescents. *Biological Psychiatry, 47*(4), 338–350.

Armitage, R., Hoffmann, R., Emslie, G., Rintelmann, J., & Robert, J. (2006). Sleep microarchitecture in childhood and adolescent depression: Temporal coherence. *Clinical EEG and Neuroscience, 37*(1), 1–9.

Armitage, R., Hoffmann, R. F., Emslie, G. J., Weinberg, W. A., Mayes, T. L., & Rush, A. J. (2002). Sleep microarchitecture as a predictor of recurrence in children and adolescents with depression. *International Journal of Neuropsychopharmacology, 5*(3), 217–228.

Asarnow, J. R., Tompson, M., Woo, S., & Cantwell, D. P. (2001). Is expressed emotion a specific risk factor for depression or a nonspecific correlate of psychopathology? *Journal of Abnormal Child Psychology, 29*(6), 573–583.

Austin, M. P., Leader, L. R., & Reilly, N. (2005). Prenatal stress, the hypothalamic-pituitary-adrenal axis, and fetal and infant neurobehaviour. *Early Human Development, 81*, 917–926.

Avenevoli, S., & Steinberg, L. (2001). The continuity of depression across the adolescent transition. *Advances in Child Development and Behavior, 28*, 139–173.

Bagot, R. C., & Meaney, M. J. (2010). Epigenetics and the biological basis of gene x environment interactions. *Journal of the American Academy of Child and Adolescent Psychiatry, 49*(8), 752–771.

Barber, B. K., & Xia, M. (2013). The centrality of control to parenting and its effects. In A. S. Morris, R. E. Larzelere, & A. W. Harrist (Eds.), *New directions for authoritative parenting* (pp. 61–87). Washington, DC: American Psychological Association.

Bartels, M., van den Oord, E. J., Hudziak, J. J., Rietveld, M. J., van Beijsterveldt, C. E., & Boomsma, D. I. (2004). Genetic and environmental mechanisms underlying stability and change in problem behaviors at ages 3, 7, 10, and 12. *Developmental Psychology, 40*(5), 852–867.

Beck, A. T. (1967). *Depression: Clinical, experiential, and theoretical aspects.* New York: Harper & Row.

Beck, A. (2008). The evolution of the cognitive model of depression and its neurobiological correlates. *American Journal of Psychiatry, 165*(8), 969–977.

Bifulco, A. T., Moran, P. M., Ball, C., Jacobs, C., Baines, R., Bunn, A., et al. (2002). Child adversity, parental vulnerability and disorder: Examination of intergenerational transmission of risk. *Journal of Child Psychology and Psychiatry, and Allied Disciplines, 43*, 1075–1086.

Birmaher, B., Ryan, N. D., Williamson, D. E., Brent, D. A., Kaufman, J., & Nelson, B. (1996). Childhood and adolescent depression: A review of the past ten years. Part I. *Journal of the American Academy of Child and Adolescent Psychiatry, 35*, 1427–1439.

Birmaher, B., Williamson, D. E., Dahl, R. E., Axelson, D. A., Kaufman, J., Dorn, L., et al. (2004). Clinical presentation and course of depression in youth: Does onset in childhood differ from onset in adolescence? *Journal of the American Academy of Child and Adolescent Psychiatry, 43*, 63–70.

Bohon, C., Stice, E., Burton, E., Fudell, M., & Nolen-Hoeksema, S. (2008). A prospective test of cognitive vulnerability models of depression with adolescent girls. *Behavior Therapy, 39*(1), 79–90.

Boomsma, D. I., van Beijsterveldt, C. E., & Hudziak, J. J. (2005). Genetic and environmental influences on Anxious/Depression during childhood: A study from the Netherlands Twin Register. *Genes, Brain, and Behavior, 4*(8), 466–481.

Borelli, J. L., & Prinstein, M. J. (2006). Reciprocal, longitudinal associations between adolescents' negative feedback-seeking, depressive symptoms, and friendship perceptions. *Journal of Abnormal Child Psychology, 34*, 159–169.

Borowsky, I. W., Ireland, M., & Resnick, M. D. (2001). Adolescent suicide attempts: Risks and protectors. *Pediatrics, 107*, 485–493.

Botteron, K. N., Raichle, M. E., Drevets, W. C., Heath, A. C., & Todd, R. D. (2002). Volumetric reduction in left subgenual prefrontal cortex in early onset depression. *Biological Psychiatry, 51*(4), 342–344.

Bowlby, J. (1980). *Attachment and loss: Vol 3. Loss, sadness, and depression.* New York: Basic Books.

Brendgen, M., Vitaro, F., & Bukowski, W. (2000). Deviant friends and early adolescents' emotional and behavioral adjustment. *Journal of Research on Adolescence, 10*, 173–189.

Brendgen, M., Vitaro, F., Turgeon, L., & Poulin, F. (2002). Assessing aggressive and depressed children's social relations with classmates and friends: A matter of perspective. *Journal of Abnormal Child Psychology, 30*, 609–624.

Brendgen, M., Wanner, B., Morin, A. J. S., & Vitaro, F. (2005). Relations with parents and with peers, temperament, and trajectories of depressed mood during early adolescence. *Journal of Abnormal Child Psychology, 33*, 579–594.

Brown, G. W. (1993). Life events and affective disorder: Replications and limitations. *Psychosomatic Medicine, 55*, 248–259.

Brumariu, L. E., & Kerns, K. A. (2010). Parent–child attachment and internalizing symptoms in childhood and adolescence: A review of empirical findings and future directions. *Development and Psychopathology, 22*(1), 177–203.

Bufferd, S. J., Dougherty, L. R., Carlson, G. A., & Klein, D. N. (2011). Parent-reported DSM-IV disorders in a community sample of preschoolers. *Comprehensive Psychiatry, 52*, 359–369.

Busby, K. A., Mercier, L., & Pivik, R. T. (1994). Ontogenetic variations in auditory arousal threshold during sleep. *Psychophysiology, 31*(2), 182–188.

Campbell, S., & Macqueen, G. (2004). The role of the hippocampus in the pathophysiology of major depression. *Journal of Psychiatry and Neuroscience, 29*(6), 417–426.

Campbell, S., Marriott, M., Nahmias, C., & MacQueen, G. M. (2004). Lower hippocampal volume in patients suffering from depression: A meta-analysis. *American Journal of Psychiatry, 161*(4), 598–607.

Canino, G., Shrout, P. E., Rubio-Stipec, M., Bird, H. R., Bravo, M., & Martinez-Taboas, A. (2004). DSM-IV rates of child and adolescent disorders in Puerto Rico: Prevalence, correlates, service use, and the effects of impairment. *Archives of General Psychiatry, 61*, 85–93.

Carskadon, M. A., Orav, E. J., & Dement, W. C. (1983). Evolution of sleep and daytime sleepiness in adolescents. In C. G. Lugaresi (Ed.), *Sleep/wake disorders: Natural history, epidemiology, and long-term evolution* (pp. 201–216). New York: Raven.

Carter, J., & Garber, J. (2011). Predictors of the first onset of a major depressive episode and changes in depressive symptoms across adolescence: Stress and negative cognitions. *Journal of Abnormal Psychology, 120*, 779–796.

Carter, J. S., Garber, J., Ciesla, J. A., & Cole, D. A. (2006). Modeling relations between hassles and internalizing and externalizing symptoms in adolescents: A four-year prospective study. *Journal of Abnormal Psychology, 115*, 428–442.

Carver, C. S., Johnson, S. L., & Joormann, J. (2008). Serotonergic function, two-mode models of self-regulation, and vulnerability to depression: What depression has in common with impulsive aggression. *Psychological Bulletin, 134*, 912–943.

Caspi, A., Moffitt, T. E., Newman, D. L., & Silva, P. A. (1996). Behavioral observations at age 3 years predict adult psychiatric disorders: Longitudinal evidence from a birth cohort. *Archives of General Psychiatry, 53*, 1033–1039.

Caspi, A., Sugden, K., Moffitt, T. E., Taylor, A., Craig, I. W., Harrington, H., et al. (2003). Influence of life stress on depression: Moderation by a polymorphism in the 5-HTT gene. *Science, 301*(5631), 386–389.

Caverzasi, E., Pichiecchio, A., Poloni, G. U., Calligaro, A., Pasin, M., Palesi, F., et al. (2012). Magnetic resonance spectroscopy in the evaluation of treatment efficacy in unipolar major depressive disorder: A review of the literature. *Functional Neurology, 27*(1), 13–22.

Chen, M. C., Joormann, J., Hallmayer, J., & Gotlib, I. H. (2009). Serotonin transporter polymorphism predicts waking cortisol in young girls. *Psychoneuroendocrinology, 34*(5), 681–686.

Cicchetti, D., & Dawson, G. (2002). Multiple levels of analysis. *Development and Psychopathology, 14*, 581–611.

Cicchetti, D., & Schneider-Rosen, K. (Eds.). (1984). *Childhood depression. New directions in child development* (pp. 5–27). San Francisco: Jossey-Bass.

Cicchetti, D., & Toth, S. L. (1998). The development of depression in children and adolescents. *American Psychologist, 53*, 221–241.

Clark, L. A., & Watson, D. (1991). Tripartite model of anxiety and depression: Psychometric evidence and taxonomic implications. *Journal of Abnormal Psychology, 100*, 316–336.

Clarke, G., & Harvey, A. G. (2012). The complex role of sleep in adolescent depression. *Child and Adolescent Psychiatric Clinics of North America, 21*(2), 385–400.

Cole, D. A., Ciesla, J., Dallaire, D. H., Jacquez, F. M., Pineda, A., LaGrange, B., et al. (2008). Emergence of attributional style and its relation to depressive symptoms. *Journal of Abnormal Psychology, 117*, 16–31.

Cole, D. A., Martin, J. M., Peeke, L. G., Seroczynski, A. D., & Hoffman, K. (1998). Are cognitive errors of underestimation predictive or reflective of depressive symptoms in children?: A longitudinal study. *Journal of Abnormal Psychology, 107*, 481–496.

Cole, D. A., Martin, J. M., Powers, B., & Truglio, R. (1996). Modeling causal relations between academic and social competence and depression: A multi-trait-multimethod longitudinal study of children. *Journal of Abnormal Psychology, 105*, 258–270.

Cole, D. A., Nolen-Hoeksema, S., Girgus, J., & Paul, G. (2006). Stress exposure and stress generation in child and adolescent depression: A latent trait-state-error approach to longitudinal analyses. *Journal of Abnormal Psychology, 115*, 40–51.

Cole, D. A., Truglio, R., & Peeke, L. (1997). Relation between symptoms of anxiety and depression in children: A multitrait-multimethod-multigroup assessment. *Journal of Consulting and Clinical Psychology, 65*, 110–119.

Compas, B. E., Connor-Smith, J., & Jaser, S. S. (2004). Temperament, stress reactivity, and coping: Implications for depression in childhood and adolescence. *Journal of Clinical Child and Adolescent Psychology, 33*, 21–31.

Compas, B. E., Connor-Smith, J. K., Saltzman, H., Thomsen, A. H., & Wadsworth, M. E. (2001). Coping with stress during childhood and adolescence: Problems, progress, and potential in theory and research. *Psychological Bulletin, 127*, 87–127.

Compas, B. E., Forehand, R., Keller, G., Champion, J., Rakow, A., & Cole, D. A. (2009). Randomized controlled trial of a family cognitive-behavioral preventive intervention for children of depressed parents. *Journal of Consulting and Clinical Psychology, 77*(6), 1007–1020.

Conley, C., & Rudolph, K. (2009). The emerging sex difference in adolescent depression: Interacting contributions of puberty and peer stress. *Development and Psychopathology, 21*(2), 593–620.

Connell, A. M., & Dishion, T. J. (2006). The contribution of peers to monthly variation in adolescent depressed mood: A short-term longitudinal study with time-varying predictors. *Development and Psychopathology, 18*, 139–154.

Conway, C. C., Hammen, C., Brennan, P. A., Lind, P. A., & Najman, J. M. (2010). Interaction of chronic stress with serotonin transporter and catechol-O-methyltransferase polymorphisms in predicting youth depression. *Depression and Anxiety, 27*(8), 737–745.

Copeland, W. E., Shanahan, L., Costello, J., & Angold, A. (2009). Child and adolescent psychiatric disorders as predictors of young adult disorders. *Archives of General Psychiatry, 66*, 764–772.

Copeland, W., Shanahan, L., Miller, S., Costello, E. J., Angold, A., & Maughan, B. (2010). Outcomes of early pubertal timing in young women: A prospective population-based study. *American Journal of Psychiatry, 167*, 1218–1225.

Coplan, J. D., Wolk, S. I., Goetz, R. R., Ryan, N. D., Dahl, R. E., Mann, J. J., et al. (2000). Nocturnal growth hormone secretion studies in adolescents with or without major depression re-examined: Integration of adult clinical follow-up data. *Biological Psychiatry, 47*(7), 594–604.

Costello, E. J., Angold, A., Burns, B. J., Stangl, D. K., Tweed, D. L., Erkanli, A., et al. (1996). The Great Smoky Mountains study of youth: Goals, design, methods, and prevalence of DSM-III-R disorders. *Archives of General Psychiatry, 53*, 1129–1136.

Costello, E. J., Foley, D. L., & Angold, A. (2006). 10-year research update review: The epidemiology of child and adolescent psychiatric disorders: II. Developmental epidemiology. *Journal of the American Academy of Child and Adolescent Psychiatry, 45*, 8–25.

Costello, E. J., Mustillo, S., Erkanli, A., Keeler, G., & Angold, A. (2003). Prevalence and development of psychiatric disorders in childhood and adolescence. *Archives of General Psychiatry, 60*, 837–844.

Coyne, J. C. (1976). Toward an interactional description of depression. *Psychiatry, 39*, 28–40.

Cullen, K. R., Klimes-Dougan, B., Muetzel, R., Mueller, B. A., Camchong, J., Houri, A., et al. (2010). Altered white matter microstructure in adolescents with major depression: A preliminary study. *Journal of the American Academy Child and Adolescent Psychiatry, 49*(2), 173–183 e171.

Cusi, A. M., Nazarov, A., Holshausen, K., Macqueen, G. M., & McKinnon, M. C. (2012). Systematic review of the neural basis of social cognition in patients with mood disorders. *Journal of Psychiatry and Neuroscience, 37*(3), 154–169.

Cyranowski, J. M., Frank, E., Young, E., & Shear, M. K. (2000). Adolescent onset of the gender difference in lifetime rates of major depression. *Archives of General Psychiatry, 57*, 21–27.

Dahl, R. E., Puig-Antich, J., Ryan, N. D., Nelson, B., Dachille, S., Cunningham, S. L., et al. (1990). EEG sleep in adolescents with major depression: The role of suicidality and inpatient status. *Journal of Affective Disorders, 19*(1), 63–75.

Davidson, R. J., Pizzagalli, D., Nitschke, J. B., & Putnam, K. (2002). Depression: Perspectives from affective neuroscience. *Annual Review of Psychology, 53*, 545–574.

Davila, J., Hammen, C., Burge, D., Paley, B., & Daley, S. E. (1995). Poor interpersonal problem solving as a mechanism of stress generation in depression among adolescent women. *Journal of Abnormal Psychology, 104*, 592–600.

Dawson, G., Klinger, L. G., Panagiotides, H., Hill, D., & Spieker, S. (1992). Frontal lobe activity and affective behavior of infants of mothers with depressive symptoms. *Child Development, 63*(3), 725–737.

Dinan, T. G. (1998). Psychoneuroendocrinology of depression. Growth hormone. *Psychiatric Clinics of North America, 21*(2), 325–339.

Dunn, V., & Goodyer, I. M. (2006). Longitudinal investigation into childhood- and adolescence-onset depression: Psychiatric outcome in early adulthood. *British Journal of Psychiatry, 188*, 216–222.

Eaves, L. J., Silberg, J. L., Meyer, J. M., Maes, H. H., Simonoff, E., Pickles, A., et al. (1997). Genetics and developmental psychopathology: 2. The main effects of genes and environment on behavioral problems in the Virginia Twin Study of Adolescent Behavioral Development. *Journal of Child Psychology and Psychiatry, 38*(8), 965–980.

Egger, H. L., & Angold, A. (2006). Common emotional and behavioral disorders in preschool children: Presentation, nosology, and epidemiology. *Journal of Child Psychology and Psychiatry, and Allied Disciplines, 47*, 313–337.

Eisenberg, N., Spinrad, T. L., & Eggum, N. D. (2010). Emotion-related self-regulation and its relation to children's maladjustment. *Annual Review of Clinical Psychology, 6*, 495–525.

Eley, T. C., & Stevenson, J. (1999). Exploring the covariation between anxiety and depression symptoms: A genetic analysis of the effects of age and sex. *Journal of Child Psychology and Psychiatry, 40*(8), 1273–1282.

Else-Quest, N., Hyed, J., Goldsmith, H., & van Hulle, C. (2006). Gender differences in temperament: A meta-analysis. *Psychological Bulletin, 132*, 33–72.

Emslie, G. J., Armitage, R., Weinberg, W. A., Rush, A. J., Mayes, T. L., & Hoffmann, R. F. (2001). Sleep polysomnography as a predictor of recurrence in children and adolescents with major depressive disorder. *The International Journal of Neuropsychopharmacology, 4*(2), 159–168.

Emslie, G. J., Rush, A. J., Weinberg, W. A., Kowatch, R. A., Hughes, C. W., Carnody, T., et al. (1997). A double-blind, randomized, placebo-controlled trial of Fluoxetine in children and adolescents with depression. *Archives of General Psychiatry, 54*, 1031–1037.

Ende, G., Demirakca, T., & Tost, H. (2006). The biochemistry of dysfunctional emotions: Proton MR spectroscopic findings in major depressive disorder. *Progress in Brain Research, 156*, 481–501.

Essex, M. J., Klein, M. H., & Kalin, N. H. (2002). Maternal stress beginning in infancy may sensitize children to later stress exposure: Effects on cortisol and behavior. *Biological Psychiatry, 52*, 776–784.

Eysenck, H. J., & Eysenck, M. W. (1985). *Personality and individual differences: A natural science approach.* New York: Plenum.

Ezpeleta, L., Domenech, J. M., & Angold, A. (2006). A comparison of pure and comorbid CD/ODD and depression. *Journal of Child Psychology and Psychiatry, 47,* 704–712.

Fergusson, D. M., Horwood, L. J., Miller, A. L., & Kennedy, M. A. (2011). Life stress, 5-HTTLPR and mental disorder: Findings from a 30-year longitudinal study. *British Journal of Psychiatry, 198*(2), 129–135.

Fergusson, D. M., & Woodward, L. J. (2002). Mental health, educational, and social role outcomes of adolescents with depression. *Archives of General Psychiatry, 59,* 225–331.

Fleming, J., Offord, D., & Boyle, M. (1989). Prevalence of childhood and adolescent depression in the community. Ontario child health study. *British Journal of Psychiatry, 155*(5), 647–654.

Flynn, M., & Rudolph, K. D. (2007). Perceptual asymmetry and youths' responses to stress: Understanding vulnerability to depression. *Cognition and Emotion, 21,* 773–788.

Forbes, E. E., Christopher May, J., Siegle, G. J., Ladouceur, C. D., Ryan, N. D., Carter, C. S., et al. (2006). Reward-related decision-making in pediatric major depressive disorder: An fMRI study. *Journal of Child Psychology and Psychiatry, 47*(10), 1031–1040.

Forbes, E. E., Fox, N. A., Cohn, J., Galles, S., & Kovacs, M. (2006). Children's affect regulation during a disappointment: Psychophysiological responses and relation to parent history to parent history of depression. *Biological Psychiatry, 71,* 264–277.

Forbes, E. E., Hariri, A. R., Martin, S. L., Silk, J. S., Moyles, D. L., Fisher, P. M., et al. (2009). Altered striatal activation predicting real-world positive affect in adolescent major depressive disorder. *American Journal of Psychiatry, 166*(1), 64–73.

Frodl, T. S., Koutsouleris, N., Bottlender, R., Born, C., Jager, M., Scupin, I., et al. (2008). Depression-related variation in brain morphology over 3 years: Effects of stress? *Archives of General Psychiatry, 65*(10), 1156–1165.

Gale, C. R., & Martyn, C. N. (2004). Birthweight and later risk of depression in a national birth cohort. *British Journal of Psychiatry, 184,* 28–33.

Garber, J. (2005). Depression and the family. In J. L. Hudson & R. M. Rapee (Eds.), *Psychopathology and the family* (pp. 227–283). Oxford, UK: Elsevier.

Garber, J. (2007). Depression in youth: A developmental psychopathology perspective. In A. Masten & A. Sroufe (Eds.), *Multilevel dynamics in developmental psychopathology: Pathways to the future* (Vol. 34, pp. 181–242). New York: Erlbaum.

Garber, J., & Flynn, C. (2001). Predictors of depressive cognitions in young adolescents. *Cognitive Therapy and Research, 25,* 353–376.

Garber, J., & Hollon, S. D. (1991). What can specificity designs say about causality in psychopathology research? *Psychological Bulletin, 110,* 129–136.

Garber, J., & Martin, N. C. (2002). Negative cognitions in offspring of depressed parents: Mechanisms of risk. In S. H. Goodman & I. H. Gotlib (Eds.), *Children of depressed parents: Mechanisms of risk and implications for treatment* (pp. 121–153). Washington, DC: APA.

Garber, J., & Robinson, N. S. (1997). Cognitive vulnerability in children at risk for depression. *Cognitions and Emotions, 11,* 619–635.

Garber, J., Robinson, N. S., & Valentiner, D. (1997). The relation between parenting and adolescent depression: Self-worth as a mediator. *Journal of Adolescent Research, 12,* 12–33.

Gazelle, H., & Rudolph, K. D. (2004). Moving toward and away from the world: Social approach and avoidance trajectories in anxious solitary youth. *Child Development, 75,* 829–849.

Ge, X., Best, K. M., Conger, R. D., & Simons, R. L. (1996). Parenting behaviors and the occurrence and co-occurrence of adolescent depressive symptoms and conduct problems. *Developmental Psychology, 32,* 717–731.

Ge, X., Lorenz, F. O., Conger, R. D., Elder, G. H., & Simons, R. L. (1994). Trajectories of stressful life events and depressive symptoms in young adults: Gender differences in developmental trajectories. *Developmental Psychology, 30,* 467–483.

Geller, B., Zimerman, B., Williams, M., Bolhofner, K., & Craney, J. L. (2001). Bipolar disorder at prospective follow-up of adults who had prepubertal major depressive disorder. *American Journal of Psychiatry, 158,* 125–127.

Gerber, A. J., & Peterson, B. S. (2008). Applied brain imaging. *Journal of the American Academy of Child and Adolescent Psychiatry, 47*(3), 239.

Gibb, B. E. (2002). Childhood maltreatment and negative cognitive styles: A quantitative and qualitative review. *Clinical Psychology Review, 22,* 223–246.

Gibb, B. E., & Alloy, L. B. (2006). A prospective test of the hopelessness theory of depression in children. *Journal of Clinical Child and Adolescent Psychology, 35,* 264–274.

Gibb, B. E., Alloy, L. B., Abramson, L. Y., Rose, D. T., Whitehouse, W. G., & Tierney, S. (2001). History of childhood maltreatment, negative cognitive styles, and episodes of depression in adulthood. *Cognitive Therapy and Research, 25,* 425–446.

Gilman, S. E., Kawachi, I., Fitzmaurice, G. M., & Buka, S. L. (2003). Family disruption in childhood and risk of adult depression. *American Journal of Psychiatry, 160,* 939–946.

Gjerde, P. F. (1995). Alternative pathways to chronic depressive symptoms in young adults: Gender differences in developmental trajectories. *Child Development, 66,* 1277–1300.

Glowinski, A. L., Madden, P. A., Bucholz, K. K., Lynskey, M. T., & Heath, A. C. (2003). Genetic epidemiology of self-reported lifetime DSM-IV major depressive disorder in a population-based twin sample of female adolescents. *Journal of Child Psychology and Psychiatry, 44*(7), 988–996.

Gonzalez-Tejera, G., Canino, G., Ramirez, R., Chavez, L., Shrout, P., Bird, H., et al. (2005). Examining minor and major depression in adolescents. *Journal of Child Psychology and Psychiatry, 46*, 888–899.

Goodman, S. (2007). Depression in mothers. *Annual Review of Clinical Psychology, 3*, 107–135.

Goodman, S. H., Schwab-Stone, M., Lahey, B. B., Shaffer, D., & Jensen, P. S. (2000). Major depression and dysthymia in children and adolescents: Discriminant validity and differential consequences in a community sample. *Journal of the American Academy of Child and Adolescent Psychiatry, 36*, 761–770.

Goodwin, R. D., Fergusson, D. M., & Horwood, L. J. (2004). Early anxious/withdrawn behaviours predict later internalizing disorders. *Journal of Child Psychology and Psychiatry, and Allied Disciplines, 45*, 874–883.

Goodyer, I. M., Bacon, A., Ban, M., Croudace, T., & Herbert, J. (2009). Serotonin transporter genotype, morning cortisol and subsequent depression in adolescents. *British Journal of Psychiatry, 195*(1), 39–45.

Goodyer, I. M., Croudace, T., Dudbridge, F., Ban, M., & Herbert, J. (2010). Polymorphisms in BDNF (Val66Met) and 5-HTTLPR, morning cortisol and subsequent depression in at-risk adolescents. *British Journal of Psychiatry, 197*(5), 365–371.

Goodyer, I. M., Herbert, J., Tamplin, A., & Altham, P. M. (2000). Recent life events, cortisol, dehydroepiandrosterone and the onset of major depression in high-risk adolescents. *British Journal of Psychiatry, 177*, 499–504.

Goodyer, I. M., Park, R. J., & Herbert, J. (2001). Psychosocial and endocrine features of chronic first-episode major depression in 8–16 year olds. *Biological Psychiatry, 50*(5), 351–357.

Gotlib, I. H., Hamilton, J. P., Cooney, R. E., Singh, M. K., Henry, M. L., & Joormann, J. (2010). Neural processing of reward and loss in girls at risk for major depression. *Archives of General Psychiatry, 67*(4), 380–387.

Gotlib, I. H., Joormann, J., Minor, K. L., & Cooney, R. E. (2006). Cognitive and biological functioning in children at risk for depression. In T. Canli (Ed.), *Biology of personality and individual differences* (pp. 353–382). New York, NY: Guilford.

Gotlib, I. H., Joormann, J., Minor, K. L., & Hallmayer, J. (2008). HPA axis reactivity: A mechanism underlying the associations among 5-HTTLPR, stress, and depression. *Biological Psychiatry, 63*(9), 847–851.

Grant, K. E., Compas, B. E., Thurm, A. E., McMahon, S. D., Gipson, P. Y., & Westerholm, R. I. (2006). Stressors and child and adolescent psychopathology: Evidence of moderating and mediating effects. *Clinical Psychology Review, 26*, 257–283.

Gray, J. A. (1991). The neuropsychology of temperament. In J. Strelau & A. Angleitner (Eds.), *Explorations in temperament: International perspectives on theory and measurement* (pp. 105–128). New York: Plenum.

Guedeney, N., Guedeney, A., Rabouam, C., Mintz, A. S., Danon, G., Huet, M. M., et al. (2003). The Zero-to-Three diagnostic classification: A contribution to the validation of this classification from a sample of 85 under-threes. *Infant Mental Health Journal, 24*, 313–336.

Hammen, C. (1991). The generation of stress in the course of unipolar depression. *Journal of Abnormal Psychology, 100*, 555–561.

Hammen, C. (2002). The context of stress in families of children with depressed parents. In S. Goodman & I. Gotlib (Eds.), *Children of depressed parents: Mechanisms of risk and implications for treatment* (pp. 175–199). Washington, D.C.: American Psychological Association.

Hammen, C. (2006). Stress generation in depression: Reflections on origins, research, and future directions. *Journal of Clinical Psychology, 62*, 69–82.

Hammen, C., & Brennan, P. A. (2001). Depressed adolescents of depressed and nondepressed mothers: Tests of an interpersonal impairment hypothesis. *Journal of Consulting and Clinical Psychology, 69*, 284–294.

Hammen, C., Brennan, P. A., Keenan-Miller, D., Hazel, N. A., & Najman, J. M. (2010). Chronic and acute stress, gender, and serotonin transporter gene-environment interactions predicting depression symptoms in youth. *Journal of Child Psychology and Psychiatry, 51*(2), 180–187.

Hammen, C., Henry, R., & Daley, S. E. (2000). Depression and sensitization to stressors among young women as a function of childhood adversity. *Journal of Consulting and Clinical Psychology, 68*, 782–787.

Hammen, C., Shih, J. H., & Brennan, P. A. (2004). Intergenerational transmission of depression: Test of an interpersonal stress model in a community sample. *Journal of Consulting and Clinical Psychology, 72*, 511–522.

Hankin, B. L. (2005). Childhood maltreatment and psychopathology: Prospective tests of attachment, cognitive vulnerability, and stress as mediating processes. *Cognitive Therapy and Research, 29*, 645–671.

Hankin, B. L. (2012). Future directions in vulnerability to depression among youth: Integrating risk factors and processes across multiple levels of analysis. *Journal of Clinical Child and Adolescent Psychology, 41*(5), 695–718.

Hankin, B. L., & Abramson, L. (2001). Development of gender differences in depression: An elaborated cognitive vulnerability-transactional stress theory. *Psychological Bulletin, 127*, 773–796.

Hankin, B. L., Abramson, L., Miller, N., & Haeffel, G. (2004). Cognitive vulnerability-stress theories of depression: Examining affective specificity in the prediction of depression versus anxiety in three prospective studies. *Cognitive Therapy & Research, 28*, 309–345.

Hankin, B. L., Abramson, L. Y., Moffitt, T. E., Silva, P. A., McGee, R., & Angell, K. E. (1998). Development of depression from preadolescence to young adulthood: Emerging gender differences in a 10-year longitudinal study. *Journal of Abnormal Psychology, 107*, 128–140.

Hankin, B. L., Fraley, R. C., Lahey, B. B., & Waldman, I. D. (2005). Is depression best viewed as a continuum or discrete category? A taxometric analysis of childhood and adolescent depression in a population-based sample. *Journal of Abnormal Psychology, 114*, 96–110.

Hankin, B. L., Mermelstein, R., & Roesch, L. (2007). Sex differences in adolescent depression: Stress exposure and reactivity models in interpersonal and achievement contextual domains. *Child Development, 78*, 279–295.

Happonen, M., Pulkkinen, L., Kaprio, J., Van der Meere, J., Viken, R. J., & Rose, R. J. (2002). The heritability of depressive symptoms: Multiple informants and multiple measures. *Journal of Child Psychology and Psychiatry, 43*(4), 471–479.

Harkness, K. L., Bruce, A. E., & Lumley, M. N. (2006). The role of childhood abuse and neglect in the sensitization to stressful life events in adolescent depression. *Journal of Abnormal Psychology, 115*, 730–741.

Harkness, K. L., & Lumley, M. N. (2008). Child abuse and neglect and the development of depression in children and adolescents. In J. R. Z. Abela & B. L. Hankin (Eds.), *Handbook of depression in children and adolescents* (pp. 466–488). New York: Guilford.

Harrington, R., Fudge, H., Rutter, M., Pickles, A., & Hill, J. (1990). Adult outcomes of childhood and adolescent depression. *Archives of General Psychiatry, 47*, 465–473.

Harrington, R., Peters, S., Green, J., Byford, S., Woods, J., & McGowan, R. (2000). Randomised comparison of the effectiveness and costs of community and hospital based mental health services for children with behavioral disorders. *British Journal of Medicine, 321*, 1–5.

Hasler, G., & Northoff, G. (2011). Discovering imaging endophenotypes for major depression. *Molecular Psychiatry, 16*(6), 604–619.

Hayden, E. P., Klein, D. N., & Durbin, C. E. (2005). Parent reports and laboratory assessments of child temperament: A comparison of their associations with risk for depression and externalizing disorders. *Journal of Psychopathology & Behavioral Assessment, 27*, 89–100.

Hoffman, K. B., Cole, D. A., Martin, J. M., Tram, J., & Serocynski, A. D. (2000). Are the discrepancies between self- and others' appraisals of competence predictive or reflective of depressive symptoms in children and adolescents?: A longitudinal study, Part II. *Journal of Abnormal Psychology, 109*, 651–662.

Hofstra, M. B., van der Ende, J., & Verhulst, F. C. (2000). Continuity and change in psychopathology from childhood into adulthood: A 14-year follow-up study. *Journal of the American Academy of Child and Adolescent Psychiatry, 39*, 850–858.

Hu, X. Z., Lipsky, R. H., Zhu, G., Akhtar, L. A., Taubman, J., Greenberg, B. D., et al. (2006). Serotonin transporter promoter gain-of-function genotypes are linked to obsessive-compulsive disorder. *American Journal of Human Genetics, 78*(5), 815–826.

Huang, H., Fan, X., Williamson, D. E., & Rao, U. (2011). White matter changes in healthy adolescents at familial risk for unipolar depression: A diffusion tensor imaging study. *Neuropsychopharmacology, 36*(3), 684–691.

Huang, H., Gundapuneedi, T., & Rao, U. (2012). White matter disruptions in adolescents exposed to childhood maltreatment and vulnerability to psychopathology. *Neuropsychopharmacology, 37*(12), 2693–2701.

Hulvershorn, L. A., Cullen, K., & Anand, A. (2011). Toward dysfunctional connectivity: A review of neuroimaging findings in pediatric major depressive disorder. *Brain Imaging and Behavior, 5*(4), 307–328.

Hyde, J. S., Mezulis, A. H., & Abramson, L. Y. (2008). The ABCs of depression: Integrating affective, biological, and cognitive models to explain the emergence of the gender difference in depression. *Psychological Review, 115*, 291–313.

Ingram, R. E., Miranda, J., & Segal, Z. V. (1998). *Cognitive vulnerability to depression.* New York: Guilford.

Insel, T. (2013, April 29). *Transforming diagnosis* [Web log post]. Retrieved from http://www.nimh.nih.gov/about/director/index.shtml

Ivanenko, A., & Johnson, K. (2008). Sleep disturbances in children with psychiatric disorders. *Seminars in Pediatric Neurology, 15*(2), 70–78.

Ivarsson, T., Broberg, A. G., Arvidsson, T., & Gillberg, C. (2005). Bullying in adolescence: Psychiatric problems in victims and bullies as measured by the youth self report (YSR) and the depression self-rating scale (DSRS). *Nordic Journal of Psychiatry, 59*, 365–373.

Jacobs, R. H., Reinecke, M. A., Gollan, J. K., & Kane, P. (2008). Empirical evidence of cognitive vulnerability for depression among children and adolescents: A cognitive science and development perspective. *Clinical Psychology Review, 28*, 759–782.

Jaffee, S. R., Moffitt, T. E., Caspi, A., Fombonne, E., Poulton, R., & Martin, J. (2002). Differences in early childhood risk factors for juvenile-onset and adult-onset depression. *Archives of General Psychiatry, 59*, 215–222.

Jenness, J. L., Hankin, B. L., Abela, J. R., Young, J. F., & Smolen, A. (2011). Chronic family stress interacts with 5-HTTLPR to predict prospective depressive symptoms among youth. *Depression and Anxiety, 28*(12), 1074–1080.

Joiner, T. E., & Coyne, J. C. (Eds.). (1999). *The interactional nature of depression.* Washington, DC: American Psychological Association.

Jones, D. J., Forehand, R., & Neary, E. M. (2001). Family transmission of depressive symptoms: Replication across Caucasian and African American mother-child dyads. *Behavior Therapy, 32*, 123–138.

Joormann, J., Talbot, L., & Gotlib, I. H. (2007). Biased processing of emotional information in girls at risk for depression. *Journal of Abnormal Psychology, 116*, 135–143.

Kaltiala-Heino, R., Rimpela, M., Rantanen, P., & Rimpela, A. (2000). Bullying at school: An indicator of adolescents at risk for mental disorders. *Journal of Adolescence, 23*, 661–674.

Kapoor, A., Dunn, E., Kostaki, A., Andrews, M. H., & Matthews, S. G. (2006). Fetal programming of hypothalamo-pituitary-adrenal function: Prenatal stress and glucocorticoids. *Journal of Physiology, 572*, 31–44.

Kashani, J. H., Rosenberg, T. K., & Reid, J. C. (1989). Developmental perspectives in child and adolescent depressive symptoms in a community sample. *American Journal of Psychiatry, 146*, 871–875.

Katainen, S., Raikkonen, K., Keskivaara, P., & Keltikangas-Jarvinen, L. (1999). Maternal child-rearing attitudes and role satisfaction and children's temperament as antecedents of adolescent depressive tendencies: Follow-up study of 6- to 15-year olds. *Journal of Youth and Adolescence, 28*, 139–163.

Kaufman, J., Birmaher, B., Perel, J., Dahl, R. E., Moreci, P., Nelson, B., et al. (1997). The corticotropin-releasing hormone challenge in depressed abused, depressed nonabused, and normal control children. *Biological Psychiatry, 42*(8), 669–679.

Kaufman, J., & Charney, D. (2001). Effects of early stress on brain structure and function: Implications for understanding the relationship between child maltreatment and depression. *Development and Psychopathology, 13*(3), 451–471.

Kaufman, J., Martin, A., King, R. A., & Charney, D. (2001). Are child-, adolescent-, and adult-onset depression one and the same disorder? *Biological Psychiatry, 49*(12), 980–1001.

Kaufman, J., Yang, B. Z., Douglas-Palumberi, H., Grasso, D., Lipschitz, D., Houshyar, S., et al. (2006). Brain-derived neurotrophic factor-5-HTTLPR gene interactions and environmental modifiers of depression in children. *Biological Psychiatry, 59*(8), 673–680.

Kaufman, J., Yang, B. Z., Douglas-Palumberi, H., Houshyar, S., Lipschitz, D., Krystal, J. H., et al. (2004). Social supports and serotonin transporter gene moderate depression in maltreated children. *Proceedings of the National Academy of Sciences of the United States of America, 101*(49), 17316–17321.

Kendler, K. S., Gardner, C. O., & Prescott, C. A. (2002). Toward a comprehensive developmental model for major depression in women. *American Journal of Psychiatry, 159*, 1133–1145.

Kendler, K. S., Kessler, R. C., Walters, E. E., MacLean, C., Neale, M. C., Heath, A. C., et al. (1995). Stressful life events, genetic liability, and onset of an episode of major depression in women. *American Journal of Psychiatry, 152*, 833–842.

Kennard, B. D., Emslie, G. J., Mayes, T. L., & Hughes, J. L. (2006). Relapse and recurrence in pediatric depression. *Child and Adolescent Psychiatric Clinics of North America, 15*, 1057–1079.

Kentgen, L. M., Tenke, C. E., Pine, D. S., Fong, R., Klein, R. G., & Bruder, G. E. (2000). Electroencephalographic asymmetries in adolescents with major depression: Influence of comorbidity with anxiety disorders. *Journal of Abnormal Psychology, 109*(4), 797–802.

Kessler, R., Avenevoli, S., Costello, E., Georgiades, K., Green, J., Gruber, M., et al. (2012). Prevalence, persistence, and sociodemographic correlates of DSM-IV disorders in the National Comorbidity Survey Replication Adolescent Supplement. *Archives of General Psychiatry, 69*(4), 372–380.

Kessler, R. C., Avenevoli, S., & Merikangas, K. R. (2001). Mood disorders in children and adolescents: An epidemiologic perspective. *Biological Psychiatry, 49*(12), 1002–1014.

Kessler, R. C., & Walters, E. E. (1998). Epidemiology of DSM-III-R major depression and minor depression among adolescents and young adults in the National Comorbidity Survey. *Depression and Anxiety, 7*, 3–14.

Kim, H., Capaldi, D., & Stoolmiller, M. (2003). Depressive symptoms across adolescence and young adulthood in men: Predictions from parental and contextual risk factors. *Development and Psychopathology, 15*(2), 469–495.

Kistner, J., Balthazor, M., Risi, S., & Burton, C. (1999). Predicting dysphoria in adolescence from actual and perceived peer acceptance in childhood. *Journal of Clinical Child Psychology, 28*, 94–104.

Klein, D. N., Kotov, R., & Bufferd, S. J. (2011). Personality and depression: Explanatory models and review of the evidence. *Annual Review of Clinical Psychology, 7*, 269–295.

Klein, D. N., Shankman, S. A., Lewinsohn, P. M., & Seeley, J. K. (2009). Subthreshold depressive disorder in adolescents: Predictors of escalation to full syndrome depressive disorders. *Journal of the American Academy of Child and Adolescent Psychiatry, 48*, 703–710.

Kondo, D. G., Hellem, T. L., Sung, Y. H., Kim, N., Jeong, E. K., Delmastro, K. K., et al. (2010). Review: Magnetic resonance spectroscopy studies of pediatric major depressive disorder. *Depression Research and Treatment, 2011*, 1–13.

Kovacs, M. (1994). Childhood-onset dysthymic disorder: Clinical features and prospective naturalistic outcome. *Archives of General Psychology, 51*, 365–374.

Kovacs, M. (1996a). The course of childhood-onset depressive disorders. *Psychiatric Annals, 26*, 326–330.

Kovacs, M. (1996b). Presentation and course of major depressive disorder during childhood and later years of the life span. *Journal of the American Academy of Child and Adolescent Psychiatry, 35*, 705–715.

Kovacs, M., & Lopez-Duran, N. (2010). Prodromal symptoms and atypical affectivity as predictors of major depression in juveniles: Implications for prevention. *Journal of Child Psychology and Psychiatry, 51*, 472–496.

Kovacs, M., Obrosky, D. S., & Sherrill, J. (2003). Developmental changes in the phenomenology of depression in girls compared to boys from childhood onward. *Journal of Affective Disorders, 74*, 33–48.

Kujawa, A., Torpey, D., Kim, J., Hajcak, G., Rose, S., Gotlib, I., et al. (2011). Attentional biases for emotional faces in young children of mothers with chronic or recurrent depression. *Journal of Abnormal Child Psychology, 39*, 125–135.

LaGrange, B., Cole, D. A., Jacquea, F., Ciesla, J., Dallaire, D., Pineda, A., et al. (2011). Disentangling the prospective relations between maladaptive cognitions and depressive symptoms. *Journal of Abnormal Psychology, 120*, 511–527.

Lakdawalla, Z., Hankin, B. L., & Mermelstein, R. (2007). Cognitive theories of depression in children and adolescents: A conceptual and quantitative review. *Clinical Child and Family Psychology Review, 10*, 1–24.

Lau, J. Y., & Eley, T. C. (2008). Disentangling gene-environment correlations and interactions on adolescent depressive symptoms. *Journal of Child Psychology and Psychiatry, 49*(2), 142–150.

Leinonen, J. A., Solantaus, T. S., & Punamaki, R. L. (2003). Parental mental health and children's adjustment: The quality of marital interaction and parenting as mediating factors. *Journal of Child Psychology and Psychiatry, and Allied Disciplines, 44*, 227–241.

Lengua, L. J., Sandler, I. N., West, S. G., Wolchik, S. A., & Curran, P. J. (1999). Emotionality and self-regulation, threat appraisal, and coping in children of divorce. *Development and Psychopathology, 11*, 15–37.

Lengua, L. J., Wolchik, S. A., Sandler, I. N., & West, S. G. (2000). The additive and interactive effects of parenting and temperament in predicting adjustment problems of children of divorce. *Journal of Clinical Child Psychology, 29*, 232–244.

Leppanen, J. M. (2006). Emotional information processing in mood disorders: A review of behavioral and neuroimaging findings. *Current Opinion in Psychiatry, 19*(1), 34–39.

Lesch, K. P., Bengel, D., Heils, A., Sabol, S. Z., Greenberg, B. D., Petri, S., et al. (1996). Association of anxiety-related traits with a polymorphism in the serotonin transporter gene regulatory region. *Science, 274*(5292), 1527–1531.

Lewinsohn, P. M., Allen, N. B., Seeley, J. R., & Gotlib, I. H. (1999). First onset versus recurrence of depression: Differential processes of psychosocial risk. *Journal of Abnormal Psychology, 108*, 483–489.

Lewinsohn, P. M., & Essau, C. A. (2002). Depression in adolescents. In I. H. Gotlib & C. L. Hammen (Eds.), *Handbook of depression* (pp. 541–559). New York, NY: Guilford.

Lewinsohn, P. M., Hops, H., Roberts, R. E., Seeley, J. R., & Andrews, J. A. (1993). Adolescent psychopathology: I. Prevalence and incidence of depression and other DSM-III-R disorders in high school students. *Journal of Abnormal Psychology, 102*, 133–144.

Lewinsohn, P. M., Joiner, T. E., & Rohde, P. (2001). Evaluation of cognitive diathesis-stress models in predicting major depressive disorder in adolescents. *Journal of Abnormal Psychology, 110*, 203–215.

Lewinsohn, P. M., Rohde, P. M., & Seeley, J. R. (1998). Major depressive disorder in older adolescents: Prevalence, risk factors, and clinical implications. *Clinical Psychology Review, 18*, 765–794.

Lewinsohn, P. M., Solomon, A., Seeley, J. R., & Zeiss, A. (2000). Clinical implications of "subthreshold" depressive symptoms. *Journal of Abnormal Psychology, 109*, 345–351.

Lewinsohn, P. M., Steinmetz, J. L., Larson, D. W., & Franklin, J. (1981). Depression related cognitions: Antecedent or consequence? *Journal of Abnormal Psychology, 91*, 213–219.

Lonigan, C. J., Phillips, B. M., & Hooe, E. S. (2003). Relations of positive and negative affectivity to anxiety and depression in children: Evidence from a latent variable longitudinal study. *Journal of Consulting and Clinical Psychology, 71*, 465–481.

Lovejoy, M. C., Graczyk, P. A., O'Hare, E., & Neuman, G. (2000). Maternal depression and parenting: A meta-analytic review. *Clinical Psychology Review, 20*, 561–592.

Luby, J. L., Belden, A. C., & Spitznagel, E. (2006). Risk factors for preschool depression: The mediating role of early stressful life events. *Journal of Child Psychology and Psychiatry, and Allied Disciplines, 47*, 1292–1298.

Luby, J. L., Heffelfinger, A. K., Mrakotsky, C., Hessler, M. J., Brown, K. M., & Hildebrand, T. (2002). Preschool major depressive disorder: Preliminary validation for developmentally modified DSM-IV criteria. *Journal of the American Academy of Child and Adolescent Psychiatry, 41*, 928–937.

Luby, J. L., Mrakotsky, C., Heffelfinger, A., Brown, K., Hessler, M., & Spitznagel, E. (2003). Modification of DSM-IV criteria for depressed preschool children. *American Journal of Psychiatry, 160*, 1169–1172.

Luykx, J. J., Laban, K. G., van den Heuvel, M. P., Boks, M. P., Mandl, R. C., Kahn, R. S., et al. (2012). Region and state specific glutamate downregulation in major depressive disorder: A meta-analysis of (1)H-MRS findings. *Neuroscience & Biobehavioral Reviews, 36*(1), 198–205.

MacMillan, S., Szeszko, P. R., Moore, G. J., Madden, R., Lorch, E., Ivey, J., et al. (2003). Increased amygdala: Hippocampal volume ratios associated with severity of anxiety in pediatric major depression. *Journal of Child and Adolescent Psychopharmacology, 13*(1), 65–73.

MacQueen, G., & Frodl, T. (2011). The hippocampus in major depression: Evidence for the convergence of the bench and bedside in psychiatric research? *Molecular Psychiatry, 16*(3), 252–264.

Markham, J. A., & Koenig, J. I. (2011). Prenatal stress: Role in psychotic and depressive diseases. *Development and Psychopathology, 214*(1), 89–106.

Matas, L., Arend, R. A., & Sroufe, L. A. (1978). Continuity of adaptation in the second year: The relation between quality of attachment and later competence. *Child Development, 49*, 547–556.

Mathew, S. J., Coplan, J. D., Goetz, R. R., Feder, A., Greenwald, S., Dahl, R. E., et al. (2003). Differentiating depressed adolescent 24 h cortisol secretion in light of their adult clinical outcome. *Neuropsychopharmacology, 28*(7), 1336–1343.

Mayberg, H. S. (2003). Modulating dysfunctional limbic-cortical circuits in depression: Towards development of brain-based algorithms for diagnosis and optimised treatment. *British Medical Bulletin, 65*, 193–207.

McCarty, C. A., Vander Stoep, A., & McCauley, E. (2007). Cognitive features associated with depressive symptoms in adolescence: Directionality and specificity. *Journal of Clinical Child and Adolescent Psychology, 36*, 147–158.

McEwen, B. S. (1999). Stress and hippocampal plasticity. *Annual Review of Neuroscience, 22,* 105–122.

McGinn, L. K., Cukor, D., & Sanderson, W. C. (2005). The relationship between parenting style, cognitive style, and anxiety and depression: Does increased early adversity influence symptom severity through the mediating role of cognitive style? *Cognitive Therapy and Research, 29*(2), 219–242.

McKinnon, M. C., Yucel, K., Nazarov, A., & MacQueen, G. M. (2009). A meta-analysis examining clinical predictors of hippocampal volume in patients with major depressive disorder. *Journal of Psychiatry and Neuroscience, 34*(1), 41–54.

Merikangas, K. R., He, J.-P., Brody, D., Fisher, P. W., Bourdon, K., & Koretz, D. S. (2010). Prevalence and treatment of mental disorders among U.S. children in the 2001–2004 NHANES. *Pediatrics, 125,* 75–81.

Merikangas, K. R., & Knight, E. (2009). The epidemiology of depression in adolescents. In S. Nolen-Hoeksema & L. M. Hilt (Eds.), *Handbook of depression in adolescents* (pp. 386–404). New York, NY: Taylor and Francis Group, LLC.

Mezulis, A. H., Hyde, J. S., & Abramson, L. Y. (2006). The developmental origins of cognitive vulnerability to depression: Temperament, parenting, and negative life events in childhood as contributors to negative cognitive style. *Developmental Psychology, 42,* 1012–1025.

Mitchell, A. M., & Possel, P. (2012). Frontal brain activity pattern predicts depression in adolescent boys. *Biological Psychology, 89*(2), 525–527.

Monroe, S. M., & Harkness, K. L. (2005). Life stress, the "kindling" hypothesis, and the recurrence of depression: Considerations from a life stress perspective. *Psychological Review, 112,* 417–445.

Monroe, S. M., Rohde, P., Seeley, J. R., & Lewinsohn, P. M. (1999). Life events and depression in adolescence: Relationship loss as a prospective risk factor for first-onset of major depressive disorder. *Journal of Abnormal Psychology, 108,* 606–614.

Monroe, S. M., & Simons, A. D. (1991). Diathesis-stress theories in the context of life stress research: Implications for the depressive disorders. *Psychological Bulletin, 110,* 406–425.

Moran, M. (2013). DSM-5 updates depressive, anxiety, and OCD criteria. *Psychiatric News, 48*(4), 22–43.

Morehouse, R. L., Kusumakar, V., Kutcher, S. P., LeBlanc, J., & Armitage, R. (2002). Temporal coherence in ultradian sleep EEG rhythms in a never-depressed, high-risk cohort of female adolescents. *Biological Psychiatry, 51*(6), 446–456.

Morris, M. C., Ciesla, J. A., & Garber, J. (2008). A prospective study of the cognitive-stress model of depressive symptoms in adolescents. *Journal of Abnormal Psychology, 117,* 719–734.

Mrug, S., Hoza, B., & Bukowski, W. M. (2004). Choosing or being chosen by aggressive-disruptive peers: Do they contribute to children's externalizing and internalizing problems? *Journal of Abnormal Child Psychology, 32,* 53–65.

Natsuaki, M. N., Ge, X., Brody, G. H., Simons, R. L., Gibbons, F. X., & Cutrona, C. E. (2007). African American children's depressive symptoms: The prospective effects of neighborhood disorder, stressful life events and parenting. *American Journal of Community Psychology, 39,* 163–176.

Nigg, J. T. (2006). Temperament and developmental psychopathology. *Journal of Child Psychology and Psychiatry, and Allied Disciplines, 47,* 395–422.

Nobile, M., Cataldo, M. G., Giorda, R., Battaglia, M., Baschirotto, C., Bellina, M., et al. (2004). A case–control and family-based association study of the 5-HTTLPR in pediatric-onset depressive disorders. *Biological Psychiatry, 56*(4), 292–295.

Nolan, S. A., Flynn, C., & Garber, J. (2003). Prospective relations between rejection and depression in young adolescents. *Journal of Personality and Social Psychology, 85,* 745–755.

Nolan, C. L., Moore, G. J., Madden, R., Farchione, T., Bartoi, M., Lorch, E., et al. (2002). Prefrontal cortical volume in childhood-onset major depression: Preliminary findings. *Archives of General Psychiatry, 59*(2), 173–179.

Nolen-Hoeksema, S., & Hilt, L. M. (2009). Gender differences in depression. In I. Gotlib & C. Hammen (Eds.), *Handbook of depression* (2nd ed., pp. 386–404). New York, NY: Guilford.

Oldehinkel, A. J., Veenstra, R., Ormel, J., de Winter, A. F., & Verhulst, F. C. (2006). Temperament, parenting, and depressive symptoms in a population sample of preadolescents. *Journal of Child Psychology and Psychiatry, and Allied Disciplines, 47,* 684–695.

Olino, T. M., Klein, D. N., Dyson, M. W., Rose, S. A., & Durbin, C. E. (2010). Temperamental emotionality in preschool-aged children and depressive disorders in parents: Associations in a large community sample. *Journal of Abnormal Psychology, 119,* 468–478.

Olvera, R. L., Caetano, S. C., Stanley, J. A., Chen, H. H., Nicoletti, M., Hatch, J. P., et al. (2010). Reduced medial prefrontal N-acetyl-aspartate levels in pediatric major depressive disorder: A multi-voxel in vivo(1)H spectroscopy study. *Psychiatry Research, 184*(2), 71–76.

Ormel, J., Oldehinkel, A. J., Ferdinand, R. F., Hartman, C. A., de Winter, A. F., & Verhulst, F. C. (2005). Internalizing and externalizing problems in adolescence: General and dimension-specific effects of familial loadings and preadolescent temperament traits. *Psychological Medicine, 35,* 1825–1835.

Park, I. J. K., Garber, J., Ciesla, J. A., & Ellis, B. J. (2008). Convergence among multiple methods of measuring positivity and negativity in the family environment: Relation to depression in mothers and their children. *Journal of Family Psychology, 22,* 123–134.

Park, R. J., Goodyer, I. M., & Teasdale, J. D. (2005). Self-devaluative dysphoric experience and the prediction of persistent first-episode major depressive disorder in adolescents. *Psychological Medicine, 35,* 539–548.

Phillips, B. M., Lonigan, C. J., Driscoll, K., & Hooe, E. S. (2002). Positive and negative affectivity in children: A multitrait-multimethod investigation. *Journal of Clinical Child and Adolescent Psychology, 31*, 465–479.

Pihlakoski, L., Sourander, A., Aromaa, M., Rautava, P., Helenius, H., & Sillanpaa, M. (2006). The continuity of psychopathology from early childhood to preadolescence. *European Child and Adolescent Psychiatry, 15*, 409–417.

Pomerantz, E. M., & Rudolph, K. D. (2003). What ensues from emotional distress? Implications for competence estimation. *Child Development, 74*, 329–346.

Posner, M. I., & Rothbart, M. K. (2007). Research on attention networks as a model for the integration of psychological science. *Annual Review of Psychology, 58*, 1–23.

Post, R. M. (1992). Transduction of psychosocial stress into the neurobiology of recurrent affective disorder. *American Journal of Psychiatry, 149*, 1006.

Price, J. L., & Drevets, W. C. (2012). Neural circuits underlying the pathophysiology of mood disorders. *Trends in Cognitive Science, 16*(1), 61–71.

Prinstein, M. J., Borelli, J. L., Cheah, C. S. L., Simon, V. A., & Aikins, J. W. (2005). Adolescent girls' interpersonal vulnerability to depressive symptoms: A longitudinal examination of reassurance-seeking and peer relationships. *Journal of Abnormal Psychology, 114*, 676–688.

Rajkowska, G., & Miguel-Hidalgo, J. J. (2007). Gliogenesis and glial pathology in depression. *Current Drug Targets – CNS and Neurological Disorders, 6*(3), 219–233.

Rao, U. (2011). Sleep disturbances in pediatric depression. *Asian Journal of Psychiatry, 4*(4), 234–247.

Rao, U., & Chen, L. A. (2009). Characteristics, correlates, and outcomes of childhood and adolescent depressive disorders. *Dialogues in Clinical Neuroscience, 11*(1), 45–62.

Rao, U., Chen, L. A., Bidesi, A. S., Shad, M. U., Thomas, M. A., & Hammen, C. L. (2010). Hippocampal changes associated with early-life adversity and vulnerability to depression. *Biological Psychiatry, 67*(4), 357–364.

Rao, U., Dahl, R. E., Ryan, N. D., Birmaher, B., Williamson, D. E., Giles, D. E., et al. (1996). The relationship between longitudinal clinical course and sleep and cortisol changes in adolescent depression. *Biological Psychiatry, 40*(6), 474–484.

Rao, U., Dahl, R. E., Ryan, N. D., Birmaher, B., Williamson, D. E., Rao, R., et al. (2002). Heterogeneity in EEG sleep findings in adolescent depression: Unipolar versus bipolar clinical course. *Journal of Affective Disorders, 70*(3), 273–280.

Rao, U., Hammen, C., Ortiz, L. R., Chen, L. A., & Poland, R. E. (2008). Effects of early and recent adverse experiences on adrenal response to psychosocial stress in depressed adolescents. *Biological Psychiatry, 64*(6), 521–526.

Rao, U., Hammen, C. L., & Poland, R. E. (2009a). Ethnic differences in electroencephalographic sleep patterns in adolescents. *Asian Journal of Psychiatry, 2*(1), 17–24.

Rao, U., Hammen, C. L., & Poland, R. E. (2009b). Risk markers for depression in adolescents: Sleep and HPA measures. *Neuropsychopharmacology, 34*(8), 1936–1945.

Rao, U., Hammen, C. L., & Poland, R. E. (2010). Longitudinal course of adolescent depression: Neuroendocrine and psychosocial predictors. *Journal of the American Academy of Child and Adolescent Psychiatry, 49*, 141–151.

Raynor, P., & Rudolf, M. (1996). What do we know about children who fail to thrive? *Child: Care, Health and Development, 22*(4), 241.

Resnick, M. D., Bearman, P. S., Blum, R. W., Bauman, K. E., Harris, K. M., & Udry, R. (1997). Protecting adolescents from harm: Findings from the National Longitudinal Study on Adolescent Health. *Journal of American Medical Association, 278*, 823–832.

Rice, F. (2010). Genetics of childhood and adolescent depression: Insights into etiological heterogeneity and challenges for future genomic research. *Genome Medicine, 2*(9), 68.

Rice, F., Harold, G. T., & Thapar, A. (2002). Assessing the effects of age, sex and shared environment on the genetic aetiology of depression in childhood and adolescence. *Journal of Child Psychology and Psychiatry, 43*(8), 1039–1051.

Rice, F., Harold, G. T., & Thapar, A. (2003). Negative life events as an account of age-related differences in the genetic aetiology of depression in childhood and adolescence. *Journal of Child Psychology and Psychiatry, 44*(7), 977–987.

Richey, J., Schmidt, N., Lonigan, C., Phillips, B., Catanzaro, S., & Kotov, R. (2009). The latent structure of child depression: A taxometric analysis. *Journal of Child Psychology and Psychiatry, and Allied Disciplines, 50*(9), 1147–1155.

Rizzo, C. J., Daley, S. E., & Gunderson, B. H. (2006). Interpersonal sensitivity, romantic stress, and the prediction of depression: A study of inner-city, minority adolescent girls. *Journal of Youth and Adolescence, 35*, 444–453.

Roberson-Nay, R., McClure, E. B., Monk, C. S., Nelson, E. E., Guyer, A. E., Fromm, S. J., et al. (2006). Increased amygdala activity during successful memory encoding in adolescent major depressive disorder: An FMRI study. *Biological Psychiatry, 60*, 966–973.

Robert, J. J., Hoffmann, R. F., Emslie, G. J., Hughes, C., Rintelmann, J., Moore, J., et al. (2006). Sex and age differences in sleep macroarchitecture in childhood and adolescent depression. *Sleep, 29*(3), 351–358.

Rohde, P., Lewinsohn, P. M., & Seeley, J. R. (1991). Comorbidity of unipolar depression: II. Comorbidity with other mental disorders in adolescents and adults. *Journal of Abnormal Psychology, 100*, 214–222.

Rosso, I. M., Cintron, C. M., Steingard, R. J., Renshaw, P. F., Young, A. D., & Yurgelun-Todd, D. A. (2005). Amygdala and hippocampus volumes in pediatric major depression. *Biological Psychiatry, 57*(1), 21–26.

Rothbart, M. K., & Bates, J. E. (2006). Temperament. In W. Damon, R. M. Lerner, & N. Eisenberg (Eds.),

Handbook of child psychology: Vol. 3. Social, emotional, and personality development (6th ed., pp. 99–166). New York: Wiley.

Rubio-Stipec, M., Fitzmaurice, G., Murphy, J., & Walker, A. (2003). The use of multiple informants in identifying the risk factors of depressive and disruptive disorders: Are they interchangeable? *Social Psychiatry and Psychiatric Epidemiology, 38,* 51–58.

Rudolph, K. D. (2009). The interpersonal context of adolescent depression. In S. Nolen-Hoeksema & L. Hilt (Eds.), *Handbook of depression in adolescents* (pp. 377–405). New York: Routledge.

Rudolph, K. D., & Clark, A. G. (2001). Conceptions of relationships in children with depressive and aggressive symptoms: Social-cognitive distortion or reality? *Journal of Abnormal Child Psychology, 29,* 41–56.

Rudolph, K. D., & Conley, C. S. (2005). Socioemotional costs and benefits of social-evaluative concerns: Do girls care too much? *Journal of Personality, 73,* 115–137.

Rudolph, K. D., & Flynn, M. (2007). Childhood adversity and youth depression: Influence of gender and pubertal status. *Development and Psychopathology, 19*(2), 497–521.

Rudolph, K. D., Flynn, M., & Abaied, J. L. (2008). A developmental perspective on interpersonal theories of youth depression. In J. R. Z. Abela & B. L. Hankin (Eds.), *Child and adolescent depression: Causes, treatment, and prevention.* New York: Guilford.

Rudolph, K. D., & Hammen, C. (1999). Age and gender determinants of stress exposure, generation, and reactions in youngsters: A transactional perspective. *Child Development, 70,* 660–677.

Rudolph, K. D., Hammen, C., & Burge, D. (1997). A cognitive-interpersonal approach to depressive symptoms in preadolescent children. *Journal of Abnormal Child Psychology, 25,* 33–45.

Rudolph, K. D., Hammen, C., Burge, D., Lindberg, N., Herzberg, D., & Daley, S. (2000). Toward an interpersonal life-stress model of depression: The developmental context of stress generation. *Development and Psychopathology, 12,* 215–234.

Rudolph, K. D., Kurlakowsky, K. D., & Conley, C. S. (2001). Developmental and social-contextual origins of depressive control-related beliefs and behavior. *Cognitive Therapy and Research, 25,* 447–475.

Rudolph, K. D., Troop-Gordon, W., & Llewellyn, N. (2013). Interactive contributions of self-regulation deficits and social motivation to psychopathology: Unraveling divergent pathways to aggressive behavior and depressive symptoms. *Development and Psychopathology, 25*(2), 407–418.

Rueter, M. A., Scaramella, L., Wallace, L. E., & Conger, R. D. (1999). First onset of depressive or anxiety disorders predicted by the longitudinal course of internalizing symptoms and parent-adolescent disagreements. *Archives of General Psychiatry, 56,* 726–732.

Rutter, M., & Sroufe, L. A. (2000). Developmental psychopathology: Concepts and challenges. *Development and Psychopathology, 12*(3), 265–296.

Ryan, N. D., Puig-Antich, J., Ambrosini, P., Rabinovich, H., Robinson, D., Nelson, B., et al. (1987). The clinical picture of major depression in children and adolescents. *Archives of General Psychiatry, 44*(10), 854–861.

Sandstrom, M. J., Cillessen, A. H. N., & Eisenhower, A. (2003). Children's appraisal of peer rejection experiences: Impact on social and emotional adjustment. *Social Development, 12,* 530–550.

Sapolsky, R. M. (2003). Stress and plasticity in the limbic system. *Neurochemical Research, 28*(11), 1735–1742.

Schneider, M. L., Moore, C. F., & Kraemer, G. W. (2003). On the relevance of prenatal stress to developmental psychopathology: A primate model. In D. Cicchetti & E. Walker (Eds.), *Neurodevelopmental mechanisms in psychopathology* (pp. 155–186). New York, NY: Cambridge University Press.

Schrepferman, L. M., Eby, J., Snyder, J., & Stropes, J. (2006). Early affiliation and social engagement with peers: Prospective risk and protective factors for childhood depressive behaviors. *Journal of Emotional and Behavioral Disorders, 14,* 50–61.

Scourfield, J., Rice, F., Thapar, A., Harold, G. T., Martin, N., & McGuffin, P. (2003). Depressive symptoms in children and adolescents: Changing aetiological influences with development. *Journal of Child Psychology and Psychiatry, 44*(7), 968–976.

Shad, M. U., Bidesi, A. P., Chen, L. A., Ernst, M., & Rao, U. (2011). Neurobiology of decision making in depressed adolescents: A functional magnetic resonance imaging study. *Journal of American Academy of Child and Adolescent Psychiatry, 50*(6), 612–621.

Shad, M. U., Muddasani, S., & Rao, U. (2012). Gray matter differences between healthy and depressed adolescents: A voxel-based morphometry study. *Journal of Child and Adolescent Psychopharmacology, 22*(3), 190–197.

Sheeber, L., Hops, H., Alpert, A., Davis, B., & Andrews, J. A. (1997). Family support and conflict: Prospective relations to adolescent depression. *Journal of Abnormal Child Psychology, 25,* 333–344.

Sheeber, L., Hops, H., & Davis, B. (2001). Family processes in adolescent depression. *Clinical Child and Family Psychology Review, 4,* 19–35.

Shih, J. H., Eberhart, N. K., Hammen, C. L., & Brennan, P. A. (2006). Differential exposure and reactivity to interpersonal stress predict sex differences in adolescent depression. *Journal of Clinical Child and Adolescent Psychology, 35,* 103–115.

Shiner, R. L., & Masten, A. S. (2012). Childhood personality as a harbinger of competence and resilience in adulthood. *Development and Psychopathology, 24*(2), 507–528.

Silberg, J., Pickles, A., Rutter, M., Hewitt, J., Simonoff, E., Maes, H., et al. (1999). The influence of genetic factors and life stress on depression among adolescent girls. *Archives of General Psychiatry, 56*(3), 225–232.

Silk, J. S., Shaw, D. S., Forbes, E. E., Lane, T. L., & Kovacs, M. (2006). Maternal depression and child internalizing: The moderating role of child emotion regulation. *Journal of Clinical Child and Adolescent Psychology, 35*, 116–126.

Solomon, A., Ruscio, J., Seeley, J. R., & Lewinsohn, P. M. (2006). A taxometric investigation of unipolar depression in a large community sample. *Psychological Medicine, 36*, 973–985.

Sorensen, M. J., Nissen, J. B., Mors, O., & Thomsen, P. H. (2005). Age and gender differences in depressive symptomatology and comorbidity: An incident sample of psychiatrically admitted children. *Journal of Affective Disorders, 84*, 85–91.

Stein, D., Williamson, D. E., Birmaher, B., Brent, D. A., Kaufman, J., Dahl, R. E., et al. (2000). Parent–child bonding and family functioning in depressed children and children at high risk and low risk for future depression. *Journal of the American Academy of Child and Adolescent Psychiatry, 39*, 1387–1395.

Steingard, R. J., Renshaw, P. F., Hennen, J., Lenox, M., Cintron, C. B., Young, A. D., et al. (2002). Smaller frontal lobe white matter volumes in depressed adolescents. *Biological Psychiatry, 52*(5), 413–417.

Steinhausen, H. C., & Winkler, M. C. (2003). Prevalence of affective disorders in children and adolescents: Findings from the Zurich epidemiological studies. *Acta Psychiatrica Scandinavica, 108*, 20–23.

Stice, E., Hayward, C., Cameron, R. P., Killen, J. D., & Taylor, C. B. (2000). Body-image and eating disturbances predict onset of depression among female adolescents: A longitudinal study. *Journal of Abnormal Psychology, 109*, 438–444.

Strauman, T. J., Costanzo, P. R., & Garber, J. (Eds.). (2011). *Depression in adolescent girls: Science and prevention*. New York: Guilford.

Sugimura, N., & Rudolph, K. (2012). Temperamental differences in children's reactions to peer victimization. *Journal of Clinical Child and Adolescent Psychology, 41*(3), 314–328.

Sullivan, P. F., Neale, M. C., & Kendler, K. S. (2000). Genetic epidemiology of major depression: Review and meta-analysis. *American Journal of Psychiatry, 157*(10), 1552–1562.

Tackett, J. L. (2006). Evaluating models of the personality-psychopathology relationship in children and adolescents. *Clinical Psychology Review, 26*, 584–599.

Taylor, L., & Ingram, R. E. (1999). Cognitive reactivity and depressotypic information processing in children of depressed mothers. *Journal of Abnormal Psychology, 108*, 202–210.

Teasdale, J. D. (1983). Negative thinking in depression: Cause, effect or reciprocal relationship? *Advances in Behavior Research and Therapy, 5*, 3–25.

Teasdale, J. D. (1988). Cognitive vulnerability to persistent depression. *Cognition and Emotion, 2*, 247–274.

Teunissen, H. A., Adelman, C. B., Prinstein, M. J., Spijkerman, R., Poelen, E. A. P., Engels, R. C. M. E., et al. (2011). The interaction between pubertal timing and peer popularity for boys and girls: An integration of biological and interpersonal perspectives on adolescent depression. *Journal of Abnormal Child Psychology, 39*, 413–423.

Thomas, A., & Chess, S. (1977). *Temperament and development*. Oxford, UK: Brunner/Mazel.

Thomson, R. A. (1994). Emotion regulation: A theme in search of definition. *Monographs of the Society for Research in Child Development, 59*, 25–52.

Timbremont, B., & Braet, C. (2004). Cognitive vulnerability in remitted depressed children and adolescents. *Behaviour Research and Therapy, 42*, 423–437.

Tomarken, A. J., Dichter, G. S., Garber, J., & Simien, C. (2004). Resting frontal brain activity: Linkages to maternal depression and socio-economic status among adolescents. *Biological Psychology, 67*(1–2), 77–102.

Twenge, J. M., & Nolen-Hoeksema, S. (2002). Age, gender, race, socioeconomic status, and birth cohort differences on the Children's Depression Inventory: A meta-analysis. *Journal of Abnormal Psychology, 111*(4), 578–588.

Uhrlass, D. J., & Gibb, B. E. (2007). Childhood emotional maltreatment and the stress generation model of depression. *Journal of Social and Clinical Psychology, 26*, 119–130.

van Leeuwen, K. G., Mervielde, I., De Clercq, B. J., & De Fruyt, F. (2007). Extending the spectrum idea: Child personality, parenting and psychopathology. *European Journal of Personality, 21*, 63–89.

Wagner, K. D. (2003). Major depression in children and adolescents. *Psychiatric Annals, 33*, 266–270.

Waller, N. G., & Meehl, P. E. (1998). *Multivariate taxometric procedures: Distinguishing types from continua*. Thousand Oaks, CA: Sage.

Weinstock, M. (2005). The potential influence of maternal stress hormones on development and mental health of the offspring. *Brain, Behavior, and Immunity, 19*, 296–308.

Weir, J. M., Zakama, A., & Rao, U. (2012). Developmental risk I: Depression and the developing brain. *Child and Adolescent Psychiatric Clinics of North America, 21*(2), 237–259.

Weiss, B., & Garber, J. (2003). Developmental differences in the phenomenology of depression. *Development and Psychopathology, 15*, 403–430.

Weissman, M. M., & Olfson, M. (1995). Depression in women: Implications for health care research. *Science, 269*, 799–801.

Weissman, M. M., Wolk, S., Goldstein, R. B., Moreau, D., Adams, P., Greenwald, S., et al. (1999). Depressed adolescents grown up. *Journal of American Medical Association, 281*, 1707–1713.

Weisz, J. R., Southam-Gerow, M. A., & McCarty, C. A. (2001). Control-related beliefs and depressive symptoms in clinic-referred children and adolescents: Developmental differences and model specificity. *Journal of Abnormal Psychology, 110*, 97–109.

Wetter, E. K., & Hankin, B. L. (2009). Mediational pathways through which positive and negative emotionality contribute to anhedonic symptoms of depression: A prospective study of adolescents. *Journal of Abnormal Child Psychology, 37*, 507–520.

Wigg, K., Feng, Y., Gomez, L., Kiss, E., Kapornai, K., Tamás, Z., et al. (2009). Genome scan in sibling pairs with juvenile-onset mood disorders: Evidence for linkage to 13q and Xq. *American Journal of Medical Genetics Part B: Neuropsychiatric Genetics, 150*(5), 638–646.

Williamson, D. E., Birmaher, B., Dahl, R. E., al-Shabbout, M., & Ryan, N. D. (1996). Stressful life events influence nocturnal growth hormone secretion in depressed children. *Biological Psychiatry, 40*(11), 1176–1180.

World Health Organization. (2008). *The global burden of disease: 2004 Update.* Geneva, Switzerland: World Health Organization Press.

Yildiz-Yesiloglu, A., & Ankerst, D. P. (2006). Review of 1H magnetic resonance spectroscopy findings in major depressive disorder: A meta-analysis. *Psychiatry Research, 147*(1), 1–25.

Yorbik, O., Birmaher, B., Axelson, D., Williamson, D. E., & Ryan, N. D. (2004). Clinical characteristics of depressive symptoms in children and adolescents with major depressive disorder. *Journal of Clinical Psychiatry, 65*, 1654–1659.

Zalsman, G., Oquendo, M. A., Greenhill, L., Goldberg, P. H., Kamali, M., Martin, A., et al. (2006). Neurobiology of depression in children and adolescents. *Child and Adolescent Psychiatric Clinics of North America, 15*(4), 843–868.

A Developmental Model of Self-Inflicted Injury, Borderline Personality, and Suicide Risk

26

Christina M. Derbidge and Theodore P. Beauchaine

Human fascination with life and death needs little explanation. We are confronted with our own and others' mortality from very early in life. Yet we find self-injury and suicide, which have been observed throughout recorded history, to be confusing and uncomfortable to discuss (for a review, see van Hooff, 2000). In part, our discomfort derives from historical conceptions of immorality that have been associated with suicide and related behaviors for centuries. As far back as anthropologists can trace, across all cultures, humans with tools appear to have used those tools to hurt and kill themselves. Presently, over one million people worldwide die by suicide each year (World Health Organization [WHO], 2012). Why, we ask? Published works have explored this question for centuries (e.g., Durkheim, 1951; Merian, 1763; Shneidman, 1985), yet the answer eludes us.

Over the course of the twentieth century, substantive gains in longevity were observed, with people living 30 years longer in 1999 than in 1900 (Centers for Disease Control and Prevention

C.M. Derbidge, Ph.D.
George E. Wahlen, Department of Veterans Affairs
Medical Center, 500 Foothill Drive, Salt Lake City,
UT 84148, USA
e-mail: christina.derbidge@va.gov

T.P. Beauchaine, Ph.D. (✉)
Department of Psychology, The Ohio State
University, 233 Psychology Building,
1835 Neil Avenue, Columbus, OH 43201, USA
e-mail: beauchaine.1@osu.edu

[CDC], 1999). Although this trend has slowed, year-to-year increases in longevity continue (Kochanek, Xu, Murphy, Miniño, & Kung, 2011). Between 1999 and 2009, life expectancy increased by 1.8 years. This increased longevity follows from reduced mortality for many leading causes of death including heart disease, several forms of cancer, cerebrovascular disease, diabetes, influenza, and pneumonia, among others. In contrast, age-adjusted suicide mortality rates have increased from 10.5 per 100,000 in 1999 to 11.8 per 100,000 in 2009. However, overall mortality rates obscure differences in suicide rates among those with particular characteristics, across cohorts, and in different geographical locals (Gunnell, 2000). Alarming rates of suicide in certain subpopulations, and its resistance to intervention, make it a major public health concern (U.S. Public Health Service, 1999).

In this chapter, we describe a developmental model of self-inflicted injury (SII), the single best prospective predictor of suicide risk (e.g., Joiner et al., 2005). We state at the outset that our model is not meant to capture all causes of suicide. Such causes are diverse and cannot possibly be accounted for by a single etiological model. Indeed, increased suicide rates are observed among those afflicted with a wide range of psychiatric disorders (e.g., unipolar depression, bipolar depression, antisocial personality disorder, borderline personality disorder, substance use disorders, eating disorders) and medical conditions (e.g., amyotrophic lateral sclerosis, cancer, diabetes), and among those confronted with

M. Lewis and K.D. Rudolph (eds.), *Handbook of Developmental Psychopathology*,
DOI 10.1007/978-1-4614-9608-3_26, © Springer Science+Business Media New York 2014

traumatic life experiences and other untoward environmental events (e.g., child sexual abuse, death of a family member, prolonged unemployment). Thus, many routes to suicide exist, some of which overlap and others of which do not overlap with the pathway discussed below.

In the sections to follow, we first review the history of studying suicide, or suicidology as it is commonly called today, as it has strong reverberations for current theoretical perspectives and knowledge (Shneidman, 1985). We follow this with a discussion of definitions necessary to understand research in the field today. Next, we examine current knowledge about self-injury and suicide and identify commonalities and variations in the course and etiology of suicide across the lifespan. In addition to asking why people hurt themselves, we ask "Why now?" and in doing so, we explicate our developmental model of self-injury and suicide risk (Beauchaine, Klein, Crowell, Derbidge, & Gatzke-Kopp, 2009; Crowell, Beauchaine, & Linehan, 2009; Crowell, Derbidge, & Beauchaine, in press), in hopes of influencing future research to focus on underlying mechanisms rather than correlates. Finally, we comment on potential implications of a developmental psychopathology perspective for advancing suicide prevention research. Given the scope of suicide research, we acknowledge at the outset that some topics cannot be explored in full detail. However, our reference list includes many original sources for interested readers.

Suicide, Morality, and History

The value placed on human life and the control afforded to individuals over their own lives are deeply embedded in Western conceptualizations of morality, culture, and society (for a review, see van Hooff, 2000). In ancient Rome and Greece, suicide was sometimes a way to reclaim or maintain one's honor in the face of shame, or a means for a victim to transform into a tragic hero. In contrast, other cultures have viewed suicide as an indication of personal weakness, cowardice, or sin. For example, in the Middle Ages, suicide was condemned by the Roman Catholic Church,

and suicide completers were denied proper burials, or buried with stakes in their hearts after being dragged through the street (Farberow, 1975). In modern Western society, we often see suicidal wishes as responses to suffering from psychological pain (e.g., King, 1998). Nevertheless, many still hold the belief that suicidal impulses reflect moral deficiency.

Despite an established tradition of research, attempts to define suicide still incite impassioned debate (e.g., Linehan, Comtois, Brown, Heard, & Wagner, 2006; Silverman, Berman, Sanddal, O'Carroll, & Joiner, 2007a, 2007b). For example, is martyrdom really suicide? Is passive acceptance of death and refusal for treatment suicide? Is euthanasia, where an individual prepares the circumstances for his/her death, but someone else takes the final steps, suicide? People among different nations, cultures, and states feel differently about this, but as a rule of thumb when a behavior is widely accepted by a society, it is not usually considered to be suicide. Assisted suicide and euthanasia in the face of intractable suffering and terminal illness are condoned or condemned to varying degrees across nations and remain active areas of controversy within bioethics (Borry, Schotsmans, & Dierickx, 2006). Assisted suicides are legal in several countries such as the Netherlands and Switzerland and in US states including Oregon, Montana, and Washington (Borry et al., 2006; Cohen-Almagor, 2001). Euthanasia is less often legal. Although supporters claim compassion, research conducted among elderly with terminal illnesses suggests that wishes to die are often transient, correlated with depressive states, and treatable (e.g., Ganzini, Goy, & Dobscha, 2008). One lesson to be learned from reviewing this history is that individual suicides occur in broader sociopolitical contexts. Decisions to suicide are affected not only by unique struggles faced by individuals living in certain times, but also by unique sociopolitical and moral influences. In today's multicultural societies, moral codes are more complex, fluid, and nuanced than in monocultural societies.

The modern lifespan approach to studying suicide embraces the importance of context, particularly through evaluation of groups of people within particular age cohorts (e.g., those born in the USA during the Great Depression, World War II, or following 9/11). We discuss this approach further below. Yet, as those who study lifespan development agree, moral codes and historical context alone cannot explain suicide, for not every shamed Roman took his or her life and not every terminally ill person with the option of assisted suicide or euthanasia chooses it. However, the meaning of life and death to a person and the context in which a person lives (including historical epoch) clearly matter. These factors affect public discourses around suicide, stigma, funds for research, and willingness to accept treatment or disclose suicidal thoughts and urges. In the next section, we expand on the historical foundations for modern Western perspectives of the meaning of suicide.

Empirical Foundations of Suicidology

Despite varied moral and cultural influences on the meaning of suicide, contemporary conceptualizations usually emphasize psychological distress and/or psychiatric impairment. As noted above, various forms of psychopathology confer elevated risk of self-injury and suicide (e.g., Haw, Hawton, Houston, & Townsend, 2001). However, most who are afflicted by psychopathology do not engage in self-injury or suicide, and many who suicide do not suffer from psychiatric impairment (see above). Accordingly, additional influences must be considered. From this standpoint, the perspectives of Durkheim (e.g., 1951) and Shneidman (e.g., 1985) are central to modern conceptualizations of suicide risk.

The empirical study of suicide originates with Durkheim (ca. 1858–1917) and some of his predecessors (e.g., Thomas Masaryk, ca. 1850–1937). Durkheim, widely regarded as the founder of empirical sociology, focused his study of suicide on societal or group-level phenomena (e.g., Durkheim, 1951). Durkheim was the first to discover several correlates of suicide risk. Among these, he noted that suicide rates are

higher for (1) men than women, (2) people without children than people with children, (3) single than married people, (4) soldiers than civilians, and (5) nonreligious than religious people. Durkheim identified four types of suicide along two continua. On the first continuum, suicide is related to individuality versus group cohesion. Durkheim believed that when social bonds are too thin, people become too individualized, which gives rise to a sense of meaninglessness, apathy, depression, and what he termed *egoistic* suicide. He believed that religious affiliation and nationalism (e.g., war time decreases in suicide) protected people from suicide so long as bonds were not too tight such that a person was likely to place his/her life secondary to the whole and perform *altruistic* suicide. The second continuum concerned the degree to which a society regulates individuals and businesses. Durkheim stated that unregulated businesses can result in boom and bust cycles that produce extreme fluctuations in wealth for societies and individuals, both of which can lead to a dramatic sense of instability and *anomic* suicide. Oppressive regulation, on the other hand, leads to hopelessness and what is termed *fatalistic* suicide (e.g., slaves who suicide). Durkheim devoted most of his attention to *egoistic* suicide, which he believed stems from social disintegration. Durkheim's theoretical paradigm of disintegration foreshadowed concepts such as thwarted belongingness (e.g., Joiner et al., 2005) and lack of connectedness, espoused as key factors in suicide research and prevention today. Although he tended to view suicide as a phenomenon caused by environmental forces and independent of psychopathology, Durkheim's work has been credited as a precursor to the psychosocial view of suicide often espoused in modern perspectives.

Edwin Shneidman (ca. 1918–2009), a clinical psychologist, revered Durkheim's work (see Leenaars, 2010, for a review of Shneidman's life work). As an intern at the Los Angeles Veterans Administration, Shneidman was asked to write letters to two widows of individuals who killed themselves. In researching those cases, he discovered hundreds of files of individuals who died by suicide and many suicide notes. He quickly realized that rigorous and systematic scientific evaluation of those notes could be invaluable toward furthering understanding of suicide. In a controlled double-blind experiment, Shneidman evaluated differences and similarities between those notes and simulated notes created by non-suicidal individuals. He identified several characteristics common to suicide notes, which we review briefly below. The discovery of these notes sparked an immensely fruitful career and a new field of research devoted to studying suicide and suicide prevention, which he termed suicidology. In addition to his widely cited "ten commonalities" (see below), Shneidman observed a general characteristic of suicidal individuals, which helped change societal perspectives on suicide: ambivalence. Even in the end stages of planning to suicide, most people still have some desire to live or be rescued. This discovery led Shneidman, along with Roman Farberow and Robert Litman, to found the Los Angeles Suicide Prevention Center in the late 1950s, which became the first suicide crisis call center in the USA. From there, Shneidman worked tirelessly with the National Institute of Mental Health to create a network of crisis centers across the nation. In 1964, Shneidman founded the American Association of Suicidology, which remains active today.

Shneidman (1985) believed that suicide was a result of "psychache" or psychological pain. He asserted that the vast majority of committed suicides, "95 of 100" (Shneidman, 1996, p. 129), have 10 commonalities. Because Shneidman's work is so fundamental to the modern psychological perspective on suicide, we list these commonalities here: (1) a common *purpose* is to seek a solution to a problem that generates unbearable suffering and eludes an acceptable alternative solution; (2) a common *goal* is the cessation of consciousness in order to stop unbearable suffering; (3) a common *stimulus* is psychological pain or psychache, from which the person seeks escape; (4) a common *stressor* is frustrated psychological need (e.g., achievement, affiliation); (5) a common *emotion* is hopelessness-helplessness, such that nothing can be done to escape the situation; (6) a common *cognitive state*

is ambivalence, wishing both to die and be rescued (reminiscent of Freud's (1965) Thanatos and Eros); (7) a common *perception* is constriction, a transient psychological state in which the individual experiences "tunnel vision," or a narrowing of plausible solutions; (8) a common *action* is escape from the problem and the pain; (9) a common *interpersonal act* is communication of intention, or exhibition of signs of intent, signals of distress or helplessness, or pleas for help; and (10) a common *pattern* is consistent with lifelong styles of coping, such that the act and manner of suicide is consistent with prior coping patterns. Shneidman (1991) suggested that suicide happens for a given individual at a given time because he or she has reached a peak, or intolerable level, of press (high psychosocial pressures), pain (psychological distress), and perturbation (cognitive constriction leading to "precipitous or ill-advised action" or self-destructive tendencies when coping; p. 47). Notably, Shneidman defined pain similar to modern definitions of emotion dysregulation and perturbation similar to modern definitions of impulsivity; two commonly discussed vulnerabilities for suicide that we propose interact with psychosocial stressors to potentiate suicide risk (Beauchaine et al., 2009; Crowell et al., 2009, in press). We discuss these vulnerabilities in further detail in later sections.

In his writings and interviews, Shneidman seemed to struggle between his support of scientific inquiry, which has identified several biological and social correlates of suicide, with his ultimate belief that suicide is primarily a psychological phenomenon, the result of *psychache*, largely influenced by personality characteristics determined by events in childhood (for a review, see Leenaars, 2010). He likened the suicidal person to a tree, with surrounding soil, roots, branches, and leaves that have several plausible influences. The most prominent feature, the trunk, he asserted was the *psychache*. He noted how a true understanding of the individual, their history, and lifelong modes of coping illuminate the inevitability of suicide when in a particular circumstance without external intervention. The solution to *psychache* is to resolve or alter needs and coping of individuals in pain (Shneidman, 1996). His perspective was to alter the character or personality of individuals, thus altering their approaches to obtaining unmet needs. Despite obvious psychodynamic underpinnings, Shneidman's work led to cognitive-behavioral theories of suicide given identification of the interplay among cognitions, behaviors, and emotions common to suicidal individuals (e.g., Ellis, 2006).

Definitional Considerations: Suicide and Self-Inflicted Injury

Despite a well-established tradition of research on suicide and Shneidman's (1985) extensive work on delineating the construct, defining and conceptualizing suicide remains a challenge (e.g., Linehan et al., 2006; Silverman et al., 2007a, 2007b). Early definitions of suicide proposed by Durkheim and Shneidman are often quoted. Durkheim (1951) defined suicide as follows: "…all cases of death resulting directly or indirectly from a positive or negative act of the victim himself, which he knows will produce this result" (p. 44). Although Durkheim's (1951) focus was consistent with lay terminology, Shneidman (1985) defined suicide in psychological terms as "a conscious act of self-induced annihilation, best understood as a multidimensional malaise in a needful individual who defines an issue for which the suicide is perceived as the best solution" (p. 203). Much of Shneidman's theoretical perspective is embedded in this definition, something most modern researchers tend to avoid in order to promote clarity across areas and fields invested in suicide research (e.g., Linehan et al., 2006).

Much of the challenge in defining suicide derives from our inability to know for certain, without a suicide note, the intention of the individual (for a review, see Maris, Berman, & Silverman, 2000). In addition, surviving friends and relatives often have a vested interest in keeping the death from being classified as suicide, for reasons of avoiding stigma, claiming insurance benefits, etc. Furthermore, governments that report low suicide rates and strongly disapprove of suicide may not adequately investigate or accept suicide as a possibility when it exists. It is widely believed that these and other challenges result in an underestimation of the number of suicides worldwide by at least 10 %.

These issues notwithstanding, much of the definitional controversy today concerns the scope of behaviors that should be included in research on suicide, and whether categorization of suicide and suicide-related behaviors including self-inflicted injury (SII) would be better served by a focus on lethality, intention, method, consequence, or some combination of these factors (e.g., Linehan et al., 2006; Silverman et al. 2007a, 2007b). For example, some question whether various suicide-related behaviors should be classified together (e.g., attempted suicide, suicidal ideation without attempt or injury, nonfatal self-injury without suicidal intent). Can an attempt with very little or no chance of resulting in death be considered a suicide attempt? Some propose the use of the term suicidal gesture in this situation. What about self-inflicted injuries enacted without intent to die and without medical purpose, but for some psychological purpose? Are these acts related or qualitatively different? Although he clearly believed in the value of separating various suicide-related behaviors across studies, Shneidman (1985) argued that the broad scope of suicide-related behaviors is relevant to prevention efforts and therefore should be included in the field of suicidology.

Researchers who focus primarily on completed suicide often note the widely different demographic correlates and prevalence rates of completed suicide versus attempted suicides and other nonfatal self-injuries (for a review, see Maris et al., 2000). For example, in the US, the male-to-female suicide ratio is 4:3, yet females attempt suicide three times more often than males and are 1.5 times more likely to self-inflict injury (Hawton & Harris, 2008). In fact, with a 13 % prevalence rate among adolescents (Lloyd-Richardson, Perrine, Dierker, & Kelley, 2007) self-inflicted injury (SII) is much more common than suicide, which is observed in only about 12 of 100,000 individuals (Kochanek et al., 2011). Based on such data and concerns expressed by some experts that individuals who study mostly attempters or nonsuicidal self-injurers identify their work primarily as studying suicide (Maris et al., 2000), some have begun to focus on particular subtypes of self-injury, such as nonsuicidal self-injury (e.g., Crowell et al., 2005, 2008, 2012; Nock, Joiner, Gordon, Lloyd-Richardson, & Prinstein, 2006). However, as Linehan et al. (2006) proposed, although agreement and usage of terms would be ideal for promoting scientific advancement, comparability across samples would be vastly improved if researchers simply categorized acts according to a few key features, namely, method, potential for lethality, intention, and consequence.

Differences notwithstanding, suicidal ideation and attempts are often precursors to suicide (e.g., Caspi et al., 2003). Approximately 15 % of suicide attempters eventually die by suicide (Bongar, 2002). Moreover, despite large discrepancies among rates of self-injury, suicide attempts, and suicide completion, self-inflicted injury remains the single best predictor of later suicide across all ages, regardless of whether the injury was enacted with intent to die (Hawton et al., 2012; Joiner et al., 2005). In addition, there is substantial overlap between biological vulnerabilities to and environmental risk factors for suicide-related behaviors (Joiner et al., 2005). This has led our research group and others to propose that, among vulnerable individuals, there is a developmental progression from ideation or mild self-injury (e.g., scratching self, poking self with pins, picking at wounds) to behaviors that increase in lethality and degree of suicidal intent (Beauchaine et al., 2009; Crowell et al., 2009, in press).

For these reasons, we conceptualize SII as a spectrum of thoughts and behaviors (e.g., Crowell et al., 2009; Nock et al., 2006) including suicidal ideation, nonsuicidal SII, and suicidal SII or suicide attempts (Crowell et al., in press). Self-inflicted injury is defined as a purposeful act of self-injury accompanied by intent to cause acute physical injury or death. Self-inflicted injury can be subdivided into (1) suicidal SII, including all deliberate acts of acute physical injury enacted with some degree of suicidal intent, including those characterized by ambivalence, and (2) nonsuicidal SII, including all deliberate acts of acute physical injury enacted without any degree of suicidal intent. We consider these overt acts separately from the covert cognitive process of suicidal ideation.

Demographics of Suicide Risk: A Statistical Snapshot

With a few key exceptions (e.g., Caspi, 2000), two methods dominate the study of suicide across the lifespan: epidemiological and cohort studies (Stillion & McDowell, 1996). Epidemiological studies have been helpful in discovering population rates of suicide associated with key demographic variables (e.g., age, sex, race, ethnicity). However, given the broad scope and expense of such studies, they often cannot include key psychological, social, or biological variables that represent mechanisms of vulnerability and risk. In contrast, although the cohort method does an excellent job of explicating risk factors unique to groups of people living in particular historical epochs, it requires constant updating as cohorts move through new developmental stages. In addition, the cohort approach confounds cohort-specific factors with age. It may also miss common factors associated with suicide, regardless of age (e.g., Shneidman, 1985). Methodological considerations aside, there are some characteristics of suicide of which readers should be aware.

Suicidal behaviors are observed across most of the lifespan, beginning in mid- to late childhood (Stillion & McDowell, 1996). However, suicide rates vary dramatically across geographical locals, economic conditions, and according to several additional personal factors such as age, ethnicity, sex, and marital status (Gunnell, 2000). We summarize several of these factors below.

First, as noted above, males exhibit higher suicide rates than females, at least in part because they use more lethal means. Across the world, with the exception of China, males are much more likely to die by suicide than females (WHO, 2011). For each racial and ethnic group within the US, males exhibit higher rates of suicide than females, with a sex ratio of approximately 4:1.

However, females attempt suicide three times more often than males (Krug & WHO, 2002). In addition, Whites tend to have higher rates of suicide than other racial and ethnic groups except during young adulthood when rates are highest among American Indians and Alaskan Natives.

Second, rates of suicide peak at different times in life depending on sex, race, and ethnicity. The rate of White male suicide increases with age, peaking in older adulthood. Older adult White males (80+) have higher suicide rates than any other age, racial, or ethnic group in the US. Rates of suicide also increase with age for Asian/ Pacific Islander males and females, and for Latino males. However, for Native Americans and Alaskan Natives (combined data), suicide rates for both sexes peak in adolescence and early adulthood (between ages 15 and 24) and decline thereafter. In contrast, White, Black, and Latina suicide rates are highest in midlife (ages 25–44). Notably, however, lifespan suicide rates are much lower among Blacks and Latinas than among any other aforementioned group.

Third, although suicide rates have increased over the last decade (see above), the overall rate of suicide across the 20th Century has not changed much, yet the distribution of suicides across the lifespan has changed. Rates of elderly suicides have decreased, whereas rates of adolescent and young adult suicides have increased.

Fourth, access to, knowledge of, and use of more lethal means may moderate differences in suicide rates observed across groups (e.g., sex, nationality/geographical region). Recall that males are likely to use more lethal means (e.g., Elnour & Harrison, 2008) and to die by suicide despite much higher rates of attempts among females (Krug, 2002). Firearms are a highly lethal means of suicide, and positive correlations between gun ownership and overall suicide rates have been reported (Miller & Hemenway, 2008). Moreover, some occupations confer greater risk than others (e.g., healthcare workers, pharmacists, farmers), perhaps due to increased access and knowledge of lethal means (Kelly & Bunting, 1998).

Suicide Across the Lifespan

Childhood Suicide

Although rare, childhood suicide does occur. Because of its rarity and ethical considerations of discussing suicide with community samples of young children, data beyond basic descriptive statistics are sparse. From 1999 to 2009, approximately 279 US children per year died by suicide. Approximately 5 per year were between ages of 5 and 9 years old. In these rare cases, children are often profoundly impaired intellectually and/or psychologically (Hawton, 1982). Children seem to be protected by their limited lifespan and cognitive capacities in terms of not having had much time to accumulate life stressors and knowledge about suicide means and methods (Stillion & McDowell, 1996). Yet for those who have experienced extreme loss, abuse, or neglect, cognitive immaturity may put them at risk for suicide. Children may not understand that death is permanent, an insight that usually develops somewhere between ages of 7 and 12 years. In this age group, attempts appear to be extremely impulsive, highly lethal (e.g., jumping out of a window), yet set off by seemingly minor events (e.g., criticism by a teacher). Warning signs include trouble in school, low frustration tolerance, aggressiveness, and impulsiveness, among others (Maris et al., 2000; Stillion & McDowell, 1996). We should note, however, that accurate prediction of child suicide is impossible statistically given the large number of children who exhibit such signs compared with the exceedingly small number of children who suicide.

Adolescent and Young Adulthood Suicide

Many adolescents and young adults who suicide suffer from severe psychopathology (e.g., comorbid affective disorders and substance use or antisocial behavior), trouble in school, and emotional lability (e.g., Maris et al., 2000; Stillion & McDowell, 1996). Families of these youth tend to be chaotic, unresponsive to their children's needs, and suffer from numerous problems, such as parental alcohol and other drug abuse. A major challenge of adolescence is to develop a sense of identity within society, not unlike Durkheim's (1951) description of a need to belong. If this need is unmet or achieving it exceeds a teen's ability to cope, he or she may be at increased risk for suicide. Unsuccessful navigation may also portend difficulties meeting future developmental challenges that ordinarily build upon a strong self-identity (e.g., successful marriage and child relationships), conferring additional risk. Indeed, the large degree of culture loss experienced by indigenous populations may contribute to heightened rates of suicide among Native Americans and Alaskan Natives (Joiner, 2005; Wexler & Gone, 2012). Individuals who commit suicide tend to have less interpersonal support and less satisfying relationships both within and outside the home.

Suicide among vulnerable adolescents often follows stressful life events that are interpersonal in nature such as romantic rejection, arguments about discipline, or separation from home and friends (e.g., Lewinsohn, Rohde, & Seeley, 1995). However, past suicidal behavior is more predictive of future suicidal behavior than any of these factors (e.g., Hawton et al., 2012). Nevertheless, stressful life events likely function as triggers (proximal risk factors), perhaps nudging vulnerable youth past their threshold of coping ability (e.g., King, 1998). Another common trigger is suicide by a first- or second-degree relative and to a lesser extent a close friend (e.g., Voracek & Loibl, 2007). In addition, suicides sometimes cluster among teens, yet this accounts for only 1 % of teen suicides (Gould, Wallenstein, & Kleinman, 1990).

Alcohol use is especially concerning among vulnerable adolescents. Studies of adolescent-completed suicides reveal that half or more have alcohol use problems. Moreover, both adolescents and adults often consume alcohol just hours prior to their attempt (e.g., Hawton, Fagg, & McKeown, 1989).

As adolescents transition to young adulthood, seek employment, marry, and have children,

specific stressors may change, yet difficulties with coping still precipitate suicidal behaviors (Stillion & McDowell, 1996). Interpersonal stressors remain important (e.g., lack of social support combined with young children and marital conflict; Brown & Harris, 1978), especially for women. For young adult women, moves are often perceived as highly stressful even if they result in greater opportunity, better employment, and higher standard of living. In contrast, risk of suicide for young men is associated more with occupational stress, although marital stress also contributes (Illfeld, 1977). Some have suggested that the rates of suicide in this age range result from cohort effects, with suicide rates increasing proportionally with the number of individuals of that age who are competing for jobs, spouses, and other resources (e.g., Easterlin, 1980).

Midlife Suicide

Like young adults, suicidal behaviors among middle-aged adults most commonly follow accumulated stressors among those with some form of affective disorder and/or alcoholism (Stillion & McDowell, 1996). Middle adulthood presents several new challenges. Particular stressors for this age group sometimes include declining health, financial pressures, and interpersonal losses or death of loved ones. For some, there is professional stagnation, such that they have reached the height of their careers and yet remain unfulfilled (Maris, 1981). Maris calls this the "suicidal career." As previously noted, the suicide rate among White females does not exhibit the same linear increase observed among White males. Rather, White females are at highest risk between ages 45 and 64, with a rate of 9.4 per 100,000. This is paralleled by a drop in nonfatal self-injuries (Nock et al., 2008). Longitudinal follow-up studies are needed, but perhaps the declining rate of nonfatal SII is in part because at least some women who previously attempted or self-injured have completed suicide. Multiple life transitions may enhance stress within this age group, including "empty nest" syndrome. Alternatively, with the increase of women in the workforce, and a slightly later career peak, perhaps the increased suicide rate is also influenced by the so-called suicidal career. Regardless, coping mechanisms developed at younger ages may either prepare people well for this stage of life or place them at risk of failing to navigate midlife transitions. Indeed, "baby boomers" were the first cohort to present with a dramatically increased adolescent suicide rate (e.g., Easterlin, 1980; Maris et al., 2000). When baby boomers again reached a developmental stage marked with new challenges and demands, the suicide rate for the middle-aged group increased.

Older-Age Suicide

Since the early 1900s, an overall decrease in rates of suicide among older adults has been observed (CDC, 1999). For the purposes of this discussion, however, we consider elderly to be over age 65 years. Among this group, the rate of suicide for White males over age 85 years is three times that observed among White males of ages 15 to 24. Risk factors associated with suicide among the elderly include alcohol abuse, psychiatric illness, availability of firearms, declining health, loss of loved ones, and failure to adapt to or accept changing life circumstances (Fiske, O'Riley, & Widow, 2008). Depression is related more strongly to suicide among older adults than younger adults. Although mechanisms through which age interacts with depression are unclear, physical illness has been linked consistently to suicide among older adults. Risk is especially elevated the first few years after diagnosis and during times of decreased functioning.

Interim Summary

To summarize, suicide appears to be the end result of a complex set of developmental pathways, a phenomenon known as equifinality. Reasons for taking one's life vary considerably across time periods, cultures, and age groups. However, these factors alone do not explain suicide risk fully. Within given time periods, cultures,

and age groups, several psychological (e.g., affective, cognitive), biological (e.g., genetic, neural, hormonal), and environmental (e.g., familial, social, contextual) factors increase risk. We review these factors further in the context of our developmental model, presented below.

Both psychiatric impairment and environmental risk factors also confer vulnerability to SII and suicide (Maris et al., 2000). Indeed, elevated suicide risk is observed among those with unipolar depression, bipolar depression, schizophrenia, borderline personality disorder, antisocial personality disorder, substance use disorders, and eating disorders, and among those who experience low social support, histories of childhood physical and sexual abuse, death of loved ones, and certain occupations (e.g., healthcare workers).

As noted by King (1998), "At the moment a human being engages in suicidal behavior, he or she has crossed the threshold for suffering and adaptive coping" (p. 329). This is consistent with Shneidman's assertion that psychache is common and necessary for suicide but also highlights a need for an organizing framework to explain why different individuals reach this threshold for coping at different times in life and why some specific risk factors vary across the lifespan but are common to life stages. We believe that developmental context is the key to identifying these common pathways and that understanding how development interacts with biological and psychosocial factors will result in new directions for intervention.

Modern Models of Suicide Across the Lifespan

Lifespan/developmental approaches to understanding suicide have existed for several decades (Leenaars, 1991; Stillion & McDowell, 1996). Proponents of lifespan approaches propose complex reciprocal interactions among psychological, biological, and environmental mechanisms over time in affecting risk for SII and suicide (e.g., Beauchaine et al., 2009; Crowell et al., 2009). To date, however, these models outstrip available data, since longitudinal research on suicide is sparse, and predominant models are fraught with limitations (Crowell et al., in press).

Developmental models have often focused on adolescents and young adults, neglecting large portions of the population and important processes that influence increasing risk for suicide with age (Leenaars, 1991; Stillion & McDowell, 1996). Furthermore, many models are based on clinical impressions and have not been tested empirically (Crowell et al., in press). Clinical impressions are derived primarily from individuals who are at high risk for suicide (e.g., borderline personality disorder and major depressive disorder), most of whom are not or have not been suicidal (e.g., Crowell et al., 2009). In addition, many existing models emphasize biological, psychological, or environmental factors as etiologically dominant and rarely examine interactions across levels of analysis. As noted above, lifespan research approaches have often used cohort designs, with limited follow-up periods, rather than longitudinal designs. The cohort approach assumes that unique qualities of a given historical epoch interact adversely with normative developmental challenges/stressors to predict negative mental health outcomes. Cohort studies inherently confound age with cohort. Cohort studies of baby boomers, for example, may leave us wondering whether adolescence and midlife are really times of increased suicide risk or whether factors specific to that cohort enhance risk at those ages. Only longitudinal research can disambiguate such questions.

Methodological limitations of current research make any comprehensive lifespan model of SII and suicide premature. Nevertheless, developmental models that propose plausible interacting mechanisms for suicide-related behaviors may be uniquely suited to answering the critically important question, "Why now?" (Crowell et al., in press).

Developmental Conceptualizations of Suicide

Despite the aforementioned limitations in our knowledge, there have been several recent attempts to specify developmental models of SII (Blumenthal & Kupfer, 1990; Crowell et al.,

2009, 2014; Leenaars, 1991; Stillion & McDowell, 1996). Following a developmental psychopathology perspective, our research group has recently proposed a model whereby many cases of SII and borderline personality disorder (BPD) emerge from common etiological/ developmental mechanisms (Beauchaine et al., 2009; Crowell et al., 2009). This model specifies how biological vulnerabilities interact with environmental adversity or protection to amplify or mollify risk of suicide among liable individuals, thereby accommodating the observation that not all who engage in SII go on to develop BPD.

The developmental psychopathology perspective emphasizes interactions among biological vulnerabilities and environmental risk factors in shaping trajectories to psychopathology (e.g., Hinshaw, 2013). In our view, SII results from interactions among (1) predisposing genetic vulnerabilities that give rise to both serotonergic and dopaminergic dysfunction (Crowell et al., 2005, 2009) and downstream other biological/behavioral vulnerabilities (e.g., trait impulsivity; Beauchaine et al., 2009) and (2) familial risk factors such as invalidating and coercive family environments (Beauchaine et al., 2009; Crowell et al., 2012). As articulated below, confluence of and interactions among these vulnerabilities and risk factors can produce enduring patterns of emotion dysregulation, for which SII is used by some to cope (Crowell et al., 2009). Importantly, none of these vulnerabilities or risk factors account for SII in isolation. Our developmental model, which we expand upon in sections to follow, can be summarized as follows (Beauchaine et al., 2009; Crowell et al., 2009, in press):

1. Trait impulsivity is a principle predisposing vulnerability to SII and BPD. It is present very early in life, is almost entirely heritable, and arises from central dopaminergic and serotonergic dysfunction.
2. Coercive and invalidating family interaction patterns reinforce emotional lability among trait-impulsive and therefore vulnerable individuals through operant reinforcement.
3. Across development, these interaction patterns produce enduring patterns of emotion dysregulation, poor behavioral control, and maladaptive cognitive coping styles, resulting

in rigidity, loneliness, hopelessness, low self-worth, difficulties with conflict resolution, and social withdrawal.

4. Affected individuals affiliate with deviant peer groups, within which contagion effects and social reinforcement act as mechanisms through which SII is acquired and maintained as a maladaptive emotion regulation strategy.

5. Over time, SII and related behaviors become canalized, contributing to development of BPD and related forms of psychopathology such as antisocial personality disorder (ASPD).

Below we review briefly each of these suppositions in light of recent research on the development of SII.

Impulsivity, SII, and BPD

Trait impulsivity, present very early in life and derived largely from central dopaminergic and serotonergic dysfunction, is a principle predisposing vulnerability to SII and BPD. Impulsivity is a term that is used widely in psychology to describe a broad range of behavioral phenomena, from very specific acts such as errors in maze solving to scores on factor analytically derived ADHD scales (Beauchaine & Gatzke-Kopp, 2012). Given space constraints, we cannot review these different conceptualizations of impulsivity here. Our model focuses on *trait* impulsivity, a highly heritable and enduring component of personality that is shaped by environment to predispose individuals to various forms of psychopathology across development (Beauchaine, Hinshaw, & Pang, 2010; Beauchaine & McNulty, 2013). Behavioral genetics studies indicate that trait impulsivity is over 80 % heritable and predisposes to externalizing behavior disorders including ADHD, conduct disorder, substance use disorders, and ASPD (Tuvblad, Zheng, Raine, & Baker, 2009). In fact, trait impulsivity early in life, as indicated by severe ADHD, often marks the initial step in the development of ASPD via a heterotypic trajectory of externalizing problems beginning with ADHD and progressing to oppositionality, conduct problems, delinquency, and antisocial personality development (Beauchaine et al., 2010).

Furthermore, recent research indicates that girls who are diagnosed with ADHD in childhood are increased risk for self injury as young adults (Hinshaw et al., 2012).

Individuals with BPD, many of whom engage in SII, share much in common with those who develop ASPD (Paris, 1997). Both disorders are characterized by trait impulsivity (Beauchaine et al., 2009), and affected individuals often come from the same families, where males are more likely to be diagnosed with ASPD and females are more likely to be diagnosed with BPD (Goldman, D'Angelo, & DeMaso, 1993). Given this, it is not surprising that increased prevalence of ASPD is observed in the first-degree relatives of those with BPD (Schulz et al., 1989) and that comorbidity rates between the disorders are quite high (e.g., McGlashan et al., 2000). In addition, disturbed parent–child relationships, disrupted attachment, family discord, and traumatic experiences including abuse are common in the life histories of those with ASPD and those with BPD (e.g., Lyons-Ruth, 2008). Moreover, both disorders are characterized by significant risk for depression and suicide. Among those with BPD, 8–10 % eventually die by suicide (APA, 2000). Those with ASPD are also at much higher suicide risk than the general population (Dyck, Bland, Newman, & Orn, 1988; Robins, 1966). Finally, ASPD and BPD have similar prevalence rates in the community and nearly identical sex distributions of about 3–4:1 favoring males for ASPD and females for BPD. This set of observations led Paris (1997) to suggest that ASPD and BPD are sex-moderated manifestations of a single underlying pathology (see also Beauchaine et al., 2009; Lyons-Ruth, 2008).

Although not all adolescents who self-injure develop BPD, the two groups overlap substantially. About 40–90 % of those who self-injure make a suicide attempt during their lifetime (APA, 2000), and many self-injurious behaviors are themselves impulsive acts (Klonsky, 2007). Behavioral genetics studies consistently yield very high heritabilities for trait impulsivity, as discussed above, yet this tells us nothing about specific genes implicated. Discovering such genes requires molecular genetics studies (for a discussion of the advantages and disadvantages of molecular and behavioral genetics approaches, see Beauchaine & Gatzke-Kopp, 2013). Among these, genetic association studies, in which frequencies of a candidate genetic polymorphism among individuals with and without a disorder are compared, are particularly helpful. This is because association studies carry far greater statistical power than linkage studies in which broad sections of the genome are scanned. However, the downside of association studies is that a well-articulated theory is needed to know what candidate polymorphisms to analyze. We are fortunate in this regard given a very rich tradition of neurobiological research on the reward circuitry of impulse control and impulsivity.

It has long been known that those with externalizing conditions including ADHD, ODD, CD, ASPD, and substance use disorders (SUDs) respond to reward differently than controls. Behaviorally, males with externalizing spectrum disorders perseverate longer than their peers in responding to reward contingencies that have been either discontinued or turned against them such that they lose money (e.g., Giancola, Peterson, & Pihl, 1993; Matthys, van Goozen, Snoek, & van Engeland, 2004). This has been shown repeatedly using multiple monetary incentive paradigms. Neuroimaging studies indicate that the central nervous system (CNS) substrates of deficient reward responding are likely (1) underactivation in the mesolimbic (striatal) and mesocortical (anterior and prefrontal cortical) dopamine (DA) systems (Gatzke-Kopp & Beauchaine, 2007) and (2) reduced functional connectivity between these brain regions (Shannon, Sauder, Beauchaine, & Gatzke-Kopp, 2009). Projections from the ventral tegmental area to the nucleus accumbens (housed within the ventral striatum) are activated during all approach behaviors, including impulsive behaviors (Berridge & Robinson, 2003; Sagvolden, Aase, Johansen, Russell, 2005). Although early theories linked impulsivity to overactivity in the central DA system (Quay, 1993), overwhelming evidence from neuroimaging studies now links both underactive mesolimbic and mesocortical responding and volumetric abnormalities in these structures to disorders of impulse control (e.g., Sauder,

Beauchaine, Gatzke-Kopp, Shannon, Aylward, 2012; Volkow et al., 2009). We have argued that individuals with impulse control disorders engage in excessive reward-seeking behaviors in an effort to upregulate their chronically underactive mesolimbic reward system (Gatzke-Kopp & Beauchaine, 2007), which is experienced psychologically as an aversive, irritable mood state (e.g., Laakso et al., 2003).

Given that the mesolimbic and mesocortical pathways are dopaminergically mediated, DA genes are logical foci for genetic association studies of impulsivity. Perhaps not surprisingly, several genetic polymorphisms that affect DA neurotransmission are associated with impulse control disorders. Replicated findings exist for the DRD_4 receptor, the DAT_1 transporter, the dopamine-β-hydroxylase gene, the monoamine oxidase gene, and the catechol-O-methyltransferase gene (Beauchaine et al., 2009; Beauchaine, Neuhaus, Zalewski, Crowell, & Potapova, 2011; Waldman & Lahey, 2013). Each of these genes affect either synthesis, turnover, or metabolism of DA, thereby contributing to individual differences in trait impulsivity. However, considerable work on the molecular genetics of impulsivity remains, because candidate polymorphisms account for only a small fraction of the large heritability coefficients for impulsivity observed in behavioral genetics studies, a problem that plagues psychiatric genetics (see e.g., Beauchaine & Gatzke-Kopp, 2013).

Until recently, most studies of suicide and related behaviors followed from the serotonin hypothesis, described below. Thus, examination of DA in relation to SII and suicide is a recent development (Sher et al., 2006). As with psychiatric genetics in general, findings have not always been consistent (Currier & Mann, 2008). In all likelihood, small sample sizes and inconsistencies in defining phenotypes contribute to nonreplications (Bosker et al., 2011). Furthermore, multiple gene interactions with the environment are more likely the norm when dealing with complex human behaviors such as SII and suicide (Moore & Williams, 2002), yet multifactorial designs in genetics research are notoriously underpowered (Lou et al., 2008). Nevertheless, emerging findings suggest links between low central DA function, SII, and suicide, consistent with our impulsivity hypothesis. In DA challenge tests, decreased responding is observed among suicide attempters and victims, independent of depression (e.g., Pitchot, Hansenne, & Ansseau, 2001). Moreover, suicide attempters exhibit reduced DA transporter binding compared to controls, a finding associated with individual differences in impulsivity (Ryding, Ahnlide, Lindström, Rosén, & Träskman-Bendz, 2006), and polymorphisms in both the DAT_1 gene and the DRD_5 gene have been associated with BPD (Fernández-Navarro et al., 2012; Joyce et al., 2006). Also consistent with the DA hypothesis, recent findings from the Multimodal Treatment of ADHD (MTA) trial indicate that middle school girls diagnosed with ADHD are at increased risk of self-harm as they move into adolescence and young adulthood (Hinshaw et al., 2012).

As alluded to above, deficiencies in central serotonin function have also been linked to impulsivity, particularly impulsive suicide. Serotonergic neurons project from the dorsal raphe nuclei to the septohippocampal system, amygdala, and frontal cortex. The septohippocampal system exerts inhibitory effects on behavior in the presence of competing motivational goals, producing anxiety, which is expressed behaviorally as passive avoidance of threat (Corr, 2004). Septohippocampal dysfunction is associated with difficulties halting prepotent behaviors when environmental cues indicate better and safer alternatives. For example, studies with rats illustrate that lesions to the raphe nuclei result in uninhibited preferences for reward (Bizot, Le Bihan, Puech, Hamon, & Thiébot, 1999), whereas serotonin agonists promote delay of gratification for larger rewards (Evenden & Ryan, 1996). Several findings link deficits within the 5-HT and DA systems to SII, providing further evidence for the role of impulsivity in self-harming behaviors (Beauchaine et al., 2009; Crowell et al., 2009).

There is also a long history of studying the role of 5-HT dysfunction in the prefrontal cortex (PFC) and suicide (Mann et al., 2009). Several studies indicate decreased presynaptic serotonin transporter (5-HTT) binding sites and increased postsynaptic 5-HT receptors among those who complete suicide (Mann, Brent, & Arango, 2001). Furthermore, reduced 5-HT_{2A} receptor binding is observed in the PFC among depressed suicide attempters relative to controls (Audenaert et al., 2001). The ventral PFC is also involved in behavioral and cognitive inhibition. Individuals who attempt suicide perform poorly on cognitive tasks relying on the PFC (e.g., Jollant et al., 2005).

Based on the serotonin hypothesis, molecular geneticists have identified candidate alleles for association studies of SII (Mann et al., 2009). Among others, these include 5-HTR_{1A}, 5-HTR_{2A}, TPH_1, TPH_2, and 5-HTTLPR genes. This area has been plagued by inconsistent results, again likely due to small sample sizes and inconsistencies in defining phenotypes (Bosker et al., 2011). Nevertheless, a few studies with clearly defined phenotypes have identified genes associated with suicidal behavior across different forms of psychiatric illness. For example, Brezo and colleagues (2010) followed over 1,000 individuals in a prospective longitudinal study over 22 years. A variation of the tryptophan 5-monooxygenase (TPH_1) gene was associated with suicide attempts but not depression. The TPH_1 gene affects rate of serotonin synthesis. In addition, three different variants of the $5HTR_{2A}$ gene predict suicidal behavior in interaction with childhood sexual or physical abuse assessed 22 years prior. These were different genes than those that interacted with abuse to predict depression. Finally, the short allele on the promoter region of the 5-HTT gene (5-HTTLPR) confers risk for psychopathology and SII following adverse life experiences (Karg, Burmeister, Shedden, & Sen, 2011). The 5-HTTLPR gene has two common allelic variations (short and long), resulting in three genotypes: homozygous long (ll), homozygous short (ss), and heterozygous (sl). Carriers of the short allele are at higher risk for a number of psychopathological outcomes, including violent suicide attempts among those with major depression (Bellivier et al., 2000), especially following adverse life events (e.g., Caspi et al., 2003).

To summarize, mounting evidence from neuroimaging and molecular genetics studies indicates that trait impulsivity is conferred through both dopaminergic and serotonergic mechanisms and that these vulnerabilities confer risk for SII and suicide (for more detailed accounts, see Beauchaine et al., 2009; Crowell et al., 2009). However, most trait-impulsive individuals do not engage in self-injury. Any developmental model of SII and suicide must account for this observation and provide a mechanism or mechanisms through which trait impulsivity either interacts with or is shaped by other influences, whether endogenous or exogenous, in elevating risk.

Emotion Dysregulation and Developmental Context

Coercive and invalidating family interaction patterns reinforce emotional lability among trait-impulsive, and therefore vulnerable, individuals through operant reinforcement (Beauchaine et al., 2009; Snyder, Schrepferman, & St. Peter, 1997). According to coercion theory (Patterson, 1982; Patterson, DeBaryshe, & Ramsey, 1989), trajectories toward antisocial behavior have roots in aversive dyadic interaction patterns that are enacted thousands of times between parents and children in at-risk families. During such coercive exchanges, aggression and emotional lability are negatively reinforced as children and parents match and oftentimes exceed one another's aversiveness, thereby escalating anger, antagonism, and physiological arousal. High levels of aversiveness eventually result in escape, which is experienced as rewarding since it terminates the unpleasant interaction (hence the term escape conditioning). Over time, emotional lability and aggression generalize and become primary means through which individuals cope with interpersonal stress (see e.g., Beauchaine & Zalewski, in press).

Evidence for the role of coercive family processes in shaping antisocial outcomes is considerable. In a series of studies using painstaking microanalytic coding procedures, Snyder and colleagues (e.g., Snyder et al., 1997) demonstrated

how parents of aggressive children tend to match or exceed the level of arousal and aversiveness displayed by their children, who in turn match and exceed the arousal and aversiveness of their parents. These exchanges often begin in the first 5 years of life and occur throughout development, solidifying aversive behaviors and emotional lability (Beauchaine, Gatzke-Kopp, & Mead, 2007). Notably, impulsive children are more likely than nonimpulsive children to evoke such reactions from their caregivers, thus exacerbating their preexisting genetic vulnerabilities (O'Connor, Deater-Deckard, Fulker, Rutter, & Plomin, 1998).

Although Linehan's (1993) model emphasizes emotional invalidation by parents and escape conditioning as etiological factors in the development of borderline personality, very little empirical research has been conducted on interaction patterns among families of those with BPD or those who self-injure. Recently, we hypothesized a negative reinforcement model of emotional lability and emotion dysregulation in borderline personality development, following from several sources of evidence outlined briefly above for a common etiology for ASPD and BPD (Beauchaine et al., 2009; Crowell et al., 2009). Perhaps most importantly, given that males who develop ASPD and females who develop BPD are often reared in the same families (Goldman et al., 1993), similar socialization mechanisms might be expected.

Accordingly, we compared interaction patterns among mother–daughter dyads in which daughters self-injured versus control dyads (Crowell et al., 2012). As expected, microanalytic coding indicated that self-injuring dyads were more likely to escalate conflict, suggesting a potential mechanism through which emotion dysregulation is shaped and maintained over time. Furthermore, mother–teen aversiveness interacted to predict adolescent resting respiratory sinus arrhythmia, a well validated physiological marker of emotion regulation capability (Beauchaine, 2001; Beauchaine et al., 2007). For daughters, the lowest levels of RSA were observed when both dyad members scored high on aversiveness. Finally, maternal invalidation (eschewing/ rejecting daughters' emotional expressions) was associated with higher levels of anger on the part of adolescents, consistent with Linehan's (1993) theory.

At this point, it is important to reemphasize the interactive nature of our model. Trait impulsivity—a preexisting vulnerability—is insufficient, in and of itself, to result in SII, BPD, or suicide. Rather, it interacts with socialized deficiencies in emotion regulation to amplify risk for these and other (e.g., CD, ASPD) outcomes. Mechanisms of socialization include coercive processes and invalidation. It is also important to note that given the high heritability of trait impulsivity, impulsive children often, if not usually, have impulsive parents, who are more likely to react in these ways (e.g., Patterson, 1982; Patterson et al., 1989). Consistent with our biological vulnerability×environmental risk perspective, we also found that the interaction between observed family conflict and low peripheral serotonin accounted for 64 % of the variance in SII behaviors in a female adolescent sample (Crowell et al., 2008), even though main effects were negligible.

One limitation in the literature on emerging SII and BPD is a scarcity of longitudinal studies. However, this state of affairs has been slowly improving. Currently, longitudinal studies indicate that suicide-related behaviors are often chronic and often continue following remission of psychiatric impairment (Mehlum, Friis, Vaglum, & Karterud, 1994). Wichstrom (2000) found that adolescents with previous attempts, suicidal ideation, alcohol use problems, poor self-worth, and early pubertal development, and who were raised by single parents, were at increased risk for suicide attempts two years later. In addition, impulsive and emotionally labile youth are vulnerable to psychopathology, and when life stressors accumulate, they are at greater risk for suicide (Caspi, 2000; Caspi et al., 2003). Furthermore, comorbid internalizing and externalizing problems in early childhood predict later suicide among male youth, ages 8 to 24 years (Sourander, Helstelä, & Helenius, 1999). In a recent longitudinal study by Belsky et al. (2012), a strong relationship was observed between behavioral and affective dysregulation

at age 5, and borderline features at age 12. Moreover, harsh treatment (i.e., physical maltreatment and maternal negative expressed emotion) moderated the relationship between family history of psychiatric disorder and borderline personality-related characteristics. This is consistent with studies indicating that child abuse increases risk for both borderline personality disorder and suicide-related behaviors (e.g., Lyons-Ruth, 2008).

Across development, coercive and invalidating interaction patterns produce enduring patterns of emotion dysregulation, poor behavioral control, and maladaptive cognitive coping styles, resulting in rigidity, loneliness, hopelessness, low self-worth, difficulties with conflict resolution, and social withdrawal. Extensive research conducted in the last decade indicates that those who self-injure exhibit extreme emotion dysregulation. Emotion *regulation* refers to processes through which emotional experience (e.g., sadness) and expression (e.g., crying) are shaped in the service of adaptive functioning (Thompson, 1994). Some of these processes are automatic whereas others are volitional (see e.g., Goldsmith & Davidson, 2004). In contrast, emotion *dysregulation* refers to patterns of emotional experience and expression that interfere with adaptive functioning. Following from this definition, individuals affected by diverse forms of psychopathology exhibit some dysregulated emotion of some kind (e.g., panic, sadness, rage, anxiety; Beauchaine, 2001; Beauchaine et al., 2007). Individuals who engage in SII tend to (1) be more anxious, depressed, and aggressive than both clinical controls and healthy peers (Ross & Heath, 2002), (2) score higher on self-report measures of emotion dysregulation (e.g., Crowell et al., 2005), and (3) report emotion dysregulation as a core precipitant of self-injury (Linehan, Rizvi, Welch, & Page, 2000).

Although little empirical data exist describing how coercive processes may be associated with development of poor ER, SII, and borderline personality (Crowell et al., 2012), Linehan (1993) proposed similar mechanisms underlying development of emotion dysregulation. According to Linehan, emotion dysregulation is developed in the context of an invalidating environment. Invalidating environments are characterized by rejection of internal emotional experience and oversimplification of problems. A child who is reared in such a context is not taught how to cope with distress or modulate emotional arousal. Ever-increasing displays of emotion are often required for the child to promote helpful responses from his or her caregivers. Thus, the family both punishes communication of negative emotions, and intermittently reinforces extreme emotional reactions. As a consequence, the child vacillates between emotional inhibition and extreme emotional lability. Together, these coercive and invalidating interactions occur thousands of times over the course of development, potentiating inherited vulnerability and leading to chronic dysregulated emotions, interpersonal conflict, and generally negative affect (for further reviews, see Beauchaine et al., 2009; Crowell et al., 2009).

It seems face valid to assert that poor interpersonal problem solving, a consequence of coercive and invalidating developmental contexts, could result in social problems. Among other possible mechanisms, we propose that social withdrawal begins as an adaptation to anticipated rejection (Crowell et al., in press). For example, children who develop SII and BPD often have histories of abuse, neglect, or chronic invalidation (e.g., Beauchaine et al., 2009). In addition, parental, peer, institutional, and/or other rejections are commonly experienced by those who engage in SII and suicide (e.g., Ryan, Huebner, Diaz, & Sanchez, 2009). Since belonging is a basic human need, this leads to psychological distress (Durkheim, 1951). The tendency to isolate socially has also been linked consistently to completed suicide (Negron, Piacentini, Graae, Davies, & Shaffer, 1997).

Deviant Peer Group Affiliations and Contagion Effects

Impulsive and dysregulated individuals are likely to affiliate with deviant peer groups, within which contagion effects and social reinforcement

may act as mechanisms through which SII is acquired and maintained as a maladaptive emotion regulation strategy (Nock & Prinstein, 2004; Prinstein, Boergers, Spirito, Little, & Grapentine, 2000). High-risk environments extend beyond the family to classrooms, peer groups, and neighborhoods. An extensive body of research indicates that impulsive boys and girls are especially vulnerable to effects of both deviant peer groups and neighborhood disadvantage (e.g., violence, crime), which increase their risk for delinquency (e.g., Dishion, McCord, & Poulin, 1999; Meier, Slutske, Arndt, & Cadoret, 2008). In fact, impulsive youth are more likely to engage in status and violent crimes than nonimpulsive youth when they live in neighborhoods characterized by low socioeconomic status and high rates of delinquency (Meier et al., 2008). Links between high-risk neighborhoods and behavior problems may be mediated by exposure to violence (Ingoldsby & Shaw, 2002) and deviant peer group affiliations (e.g., Dishion et al., 1999). Prinstein and colleagues (2000) demonstrated that self-injury is also transmitted among depressed teens through contagion within deviant peer groups. Indeed, some adolescents report engaging in self-injury in part because it is reinforced socially (e.g., Nock & Prinstein, 2004). Whitlock, Powers, and Eckenrode (2006) demonstrated a plausible link between increased presence of SII in the media and increasing rates of SII in society at large, also suggesting contagion (see also Whitlock, Purington & Gershkovich, 2009). Perhaps more importantly, several investigators have found that one or two individuals engaging in SII (or committing suicide) can result in dramatic spread of these behaviors throughout inpatient hospitals and detention centers (e.g., Rosen & Walsh, 1989). Thus, a picture emerges in which delinquency and self-injury are both transmitted via contagion effects. Delinquency may be transmitted more strongly in males, whereas self-injury may be transmitted more strongly in females, which may explain in part the sex differences observed in these behaviors (Beauchaine et al., 2009).

Over time, SII and related behaviors become canalized, contributing to development of BPD and related forms of psychopathology such as anti-social personality disorder (Beauchaine et al., 2009). To this point, our model can be summarized as follows: Children in high-risk environments acquire automated response patterns characterized by emotion dysregulation, which is overlaid onto heritable impulsivity. In later childhood and adolescence, the combinations of impulsivity, mood lability, and disrupted interpersonal relationships combine with the effects of deviant peer groups to increase risk for extremely maladaptive coping responses such as SII. Over time, engaging in such maladaptive coping strategies may enhance invalidation of adolescent's emotional experience by the family as they further exacerbate dysregulated emotional responding, making SII more likely. Thus, SII and other maladaptive coping strategies (e.g., coercion) are used to cope with extreme negative affect, thereby increasing risk for development of future borderline psychopathology.

Model Summary

In sum, we propose that several interacting, parallel processes contribute to development of SII and risk for suicide. In this model, SII is one of the many possible outcomes for a vulnerable (i.e., trait-impulsive) individual who is raised in a high-risk environment characterized by coercion, invalidation, and deviant peer group affiliations. Many individuals who meet this description become dysregulated emotionally, and it is therefore easier for them to reach their capacity to cope with environmental stressors (Crowell et al., in press). Certain developmental challenges may increase risk for specific age and demographic groups, such as adolescents, middle-aged females, and older White males. Indeed, problematic coping strategies characterized by both passive and active avoidance of emotional distress are especially linked to self-injury across the lifespan (e.g., Pollard, & Kennedy, 2007). Different individuals may reach their coping capacity at different times in life, contributing to dramatic variations in the prevalence of suicide-related behaviors across the lifespan.

Conclusions

In our model, we propose that suicide and self-injury are multifinal outcomes. Multifinality refers to the notion that a given risk or vulnerability factor (e.g., temperamental impulsivity) may lead to a diversity of outcomes (e.g., BPD, ASPD, substance use, suicide) through its interactions with other interconnected processes across development (Cicchetti & Rogosch, 1996). However, the number of risk factors associated with suicide is vast, illustrating the principle of equifinality, which holds that a particular outcome (e.g., suicide) is the common endpoint of several converging developmental pathways (see above). Consistent with a developmental psychopathology approach, it is essential that researchers continue to examine possible individual differences, attending to both continuities and discontinuities across development. Unfortunately, despite clear advantages to conceptualizing self-injury from a developmental perspective, research on suicide from this perspective is quite sparse.

The majority of research conducted to date has addressed main effects of either biology or environment on SII and suicide risk. However, it is often the case that interactions between biology and environment account for more variance in negative health outcomes than the addition of their main effects alone (Beauchaine, Neuhaus, Brenner, & Gatzke-Kopp, 2008; Crowell et al. 2005). This is why ours and other contemporary models of psychopathology have emphasized the importance of both neurobiological and contextual influences on behavior (e.g., Beauchaine et al., 2009, 2010; Cicchetti & Toth, 1998; Crowell et al., 2009; Dawson, 2008).

In addition, studying biological × environmental interactions in the development of SII and suicide should increase our understanding of causal mechanisms for the behaviors (e.g., Beauchaine & Marsh, 2006). In turn, interventions that target causal mechanisms directly are likely to be more effective. This has been the case in other areas of research. For example, understanding the role of coercive family processes in the development of delinquency has led to much more effective interventions for conduct problems that target the specific parent–child interaction styles that potentiate aggressive tendencies associated with ASPD (e.g., Webster-Stratton & Hammond, 1997). Indeed, future research on suicide-related behaviors should reach beyond the basic topographical description of the behaviors and their diagnostic, psychosocial, and biological correlates. Such descriptive approaches allow us to characterize psychological problems but are much less effective for predicting individual health outcomes (Crowell et al., in press). Whether or not our particular model realizes the ideal of predicting individual health outcomes, we hope it provides a useful organizing framework for future research leading to advanced knowledge about an urgent and devastating health problem.

References

American Psychiatric Association. (2000). *Diagnostic and statistical manual of mental disorders* (4th ed., text rev.). Washington, DC: Author.

Audenaert, K., Van Laere, K., Dumont, F., Slegers, G., Mertens, J., van Heeringen, C., et al. (2001). Decreased frontal serotonin 5-HT2a receptor binding index in deliberate self-harm patients. *European Journal of Nuclear Medicine and Molecular Imaging, 28,* 175–182.

Beauchaine, T. P. (2001). Vagal tone, development, and Gray's motivational theory: Toward an integrated model of autonomic nervous system functioning in psychopathology. *Development and Psychopathology, 13,* 183–214.

Beauchaine, T. P., & Gatzke-Kopp, L. M. (2012). Instantiating the multiple levels of analysis perspective into a program of study on the development of antisocial behavior. *Development and Psychopathology, 24,* 1003–1018.

Beauchaine, T. P., & Gatzke-Kopp, L. M. (2013). Genetic and environmental influences on behavior. In T. P. Beauchaine & S. P. Hinshaw (Eds.), *Child and adolescent psychopathology* (2nd ed., pp. 111–140). Hoboken, NJ: Wiley.

Beauchaine, T. P., Gatzke-Kopp, L. M., & Mead, H. K. (2007). Polyvagal theory and developmental psychopathology: Emotion dysregulation and conduct problems from preschool to adolescence. *Biological Psychology, 74,* 174–184.

Beauchaine, T. P., Hinshaw, S. P., & Pang, K. L. (2010). Comorbidity of attention-deficit/hyperactivity disorder and early-onset conduct disorder: Biological, environmental, and developmental mechanisms. *Clinical Psychology: Science and Practice, 17,* 327–336.

Beauchaine, T. P., Klein, D. N., Crowell, S. E., Derbidge, C. M., & Gatzke-Kopp, L. M. (2009). Multifinality in the development of personality disorders: A biology × sex × environment interaction model of antisocial and borderline traits. *Development and Psychopathology, 21,* 735–770.

Beauchaine, T. P., & Marsh, P. (2006). Taxometric methods: Enhancing early detection and prevention of psychopathology by identifying latent vulnerability traits. In D. Cicchetti & D. Cohen (Eds.), *Developmental psychopathology* (2nd ed., pp. 931–967). Hoboken, NJ: Wiley.

Beauchaine, T. P., & McNulty, T. (2013). Comorbidities and continuities as ontogenic processes: Toward developmental spectrum model of externalizing behavior. *Development and Psychopathology, 25,* 1505–1528.

Beauchaine, T. P., Neuhaus, E., Brenner, S. L., & Gatzke-Kopp, L. (2008). Ten good reasons to consider biological processes in prevention and intervention research. *Development and Psychopathology, 20,* 745–774.

Beauchaine, T. P., Neuhaus, E., Zalewski, M., Crowell, S. E., & Potapova, N. (2011). The effects of allostatic load on neural systems subserving motivation, mood regulation, and social affiliation. *Development and Psychopathology, 23,* 975–999.

Beauchaine, T. P., & Zalewski, M. (in press). Physiological and developmental mechanisms of emotional lability in coercive relationships. In T. J. Dishion & J. J. Snyder (Eds.), *Oxford handbook of coercive relationship dynamics.* New York: Oxford University Press.

Bellivier, F., Szöke, A., Henry, C., Lacoste, J., Bottos, C., Nosten-Bertrand, M., et al. (2000). Possible association between serotonin transporter gene polymorphism and violent suicidal behavior in mood disorders. *Biological Psychiatry, 48,* 319–322.

Belsky, D., Caspi, A., Arseneault, L., Bleidorn, W., Fonagy, P., Goodman, M., et al. (2012). Etiological features of borderline personality-related characteristics in a birth cohort of 12-year-old children. *Development and Psychopathology, 24,* 251–265.

Berridge, K. C., & Robinson, T. E. (2003). Parsing reward. *Trends in Neurosciences, 26,* 507–513.

Bizot, J. C., Le Bihan, C., Puech, A. J., Hamon, M., & Thiébot, M. H. (1999). Serotonin and tolerance to delay of reward in rats. *Psychopharmacology, 146,* 400–412.

Blumenthal, S. J., & Kupfer, D. J. (Eds.). (1990). *Suicide over the life cycle.* Washington, DC: American Psychiatric Press.

Bongar, B. (2002). *The suicidal patient: Clinical and legal standards of care* (2nd ed.). Washington, DC: American Psychological Association.

Borry, P., Schotsmans, P., & Dierickx, K. (2006). Empirical research in bioethical journals. A quantitative analysis. *Journal of Medical Ethics, 32,* 240–245.

Bosker, F. J., Hartman, C. A., Nolte, I. M., Prins, B. P., Terpstra, P., Posthuma, D., et al. (2011). Poor replication of candidate genes for major depressive disorder using genome-wide association data. *Molecular Psychiatry, 16*, 516–32.

Brezo, J., Bureau, A., Merette, C., Jomphe, V., Barker, E. D., Vitaro, F., et al. (2010). Differences and similarities in the serotonergic diathesis for suicide attempts and mood dis-orders: A 22-year longitudinal gene-environment study. *Molecular Psychiatry, 15*, 831–843.

Brown, G. W., & Harris, T. (1978). *Social origins of depression*. London: Tavistock.

Caspi, A. (2000). The child is the father of the man: Personality continuities from childhood to adulthood. *Journal of Personality and Social Psychology, 78*, 158–172.

Caspi, A., Sugden, K., Moffitt, T. E., Taylor, A., Craig, I. W., Harrington, H., et al. (2003). Influence of life stress on depression: Moderation by a polymorphism in the 5-HTT gene. *Science, 301*, 386–389.

Centers for Disease Control and Prevention. (1999, April 02). *MMWR weekly: Ten great public health achievements—United States, 1900–1999*. Retrieved July 11, 2012, from source.

Centers for Disease Control and Prevention, National Center for Injury Prevention and Control. (2009). *Web-based injury statistics query and reporting system (WISQARS)* [online]. [cited 2012 Aug 04]. Available from http://www.cdc.gov/ncipc/wisqars

Cicchetti, D., & Rogosch, F. A. (1996). Equifinality and multifinality in developmental psychopathology. *Development and Psychopathology, 8*, 597–600.

Cicchetti, D., & Toth, S. L. (1998). The development of depression in children and adolescents. *American Psychologist, 53*, 221–241.

Cohen-Almagor, R. (2001). "Culture of Death" in the Netherlands: Dutch perspectives. *Issues in Law and Medicine, 17*, 167–179.

Corr, P. J. (2004). Reinforcement sensitivity theory and personality. *Neuroscience and Biobehavioral Reviews, 28*, 317–332.

Crowell, S. E., Beauchaine, T. P., Hsiao, R. C. J., Vasilev, C. A., Yaptangco, M., Linehan, M. M., et al. (2012). Differentiating adolescent self-injury from adolescent depression: Possible implications for borderline personality development. *Journal of Abnormal Child Psychology, 40*, 45–57.

Crowell, S. E., Beauchaine, T. P., & Linehan, M. M. (2009). A biosocial developmental model of borderline personality: Elaborating and extending Linehan's theory. *Psychological Bulletin, 135*, 495–510.

Crowell, S. E., Beauchaine, T. P., McCauley, E., Smith, C., Stevens, A. L., & Sylvers, P. D. (2005). Psychological, physiological, and serotonergic correlates of parasuicidal behavior among adolescent girls. *Development and Psychopathology, 17*, 1105–1127.

Crowell, S. E., Beauchaine, T. P., McCauley, E., Smith, C., Vasilev, C., & Stevens, A. L. (2008). Parent–child interactions, peripheral serotonin, and intentional self-injury in adolescents. *Journal of Consulting and Clinical Psychology, 76*, 15–21.

Crowell, S. E., Derbidge, C. M., & Beauchaine, T. P. (in press). Developmental approaches to understanding self-injury and suicidal behaviors. In M. K. Nock (Ed.), *Oxford handbook of suicide and self-injury*. New York: Oxford University Press.

Currier, D., & Mann, J. J. (2008). Stress, genes and the biology of suicidal behavior. *Psychiatric Clinics of North America, 31*, 247–269.

Dawson, G. (2008). Early behavioral intervention, brain plasticity, and the prevention of autism spectrum disorder. *Development and Psychopathology, 20*, 775–803.

Dishion, T. J., McCord, J., & Poulin, F. (1999). When interventions harm. *American Psychologist, 54*, 755–764.

Durkheim, E. (1951). *Suicide: A study in sociology*. (J. Spaulding, & G. Simpson, Trans.) New York: Free Press. (Original work published 1897).

Dyck, R. J., Bland, R. C., Newman, S. C., & Orn, H. (1988). Suicide attempts in psychiatric disorders in Edmonton. *Acta Psychiatrica Scandinavica, 77*, 64–71.

Easterlin, R. A. (1980). *Birth and fortune*. New York: Basic Books.

Ellis, T. A. (2006). *Cognition and suicide: Theory, research, and therapy*. Washington, DC: American Psychological Association.

Elnour, A. A., & Harrison, J. (2008). Lethality of suicide methods. *Injury Prevention, 14*, 39–45.

Evenden, J. L., & Ryan, C. N. (1996). The pharmacology of impulsive behaviour in rats: The effects of drugs on response choice with varying delays of reinforcement. *Psychopharmacology, 128*, 161–170.

Farberow, N. L. (Ed.). (1975). *Suicide in different cultures*. Baltimore, MD: University Park Press.

Fernández-Navarro, P., Vaquero-Lorenzo, C., Blasco-Fontecilla, H., Díaz-Hernández, M., Gratacòs, M., Estivill, X., et al. (2012). Genetic epistasis in female suicide attempters. *Progress in Neuro-Psychopharmacology and Biological Psychiatry, 38*, 294–301.

Fiske, A., O'Riley, A. A., & Widow, R. K. (2008). Physical health and suicide late in life. *Clinical Gerontologist, 31*, 31–50.

Freud, S. (1965). Beyond the pleasure principle. In J. Starchey (Ed. and Trans.), *The standard edition of the complete psychological works of Sigmund Freud* (Vol. 18). London: Hogarth Press. (Original work published 1917).

Ganzini, L., Goy, E. R., & Dobscha, S. K. (2008). Prevalence of depression and anxiety in patients requesting physicians' aid in dying: Cross sectional survey. *British Medical Journal, 337*, a1682.

Gatzke-Kopp, L., & Beauchaine, T. P. (2007). Central nervous system substrates of impulsivity: Implications for the development of attention-deficit/hyperactivity disorder and conduct disorder. In D. Coch, G. Dawson, & K. Fischer (Eds.), *Human behavior, learning, and the developing brain: Atypical development* (pp. 239–263). New York: Guilford Press.

Giancola, P. R., Peterson, J. B., & Pihl, R. O. (1993). Risk for alcoholism, antisocial behavior, and response perseveration. *Journal of Clinical Psychology, 49*(3), 423–428.

Goldman, S. J., D'Angelo, E. J., & DeMaso, D. R. (1993). Psychopathology in the families of children and adolescents with borderline personality disorder. *American Journal of Psychiatry, 150*, 1832–1835.

Goldsmith, H. H., & Davidson, R. J. (2004). Disambiguating the components of emotion regulation. *Child Development, 72*, 361–365.

Gould, M. S., Wallenstein, S., & Kleinman, M. (1990). Time-space clustering of teenage suicide. *American Journal of Epidemiology, 131*, 71–78.

Gunnell, D. J. (2000). The epidemiology of suicide. *International Review of Psychiatry, 12*, 21–26.

Haw, C., Hawton, K., Houston, K., & Townsend, E. (2001). Psychiatric and personality disorders in deliberate self-harm patients. *British Journal of Psychiatry, 178*, 48–54.

Hawton, K. (1982). Attempted suicide in children and adolescents. *Journal of Child Psychology and Psychiatry, 23*, 497–503.

Hawton, K., Bergen, H., Kapur, N., Cooper, J., Steeg, S., Ness, J., et al. (2012). Repetition of self-harm and suicide following self-harm in children and adolescents: Findings from the multicentre study of self-harm in England. *Journal of Child Psychology and Psychiatry, 53*(12), 1212–1219.

Hawton, K., Fagg, J., & McKeown, S. P. (1989). Alcoholism, alcohol, and attempted suicide. *Alcohol and Alcoholism, 24*, 3–9.

Hawton, K., & Harris, L. (2008). The changing gender ratio in occurrence of deliberate self-harm across the lifecycle. *Journal of Crisis Intervention and Suicide Prevention, 29*, 4–10.

Hinshaw, S. P. (2013). Developmental psychopathology as a scientific discipline: Rationale, principles, and advances. In T. P. Beauchaine & S. P. Hinshaw (Eds.), *Child and adolescent psychopathology* (2nd ed., pp. 3–27). Hoboken, NJ: Wiley.

Hinshaw, S. P., Owens, E. B., Zalecki, C., Huggins, S. P., Montenegro-Nevado, A., Schrodek, E., & Swanson, E. N. (2012). Prospective follow-up of girls with attention-deficit/ hyperactivity disorder into young adulthood: Continuing impairment includes elevated risk for suicide attempts and self-injury. *Journal of Consulting and Clinical Psychology, 80*, 1041–1051.

Illfeld, F. W. (1977). Current social stressors and symptoms of depression. *American Journal of Psychiatry, 135*, 161–166.

Ingoldsby, E. M., & Shaw, D. S. (2002). Neighborhood contextual factors and early-starting antisocial pathways. *Clinical Child and Family Psychology Review, 5*, 21–55.

Joiner, T. E. (2005). *Why people die by suicide.* Cambridge, MA: Harvard University Press.

Joiner, T. E., Jr., Conwell, Y., Fitzpatrick, K. K., Witte, T. K., Schmidt, N. B., Berlim, M. T., et al. (2005). Four studies on how past and current suicidality relate even when "everything but the kitchen sink" is covaried. *Journal of Abnormal Psychology, 114*, 291–303.

Jollant, F., Bellivier, F., Leboyer, M., Astruc, B., Torres, S., Verdier, R., et al. (2005). Impaired decision making in suicide attempters. *American Journal of Psychiatry, 162*, 304–310.

Joyce, P. R., McHugh, P. C., McKenzie, J. M., Sullivan, P. F., Mulder, R. T., Luty, S. E., et al. (2006). A dopamine transporter polymorphism is a risk factor for borderline personality disorder in depressed patients. *Psychological Medicine, 36*, 807–813.

Karg, K., Burmeister, M., Shedden, K., & Sen, S. (2011). The serotonin transporter variant (5-HTTLPR), stress, and depression meta-analysis revisited. *Archives of General Psychiatry, 68*, 444–454.

Kelly, S., & Bunting, J. (1998). Trends in suicide in England and Wales, 1982–96. *Population Trends, 92*, 29–41.

King, C. (1998). Suicide across the life span: Pathways to prevention. *Suicide and Life-Threatening Behavior, 28*, 328–337.

Klonsky, E. D. (2007). The functions of deliberate self-injury: A review of the evidence. *Clinical Psychology Review, 27*, 226–239.

Kochanek, K. D., Xu, J. Q., Murphy, S. L., Miniño, A. M., & Kung, H. (2011). Deaths: Final data for 2009. *National Vital Statistics Reports, 60*, 3.

Krug, E. G., & World Health Organization. (2002). *World report on violence and health.* Geneva, Switzerland: World Health Organization.

Laakso, A., Wallius, E., Kajander, J., Bergman, J., Eskola, O., Solin, O., et al. (2003). Personality traits and striatal dopamine synthesis capacity in healthy subjects. *American Journal of Psychiatry, 160*, 904–910.

Leenaars, A. A. (Ed.). (1991). *Life span perspectives of suicide: Timelines in the suicide process.* New York: Plenum Press.

Leenaars, A. A. (2010). Edwin Shneidman on suicide. *Suicidology Online, 1*, 5–18.

Lewinsohn, P. M., Rohde, P., & Seeley, J. R. (1995). Adolescent psychopathology: III. The clinical consequences of comorbidity. *Journal of the American Academy of Child and Adolescent Psychiatry, 34*, 510–519.

Linehan, M. M. (1993). *Cognitive-behavioral treatment of borderline personality disorder.* New York: Guilford Press.

Linehan, M. M., Comtois, K. A., Brown, M. Z., Heard, H. L., & Wagner, A. (2006). Suicide attempt self-injury interview (SASII): Development, reliability, and validity of a scale to assess suicide attempts and intentional self-injury. *Psychological Assessment, 18*, 303–312.

Linehan, M. M., Rizvi, S. L., Welch, S. S., & Page, B. (2000). Suicide and personality disorders. In K. Hawton & K. van Heeringen (Eds.), *International handbook of suicide and attempted suicide* (pp. 147–178). Chichester: Wiley.

Lloyd-Richardson, E. E., Perrine, N., Dierker, L., & Kelley, M. L. (2007). Characteristics and functions of non-suicidal self-injury in a community sample of adolescents. *Psychological Medicine, 37*, 1183–1192.

Lou, X. Y., Chen, G. B., Yan, L., Ma, J. Z., Mangold, J. E., Zhu, J., et al. (2008). A combinatorial approach to detecting gene-gene and gene-environment interactions in 6 family studies. *American Journal of Human Genetics, 83*, 457–467.

Lyons-Ruth, K. (2008). Contributions of the mother-infant relationship to dissociative, border-line, and conduct symptoms in young adulthood. *Infant Mental Health Journal, 29*, 203–218.

Mann, J. J., Arango, V. A., Avenevoli, S., Brent, D. A., Champagne, F. A., Clayton, P., et al. (2009). Candidate endophenotypes for genetic studies of suicidal behavior. *Biological Psychiatry, 65*, 556–563.

Mann, J. J., Brent, D. A., & Arango, V. (2001). The neurobiology and genetics of suicide and attempted suicide: A focus on the serotonergic system. *Neuropsychopharmacology, 24*, 467–477.

Maris, R. W. (1981). *Pathways to suicide.* Baltimore, MD: Johns Hopkins University Press.

Maris, R. W., Berman, A. L., & Silverman, M. M. (2000). *Comprehensive textbook of suicidology.* New York: Guilford Press.

Matthys, W., Van Goozen, S., Snoek, H., & Van Engeland, H. (2004). Response perseveration and sensitivity to reward and punishment in boys with oppositional defiant disorder. *European Child and Adolescent Psychiatry, 13*, 362–364.

McGlashan, T. H., Grilo, C. M., Skodol, A. E., Gunderson, J. G., Shea, M. T., Morey, L. C., et al. (2000). The collaborative longitudinal personality disorders study: Baseline axis I/II and II/II diagnostic co-occurrence. *Acta Psychiatrica Scandinavica, 102*, 256–264.

Mehlum, L., Friis, S., Vaglum, P., & Karterud, S. (1994). The longitudinal pattern of suicidal behaviour in borderline personality disorder: A prospective follow-up study. *Acta Psychiatrica Scandinavica, 90*, 124–130.

Meier, M. H., Slutske, W. S., Arndt, S., & Cadoret, R. J. (2008). Impulsive and callous traits are more strongly associated with delinquent behavior in higher risk neighborhoods among boys and girls. *Journal of Consulting and Clinical Psychology, 117*, 377–385.

Merian, J. (1763). Memoir sur le suicide [A memoir on suicide]. In *Historie de l'Academie Royales des Sciences et Belles-Lettres de Berlin* (Vol. 19). Berlin: Haude et Spener.

Miller, M., & Hemenway, D. (2008). Guns and suicide in the United States. *New England Journal of Medicine, 359*, 989–91.

Moore, J. H., & Williams, S. M. (2002). New strategies for identifying gene-gene interactions in hypertension. *Annals of Medicine, 34*, 88–95.

Negron, R., Piacentini, J., Graae, F., Davies, M., & Shaffer, D. (1997). Microanalysis of adolescent suicide attempters and ideators during the acute suicidal episode. *Journal of the American Academy of Child and Adolescent Psychiatry, 36*, 1512–1519.

Nock, M. K., Borges, G., Bromet, E. J., Cha, C. B., Kessler, R. C., & Lee, S. (2008). Suicide and suicidal behavior. *Epidemiologic Reviews, 30*, 133–154.

Nock, M. K., Joiner, T. E., Gordon, K. H., Lloyd-Richardson, E., & Prinstein, M. J. (2006). Non-suicidal self-injury among adolescents: Diagnostic correlates and relation to suicide attempts. *Psychiatry Research, 144*, 65–72.

Nock, M. K., & Prinstein, M. J. (2004). A functional approach to the assessment of self-mutilative behavior. *Journal of Consulting and Clinical Psychology, 72*, 885–890.

O'Connor, T. G., Deater-Deckard, K., Fulker, D., Rutter, M., & Plomin, R. (1998). Genotype–environment correlations in late childhood and adolescence: Antisocial behavior problems and coercive parenting. *Developmental Psychology, 34*, 970–981.

Paris, J. (1997). Antisocial and borderline personality disorders: Two separate diagnoses or two aspects of the same psychopathology? *Comprehensive Psychiatry, 38*, 237–242.

Patterson, G. R. (1982). *Coercive family process.* Eugene, OR: Castalia.

Patterson, G. R., DeBaryshe, B. D., & Ramsey, E. (1989). A developmental perspective on antisocial behavior. *American Psychologist, 44*, 329–335.

Pitchot, W., Hansenne, M., & Ansseau, M. (2001). Role of dopamine in non-depressed patients with a history of suicide attempts. *European Psychiatry, 16*, 424–427.

Pollard, C., & Kennedy, P. (2007). A longitudinal analysis of emotional impact, coping strategies and post-traumatic psychological growth following spinal cord injury: A 10-year review. *British Journal of Health Psychology, 12*, 347–362.

Prinstein, M. J., Boergers, J., Spirito, A., Little, T. D., & Grapentine, W. L. (2000). Peer functioning, family dysfunction, and psychological symptoms in a risk factor model for adolescent inpatients' suicidal ideation severity. *Journal of Clinical Child Psychology, 29*, 392–405.

Quay, H. C. (1993). The psychobiology of undersocialized aggressive conduct disorder: A theoretical perspective. *Development and Psychopathology, 5*, 165–180.

Robins, L. N. (1966). *Deviant children grown up.* Baltimore, MD: Williams & Wilkins.

Rosen, P. M., & Walsh, B. W. (1989). Patterns of contagion in self mutilation epidemics. *American Journal of Psychiatry, 146*, 656–658.

Ross, S., & Heath, N. (2002). A study of the frequency of self-mutilation in a community sample of adolescents. *Journal of Youth and Adolescence, 31*, 67–77.

Ryan, C., Huebner, D., Diaz, R. M., & Sanchez, J. (2009). Family rejection as a predictor of negative health outcomes in White and Latino lesbian, gay, and bisexual young adults. *Pediatrics, 123*, 346–352.

Ryding, E., Ahnlide, J.-A., Lindström, M., Rosén, I., & Träskman-Bendz, L. (2006). Regional brain serotonin and dopamine transporter binding capacity in suicide attempters relate to impulsiveness and mental energy. *Psychiatry Research: Neuroimaging, 148*, 195–203.

Sagvolden, T., Aase, H., Johansen, E. B., & Russell, V. A. (2005). A dynamic developmental theory of attention-deficit/hyperactivity disorder (ADHD) predominantly hyperactive/impulsive and combined subtypes. *Behavioral and Brain Sciences, 28*, 397–468.

Sauder, C., Beauchaine, T. P., Gatzke-Kopp, L. M., Shannon, K. E., & Aylward, E. (2012). Neuroanatomical correlates of heterotypic comorbidity in externalizing male adolescents. *Journal of Clinical Child and Adolescent Psychology, 41*, 346–352.

Schulz, P. M., Soloff, P. H., Kelly, R., Morgenstern, M., Di-Franco, R., & Schulz, S. C. (1989). A family history study of borderline subtypes. *Journal of Personality Disorders, 3*, 217–229.

Shannon, K. E., Sauder, C., Beauchaine, T. P., & Gatzke-Kopp, L. (2009). Disrupted effective connectivity between the medial frontal cortex and the caudate in adolescent boys with externalizing behavior disorders. *Criminal Justice and Behavior, 36*, 1141–1157.

Sher, L., Mann, J. J., Traskman-Bendz, L., Winchel, R., Huang, Y., Fertuck, E., et al. (2006). Lower cerebrospinal fluid homovanillic acid levels in depressed suicide attempters. *Journal of Affective Disorders, 90*, 83–89.

Shneidman, E. S. (1985). *Definition of suicide*. New York: Wiley.

Shneidman, E. S. (1991). The commonalities of suicide across the life span. In A. A. Leenaars (Ed.), *Life span perspectives of suicide: Timelines in the suicide process* (pp. 39–52). New York: Plenum Press.

Shneidman, E. S. (1996). *The suicidal mind*. New York: Oxford University Press.

Silverman, M. M., Berman, A. L., Sanddal, N. D., O'Carroll, P. W., & Joiner, T. E. (2007a). Rebuilding the tower of Babel: A revised nomenclature for the study of suicide and suicidal behaviors. Part 1: Background, rationale, and methodology. *Suicide and Life-Threatening Behavior, 37*, 264–277.

Silverman, M. M., Berman, A. L., Sanddal, N. D., O'Carroll, P. W., & Joiner, T. E. (2007b). Rebuilding the tower of Babel: A revised nomenclature for the study of suicide and suicidal behaviors. Part 2: Suicide-related ideations, communications, and behaviors. *Suicide and Life-Threatening Behavior, 37*, 264–277.

Snyder, J., Schrepferman, L., & St. Peter, C. (1997). Origins of antisocial behavior: Negative reinforcement and affect dysregulation of behavior as socialization mechanisms in family interaction. *Behavior Modification, 21*, 187–215.

Sourander, A., Helstelä, L., & Helenius, H. (1999). Parent-adolescent agreement on emotional and behavioral problems. *Social Psychiatry and Psychiatric Epidemiology, 34*, 657–663.

Stillion, J. M., & McDowell, E. E. (1996). *Suicide across the life span: Premature exits* (2nd ed.). Washington, DC: Taylor and Francis.

Thompson, R. (1994). Emotion regulation: A theme in search of definition. *Monographs of the Society for Research in Child Development, 59*, 25–52.

Tuvblad, C., Zheng, M., Raine, A., & Baker, L. (2009). A common genetic factor explains the covariation among ADHD ODD and CD symptoms in 9–10 year old boys and girls. *Journal of Abnormal Child Psychology, 37*, 153–167.

U.S. Public Health Service. (1999). *The surgeon general's call to action to prevent suicide*. Washington, DC: U.S. Public Health Service.

van Hooff, A. J. L. (2000). A historical perspective on suicide. In R. W. Maris, A. L. Berman, & M. M. Silverman (Eds.), *Comprehensive textbook of suicidology* (pp. 96–123). New York: Guilford Press.

Volkow, N. D., Wang, G. J., Kollins, S. H., Wigal, T. L., Newcorn, J. H., Telang, F., et al. (2009). Evaluating dopamine reward pathway in ADHD: Clinical implications. *Journal of the American Medical Association, 302*, 1084–1091.

Voracek, M., & Loibl, L. M. (2007). Genetics of suicide: A systematic review of twin studies. *Wiener Klinische Wochenschrift, 119*, 463–475.

Waldam, I. D., & Lahey, B. B. (2013). Oppositional defiant disorder, conduct disorder, and juvenile delinquency. In T. P. Beauchaine & S. P. Hinshaw (Eds.), *Child and adolescent psychopathology* (2nd ed., pp. 411–452). Hoboken, NJ: Wiley.

Webster-Stratton, C., & Hammond, M. (1997). Treating children with early-onset conduct problems: A comparison of child and parent training interventions. *Journal of Consulting and Clinical Psychology, 65*, 93–109.

Wexler, L. M., & Gone, J. P. (2012). Culturally responsive suicide prevention in indigenous communities: Unexamined assumptions and new possibilities. *American Journal of Public Health, 102*, 800–806.

Whitlock, J. L., Powers, J. L., & Eckenrode, J. E. (2006). The virtual cutting edge: Adolescent self-injury and the Internet. *Developmental Psychology, 42*(3), 407–417.

Whitlock, J. L., Purington, A., & Gershkovich, M. (2009). Influence of the media on self injurious behavior. In M. Nock (Ed.), *Understanding non-suicidal self-injury: Current science and practice* (pp. 139–156). Washington, DC: American Psychological Association Press.

Wichstrom, L. (2000). Predictors of adolescent suicide attempts: A nationally representative longitudinal study of Norwegian adolescents. *Journal of the American Academy of Child and Adolescent Psychiatry, 39*, 603–610.

World Health Organization. (2011). *Suicide rates per 100,000 by country, year, and sex* (table). Retrieved August 6, 2012, from source.

World Health Organization. (2012). *Mental health*. Retrieved April 17, 2012, from source.

World Health Organization Suicide Prevention [SUPRE]. (2012). Retrieved August 6, 2012, from http://www.who.int/mental_health/prevention/suicide/suicideprevent/en/index.html

The Developmental Psychopathology of Anxiety

27

Michael W. Vasey, Guy Bosmans, and Thomas H. Ollendick

Anxiety and fear are common in childhood and adolescence, with their focus typically reflecting important developmental themes and challenges (Muris & Field, 2011) that are largely consistent across cultures (Ollendick, Yang, King, Dong, & Akande, 1996). As such, anxiety is an adaptive emotion that prepares the individual to detect and deal with threats, thereby fostering survival (Marks & Nesse, 1994). However, high levels of anxiety have strong potential to interfere with development, raising risk for a wide range of maladaptive outcomes, including impaired interpersonal and academic functioning (Rapee, Schniering, & Hudson, 2009). Consequently, such problems have strong potential to initiate negative developmental cascades.

Anxiety disorders are the most prevalent form of psychopathology in youth (Lepine, 2002). Furthermore, these disorders often persist and carry risk for other disorders in adolescence and adulthood, particularly depression (Rapee et al., 2009). Thus, there is a need for improved understanding of such disorders and the factors contributing to their development, persistence, and amelioration so as to foster their early detection, treatment, and prevention.

In this chapter we provide a roadmap to research on the central issues in understanding the developmental psychopathology of youth anxiety. First, we consider issues in the definition of anxiety disorders and their epidemiology, with particular emphasis in each case on the implications of development. Second, we consider factors contributing to the etiology of such problems, again with emphasis on the impact of development. Unfortunately, space does not permit discussion of developmental issues in the assessment, treatment, and prevention of childhood anxiety disorders. Interested readers are directed to recent reviews of these issues (e.g., Lyneham & Rapee, 2011; Rapee et al., 2009; Silverman & Ollendick, 2008).

Definitional Issues

Progress toward understanding anxiety disorders in youth hinges on being able to recognize and distinguish between different anxiety pathology phenotypes. However, efforts to define anxiety disorders in youth are complicated by a range of issues (Bernstein & Zvolensky, 2011). First, the high normative frequency of anxiety in youth raises questions about where to draw the boundaries between normal and pathological forms. However, it is also unclear if pathological and

M.W. Vasey, Ph.D. (✉)
Department of Psychology, The Ohio State University, Columbus, OH 43210, USA
e-mail: vasey@psy.ohio-state.edu

G. Bosmans, Ph.D.
Parenting and Special Education Research Group, University of Leuven, 3000 Leuven, Belgium

T.H. Ollendick, Ph.D.
Department of Psychology, Child Study Center, Virginia Polytechnic Institute and State University, Blacksburg, VA 24061, USA

M. Lewis and K.D. Rudolph (eds.), *Handbook of Developmental Psychopathology*, DOI 10.1007/978-1-4614-9608-3_27, © Springer Science+Business Media New York 2014

normal anxieties are best thought of as different forms (i.e., categories) or as different only in degree (i.e., dimensions). Bernstein and Zvolensky (2011) suggest that future work will likely converge on hybrid models including both categorical and dimensional aspects, and it was expected that the fifth edition of the Diagnostic and Statistical Manual (DSM-5; American Psychiatric Association [APA], 2013) would take the first steps toward such a hybrid model. For example, dimensional assessments could be used to supplement categorical diagnosis. This would allow clinicians and researchers to capture not only the level of severity of a given disorder's symptoms but also the full range of symptoms an individual experiences regardless of diagnosis (e.g., levels of other forms of anxiety or of depressive or attention deficit hyperactivity disorder symptoms). Such definitional changes were ultimately deemed premature by the DSM-5 Task Force but remain an important emphasis for future research (APA, 2013). Finally, it is unclear how anxiety disorders should be differentiated. Should they be organized based on their descriptive psychopathology (as in the DSM), etiology, or the function served by symptoms (see, e.g., Kearney & Silverman, 1990)?

There is also ambiguity as to what is the best approach to answering these questions (Bernstein & Zvolensky, 2011). Should we proceed empirically, with a minimum of assumptions (i.e., a bottom-up approach) or should we begin by defining anxiety disorders based on consensus or theory (i.e., a top-down approach). Although bottom-up approaches have a long history in the study of child psychopathology (Achenbach, 1982), top-down approaches have predominated since the introduction of DSM-III (APA, 1980).

The anxiety disorder categories defined in DSM-5 (APA, 2013) reflect a largely top-down approach to distinguishing among types of anxiety problems. Very little bottom-up research has been done. However, there is factor analytic evidence that generally supports many of the DSM-5 anxiety disorders. Spence (1997) used confirmatory factor analysis of children's self-reports regarding the major symptoms of each of six DSM-IV anxiety disorder subcategories: panic disorder (PD) with agoraphobia (AG), separation anxiety disorder (SAD), social phobia (SoP),

generalized anxiety disorder (GAD), obsessive–compulsive disorder (OCD), and a specific phobia (SP, i.e., fear of injury). The best-fitting model was a single, higher order anxiety factor associated with these six subdimensions. Thus, these results converge fairly well with DSM-5. However, consistent with the high rates of comorbidity among these disorders, they also show that these anxiety disorders share much in common (i.e., a higher order factor). This overlap may stem from inadequacies in our current nosology but also likely reflects a high degree of commonality in the risk factors and causal processes involved in these disorders' etiology and maintenance.

Diagnostic Categories

DSM-IV described seven major anxiety disorders commonly diagnosed in youth: (1) SAD, (2) SP, (3) SoP, (4) PD with and without agoraphobia AG, (5) GAD, (6) OCD, and (7) post-traumatic stress disorder (PTSD). DSM-5 largely retained these diagnoses although AG was promoted to a standalone diagnosis and OCD and PTSD were moved to separate sections. Below, we discuss the major features and epidemiology of each of these except OCD and PTSD, which are not considered because they are addressed in separate chapters in this volume.

Separation Anxiety Disorder

The hallmark of SAD is developmentally inappropriate, recurrent, and excessive anxiety concerning separation from home or attachment figures. Affected children experience excessive worry about losing or harm befalling major attachment figures or that events will separate them from caregivers. Associated features include reluctance or refusal to attend school, fear of being alone, nightmares concerning separation, and physical symptoms (e.g., stomach aches) in anticipation of or following separation. The disorder must persist for at least 4 weeks and cause clinically significant distress and/or interference with functioning in academic, social, or other important domains.

SAD changed only slightly from DSM-IV to DSM-5. The main change was to allow onset after age 18 years. Such a change is consistent with research showing that SAD may have onset in adulthood (Cyranowski et al., 2002). However, in such cases (i.e., ages ≥ 18 years) duration is required to be at least 6 months). Adults with SAD are described as tending to be overconcerned about loved ones (e.g., a spouse) and intensely anxious when separated from them (APA, 2013).

Specific Phobia

SPs involve marked, persistent fear of specific objects or situations lasting at least 6 months. In children, this fear may take the form of tantrums, crying, freezing, or clinging (APA, 2013). To distinguish phobias from normal fears, particularly in children, severity must be sufficient to interfere significantly with normal functioning. Like DSM-IV, DSM-5 distinguishes among five foci: animals, situations (e.g., elevators, flying), blood-injection-injury, natural environment (e.g., storms, heights), and other. These fear foci are avoided or endured with intense distress. Whereas adults may recognize their fears are excessive or unreasonable, children typically do not.

Changes to the specific phobia category under DSM-5 are minor (APA, 2013), largely involving wording changes intended to reduce ambiguity (e.g., the term "marked" was operationalized as "intense").

Social Phobia

SoP is characterized by pronounced, persistent (at least 6 months) fear of one or more social performance situations in which embarrassment and negative social evaluation may occur or in which the individual encounters unfamiliar people. This phobia can be limited to specific contexts (e.g., public speaking) or generalized across social situations. In the feared situation intense anxiety is experienced, often taking the form of a panic attack. In children, this anxiety may take the form of crying, tantrums, freezing,

or retreating from the feared stimulus. Typically this distress leads to efforts to avoid, although some individuals endure feared situations despite intense distress. The avoidance and/or distress must interfere with normal functioning or there must be marked distress about having the phobia. Also, in children there must be evidence of the capacity for age-appropriate social relationships with familiar people, and the anxiety must occur with peers and not just in interactions with adults.

DSM-5 made few changes to SoP. One change which had been proposed was to make selective mutism a behavioral specifier to SoP rather than a disorder in its own right. Although this change ultimately was not made, such a change would be consistent with evidence of high comorbidity between selective mutism (SM) and SoP, which suggests that SM is best regarded as an avoidance pattern that is particularly relevant to the expression of social anxiety in young children (Bögels et al., 2010).

Panic Disorder with or Without Agoraphobia

Recurrent, unexpected panic attacks are the hallmark of PD. Such attacks involve intense fear accompanied by somatic symptoms of sympathetic nervous system arousal and by catastrophic cognitions (e.g., fear of having a heart attack). PD is often associated with AG, which involves pronounced anxiety about being in places or situations where escape may be difficult or embarrassing in the event that a panic attack were to occur. These situations are avoided or endured with significant distress.

Few changes were made to PD under DSM-5 but AG became codeable as a separate disorder (APA, 2013). This change is in keeping with evidence showing that panic and AG are not closely linked in youth. For example, Wittchen et al. (2008) found that adolescents with panic disorder or panic attacks were only moderately more likely to develop agoraphobia than those without. Furthermore, the majority meeting criteria for agoraphobia had never experienced a panic attack.

Generalized Anxiety Disorder

The definition of GAD changed little from DSM-IV to DSM-5 (APA, 2013). GAD is characterized by frequent, uncontrollable, and persistent (at least 6 months) worry that causes significant distress or impaired function. This worry typically includes a broad range of topics and is associated with at least three (only one among children) of the following somatic symptoms: feeling restless or keyed up, becoming easily fatigued, poor concentration, irritability, muscle tension, and sleep difficulties. Children with GAD are described as tending to be overly compliant, perfectionistic, and prone to excessively seek reassurance (APA, 2013).

Developmental Issues

Development poses serious challenges for defining anxiety disorders because the normative base rate of any potentially symptomatic behavior, and hence its diagnostic utility, is likely to vary substantially with age. Furthermore, the clinical manifestations of anxiety disorders are likely to show considerable developmental variation in focus, severity, and form, making continuity from early childhood through adolescence and into adulthood at the level of molecular anxiety symptoms very unlikely (Fonseca & Perrin, 2011). For example, the typical presentation of SAD shifts from nightmares at ages 5–8, to somatic complaints at ages 9–12, to school refusal in adolescence (Whiteside & Ollendick, 2009). Thus, definitions must reflect developmental changes in the content of children's fears as well as how severe they must be to be judged outside the normal range of anxiety (Whiteside & Ollendick, 2009).

Although DSM-IV specified developmental variations in the criteria that define some anxiety disorders, for many of the disorders such variations were notably lacking (see Whiteside & Ollendick, 2009). For example, none is provided for PD despite there being considerable evidence for important developmental variations in its presentation (e.g., Ollendick, Mattis, & King, 1994).

Consequently, there was significant risk that researchers may focus their attention too narrowly on those children who meet adult criteria while missing others who display developmental variants of symptoms (Costello, Egger, Copeland, Erkanli, & Angold, 2011). Furthermore, even when such variations were provided, rarely were they grounded in research, leaving their validity open to question.

In light of such deficiencies in DSM-IV, Whiteside and Ollendick (2009) made several recommendations for developmentally informed changes to the anxiety disorders section in DSM-5. Most importantly, they argued that it should incorporate recent findings regarding the somatic, cognitive, and behavioral manifestations of anxiety in children. Specifically, they concluded that somatic symptoms should be considered for all anxiety disorders and, because evidence suggests that the list of applicable symptoms is not the same in children as in adults, those symptoms should specify expected developmental variations. For example, of the symptoms found by Ginsburg, Riddle, and Davies (2006) to differentiate children with GAD from those without (i.e., restlessness, stomachaches, and hot flashes), only one is included in the criteria for GAD (i.e., restlessness). Poor fit was also seen for the somatic symptoms of PD.

Whiteside and Ollendick (2009) also called for the role of cognitive factors to be reconsidered in DSM-5, especially for young children. For example, they noted that in PD children typically report non-catastrophic, external attributions regarding panic symptoms rather than the catastrophic, internal attributions that characterize the disorder in adults (Ollendick et al., 1994). They argued that an emphasis on cognitions is particularly inappropriate for young children, who are more likely to exhibit behavioral manifestations of anxiety such as those included for some PTSD criteria (e.g., instead of recurrent thoughts or images, children may reexperience the trauma through repetitive play in which traumatic themes appear). Indeed, they noted that many of the problems in assessing physical and cognitive symptoms of anxiety in children could be circumvented through the specification of behavioral manifestations of such disorders in childhood. Parents and teachers can easily observe such behaviors whereas they must infer cognitive and somatic symptoms when children are too young to adequately report on such symptoms. How this might be done is illustrated by the International Classification of Diseases (10th revision [ICD-10], World Health Organization, 1992). For example, to accommodate developmental variation in GAD symptoms, ICD-10 offers an alternative set of criteria for use in children that permit GAD to be diagnosed in the absence of cognitive symptoms. Similarly, the ICD-10 criteria for SoP can be met in the absence of fear of negative evaluation. Unfortunately, of the changes to the anxiety disorders in DSM-5, few appear likely to enhance their developmental sensitivity (see APA, 2013).

Epidemiology

Based on a meta-analysis of community samples, Costello et al. (2011) report a mean of 10.2 % (95 % confidence interval [CI]: 9.3 %–11.3 %) for the prevalence of any anxiety disorder among individuals ages 2–21 years. Rates are somewhat higher and more variable among children ages 6–12 (mean: 12.3 %, CI: 7.1–28.2 %) than among adolescents ages 13–18 (mean: 11.0 %, CI: 10.3–12.2 %). Finally, the prevalence of some anxiety disorders varies with age and gender. Such differences raise questions about age and gender differences in the validity of diagnostic categories but also may provide important clues regarding the role of developing biological, social, cognitive, and emotional capacities in the etiology of these disorders.

Prevalence of Specific Disorders

SAD

Average age of onset for SAD is 6.5 years (Costello et al., 2011). Costello and colleagues found average prevalence ranged from 3.9 % (ages 6–12) to 2.4 % (ages 12–18). SAD appears to be substantially more common in girls than boys (Crozier, Gillihan, & Powers, 2011).

SP

Average age of onset for specific phobia is also 6.5 years (Costello et al., 2011). Prevalence estimates average 5 %–6.7 % (Costello et al., 2011; Ollendick, King, & Muris, 2002), with rates being similar across age [6 to 18 years (Costello et al., 2011)]. However, many cases of SP involve little functional impairment; prevalence rates appear to be reduced by about 50 % if significant impairment is required (Shaffer et al., 1996). Evidence suggests phobias are also more common in girls than boys (Crozier et al., 2011).

SoP

Average age of onset for SoP is about 9.5 years (Costello et al., 2011). Prevalence estimates for SoP range from 1 % to 6 % in youth samples (Crozier et al., 2011). Based on their meta-analysis, Costello et al. (2011) report that the average prevalence of social anxiety disorder ranges from 2.2 % (ages 6–12) to 5 % (ages 12–18). Unlike most anxiety disorders, prevalence rates are similar among males and females (Crozier et al., 2011).

PD and AG

Average age of onset for PD is about 19 years, with few cases appearing before mid-adolescence. In contrast, typical onset for AG is around 11.5 years. Costello et al. (2011) report that the average prevalence of PD ranges from 1.5 % (ages 6–12) to 1.1 % (ages 12–18). The prevalence of AG is about 1.5 % (Costello, Egger, & Angold, 2004). Panic attacks and PD are more prevalent among girls than boys (Ollendick et al., 1994).

GAD

Average age of onset for GAD is 8.5 years (Costello et al., 2011). Costello et al. (2011) report that average prevalence ranges from 1.7 % (ages 6–12) to 1.9 % (ages 12–18). In adulthood, GAD is twice as common in females as males (Wittchen, Zhao, Kessler, & Eaton, 1994). However, as is the case for depression, this disparity does not appear to emerge until adolescence. In childhood, GAD has similar prevalence in boys and girls (Costello et al., 2011).

Comorbidity

There is a high degree of comorbidity among the anxiety disorders, especially among the phobias [i.e., SP, SoP, and AG (Costello et al., 2011)]. However, there is also evidence supporting the distinctiveness of at least some of these disorders. For example, Costello et al. (2011) found no connection between SAD and the group of phobias or between SAD and GAD.

Comorbidity with other disorders is also common, especially depression [particularly with GAD (Whiteside & Ollendick, 2009)], disruptive behavior problems (Costello et al., 2011), and substance abuse (Fonseca & Perrin, 2011). However, Costello et al. (2011) note that there are very few published studies adequate to speak to questions of comorbidity. Insofar as the available evidence suggests important differences among the anxiety disorders in terms of overlap with or risk for other disorders (e.g., see Kaplow, Curran, Angold, & Costello, 2001), there is clearly a need for further research on the question.

Continuity Across Age

Prospective studies generally support continuity at the broad level of any anxiety disorder but not at the level of individual diagnoses (Costello et al., 2011; Whiteside & Ollendick, 2009). There is some evidence for continuity of specific anxiety disorders from childhood to adolescence (Costello et al., 2003). However, there is less evidence for such continuity into adulthood: Adult anxiety disorders are similarly associated with childhood GAD, SAD, and SoP (Gregory et al., 2007). However, whereas most adult anxiety disorders appear to have been preceded by a child or adolescent anxiety disorder, most childhood disorders do not persist to adulthood—instead resolving or changing to another disorder (Costello et al., 2011).

Etiological Factors

In this section we provide an overview of the major biological, environmental, and psychological factors playing roles in the etiology and maintenance of clinical forms of anxiety in youth. Where possible we consider developmental variations in these factors, their operation, and the roles they may play. Also, although we discuss them separately, these factors invariably operate through complex transactions with one another (Vasey & Dadds, 2001). Depending on the configuration of other factors in play, a given factor may lead to different anxiety disorders, other forms of psychopathology, or to no disorder at all. Therefore, where possible we emphasize demonstrated (or likely) interactions with other factors. Furthermore, because few disorder-specific factors have been identified, we mainly focus on factors that contribute broadly to anxiety pathology rather than to specific disorders. Finally, we conclude by offering an integrative perspective on the etiology of such disorders.

Genetics

Several issues complicate research on genetic factors in anxiety. First, the genetic underpinnings of anxiety problems are complex, involving the additive and interactive impact of many genes, each having only small effects in isolation (Arnold & Taillefer, 2011). This limits statistical power to identify specific risk-related genes. Second, as discussed above, there is considerable phenotypic variability in anxiety symptoms, and it is unlikely that it is optimally divided by current diagnostic categories (Arnold & Taillefer, 2011). Such ambiguity weakens research seeking to understand the genes involved in specific anxiety disorders.

Despite these challenges, research clearly shows that anxiety and anxiety disorders run in families (Hettema, Neale, & Kendler, 2001) and they do so, in part, because of heritable genetic effects (Gregory & Eley, 2011). Although clarity is lacking regarding genetic effects on specific disorders, twin studies of youth suggest that anxiety symptoms are moderately heritable. Approximately 30 % of the variance in anxiety problems is attributable to additive genetic effects (Gregory & Eley, 2011) with 20 % attributable to shared environmental effects and 50 %

to non-shared environmental factors (Muris, 2007). However, the magnitude of genetic and shared environmental effects varies with age (Gregory & Eley, 2011). Specifically, heritability of anxiety appears to increase and the influence of shared environment to decrease with age (Gregory & Eley, 2011). This is consistent with the increasing potential for individuals to select their own environment as they get older, thereby increasing the potential for anxiety-promoting gene–environment correlations.

Most studies of genetic effects to date assume that genes and environments have additive effects. However, it is clear that interactive (e.g., gene×environment [G×E]) effects should be expected and research has begun to isolate them (Lau, Gregory, Goldwin, Pine, & Eley, 2007). For example, Silberg, Rutter, Neale, and Eaves (2001) found that genetic effects on GAD symptoms were strongest among girls exposed to high levels of negative life events.

Although a number of gene-linkage and association studies of youth anxiety have begun to appear, few consistent findings have yet emerged. However, there are several likely candidate genes or gene regions, among the most promising of which are the serotonin transporter polymorphism (5-HTTLPR) and the gene for catechol-O-methyltransferase (COMT), an enzyme involved in the metabolism of dopamine and other catecholamines (Arnold & Taillefer, 2011; Gregory & Eley, 2011). The s-allele of the 5-HTTLPR has been linked to heightened fear conditionability (Lonsdorf et al., 2009) and vulnerability to anxiety (and depression), although results in youth studies thus far have been mixed (Gregory & Eley, 2011). Homozygosity for the met-allele of the COMT gene has been linked to poor fear extinction learning (especially in individuals with the 5-HTTLPR s-allele (Lonsdorf et al., 2009) and to increased odds for phobic anxiety disorder in youth (McGrath et al., 2004). Future research will likely specify other genes linked to these and other neurotransmitters, including the gamma-aminobutyric (GABA), corticotropin-releasing hormone (CRH), and estrogen systems (Gregory & Eley, 2011).

Also holding considerable promise is research focused on endophenotypes and epigenetic factors (Gregory & Eley, 2011). Endophenotypes are characteristics that are presumed to be closer to the genotype than a disorder phenotype and therefore they permit easier identification of genetic effects. Several recent studies reveal the promise of research focused on such characteristics (e.g., Battaglia, Pesenti-Gritti, Medland, Ogliari, & Spatola, 2009; Eley et al., 2007). For example, Battaglia et al. (2009) studied an endophenotype presumed to be linked to PD—hypersensitivity to a CO_2 inhalation challenge—and found that the variance it shared with diagnoses of PD and SAD was largely (89 %) a function of shared genes, with the remaining 11 % linked to childhood parental loss. Epigenetic effects reflect factors that regulate gene expression and thus are the processes by which genes are turned on or off over time. For example, a growing body of animal research shows there is significant potential for early experiences to impact risk for anxiety disorders (Nolte, Guiney, Fonagy, Mayes, & Luyten, 2011). Weaver et al. (2004) found that rat pups licked and groomed to a greater extent by their mothers were more stress resistant as adults and that difference was mediated by methylation changes in the promoter region of a gene linked to a glucocorticoid receptor in the hippocampus.

Neurobiology

A rapidly growing body of animal and human research provides an increasingly clear picture of the brain circuits underlying anxiety and fear responses and their regulation, with particular emphasis on bidirectional connections between the amygdala and the prefrontal cortex (PFC; LeDoux, 2000). Although undoubtedly an oversimplification, pathological anxiety appears to involve hypersensitivity of the amygdala interacting with deficient regulatory processes mediated by the PFC (Nolte et al., 2011). The former is shown by hypervigilance characterized by rapid orienting to threat stimuli presented for very brief intervals whereas the latter is shown by delayed disengagement of attention from threat stimuli presented for longer intervals (Pine, 2011). As discussed below (see Cognitive Factors), such effects have been documented in relation to a range of anxiety-related individual differences including BI temperament, trait anxiety, and anxiety disorders.

The functioning of this fear circuitry changes with development. For example, Lau et al. (2011) report evidence of developmental change in threat learning between early adolescence and adulthood. Young adolescents were less able than adults to discriminate threat and safety cues in their verbal ratings of fear and these results were mirrored by fMRI results. Specifically, whereas both groups showed a similar pattern of amygdala response to threat versus safety cues, only adults showed evidence of activation in the dorsolateral (dl)PFC in response to safety cues. Lau et al. (2011) interpret their findings as being consistent with maturation of the dlPFC, which likely supports the capacity for reappraisal of potentially threatening stimuli. Failures to develop this capacity may contribute to persistent anxiety disorders (Britton et al., 2011).

Temperament

The genetic risk for anxiety disorders is mediated by temperamental factors, particularly early emerging individual differences in negative affectivity (NA, Clark, Watson, & Mineka, 1994) and associated constructs such as behavioral inhibition (BI) to the unfamiliar (Degnan & Fox, 2007). BI temperament, both as a dimension and as a categorical construct, has received the most attention, with research consistently supporting its link to heightened risk for anxiety problems in childhood, especially SoP (e.g., Hirschfeld-Becker et al., 2007). This is particularly true for that subset of children who show stable BI from infancy through middle childhood. Lonigan, Phillips, Wilson, and Allan (2011) suggest that such stable BI likely reflects not only high levels of NA but also deficient competence at regulating emotional reactions. Indeed, a second aspect of temperament thought to contribute to anxiety pathology is effortful control (EC), which is the capacity for self-regulation (i.e., the capacity to override one's automatic, reactive tendencies and substitute more adaptive responses). Deficits in

EC are associated with heightened risk for anxiety and depression (Muris, 2007). Furthermore, Lonigan and Phillips (2001) postulated an interactive relation between NA and EC such that heightened NA is most likely to lead to anxiety problems when coupled with deficits in EC. A growing body of evidence supports this model (Lonigan et al., 2011). For example, Lonigan and Vasey (2009) showed that high NA was associated with an attentional bias toward threat only when EC was low, and Lonigan et al. (2011) report finding the NA × EC interaction to be significant in relation to concurrent symptoms of SAD, GAD, and PD/AG.

There are at least four ways in which temperament can influence anxiety problems, often in transaction with environmental influences (Lonigan et al., 2011). First, temperament may predispose to the development of anxiety disorders in interaction with environmental stressors (i.e., the *diathesis-stress model*). Second, the *pathoplasticity model* postulates that temperament may influence the symptoms or course of an anxiety disorder without having a direct causal role in its onset. For example, even before the onset of a phobia, children with BI temperament are likely to have taught their parents to protect them from anxiety-provoking experiences, thereby fostering the persistence of a phobia following its onset. Third, under the *complication* or *scar model*, enduring changes to temperament that foster anxiety emerge as a complication of developing an anxiety disorder. For example, an anxious child's avoidance and protective responses to the child's anxiety by parents and others may increase a child's level of NA. Fourth, under the *continuity model*, anxiety disorders and temperament are seen as reflecting the same underlying processes. Of course, these models are not mutually exclusive.

Parental Influences

Many of the experiences through which children's fears are acquired and shaped involve their parents (Dadds & Roth, 2001). Murray, Creswell, and Cooper (2009) described three paths by which parents may contribute to their child's anxiety problems. First, parents may adopt approaches to socialization that lead their child to perceive the world as full of uncontrollable dangers, with which he or she is incompetent to cope. Second, if anxious themselves, parents may promote anxiety through modeling and verbal information transmission, as discussed below in the context of respondent conditioning influences. Third, whether they are anxious or not, parents may respond to their child's anxious responses in ways that contribute to their maintenance and intensification, as discussed below in the context of operant conditioning influences. However, next to these direct paths, research also suggests indirect effects of interactions with parents through trust in parental support (Bosmans, Braet, Beyers, Van Leeuwen, & Van Vlierberghe, 2011; Brumariu & Kerns, 2010).

Direct Parental Influences

Based on a recent meta-analysis, the effects of parental influences are small on average (McLeod, Wood, & Weisz, 2007). However, their magnitude varies substantially, with the strongest effects being seen in studies of younger children, clinical samples, and studies which use behavioral observations rather than questionnaires (Creswell, Murray, Stacey, & Cooper, 2011). However, parenting influences do not operate in isolation, and evidence suggests that such effects are likely to be substantially larger in interaction with other factors. For example, their impact is stronger among temperamentally vulnerable children (e.g., Murray et al., 2008; Thirlwall & Creswell, 2010). Other research has begun to reveal the processes that mediate the effect of parental influences on anxiety. For example, Perez-Olivas, Stevenson, and Hadwin (2008) found evidence that the impact of parental control on child anxiety is mediated by a tendency to interpret ambiguous information as threatening.

Parents may also foster anxiety in their child by being over-involved and exerting intrusive control over the child's experiences and behavior (Cresswell et al., 2011). For example, parents may limit their child's exposure to fear-provoking stimuli, thereby interfering with the normal process of fear habituation or mastery (Vasey & Dadds, 2001). Similarly, they may foster vulnerability by failing to grant and support the child's autonomy, instead limiting contact with challenging situations or exerting intrusive control as the child copes with such challenges. A growing body of evidence supports an association between parental control and child anxiety (Creswell, Shildrick, & Field, 2011). For example, in their meta-analysis, McLeod et al. (2007) found an average correlation of $r = -0.42$ between parental autonomy granting and child anxiety.

Anxious parents, specifically mothers, have long been viewed as likely to behave in ways that promote anxiety in their offspring. Evidence suggests they do indeed display more anxiety to their children and that doing so increases the likelihood of later anxious responses by the child (Rapee et al., 2009). For example, Murray, Cooper, Creswell, Schofield, and Sack (2007) observed mothers with SoP to exhibit more anxiety toward a stranger and to be less likely to encourage their 10-month-old infants to engage with the stranger. Furthermore, such behavior was shown to increase the likelihood that infants would later show stranger avoidance.

Whereas early studies left it unclear if this association meant parental behaviors causally contribute to child anxiety or if anxious children lead their parents to exert more control, recent evidence suggests both are true. Experimental studies suggest that parental control does indeed promote anxiety and related responses from children (De Wilde & Rapee, 2008; Thirlwall & Creswell, 2010). However, Gar and Hudson (2008) conducted an experimental study in which mothers of children with and without anxiety disorders interacted with two unrelated children, one anxious and the other non-anxious. Mothers were observed to be more involved and controlling with the anxious versus control child regardless of the anxiety status of their own children, suggesting that anxious children engender controlling responses from their parents.

Parents may also exert control by fostering their child's selection of avoidant responses to anxiety-provoking situations. Barrett, Rapee, Dadds, and Ryan (1996) found that anxious children chose avoidant solutions to challenging situations more often than normal controls, and this tendency was fostered by their parents in family problem-solving discussions. Dadds, Barrett, Rapee, and Ryan (1996) found that parents of anxious children were significantly more likely than parents of normal controls to differentially reinforce their children's mention of avoidance during problem-solving discussions. Further, rates of such reinforcement were positively correlated with the child's selection of avoidant responses following the discussion.

Indirect Parental Effects (Attachment)

Research suggests that parenting effects on child anxiety are at least partly mediated by the child's lack of confidence in parental support. Moreover, in keeping with the finding that shared environment matters less with increasing age (Gregory & Eley, 2011), the direct effect of parenting declines during adolescence. In contrast, confidence in parental support appears to remain important (Bosmans et al., 2011).

These findings are unsurprising in light of attachment research. Multiple studies have shown that lack of confidence in parental support, or insecure attachment, is an important predictor of child anxiety problems (Brumariu & Kerns, 2010; Groh, Roisman, van IJzendoorn, Bakermans-Kranenburg, & Fearon, 2012). According to attachment theory, perceived threats activate the attachment system, triggering a cascade of processes targeted at reducing the threat and also serving to regulate the stress response itself (Nolte et al., 2011). Key among these threat responses in infancy and childhood is the seeking of proximity to and support from one's caregiver (Cassidy, 2008). Over time however, the child develops expectations regarding the caregiver's reliability as a source of support depending on whether or not the caregiver is sensitive and responsive to the child's needs. A securely attached child builds an internal working model of a sensitive caregiver that enables the child to feel safe while exploring the world (Cassidy, 2008). In contrast, the insecurely attached child's model of an insensitive and unreliable caregiver leads to feeling unsafe in navigating the world (Bowlby, 1973). Such children

should therefore face increased risk for the development of anxiety disorders.

Insecure attachment fundamentally alters children's abilities to regulate distress, explaining links between attachment and anxiety (Nolte et al., 2011). When distressed, securely attached children readily seek caregiver support and derive comfort from it. However, because insecurely attached children lack confidence in the caregiver, they must rely on less adaptive, secondary coping strategies (Brenning, Soenens, Braet, & Bosmans, 2011; Mikulincer & Shaver, 2007). The nature of these strategies depends on the child's insecure attachment style. Avoidantly attached children distance themselves from their caregivers and do not seek support, instead adopting a "deactivating" strategy involving emotional suppression. In contrast, children with an anxious/ambivalent attachment are highly dependent on caregiver support, but fear abandonment and rejection. Consequently, they adopt a "hyperactivating" strategy associated with pronounced anxiety reactions in response to, and hypervigilance for, threats (Nolte et al., 2011). Finally, children exposed to highly unpredictable and negative caregiver interactions are at risk to develop a disorganized pattern of coping behavior characterized by chaotic swings between hyperactivating and deactivating responses (Groh et al., 2012).

Across age-groups, cross-sectional and prospective research has confirmed that anxiety problems are linked to insecure attachment, especially the anxious/ambivalent pattern (Colonnesi et al., 2011), although some evidence also supports a link to the disorganized pattern (e.g., Brumariu & Kerns, 2010; Groh et al., 2012). Furthermore, evidence suggests that attachment interacts with other factors in association with anxiety problems, including BI temperament (Brumariu & Kerns, 2010) and stressful life events (Dallaire & Weinraub, 2007).

Learning Influences

Respondent conditioning processes undoubtedly play an important role in precipitating the onset of phobic anxiety but can contribute to anxiety disorders in other ways as well (Dadds, Davey, & Field, 2001). Modern respondent conditioning theories (see Field & Purkis, 2011) emphasize the acquisition of an expectation that a previously neutral stimulus (i.e., the conditioned stimulus [CS]) predicts the occurrence of a second stimulus that is appraised as aversive (i.e., the unconditioned stimulus [UCS]), thereby provoking a fear response. By virtue of that expectation, the CS comes to elicit a conditioned fear response (CR). It is important to emphasize that direct experiences pairing the CS and UCS are not necessary; the requisite expectancy can be learned indirectly. Indeed, direct conditioning experiences may account for only a minority of childhood phobias, with a basis in vicarious learning and verbal information transmission being more common (Ollendick & King, 1991). Similarly, the aversive stimulus need not be truly dangerous; it need only be appraised as such. Indeed, it need not even be real: an imagined aversive event is sufficient (Field & Purkis, 2011).

There are one direct and two indirect paths by which such conditioning occurs: (1) direct traumatic conditioning, (2) vicarious (i.e., observational) learning, and (3) verbal information transmission (Field & Purkis, 2011). Experimental evidence from child samples shows that all three paths are sufficiently powerful as to produce conditioned fear responses to novel, neutral stimuli as expressed through cognitive, behavioral, and physiological response channels (see Field & Purkis, 2011). Furthermore, such conditioned responses persist over time (Field & Purkis, 2011). However, as should be expected given that even direct traumatic conditioning episodes often do not result in phobias (Dadds et al., 2001), evidence shows that respondent conditioning processes interact with other factors such as parental characteristics (e.g., negative interactions with parents, e.g., Field, Ball, Kawycz, & Moore, 2007) and temperament (e.g., trait anxiety, e.g., Field & Price-Evans, 2009) to produce heightened fear conditioning and resistance to extinction in vulnerable individuals (e.g., Waters, Henry, & Neumann, 2009).

Although respondent conditioning processes are most commonly discussed as precipitating factors, they may also play predisposing, protective, maintaining, exacerbating, and ameliorating roles. For example, the phenomenon of sensory preconditioning may explain why some children develop phobias despite lacking any apparent history of direct conditioning involving the feared stimulus (see Dadds et al., 2001). Similarly, to the extent that children have non-traumatic experiences with a stimulus, they may be less likely to acquire a fear of that stimulus subsequent to a conditioning episode [i.e., latent inhibition, see Dadds et al. (2001)]. Finally, such processes may contribute to the maintenance, intensification, or amelioration of phobic responses through stimulus revaluation (see Dadds et al., 2001).

Operant conditioning also may play a role in the acquisition of anxiety disorders [e.g., inept social behavior may bring negative social evaluation and thus lead to social anxiety (Ollendick, Vasey, & King, 2001)]. However, the impact of such factors is perhaps greatest with regard to the maintenance, exacerbation, and amelioration of such problems. Subsequent to the onset of anxiety symptoms, there are numerous opportunities for such responses to be shaped by their consequences (Ollendick et al., 2001). For example, by virtue of their extreme distress, anxious children are likely to be effective at punishing those around them for not accommodating their desire for avoidance. Simultaneously, relief from the child's intense reactions is likely to be a potent source of negative reinforcement when others permit or foster such avoidance. Thus, those around the anxious child may come to be controlled by the short-term reduction of the child's anxiety, at the expense of the child's ultimate mastery of anxiety and the demands of anxiety-provoking situations (Vasey & Dadds, 2001).

Stress

Stressful life events appear to increase risk for anxiety disorders in youth (Muris, 2007). For example, the onset of SAD often follows a major stressor such as a move to a new school (Gittelman-Klein & Klein, 1980). Although most of the evidence for this association is cross sectional and relies on retrospective reports of stress, a few prospective studies also support the link. For example, Grover, Ginsburg and Ialongo (2005) found that total negative life events at baseline predicted anxiety levels six years later in a high-risk sample of African-American children. However, it is important to note that evidence also shows that anxiety disorders predict the occurrence of such events (Kim, Conger, Elder, & Lorenz, 2003).

The controllability of environmental events, especially early in childhood, may be particularly important in the development of anxiety disorders (Chorpita & Barlow, 1998). Specifically, early exposure to controllable environments appears to protect against anxiety, whereas uncontrollable environments predispose to anxiety. For example, infant rhesus monkeys exposed to chronically uncontrollable environments responded to novel stimuli with greater fear and less exploration than monkeys having control over their environment (Mineka, Gunnar, & Champoux, 1986). The predisposing effects of uncontrollable environments may be mediated, in part, by changes in the endocrine systems associated with stress responses that may increase reactivity to stress (Nachmias, Gunnar, Mangelsdorf, Parritz, & Buss, 1996). However, such effects are also likely to be mediated by control-related cognitions formed through experiences with controllable and uncontrollable events (Weems & Silverman, 2006).

Relationship problems, especially peer rejection and victimization, are potent stressors that can contribute to the development of anxiety disorders (La Greca & Landoll, 2011). In their most extreme forms (e.g., bullying), such social stressors can provoke onset of SoP, PTSD, or other anxiety disorders (Hawker & Boulton, 2000). Furthermore, once anxiety symptoms develop, especially social anxiety symptoms, they can lead to further relationship difficulties. For example, Blöte, Kint, and Westenberg (2007) found that higher levels of social anxiety in adolescents predicted more negative treatment by their peers.

Cognitive Factors

Anxiety disorders in youth are associated with a wide range of cognitive factors that may play important etiological and maintaining roles. These include anxiety-promoting beliefs such as low self-efficacy, lack of control, and anxiety sensitivity (see Muris, 2007) as well as information processing biases. Despite some inconsistencies, the extant evidence shows that such cognitive factors characterize anxious youth just as they do anxious adults (see Field, Hadwin, & Lester, 2011). For example, studies using a variety of paradigms show that anxious children exhibit an attentional bias in favor of threat-relevant stimuli relative to controls and that effect sizes are generally comparable to those seen among adults (see Bar-Haim et al., 2007). Similarly, compared to controls, anxious children show a bias toward interpreting ambiguous information as threatening (see Field et al., 2011).

To the extent that such biases are shown by children prior to the onset of problematic anxiety, they may contribute significantly to risk for its development. Unfortunately, prospective studies addressing this possibility remain largely lacking. However, whether such cognitive biases predispose to, or result from anxiety, a growing body of experimental evidence suggests they are causally involved in its maintenance. Studies in youth and adult samples show that the attentional and interpretive biases can be modified through computer-based training procedures and that the resulting reductions in bias lead to commensurate reductions in anxiety symptoms (e.g., Rozenmann, Weersing, & Amir, 2011; Vassilopoulos, Banerjee, & Prantzalou, 2009). Similarly, evidence suggests that risk for anxiety disorders in adolescents can be substantially reduced through a program designed to reduce anxiety sensitivity (Schmidt et al., 2007).

How such cognitive biases develop remains poorly understood. With regard to the attentional and interpretational biases, Field et al. (2011) consider three possibilities. First, such biases may be innate or emerge very early, distinguishing anxiety-prone children even in infancy. Second, all young children may show biases favoring threat, which normally diminish with increasing age but fail to do so in anxious children. Third, such biases may be acquired, emerging only as children get older. However, these possibilities are not mutually exclusive. Indeed, although the situation is less clear for the interpretation bias (Field et al., 2011), in the case of the attentional bias, evidence supports all three. Not surprisingly given their likely adaptive advantage, attentional biases toward threat are present even in infancy (e.g., LoBue & DeLoache, 2010) and can be found in non-anxious children (Field et al., 2011). However, there is also evidence that this bias is larger in anxious versus non-anxious samples among children as young as 3 to 4 years (e.g., Martin & Jones, 1992). Similarly, Perez-Edgar et al. (2011) found a link between an attentional bias toward angry faces and social withdrawal in 5-year-olds. Finally, it appears that such biases can be acquired through experience (e.g., Field, 2006). Thus, although it remains unclear if the bias is larger in anxiety-prone children even in infancy, it appears that the difference emerges early in childhood and thus has significant potential to contribute to the etiology of anxiety disorders. Nevertheless, evidence also suggests that the bias becomes stronger with age in anxious children and weaker in non-anxious children, presumably reflecting developing capacity for executive control of attention (Lonigan et al., 2004) and the operation of other factors promoting anxiety. For example, the attentional bias appears to mediate the link between maternal over-involvement and symptoms of SAD (Perez-Olivas et al., 2008). Furthermore, it appears that the attentional bias promotes the interpretation bias (White, Suway, Bar-Haim, Pine, & Fox, 2011).

An Integrative Perspective

It is highly unlikely that any one of the etiological influences reviewed above is sufficient to produce clinical levels of anxiety by itself. Rather, anxiety disorders in youth emerge via developmental pathways involving many and varied combinations of these influences, each operating in transaction with the others (Vasey & Dadds, 2001). Depending upon the configuration and timing with which they occur, any given factor may lead to several different anxiety disorders, to other forms of psychopathology, or to no disorder at all.

In keeping with this view, once typically studied in isolation, etiological factors are now often considered in the context of or in interaction with one another. Indeed, numerous scholars have offered complex, integrative developmental models of youth anxiety (e.g., Degnan & Fox, 2007; Lau & Pine, 2009; Muris, 2007; Nolte et al., 2011; Vasey & Dadds, 2001), and prospective tests of predictions from such models are increasingly common in the literature (e.g., Barrocas & Hankin, 2011; Bosquet & Egeland, 2006; Creswell, Shildrick, & Field, 2011; White, McDermott, Degnan, Henderson, & Fox, 2011).

For example, drawing on research on biological, temperamental, and cognitive biases, growing evidence suggests that hypersensitivity of the amygdala to threat cues and deficient regulation of the fear circuit by the PFC reflect genetic influences and manifest in an anxiety-prone temperament reflecting high levels of NA and low levels of EC (Bosquet & Egeland, 2006; Lau & Pine, 2008). This combination elevates risk for stable difficulties regulating anxiety (e.g., stable BI temperament) that are associated with heightened vigilance for and orienting to threat cues coupled with deficient ability to disengage attention from such cues (Lonigan & Vasey, 2009; White et al., 2011). Such biases are further instilled and fostered by attachment insecurity (Nolte et al., 2011) as well as parental modeling, verbal information transmission, and reinforcement of threatening interpretations of ambiguous information (Creswell et al., 2011; Perez-Olivas et al., 2008). Parents respond by limiting the child's autonomy, likely leaving the child deficient in skills needed to master the challenges posed by threatening situations and the anxiety they produce (Creswell et al., 2011). Children following such a path have a low sense of control and view anxiety itself as dangerous and themselves as incompetent to cope with threatening situations and the anxiety they trigger (Weems & Silverman, 2006). Furthermore, it is easy to see the potential for reciprocal links among these influences, with each promoting the other in a negative developmental cascade (Vasey & Dadds, 2001). Evidence for such a cascade can be found in recent prospective studies (e.g., Barrocas & Hankin, 2011; Bosquet & Egeland, 2006).

Summary

In this chapter, we have attempted to provide a glimpse into the complex, unfolding nature of anxiety and its disorders in children and adolescents. This is a particularly exciting time in the study of anxiety insofar as research on anxiety problems in youth is advancing at a rapid pace (Grills-Taquechel & Ollendick, 2012; Muris & Broeren, 2009). Development in its many forms is at center stage in this quickly evolving and exciting area of study.

We began this chapter with a brief foray into definitional issues associated with the study of anxiety in children. The definition of childhood anxiety disorders is made difficult by a range of issues (see Bernstein & Zvolensky, 2011), especially the fact that clinical manifestations of anxiety disorders in children are likely to show considerable variation in focus, severity, and form as a function of development (see Whiteside & Ollendick, 2009). Unfortunately, such developmental variations were poorly represented in DSM-IV and largely remain so in DSM-5.

Development also plays a central role in the epidemiology of anxiety disorders. Age of onset varies greatly across the anxiety disorders, as does prevalence of the various disorders. Such differences in age of onset and prevalence of childhood anxiety disorders may provide important clues regarding the role of developing biological, social, cognitive, and emotional capacities and processes in the etiology and maintenance of these disorders.

Finally, the development of anxiety disorders reflects the influence of a wide range of biological, environmental, and psychological factors operating in complex transaction over time. Depending upon the configuration with which these factors occur, any given factor may lead to several different anxiety disorders, to other forms of psychopathology, or to no disorder at all. Moreover, it is becoming increasingly clear that there are multiple pathways associated with many anxiety disorders. However, although we understand much regarding the broad outlines of these pathways, the developmentally informed study of anxiety disorders in youth remains early in its own development. Although it is happily well past its infancy and maturing rapidly, many challenges remain.

References

Achenbach, T. M. (1982). *Developmental psychopathology* (2nd ed.). New York: Wiley.

American Psychiatric Association. (1980). *Diagnostic and statistical manual of mental disorders* (3rd ed.). Washington, DC: American Psychiatric Association.

American Psychiatric Association. (2013). *Diagnostic and statistical manual of mental disorders* (5th ed.). Arlington, VA: American Psychiatric Publishing.

Arnold, P. D., & Taillefer, S. (2011). Genetics of childhood and adolescent anxiety. In D. McKay & E. A. Storch (Eds.), *Handbook of child and adolescent anxiety disorders* (pp. 49–73). New York: Springer.

American Psychiatric Association. (2000). *Diagnostic and statistical manual of mental disorders* (4th ed., text revision). Washington, DC: American Psychiatric Association.

Bar-Haim, Y., Lamy, D., Pergamin, L., Bakermans-Kranenburg, M. J., & van IJzendoorn, M. H. (2007). Threat-related attentional bias in anxious and non-anxious individuals: A meta-analytic study. *Psychological Bulletin, 133*, 1–24.

Barrett, P. M., Rapee, R. M., Dadds, M. R., & Ryan, S. M. (1996). Family enhancement of cognitive style in anxious and aggressive children: Threat bias and the FEAR effect. *Journal of Abnormal Child Psychology, 24*, 187–203.

Barrocas, A. L., & Hankin, B. L. (2011). Developmental pathways to depressive symptoms in adolescence: A multi-wave prospective study of negative emotionality, stressors, and anxiety. *Journal of Abnormal Child Psychology, 39*, 489–500.

Battaglia, M., Pesenti-Gritti, P., Medland, S. E., Ogliari, A. K., & Spatola, C. A. M. (2009). A genetically informed study of the association between childhood separation anxiety, sensitivity to CO2, panic disorder, and the effect of childhood parental loss. *Archives of General Psychiatry, 66*, 64–71.

Bernstein, A., & Zvolensky, M. J. (2011). Empirical approaches to the study of latent structure and classification of child and adolescent anxiety pathology. In D. McKay & E. A. Storch (Eds.), *Handbook of child and adolescent anxiety disorders* (pp. 91–104). New York: Springer.

Blöte, A. W., Kint, M. J. W., & Westenberg, P. M. (2007). Peer behavior toward socially anxious adolescents: Classroom observations. *Behaviour Research and Therapy, 45*, 2773–2779.

Bögels, S. M., Alden, L., Beidel, D. C., Clark, L. A., Pine, D. S., Stein, M. B., & Voncken, M. (2010). Social anxiety disorder: Questions and answers for the DSM-V. *Depression and Anxiety, 27*, 168–189.

Bosmans, G., Braet, C., Beyers, W., Van Leeuwen, K., & Van Vlierberghe, L. (2011). Parents' power assertive discipline and internalizing problems in adolescents: The role of attachment. *Parenting, 11*, 34–55.

Bosquet, M., & Egeland, B. (2006). The development and maintenance of anxiety symptoms from infancy through adolescence in a longitudinal sample. *Development and Psychopathology, 18*, 517–550.

Bowlby, J. (1973). *Attachment and loss: Separation* (Vol. 2). New York: Basic Books.

Brenning, K., Soenens, B., Braet, C., & Bosmans, G. (2011). Attachment and depressive symptoms in middle childhood and early adolescence: Testing the validity of the emotion regulation model. *Personal Relationships, 19*, 445–464.

Britton J. C, Lissek, S., Grillon, C., Norcross, M.A., & Pine, D. S. (2011). Development of anxiety: The role of threat appraisal and fear learning. *Depression and Anxiety, 28*, 5–17.

Brumariu, L. E., & Kerns, K. A. (2010). Mother-child attachment and social anxiety symptoms in middle childhood. *Journal of Applied Developmental Psychology, 29*, 393–402.

Cassidy, J. (2008). The nature of the child's ties. In J. Cassidy & P. R. Shaver (Eds.), *Handbook of attachment: Theory, research, and clinical applications* (2nd ed.). New York: Guilford Press.

Chorpita, B., & Barlow, D. (1998). The development of anxiety: The role of control in the early environment. *Psychological Bulletin, 124*, 3–21.

Clark, L. A., Watson, D., & Mineka, S. (1994). Temperament, personality, and the mood and anxiety disorders. *Journal of Abnormal Psychology, 103*, 103–116.

Colonnesi, C., Draijer, E. M., Stams, G. J. J. M., Van der Bruggen, C. O., Bögels, S. M., & Noom, M. J. (2011). The relation between insecure attachment and child anxiety: A meta-analytic review. *Journal of Clinical Child and Adolescent Psychology, 40*, 630–645.

Costello, E. J., Egger, H. L., & Angold, A. (2004). The developmental epidemiology of anxiety disorders. In T. H. Ollendick & J. S. March (Eds.), *Phobic and anxiety disorders in children and adolescents: A clinician's guide* (pp. 61–91). Oxford: Oxford University Press.

Costello, E. J., Egger, H. L., Copeland, W., Erkanli, A., & Angold, A. (2011). The developmental epidemiology of anxiety disorders: Phenomenology, prevalence, and comorbidity. In W. K. Silverman & A. P. Field (Eds.), *Anxiety disorders in children and adolescents* (2nd ed., pp. 56–75). New York: Cambridge University Press.

Costello, E. J., Mustillo, S., Erkanli, A., Keeler, G., & Angold, A. (2003). Prevalence and development of psychiatric disorders in childhood and adolescence. *Archives of General Psychiatry, 60*, 837–844.

Creswell, C., Murray, L., Stacey, J., & Cooper, P. (2011). Parenting and child anxiety. In W. K. Silverman & A. P. Field (Eds.), *Anxiety disorders in children and adolescents* (2nd ed., pp. 299–322). New York: Cambridge University Press.

Creswell, C., Shildrick, S., & Field, A. P. (2011). Interpretation of ambiguity in children: A prospective study of associations with anxiety and parental interpretations. *Journal of Family Studies, 20*, 240–250.

Crozier, M., Gillihan, S. J., & Powers, M. B. (2011). Issues in differential diagnosis: Phobias and phobic conditions. In D. McKay & E. A. Storch (Eds.), *Handbook of child and adolescent anxiety disorders* (pp. 7–22). New York: Springer.

Cyranowski, J. M., Shear, M. K., Rucci, P., Fagiolini, A., Frank, E., Grochocinski, V. J., et al. (2002). Adult separation anxiety: Psychometric properties of a new structured interview. *Journal of Psychiatric Research, 36*, 77–86.

Dadds, M. R., Barrett, P. M., Rapee, R. M., & Ryan, S. (1996). Family process and child psychopathology: An observational analysis of the FEAR effect. *Journal of Abnormal Child Psychology, 24*, 715–734.

Dadds, M. R., Davey, G. C. L., & Field, A. P. (2001). Developmental aspects of conditioning processes in anxiety disorders. In M. W. Vasey & M. R. Dadds (Eds.), *The developmental psychopathology of anxiety* (pp. 205–230). New York: Oxford University Press.

Dadds, M. R., & Roth, J. H. (2001). Family processes in the development of anxiety problems. In M. W. Vasey & M. R. Dadds (Eds.), *The developmental psychopathology of anxiety* (pp. 278–303). New York: Oxford University Press.

Dallaire, D. H., & Weinraub, M. (2007). Infant-mother attachment security and children's anxiety and aggression at first grade. *Journal of Applied Developmental Psychology, 28*, 477–492.

De Wilde, A., & Rapee, R. M. (2008). Do controlling maternal behaviours increase state anxiety in children's responses to a social threat? A pilot study. *Journal of Behavior Therapy and Experimental Psychiatry, 39*, 526–537.

Degnan, K. A., & Fox, N. A. (2007). Behavioral inhibition and anxiety disorders: Multiple levels of a resilience process. *Development and Psychopathology, 19*, 729–746.

Eley, T. C., Gregory, A. M., Clark, D. M., & Ehlers, A. (2007). Feeling anxious: A twin study of panic/somatic symptoms, anxiety sensitivity and heart-beat perception in children. *Journal of Child Psychology and Psychiatry, 48*, 1184–1191.

Field, A. P. (2006). Watch out for the beast: Fear information and attentional bias in children. *Journal of Clinical Child and Adolescent Psychology, 35*, 431–439.

Field, A. P., Ball, J. E., Kawycz, N. J., & Moore, H. (2007). Parent-child relationship and the verbal information pathway to fear in children: A prospective paradigm and preliminary test. *Behavioural and Cognitive Psychotherapy, 35*, 473–486.

Field, A. P., Hadwin, J. A., & Lester, K. J. (2011). Information processing biases in child and adolescent anxiety: A development perspective. In W. K. Silverman & A. P. Field (Eds.), *Anxiety disorders in children and adolescents* (2nd ed., pp. 103–128). New York: Cambridge University Press.

Field, A. P., & Price-Evans, K. (2009). Temperament moderates the effect of the verbal threat information pathway on children's heart rate responses to novel animals. *Behaviour Research and Therapy, 47*, 431–436.

Field, A. P., & Purkis, H. M. (2011). Associative learning and phobias. In M. Haselgrove & L. Hogarth (Eds.), *Clinical applications of learning theory*. Hove, UK: Psychology Press.

Fonseca, A. C., & Perrin, S. (2011). The clinical phenomenology and classification of child and adolescent anxiety. In W. K. Silverman & A. P. Field (Eds.), *Anxiety disorders in children and adolescents* (2nd ed., pp. 25–55). New York: Cambridge University Press.

Gar, N., & Hudson, J. L. (2008). An observational analysis of mother-child interactions in mothers and children with anxiety disorders. *Behaviour Research and Therapy, 46*, 1266–1274.

Ginsburg, G. S., Riddle, M., & Davies, M. (2006). Somatic symptoms in children and adolescents with anxiety disorders. *Journal of the American Academy of Child and Adolescent Psychiatry, 45*, 1179–1187.

Gittelman-Klein, R., & Klein, D. F. (1980). Separation anxiety in school refusal and its treatment with drugs. In L. Hersov & I. Berg (Eds.), *Out of school* (pp. 321–341). New York: Wiley.

Gregory, A. M., Caspi, A., Moffitt, T. E., Koenen, K., Eley, T. C., & Poulton, R. (2007). Juvenile mental health histories of adults with anxiety disorders. *American Journal of Psychiatry, 164*, 301–308.

Gregory, A. M., & Eley, T. C. (2011). The genetic basis of child and adolescent anxiety. In W. K. Silverman & A. P. Field (Eds.), *Anxiety disorders in children and adolescents* (2nd ed., pp. 161–178). New York: Cambridge University Press.

Grills-Taquechel, A. E., & Ollendick, T. H. (2012). *Phobic and anxiety disorders in youth*. Cambridge, MA: Hogrefe & Huber Publishers.

Groh, A. M., Roisman, G. I., van IJzendoorn, M. H., Bakermans-Kranenburg, M. J., & Fearon, R. P. (2012). The significance of insecure and disorganized attachment for children's internalizing symptoms: A meta-analytic study. *Child Development, 83*, 591–610.

Grover, R. L., Ginsburg, G. S., & Ialongo, N. (2005). Psychosocial outcomes of anxious first graders: A seven-year follow-up. *Depression and Anxiety, 24*, 410–420.

Hawker, D. S. J., & Boulton, M. J. (2000). Twenty years' research on peer victimization and psychosocial maladjustment: A meta-analytic review of cross-sectional studies. *Journal of Child Psychology and Psychiatry, 41*(4), 441–455.

Hettema, J. M., Neale, M. C., & Kendler, K. S. (2001). A review and meta-analysis of the genetic epidemiology of anxiety disorders. *American Journal of Psychiatry, 158*, 1568–1578.

Hirschfeld-Becker, D. R., Biederman, J., Henin, A., Faraone, X. V., Davis, S., Harrington, K., et al. (2007). Behavioral inhibition in preschool children at risk is a specific predictor of middle childhood social anxiety: A five-year follow-up. *Journal of Developmental and Behavioral Pediatrics, 28*, 225–233.

Kaplow, J. B., Curran, P. J., Angold, A., & Costello, E. J. (2001). The prospective relation between dimensions of anxiety and the initiation of adolescent alcohol use. *Journal of Clinical Child Psychology, 30*, 316–326.

Kearney, C. A., & Silverman, W. K. (1990). A preliminary analysis of a functional model of assessment and treatment for school refusal behavior. *Behavior Modification, 14*, 340–366.

Kim, K. J., Conger, R. D., Elder, G. H., Jr., & Lorenz, F. O. (2003). Reciprocal influences between stressful life events and adolescent internalizing and externalizing problems. *Child Development, 74*, 127–143.

La Greca, A. M., & Landoll, R. R. (2011). Peer influences. In W. K. Silverman & A. P. Field (Eds.), *Anxiety disorders in children and adolescents* (2nd ed., pp. 323–346). New York: Cambridge University Press.

Lau, J. Y. F., Gregory, A. M., Goldwin, M. A., Pine, D. S., & Eley, T. C. (2007). Assessing gene-environment interactions on anxiety symptom subtypes across childhood and adolescence. *Development and Psychopathology, 19*, 1129–1146.

Lau, J. Y. F., Nelson, E. E., Angold, A., Britton, J., Ernst, M., Goldwin, M., Grillon, C., Lissek, S., Shiffrin, N., & Pine, D. S. (2011). Distinct neural signatures of threat learning in adolescents and adults. *Proceedings of the National Academy of Sciences, 108*, 4500–4505.

Lau, J. Y. F. & Pine, D. S. (2008). Elucidating risk mechanisms of gene-environment interactions on pediatric anxiety: integrating findings from neuroscience. *European Archives of Psychiatry and Clinical Neuroscience, 258*, 97–106.

Lau, J. Y. F., & Pine, D. S. (2009). Elucidating risk mechanisms of gene-environment interactions on pediatric anxiety: Integrating findings from neuroscience. *European Archives of Psychiatry and Clinical Neuroscience, 258*, 97–106.

LeDoux, J. E. (2000). Emotion circuits in the brain. *Annual Review of Neuroscience, 23*, 155–184.

Lepine, J. (2002). The epidemiology of anxiety disorders: Prevalence and societal costs. *Journal of Clinical Psychiatry, 63*, 4–8.

LoBue, V., & DeLoache, J. S. (2010). Superior detection of threat-relevant stimuli in infancy. *Developmental Science, 13*, 221–228.

Lonigan, C. J., & Phillips, B. M. (2001). Temperamental influences on the development of anxiety disorders. In M. W. Vasey & M. R. Dadds (Eds.), *The developmental psychopathology of anxiety* (pp. 60–91). New York: Oxford University Press.

Lonigan, C. J., Vasey, M. W., Phillips, B, & Hazen, R. (2004). Temperament, anxiety, and the processing of threat–relevant stimuli. *Journal of Clinical Child and Adolescent Psychology, 33*, 8–20.

Lonigan, C. J., Phillips, B. M., Wilson, S. B., & Allan, N. P. (2011). Temperament and anxiety in children and adolescents. In W. K. Silverman & A. P. Field (Eds.), *Anxiety disorders in children and adolescents* (2nd ed., pp. 198–224). New York: Cambridge University Press.

Lonigan, C. J., & Vasey, M. W. (2009). Negative affectivity, effortful control, and attention to threat-relevant stimuli. *Journal of Abnormal Child Psychology, 37*, 387–399.

Lonsdorf, T. B., Weike, A. I., Nikamo, P., Schalling, M., Hamm, A. O., & Öhman, A. (2009). Genetic gating of human fear learning and extinction: Possible implications for gene-environment interaction in anxiety disorder. *Psychological Science, 20*, 198–206.

Lyneham, H. J., & Rapee, R. M. (2011). Prevention of child and adolescent anxiety disorders. In W. K. Silverman & A. P. Field (Eds.), *Anxiety disorders in children and adolescents* (2nd ed., pp. 349–366). New York: Cambridge University Press.

Marks, I. M., & Nesse, R. M. (1994). Fear and fitness: An evolutionary analysis of anxiety disorders. *Ethology and Sociobiology, 15*, 247–261.

Martin, M., & Jones, G. V. (1992). Integral bias in the cognitive processing of emotionally linked pictures. *British Journal of Psychology, 86*, 419–435.

McGrath, M., Kawachi, I., Ascherio, A., Colditz, G. A., Hunter, D. J., & De Vito, I. (2004). Association between catechol-O-methyltransferase and phobic anxiety. *American Journal of Psychiatry, 161*, 1703–1705.

McLeod, B. D., Wood, J. J., & Weisz, J. R. (2007). Examining the association between parenting and childhood anxiety: A meta-analysis. *Clinical Psychology Review, 27*, 155–172.

Mikulincer, M., & Shaver, P. R. (2007). *Attachment in adulthood: Structure, dynamics, and change*. New York: Guilford Press.

Mineka, S., Gunnar, M., & Champoux, M. (1986). Control and early socioemotional development: Infant rhesus monkeys reared in controllable versus uncontrollable environments. *Child Development, 57*, 1241–1256.

Muris, P. (2007). *Normal and abnormal fear and anxiety in children and adolescents*. Amsterdam: Elsevier.

Muris, P., & Broeren, S. (2009). Twenty-five years of research on childhood anxiety disorders: Publication trends between 1982 and 2006 and a selective review of the literature. *Journal of Child and Family Studies, 18*, 388–395.

Muris, P., & Field, A. P. (2011). The "normal" development of fear. In W. K. Silverman & A. P. Field (Eds.), *Anxiety disorders in children and adolescents* (2nd ed., pp. 76–89). Cambridge: Cambridge University Press.

Murray, L., Cooper, P., Creswell, C., Schofield, E., & Sack, C. (2007). The effects of maternal social phobia on mother-infant interactions and infant social responsiveness. *Journal of Child Psychology and Psychiatry, 48*, 45–52.

Murray, L. M., Creswell, C., & Cooper, P. J. (2009). The development of anxiety disorders in childhood: An integrative review. *Psychological Medicine, 39*, 1413–1423.

Murray, L., de Rosnay, M., Pearson, J., Bergeron, C., Schofield, E., Royal-Lawson, M., et al. (2008). Intergenerational transmission of social anxiety: The role of social referencing processes in infancy. *Child Development, 79*, 1049–1064.

Nachmias, M., Gunnar, M., Mangelsdorf, S., Parritz, R. H., & Buss, K. (1996). Behavioral inhibition and stress reactivity: The moderating role of attachment security. *Child Development, 67*, 508–522.

Nolte, T., Guiney, J., Fonagy, P., Mayes, L. C., & Luyten, P. (2011). Interpersonal stress regulation and the development of anxiety disorders: an attachment-based developmental framework. *Frontiers in Behavioral Neuroscience, 5*, 1–21.

Ollendick, T. H., & King, N. J. (1991). Origins of childhood fears: An evaluation of Rachman's theory of fear acquisition. *Behaviour Research and Therapy, 29*, 117–123.

Ollendick, T. H., King, N. J., & Muris, P. (2002). Fears and phobias in children: Phenomenology, epidemiology, and aetiology. *Child and Adolescent Mental Health, 7*, 98–106.

Ollendick, T. H., Mattis, S. G., & King, N. J. (1994). Panic in children and adolescents: A review. *Journal of Child Psychology and Psychiatry, 35*, 113–134.

Ollendick, T. H., Vasey, M. W., & King, N. J. (2001). Operant conditioning influences in childhood anxiety. In M. W. Vasey & M. R. Dadds (Eds.), *The developmental psychopathology of anxiety* (pp. 231–252). New York: Oxford University Press.

Ollendick, T. H., Yang, B., King, N. J., Dong, Q., & Akande, A. (1996). Fears in American, Australian, Chinese, and Nigerian children and adolescents: A cross-cultural study. *Journal of Child Psychology and Psychiatry, 37*, 213–220.

Perez-Edgar, K., Reeb-Sutherlan, B. C., McDermott, J. M., White, L. K., Henderson, H. A., Degnan, K. A., et al. (2011). Attention biases to threat link behavioral inhibition to social withdrawal over time in very young children. *Journal of Abnormal Child Psychology, 39*, 885–895.

Perez-Olivas, G., Stevenson, J., & Hadwin, J. A. (2008). Do anxiety-related attentional biases mediate the link between maternal over involvement and separation anxiety in children? *Cognition and Emotion, 22*, 509–521.

Pine, D. S. (2011). The brain and behavior in childhood and adolescent anxiety disorders. In W. K. Silverman & A. P. Field (Eds.), *Anxiety disorders in children and adolescents* (2nd ed., pp. 179–197). New York: Cambridge University Press.

Rapee, R. M., Schniering, C. A., & Hudson, J. L. (2009). Anxiety disorders during childhood and adolescence: Origins and treatment. *Annual Review of Clinical Psychology, 5*, 311–341.

Rozenman M, Weersing V. R., Amir N. (2011). A case series of attention modification in clinically anxious youths. *Behaviour Research and Therapy, 49*, 324–330.

Schmidt, N. B., Eggleston, A. M., Woolaway-Bickel, K., Fitzpatrick, K. K., Vasey, M. W., & Richey, J. A.

(2007). Anxiety Sensitivity Amelioration Training (ASAT): A longitudinal primary prevention program targeting cognitive vulnerability. *Journal of Anxiety Disorders, 21*, 302–319.

Shaffer, D., Fisher, P., Dulcan, M. K., Davies, M., Piacentini, J., Schwab-Stone, M. E., et al. (1996). The NIMH Diagnostic Interview Schedule for Children version 2.3 (DISC-2.3): Description, acceptability, prevalence rates, and performance in the MECA study. *Journal of the American Academy of Child and Adolescent Psychiatry, 35*, 865–877.

Silberg, J., Rutter, M., Neale, M., & Eaves, L. (2001). Genetic moderation of environmental risk for depression and anxiety in adolescent girls. *British Journal of Psychiatry, 179*, 116–121.

Silverman, W. K., & Ollendick, T. H. (2008). Child and adolescent anxiety disorders. In J. Hunsley & E. J. Mash (Eds.), *A guide to assessments that work* (pp. 181–206). New York: Oxford University Press.

Spence, S. H. (1997). Structure of anxiety symptoms among children: A confirmatory factor-analytic study. *Journal of Abnormal Psychology, 106*, 280–297.

Thirlwall, K., & Creswell, C. (2010). The impact of maternal control on children's anxious cognitions, behavior and affect: An experimental study. *Behaviour Research and Therapy, 48*, 1041–1046.

Vasey, M. W., & Dadds, M. R. (2001). An introduction to the developmental psychopathology of anxiety. In M. W. Vasey & M. R. Dadds (Eds.), *The developmental psychopathology of anxiety* (pp. 3–26). New York: Oxford University Press.

Vassilopoulos, S. P., Banerjee, R., & Prantzalou C. (2009). Experimental modification of interpretation bias in socially anxious children: Changes in interpretation, anticipated interpersonal anxiety, and social anxiety symptoms. *Behaviour Research and Therapy, 47*, 1085–1089.

Waters, A. M., Henry, J., & Neumann, D. L. (2009). Aversive Pavlovian conditioning in childhood anxiety disorders: Impaired responses inhibition and resistance to extinction. *Journal of Abnormal Psychology, 118*, 311–321.

Weaver, I. C. G., Cervoni, N., Champagne, F. A., D'Alessio, A. C., Sharma, S., Seckl, J. R., et al. (2004). Epigenetic programming by maternal behavior. *Nature Neuroscience, 7*, 847–854.

Weems, C. F., & Silverman, W. K. (2006). An integrative model of control: Implications for understanding emotion regulation and dysregulation in childhood anxiety. *Journal of Affective Disorders, 91*, 113–124.

White, L. K., McDermott, J. M., Degnan, K. A., Henderson, H. A., & Fox, N. A. (2011). Behavioral inhibition and anxiety: The moderating roles of inhibitory control and attention shifting. *Journal of Abnormal Child Psychology, 39*, 735–747.

White, L. K., Suway, J. G., Bar-Haim, Y., Pine, D., & Fox, N. A. (2011). Cascading effects: The influence of attention bias to threat on the interpretation of ambiguous information. *Behavior Research and Therapy, 49*, 244–251.

Whiteside, S. P., & Ollendick, T. H. (2009). Developmental perspectives on anxiety classification. In D. McKay, J. Abramowitz, S. Taylor, & G. J. G. Asmundson (Eds.), *Current perspectives on the anxiety disorders: Implications for DSM-V and beyond* (pp. 303–325). New York: Springer.

Wittchen, H.-U., Nocon, A., Beesdo, K., Pine, D. S., Höfler, M., Lieb, R., et al. (2008). Agoraphobia and panic: Prospective-longitudinal relations suggest a rethinking of diagnostic concepts. *Psychotherapy and Psychosomatics, 77*, 147–157.

Wittchen, H., Zhao, S., Kessler, R. C., & Eaton, W. W. (1994). DSM-III-R generalized anxiety disorder in the National Comorbidity Survey. *Archives of General Psychiatry, 51*, 355–364.

World Health Organisation. (1992). *ICD-10 classifications of mental and behavioural disorder: Clinical descriptions and diagnostic guidelines*. Geneva: World Health Organization.

Obsessions and Compulsions: The Developmental and Familial Context

28

Catherine K. Kraper, Timothy W. Soto, and Alice S. Carter

Introduction

In this chapter, we describe developmental and clinical characteristics of obsessive and compulsive behaviors, highlighting both pathological and non-pathological expressions in childhood and adolescence. To provide context, we define and discuss obsessional thoughts and compulsions, ritualistic behaviors, and obsessive–compulsive disorder (OCD). Next, to present a more comprehensive picture of the clinical presentation of OCD, we briefly review empirical and theoretical literature that addresses clinical characteristics and phenomenology, epidemiological studies, neurobiology, and issues of comorbidity. However, our primary focus is to propose a developmental, family-based model of OCD that may begin as early as in the preschool years with emergence of early compulsive and ritualistic behaviors and to suggest pathways to both normative and maladaptive obsessional and compulsive outcomes. This model addresses the contribution of familial attitudes and behaviors towards the development, strengthening, and maintenance of OCD symptoms, as well as the impact of symptoms and behaviors of OCD on family relationships. In light of the emerging research on family accommodation and the impact

of OCD on family life, current family-based treatment practices will also be reviewed.

Despite recent increased research attention on obsessive–compulsive behaviors in child clinical populations (e.g., Franklin et al., 2011), the pediatric literature is still small relative to the available research on OCD in adult populations. However, given that OCD in children has unique features that are distinct from adult manifestations, it is important to focus on studies that pertain to children and adolescents to best understand the developmental experience of obsessions and compulsions in childhood. Similar to the adult literature, the vast majority of information derives from research on the disordered state. We review current knowledge about OCD in childhood and adolescence, as well as the limited number of studies that address typical variation in obsessive and compulsive behavior.

Relevant Definitions of Obsessive and Compulsive Behavior

Prior to discussing the development of and variation in these behaviors as well as individual and family experiences in more detail, it is important to understand what is meant by obsessions, compulsions, and the clinical diagnosis of obsessive–compulsive disorder.

Obsessions are repetitive, intrusive, and uncontrollable thoughts, images, and ideational impulses that can lead to significant subjective

C.K. Kraper, M.A. (✉) •T.W. Soto, M.A.
A.S. Carter, Ph.D.
Psychology Department, University of Massachusetts
Boston, Boston, MA 02125, USA
e-mail: catie.kraper@gmail.com; aliceS.carter@umb.edu

distress. The content of obsessions may appear pointless, out of sync with day-to-day tasks, and/or bizarre, inappropriate, violent, repulsive, or obscene (Rachman, 1985). The obsessional thoughts are unwanted, and individuals with frequent obsessions commonly attempt to resist or dismiss the obsessions or to neutralize them with another thought or action (Rachman, 1985). In regard to the experience of obsessions, the development of insight has previously been seen as necessary to perceive the obsessions as in conflict with one's needs or goals, although current diagnostic criteria allow an additional rating of good, poor, and absent degrees of a patient's insight into his or her disorder-related beliefs (American Psychiatric Association, 2013).

Compulsions may involve repetitive behaviors, such as checking, hoarding, hand washing, ordering objects, or cleaning, or may involve repetitive mental activities, such as counting or repeating specific words. These activities are often used as a way of decreasing the anxiety generated by obsessional thoughts, and the performance of overt or covert mental rituals may serve to relieve anxiety, restore safety in a perceived dangerous state, or prevent harm when harm is the believed inevitable outcome (Rachman, 1976). Compulsions are not necessarily directed toward a goal; even when compulsions help to relieve anxiety, maladaptive compulsive behaviors may not be functionally related to an obsessive thought (e.g., hand washing is not always preceded by a related obsessional thought, such as being exposed to germs).

When the frequency, intensity, duration, and/or distress associated with obsessions and compulsions begin to interfere with developmental progress, social relationships, and/or day-to-day functioning, the possibility of a disordered state must be considered. *Obsessive–compulsive disorder* (OCD) is the psychiatric diagnostic category, classified within Obsessive-compulsive and related disorders in the DSM-5 (APA, 2013), assigned to individuals with pathological or impairing obsessions and/or compulsions. The criteria specify that the obsessions and/or compulsions must be experienced as inappropriate, difficult to suppress, and of sufficient frequency,

intensity, or duration to cause a significant degree of distress. Children do not need to demonstrate insight to receive a diagnosis of OCD, and in both children and adults, compulsions can become over-learned and automatic such that awareness of the anxiety or efforts to resist are minimal.

Prevalence of OCD

Childhood prevalence rates of OCD range from 2 to 4 % (Flament et al., 1988; Thomsen, 1993), which is similar to the rates reported for adults (Ruscio, Stein, Chiu, & Kessler, 2008). OCD appears to be less common in the preschool period. A recent epidemiological study found that 0.3 % of preschool-aged children met criteria for OCD (with a confidence interval of 0.1–0.7 %; Wichstrom et al., 2012). Interestingly, approximately 1 in 3 adult cases had a childhood onset. The mean age of onset for childhood OCD is 9–10 years of age (Pauls, Alsobrook, Goodman, Rasmussen, & Leckman, 1995), although it can be diagnosed as early as 4 years of age (Garcia et al., 2009). More boys than girls appear to be affected, in a ratio of about 3:2, although this has not been confirmed in all of the relevant studies (Chabane et al., 2005; Geller et al., 1998). From adolescence onward, the estimated prevalence in boys and girls is the same.

Continuum of Non-pathological and Pathological Experiences

Obsessions and compulsions are common in the nonclinical population, and it is typical to experience OC symptoms despite not meeting criteria for OCD. Using longitudinal data from the Dunedin Study birth cohort, Grisham et al. (2011) noted that individuals reporting obsessive or compulsive behavior at ages 26 and 32 comprised close to 40 % of the sample. This study emphasized the difficulty with point prevalence of OCD. Although at each time point the prevalence of clinically diagnosable OCD was within the expected values of 2–4 %, only 11 % of the OCD group met full diagnostic criteria for OCD at both time points, suggesting that the symptoms of OCD change in severity over time. This is supported by a prospective, epidemiological study following children identified with OCD over 2 years: Of the 16 diagnosed youth, 31 % retained their diagnosis, an additional 25 % had subclinical OCD, and 12 % had no OCD-related disorder (Berg, Rapoport, Whitaker, & Davies, 1989). Given the apparent pervasiveness of symptoms in the general population, and the fluctuating severity of symptoms in diagnosed individuals, it is essential to describe the experience of both pathological and non-pathological forms of these behaviors.

Obsessions

Although the content of some obsessions may be extremely anxiety provoking (e.g., sexual or aggressive images involving loved ones), the content itself does not appear to discriminate pathological and non-pathological obsessions. In the adult literature, the major distinction between non-impairing and pathological obsessions involves the degree of distress and amount of time that is associated with efforts to resist, regulate, neutralize, and/or suppress the intrusive thoughts (Rachman & Hodgson, 1978). In non-pathological forms, an occasional disturbing thought may be intrusive or invasive, but it may be dismissed without lasting consequences or persistent anxiety (Flament et al., 1990). There is some evidence that the degree of distress caused by intrusive thoughts is influenced by cognitive information processing, which includes attentional biases, appraisal processes, attributions about the content of the thoughts, and the role of the self in relation to these thoughts (Bolton, 1996).

Fearful and particularly salient attributions, such as potential harm to a family member, are likely to influence the appraisal and subsequent degree of interference associated with obsessional ideation in childhood. In addition, negative information processing styles may be associated with cognitive distortions that give rise to feelings of helplessness about pathological obsessions and may contribute to risk for maintained rumination and concomitant disorders such as depression (Rehm & Carter, 1990). In pathological forms, obsessions have been associated with inflated responsibility (Farrell, Waters, & Zimmer-Gembeck, 2012); an overestimation of the importance of thoughts, including Thought–Action Fusion (TAF) (Amir, Freshman, Ramsey, Neary, & Brigidi, 2001); the need to control thoughts (Clark & Purdon, 1993); overestimation of threat (Woods, Frost, & Steketee, 2002); intolerance of uncertainty (Tolin, Abramowitz, Brigidi, & Foa, 2003); and perfectionism (Frost & Steketee, 1997). Thus, information processing styles may play a role in distinguishing pathological from non-pathological forms of obsessions.

Compulsions

Although classical depictions of OCD would suggest that compulsions are performed to minimize anxiety associated with an obsession, compulsions are not always performed in direct response to an obsessive thought, nor are they always goal directed. However, when compulsions are performed in response to an obsession, an individual may strengthen a kind of superstitious belief that the compulsions are necessary to fend off what is feared in the obsession. It has been suggested that belief in the efficacy of the compulsion to ward off or minimize anxiety associated with an obsession is akin to the kind of magical thinking that is observed in the preschool years (e.g., "If I sit very still, no one will see me") and/or superstitious beliefs typical of the early school-aged years (e.g., "Step on a crack and break your mother's back") (Bolton, 1996). Although a young child's use of magical thinking, often associated with game playing, appears developmentally appropriate, individuals engaging in compulsions are usually aware that the behaviors and mental activities are not realistically linked to the source of distress, and the compulsions are viewed neither as fun nor as a game.

Compulsions often need to be performed in a specific sequence and manner, and an individual might feel the need to start the ritual all over if it is not performed "just so." In pathological forms, the behaviors and mental activities can consume hours each day and disrupt interpersonal relationships, physical health, and occupational functioning. In non-pathological forms, compulsions are not associated with distress, and rituals are typically related to realistic obsessions. Moreover, non-pathological compulsions are brief in duration, are not performed in a repetitive or redundant manner, and may result in an experience of relief or pleasure. These behaviors often serve an adaptive, goal-directed function, such as checking each response on a math test once before moving on to the next page. When these behaviors begin to impair the child in daily activities, such a routine becomes maladaptive or pathological—for example, checking each problem seven times would likely result in an incomplete test. Non-pathological forms of checking may reflect an effort to establish control over the environment (Frost, Sher, & Geen, 1986), while non-pathological cleaning behaviors may involve restorative efforts rather than attempts to control future harm (Rachman & Hodgson, 1980).

Obsessive–Compulsive Disorder in Childhood

Phenomenology

Children and adolescents often manifest multiple OC features at the same time. The content of obsessions and compulsions often concerns contamination, aggression, symmetry and precision, and religious and sexual themes; mixed types are common (Jans et al., 2007). The most common types in childhood involve cleaning (32–87 %), followed by repetition, checking, and aggressive thoughts (Geller et al., 1998). There is evidence for symptom dimensions within the clinical presentation of OCD—namely, cleaning/washing, checking, symmetry/exactness, and hoarding/saving (Leckman, Zhang, Alsobrook, & Pauls, 2001). More recently, principal components analysis using the Yale-Brown Obsessive Compulsive Scale (Y-BOCS; Goodman, Price, Rasmussen, Mazure, Fleischmann, et al., 1989; Goodman, Price, Rasmussen, Mazure, Delgado, et al., 1989) and Child Y-BOCS (CY-BOCS; Scahill et al., 1997) revealed four dimensions of OCD symptoms that explained almost 60 % of

symptom variance in both children and adults with OCD: (1) symmetry/ordering/repeating/checking, (2) contamination/cleaning/aggressive/somatic, (3) hoarding, and (4) sexual/religious symptoms (Stewart et al., 2007). Symptom dimensions revealed in such studies have been shown to be highly stable (Delorme et al., 2006). In line with these findings that hoarding is a distinct set of behaviors within OCD, hoarding has been recognized in the DSM-5 as an OC-related disorder that can occur without the presence of other obsessive-compulsive behavior (APA, 2013).

Although OCD often makes its first appearance in childhood or adolescence, OCD is not considered a "developmental disorder" (Bolton, 1996). Clinical work and diagnosis does, however, acknowledge the role of development in assigning a diagnosis of OCD. Although current diagnostic criteria recognizes that adults with OCD may also lack insight into their obsessions, children with OCD may not be developmentally prepared to acknowledge that their obsessions and compulsions are either excessive or senseless. As the definitive symptoms of OCD involve cognitive ideation, the clinician determining whether an individual meets criteria for a diagnosis of OCD must obtain subjective accounts of the individual's cognitive and affective experiences. With young children, obtaining information about mental processes such as resistance, interference, and ego-dystonicity (i.e., whether or not the thoughts are part of the self) can be extremely difficult (Carter, Pauls, & Leckman, 1995).

Indeed, even children who exhibit severe OC symptoms may have no explanation for the source(s) of their compulsions, and instead, the obsessions they report subsequent to the onset of the compulsions may serve to give meaning to their otherwise senseless behavior (Carter et al., 1995). Young children may have difficulty answering questions that require them to reflect on their own behaviors, cognitions, and emotions and may not fully grasp the meaning of relevant but abstract constructs (e.g., interference). Thus, it is not surprising that young children with OCD show more compulsions without obsessions than do adults (Rettew, Swedo, Leonard, Lenane, & Rapoport, 1992).

Features of Early-Onset OCD

An important distinction within individuals with OCD is the timing of the onset of symptoms, in that a bimodal age distribution—with a first peak of onset at age 11 and a second one in early adulthood (Delorme et al., 2005)—often distinguishes the course and experience of comorbid symptoms and disorders. Obsessive–compulsive disorder has been characterized as early onset if symptoms present before puberty (Kalra & Swedo, 2009). The nature of the obsessive–compulsive symptoms reported for childhood-onset OCD is generally similar to adult-onset OCD (e.g., Mancebo et al., 2008; Reddy et al., 2003), with some potentially important differences. For instance, childhood-onset OCD occurs predominantly in males, though beginning in puberty there is equal gender representation (Castle, Deale, & Marks, 1995). Further, a substantial proportion of individuals with early-onset OCD have symptoms that remit before early adulthood (e.g., Stewart et al., 2004), although early-onset OCD is also associated with longer duration of illness and greater psychosocial difficulties than adult-onset OCD (Nakatani et al., 2011). Moreover, compared to later-onset OCD, early-onset OCD has a higher rate of comorbidity with chronic tic disorders and attention-deficit hyperactivity disorder (ADHD; Peterson, Pine, Cohen, & Brook, 2001).

Biological Roots of OCD: Genetics and Neurobiology

Genetics plays a clear role in the etiology of OCD with some candidate genes identified; no single gene appears to be responsible for the full presentation of the disorder (Pauls, 2008). In a recent genome-wide association study of OCD (Stewart et al., 2012), no significant genome-wide associations were observed in the overall sample, but several genes with known important functions in the brain (e.g., methylation, glutamate receptor function) were identified that warrant future research.

Advances in neuroscience, particularly neuroimaging, suggest neurobiological involvement in OCD in adults indicating a series of cortico-striato-thalamo-cortical loops in the pathogenesis of OCD (Saxena & Rauch, 2000). Neuroimaging studies suggest atypical activity in various brain regions related to deficits in response inhibition (ventral medial orbitofrontal cortex) and set-shifting (dorsolateral prefrontal cortex) in patients with OCD, as well as heightened error detection (anterior cingulate cortex) (Evans, Lewis, & Iobst, 2004). In a study of children with OCD onset prior to age 10 years, additional differences in brain activity were observed: decreased blood flow in the right thalamus, left anterior cingulate cortex, and bilateral inferior prefrontal cortex relative to late-onset patients (Busatto et al., 2001).

Neuropsychological deficits in executive function related to these brain regions, specifically response inhibition and set-shifting, are fairly well documented in the OCD literature (Evans et al., 2004; Pietrefesa & Evans, 2007). Moreover, although often performed at a similar overall level of achievement to nonclinical comparison groups, executive performances in attentional set-shifting, verbal fluency, planning, and decision making are often characterized by increased response latencies, perseveration of previous responses, and difficulties in effectively utilizing feedback to adapt to changing conditions and environments that can compromise school performance (for a review, see Olley, Malhi, & Sachdev, 2007).

It has been hypothesized that some susceptible individuals develop OCD symptoms and tic disorders as a result of post-infectious autoimmune processes. Swedo et al. (1998) have proposed that this subgroup, identified by the acronym PANDAS, follows a clinical course that is closely temporally linked to group A beta hemolytic streptococci (GABHS) infections. Strong evidence that GABHS may be involved in the onset of Tourette syndrome (TS) and OCD comes from a report by Mell, Davis, and Owens (2005), who found that children with OCD, TS, or tic disorder were significantly more likely than those in the nonclinical comparison group to have had streptococcal infection in the 3 months before onset date, with risk highest among children with multiple streptococcal infections within 12 months. Although encompassing a small subset of individuals with OCD, better understanding PANDAS may help identify the mechanisms and neural substrates involved in obsessive and compulsive behavior, potentially offering insights into genetic and nongenetic pathways involved in the etiology of OCD.

Comorbidity

As previously mentioned, it is common for OCD to co-occur with other disorders, both in children and adults (Costello, Egger, & Angold, 2005). Childhood-onset OCD has a particularly high rate of comorbid disorders, which affect both the individual and the family. As many as 80 % of children affected by OCD meet criteria for an additional diagnosis (Geller, 2006), including anxiety disorders (26–70 %), major depression (10–73 %), tic disorders (17–59 %), ADHD (10–50 %), and disruptive behavior disorders (10–53 %) based on clinical pediatric OCD samples (cf. Storch et al., 2008). Early-onset OCD also appears to have a distinctive pattern of comorbidity from later-onset OCD. For example, Hemmings et al. (2004) reported that early onset of OCD (<15 years vs. >15 years) was associated with an increased frequency of chronic tic disorders and trichotillomania. Carter, Pollock, Suvak, and Pauls (2004) reported that early age at onset (<10 years vs. >10 years) in adults and adolescents with OCD was associated with higher rates of anxiety and depression among relatives with OCD but not among relatives without OCD. Within the affected child's family, different rates of morbidity of psychiatric illness among family members have been reported, ranging from 3.4 % morbidity among family members of adult patients (Bellodi, Sciuto, Diaferia, Ronchi, & Smeraldi, 1992) to 25 % of pediatric patients (Lenane et al., 1990). In the Bellodi et al. study, the familial morbidity rates more than doubled (8.8 %) when considering only individuals with an onset under age 14. The apparent greater

genetic loading in childhood-onset OCD and the high rate of comorbid diagnoses suggest that there is a particularly high degree of stress and complex family dynamics in pediatric OCD.

The co-occurrence of certain disorders and symptoms characterized by repetitive thoughts or behaviors has influenced the diagnostic criteria for the recently published DSM-5 such that there is now a category for obsessive-compulsive and related disorders (APA, 2013). Included in this group of disorders are body dysmorphic and hoarding disorders, trichotillomania, and skin picking disorder. These have been observed to co-occur with OCD more frequently than in non-clinical comparison subjects (Bienvenu et al., 2000); research regarding their shared phenomenology and clinical features is ongoing (for a review, see Phillips et al., 2010). Changes in the DSM-5 also include distinctions between substance-induced OC or related disorders, OC or related disorders attributable to other medical conditions, and OC or related disorders not elsewhere classified. Moreover, as previously mentioned, for the diagnoses of OCD, hoarding disorder, and body dysmorphic disorder, which have a cognitive component, the DSM-5 allows for patients' degree of insight to be rated by the clinician.

Developmental Model and Familial Context

Cognitive Developmental Concepts Related to Obsessions and Compulsions

In this section, we offer a brief review of the historical context of cognitive developmental theories regarding repetitive and ritualistic behavior in childhood and describe pathways from normative childhood behavior to maladaptive obsessive and compulsive behavior. From a cognitive developmental perspective, repeating behaviors and activities, adhering to rules, and enacting rituals are important components of typical development. Piaget (1962) discussed the critical role that repetition serves in the first year of life and that, along with imitation, repetition forms the basis for acquiring many functional skills (e.g., waving goodbye). Viewing adaptive repetitive behaviors as goal oriented informs a definition of maladaptive compulsive behavior, in which rituals are identified as lacking a goal direction.

Cognitive developmental studies of repetition or response inhibition have viewed perseveration as a component of the broader set of executive functions associated with frontal lobe development and dysfunction (e.g., Zelazo, Carter, Reznick, & Frye, 1997). Although it is not clear whether individual variation in the acquisition of normative cognitive and motor inhibition skills is associated with the development of obsessions and compulsions, Gesell, Ames, and Ilg (1974) noted that at 2.5 years of age there appears a qualitative shift in toddlers' interest in maintaining routines and insistence on sameness during stressful transitions. The authors described toddlers' use of rituals (e.g., insisting a bedtime story be read "just so") to minimize anxiety and heighten feelings of mastery and control. In the same manner that young children's rituals serve to organize a sense of efficacy in the environment, non-pathological adult compulsive behaviors may be employed adaptively to gain control over the environment (Frost et al., 1986) and prevent future harm (Rachman & Hodgson, 1978).

Evans, Leckman, King, Henshaw, and Alsobrook (1995) examined developmental changes between 8 and 72 months of age in the frequency, intensity, and age of onset of specific ritualistic and repetitive behaviors. Supporting Gesell et al.'s (1974) observations, children aged 2, 3, and 4 years had the highest frequency/intensity ratings compared to younger and older children. Further, two salient dimensions of childhood routines were observed: (1) things being "just right" (e.g., "arranges objects in straight lines or symmetrical patterns") and (2) repetitive behaviors and insistence on sameness (e.g., "prefers the same household schedule every day"). In addition, normative variation in parent ratings of child repetitive and compulsive behaviors is correlated with anxiety symptoms, executive functioning, and brain processing corresponding to detection of visual asymmetry (Evans & Maliken, 2011; Pietrefesa & Evans, 2007).

The preschool years are a time of dramatic change in cognitive aspects of inhibition and perseveration (Zelazo et al., 1997). In typical development, a significant increase in the performance of repetitive behaviors during these years is followed by a decrease in the ensuing developmental time period (Evans et al., 1995). Attention to adaptive and maladaptive perseveration in the preschool years is warranted, as maladaptive perseverative behavior may predict later developmental pathology or may be an important signal of a very early onset OCD, as children as young as age 4 meet criteria for OCD (Garcia et al., 2009).

As children enter elementary school, they engage in complex ritualistic, rule-based games and superstitious behaviors (Carter et al., 1995). Normally emerging superstitious beliefs appear similar to adaptive compulsions in that they may minimize anxiety associated with disturbing thoughts or impulses (Leonard, Goldberger, Rapoport, Cheslow, & Swedo, 1990). These typical superstitions may be viewed on a continuum with maladaptive compulsions, with the primary distinctions being duration, distress, and interference with routine activities (Leonard et al., 1990). Commonly occurring patterns of OC behavior in school-aged children decline as children approach puberty (Zohar & Bruno, 1997).

Temperament and Obsessive–Compulsive Symptoms in Childhood

Investigators studying nonclinical populations from early childhood through high school demonstrate wide individual variation in the expression of obsessional ideation or ritualistic behaviors (e.g., Flament et al., 1990; Zohar & Bruno, 1997). Individual childhood traits appear to contribute to the development of OC behaviors in children, and some temperamental styles may place children at higher risk for maladaptive variants of obsessions and compulsions. Specifically, highly emotionally reactive children (Rothbart, 1989) may become hypervigilant and increasingly distressed when confronted by anxiety-provoking ideation and/or more frustrated when unable to inhibit a repetitive behavior, thus indicating that heightened reactivity may determine whether a child's behavior crosses the threshold to malad-aptation. Consistent with this theory, a recent prospective study of risk for OCD in a large epidemiological sample found that difficulty and sluggishness assessed at age 3 were associated with subthreshold obsessive symptoms in adults, and both social isolation and internalizing symptoms between ages 5 and 11 years were associated with adult OCD diagnosis (Grisham et al., 2011). It is also important to note that children's temperamental styles may both influence and be influenced by their parenting environments (Arcus & McCartney, 1989), which further complicates the clinical picture of how temperament contributes to the development of both normative and pathological forms of obsessions and compulsions.

Familial Contribution in the Development of OCD

A model for the development of OCD that takes into account both genetic loading and familial risk factors may best explain the occurrence of this disorder. Genetic concordance rates in monozygotic twins, estimated to be 60 % (Billet, Richter, & Kennedy, 1998), support the critical role that environment plays in the development and maintenance of this disorder. In fact, as mentioned previously, although candidate genes linked to OCD have been identified, none explains the entirety of OCD's expression in the population (Pauls, 2008). Thus, the role of the family in OCD is critical to understand in building models of symptom development, prevention, and treatment.

Given that children often depend on their parents to interpret their experiences, especially prior to the development of symbolic thought and enhanced linguistic abilities, studying parental cognitive information processing styles may help to identify critical predictors of child adaptation and information processing styles. Indeed, Farrell et al. (2012) showed a significant relation between parental cognitive style (specifically, inflated sense of responsibility and overestimation of the importance of thoughts) and child OCD severity. Age significantly moderated this relationship,

with younger children particularly susceptible to parental cognitive styles. Although observed in a clinical population, parental response to and management of early emerging and potentially maladaptive ideation may influence the subsequent severity and maintenance of similar, or even pathological, thoughts in the child.

Additionally, parental patterns of behavior may shape the development of both normative and pathological obsessive and compulsive behaviors. For instance, a well-intentioned parent may comply with a request to participate in a ritual to pacify their distressed child, thus reinforcing the ritual. Parents may also unknowingly become incorporated into a child's ritual. For example, as part of a long sequence of behaviors, a child may require the parent to provide a goodnight kiss on the cheek. Unbeknownst to the parent, prior to requesting the kiss, the child may have rearranged his or her bedding, checked under the bed, flipped the lights on and off 7 times, put clothing out for the next morning, and set up stuffed animals in a very particular, "just right" arrangement. Once the child completes this sequence of events in a satisfactory manner, the ritual is sealed for the night with a parent's goodnight kiss. Thus, parental behavioral responses can range from active to passive.

In their transactional model of child behaviors and parent responses, Van Noppen, Rasumussen, Eisen, and McCartney (1991) suggest that the emotional response and attitude of family members to OCD symptoms fall on a continuum from overly accommodating to harshly antagonistic and that both family extremes lead to worsening of OCD behaviors. Van Noppen et al. suggest that falling in the middle of the continuum—by neither engaging in the ritual nor rejecting the individual—is most beneficial to lessening OCD symptoms. Indeed, the relationship of expressed emotion (EE) to the severity of OCD was demonstrated when this conceptual model was tested, revealing that individuals with OCD who reported greater levels of hostility and criticism in their relatives showed more severe OCD symptoms (Van Noppen & Steketee, 2009).

This model of family contribution to obsessive and compulsive behavior is further complicated when the parent has a diagnosis of anxiety or

OCD themselves. Parent modeling of fear and avoidance may encourage nonadaptive coping styles in the child, such as avoidance or rituals in response to intrusive thoughts (Waters & Barrett, 2000). Consistent with modeling, Ettelt et al. (2008) reported that both individuals with OCD and their family members reported higher levels of harm avoidance than individuals in a nonclinical comparison group. In addition to modeling, this finding could be accounted for by accommodation, described below.

Family Accommodation of OCD Symptoms

As a result of the obvious impact that OCD symptoms have on both the child and his or her family, there are substantial and unique ways that families manage a child's OCD diagnosis. A commonly used strategy is termed "accommodation," or participation in the compulsions and rituals that are part of the affected individual's symptoms, and modification of family routines. Examples include altering an outing to avoid places that cause anxiety for the affected individual or altering household activities to minimize the affected individual's contamination fears. Such accommodations often function to decrease stress associated with the affected individual's symptoms in all family members. In this way, accommodation behaviors begin as well-intentioned, adaptive actions on the part of the family to relieve the affected individual's anxiety and stress. Accommodation may also result from a parent's inability to manage his or her own stress related to their child's symptoms and is used as a way of eliminating (or avoiding) the problem, especially among parents who suffer from depression or anxiety themselves. Therefore, helping a parent first to manage his or her own depression and anxiety may be an important factor in decreasing family accommodation of a child's OCD symptoms. Accommodation may also be elicited from the child as "reassurance seeking," which has been commonly observed in young children with OCD (Rettew et al., 1992).

Family accommodation was first described in families in which an adult carried the diagnosis of OCD. Among 34 relatives of individuals with a diagnosis of OCD, ages 26–78, 88 % reported accommodating the individual's symptoms at least some of the time (Calvocoressi et al., 1995). Interestingly, although accommodation behaviors are adopted as a way for the family to reduce and avoid stress, the degree of accommodation was correlated with relatives' ratings of distress and poor family functioning, as well as rejecting attitudes toward the affected individual. This was corroborated by observations of a significant, positive correlation between escape-avoidant coping strategies and levels of both accommodation and negative affect in parents of children with OCD (Futh, Simonds, & Micali, 2012). Thus, it appears that significant accommodation exists in families affected by OCD and that accommodation does not necessarily reduce family stress.

In a larger study of family accommodation comparing children and adults, there was significantly more accommodation reported of a child's symptoms and rituals (under 18 years) than of an adult's—more than 75 % versus 58 % (Cooper, 1996). This difference suggests either that the impact is greater on the family when a child is diagnosed with OCD or that a child's relative developmental needs make it more difficult for family members to not "help."

As described earlier, family accommodation may involve a wide range of behaviors, and specific accommodation patterns likely differ between families. A study examining subscale-level responses to the Family Accommodation Scale, a commonly used measure for understanding the familial impact of OCD, revealed that some types of accommodation occur with greater frequency: Reassurance of the patient occurred daily in 56 % of the sample, participation in the compulsion or ritual itself occurred in 46 % of the sample, and assisting the affected child in his or her avoidance of an object or place daily only occurred in 22 % of the sample (Peris et al., 2008). Child symptom severity was also positively correlated with more frequent participation in rituals, and both child symptom severity and externalizing behavior were correlated with greater modification of family routines and with more negative child behavior in response to non-accommodation (e.g., distress, aggression, and increased duration of rituals). Higher rates of accommodation and involvement in rituals were also correlated with parental anxiety and parental diagnosis of OCD, and greater family conflict was associated with increased parental distress when accommodating children's behaviors, as well as with more negative child behavior when not accommodated. These findings support the notion that parents with OCD or high anxiety may be modeling avoidance and rituals or may find it harder to not accommodate their child's OC behaviors. Conversely, higher reported family organization was associated with lower parental distress when accommodating child OCD behavior and fewer child consequences when not accommodating.

The Peris et al. (2008) finding regarding family conflict and accommodation highlights that the mechanism for the development of accommodation within a family remains unclear. For example, accommodation might emerge in response to the stress felt in a family as a result of the OCD, or accommodation-like behaviors and over-involvement in a child's behaviors might precede the full OCD symptoms. Similarly, it is unclear whether, as reported in the Peris et al. (2008) study, a more organized family leads to less child distress when not being accommodated or whether the family is able to retain organization because the child does not show significant distress when not accommodated.

Developmentally, the process of accommodation and the development and maintenance of OCD within the family context may vary based on the age at which a child is diagnosed. Although still considered "early onset," a child who first experiences OCD's emergence at 11 years of age will have a different experience within the family context than a child with preschool onset, when it may be more challenging to distinguish a normative desire for sameness or routine from that which is atypically rigid and compulsive. When a family begins to cope with the compulsions and obsessions associated with their child's OCD at a younger age, accommodation may occur to a greater extent and more naturally because of the child's dependence on their parents. Families may be less inclined to incorporate the child's

OCD behaviors into family routines when the disorder emerges in later childhood, at which point family routines have been established and the child is less dependent on the parent for self-care. In addition to the added stress that a family experiences when accommodating an individual's OCD symptoms, accommodation can lead to worse treatment outcomes. The degree of accommodation in a family has been correlated with posttreatment OCD severity, even when controlling for pretreatment severity (Amir, Freshman, & Foa, 2000). In this study, treatment appeared to be hindered when the family reported greater accommodation and modification of routine, and conversely, individuals with less family accommodation showed the greatest improvement in OCD severity in the course of treatment. This appears to be true for children as well: Reduction in OCD symptoms was related to decreases in family accommodation following 14 sessions of cognitive-behavioral family therapy (Merlo, Lehmkuhl, Geffken, & Storch, 2009). The results of these studies imply a crucial mechanism of family processes in relation to OC symptom presentation and demonstrate the importance of including families in the planning of treatment, which will be discussed later in more depth.

Quality of Life and Family Relationships

OCD has been found to be the 10th leading cause of disability among all medical conditions (Murray & Lopez, 1996). In regard to the psychosocial impact of the disorder, OCD can cause clinically significant functional impairment, generally defined as the inability to perform age-appropriate and routine tasks and engage in developmentally appropriate relationships. OCD-related impairment is sensitive to development, as different developmental stages bring about varying adaptational demands. In children with OCD, functional impairment includes impaired social and academic functioning. In one study of 151 pediatric patients with OCD examining the impact of the disorder on academic, family, and social functioning, 90 % of participants reported at least one dysfunction related to OCD (Piacentini, Bergman, Keller, & McCracken, 2003). Lack of ability to concentrate on schoolwork as a result of obsessions and compulsions was the most commonly occurring area of dysfunction.

In addition to functional impairment, recent research has focused on the specific impact of OCD on the related domain of quality of life (QoL), although relatively little work has been done in this area for pediatric populations. QoL may be defined as an individual's *perception* of the impact of the disorder on various aspects of life and has been found to be significantly lower in individuals with OCD (Eisen et al., 2006). QoL is even more impacted when comorbid disorders are present (Huppert, Simpson, Nissenson, Liebowitz, & Foa, 2009). Among youth affected by the disorder, QoL appears to be impaired relative to nonclinical comparison subjects (Lack et al., 2009), though QoL was better predicted by the presence of internalizing symptoms—reported more frequently in girls—than by OCD symptom severity. Recent results from a longitudinal study suggest that children whose symptoms remit by adulthood report no impact on QoL (Palermo et al., 2011). Surprisingly, Palermo et al. also found that individuals diagnosed with OCD in childhood who continued to show symptoms into adulthood reported only mild impact on QoL, although individuals who displayed hoarding symptoms in childhood reported the greatest symptom persistence and the greatest impact on QoL.

Fewer studies have utilized QoL constructs to examine the impact on family relationships when a child receives a diagnosis of OCD. However, one study used the Parent Experience of Chronic Illness (PECI; Bonner et al., 2006) measure, developed for parents of children with brain tumors, to examine the domains of Guilt and Worry, Emotional Resources, Unresolved Sorrow and Anger, and Long-term Uncertainty that parents may feel in regard to their child's OCD diagnosis (Storch et al., 2009). Storch et al. found that higher scores on the scales most related to distress (Guilt and Worry, Unresolved Sorrow and Anger, and Long-term Uncertainty) were associated with more OCD symptoms and greater OCD-related

impairment as well as greater caregiver distress and strain. Of note, co-occurring child internalizing symptoms mediated the relation between parent distress and the domains of Guilt and Worry and Unresolved Sorrow and Anger, suggesting that treatments that target child internalizing symptoms may most effectively ease parent distress and emotional demand on the parent.

Though lacking in standardized measures, qualitative studies that include parents with a child with OCD support these themes of guilt and uncertainty, as well as stigma related to the child's diagnosis. Parents often reported feeling that it was their role to promote child progress and reported ruminating over strategies for helping their child and their ability to affect change in their child's disorder (Stengler-Wenzke, Trosbach, Dietrich, & Angermeyer, 2004b). Parents also frequently described the need to conceal the child's symptoms from others, suggesting that they felt stigma related to the OCD. In a separate thematic analysis of interviews, parents reported feeling stigma when interacting with the medical community in the process of the child's treatment and also described feeling excluded from the treatment process, which was associated with feelings of blame and guilt for the child's symptoms (Stengler-Wenzke, Trosbach, Dietrich, & Angermeyer, 2004a). Although current studies focus on families who have pursued treatment, it is possible that a parent's experience of stigmatization could be an obstacle to pursuing treatment.

Communication and interactions between parents and children with OCD also appear to be affected by the diagnosis. Barrett, Shortt, and Healy (2002) compared interactions of families with children with OCD, anxiety disorders (generalized anxiety disorder, separation anxiety disorder, and social phobia), externalizing disorders (oppositional defiant disorder, ADHD, and conduct disorder), and no psychiatric disorders. When observing parents and their children involved in family discussions of hypothetical difficult situations, parents of children with OCD were less positive overall during the interaction, used less positive problem solving, rewarded their children's independence less, and were less confident in their children's abilities than parents in any of the other groups. Children with OCD could also be differentiated from children in other groups. They showed the least confidence, were least likely to use positive problem solving, and displayed less warmth in their interactions. The authors suggest a link between a lack of encouragement to use problem solving and a child's reliance on rituals and compulsive behaviors. Parent psychopathology was an influential factor, as well. Depression and anxiety were highest in the OCD group, and depression was related to greater stress, lower confidence in their children, and less reward of their children's independence across the groups. The direct observation of these interactions allows for a unique window into family dynamics but does not address the direction of influence. In other words, it is unclear whether the parent's behaviors have shaped the child's characteristics and behaviors or if the child's disorder has shaped the parent's behaviors.

Treatment of Child and Adolescent OCD

This section will discuss the current treatments of OCD, as well as the potential role of the family in interventions. Current treatment of OCD in children often involves a combination of approaches, with empirical support for both pharmacological treatment—including selective serotonin reuptake inhibitors (SSRIs)—and psychotherapy (Abramowitz, Franklin, & Foa, 2002; Ercan, Kandulu, & Ardic, 2012). Among psychotherapies, cognitive-behavioral therapy (CBT), particularly exposure and response prevention (ERP), has been most commonly studied and recommended for OCD. Although both produce clinically significant change in the child or adolescent, ERP treatment appears to be superior to SSRIs, showing greater reduction in OCD symptoms (Abramowitz, Whiteside, & Deacon, 2005). Moreover, one intensive study showed that children who underwent combined CBT and drug therapy showed greater remission of their OCD symptoms than either CBT or drug therapy alone (The Pediatric OCD Treatment Study Team, 2004).

The benefits of family involvement in the treatment process are highlighted in a study comparing individuals (children and adults) receiving only ERP therapy with individuals receiving ERP who also had a family member involved in an 8-week family intervention group (Grunes, Neziroglu, & McKay, 2001). Participants in the family intervention group (receiving psychoeducation, support, and instruction for aiding in the practice of ERP) showed greater reduction in their OCD symptoms—an improvement that was maintained at the 1-month follow-up. Additionally, family members reported lower anxiety and depression following treatment and significantly lower EE than family members of individuals in the ERP group only.

The effectiveness of family involvement has also been shown in pediatric-specific populations. In a study of the effectiveness of family-based CBT, children between the ages of 6 and 18 with a diagnosis of OCD participated in 14 sessions of CBT that included their parents (Merlo et al., 2009). Similar to the Amir et al. (2000) study, pretreatment measures of OCD symptoms were positively correlated with the degree of family accommodation reported at baseline. At the completion of treatment, change in the degree of family accommodation was significantly correlated with both parent- and clinician-rated severity of OCD symptoms in the child, even when controlling for pretreatment OCD severity. Not only does family-based CBT promote positive changes in accommodation levels (e.g., Merlo et al., 2009), but family relationships also appear to be positively impacted. A recent study showed that, following family-based CBT, mother–child interactions were rated by clinicians as significantly more positive (e.g., greater warmth, confidence, and positive problem solving) than prior to treatment (Schlup, Farrell, & Barrett, 2011).

Family interventions that meet criteria for evidence-based treatments are particularly compelling in support of including parents and family in the treatment process. In a review of studies that were identified as meeting at least partial criteria for evidence-based treatments, CBT with a family component was found to be possibly efficacious according to criteria established by

Chambless et al. (1996) (Barrett, Farrell, Pina, Peris, & Piacentini, 2008). Although none of the interventions with a family component met criteria for a well-established treatment, Barrett, Healy-Farrell, and March's (2004) study met the greatest number of criteria (e.g., the study was randomized, had a wait-list control condition, and was driven by a manualized protocol). However, it is not possible to parse out the additive family benefit, as the groups being compared both contained a family component. The same is true of Storch et al. (2007), who compared intensive and weekly formats of a cognitive-behavioral family therapy. Although both formats contributed to significant improvement in child OCD symptoms, there was not a control group to discern the specific contribution of family involvement.

Two additional smaller scale studies described by Barrett et al. (2008) met criteria for possibly efficacious studies. Martin and Thienemann (2005) included 14 families in 14 sessions of group cognitive-behavioral therapy and observed significant improvement in OCD symptom severity, child-rated depression symptoms, and parent-rated negative impact of the disorder. In a sample of 18 adolescents, Thienemann, Martin, Cregger, Thompson, and Dyer-Friedman (2001) included a parent component in group cognitive-behavioral therapy, though parents attended only the last 15 minutes to review important topics from the session. Although the adolescents' OCD symptom severity had decreased at posttreatment, scores on the Parenting Stress Index did not decrease, indicating that a child's improvement in OCD symptoms might be separate from perceived stress of parents and suggesting that a threshold of parental involvement in treatment must be reached to affect family processes. Waters, Barrett, and March (2001) included the most thorough pre- and posttreatment measures of family functioning and accommodation but had the smallest sample (seven children). At the conclusion of 14 weeks of cognitive-behavioral family therapy, all of the children had improved in OCD symptom severity, and six of the seven children no longer met criteria for the disorder. Family accommodation had decreased in each of the families participating in the study. Notably, Waters

et al. also taught strategies for parents to manage their own stress and anxiety associated with their child's OCD behaviors, which could be an especially crucial therapeutic skill to gain within families with comorbid psychiatric illness.

These findings across a variety of treatment modalities suggest the importance of including family members in treatment of children with OCD. Further, a child's inherent dependence upon parents yields a unique vulnerability to factors such as parent mental health and general family dynamics, such that both a child's symptom presentation and response to intervention are likely to impact and be impacted by the family. Further research is needed to fully understand the unique contribution of family involvement in the treatment of children and adolescents with OCD, in that most of the reviewed studies lacked a comprehensive control.

Summary and Future Directions

Given the high prevalence of obsessions and compulsions reported in nonclinical studies and the association at particular ages of elevated symptoms with greater anxiety (e.g., Zohar & Bruno, 1997), it would be useful to assess children with subclinical manifestations of OCD prior to significant developmental transitions and follow them through periods of highest risk. Taking into consideration the recent findings discussed in this chapter may help identify children with known risk factors who may be at particularly elevated risk for developing OCD—e.g., children who have a family history of OCD, present with negative emotionality, or demonstrate neuropsychological profiles common to OCD. Repeated assessment of information processing and qualities of parent–child interactions may aid in determining predictors of pathological obsessional states and appropriate windows of opportunity for prevention and intervention. For example, the transition to middle school or high school presents unique challenges with increased responsibility and unpredictability as well as a wide range of other stressors that may lower an individual's threshold for OC behavior. Such high-risk studies may also improve the early identification of children who are suffering, which is critical due to the secretiveness typically associated with OC pathology, chronicity of symptoms, and vulnerability to impairment in multiple developmental domains.

Although there is a body of research that has focused on the profound impact that a child's diagnosis of OCD can have on the family, there are still significant gaps to address in the current literature. Assessment of OCD symptoms is largely consistent across studies, but comparison of specific family factors is more difficult across studies due to variations in measures. Especially within intervention research, a lack of equivalent measures across studies limits the comparability of study outcomes and effectiveness. For example, studies vary in their use of measures of family variables that address either family functioning (e.g., the Family Environment Scale; Moos & Moos, 1986), family accommodation (e.g., the Family Accommodation Scale; Calvocoressi et al., 1999), or specific parent variables such as levels of depression, stress, or anxiety (e.g., Parenting Stress Index; Abidin, 1995). Alternatively, some studies include a family component in the treatment but do not specifically measure family outcomes. In terms of the applied utility of these scales, however, clinical practice can benefit from the additional information that subscale responses can provide (Peris et al., 2008), and this information can serve to better address individual family needs in treatment planning.

Additional issues in comparing outcomes across studies include uneven inclusion criteria for children. Although most studies require a child to have carried a diagnosis for a minimum of 1 year, and they report the range of years that children have been affected by the disorder, there is likely a vast difference in the family patterns and processes when a child has been diagnosed with OCD for 1 year versus 5 years, for instance. Family accommodation patterns might significantly vary with the amount of time they have been established, which may be particularly true when a very young, dependent child is diagnosed

with OCD as opposed to an older, more independent adolescent. An additional factor limiting our understanding of the development of family processes in OCD is that, currently, most literature treats all children diagnosed with OCD as part of the early-onset category, despite previously discussed findings that demonstrate distinctive patterns of symptom expression and comorbidity associated with early-onset versus late-onset OCD (e.g., Carter et al., 2004; Hemmings et al., 2004). This type of broad categorization of childhood OCD does not sufficiently describe the developmental differences proposed here that likely impact the family differently across the childhood years. Research thus far does not adequately reflect these differences and would benefit from greater attention to these developmental distinctions.

Lastly, treatment for children with OCD has appeared to lag behind the findings of intervention research in regard to family involvement. Although research suggests that family involvement in therapy is helpful in improving both child OCD symptoms and family accommodation and distress, only one manual exists that thoroughly specifies the role of parents in each session. In addition to greater improvement in OCD symptoms and family processes, more consistent and thorough parental involvement in treatment could decrease some of the stigma and guilt that parents report in relation to being excluded from their child's treatment sessions (Stengler-Wenzke et al., 2004a). Further, severity and chronicity of parental psychopathology may interfere with parental availability, positive emotional expressivity, appropriate structuring, and response to the child's difficulties more than any specific disorder (March & Curry, 1998). Given the high incidence of parental psychiatric illness when a child has been diagnosed with OCD, parents would also benefit from specific instruction on managing their own anxiety, both when faced with children's OCD symptoms and in everyday modeling of adaptive responses to stress and anxiety. Although some interventions have included strategies for managing parental stress specifically associated with a child's OCD (Waters et al., 2001), the relationship described by Farrell et al. (2012) between broader parental cognitive styles (e.g., inflated sense of responsibility, overestimation of the importance of thoughts) and severity of OCD in children suggests that more intensive, early management of maladaptive parental cognitive styles may have a positive impact on both child OCD symptoms and parent mental health.

In conclusion, obsessive–compulsive behavior reflects a heterogeneous pattern of repetitive and intrusive thoughts and behaviors. Throughout development, both pathological and non-pathological repetitive forms are observed, with maladaptive behaviors characterized by heightened distress and an inability to suppress or inhibit thoughts and actions leading to significant interference with daily functioning. Studies are beginning to address the developmental course and correlates of typical obsessive behaviors, and findings to date support the notion that adaptive and maladaptive manifestations of obsessions and compulsions may occur on a continuum. Although obsessive–compulsive behaviors appear quite common at various points in childhood and adolescence, particularly for compulsive behaviors in the preschool period, extreme rates of these behaviors are usually associated with anxiety and most likely reflect a disordered state. Further attention to the developmental and familial context of obsessive–compulsive behavior is warranted in both research and clinical endeavors.

References

Abidin, R. (1995). *Professional manual for the parenting stress index* (3rd ed.). Odessa, FL: Psychological Assessment Resources.

Abramowitz, J. S., Franklin, M. E., & Foa, E. B. (2002). Empirical status of cognitive-behavioral therapy for obsessive-compulsive disorder: A meta-analytic review. *Romanian Journal of Cognitive and Behavioral Psychotherapies, 2,* 89–104.

Abramowitz, J. S., Whiteside, S. P., & Deacon, B. J. (2005). The effectiveness of treatment for pediatric obsessive-compulsive disorder: A meta-analysis. *Behavior Therapy, 36,* 55–63.

American Psychiatric Association. (2013). *Diagnostic and statistical manual of mental disorders (5th ed.).* Arlington, VA: American Psychiatric Publishing.

Amir, N., Freshman, M., & Foa, E. B. (2000). Family distress and involvement in relatives of obsessive-compulsive disorder patients. *Journal of Anxiety Disorders, 14,* 209–217.

Amir, N., Freshman, M., Ramsey, B., Neary, E., Brigidi, B. (2001). Thought-action fusion in individuals with OCD symptoms. *Behavioral Research and Therapy, 39,* 765–776.

Arcus, D., & McCartney, K. (1989). When baby makes four: Family influences in the stability of behavioral inhibition. In J. Reznick (Ed.), *Perspectives on behavioral inhibition* (pp. 197–218). Chicago: University of Chicago Press.

Barrett, P. M., Farrell, L., Pina, A. A., Peris, T. S., & Piacentini, J. (2008). Evidence-based psychological treatments for child and adolescent obsessive-compulsive disorder. *Journal of Clinical Child and Adolescent Psychology, 37,* 131–155.

Barrett, P., Healy-Farrell, L., & March, J. S. (2004). Cognitive-behavioral family treatment of childhood obsessive-compulsive disorder: A controlled trial. *Journal of the American Academy of Child and Adolescent Psychiatry, 43,* 46–62.

Barrett, P., Shortt, A., & Healy, L. (2002). Do parent and child behaviours differentiate families whose children have obsessive-compulsive disorder from other clinic and non-clinic families? *Journal of Child Psychology and Psychiatry, 43,* 597–607.

Bellodi, L., Sciuto, G., Diaferia, G., Ronchi, P., & Smeraldi, E. (1992). Psychiatric disorders in the families of patients with obsessive-compulsive disorder. *Psychiatry Research, 42,* 111–120.

Berg, C. Z., Rapoport, J. L., Whitaker, A., & Davies, M. (1989). Childhood obsessive compulsive disorder: A two-year prospective follow-up of a community sample. *Journal of the American Academy of Child & Adolescent Psychiatry, 28*(4), 528–533.

Bienvenu, O. J., Samuels, J. F., Riddle, M. A., Hoehn-Saric, R., Liang, K. Y., Cullen, B. A., et al. (2000). The relationship of obsessive-compulsive disorder to possible spectrum disorders: Results from a family study. *Biological Psychiatry, 48,* 287–293.

Billet, E. A., Richter, M. A., & Kennedy, J. L. (1998). Genetics of obsessive-compulsive disorder. In R. P. Swinson, M. M. Antony, S. Rachman, & M. A. Richter (Eds.), *Obsessive-compulsive disorder: Theory, research, and treatment* (pp. 120–140). New York: Guilford Press.

Bolton, D. (1996). Annotation: Developmental issues in obsessive compulsive disorder. *Journal of Child Psychology and Psychiatry, 37,* 131–137.

Bonner, M. J., Hardy, K. K., Guill, A. B., McLaughlin, C., Schweitzer, H., & Carter, K. (2006). Development and validation of the parent experience of child illness. *Journal of Pediatric Psychology, 31,* 310–321. doi:10.1093/jpepsy/jsj034.

Busatto, G. F., Buchpiguel, C. A., Zamignani, D. R., Garrido, G. E. J., Glabus, M. F., Rosario-Campos, M., et al. (2001). Regional cerebral blood flow abnormalities in early-onset obsessive- compulsive disorder: An exploratory SPECT study. *Journal of American Academy of Child and Adolescent Psychiatry, 40,* 347–354.

Calvocoressi, L., Lewis, B., Harris, M., Trufan, S. J., Goodman, W. K., McDougle, C. J., et al. (1995). Family accommodation in obsessive-compulsive disorder. *The American Journal of Psychiatry, 152*, 441–443.

Calvocoressi, L., Mazure, C. M., Kasl, S. V., Skolnick, J., Fisk, D., Vegso, S. J., et al. (1999). Family accommodation of obsessive-compulsive symptoms: Instrument development and assessment of family behavior. *Journal of Nervous and Mental Disease, 187*, 636–642.

Carter, A., Pauls, D., & Leckman, J. (1995). The development of obsessionality: Continuities and discontinuities. In D. Cicchetti & D. Cohen (Eds.), *The manual of developmental psychopathology* (pp. 609–632). New York: Wiley.

Carter, A. S., Pollock, R. A., Suvak, M. K., & Pauls, D. L. (2004). Anxiety and major depression comorbidity in a family study of obsessive-compulsive disorder. *Depression & Anxiety, 20*, 165–174.

Castle, D. J., Deale, A., & Marks, I. M. (1995). Gender differences in obsessive-compulsive disorder. *Australian and New Zealand Journal of Psychiatry, 29*, 114–117.

Chabane, N., Delorme, R., Millet, B., Mouren, M. C., Leboyer, M., & Pauls, D. (2005). Early-onset obsessive-compulsive disorder: A subgroup with a specific clinical and familial pattern? *Journal of Child Psychology and Psychiatry, 46*, 881–887.

Chambless, D. L., Sanderson, W. C., Shoham, V., Johnson, S. B., Pope, K. S., Crits-Christoph, P., et al. (1996). An update on empirically validated therapies. *The Clinical Psychologist, 49*, 5–18.

Clark, D. A., & Purdon, C. (1993). New perspectives for a cognitive theory of obsessions. *Australian Psychologist, 28*, 161–167.

Cooper, M. (1996). Obsessive-compulsive disorder: Effects on family members. *American Journal of Orthopsychiatry, 66*, 296–304.

Costello, E., Egger, H. L., & Angold, A. (2005). The developmental epidemiology of anxiety disorders: Phenomenology, prevalence, and comorbidity. *Child and Adolescent Psychiatric Clinics of North America, 14*(4), 631–648. doi:10.1016/j.chc.2005.06.003.

Delorme, R., Bille, A., Betancur, C., Mathier, F., Chabane, N., Mouren-Simeoni, M., et al. (2006). Exploratory analysis of obsessive compulsive symptom dimensions in children and adolescents: A prospective follow-up study. *BMC Psychiatry, 6*, doi: 10.1186/1471-244X-6-1.

Delorme, R., Golmard, J. L., Chabane, N., Millet, B., Krebs, M. O., Mouren-Simeoni, M. C., et al. (2005). Admixture analysis of age at onset in obsessive-compulsive disorder. *Psychological Medicine, 35*, 237–243.

Eisen, J. L., Mancebo, M. A., Pinto, A., Coles, M. E., Pagano, M. E., Stout, R., et al. (2006). Impact of obsessive-compulsive disorder on quality of life. *Comprehensive Psychiatry, 47*, 270–275.

Ercan, E. S., Kandulu, R., & Ardic, U. A. (2012). Preschool children with obsessive-compulsive disorder and fluoxetine treatment. *European Child and Adolescent Psychiatry, 21*, 169–172.

Ettelt, S., Grabe, H. J., Ruhrmann, S., Buhtz, F., Hochrein, A., Kraft, S., et al. (2008). Harm avoidance in subjects with obsessive-compulsive disorder and their families. *Journal of Affective Disorders, 107*, 265–269.

Evans, D., Leckman, J., King, R., Henshaw, D., & Alsobrook, K. (1995). *The development of compulsive-like behaviors in young children*. Indianapolis, IN: Presented at the Society for Research in Child Development.

Evans, D. W., Lewis, M. D., & Iobst, E. (2004). The role of the orbito-frontal cortex in normally developing compulsive-like behavior and obsessive–compulsive disorder. *Brain and Cognition, 55*(1), 220–34.

Evans, D. W., & Maliken, A. (2011). Cortical activity and children's rituals, habits and other repetitive behavior: A visual P300 study. *Behavioural Brain Research, 224*, 174–179.

Farrell, L. J., Waters, A. M., & Zimmer-Gembeck, M. J. (2012). Cognitive biases and obsessive-compulsive symptoms in children: Examining the role of maternal cognitive bias and child age. *Behavior Therapy, 43*, 593–605.

Flament, M., Koby, E., Rapoport, J., Berg, C., Zahn, T., Cox, C., et al. (1990). Childhood obsessive compulsive disorder: A prospective follow-up study. *Journal of Child Psychology and Psychiatry, and Allied Disciplines, 13*, 363–380.

Flament, M. F., Whitaker, A., Rapoport, J. L., Davies, M., Berg, C. Z., Kalikow, K., et al. (1988). Obsessive compulsive disorder in adolescence: An epidemiological study. *Journal of the American Academy of Child & Adolescent Psychiatry, 27*(6), 764–771.

Franklin, M. E., Saptya, J., Freeman, J. B., Khanna, M., Compton, S., Almirall, D., et al. (2011). Cognitive behavior therapy augmentation of pharmacotherapy in pediatric obsessive-compulsive disorder: The Pediatric OCD Treatment Study II (POTS II) randomized controlled trial. *Journal of the American Medical Association, 306*, 1224–1232.

Frost, R., Sher, K., & Geen, T. (1986). Psychopathology and personality characteristics of nonclinical compulsive checkers. *Behavior Research and Therapy, 24*, 133–143.

Frost, R. O., & Steketee, G. (1997). Perfectionism in obsessive-compulsive disorder patients. *Behaviour Research and Therapy, 35*, 291–296.

Futh, A., Simonds, L. M., & Micali, N. (2012). Obsessive-compulsive disorder in children: Parental understanding, accommodation, coping and distress. *Journal of Anxiety Disorders, 26*, 624–632.

Garcia, A., Freeman, J. B., Himle, M. B., Berman, N. C., Ogata, A. K., Ng, J., et al. (2009). Phenomenology of Early Childhood Onset Obsessive Compulsive Disorder. *Journal of Psychopathology and Behavioral Assessment, 31*, 104–111.

Geller, D. A. (2006). Obsessive-compulsive and spectrum disorders in children and adolescents. *Psychiatric Clinics of North America, 29*, 353–370.

Geller, D., Biederman, J., Jones, J., Park, K., Schwartz, S., Shapiro, S., et al. (1998). Is juvenile obsessive-compulsive disorder a developmental subtype of the disorder? A review of the pediatric literature. *Journal of American Academy of Child and Adolescent Psychiatry, 37*, 420–427.

Gesell, A., Ames, L., & Ilg, F. (1974). *Infant and child in the culture of today*. New York: Harper & Row.

Goodman, W. K., Price, L. H., Rasmussen, S. A., Mazure, C., Delgado, P., Heninger, G. R., et al. (1989). The Yale-Brown Obsessive Compulsive Scale II: Validity. *Archives of General Psychiatry, 46*, 1012–1016.

Goodman, W. K., Price, L. H., Rasmussen, S. A., Mazure, C., Fleischmann, R. L., Hill, C. L., et al. (1989). The Yale-Brown Obsessive Compulsive Scale I: Development, use, and reliability. *Archives of General Psychiatry, 46*, 1006–1011.

Grisham, J. R., Fullana, M. A., Mataix-Cols, D., Moffitt, T. E., Caspi, A., & Poulton, R. (2011). Risk factors prospectively associated with adult obsessive-compulsive symptom dimensions and obsessive-compulsive disorder. *Psychological Medicine, 41*, 2495–2506.

Grunes, M. S., Neziroglu, F., & McKay, D. (2001). Family involvement in the behavioral treatment of obsessive-compulsive disorder: A preliminary investigation. *Behavior Therapy, 32*, 803–820.

Hemmings, S. M., Kinnear, C. J., Lochner, C., Nieuhaus, D. J., Knowles, J. A., Moolman-Smook, J. C., et al. (2004). Early- versus late-onset obsessive compulsive disorder: Investigating genetic and clinical correlates. *Psychiatry Research, 128*, 175–182.

Huppert, J. D., Simpson, H. B., Nissenson, K. J., Liebowitz, M. R., & Foa, E. B. (2009). Quality of life and functional impairment in obsessive-compulsive disorder: A comparison of patients with and without comorbidity, patients in remission, and healthy controls. *Depression and Anxiety, 26*, 39–45.

Jans, T., Wewetzer, C., Klampfl, K., Schulz, E., Herpertz-Dahlmann, B., Remschmidt, H., et al. (2007). Phenomenology and co-morbidity of childhood onset obsessive compulsive disorder. *Zeitschrift für Kinder- und Jugendpsychiatrie und Psychotherapie, 35*, 41–50.

Kalra, S.K., & Swedo, S.E. (2009). Children with obsessive-compulsive disorder: are they just "little adults"? *Journal of Clinical Investigation, 119*, 737–746.

Lack, C. W., Storch, E. A., Keeley, M. L., Geffken, G. R., Ricketts, E. D., Murphy, T. K., et al. (2009). Quality of life in children and adolescents with obsessive-compulsive disorder: Base rates, parent–child agreement, and clinical correlates. *Social Psychiatry and Psychiatric Epidemiology, 44*, 935–942.

Leckman, J. F., Zhang, H., Alsobrook, J. P., & Pauls, D. L. (2001). Symptom dimensions in obsessive-compulsive disorder: Toward quantitative phenotypes. *American Journal of Medical Genetics, 105*, 28–30.

Lenane, M. C., Swedo, S. E., Leonard, H., Pauls, D. L., Sceery, W., & Rapoport, J. L. (1990). Psychiatric disorders in first degree relatives of children and adolescents with obsessive compulsive disorder. *Journal of the American Academy of Child and Adolescent Psychiatry, 29*, 407–412.

Leonard, H., Goldberger, E., Rapoport, J., Cheslow, D., & Swedo, S. (1990). Childhood rituals: Normal development or obsessive-compulsive symptoms? *Journal of the American Academy of Child and Adolescent Psychiatry, 29*, 17–23.

Mancebo, M. C., Garcia, A. M., Pinto, A., Freeman, J. B., Przeworski, A., Stout, R., et al. (2008). Juvenile-onset OCD: Clinical features in children, adolescents and adults. *Acta Psychiatrica Scandinavica, 118*, 149–159.

March, J. S., & Curry, J. F. (1998). Predicting the outcome of treatment. *Journal of Abnormal Child Psychology, 26*, 39–51.

Martin, J. L., & Thienemann, M. (2005). Group cognitive behavior therapy with family involvement for middle-school-age children with obsessive-compulsive disorder: A pilot study. *Child Psychiatry and Human Development, 36*, 113–127.

Mell, L. K., Davis, R. L., & Owens, D. (2005). Association between streptococcal infection and obsessive-compulsive disorder, Tourette's syndrome, and tic disorder. *Pediatrics, 116*, 56–60.

Merlo, L. J., Lehmkuhl, H. D., Geffken, G. R., & Storch, E. A. (2009). Decreased family accommodation associated with improved therapy outcome in pediatric obsessive-compulsive disorder. *Journal of Consulting and Clinical Psychology, 77*, 355–360.

Moos, R. H., & Moos, B. M. (1986). *Family environment scale manual*. Palo Alto, CA: Consulting Psychologists Press.

Murray, C. J. L., & Lopez, A. D. (1996). *The global burden of disease*. Boston, MA: Harvard University Press.

Nakatani, E., Krebs, G., Micali, N., Turner, C., Heyman, I., & Mataix-Cols, D. (2011). Children with very early onset obsessive compulsive disorder: Clinical features and treatment outcome. *Journal of Child Psychology and Psychiatry, 52*, 1261–1268.

Olley, A., Malhi, G., & Sachdev, P. (2007). Memory and executive functioning in obsessive-compulsive disorder: A selective review. *Journal of Affective Disorders, 104*, 15–23.

Palermo, S. D., Bloch, M. H., Craiglow, B., Landeros-Weisenberger, A., Dombrowski, P. A., Panza, K., et al. (2011). Predictors of early adulthood quality of life in children with obsessive-compulsive disorder. *Social Psychiatry and Psychiatric Epidemiology, 46*, 291–297.

Pauls, D. L. (2008). The genetics of obsessive compulsive disorder: A review of the evidence. *American Journal of Medical Genetics Part C: Seminars in Medical Genetics, 148C*, 133–139.

Pauls, D., Alsobrook, J. I., Goodman, W., Rasmussen, S., & Leckman, J. (1995). A family study of obsessive compulsive disorder. *American Journal of Psychiatry, 143*, 76–84.

Peris, T. S., Bergman, L., Langley, A., Chang, S., McCracken, J. T., & Piacentini, J. (2008). Correlates of accommodation of pediatric obsessive-compulsive disorder: Parent, child, and family characteristics. *Journal of the American Academy of Child and Adolescent Psychiatry, 47*, 1173–1181.

Peterson, B. S., Pine, D. S., Cohen, P., & Brook, J. S. (2001). Prospective, longitudinal study of tic, obsessive-compulsive, and attention-deficit/hyperactivity disorders in an epidemiological sample. *Journal of the American Academy of Child & Adolescent Psychiatry, 40*, 685–695.

Phillips, K. A., Stein, D. J., Rauch, S. L., Hollander, E., Fallon, B. A., Barsky, A., et al. (2010). Should an obsessive-compulsive spectrum grouping of disorders be included in DSM-V? *Depression & Anxiety, 27*, 528–555.

Piacentini, J., Bergman, L., Keller, M., & McCracken, J. (2003). Functional impairment in children and adolescents with obsessive-compulsive disorder. *Journal of Child and Adolescent Psychopharmacology, 13*, S61–S69.

Piaget, J. (1962). *Play, dreams and imitation in childhood.* New York: Norton.

Pietrefesa, A., & Evans, D. W. (2007). Affective and neuropsychological correlates of children's compulsive-like behaviors: Continuities and discontinuities with obsessive–compulsive disorder. *Brain & Cognition, 65*(1), 36–46.

Rachman, S. (1976). The modification of obsessions: A new formulation. *Behaviour Research and Therapy, 14*, 437–443.

Rachman, S. (1985). An overview of clinical and research issues in obsessive-compulsive disorders. In M. Mavissakalian, S. Turner, & L. Michelson (Eds.), *Obsessive-compulsive disorders: Psychological and pharmacological treatment* (pp. 1–47). New York: Plenum.

Rachman, S., & Hodgson, R. (1978). Abnormal and normal obsessions. *Behavior Research and Therapy, 16*, 233–248.

Rachman, S., & Hodgson, R. (1980). *Obsessions and compulsions.* Englewood Cliffs, NJ: Prentice-Hall.

Reddy, Y. C., Srinath, S., Prakash, H. M., Girimaji, S. C., Sheshadri, S. P., Khanna, S., et al. (2003). A follow-up study of juvenile obsessive-compulsive disorder from India. *Acta Psychiatrica Scandinavica, 107*, 457–464.

Rehm, L., & Carter, A. (1990). Cognitive components of depression. In M. Lewis & S. Miller (Eds.), *Handbook of developmental psychopathology* (pp. 341–351). New York: Plenum Press.

Rettew, D., Swedo, S., Leonard, H., Lenane, M., & Rapoport, J. (1992). Obsessions and compulsions across time in 79 children and adolescents with obsessive compulsive disorder. *Journal of the American Academy of Child and Adolescent Psychiatry, 31*, 1050–1056.

Rothbart, M. K. (1989). Behavioral approach and inhibition. In S. J. Reznick (Ed.), *Perspectives on behavioral inhibition* (pp. 139–157). Chicago, IL: University of Chicago Press.

Ruscio, A. M., Stein, D. J., Chiu, W. T., & Kessler, R. C. (2008). The epidemiology of obsessive-compulsive disorder in the National Comorbidity Survey Replication. *Molecular Psychiatry, 15*, 53–63.

Saxena, S., & Rauch, S. L. (2000). Functional neuroimaging and the neuroanatomy of obsessive–compulsive disorder. *Psychiatric Clinics of North America, 23*, 563–86.

Scahill, L., Riddle, M. A., McSwiggin-Hardin, M., Ort, S. I., King, R. A., Goodman, W. K., et al. (1997). Children's Yale-Brown Obsessive Compulsive Scale: Reliability and validity. *Journal of the American Academy of Child & Adolescent Psychiatry, 36*, 844–852.

Schlup, B., Farrell, L., & Barrett, P. (2011). Mother-child interactions and childhood OCD: Effects of CBT on mother and child observed behaviors. *Child & Family Behavior Therapy, 33*, 322–336.

Stengler-Wenzke, K., Trosbach, J., Dietrich, S., & Angermeyer, M. C. (2004a). Coping strategies used by the relatives of people with obsessive-compulsive disorder. *Journal of Advanced Nursing, 48*, 35–42.

Stengler-Wenzke, K., Trosbach, J., Dietrich, S., & Angermeyer, M. C. (2004b). Experience of stigmatization by relatives of patients with obsessive compulsive disorder. *Archives of Psychiatric Nursing, 18*, 88–96.

Stewart, S. E., Geller, D. A., Jenike, M., Pauls, D. L., Shaw, D., Mullin, B., et al. (2004). Long-term outcome of pediatric obsessive-compulsive disorder: A meta-analysis and qualitative review of the literature. *Acta Psychiatrica Scandinavica, 110*, 4–13.

Stewart, S. E., Rosario-Campos, M. C., Brown, T. A., Carter, A., Leckman, J. F., Sukhdolsky, D., et al. (2007). Principal Components Analysis of Obsessive-Compulsive Disorder Symptoms in Children and Adolescents. *Biological Psychiatry, 61*, 285–291.

Stewart, S. E., Yu, D., Scharf, J. M., Neale, B. M., Fagerness, J. A., Mathews, C. A., et al. (2012). Genome-wide association study of obsessive-compulsive disorder. *Molecular Psychiatry, 1*–11, doi 10.1038/mp.2012.85.

Storch, E. A., Geffken, G. R., Merlo, L. J., Mann, G., Duke, D., Munson, M., et al. (2007). Family-based cognitive behavioral therapy for pediatric obsessive-compulsive disorder: Comparison of intensive and weekly approaches. *Journal of the American Academy of Child and Adolescent Psychiatry, 46*, 469–478.

Storch, E. A., Lehmkuhl, H., Pence, S. L., Geffken, G. R., Ricketts, E., Storch, J. F., et al. (2009). Parental experiences of having a child with obsessive-compulsive disorder: Associations with clinical characteristics and caregiver adjustment. *Journal of Child and Family Studies, 18*, 249–258.

Storch, E. A., Merlo, L. J., Larson, M. J., Marien, W. E., Geffken, G. R., Jacob, M. L., et al. (2008). Clinical features associated with treatment-resistant pediatric obsessive-compulsive disorder. *Comprehensive Psychiatry, 49*, 35–42.

Swedo, S. E., Leonard, H. L., Garvey, M., Mittleman, B., Allen, A. J., Perlmutter, S., et al. (1998). Pediatric autoimmune neuropsychiatric disorders associated with streptococcal infections: Clinical description of the first 50 cases. *The American Journal of Psychiatry, 155*, 264–271.

The Pediatric OCD Treatment Study (POTS) Team. (2004). Cognitive-behavior therapy, sertraline, and their combination for children and adolescents with obsessive-compulsive disorder: The Pediatric OCD Treatment Study (POTS) randomized controlled trial. *Journal of the American Medical Association, 292*, 1969–1976.

Thienemann, M., Martin, J., Cregger, B., Thompson, H., & Dyer-Friedman, J. (2001). Manual-driven group cognitive-behavioral therapy for adolescents with obsessive-compulsive disorder: A pilot study. *Journal of the American Academy of Child and Adolescent Psychiatry, 10*, 1254–1260.

Thomsen, P. (1993). Obsessive-compulsive disorder in children and adolescents: Self-reported obsessive-compulsive behaviour in pupils in Denmark. *Acta Psychiatrica Scandinavica, 88*, 212–217.

Tolin, D. F., Abramowitz, J. S., Brigidi, B. D., & Foa, E. B. (2003). Intolerance of uncertainty in obsessive-compulsive disorder. *Journal of Anxiety Disorders, 17*, 233–242.

Van Noppen, B., Rasumussen, S. A., Eisen, J., & McCartney, L. (1991). A multifamily group approach as an adjunct to treatment of obsessive compulsive disorder. In M. T. Pato & J. Zohar (Eds.), *Current treatments of obsessive compulsive disorder* (pp. 115–134). Washington, DC: American Psychological Press.

Van Noppen, B., & Steketee, G. (2009). Testing a conceptual model of patient and family predictors of obsessive compulsive disorder (OCD) symptoms. *Behaviour Research and Therapy, 47*, 18–25.

Waters, T. L., & Barrett, P. M. (2000). The role of the family in childhood obsessive-compulsive disorder. *Clinical Child and Family Psychology Review, 3*, 173–184.

Waters, T. L., Barrett, P. M., & March, J. S. (2001). Cognitive-behavioral family treatment of childhood obsessive-compulsive disorder: Preliminary findings. *American Journal of Psychotherapy, 55*, 372–387.

Wichstrøm, L., Berg-Nielsen, T., Angold, A., Egger, H., Solheim, E., & Sveen, T. (2012). Prevalence of psychiatric disorders in preschoolers. *Journal Of Child Psychology And Psychiatry, 53*(6), 695–705. doi:10.1111/j.1469-7610.2011.02514.x.

Woods, C. M., Frost, R. O., & Steketee, G. (2002). Obsessive compulsive (OC) symptoms and subjective severity, probability, and coping ability estimations of future negative event. *Clinical Psychology and Psychotherapy, 9*, 104–111.

Zelazo, P., Carter, A., Reznick, J., & Frye, D. (1997). Early development of executive function: A problem-solving framework. *Review of General Psychology, 1*, 198–226.

Zohar, A., & Bruno, R. (1997). Normative and pathological obsessive-compulsive behavior and ideation in childhood: A question of timing. *Journal of Child Psychology and Psychiatry, and Allied Disciplines, 38*, 993–999.

Part VII

Control Disorders

Alcoholism: A Life Span Perspective on Etiology and Course

29

Brian M. Hicks and Robert A. Zucker

Alcoholism is a disorder involving problems with the use of alcohol such that the consumption becomes compulsive and/or negatively affects the person's health, personal relationships, and ability to fulfill major role obligations (e.g., work, family). For over 30 years, the disorder was defined by the Diagnostic and Statistical Manual (DSM) disorders of *alcohol dependence* and *abuse*. Dependence involves physiological addiction (tolerance or withdrawal) and/or compulsive alcohol use, where use is continued despite problems of physical and mental health as well as impairment in social, family, and job responsibilities. Alcohol abuse involves less severe drinking problems, including hazardous use (e.g., drunk driving) and social problems (e.g., legal problems due to drinking), but not physiological dependence. There is little evidence, however, to justify the distinction between symptoms of abuse and dependence (Borges et al., 2010).

Rather, problematic alcohol use seems best conceptualized as a continuum ranging from heavy use to severe symptoms. As such, the broader term alcohol use disorder (AUD) is now used in the recently published, latest edition of the DSM (DSM-5), which we also use to refer to the general condition of problematic alcohol use over time.

From a developmental psychopathology perspective, AUD occupies a special place among other disorders for a number of reasons. The first is common to all substance use disorders, but not other forms of psychopathology, namely, that the deviant behavior occurs in conjunction with an external object. As such, a distinguishing feature of AUD is that the availability, regulation of use, and patterns of use within the social context have direct impact upon the development of the disorder. For example, AUD is not a high-prevalence disorder in abstinent Muslim countries, but it may become a problem for those with high-risk profiles who emigrate or travel. Related to availability, prevalence of AUD has been shown to vary with the overall the use structure of the larger social system in which it is embedded (Reich, Cloninger, Van eerdewegh, Rice, & Mullaney, 1988). Thus, when consumption rates are higher, there is a lower threshold for moving into problem activity because access is easy and the cue structure for continued use is also more common. Under these conditions, population rates for AUD increase. Conversely, when social controls are tighter and the normative structure is more abstinence orientated, rates of AUD decrease.

B.M. Hicks, Ph.D. (✉)
Department of Psychiatry, Addiction Research Center, University of Michigan, 4250 Plymouth Rd., Ann Arbor MI 48109-2700, USA
e-mail: brianhic@med.umich.edu

R.A. Zucker, Ph.D.
Departments of Psychiatry and Psychology, Addiction Research Center, University of Michigan Medical School, Ann Arbor MI 48109, USA
e-mail: zuckerra@umich.edu

M. Lewis and K.D. Rudolph (eds.), *Handbook of Developmental Psychopathology*, DOI 10.1007/978-1-4614-9608-3_29, © Springer Science+Business Media New York 2014

Second, alcohol is a drug of everyday use and occupies a special place in the social order that ties patterns of use and abuse to other stages of the life cycle more tightly than most other psychiatric disorders. Ethanol is the world's most domesticated psychoactive drug. It is heavily sought after for its pharmacological effects and in the form of beer and wine is one of the world's most common foods and celebratory substances. Thus, alcohol's use structure is heavily embedded in the fabric of the majority of modern societies. It is a drug of courting, recreation, and relaxation and also the drug with which we sometimes mourn.

Third, because alcohol is embedded in the fabric of everyday life, both alcohol use and AUD are superimposed upon the ongoing life structure. Therefore, patterns of AUD differ as a function of life course variations upon which alcohol involvement is overlaid (Zucker, 1998). Therefore, an understanding of AUD needs to take account of the life cycle variations that co-occur with age, affect availability, and to a degree either proscribe or prescribe use with shifts in role structure. Thus, many of the trends in epidemiological data are explained by this life cycle variation, but this underlying variation is often not sufficiently emphasized.

Finally, a notable advantage in understanding etiological course is that AUD cannot occur prior to the discrete event of initiation of alcohol use. This allows for a clear separation between preexisting risk factors and factors that may either be confounded with the symptoms of the disorder or involve different expressions of the same underlying risk structure. Also, substance use disorders have a relatively late onset, with early-onset cases typically emerging in middle to late adolescence. By that point in the life course, there has been substantial development of personality structure and exposure to environmental risks. This provides the opportunity to track individual differences in the underlying risk structure for lengthy periods both before and after initiation, which assists in delineating the causal role of various risk factors contributing to the development and maintenance of AUD.

To do justice to the complexity of the biopsychosocial matrix of risk obviously requires more space than is available here. To manage this limitation, after a brief review of epidemiology, we address several topics critical to understanding AUD including heterogeneity of course, developmental trends, early risk factors with a focus on behavioral disinhibition/dysregulation, and genetic and environmental influences including gene–environment interplay. We also provide a brief discussion of the neurobiology of addiction. A recurrent theme is the need to disaggregate risk into two domains: one involving nonspecific risk factors shared between AUD and other impulse control disorders, and the other involving risks that are specific to AUD.

Epidemiology

Table 29.1 summarizes findings from the National Epidemiologic Survey on Alcohol and Related Conditions (NESARC) for the 12-month and lifetime prevalence rates for DSM-IV alcohol abuse and dependence (Hasin, Stinson, Ogburn, & Grant, 2007). NESARC was conducted in 2001–2002 and included 43,093 respondents age 18 to over 65. In order to give a broader perspective on the alcohol problem, we also present rates for illicit drug abuse and dependence (Compton, Thomas, Stinson, & Grant, 2007). A number of points about these prevalence rates are of importance:

1. Alcohol abuse and dependence are much more common than illicit drug use disorders.
2. Among males, 4 in 10 have at some point in their lives met abuse or dependence criteria.
3. Gender differences are significant and approximate 2:1 for both abuse and dependence.
4. Illicit drug use disorders are substantially less of an issue than alcohol abuse/dependence with a ratio of 12-month alcohol to drug disorder of over 4:1.
5. Illicit drug use disorders are to a large degree superimposed upon AUDs given that a minority of 12-month drug disorders occur without a concomitant AUD diagnosis.

Table 29.1 Lifetime and 12-month prevalence of DSM-IV substance use disorders

Disorder	Total		Male		Female	
	Lifetime	12 months	Lifetime	12 months	Lifetime	12 months
Alcohol abuse without dependence	17.8	4.7	24.6	6.9	11.5	2.6
Alcohol dependence	12.5	3.8	17.4	5.4	8.0	2.3
Alcohol abuse/dependence combined	30.3	8.5	42.0	12.4	19.5	4.9
Drug abuse	7.7	1.4	10.6	2.0	5.2	0.8
Drug dependence	2.6	0.6	3.3	0.9	2.0	0.4
Drug abuse/dependence combined	10.3	2.0	13.8	2.8	7.1	1.2

Source from Hasin et al. (2007) and Compton et al. (2007) National Epidemiologic Survey on Alcohol and Related Conditions and are weighted non-institutionalized United States population percentage estimates for persons 18 years or older

6. The visibility of illicit drug use disorders is likely because they are more dramatic, hence socially compelling; because they appear more of a threat to the social order (e.g., because of their links with crime and the belief that they may be less responsive to treatment); and because societal costs involved in interdiction and treatment are proportionately much larger.

Related to the these points, AUD is nationally one of the most prevalent psychiatric disorders with approximately 30 % of the population reporting symptoms sufficient for either an abuse or dependence diagnosis at some point during their lives. Thus, the set of problems encompassed by this disorder is an extraordinarily large one. At the same time, when examining the disorder from a developmental perspective, among all those who meet the AUD criterion, there is substantial heterogeneity of onset and course. Such variation has been identified at least as far back as Carpenter (1850), and because the variation continues to emphasize the point that "one size does not fit all," there have been periodic attempts to classify the heterogeneity.

Heterogeneity of Course and Phenotype

Babor's (1996) review of this literature noted that different classification schemes identify two consistent "types," with different etiologies and symptom presentations. One type is characterized by early onset, physical aggression, more severe dependence symptoms, a denser positive family history—suggesting a stronger genetic basis—and more personality disturbance. The other is characterized by later onset of alcohol dependence, a slower disease course, fewer social complications, less psychological impairment, and a better prognosis. More recent studies using factor analytic and cluster analytic techniques continue to identify these two forms, but a number of others have also been identified. The unearthing of this larger spectrum of course heterogeneity is due to the newer studies' use of samples that are less chronic, improved statistical methodology, and utilization of functional characteristics rather than symptoms to make the differentiation. Leggio, Kenna, Fenton, Bonefant and Swift (2009) provide a comprehensive tally of the current array.

Developmental Trends

Only in the past generation has significant attention been paid to the earlier developmental manifestations of these course variations by utilizing prospective course information to more accurately characterize course variation. This work has focused more on course of heavy drinking than on AUD symptoms. Reviewing this literature, Maggs and Schulenberg (2005) note that virtually all of the studies identify four pathways of heavy use: a chronic/severe and continuing trajectory, a mild low-level binging and symptom group, an initially severe use group that drops off with entry

Fig. 29.1 Prevalence of alcohol, nicotine, and cannabis use disorder by chronological age in the longitudinal twin, adoption, and family studies of the Minnesota Center for Twin and Family Research (*N*=5,001). Each substance use disorder was defined as the presence of three or more symptoms of abuse or dependence according to DSM-III-R criteria, the current diagnostic system when the earliest studies began. Participants reported on the symptoms over the past 3 years

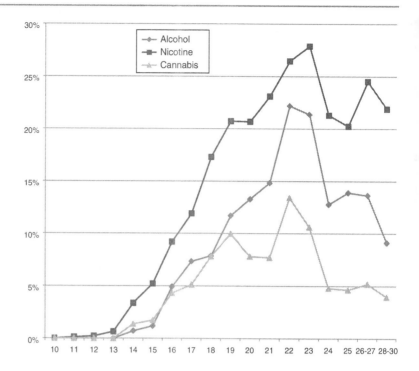

into early adulthood, and one that begins in adolescence and escalates over time into adulthood. The later-onset path for this last group is not well understood.

There are also normative developmental trends in age of onset, escalation, and decline of the prevalence of AUD over the life course. To illustrate this patterning, we report data from the longitudinal Minnesota Twin Family Study (Iacono, McGue, & Krueger, 2006). Approximately 5,000 individuals began participating in this study as either children or adolescents and have been followed until about age 30 reporting on patterns of substance use every 3–5 years. Fairly large and representative samples are available for almost each year between ages 10 and 30 to track developmental trends in the prevalence of substance use disorders.

In Fig. 29.1, the prevalence rates of substance use disorders in the Minnesota Twin Family Study sample are presented for the three most widely used substances in the United States: alcohol, nicotine, and cannabis. Substance use disorders were defined as 3 symptoms of abuse or dependence according to DSM-III-R criteria (the

diagnostic system that was current when the study began). Based on these data, substance use disorders first emerge in a small subset of people around ages 14–15, followed by a steep rise in the prevalence rates of each disorder through adolescence until rates peak at ages 21–23. Around age 24, there is a notable decline in the prevalence of each disorder. Nicotine dependence is always the most common substance use disorder. AUD and cannabis use disorder have similar prevalence rates until about age 20, whereupon there is a dramatic increase in AUD that outpaces that of cannabis use disorder. During the late 20s, nicotine dependence and cannabis use disorder decline to relatively stable prevalence rates of slightly over 20 % and about 5 %, respectively. In contrast, AUD continues to decline out to age 30 to a prevalence rate of slightly less than 10 %. Given the lifetime prevalence rates reported from the NESARC, it would appear that the vast majority of people who meet criteria for a substance use disorder will first do so before age 30.

These patterns suggest that (1) nonspecific risk processes likely underlie the emergence and rapid escalation of each substance use disorder

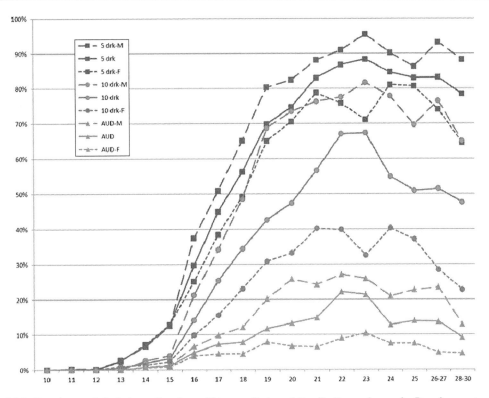

Fig. 29.2 Prevalence of alcohol use disorder and binge drinking defined as 5+ and 10+ drinks in a 24-h period as function of chronological age in the Minnesota Center for Twin and Family Research sample. Prevalence rates are also provided separately for men and women

in late adolescence and young adulthood and (2) similar general processes likely underlie the reductions in substance use disorders beginning in the mid-20s, though the rate of this decline differs across substances. Differences in legal status and psychoactive effect across the substances undoubtedly account for many of the differences in prevalence. Specifically, the sale and purchase of tobacco and alcohol are both legal, which contributes to their higher prevalence rates relative to cannabis. In terms of psychoactive effects, nicotine is associated with greater physiological dependence than alcohol, but persistent nicotine dependence has weaker associations with psychosocial impairment than persistent AUD. As such, tobacco is harder to quit using than alcohol, but nicotine dependence is easier to live with than AUD, hence the higher prevalence rate for nicotine dependence than AUD, especially as people transition into middle adulthood.

A major premise of this volume is that adult disorders do not emerge full-blown in adulthood, but rather are the endpoint of a process that culminates over time for which childhood precursors and risk factors can be identified. To illustrate this, Fig. 29.2 presents the rates for two measures of binge drinking (consuming either 5 or 10 drinks in a 24-h period)—markers of problematic alcohol use that typically precede AUD symptoms—along with the prevalence rates for AUD. Rates are reported separately for males and females to illustrate the large gender differences for both use and disorder.

These data illustrate that by middle adolescence there is a subset of individuals who are already exhibiting problematic alcohol use that portends later AUDs. For example, by age 15 over 10 % of the sample reported consuming 5 drinks on one occasion, and by age 16 over 20 % of males reported consuming 10 drinks on one occasion. The increases in drinking are so dramatic that heavy drinking is essentially normative by age 19 and ubiquitous by age 23. While not everyone who engages in heavy drinking goes on to develop AUD, heavy drinking provides the necessary context as the rates of AUD closely track those of binge drinking, especially binges of 10 or more drinks. Also note the dramatic gender differences in the rates of larger binges and AUD. By age 18, the rate for women who reported a binge of 5 drinks is equal to the rate for men who reported a binge of 10 drinks, and the rate of AUD in men is over twice that of women; these gender differences persist at least to age 30. Men it seems literally drink twice as much as women.

Early Risk Factors

I. Behavioral Disinhibition

Although the prevalence of AUD begins its ascent in late adolescence, increased risk for AUD can be detected at much younger ages. Like many disorders, a family history of AUD is a robust predictor of AUD and also suggestive of genetic influences. Family history, however, does not rule out environmental influences, as genetic and environmental influences are confounded when biological parents raise their own children. Family history then is only a proxy for risk, the mechanisms of which require further explication. Moreover, not all families with an alcoholic parent contain the same levels of risk, and in some, the vulnerability components may be largely absent. Designs that leverage family history—most notably children of alcoholic parents studies—can be especially helpful by comparing individuals who differ on family history of AUD on a number of variables to identify potential risk pathways. One long-term high-risk study, the Michigan Longitudinal Study, has been following a large number of families with either an alcoholic father or control families in which neither parent had an alcohol or illicit drug use disorder, for over 25 years beginning when the children were 3–5 years old (Zucker et al., 2000). They found that even at ages 3–5, children of an alcoholic parents exhibited significantly more

internalizing (anxiety, depression) and externalizing (aggression, rule breaking) problems than children of nonalcoholic parents, indicating risk mechanisms for AUD are present long before even the initiation of alcohol use.

Several lines of evidence including long-term longitudinal studies of high-risk (e.g., children of alcoholic parents) and epidemiological samples have demonstrated a robust association between childhood externalizing behavior and an earlier age of initiation of substance use, heavy use, and onset of substance use disorders in general, not just for alcohol (Armstrong & Costello, 2002). At the diagnostic level, externalizing behavior is typically operationalized as one of the disruptive behavior disorders (conduct disorder, oppositional defiant disorder, attention deficit hyperactivity disorder) or as scores on problem behavior checklists (aggression, rule breaking). As such, rather than antisocial behavior per se, the broader temperament trait of **behavioral disinhibition**—defined as an inability to inhibit socially undesirable or restricted behavior—is the key childhood risk factor for later problematic substance use (Iacono, Malone, & McGue, 2008; Zucker, Heitzeg, & Nigg, 2011). The phenotypic or observable manifestations of behavioral disinhibition are typically referred to as **"externalizing,"** which includes disinhibited personality traits, disruptive behavior disorders, substance use disorders, and antisocial behavior.

The conceptualization of a behavioral disinhibition liability provides a model of general and specific risk processes for AUD. Most notably, this model helps to account for the high rates of co-occurrence or comorbidity between AUD and other substance use disorders as well as with antisocial behavior and disinhibited personality traits. AUD and other addictions rarely occur in isolation, but rather tend to be part of a profile of correlated externalizing features. Conceptually then, persons who exhibit multiple externalizing disorders are simply higher on the behavioral disinhibition dimension. A meta-analysis of several epidemiological studies comprising over 23,000 individuals that modeled the structure of 10 common mental disorders found that the covariance among AUD, illicit drug use disorders, and the child and adult symptoms of antisocial personality disorder was best modeled by a single underlying externalizing factor (Krueger & Markon, 2006; also see Kendler, Prescott, Myers, & Neale, 2003). Juxtaposed to this externalizing factor was a latent "internalizing" factor that accounted for the comorbidity among unipolar mood and anxiety disorders. Specific risk processes then differentiate these general liability dimensions into the specific disorders and accounts for why people manifest some disorders and not others.

II. Early Onset of Use

Another early risk factor for AUD is the age at which individuals first use alcoholic beverages. Persons who have their first use before age 15 are approximately four times more likely to meet criteria for alcohol dependence in adulthood relative to persons who first tried alcohol at age 20 or later (Grant & Dawson, 1997). Consistent with a model of nonspecific risk processes, earlier age of first use (<15 years old) has frequently been identified as an intermediate outcome associated with behavioral undercontrol, disruptive behavior disorders, and academic problems in preadolescence, which then predicts not only AUD but also nicotine dependence, illicit drug dependence, and antisocial personality disorder in adulthood (McGue, Iacono, Legrand, Malone, & Elkins, 2001). It also is associated with a more rapid progression to and longer duration of alcoholism, greater difficulty achieving abstinence, and more severe symptom profiles of AUD.

III. Negative Affectivity/Internalizing

In addition to behavioral disinhibition, there is a long history of work indicating an internalizing or negative affect pathway to AUD (Hussong, Jones, Stein, Baucom, & Boeding, 2011; Zucker, 2006). The major evidence for an internalizing pathway comes from a small number of prospective studies showing a relationship between internalizing symptoms in childhood and an AUD outcome in adulthood (Caspi, Moffitt, Newman,

& Silva, 1996; Hawkins, Catalano, & Miller, 1992; Kellam, Brown, Rubin, & Ensminger, 1983; Kellam, Ensminger, & Simon, 1980). Indirect evidence for an internalizing pathway is also suggested by the elevated rates of comorbidity between AUD, major depression, and some anxiety disorders (Hasin et al., 2007), as well as the moderate correlation ($r=0.50$) between the latent internalizing and externalizing dimensions (Krueger & Markon, 2006). Also, personality traits that tap negative emotionality such as neuroticism are elevated in both internalizing disorders and AUD (Krueger, Caspi, Moffitt, Silva, & McGee, 1996). The longitudinal evidence for a direct childhood internalizing pathway, however, is mixed, especially after controlling for comorbid externalizing (Chassin, Pitts, DeLucia, & Todd, 1999; Costello, Erkanli, Federman, & Angold, 1999; Kaplow, Curran, Angold, & Costello, 2001). Although the prospective studies already noted find a positive association between internalizing and substance use disorders, others find a null or negative association (Kaplow et al., 2001; Masse & Tremblay, 1997). Possibly the association between internalizing and AUD is a function of greater symptom severity, or it may only operate as a moderator of externalizing characteristics.

Genetic Influences

Twin and adoption studies have demonstrated that genetic influences play an important role in the development of AUD (Goldman, Oroszi, & Ducci, 2005). For such biometric analyses, the variance of a trait is partitioned into additive genetic (a^2), shared or common environment (c^2), and non-shared or unique environment (e^2) components by comparing the similarity of individuals on the trait who differ in genetic relatedness (e.g., by comparing the similarity of monozygotic twins to that of dizygotic twins). The ratio of genetic variance to total variance is called the heritability estimate. The shared environment refers to environmental influences that contribute to similarity among relatives (e.g., being part of the same peer group that encourages drinking). The non-shared environment refers to environmental influences that contribute to differences among relatives (e.g., having romantic partners that differ in attitudes toward substance use).

Twin studies consistently find that genetic influences account for approximately 45 % of the variance of AUD and measures of quantity and frequency in adulthood (Dick, Latendresse, et al., 2009; Dick, Prescott, & McGue, 2009; Goldman et al., 2005). The relative genetic and environmental influences are moderated by age, however, as initiation of alcohol use exhibits both moderate genetic and shared environmental influences as does quantity/frequency and AUD in adolescence (Dick, Latendresse, et al., 2009; Dick, Prescott, & McGue, 2009). Further, longitudinal studies have found that genetic influences increase and shared environmental influences decrease with age (Bergen, Gardner, & Kendler, 2007). This suggests that shared environmental influences are important to initiation and early drinking, but that genetic and non-shared environmental influences are determinative for long-term problematic alcohol use in adulthood.

Several multivariate twin studies have also established that there is substantial common variance in genetic influences among AUD, nicotine dependence, and illicit drug dependence, as well as with their precursive nonspecific risk components, namely, antisocial behavior and disinhibited personality traits (Button et al., 2006; Kendler, Meyers, & Prescott, 2007; Slutske et al., 1998, True et al., 1999). This work prompted the fitting of biometric factor models to estimate the heritability of the externalizing factor, which would identify the extent to which comorbidity among externalizing phenotypes was due to common genetic and environmental influences. These studies find that externalizing is highly heritable (70 % to 85 %) in late adolescence and young adulthood, with little or no shared environmental influences (Kendler et al., 2003; Krueger et al., 2002; McGue, Iacono, & Krueger, 2006). These estimates are typically higher than for any individual disorder, with the externalizing factor accounting for the majority of genetic variance in each disorder. Each substance use disorder,

however, also exhibited specific genetic and non-shared environmental variance. These findings are consistent with a hierarchical model of risk, involving a highly heritable nonspecific risk factor, but with the final phenotypic expression of the nonspecific risk determined by environmental and genetic influences that are unique to each disorder.

Genetic influences on nonspecific risk also shift over the course of development. McGue et al. (2006) found that the covariance among five trait indicators of early adolescent problem behavior was only modestly heritable ($a^2 = 0.18$) with moderate shared environmental influences ($c^2 = 0.39$). However, the association between problem behavior at age 15 and the more heritable externalizing factor underlying adult disorders at age 20 ($a^2 = 0.75$) was entirely due to common genetic influences, suggesting genetic influences are particularly important to the stability of externalizing over time. Also, the impact of the general externalizing factor on individual substance use disorders appears to peak in late adolescence and decline thereafter as disorder-specific effects increase (Vrieze, Hicks, Iacono, & McGue, 2012). Most of the decline is attributable to the fact that externalizing accounts for less heritable variance of the individual disorders, while disorder-specific genetic and environmental effects increase with age. These findings are consistent with the interpretation that a highly heritable behavioral disinhibition liability leads to nonspecific substance use and externalizing behaviors in late adolescence, but that substance-specific risk factors increase in importance as people age, leading to a specialization in substance use and abuse over time.

Identifying specific genes that reliably account for this nonspecific genetic risk for externalizing disorders and for AUD is high on the current research agenda, but the actuality has yet to be fully realized. The most promising candidate gene may be the $GABA_A$ receptor α2 subunit (*GABRA2*) on chromosome 4. GABA is a major inhibitory neurotransmitter that is sensitive to ethanol including its anxiolytic effects (Grobin, Matthews, Devaud, & Morrow, 1998). *GABRA2* has now been associated with several externalizing phenotypes including alcohol and drug dependence, antisocial personality disorder and conduct disorder, and an electrophysiological endophenotype. There is also some evidence that the effects of *GABRA2* are moderated by environmental context including parental monitoring and marital status (Dick, Latendresse, et al., 2009; Dick, Prescott, & McGue, 2009).

Given the abundant nonspecific genetic risk, it is somewhat ironic that the most replicable genes associated with risk for AUD are specific to alcohol sensitivity (Higuchi et al., 1994). Aldehyde dehydrogenase (ALDH) is the rate-limiting enzyme in the metabolism of ethanol, and the rate of its production varies as a function of ALDH genotype. The mutant form of *ALDH2* (*ALDH2*2* allele) is inefficient at converting acetaldehyde—a toxin and the initial metabolite of ethanol—into acetate. After consuming alcohol, carriers of the *ALDH2*2* allele experience flushing, nausea, and headaches due to the accumulation of acetaldehyde. As a result, individuals with more acetaldehyde inefficient alleles exhibit lower rates of AUD. Notably, the frequency of the *ALDH2*2* variant differs widely across ancestral populations, being common in certain East Asian populations but virtually absent in European populations, which helps to account for some of the historic differences in rates of AUD across world populations. Also, this genetic mechanism is specific to AUD, as demonstrated in a study that showed East Asian adoptees in the United States who carried the *ALDH2*2* allele were less likely to have problems with alcohol use, but not less likely to have ever tried alcohol; they also exhibited similar levels of nicotine and marijuana use and antisocial behavior as those without the *ALDH2*2* allele (Irons, McGue, Iacono, & Oetting, 2007).

A recent advance in gene association methodology has been the advent of genome-wide association studies that are able to interrogate a target phenotype on over one million single nucleotide polymorphisms (SNPs) of common variation (minor allele frequency >0.01). Findings from genome-wide association studies show that the effect for any individual SNP is small, and sample sizes in the many thousands are necessary to detect even a small number of risk SNPs that exceed genome-wide significance ($p < 5^{-8}$). An early genome-wide association study of alcohol dependence included over 1,500 male cases and 2,300 matched controls detected two SNPs on chromosome 2 in linkage disequilibrium with the peroxisomal trans-2-enoyl-coenzyme A reductase (*PECR*) gene, which is involved in fatty acid metabolism and primarily expressed in the liver (Treutlein et al., 2009). A much larger study of alcohol consumption ($N > 47,000$) detected an association with the autism susceptibility candidate 2 gene (*AUTS2*) (Schumann et al., 2011). The mechanism by which *AUTS2* effects alcohol consumption is unclear, but it has been linked with other neurobehavioral disorders in humans and alcohol sensitivity in animals. Of note, this study failed to detect an association with the *PECR* gene. Despite the advantage of scanning the whole genome and the possibility of generating novel leads for etiology then, it is clear that genome-wide association studies for alcohol use phenotypes are in their early stages, and extensive follow-up studies will be needed to delineate the causal chain from genotype to phenotype.

Environmental Risk and Person–Environment Transactions

AUD is also affected by a variety of environmental influences related to family, peer, school, and neighborhood contexts (Hawkins et al., 1992; Zucker, 2006). A family history of AUD, especially in combination with antisocial behavior, is associated with increased risk via various mechanisms involving both inherited risk and disorganization of the social environment (Puttler, Zucker, Fitzgerald, & Bingham, 1998). The link between externalizing and these contextual risk factors tends to follow a typical developmental sequence culminating in early initiation of substance use and escalation to substance use disorders by late adolescence (Granic & Patterson, 2006). This sequence has been called a developmental cascade, as exposure to one contextual risk factor increases the likelihood of exposure to another, and involves transactions with person-level risk factors. Specifically, high-risk rearing environments are characterized by poor parent–child relationships, harsh and inconsistent discipline, lax parental monitoring, and parental substance abuse that provides children with access and models for use. Such ineffective parenting and family management practices combined with undercontrolled temperament traits then result in child conduct problems, which in turn are often followed by academic failure and disengagement and rejection by prosocial peers. Failure to bond with these socializing agents then increases the likelihood of depressed mood and hostility and deviant peer affiliation. Deviant peer affiliation sets the stage for an early initiation and rapid escalation of substance use in adolescence, as well as with concomitant adolescent problem behaviors (e.g., delinquency, precocious and risky sexual behavior; Jessor & Jessor, 1977). Reinforcing these processes are contextual factors such as family, money, and legal problems, parental conflict and divorce, and residence in neighborhoods characterized by high rates of poverty, crime, and residential instability, all of which have been associated with high rates of adolescent substance abuse (Appleyard, Egeland, van Dulmen, & Sroufe, 2005; Buu et al., 2009; Hawkins et al., 1992). Importantly, these contextual risk factors are nested, and exposure is disproportionately spread across the population, such that youth are typically exposed to not one but several of these risk factors (Appleyard et al., 2005; Hicks, South, DiRago, Iacono, & McGue, 2009; Zucker, 2006).

Exposure to environmental risk is also not independent of the child's characteristics, as the child's behavior both elicits responses from others and moves the child into circumstances that increase exposure to risk. For example, using an empirical approach, Hicks, Iacono, and McGue (2014) identified the childhood personality trait of socialization (conformity to rules and adult supervision and endorsement of conventional moral and ethical values) was most predictive of later substance use disorders in the Minnesota Twin Family Study sample. Additionally, socialization at age 11 was strongly correlated with

several concurrent contextual risk factors associated with substance use disorders including deviant peer affiliation, academic failure and disengagement, poor parent–child relationships, and stressful life events.

Such person–environment transactions continue to be played out over the life course. A study by Buu et al. (2007) provides an example of this transactional process, wherein the residential migration patterns of sociodemographically matched families with or without an alcoholic father were tracked over a 12-year interval. Families with an alcoholic father were more likely to either remain in or migrate into a disadvantaged neighborhood (high crime, poverty, and residential instability). Conversely, men whose AUD was in remission tended to live in neighborhoods whose residential characteristics were indistinguishable from those of non-AUD men. Shifting the focus to the children of these men, Buu et al. (2009) found that these same characteristics of neighborhood disadvantage during early childhood (ages 3–5) predicted alcohol, nicotine, and marijuana symptoms as well as antisocial personality disorder and major depression in young adulthood (ages 18–20) even after controlling for family history of AUD.

While we have focused on nonspecific processes of both person-level and environmental risk, there are also alcohol-specific risk processes that are present at a young age. Social cognition studies have found that preschoolers in the general population have already learned two core alcohol use schemas of the larger culture, namely, that alcohol consumption is age graded (alcohol use is acceptable for adults but not for children) and also is sex typed (use is more common for adult males than for adult females) (Noll, Zucker, & Greenberg, 1990; Zucker, Kincaid, Fitzgerald, & Bingham, 1995). Noll et al. (1990) also established that the knowledge of alcoholic beverage use patterns is acquired in the home rather than through media exposure. Zucker et al. (1995) later showed this effect is heightened among high-risk families by virtue of a resident alcoholic parent; children of alcoholic parents were better than children of nonalcoholic parents in correctly identifying specific alcoholic beverages. Also, the extent to which children attributed alcohol use to common life situations (picnics, family meals, school lunch, adult parties) was predicted by their parents' level of alcohol consumption. In short, children's alcohol schemas relating to both knowledge and use were more sophisticated in the families with an alcoholic parent and were more salient in families where the drinking was more common and therefore more visible.

Gene–Environment Interplay

The foregoing not only illustrates the importance of both genetic and environmental influences on the development of AUD but also indicates that the underlying mechanisms of risk are a function of gene–environment interplay rather than simply main effects of genes and environments. Two mechanisms of gene–environment interplay are gene–environment correlation and gene × environment interaction. Gene–environment correlation refers to the nonindependence between a person's genotype and the likelihood of exposure to environmental risk, such that those with higher genetic risk also tend to experience greater environmental risk exposure (Scarr & McCartney, 1983). Passive gene–environment correlations arise from parents providing both the genes and the rearing environments. The Buu et al. (2009) study finding that parental AUD was associated with residence in disadvantaged neighborhoods, which in turn increased risk for negative outcomes in offspring, is an example of such a passive gene–environment correlation.

As children transition into adolescence and gain greater autonomy in selecting their environments, active gene–environment correlations become more relevant mechanisms to the development of substance use and abuse, which also emerge during the same period (Bergen et al., 2007; Scarr & McCartney, 1983). Active gene–environment correlations primarily arise because heritable individual differences increase exposure to trait-congruent environments that then increase risk for substance use disorders. Hicks et al. (2013) used a longitudinal-twin design to

delineate active gene–environment correlation processes over time, between the nonspecific risk (under)socialization trait at age 11, an environmental risk composite at age 14, and a composite of substance use disorders at age 17 involving alcohol, nicotine, and marijuana disorders. Low socialization predicted substance use disorders at age 17 but was also strongly correlated with environmental risk at age 14. Moreover, low socialization at age 11 predicted greater environmental risk at age 14, even after controlling for the stability of environmental risk from ages 11 to 14. In turn, environmental risk at age 14 mediated some—but not all—of the effect of low socialization at age 11 on substance use disorders at age 17. In fact, 78 % of the genetic correlation between childhood socialization and adolescent substance use disorders was mediated by environmental risk at age 14. That is, to the extent that (under)socialization accounts for heritable risk in substance use disorders, the mechanism is indirect, via increased exposure to high-risk environments.

Gene × environment interactions have also been documented for alcohol use and AUD and again emphasize that the importance of + genetic influences on alcohol use outcomes varies as a function of the environmental context. For example, in a Finnish study, Dick, Rose, Viken, Kaprio, and Koskenvuo (2001) demonstrated gene × environment interactions for areas with more young adults (more role modeling), greater social mobility, and higher regional alcohol sales, all of which encouraged a greater expression of genetic disposition to heavier use. Other investigators have found that genetic influences on alcohol initiation and alcohol use were weaker for adolescents who were highly religious (Koopmans, Slutske, van Baal, & Boomsma, 1999) and for women who were married (Heath, Jardine, & Martin, 1989), respectively. A common thread that may be operating across these environments is one of the greater social controls, such that more constrained environments depress the influence of genetic factors. Such an effect is not limited to alcohol; for example, genetic influences on smoking are attenuated in the context of high parental monitoring (Dick et al., 2007). A comprehensive test of this hypothesis was carried out by examining the impact of six different environmental variables on the genetic influences of a composite of externalizing disorders in late adolescence (Hicks et al., 2009). For each environmental variable, genetic influences on externalizing were greatest in the context of greater environmental adversity. These findings are consistent with a general mechanism of gene–environment interplay for externalizing disorders, such that those with the greatest genetic risk were the mostly likely both to be exposed to environmental risk (gene–environment correlation) and to be most sensitive to the influences of environmental risk factors (gene×environment interaction).

Neurobiology of Addiction

AUD and problems of undercontrol more generally are associated with a number of neurocognitive deficits (Oscar-Berman, 2000). While prolonged substance use—especially chronic and heavy alcohol use—has neurotoxic effects, some neurocognitive deficits, most notably those involving deficits in control and inhibition, are present in those at high risk for substance use disorders even before symptoms are present and thus are indicative of an etiological role rather than a consequence of use (Corral, Holguin, & Cadaveira, 2003; Tarter et al., 2003). The neural underpinnings of these deficits involve regions of the brain that regulate the incentive motivation and effortful control networks (Bechara, 2005; Kalivas & Volkow, 2005; Robinson & Berridge, 2003; Wiers et al., 2007; Zucker et al., 2011). These systems are interconnected and exist in a dynamic tension such that an imbalance between the two provides a model for addictive behavior.

The incentive motivation network is responsible for scanning the environment for the anticipation of reward and detection of potential danger (Berridge & Robinson, 2008; Kalivas & Volkow, 2005). The network centrally involves the anterior cingulate cortex, as well as other structures including the ventral striatum, nucleus accumbens, and ventral tegmental area that are major dopaminergic or reward structures of the brain.

The processes of the incentive motivation network are relatively automatic in that they do not require higher order mental resources and operate rapidly. It is sensitive to novelty and incentive cues that signal potential near-term reward or loss, orientating the organism by interrupting ongoing behavior. The incentive motivation network is distinct from the more basic appetitive systems that underlie motivations and emotions such as hunger or fear, which are sensitive to actual reward or loss rather than cues that signal their potential. The system orientates the organism to the incentive stimulus by inducing high arousal or excitement rather than by inhibiting previous behavior, while also activating attentional resources to the novel stimulus. The basic appetitive systems are sensitive to the psychopharmacological effects of drugs including addiction following drug ingestion. In contrast, the incentive motivation network becomes excessively activated following repeated failures to obtain the drug; thus, it is a liability marker for drug problems.

The incentive motivation network is functionally integrated with other brain structures that collectively constitute the effortful control network, notably the dorsolateral and orbitofrontal prefrontal cortex and inferior frontal gyrus (Miller & Cohen, 2001). Functionally, the effortful control network uses the information obtained from the incentive motivation network to guide responses, often by modifying an ongoing behavioral set. Effortful control involves the ability to regulate behavior to fit contextual demands and maintain a goal set by way of forming mental representations of a distal goal via working memory processes rather than by immediate incentives and cues. Effortful control likely reflects both activation in prefrontal cortical regions and suppression of activation in limbic regions, particularly the ventral striatum-nucleus accumbens structures.

Heuristically, the incentive motivation network can be thought of as a "bottom-up" process, while the effortful control network functions via "top-down" processes. As such the two systems are in dynamic tension to generate and modulate behavior (Zucker et al., 2011). An imbalance in activation between the two systems then leads to the loss of control of drug use and addictive behavior. For example, especially strong activation of incentive motivation processes can overcome the inhibiting processes of the effortful control network. Alternatively, weak control processes will fail to inhibit or modulate even relatively modest incentive motivation drives. When modulation of incentive drives fails, undercontrolled behavior occurs and the individual goes forward with behavior despite a signal of potential problems (Heitzeg, Nigg, Yau, Zubieta, & Zucker, 2008). Ultimately, the extent to which drug (or other) cues provide greater activation of the incentive motivation network with relatively less activation of the effortful control network, an individual has less control over drug use behavior.

Developmentally, the reason adolescence is a period of high risk for substance use and abuse may be because maturation (or at least levels of activation) of the incentive motivation network outpaces that of the effortful control network (Spear, 2000). Limbic and striatal systems are relatively mature and responsive to cues, biasing behavior during adolescence. Thus, adolescents are especially sensitive to rewards and engage in high levels of exploratory and risk-taking behaviors, increasing risk for substance use and abuse. In contrast, areas such as the dorsolateral prefrontal cortex are some of the last brain regions to mature, contributing to the tendency to act impulsively and fail to delay gratification, appropriately modulate emotional reactivity, and consider the consequences of risky behavior. As prefrontal structures mature, nonspecific substance use and externalizing behavior decline, and substance-specific processes become more determinative in the persistence of problematic substance use.

Summary and Conclusion

Why some people lack the ability to moderate their intake of alcohol to the point that their use is compulsive and disrupts their ability to meet major life roles and responsibilities remains a complex question, but one where substantial progress has been made in finding an answer. AUD is an endpoint that will always be preceded by the initiation of alcohol use and regular drinking and that will only manifest after a period of heavy use. These are discrete mileposts, objectively assessed, and they occur relatively late in psychosocial development, all of which are advantages in identifying risk factors, developmental sequencing, contextual triggers and moderators, and causal structure. Much of the risk in childhood is nonspecific and is primarily the consequence of a broad and highly heritable behavioral disinhibition liability that increases risk not just for AUD, but for a spectrum of externalizing phenotypes including other substance use disorders, antisocial behavior, and disinhibited personality traits.

The behavioral disinhibition liability is expressed as several developmentally intermediate phenotypes prior to full-blown AUD in adulthood. At the personality level, early in life, it involves the trait of (under)socialization. At the behavioral level, its extreme phenotypic manifestation is in the form of the disruptive behavior disorders of childhood. In adolescence, the phenotype continues to involve disruptive behavior and rule breaking, but it also involves precocious substance use, usually including other drugs in addition to alcohol.

This liability also has a contextual parallel involving heightened exposure to conflictful and socially disorganized environments, which in turn provide poorer parental monitoring and a greater probability of parental abuse. Some of this elevated exposure is a direct outcome of niche seeking by individuals high in behavioral disinhibition. It also occurs as a result of passive, correlated environment effects which create a higher probability of exposure to the exacerbating environmental circumstances. We have elsewhere referred to this interconnected and overdetermined risk matrix as a "nesting structure" (Zucker et al., 2006), which changes the process model because the variable network is more likely to produce overlearning and coalescence of a risky behavioral repertoire.

At the neurobiological level, these disorders are largely a function of two interconnected brain systems, one of effortful control (primarily localized in the prefrontal cortex) and the other involving incentive motivation (localized in the subcortical reward systems of the brain). These systems mature at different rates, and their imbalance in adolescence, as well as major changes in arousal regulation that occur during this interval, likely accounts for much of the dramatic increase in substance use and abuse in adolescence and young adulthood (Windle et al., 2008). The extent to which preadolescent differences in strength of these systems also play a role in creating individual differences in susceptibility to drug involvement remains unknown, but it is an issue of major interest to the research community at this time.

The generalized risk conferred by behavioral disinhibition and early environmental risk eventually gives way to substance-specific risk factors as people begin to specialize in their substance use and exhibit long-term problematic use. Though behavioral disinhibition is a core, early emerging pathway to AUD, the adult manifestations of the disorder are etiologically heterogeneous. Developmental specifiers of onset and persistence of AUD are helpful in identifying distinct etiological groups, with adolescent onset and persistent course past young adulthood indicative of severe psychopathology. Desistence, however, has substantial ameliorative effects, providing for recovery after even relatively severe substance abuse. Some of the correlates of desistence are known (e.g., marriage, parenthood, treatment), but the underlying mechanisms of effect require elaboration.

It is also instructive to note that when examining AUD as it occurs across the population, a substantial proportion of AUD individuals exhibit a "developmentally limited" form of the disorder (Zucker, 2006), where return to normative levels of use takes place without the assistance of treatment. At the same time, another subset of those moving into diagnosis in adolescence/early adulthood will remain involved in recurring and severe alcohol abuse throughout the life span and will leave a trail of personal and collateral damage that creates tragedy at the individual level and is responsible for major social and health costs at the societal level. For this subset, a return to moderate levels of consumption is not an option; the disorder needs to be regarded as a chronic and recurring disease, requiring monitoring and periodic intervention thereafter (McLellan, Lewis, O'Brien, & Kleber, 2000). The ability to identify these different developmental trajectories prior to the onset of first diagnosis is an essential task, which will bring the ultimate practicality of developmental science into the clinic and the community. Such work is currently under way, but still in its infancy (see NIAAA, 2011).

References

Appleyard, K., Egeland, B., van Dulmen, M. H. M., & Sroufe, L. A. (2005). When more is not better: The role of cumulative risk in child behavior outcomes. *Journal of Child Psychology and Psychiatry, 46*, 235–245.

Armstrong, T. D., & Costello, E. J. (2002). Community studies on adolescent substance use, abuse, or dependence and psychiatric comorbidity. *Journal of Consulting and Clinical Psychology, 70*, 1224–1239.

Babor, T. F. (1996). The classification of alcoholics: Typology theories from the 19th century to the present. *Alcohol Health and Research World, 20*, 6–14.

Bechara, A. (2005). Decision making, impulse control, and loss of willpower to resist drugs: A neurocognitive perspective. *Nature Neuroscience, 8*, 1458–1463.

Bergen, S. E., Gardner, C. O., & Kendler, K. S. (2007). Age-related changes in heritability of behavioral phenotypes over adolescence and young adulthood: A meta-analysis. *Twin Research and Human Genetics, 10*, 423–433.

Berridge, K. C., & Robinson, T. E. (2008). What is the role of dopamine in reward: Hedonic impact, reward learning, or incentive salience? *Brain Research Reviews, 28*, 309–369.

Borges, G., Ye, Y., Bond, J., Cherpitel, C. J., Cremonte, M., Moskalewicz, J., et al. (2010). The dimensionality of alcohol use disorders and alcohol consumption in a cross-national perspective. *Addiction, 105*, 240–254.

Button, T. M. M., Hewitt, J. K., Rhee, S. H., Young, S. E., Corley, R. P., & Stallings, M. C. (2006). Examination of the causes of covariation between conduct disorder symptoms and vulnerability to drug dependence. *Twin Research and Human Genetics, 9*, 38–45.

Buu, A., DiPiazza, C., Wang, J., Puttler, L. I., Fitzgerald, H. E., & Zucker, R. A. (2009). Parent, family, and neighborhood effects on the development of child substance use and other psychopathology from preschool to the start of adulthood. *Journal of Studies on Alcohol and Drugs, 70*, 489–498.

Buu, A., Mansour, M. A., Wang, J., Reifor, S. K., Fitzgerald, H. E., & Zucker, R. A. (2007). Alcoholism effects on social migration and neighborhood effects on alcoholism over the course of 12 years. *Alcoholism, Clinical and Experimental Research, 31*, 1545–1551.

Carpenter, W. B. (1850). *On the use and abuse of alcoholic liquors in health and disease*. Philadelphia: Lea and Blanchard.

Caspi, A., Moffitt, T. E., Newman, D. L., & Silva, P. A. (1996). Behavioral observations at age 3 years predict adult psychiatric disorders: Longitudinal evidence from a birth cohort. *Archives of General Psychiatry, 53*, 1033–1039.

Chassin, L., Pitts, S. C., DeLucia, C., & Todd, M. (1999). A longitudinal study of children of alcoholics: Predicting young adult substance use disorders, anxiety, and depression. *Journal of Abnormal Psychology, 108*, 106–119.

Compton, W. M., Thomas, Y. F., Stinson, F. S., & Grant, B. F. (2007). Prevalence, correlates, disability, and comorbidity of DSM-IV drug abuse and dependence in the United States: Results from the national epidemiologic survey on alcohol and related conditions. *Archives of General Psychiatry, 64*, 566–576.

Corral, M. M., Holguin, S. R., & Cadaveira, F. (2003). Neuropsychological characteristics of young children from high-density alcoholism families: A three year follow-up. *Journal of Studies on Alcohol, 64*, 1995–1999.

Costello, E. J., Erkanli, A., Federman, E., & Angold, A. (1999). Development of psychiatric comorbidity with substance abuse in adolescents: Effects of timing and sex. *Journal of Clinical Child Psychology, 28*, 298–311.

Dick, D. M., Latendresse, S. J., Lansford, J. E., Budde, J. P., Goate, A., Dodge, K. A., et al. (2009). Role of GABRA2 in trajectories of externalizing behavior across development and evidence of moderation by parental monitoring. *Archives of General Psychiatry, 66*, 649–657.

Dick, D. M., Prescott, C., & McGue, M. (2009). The genetics of substance use and substance use disorders. In Y.-K. Kim (Ed.), *Handbook of behavior genetics* (pp. 433–453). New York: Springer.

Dick, D. M., Rose, R. J., Viken, R. J., Kaprio, J., & Koskenvuo, M. (2001). Exploring gene-environment interactions: Socioregional moderation of alcohol use. *Journal of Abnormal Psychology, 110*, 625–632.

Dick, D. M., Viken, R., Purcell, S., Kaprio, J., Pulkkinen, L., & Rose, R. J. (2007). Parental monitoring moderates the importance of genetic and environmental influences on adolescent smoking. *Journal of Abnormal Psychology, 116*, 213–218.

Goldman, D., Oroszi, G., & Ducci, F. (2005). The genetics of addictions: Uncovering the genes. *Nature Reviews Genetics, 6*, 521–532.

Granic, I., & Patterson, G. R. (2006). Toward a comprehensive model of antisocial development: A dynamic systems approach. *Psychological Review, 113*, 101–131.

Grant, B. F., & Dawson, D. A. (1997). Age at onset of alcohol use and its association with DSM-IV alcohol abuse and dependence: Results from the National Longitudinal Alcohol Epidemiologic Survey. *Journal of Substance Abuse, 9*, 103–110.

Grobin, A. C., Matthews, D. B., Devaud, L. L., & Morrow, A. L. (1998). The role of GABA$_A$ receptors in the acute and chronic effects of ethanol. *Psychopharmacology, 139*, 2–19.

Hasin, D. S., Stinson, F. S., Ogburn, E., & Grant, B. F. (2007). Prevalence, correlates, disability, and comorbidity of comorbidity of DSM-IV alcohol abuse and dependence in the United States. *Archives of General Psychiatry, 64*, 830–842.

Hawkins, J. D., Catalano, R. F., & Miller, J. Y. (1992). Risk and protective factors for alcohol and other drug problems in adolescence and early adulthood: Implications for substance abuse prevention. *Psychological Bulletin, 112*, 64–105.

Heath, A. C., Jardine, R., & Martin, N. G. (1989). Interactive effects of genotype and social-environment on alcohol-consumption in female twins. *Journal of Studies on Alcohol, 50*, 38–48.

Heitzeg, M. M., Nigg, J. T., Yau, W. Y., Zubieta, J. K., & Zucker, R. A. (2008). Affective circuitry and risk for alcoholism in late adolescence: Differences in fronto-striatal responses between vulnerable and resilient children of alcoholic parents. *Alcoholism, Clinical and Experimental Research, 32*, 414–426.

Hicks, B. M., Iacono, W. G., & McGue, M. (2014). Identifying personality traits that underlie childhood risk for substance use disorders: Socialization and boldness. *Development and Psychopathology, 26*, 141–157.

Hicks, B. M., Johnson, W., Durbin, C. E., Blonigen, D. M., Iacono, W. G., & McGue, M. (2013). Gene-environment correlation in the development of adolescent substance abuse: Selection effects of child personality and mediation via contextual risk factors. *Development and Psychopathology, 25*(1), 119–32.

Hicks, B. M., South, S. C., DiRago, A. C., Iacono, W. G., & McGue, M. (2009). Environmental adversity and increasing genetic risk for externalizing disorders. *Archives of General Psychiatry, 66*, 640–648.

Higuchi, S., Matsushita, S., Imazeki, H., Kinoshita, T., Takagi, S., & Kono, H. (1994). Aldehyde dehydrogenase genotypes in Japanese alcoholics. *Lancet, 343*, 741–742.

Hussong, A. M., Jones, D. J., Stein, G. L., Baucom, D. H., & Boeding, S. (2011). An internalizing pathway to alcohol use and disorder. *Psychology of Addictive Behaviors, 25*, 390–404.

Iacono, W. G., Malone, S. M., & McGue, M. (2008). Behavioral disinhibition and the development of early-onset addiction: Common and specific influences. *Annual Review of Clinical Psychology, 4*, 12.1–12.24.

Iacono, W. G., McGue, M., & Krueger, R. F. (2006). Minnesota Center for Twin and Family Research. *Twin Research and Human Genetics, 9*, 978–984.

Irons, D. E., McGue, M., Iacono, W. G., & Oetting, W. S. (2007). Mendelian randomization: A novel test of the gateway hypothesis and models of gene-environment interplay. *Development and Psychopathology, 19*, 1181–1195.

Jessor, R., & Jessor, S. L. (1977). *Problem behavior and psychosocial development: A longitudinal study of youth.* New York: Academic.

Kalivas, P. W., & Volkow, N. D. (2005). The neural basis of addiction: A pathology of motivation and choice. *American Journal of Psychiatry, 162,* 1403–1413.

Kaplow, J. B., Curran, P. J., Angold, A., & Costello, E. J. (2001). The prospective relation between dimensions of anxiety and the initiation of adolescent alcohol use. *Journal of Clinical Child Psychology, 30,* 316–326.

Kellam, S. G., Brown, C. H., Rubin, B. R., & Ensminger, M. E. (1983). Paths leading to teenage psychiatric symptoms and substance use: Developmental epidemiological studies in Woodlawn. In S. B. Guze, F. J. Earls, & J. E. Barrett (Eds.), *Childhood psychopathology and development* (pp. 17–47). New York: Plenum Press.

Kellam, S. G., Ensminger, M. E., & Simon, M. B. (1980). Mental health in first grade and teenage drug, alcohol, and cigarette use. *Drug and Alcohol Dependence, 5,* 273–304.

Kendler, K. S., Meyers, J., & Prescott, C. A. (2007). Specificity of genetic and environmental risk factors for symptoms of cannabis, cocaine, alcohol, caffeine, and nicotine dependence. *Archives of General Psychiatry, 64,* 1313–1320.

Kendler, K. S., Prescott, C. A., Myers, J., & Neale, M. C. (2003). The structure of genetic and environmental risk for common psychiatric and substance use disorders in men and women. *Archives of General Psychiatry, 60,* 929–937.

Koopmans, J. R., Slutske, W. S., van Baal, G. C. M., & Boomsma, D. I. (1999). The influence of religion on alcohol use initiation: Evidence for genotype x environment interaction. *Behavior Genetics, 29,* 445–453.

Krueger, R. F., Caspi, A., Moffitt, T. E., Silva, P. A., & McGee, R. (1996). Personality traits are differentially linked to mental disorders: A multitrait-multidiagnosis study of an adolescent birth cohort. *Journal of Abnormal Psychology, 105,* 299–312.

Krueger, R. F., Hicks, B. M., Patrick, C. J., Carlson, S. R., McGue, M., & Iacono, W. G. (2002). Etiological relationships among substance dependence, antisocial behavior, and personality: Modeling the externalizing spectrum. *Journal of Abnormal Psychology, 111,* 411–424.

Krueger, R. F., & Markon, K. E. (2006). Reinterpreting comorbidity: A model-based approach to understanding and classifying psychopathology. *Annual Review of Clinical Psychology, 2,* 111–133.

Leggio, L., Kenna, G. A., Fenton, M., Bonefant, E., & Swift, R. M. (2009). Typologies of alcohol dependence: From Jellinek to genetics and beyond. *Neuropsychological Review, 19,* 115–129.

Maggs, J. L., & Schulenberg, J. E. (2005). Initiation and course of alcohol consumption among adolescents and young adults. *Recent Developments in Alcoholism, 17,* 29–47.

Masse, L. C., & Tremblay, R. E. (1997). Behavior of boys in kindergarten and the onset of substance use during adolescence. *Archives of General Psychiatry, 54,* 62–68.

McGue, M., Iacono, W. G., & Krueger, R. R. (2006). The association of early adolescent problem behavior and adult psychopathology: A multivariate behavioral genetic perspective. *Behavior Genetics, 36,* 591–602.

McGue, M., Iacono, W. G., Legrand, L. N., Malone, S., & Elkins, I. (2001). Origins and consequences of age at first drink. I. Associations with substance use disorders, disinhibitory behaviors and psychopathology, and P3 amplitude. *Alcoholism, Clinical and Experimental Research, 25,* 1156–1165.

McLellan, A. T., Lewis, D. C., O'Brien, C. P., & Kleber, H. D. (2000). Drug dependence, a chronic medical illness: Implications for treatment, insurance, and outcomes evaluation. *Journal of the American Medical Association, 284,* 1689–1695.

Miller, E. K., & Cohen, J. D. (2001). An integrative theory of prefrontal cortex function. *Annual Review of Neuroscience, 24,* 167–202.

National Institute on Alcohol Abuse and Alcoholism (NIAAA). (2011). *Alcohol screening and brief intervention for youth: A practitioner's guide.* Rockville, MD: Dept Health Human Services.

Noll, R. B., Zucker, R. A., & Greenberg, G. S. (1990). Identification of alcohol by smell among preschoolers: Evidence for early socialization about drugs occurring in the home. *Child Development, 61,* 1520–1527.

Oscar-Berman, M. (2000). Neuropsychological vulnerabilities in chronic alcoholism. In: Noronha, A., Eckardt, M., Warren, K. (Eds.), *Review of NIAAA's neuroscience and behavioral research portfolio* (NIAAA Research Monograph No. 34, pp. 437–471). Bethesda, MD: US Department of Health and Human Services.

Puttler, L. I., Zucker, R. A., Fitzgerald, H. E., & Bingham, C. R. (1998). Behavioral outcomes among children of alcoholics during the early and middle childhood years: Familial subtype variations. *Alcoholism, Clinical and Experimental Research, 22,* 1962–1972.

Reich, T. R., Cloninger, C. R., Van eerdewegh, P., Rice, J. P., & Mullaney, J. (1988). Secular trends in the familial transmission of alcoholism. *Alcoholism, Clinical and Experimental Research, 12,* 458–464.

Robinson, T. E., & Berridge, K. C. (2003). Addiction. *Annual Review of Psychology, 54,* 25–53.

Scarr, S., & McCartney, K. (1983). How people make their own environments: A theory of genotype greater then environment effects. *Child Development, 54,* 424–435.

Schumann, G., et al. (2011). Genome-wide association and genetic functional studies identify autism susceptibility candidate 2 gene (AUTS2) in the regulation of alcohol consumption. *Proceedings of the National Academy of Sciences, 108,* 7119–7124.

Slutske, W. S., Heath, A. C., Dinwiddie, S. H., Madden, P. A. F., Bucholz, K. K., Dunne, M. P., et al. (1998). Common genetic risk factors for conduct disorder and alcohol dependence. *Journal of Abnormal Psychology, 107,* 363–374.

Spear, L. P. (2000). The adolescent brain and age-related behavioral manifestations. *Neuroscience and Biobehavioral Reviews, 24*, 417–463.

Tarter, R. E., Kirisci, L., Mezzich, A., Cornelius, J. R., Pajer, K., Vanyukov, M., et al. (2003). Neurobehavioral disinhibition in childhood predicts early onset of substance use disorder. *American Journal of Psychiatry, 160*, 1078–1085.

Treutlein, J., Cichon, S., Ridinger, M., Wodarz, N., Soyka, M., Zill, P., et al. (2009). Genome-wide association study of alcohol dependence. *Archives of General Psychiatry, 66*, 773–784.

True, W. R., Xian, H., Scherrer, J. F., Madden, P. A., Bucholz, K. K., Heath, A. C., et al. (1999). Common genetic vulnerability for nicotine and alcohol dependence in men. *Archives of General Psychiatry, 56*, 655–661.

Vrieze, S. I., Hicks, B. M., Iacono, W. G., & McGue, M. (2012). Common genetic influences on alcohol, marijuana, and nicotine dependence symptoms declines from age 14 to 29. *American Journal of Psychiatry, 169*, 1073–1081.

Wiers, R. W., Bartholow, B. D., van den Wildenberg, E., Thush, C., Engels, R. C., Sher, K. J., et al. (2007). Automatic and controlled processes and the development of addictive behaviors in adolescents: A review. *Pharmacology, Biochemistry, and Behavior, 86*, 263–283.

Windle, M., Spear, L. P., Fuligni, A. J., Angold, A., Brown, J. D., Pine, D., et al. (2008). Transitions into underage and problem drinking: Developmental processes and mechanisms between 10 and 15 years of age. *Pediatrics, 121*(Suppl. 4), S273–S289.

Zucker, R. A. (1998). Developmental aspects of aging, alcohol involvement, and their inter-relationship. In E. S. L. Gomberg, A. M. Hegedus, & R. A. Zucker (Eds.), *Alcohol problems and aging* (NIAAA Research Monograph No. 26, pp. 255–289). Rockville, MD: U.S. Department of Health and Human Services.

Zucker, R. A. (2006). Alcohol use and the alcohol use disorders: A developmental-biopsychosocial systems formulation covering the life course. In D. Cicchetti, D. J. Cohen (Eds.), *Developmental psychopathology, vol. 3: Risk, disorder, and adaption* (2nd ed., pp. 620–656). New York: Wiley.

Zucker, R. A., Fitzgerald, H. E., Refior, S. K., Puttler, L. I., Pallas, D. M., & Ellis, D. A. (2000). The clinical and social ecology of childhood for children of alcoholics: Description of a study and implications for a differentiated social policy. In H. E. Fitzgerald, B. B. Lester, & B. S. Zuckerman (Eds.), *Children of addiction: Research, health, and policy issues* (pp. 1–30). New York: Garland Press.

Zucker, R. A., Heitzeg, M. M., & Nigg, J. T. (2011). Parsing the undercontrol-disinhibition pathway to substance use disorders: A multilevel developmental problem. *Child Development Perspectives, 5*(4), 246–255.

Zucker, R. A., Kincaid, S. B., Fitzgerald, H. E., & Bingham, C. R. (1995). Alcohol schema acquisition in preschoolers: Differences between children of alcoholics and children of non-alcoholics. *Alcoholism, Clinical and Experimental Research, 19*, 1011–1017.

John Schulenberg, Megan E. Patrick,
Julie Maslowsky, and Jennifer L. Maggs

The Epidemiology and Etiology of Adolescent Substance Use in Developmental Perspective

It is no surprise that substance use typically begins and escalates during adolescence. If there were a time in the life span that was "built" for substance use onset and escalation, it would certainly be adolescence. Individual and contextual changes are more pervasive and rapid during adolescence than during any other time of life. Infants experience more rapid physical and cognitive changes than do adolescents, but whereas infants are blissfully unaware of the rapid changes, adolescents are often acutely aware of the changes happening in their bodies, minds, and social worlds. Amidst these ubiquitous developmental changes, it is no coincidence that interest in and opportunity for alcohol and other drug use begins for most young people

J. Schulenberg, Ph.D. (✉) • M.E. Patrick, Ph.D.
Institute for Social Research, University of Michigan,
Ann Arbor, MI 48106, USA
e-mail: schulenb@umich.edu

J. Maslowsky, Ph.D.
Health Behavior and Health Education, Department
of Kinesiology and Health Education, The University
of Texas at Austin, Austin, TX 78712, USA

J.L. Maggs, Ph.D.
Human Development and Family Studies,
The Pennsylvania State University,
University Park, PA 16802, USA

(Masten, Faden, Zucker, & Spear, 2008; Schulenberg, Maggs, & Hurrelmann, 1997). Although alcohol and drug use are not without significant risks, experimentation can also serve numerous perceived positive functions during adolescence. It can provide a quick way to cope and blow off steam, indicate autonomy from parents, facilitate shared experiences and social integration with peers, and represent exploration of new sensations, experiences, and tastes of some perceived fruits of adulthood (Crosnoe, 2011; Maggs, Almeida, & Galambos, 1995). Indeed, as Baumrind (1987) concluded when considering the overwhelming array of substance use correlates, it is instructive to ponder why some adolescents refrain from initiating alcohol and other drug use.

Our purpose in this chapter is to provide a selective summary and integration of conceptualizations and empirical results regarding the epidemiology and etiology of substance use during adolescence from a developmental perspective. As illustrated by our own work, we believe that epidemiology and etiology can and should go hand in hand, together offering a more comprehensive and holistic picture of the development of adolescent substance use. There have been several recent excellent literature reviews and integrations of the multiple risk factors and developmental mechanisms of adolescent alcohol and other drug use (e.g., Brown et al., 2008, 2009; Chassin, Hussong, & Beltran, 2009; Dodge et al., 2009; Windle et al., 2008; Zucker, Donovan, Masten, Mattson, & Moss, 2008). We build on these reviews by offering integrative overviews of concepts and illustrative findings. We first frame the issues by summarizing the prevalence of use of various substances during adolescence, offering a needed historical perspective. We then consider key developmental concepts as they relate to the understanding of substance use during adolescence. Next we summarize the wide range of risk and protective factors for substance use. We conclude with implications for future research.

Adolescent Substance Use: Reasons to Worry

Substance use during adolescence is associated with numerous acute and long-term health and social effects (National Institute on Drug Abuse, 2012) and countless personal and family tragedies. Alcohol-related fatalities are responsible for the deaths of about 5,000 adolescents under the age of 21 each year due to preventable events including motor vehicle crashes, homicides, suicides, and other accidents and injuries (Hingson & Kenkel, 2004). Substance use during adolescence is also a predictor of substance-related problems and other negative health and social consequences in adulthood (Grant et al., 2004; Gunzerath, Faden, Zakhari, & Warren, 2004; Schulenberg, Maggs, & O'Malley, 2003).

The NIDA-funded Monitoring the Future (MTF) study has been collecting US nationally representative data annually from 12th graders since 1975 and from 8th and 10th graders since 1991 (Johnston, O'Malley, Bachman, & Schulenberg, 2012) and is a primary source of historical and developmental trends in substance use among American adolescents. Important strengths of epidemiological studies such as MTF include their careful attention to the representativeness of samples and consistency of methods over time, providing the basis for accurate characterization of a given problem. They can provide needed information of the broader cultural context, the macrosystem and chronosystem in Bronfenbrenner's human ecology framework (1979), in which the developing adolescent is embedded. We summarize national rates and trends of substance use, giving attention to sociodemographic variation.

Prevalence

Based on the 2011 MTF data from 8th, 10th, and 12th graders, 16 %, 35 %, and 46 %, respectively, reported using marijuana at least once in their lifetime. Corresponding rates for lifetime use of an illicit drug other than marijuana were 10 %, 16 %, and 25 %, respectively. As expected, rates of alcohol use were higher than rates of illicit drug use: Rates of lifetime alcohol use were 33 %, 56 %, and 70 % across the three grades, respectively, and corresponding rates of lifetime drunkenness were 15 %, 36 %, and 51 %. Rates of lifetime cigarette use were 18 %, 30 %, and 40 %, respectively, across the three grades. Two apparent facts are worth highlighting: (1) There is a clear developmental gradient to substance use onset across adolescence and (2) especially among 8th and 10th graders, the large majority of current US youth typically avoid substance use, and even by 12th grade, most have not tried cigarettes or an illicit drug other than marijuana (Johnston et al., 2012). That is, drug use onset increases across adolescence, but even by 12th grade, most adolescents are now avoiding cigarette and illicit drug use (a comment that does not apply to all of the recent past, as illustrated below).

When we consider heavier and more frequent substance use, rates are lower but the same developmental gradient is clear. In 2011, across the three grade levels, respectively, 30-day rates were as follows: 7 %, 18 %, and 23 % reported any marijuana use; 3 %, 5 %, and 9 % reported any illicit drug use other than marijuana; 13 %, 27 %, and 40 % reported any alcohol use; 4 %, 14 %, and 25 % reported any drunkenness; and 6 %, 12 %, and 19 % reported any cigarette use (Johnston et al., 2012). In terms of binge drinking (defined here as having 5 or more drinks in a row in the past 2 weeks), 2011 rates were 6 %, 15 %, and 22 % across the three grade levels, respectively.

In Historical and International Perspective

At the population level, adolescent substance use is best viewed as a moving target, and compared to the recent past, the 2011 rates reflect salutary movement. In considering the past two decades, illicit drug, alcohol, and cigarette use generally peaked in the middle to the late 1990s. The lifetime rates for marijuana use in 1997, a peak year, were 23 %, 42 %, and 50 %, and rates for illicit drug use other than marijuana were 18 %, 25 %, and 30 %, respectively, across 8th, 10th, and 12th graders; these 1997 rates are significantly higher than all the corresponding 2011 rates, particularly for 8th and 10th graders (Johnston et al., 2012). Rates of lifetime alcohol use and drunkenness have also declined over the past two decades, with most of this reduction occurring since 2001. In 1993, a peak year for alcohol use, lifetime rates of alcohol use were 56 %, 72 %, and 80 % and of drunkenness were 26 %, 48 %, and 63 %, respectively, across the three grade levels; all of these 1993 rates are significantly higher than the 2011 rates, especially for 8th and 10th graders. Cigarette use has dropped extensively over the past two decades; lifetime cigarette use peaked in 1996 with rates of 49 %, 61 %, and 64 %, respectively, rates over twice as high as 2011 rates for 8th and 10th graders.

One important question regarding these historical shifts pertains to the causes of such shifts. Attempting to isolate causes of historical change in adolescent substance use, or any given behavior, is complex given the likely multiple influences and the need to distinguish among cohort, period, and age effects. Nonetheless, one consistent precursor to historical changes in alcohol and marijuana use is changes in disapproval of such use (Johnston et al., 2012). In a recent analysis that contrasted age, period (year of measurement), and cohort effects of population-based social norms (based on disapproval) about heavy alcohol use on individual level heavy drinking during adolescence, cohort effects were found to predominate; being part of a birth cohort that was higher on disapproval set the stage for lower alcohol use (Keyes et al., 2012), suggesting the

power of social norms in shaping historical trends in behavior. Other likely substance-specific causes include increases in the cost of cigarettes (Tauras, O'Malley, & Johnston, 2001) and changes in legislation regarding medical use of marijuana (Cerdá, Wall, Keyes, Galea, & Hasin, 2012). More generally, adolescent substance use tends to be cyclical, with epidemics of various drugs (e.g., cocaine, ecstasy, LSD) appearing and receding. Johnston (1991) uses the term "generational forgetting" to describe why rates can increase relatively quickly following a period of low use. Pain and loss resulting from high-profile drug-related tragedies such as celebrity deaths, as well as from local accidents or overdoses, may be forgotten during periods of low use. If society in general, and new generations of youth in particular, stops viewing substance use as dangerous, this absence of caution may allow for use to come roaring back, triggering new tragic experiences, and so on.

Another important question regarding historical shifts is whether declines summarized above in the lifetime rates are also seen in rates of heavier and more frequent use. The answer is yes, that the proportions of decline from recent peaks in the past two decades have been remarkably similar across different frequencies and levels of use (Johnston et al., 2012), suggesting that historical shifts reflect similar changes for experimental and heavier use. Important exceptions pertain to adolescents at the very deep end of substance use. For example, daily marijuana use has shifted little since the late 1990s (as of 2011, rates were 1.3 %, 3.6 %, and 6.6 % across the three grade levels, respectively; Johnston et al., 2012).

A third important question regarding historical shifts is whether they pertain equally well across the different grade levels. In fact, they do not: Although most rates have declined since their recent peaks for all three grade levels, the proportional declines have generally been greater for 8th and 10th graders than 12th graders and greater for 8th graders than 10th graders (Johnston et al., 2012). That is, more adolescents are waiting longer to begin and to escalate their substance use now compared to the mid to late 1990s. Effectively, this means that the developmental

gradient noted above for both onset and continued use is stronger now than in the past. Thus,
compared to peak rates across the past two
decades, current rates of substance use among
US adolescents are all considerably lower, especially for the 8th and 10th graders.

Adolescents in the United States have considerably lower rates of cigarette and alcohol use
compared to European adolescents. Based on a
2011 cross-national survey of 15 and 16 year
olds, US adolescents were at the lowest end of
the distribution (Hibell et al., 2012). However,
rates of marijuana and other illicit drug use were
generally higher among US adolescents compared to European adolescents, with US adolescents typically being near the top of the
distribution. This unique US configuration, compared to the typical European rank-order consistency across substance use measures, likely has
many causes including the large historical decline
of cigarette use among US adolescents only, as
well as the typically higher rates of alcohol use in
many European countries due in part to lower
legal drinking ages.

Thus, the evidence suggests that currently, US
adolescents are better off than previous cohorts
and their contemporaries in Europe in terms of
cigarette and alcohol use and better off than previous US cohorts (though worse off compared to
European contemporaries) in terms of marijuana
and other illicit drugs. Nonetheless, we cannot be
complacent with the facts, for example, that
"only" one in ten 8th graders reports using an
illicit drug other than marijuana (e.g., cocaine,
heroin, hallucinogens) at least once already in
their lifetime, that one in five 10th graders reports
using marijuana at least once in the past month,
or that one in five 12th graders reports having 5
or more drinks in a row at least once in the past
two weeks (Johnston et al., 2012). Furthermore,
despite the overall decline in many substances,
some especially dangerous drugs have not
declined including the misuse of prescription
drugs. Over the past decade, 12th grade annual
rates of misuse (i.e., use not under doctor's
orders) of any prescription drug have remained
steady at about 15 %, and specifically misuse of
narcotics other than heroin (e.g., OxyContin,

Vicodin) has remained steady at about 9 %.
Of special importance, marijuana use has been
increasing again recently especially among 12th
graders (Johnston et al., 2012).

Sociodemographic Variation in Substance Use

Substance use involvement varies considerably
by sociodemographic characteristics, especially
gender, socioeconomic status (SES), and race/
ethnicity. At 12th grade, boys are more likely to
use just about every substance and at higher frequencies than girls (Johnston et al., 2012). But at
8th grade, rates are much more equivalent across
boys and girls, with girls being higher on the use
of some substances, including use of any illicit
drug other than marijuana. Thus, gender differences in substance use emerge and expand across
adolescence, with the increase in substance use
being greater for boys.

In contrast, SES differences tend to shrink
across adolescence. At 8th grade, lower SES
youth have higher rates of almost all substances,
but by 12th grade, there are far fewer SES differences in substance use (Johnston et al., 2012).
Notable exceptions include cigarette, cocaine,
and heroin use, which are still higher among
lower SES youth by 12th grade; in addition,
higher SES youth catch up with and surpass their
lower SES age-mates by 12th grade in terms of
alcohol use and drunkenness. Much of this
reflects developmental timetable variation by
SES: It has long been known that adolescents
from more working class backgrounds tend to
start earlier with risky behaviors including substance use (Ianni, 1998) and then their higher
SES age-mates catch up by the end of high school
(Bachman et al., 2008; Crosnoe, 2011).

In terms of racial/ethnic differences, African
American youth tend to have the lowest rates
of almost all substances and at all frequency/
quantity levels compared to other youth, especially at 12th grade, although differences are
typically evident at the earlier grades as well
(Johnston et al., 2012). Explanations for this
lower use include higher levels of religiosity

(e.g., Wallace et al., 2007). Hispanic youth tend to have the highest lifetime rates of substance use at 8th grade, but by 12th grade, White youth have the highest lifetime usage rates of many illicit drugs including marijuana, as well as of alcohol and cigarettes (Johnston et al., 2012; Wallace et al., 2003). Rates of substance use vary in important ways within these large sociodemographic groups. For example, rates vary significantly among Hispanic subpopulations (Delva et al., 2005). Similarly, when considering SES by race/ethnicity interactions, the SES gradient noted above generally applies more to White youth than to African American and Hispanic youth (Bachman, O'Malley, Johnston, Schulenberg, & Wallace, 2011).

Despite lower prevalence of substance use during adolescence, racial/ethnic minorities, particularly African Americans, tend to experience higher rates of negative consequences of substance use compared to Whites beginning in young adulthood, including higher rates of drug-related criminal justice involvement (Brown, Flory, Lynam, Leukefeld, & Clayton, 2004; National Institute on Drug Abuse, 2003) and psychiatric and substance use disorders (Gil, Wagner, & Tubman, 2004; Reardon & Buka, 2002). Therefore, it is important to consider the potential roots in adolescence of these racial/ethnic disparities in consequences of youth substance use despite relatively lower prevalence of use among some groups.

Developmental Concepts: Foundations for Understanding Substance Use Etiology

At the individual level, adolescent substance use is also best understood as a moving target, embedded within the many other developmental changes happening within young people and their social worlds. Through a series of conceptual papers and chapters, we have elaborated a developmental framework regarding substance use during adolescence and the transition to adulthood concerning continuity and discontinuity, trajectories of behaviors and attitudes, and intraindividual and

social transitions (e.g., Maggs & Schulenberg, 2005a, 2005b; Maggs, Schulenberg, & Hurrelmann, 1997; Patrick & Schulenberg, 2014; Patrick, Schulenberg, Maggs, & Maslowsky, in press; Schulenberg et al., 1997, 2003; Schulenberg & Maggs, 2002; Schulenberg & Maslowsky, 2009; Schulenberg & Patrick, 2012; Schulenberg, Sameroff, & Cicchetti, 2004; Schulenberg & Zarrett, 2006). Our framework, consistent with a broad interdisciplinary developmental science perspective, highlights multilevel and multidirectional changes characterized by mutual selection and accommodation of individuals and their contexts (Cairns, 2000; Elder & Shanahan, 2006; Lerner, 2006; Sameroff, 2010). We view individuals and contexts as playing strong, active roles in the process of development, highlighting the importance of the person–context match, the connection between what the developing individual needs and what the context provides. Individuals select particular contexts and activities based on opportunities and personal characteristics and competencies. Selected contexts then provide additional opportunities—and effectively limit other opportunities represented by contexts not selected—for continued socialization and further selection. This progressive accommodation suggests the qualities of coherence and continuity in development. However, consistent with our emphasis on person–context interactions and multidirectional change, development does not necessarily follow a smooth and progressive function and early experiences do not always have strong or lasting effects (Lewis, 1999; Rutter, 1996). Thus, both continuity and discontinuity are expected across adolescence and the transition to adulthood. In this subsection, we summarize broad-based developmental concepts relevant to understanding the etiology of adolescent substance use including continuity and discontinuity and developmental transitions.

Continuity and Discontinuity

Although the concepts of continuity and discontinuity are central to the understanding of development (Kagan, 1980; Werner, 1957), they are not easily defined. Stability and continuity are sometimes used interchangeably, but the two are typically viewed as distinct among developmental scientists: Stability pertains to the extent to which individuals maintain relative rank ordering over time and continuity pertains to the course of intraindividual trajectories (Lerner, 2006). Two uses of the concepts of continuity and discontinuity are common (Schulenberg et al., 2003; Schulenberg & Zarrett, 2006), and both are relevant to understanding the etiology of substance use.

First, continuity and discontinuity can be considered in terms of causative linkages across the life span (Lewis, 1999; Masten, 2001), termed ontogenetic continuity and discontinuity. Ontogenetic continuity reflects a progressive and individual coherence perspective, in which earlier events and experiences are viewed as formative and essentially causing future outcomes (Caspi, 2000). As would be expected from a development perspective, continuity tends to prevail across life, and what we see in much of adolescent substance use is "the result" of earlier difficulties and family socialization experiences (Dodge et al., 2009; Zucker et al., 2008). But it is not that simple and early functioning does not always determine later functioning (Cicchetti & Rogosch, 2002; Lewis, 1999); instead, the effects of early experiences may be neutralized or reversed by later experiences. This focus on developmentally proximal influences reflects an ontogenetic discontinuity perspective, whereby current functioning is due more to recent and current contexts and experiences than to earlier ones (Schulenberg & Zarrett, 2006). The roots of substance use for some adolescents do not go that far into the past, but rather into current social contexts and individual tasks. The distinction between ontogenetic continuity and discontinuity is important when examining the etiology of substance use. Ongoing childhood difficulties that culminate in substance use likely reflect ontogenetic continuity (e.g., life-course-persistent antisocial behavior; Moffitt & Caspi, 2001); in contrast, a positive developmental trajectory during childhood followed by involvement with substance use in adolescence likely reflects ontogenetic discontinuity (e.g., adolescence-limited antisocial behavior; Moffitt & Caspi, 2001).

Second, continuity and discontinuity can be considered as having both descriptive components (pertaining to manifest behaviors) and explanatory components (pertaining to underlying purposes, functions, and meanings; Kagan, 1980; Lerner, 2006). Homotypic continuity refers to the presence of both descriptive and explanatory continuity whereby both a given behavior (e.g., alcohol use) and the underlying purpose of that behavior (e.g., have fun with friends) remain continuous over time. Heterotypic continuity refers to when behaviors vary across time (descriptive discontinuity) while the underlying purpose or meaning of those varying behaviors remains the same (explanatory continuity). For example, although success in peer relations may be continuous from childhood into adolescence, what it takes to be successful with peers may shift over time and may cross into deviant behaviors during adolescence (Allen, Porter, McFarland, Marsh, & McElhaney, 2005). Functional discontinuity occurs when the manifested behavior appears unchanged yet the underlying function or meaning of that behavior changes over time (i.e., descriptive continuity, explanatory discontinuity). For example, a 14-year-old adolescent may first use marijuana to experiment and fit in with her friends; four years later, she still uses marijuana, but as a means of coping with stress. As we summarize later, we have found in our research such developmental shifts in substance use reasons and behaviors.

Developmental Transitions

The period between the end of childhood and the beginning of adulthood is dense with internally and externally based transitions (Schulenberg et al., 1997). Developmental transitions include transformations in individuals, their contexts, and the relations between individuals and their contexts across the life course (Bronfenbrenner, 1979; Schulenberg & Maggs, 2002). These include both global transitions (e.g., transition to adolescence) and more specific and interlinked intraindividual transitions (e.g., biological, identity-related) and socially based external ones (e.g., parent–child relations, school-related; Rutter, 1996). The power of the interlinked transitions in the individuals' lives, specifically in the course of substance use, can be understood in relation to the concepts of continuity and discontinuity discussed above. Transitions can contribute to ontogenetic discontinuity in ongoing trajectories in several ways, such as by overwhelming coping capacities or worsening the person–context match (Coleman, 1989; Schulenberg & Zarrett, 2006). By providing "shocks to the system," transitions can serve as proximal effects that can counteract developmentally distal effects.

This discontinuity in ongoing trajectories can take the form of turning points or developmental disturbances. Turning points reflect long-term changes in course (Elder & Shanahan, 2006; Rutter, 1996), such as escalating substance use during the transitions to middle and high school (Guo, Collins, Hill, & Hawkins, 2000; Jackson & Schulenberg, 2013), as well as to residential college (Schulenberg & Patrick, 2012; White et al., 2006). Transitions as turning points can also be viewed in terms of heterotypic continuity (descriptive discontinuity/explanatory continuity) and functional discontinuity (descriptive continuity/explanatory discontinuity) whereby the connection between behaviors and underlying purposes or meanings shifts. Entering high school where some forms of drinking become more normative may make alcohol use less a function of deviance and more a function of social integration (Crosnoe, 2011). In contrast to the "permanent change" associated with turning points, developmental disturbances reflect more momentary perturbations (Schulenberg & Zarrett, 2006). Once individuals are given time to adjust, they might resume their prior ongoing trajectory. In such cases, a transition may simply result in short-term deviance (e.g., increased binge drinking, affiliation with a more deviant peer group) and may not have long-term effects on developmental course or predict later functioning in adulthood (Schulenberg et al., 2003). Of course, not all discontinuity reflects maladaptation—for example, a school transition may result in a better person–context match in terms

of appropriate level of challenge and contribute to improved health and well-being.

Although the power of transitions may be more obvious in the case of discontinuity, transitions also contribute to continuity, with transitional experiences serving as proving grounds that help consolidate and strengthen ongoing behavioral and adjustment trajectories for better and worse (Schulenberg & Zarrett, 2006). Individuals tend to rely on intrinsic tendencies and known behavioral and coping repertoires in novel and ambiguous situations (Caspi, 2000; Dannefer, 1987). This accentuation effect suggests that young people already experiencing difficulties may have trouble negotiating new transitions and fall further behind their well-functioning peers; in contrast, those already doing well have the resources to deal successfully with new transitions and climb further ahead of their age-mates having difficulties (e.g., Rudolph & Troop-Gordon, 2010; Schulenberg et al., 2003). Thus, during major transitions such as puberty or the transition into high school, ongoing salutary and deviancy trajectories may become more solidified highlighting the role of transitions in perpetuating ontogenetic continuity.

Risk Factors for Adolescent Substance Use

The list of adolescent risk factors for substance use is extensive connecting to most if not all aspects of adolescent development, a fundamental premise of Problem Behavior Theory (Jessor, 1987). In a 1992 comprehensive review of the literature on risk factors for adolescent substance use, a review that remains quite useful over two decades later, Hawkins, Catalano, and Miller classified the multitude of risk factors into 17 different categories. These included contextual risk factors (e.g., availability of substances, economic deprivation, family conflict), individual risk factors (e.g., academic failure, early onset of problem behaviors), and physiological risk factors including genetic background. A few years later, Petraitis, Flay, and Miller (1995) summarized 14 theoretical models for understanding experimental substance use during adolescence, ranging from sociological theories focusing on more distal socio-structural mechanisms (e.g., an absence of commitments to conventional society) to cognitive-affective theories emphasizing more proximal processes (e.g., decision making) and mechanisms (e.g., substance-specific expectancies). Since then, the list of risk factors and mechanisms has certainly expanded (see, e.g., Brown et al., 2008; Chassin et al., 2009; Dodge et al., 2009; Windle et al., 2008; Zucker et al., 2008). The recognition of these multiple risk factors and mechanisms highlights the probabilistic nature of risk factors (Maggs & Schulenberg, 2005a)—i.e., none is sufficient or necessary for particular outcomes, thus requiring conceptualizations of explanatory processes that focus on the diversity of causal connections (Cairns, 2000). In this subsection, we provide an illustrative overview of common and interconnected risk and protective factors embedded within the multiple tasks and transitions of the second decade of life.

Biological and Physical Changes

Pubertal development during early adolescence is characterized by a rapid acceleration in growth and the development of primary and secondary sex characteristics, and by the end of high school, most adolescents have attained full adult height and reproductive capacity (Susman & Dorn, 2009). These physical and hormonal changes along with societal expectations combine to increase adolescents' interest in and tolerance of alcohol and other psychoactive substances (Spear, 2007). Adolescents who experience earlier pubertal development relative to their peers (i.e., early maturers) are more likely to associate with older and more deviant peers (Downing & Bellis, 2009; Mendle & Ferrero, 2012; Negriff & Trickett, 2012), compounding the effects of early physical transitions with earlier transitions to unsupervised time with peers. Thus, in addition to increasing access to substances, these multiple simultaneous transitions may overload the young person's coping capacity (Coleman, 1989) and

alter the person–context match (Susman & Dorn, 2009), setting the stage for discontinuities in terms of substance use onset. In contrast, through accentuation of pre-transition individual characteristics, early pubertal timing can contribute to continuities in ongoing trajectories of health and well-being (e.g., Rudolph & Troop-Gordon, 2010).

Cognitive and Neurological Changes, Sensation Seeking, and Risk Taking

Across adolescence, important normative transformations in cognitive reasoning abilities occur, including increases in the ability to think abstractly, consider theoretical possibilities, and view issues as relative rather than absolute (Keating, 2004). These changes are increasingly understood to occur in the context of functional and structural changes occurring in the adolescent brain (Blakemore, 2012; Doremus-Fitzwater, Varlinskaya, & Spear, 2010; Sturman & Moghaddam, 2011). As cognition and reasoning mature, adult-defined reality becomes viewed by the adolescent as simply one of many possible perspectives. Adolescents are able to engage in increasingly sophisticated deliberations regarding which behaviors to engage in and why, with specific end goals in mind (Gibbons, Houlihan, & Gerrard, 2009; Maslowsky, Buvinger, Keating, Steinberg, & Cauffman, 2011; Maslowsky, Keating, Monk, & Schulenberg, 2011; Reyna & Farley, 2006). It is often assumed that adolescents engage in higher levels of risk taking because they think they are invincible or invulnerable, able to avoid harm regardless of their own behavior (Elkind, 1967; Romer & Jamieson, 2001). However, research contrasting the decision making of adolescents and adults has generally not supported clear age differences in thoughts of invincibility or in downplaying risks of certain behaviors (Johnson, McCaul, & Klein, 2002). In fact, adolescents engaged in more frequent risk behavior rate their likelihood of negative consequences highest, indicating their appreciation of the relative risks involved in their behavior (Fromme, Katz, & Rivet, 1997).

Additional evidence suggests that adolescents are particularly attuned to the potential benefits of engaging in risky behavior such as substance use. Risky behavior is likely to yield social rewards salient to adolescents such as peer approval (O'Brien, Albert, Chein, & Steinberg, 2011). In addition, neurobiological evidence suggests that the development of rewards systems outpaces that of inhibitory systems during adolescence, leading to an over-prioritization of rewards during this period (Galvan, Hare, Voss, Glover, & Casey, 2007), though not all evidence suggests this mismatch (Crone & Dahl, 2012). Providing both neurophysiological and social rewards, substance use is a clear candidate for a risky behavior that yields sought-after benefits. The power of such benefit-seeking motives is evident in the extensive literature linking sensation seeking and substance use. Sensation seeking, originally defined by Zuckerman (1979) as "the need for varied, novel, and complex sensations and experiences" (p. 10), peaks in adolescence and is a strong predictor of engagement in risky behavior and substance use (Dever et al., 2012; Patrick & Schulenberg, 2010; Steinberg et al., 2008). Growing evidence demonstrates the neurological bases of heightened sensation seeking and reward seeking and their associations with substance use during adolescence (Doremus-Fitzwater et al., 2010).

Clearly, not all adolescent substance use is premeditated or executed in a deliberate search for benefits. Particularly as group-level activities, substance use and associated behaviors may not always represent planned or rationally considered choices. Decisions about how much *more* to drink or use or about whether to engage in other risky behaviors are often made when individuals do not have the benefit of being sober. Theoretically, decision-making models are useful for understanding these choices (Reyna & Farley, 2006). And practically, these choices may make the difference between light/moderate drinking and more harmful binge drinking. Consideration of contemporaneous intra- and interpersonal factors is crucial to understanding the role of new cognitive abilities and architecture in adolescents' onset and escalation of substance use (Crone & Dahl, 2012).

Identity and Motivations for Substance Use

Adolescents experience fundamental changes in their self-definition and identity (Cote, 2009; Erikson, 1968; Marcia, 1994). Although normative and part of healthy development, identity exploration may also represent a risk factor for experimentation with alcohol or other drug use (Maggs et al., 1997; Marcia, 1994). Thus, the role played by experimenting with substances in adolescents' lives can be paradoxical (Maggs et al., 1995): Despite the possibility of serious harm, substance use may serve important constructive functions, including identity exploration (Chassin, Presson, & Sherman, 1989; Jessor, 1987).

Motivations (or reasons) for substance use can provide an important window into the individual "why" of substance use, how it relates to identity exploration, to peer bonding, and to coping with pressure and disappointment. Four main types of substance use motivations—social, enhancement, coping, and conformity—have been differentiated, with research predominantly focusing on alcohol and marijuana use reasons (Bonn-Miller, Zvolensky, & Bernstein, 2007; Cooper, 1994; Simons, Correia, & Carey, 2000). Reasons for alcohol use and marijuana use change developmentally. For instance, 12th grade adolescents tend to be higher on drinking to get drunk (as well as other social and coping reasons for drinking) than young adults, but lower on drinking to relax (Patrick & Schulenberg, 2011). Motivations show important associations with current and future use. For example, an increase in binge drinking from ages 18 to 22 is most strongly correlated with concurrent reasons of using alcohol to get drunk and to relieve boredom; however, a trajectory of continued binge drinking after age 22 is most strongly related to concurrent reason of using alcohol to get away from problems (Patrick & Schulenberg, 2011). This illustrates the notion of functional discontinuity, where binge drinking remains the same but the underlying reason for binge drinking shifts toward a more problematic purpose. Reasons for use reported in 12th grade also show long-term associations with symptoms of alcohol use disorders.

Drinking to get drunk in 12th grade predicts concurrent and future increases in heavy drinking (Schulenberg, Wadsworth, O'Malley, Bachman, & Johnston, 1996) as well as alcohol use disorders at age 35 (Patrick, Schulenberg, O'Malley, Johnston, & Bachman, 2011). In contrast, peer conformity reasons for use tend to be less predictive of future alcohol use (Patrick et al., 2011), suggesting that this "why" of alcohol use has more to do with ephemeral peer connections than with the individual experience of alcohol use— i.e., a less solid connection with identity.

Externalizing Behaviors and Internalizing Symptoms

Childhood and adolescent mental health and behavioral problems, particularly externalizing behaviors and internalizing symptoms, show clear associations with adolescent substance use (Dodge et al., 2009; Zucker et al., 2008). Externalizing behaviors, like theft, property destruction, and aggression that violate social or legal norms (Hinshaw, 1987), have a strong, positive association with alcohol, cigarette, and marijuana use during adolescence (Brook, Zhang, & Brook, 2011; Ellickson, Tucker, Klein, & McGuigan, 2001; Maslowsky & Schulenberg, 2013; Reboussin, Hubbard, & Ialongo, 2007).

Empirical evidence regarding the association of internalizing symptoms (depressive symptoms, anxiety, related constructs such as self-derogation) and substance use during adolescence is inconsistent. Particularly with regard to depressive symptoms, studies have found negative, positive, and null relations to substance use during adolescence (Dodge et al., 2009; Goodman & Capitman, 2000; McCaffery, Papandonatos, Stanton, Lloyd-Richardson, & Niaura, 2008). Notably, while the main effect association of depressive symptoms and substance use is small, there are large interactions between depressive symptoms and externalizing behaviors in the prediction of substance use, particularly among younger adolescents; that is, adolescents with high levels of both are especially likely to engage in substance use (Maslowsky &

Schulenberg, 2013). Anxiety symptoms and disorders are more consistently shown to be positively associated with adolescent substance use (e.g., Costello, Mustillo, Erkanli, Keeler, & Angold, 2003), suggesting a coping or self-medicating function of substance use.

Of course, a primary issue is the direction of causality among internalizing, externalizing, and substance use. Internalizing and externalizing generally precede the onset of substance use, emerging on average 3–4 years before substance use in adolescence (Kessler et al., 2005; O'Neil, Conner, & Kendall, 2011). Thereafter, it is likely that substance use both contributes to and is caused by internalizing and externalizing behaviors. For example, substance use may relate to spending unsupervised time with peers and consequently to the onset of additional externalizing behaviors (Osgood, Wilson, O'Malley, Bachman, & Johnston, 1996). Although there is some evidence that substance use is a risk factor for onset and acceleration of depression and anxiety later in adolescence and into early adulthood (Brook, Cohen, & Brook, 1998; Stice, Burton, & Shaw, 2004), the majority of studies to date indicate that internalizing symptoms and disorders tend to precede substance use in adolescence (O'Neil et al., 2011).

Family

Adolescence is a period of significant reorganization and change in family relationships. Such normative transformations include increased autonomy and independence from parents, but ideally these changes occur in a context of continued support and attachment between developing adolescents and their parents (Laursen & Collins, 2009). The quantity of interaction often decreases, and more time is spent in contexts outside the family such as at school, with peers, and at work (Larson, Richards, Moneta, Holmbeck, & Duckett, 1996). Nonetheless, parents still play a pivotal role in adolescent experiences and in fact can sometimes counter other risk factors for alcohol and other drug use.

Parental supervision and monitoring tend to be strong predictors of lower alcohol and other drug use among adolescents (Kiesner, Poulin, & Dishion, 2010; Pilgrim, Schulenberg, O'Malley, Bachman, & Johnston, 2006) and are especially protective against substance use for high risk-taking adolescents (Dever et al., 2012). Alcohol use tends to increase as adolescents become more individuated from parents (Baer & Bray, 1999) and as parental monitoring tends to lessen (Barnes, Reifman, Farrell, & Dintcheff, 2000). Parents also protect against adolescent substance use through positive, supportive interactions and relationships with their children (Brody et al., 2006); indeed, the argument is made that parental monitoring during adolescence reflects more the quality of the relationship than actual independent monitoring by parents (Kerr & Stattin, 2000). In one study, levels of parental support during early adolescence protected against alcohol use five years later, with direct effects on alcohol use as well as indirect associations mediated by the effect of parental support on parental monitoring (Barnes et al., 2000). Parental support is particularly important in protecting against substance use for adolescents in high-risk environments as parents increase supportive behavior to protect their children from dangerous contexts (Rankin & Quane, 2002).

Parents also exert influence on substance use indirectly through their influence on their children's selection of peers and on the extent to which their children are susceptible to the influence of their peers. Adolescents who report higher levels of parental involvement in their lives also report that they are less influenced by their peers, suggesting a protective effect (Wood, Read, Mitchell, & Brand, 2004). While peers play an important in-the-moment role in substance use, it is likely that parents' influence is in effective monitoring and laying a foundation for decision making and peer selection that sets the stage for adolescent choices (Kandel, 1985; Kiesner et al., 2010; Urberg, Luo, Pilgrim, & Degirmencioglu, 2003).

Regarding sibling influences, some evidence suggests that older siblings' substance use predicts early adolescents' alcohol expectancies (D'Amico & Fromme, 1997) and subsequent substance use, above and beyond parental predictors

(Duncan, Duncan, & Hops, 1996; Kelly et al., 2011; Low, Shortt, & Snyder, 2012). Behavior genetic studies contrasting biological and adoptive siblings also suggest that, unlike many other sibling similarities and parental "influences" that can be explained by passive genotype–environment interactions, sibling similarities in the area of adolescent alcohol use involve important environmental effects (McGue & Sharma, 1995), such as sibling modeling, social influence, and access to substances (Conger & Rueter, 1996; Mercken, Candel, Willems, & de Vries, 2007). Sibling relationships can also be protective against substance use. As with parents, having a close or supportive relationship with a sibling is associated with lower rates of substance use in adolescence (East & Khoo, 2005; Samek & Rueter, 2011). In sum, despite normative transitions toward independence during adolescence, it is clear that the family context, and the sibling and parent relationships embedded within it, continues to exert both direct and indirect effects on substance use.

Peers

The importance of peer relations rises during adolescence, increasing the young person's exposure to cultural norms and influences that may or may not be compatible with the norms and values of the family of origin (Brown & Larson, 2009), providing avenues for continuity and discontinuity. Adolescent development in general, and substance use in particular, is inextricably linked to changing peer relationships (Patrick et al., in press; Prinstein & Dodge, 2008). There tends to be a shift in what is viewed as markers of status and success in peer groups toward more deviant activities (Allen et al., 2005), reflecting heterotypic continuity. Clearly, peer influences are not monolithic in their power or direction of influence (Brown & Larson, 2009). Individuals tend to seek out and be selected by peers who have similar goals, values, and behaviors (Kandel, 1985; Prinstein & Dodge, 2008), and thus peer relations relate to both using and not using substances. Peer influence tends to increase through at least middle adolescence, due to an intensification of peer relationships and a relatively immature ability to resist peer influence (O'Brien et al., 2011; Schulenberg et al., 1999; Steinberg & Monahan, 2007).

Having friends who get drunk is among the strongest risk factors for alcohol use (Patrick & Schulenberg, 2010), and perceptions of friends' use in high school predict both concurrent binge drinking and future trajectories of binge drinking (Schulenberg et al., 1996). Of course, a main issue when it comes to the correlation between peer use and individual use is whether this is due to socialization (with peers contributing to adolescents substance use) or selection (with adolescents selecting friends with similar interests); during adolescence and the transition to adulthood, it is typically both (Kandel, 1985; Patrick et al., in press). Over time, this is likely a matter of progressive accommodation, where adolescents select like-minded friends who in turn provide strong socialization influences, and so on (Cairns, 2000; Schulenberg et al., 1999).

Overall, at least four kinds of influences in the peer domain may contribute to increased substance use during adolescence (Patrick et al., in press). First, modeling is a form of indirect peer pressure. Adolescents learn by watching the substance use behaviors of peers and family members and perceiving the rewards and punishments they experience. Part of this modeling is learning how to talk about substance use, including instances of ridicule or exclusion for adolescents who do not engage in substance use (Brown & Larson, 2009; Dishion, Spracklen, Andrews, & Patterson, 1996; Patterson, Dishion, & Yoerger, 2000). Second, similarities between adolescents and their friends encourage continuity of behavior over time as peers spend time in unstructured socializing (Haynie & Osgood, 2005; Kandel, 1985; Osgood et al., 1996). The frequency of evenings out with friends (unsupervised by adults) is consistently associated with more alcohol and other drug use (Bachman et al., 2008; Kiesner et al., 2010; Patrick & Schulenberg, 2010). Third, adolescents tend to significantly overestimate the prevalence of substance use among their age-mates and then seek to match

their perceptions of others' use (Olds & Thombs, 2001). Finally, sociability that is expressed while drinking and using other drugs can be seen as indicators of successful peer relationships and markers of social group bonding (Crosnoe, 2011; Maggs et al., 1995), underscoring the role of heterotypic continuity in peer success across adolescence.

School and Work

Adolescents typically face major educational and occupational transitions every few years. These transitions represent potentially powerful risks and opportunities for young people. Successful adaptation to and performance in educational and occupational domains help define concurrent and future optimal development (Clausen, 1991; Crosnoe, 2011). In contrast, difficulties in negotiating these critical transitions can contribute to cumulative and emergent health risks (Eccles & Roeser, 2009), including substance use difficulties (Crosnoe, 2011; Schulenberg & Maggs, 2002). The transition to middle school is often marked by increased mismatch between what the developing young person expects and needs and what the context provides (Eccles & Roeser, 2009); the transition to high school can be marked by similar mismatches along with increased stress due to heightened expectations for individual responsibility for success (Guo et al., 2000; Jackson & Schulenberg, 2013), which may contribute to increased alcohol and other drug use.

Several cross-sectional and longitudinal studies provide evidence that grades, educational expectations, and school bonding are negatively related to alcohol and other drug use; likewise, school disengagement, school failure, school misbehavior, and skipping school are positively related to alcohol and other drug use (e.g., Bachman et al., 2008; Li & Lerner, 2011; McCluskey, Krohn, Lizotte, & Rodriguez, 2002; Pilgrim et al., 2006). For example, in a longitudinal multilevel regression analysis, school misbehavior and perceived peer encouragement of misbehavior in 8th grade predicted concurrent substance use and increases in substance use across high school; likewise, school bonding, school interest, and academic achievement at 8th grade predicted lower concurrent and future substance use (Bryant, Schulenberg, O'Malley, Bachman, & Johnston, 2003). Of particular importance, positive school attitudes were stronger protective factors against substance use for low-achieving students. Although it is clear that substance use can contribute to educational difficulties, broadly defined, it appears that the more common direction of influence, based on longitudinal analyses that accounted for selection factors, is that school difficulties contribute to substance use during adolescence (Bachman et al., 2008).

During high school, most US adolescents make the transition into part-time work. Although it has long been recognized that hours of work during adolescence are positively related to use of alcohol and other drugs, conclusions about causal connections have remained elusive (Mortimer, 2003; Staff, Messersmith, & Schulenberg, 2009). It is likely that some part-time work, especially in jobs that are a source of stress or mismatch between hopes and opportunities, contributes to substance use. Yet most of the evidence suggests that the positive relationship between hours of work and alcohol and other drug use is due more to selection effects—i.e., that long hours of work and substance use have a common set of causes, particularly disengagement from school (Bachman, Staff, O'Malley, Schulenberg, & Freedman-Doan, 2011; Monahan, Lee, & Steinberg, 2011).

Conclusions and Implications

As we argue in this chapter, adolescent substance use is best viewed as a moving target, both in terms of historical trends and developmental course. It is encouraging that current cohorts of adolescents are less likely than earlier cohorts to get involved with substance use; they have lower rates of initiation and escalation of most forms of substance use, especially among 8th and 10th graders (Johnston et al., 2012). Indeed, the age gradients of most substance use have become more pronounced as rates have dropped over the

years more so for younger than older youth. Nonetheless, rates of some substances have not declined and some are rising again. In particular, the misuse of prescription drugs has remained steady over recent years and marijuana use has started to increase especially among older adolescents. As we have learned through four decades of monitoring adolescent drug use, the situation can and likely will change. Thus, in terms of prevention and policy efforts, there are still plenty of reasons to worry about adolescent drug use. More generally, understanding the larger context in terms of shifting national trends in substance use and age trends in use, as well as broader sociodemographic differences in use, provides an important reference point for understanding individual adolescent development.

Broad-based concepts regarding developmental continuity, discontinuity, and transitions help highlight the dynamic aspect of functioning and adjustment during adolescence, drawing out the need to consider adolescent substance use with developmentally distal and proximal templates. For many young people, substance use during adolescence reflects a cascading effect whereby earlier difficulties in a variety of domains contribute to substance use onset and escalation, which then cascades into other difficulties (Dodge et al., 2009; Masten et al., 2008); likewise, we can view avoiding substance use during adolescence in the same way, a result of earlier positive cascades. Such cascading effects represent ontogenetic continuity (Schulenberg & Maslowsky, 2009). In contrast, partly as a function of the numerous individual and social context transitions during adolescence, this cascading flow can get interrupted or diverted, resulting in ontogenetic discontinuity whereby, for example, substance use and other risky behaviors during adolescence are more the result of developmentally proximal individual and contextual characteristics than distal ones (Moffitt & Caspi, 2001). This can be understood in terms of the peer and social integration benefits of substance use and other risky behaviors, illustrating heterotypic continuity in which the purpose of being successful in peer relations remains consistent over time but the behaviors to meet this purpose shift. In some cases, this behavioral discontinuity may prove to be a developmental disturbance (Schulenberg & Zarrett, 2006), and more salutary behavior trajectories are expected to eventually resume. But in other cases, this "detour into the dark side" that may come with the multiple transitions of adolescence is best understood as a turning point—this sort of behavioral discontinuity suggests a profound and permanent change in course (Rutter, 1996). Future advances in the understanding of the etiology of substance use rest upon our ability to distinguish among these distinct types of continuity and discontinuity within the multiple transitions that comprise the second decade of life.

It is no surprise that adolescence is the typical time for substance use onset and escalation. There are numerous risk and protective factors for substance use during adolescence—in fact, it would be difficult to find aspects of adolescence that do not relate to substance use. Based on the research over the past several decades, a reasonable assumption is that we will discover few new substance use risk or protective factors. Instead, new discoveries will come from understanding how risk and protective factors are interlinked over time and how mechanisms across levels of explanation work together or in competition to result in substance use onset, escalation, and desistence. The next waves of innovative substance use research will involve integrating multiple levels of analysis (Cicchetti & Dawson, 2002; Crone & Dahl, 2012; Hyde, Gorka, Manuck, & Hariri, 2011), spanning from brain and biology to behavior and its effects on the health and well-being of the population. Gaining a better understanding of which configurations of risk and protective factors differentiate more experimental use from more chronic use, moving the lens from point estimates to trajectories, will continue to happen. And of particular importance, the extent to which adolescent substance use and other risky behaviors set the stage for adulthood difficulties will continue to be of concern; from this line of research will be a better understanding of what matters most during adolescence in the long run.

More broadly, a better integration of epidemiological and etiological perspectives on the problem of adolescent drug use can yield needed discoveries about the universality vs. specificity of trajectories and of mechanisms. These discoveries will advance both theory and intervention. We have learned, for example, that despite changes in levels of substance use across the past three decades, common risk and protective factors (many covered in this chapter) have generally remained invariant in their effects (Brown, Schulenberg, Bachman, O'Malley, & Johnston, 2001; Patrick & Schulenberg, 2010), suggesting some consistency in etiologic mechanisms and intervention targets. In contrast, there is new evidence that the course of substance use across the transition to adulthood has changed in important ways in recent years. Specifically, although high school alcohol and marijuana use has declined for recent cohorts compared to earlier cohorts, the subsequent rates of increase in use into the early 1920s have become faster for the recent cohorts (Jager, Schulenberg, O'Malley, & Bachman, 2013). This relatively more rapid escalation of substance use following high school raises numerous questions about shifts in etiologic mechanisms and intervention targets. Simply, the multilevel context in which development is embedded is also a moving target. Such insights can only come from integrating breadth and depth in our science, allowing us to gain empirical footholds on the grand and beautifully complex ecological (Bronfenbrenner, 1979), developmental-contextual (Lerner, 2006), and systems (Sameroff, 2010) frameworks of human development.

Acknowledgments Work on this chapter was supported in part by grants from the National Institute on Drug Abuse Grant (R01 DA001411, R01 DA016575, F31 DA029335) and the National Institute on Alcohol Abuse and Alcoholism (R01 AA019606, R21 AA020045). The findings and conclusions in this report are those of the authors and do not necessarily represent the views of the NIH. We wish to thank Carola Carlier for the editorial assistance.

References

Allen, J. P., Porter, M. R., McFarland, F. C., Marsh, P., & McElhaney, K. B. (2005). The two faces of adolescents' success with peers: Adolescent popularity, social adaptation, and deviant behavior. *Child Development, 76*, 747–760.

Bachman, J. G., O'Malley, P. M., Johnston, L. D., Schulenberg, J. E., & Wallace, J. M., Jr. (2011). Racial/ethnic differences in the relationship between parental education and substance use among U.S. 8th-, 10th-, and 12th-grade students: Findings from the monitoring the future project. *Journal of Studies on Alcohol and Drugs, 72*(2), 279–285.

Bachman, J. G., O'Malley, P. M., Schulenberg, J. E., Johnston, L. D., Freedman-Doan, P., & Messersmith, E. E. (2008). *The education–drug use connection: How successes and failures in school relate to adolescent smoking, drinking, drug use, and delinquency.* New York, NY: Lawrence Erlbaum Associates/Taylor & Francis.

Bachman, J. G., Staff, J., O'Malley, P. M., Schulenberg, J. E., & Freedman-Doan, P. (2011). Twelfth-grade student work intensity linked to later educational attainment and substance use: New longitudinal evidence. *Developmental Psychology, 47*, 344–363.

Baer, P. E., & Bray, J. H. (1999). Adolescent individuation and alcohol use. *Journal of Studies on Alcohol, 13*, 52–62.

Barnes, G. M., Reifman, A. S., Farrell, M. P., & Dintcheff, B. A. (2000). The effects of parenting on the development of adolescent alcohol misuse: A six-wave latent growth model. *Journal of Marriage and the Family, 62*, 175–186.

Baumrind, D. (1987). A developmental perspective on adolescent risk taking in contemporary America. In C. E. Irwin Jr. (Ed.), *Adolescent social behavior and health* (pp. 93–125). San Francisco, CA: Jossey-Bass.

Blakemore, S. J. (2012). Imaging brain development: The adolescent brain. *NeuroImage, 61*(2), 397–406.

Bonn-Miller, M. O., Zvolensky, M. J., & Bernstein, A. (2007). Marijuana use motives: Concurrent relations to frequency of past 30-day use and anxiety sensitivity among young adult marijuana smokers. *Addictive Behaviors, 32*, 49–62.

Brody, G. H., McBride, V., Gerrard, M., Gibbons, F. X., McNair, L., Brown, A. C., et al. (2006). The strong African American Families Program: Prevention of youths' high-risk behavior and a test of a model of change. *Journal of Family Psychology, 20*, 1–11.

Bronfenbrenner, U. (1979). *The ecology of human development: Experiments by nature and design.* Cambridge, MA: Harvard University Press.

Brook, J. S., Cohen, P., & Brook, D. W. (1998). Longitudinal study of co-occurring psychiatric disorders and substance use. *Journal of the American Academy of Child and Adolescent Psychiatry, 37*, 322–330.

Brook, J. S., Zhang, C., & Brook, D. W. (2011). Developmental trajectories of marijuana use from adolescence to adulthood: Personal predictors. *Archives of Pediatrics and Adolescent Medicine, 165*(1), 55–60.

Brown, T. L., Flory, K., Lynam, D. R., Leukefeld, C., & Clayton, R. R. (2004). Comparing the developmental trajectories of marijuana use of African American and Caucasian adolescents: Patterns, antecedents, and consequences. *Experimental and Clinical Psychopharmacology, 12*(1), 47–56.

Brown, B. B., & Larson, J. (2009). Peer relationships in adolescence. In R. M. Lerner & L. Steinberg (Eds.), *Handbook of adolescent psychology* (3rd ed., pp. 74–103). Hoboken, NJ: Wiley.

Brown, S. A., McGue, M., Maggs, J. L., Schulenberg, J. E., Hingson, R., Swartzwelder, S., et al. (2008). A developmental perspective on alcohol and youths 16 to 20 years of age. *Pediatrics, 121*, S290–S310.

Brown, S. A., McGue, M., Maggs, J. L., Schulenberg, J. E., Hingson, R., Swartzwelder, S., et al. (2009). Underage alcohol use: Summary of developmental processes and mechanisms, ages 16–20. *Alcohol Research and Health, 32*, 41–52.

Brown, T. N., Schulenberg, J., Bachman, J. G., O'Malley, P. M., & Johnston, L. D. (2001). Are risk and protective factors for substance use consistent across historical time? National data from 22 consecutive cohorts of high school seniors. *Prevention Science, 2*, 29–43.

Bryant, A., Schulenberg, J., O'Malley, P. M., Bachman, J. G., & Johnston, L. D. (2003). How academic achievement, attitudes, and behaviors relate to the course of substance use during adolescence: A six-year multi-wave national longitudinal study. *Journal of Research on Adolescence, 13*, 361–397.

Cairns, R. B. (2000). Developmental science: Three audacious implications. In L. R. Bergman, R. B. Cairns, L.-G. Nilsson, & L. Nystedt (Eds.), *Developmental science and the holistic approach* (pp. 49–62). Mahwah, NJ: Lawrence Erlbaum Associates.

Caspi, A. (2000). The child is father of the man: Personality continuities from childhood to adulthood. *Journal of Personality and Social Psychology, 78*, 158–172.

Cerdá, M., Wall, M., Keyes, K., Galea, S., & Hasin, D. (2012). Medical marijuana laws in 50 states: Investigating the relationship between state legalization of medical marijuana and marijuana use, abuse and dependence. *Drug and Alcohol Dependence, 120*(1–3), 22–27.

Chassin, L., Hussong, A., & Beltran, I. (2009). Adolescent substance use. In R. M. Lerner & L. Steinberg (Eds.), *Handbook of adolescent psychology* (3rd ed., pp. 723–763). New York, NY: Wiley.

Chassin, L., Presson, C. C., & Sherman, S. J. (1989). "Constructive" vs. "destructive" deviance in adolescent health-related behaviors. *Journal of Youth and Adolescence, 18*, 245–262.

Cicchetti, D., & Dawson, G. (2002). Multiple levels of analysis. *Development and Psychopathology, 14*(3), 417–420.

Cicchetti, D., & Rogosch, F. A. (2002). A developmental psychopathology perspective on adolescence. *Journal of Consulting and Clinical Psychology, 70*, 6–20.

Clausen, J. S. (1991). Adolescent competence and the shaping of the life course. *The American Journal of Sociology, 96*(4), 805–842.

Coleman, J. C. (1989). The focal theory of adolescence: A psychological perspective. In K. Hurrelmann &

U. Engel (Eds.), *The social world of adolescents: International perspectives* (pp. 43–56). New York, NY: Walter de Gruyter.

Conger, R. D., & Rueter, M. A. (1996). Siblings, parents, and peers: A longitudinal study of social influences in adolescent risk for alcohol use and abuse. In G. H. Brody et al. (Eds.), *Sibling relationships: Their causes and consequences* (pp. 1–30). Norwood, NJ: Ablex Publishing Corp.

Cooper, M. L. (1994). Motivations for alcohol use among adolescents: Development and validation of a four-factor model. *Psychological Assessment, 6,* 117–128.

Costello, E. J., Mustillo, S., Erkanli, A., Keeler, G., & Angold, A. (2003). Prevalence and development of psychiatric disorders in childhood and adolescence. *Archives of General Psychiatry, 60,* 837–844.

Cote, J. E. (2009). Identity formation and self development in adolescence. In R. M. Lerner & L. Steinberg (Eds.), *Handbook of adolescent psychology* (3rd ed.). Hoboken, NJ: Wiley.

Crone, E. A., & Dahl, R. E. (2012). Understanding adolescence as a period of social-affective engagement and goal flexibility. *Nature Reviews Neuroscience, 13,* 636–650.

Crosnoe, R. (2011). *Fitting in, standing out: Navigating the social challenges of high school to get an education.* New York, NY: Cambridge University Press.

D'Amico, E. J., & Fromme, K. (1997). Health risk behaviors of adolescent and young adult siblings. *Health Psychology, 16,* 426–432.

Dannefer, D. (1987). Aging as intracohort differentiation: Accentuation, the Matthew effect, and the life course. *Sociological Forum, 2,* 211–236.

Delva, J., Wallace, J. M., Jr., O'Malley, P. M., Bachman, J. G., Johnston, L. D., & Schulenberg, J. E. (2005). The epidemiology of alcohol, marijuana, and cocaine use among Mexican American, Puerto Rican, Cuban American, and other Latin American 8th grade students in the United States: 1991–2002. *American Journal of Public Health, 95,* 696–702.

Dever, B. V., Schulenberg, J. E., Dworkin, J. B., O'Malley, P. M., Kloska, D. D., & Bachman, J. G. (2012). Predicting risk-taking with and without substance use: The effects of parental monitoring, school bonding, and sports participation. *Prevention Science, 13*(6), 605–615.

Dishion, T. J., Spracklen, K. M., Andrews, D. W., & Patterson, G. R. (1996). Deviancy training in male adolescents friendships. *Behavior Therapy, 27*(3), 373–390.

Dodge, K. A., Malone, P. S., Lansford, J. E., Miller, S., Pettit, G. S., & Bates, J. E. (2009). A dynamic cascade model of the development of substance use onset. *Monographs of the Society for Research in Child Development, 74*(3), 1–120.

Doremus-Fitzwater, T. L., Varlinskaya, E. I., & Spear, L. P. (2010). Motivational systems in adolescence: Possible implications for age differences in substance abuse and other risk-taking behaviors. *Brain and Cognition, 72*(1), 114–123.

Downing, J., & Bellis, M. A. (2009). Early pubertal onset and its relationship with sexual risk taking, substance use and anti-social behavior: A preliminary cross-sectional study. *BMC Public Health, 9,* 446.

Duncan, T. E., Duncan, S. C., & Hops, H. (1996). The role of parents and older siblings in predicting adolescent substance use: Modeling development via structural equation latent growth methodology. *Journal of Family Psychology, 10,* 158–172.

East, P. L., & Khoo, S. T. (2005). Longitudinal pathways linking family factors and sibling relationship qualities to adolescent substance use and sexual risk behaviors. *Journal of Family Psychology, 19*(4), 571–580.

Eccles, J. S., & Roeser, R. W. (2009). Schools, academic motivation, and stage-environment fit. In R. M. Lerner & L. Steinberg (Eds.), *Handbook of adolescent psychology* (3rd ed.). Hoboken, NJ: Wiley.

Elder, G. H., Jr., & Shanahan, M. J. (2006). The life course and human development. In W. Damon & R. M. Lerner (Eds.), *Theoretical models of human development. Volume 1 of the Handbook of child psychology* (6th ed.). Hoboken, NJ: Wiley.

Elkind, D. (1967). Egocentrism in adolescence. *Child Development, 38,* 1025–1034.

Ellickson, S. L., Tucker, J. S., Klein, D. J., & McGuigan, K. A. (2001). Prospective risk factors for alcohol misuse in late adolescence. *Journal of Studies on Alcohol, 62*(6), 773–782.

Erikson, E. H. (1968). *Identity: Youth and crisis.* New York, NY: Norton.

Fromme, K., Katz, E. C., & Rivet, K. (1997). Outcome expectancies and risk-taking behavior. *Cognitive Therapy and Research, 21*(4), 421–442.

Galvan, A., Hare, T., Voss, H., Glover, G., & Casey, B. J. (2007). Risk-taking and the adolescent brain: Who is at risk? *Developmental Science, 10,* F8–F14.

Gibbons, F. X., Houlihan, A. E., & Gerrard, M. (2009). Reason and reaction: The utility of a dual-focus, dual-processing perspective on promotion and prevention of adolescent risk behaviour. *British Journal of Health Psychology, 14,* 231–248.

Gil, A. G., Wagner, E. F., & Tubman, J. G. (2004). Associations between early-adolescent substance use and subsequent young-adult substance use disorders and psychiatric disorders among a multiethnic male sample in South Florida. *American Journal of Public Health, 94*(9), 1603–1609.

Goodman, E., & Capitman, J. (2000). Depressive symptoms and cigarette smoking among teens. *Pediatrics, 106*(4), 748–755.

Grant, B. F., Stinson, F. S., Dawson, D. A., Chou, S. P., Dufour, M. C., Compton, W., et al. (2004). Prevalence and co-occurrence of substance use disorders and independent mood and anxiety disorders: Results from the National Epidemiologic Survey on Alcohol and Related Conditions. *Archives of General Psychiatry, 61,* 807–816.

Gunzerath, L., Faden, V., Zakhari, S., & Warren, K. (2004). National Institute on Alcohol Abuse and Alcoholism report on moderate drinking. *Alcoholism, Clinical and Experimental Research, 28,* 829–847.

Guo, J., Collins, L. M., Hill, K. G., & Hawkins, J. D. (2000). Developmental pathways to alcohol abuse and dependence in young adulthood. *Journal of Studies on Alcohol, 61,* 799–808.

Hawkins, J. D., Catalano, R. F., & Miller, J. Y. (1992). Risk and protective factors for alcohol and other drug problems in adolescence and early adulthood: Implications for substance abuse prevention. *Psychological Bulletin, 112,* 64–105.

Haynie, D. L., & Osgood, D. W. (2005). Reconsidering peers and delinquency: How do peers matter? *Social Forces, 84*(2), 1109–1130.

Hibell, B., Gufformsson, U., Ahlström, S., Balakireva, O., Bjarnasson, T., Kokkevi, A., et al. (2012). *The 2011 ESPAD report (The European School Survey Project on Alcohol and Other Drugs): Substance use among students in 36 European countries.* Stockholm, Sweden: The Swedish Council for Information on Alcohol and Other Drugs, The European Monitoring Centre for Drugs and Drug Addiction, the Council of Europe, and the Co-operation Group to Combat Drug Abuse and Illicit Trafficking in Drugs.

Hingson, R., & Kenkel, D. (2004). Social, health, and economic consequences of underage drinking. In R. Bonnie & M. O'Connell (Eds.), *Reducing underage drinking: A collective responsibility* (pp. 351–382). Washington, DC: National Academies Press.

Hinshaw, S. P. (1987). On the distinction between attentional deficits/hyperactivity and conduct problems/aggression in child psychopathology. *Psychological Bulletin, 101*(3), 443–463.

Hyde, L. W., Gorka, A., Manuck, S. B., & Hariri, A. R. (2011). Perceived social support moderates the link between threat-related amygdala reactivity and trait anxiety. *Neuropsychologia, 49,* 651–656.

Ianni, F. (1998). *The search for structure: A report on American youth today.* New York, NY: Free Press.

Jackson, K. M., & Schulenberg, J. E. (2013). Alcohol use during the transition from middle school to high school: National panel data on prevalence and moderators. *Developmental Psychology, 49*(11), 2147–2158.

Jager, J., Schulenberg, J. E., O'Malley, P. M., & Bachman, J. G. (2013). Historical variation in rates of change in substance use across the transition to adulthood: The trend towards lower intercepts and steeper slopes. *Development and Psychopathology, 25*(2), 527–543.

Jessor, R. (1987). Problem-behavior theory, psychosocial development, and adolescent problem drinking. *British Journal of Addiction, 82,* 331–342.

Johnson, R. J., McCaul, K. D., & Klein, W. M. P. (2002). Risk involvement and risk perception among adolescents and young adults. *Journal of Behavioral Medicine, 25,* 67–82.

Johnston, L. D. (1991). Toward a theory of drug epidemics. In R. L. Donohew, H. Sypher, & W. Bukoski (Eds.), *Persuasive communication and drug abuse prevention* (pp. 93–132). Hillsdale, NJ: Lawrence Erlbaum Associates.

Johnston, L. D., O'Malley, P. M., Bachman, J. G., & Schulenberg, J. E. (2012). *Monitoring the Future national survey results on drug use, 1975–2011:*

Volume I, Secondary school students. Ann Arbor, MI: Institute for Social Research, University of Michigan.

Kagan, J. (1980). Perspectives on continuity. In O. G. Brim & J. Kagan (Eds.), *Constancy and change in human development* (pp. 26–74). Cambridge, MA: Harvard University Press.

Kandel, D. B. (1985). On processes of peer influences in adolescent drug use: A developmental perspective. *Advances in Alcohol & Substance Abuse, 4,* 139–163.

Keating, D. P. (2004). Cognitive and brain development. In R. M. Lerner & L. Steinberg (Eds.), *Handbook of adolescent psychology* (pp. 45–84). Hoboken, NJ: Wiley.

Kelly, A. B., O'Flaherty, M., Connor, J. P., Homel, R., Toumbourou, J. W., Patton, G. C., et al. (2011). The influence of parents, siblings and peers on pre- and early-teen smoking: A multilevel model. *Drug and Alcohol Review, 30*(4), 381–387.

Kerr, M., & Stattin, H. (2000). What parents know, how they know it, and several forms of adolescents adjustment: Further evidence for a reinterpretation of monitoring. *Developmental Psychology, 36,* 366–380.

Kessler, R. C., Berglund, P., Demler, O., Jin, R., Merikangas, K. R., & Walters, E. E. (2005). Lifetime prevalence and age-of-onset distributions of DSM-IV disorders in the National Comorbidity Survey Replication. *Archives of General Psychiatry, 62*(6), 593–602.

Keyes, K. M., Schulenberg, J. E., O'Malley, P. M., Johnston, L. D., Bachman, J. G., Li, G., et al. (2012). Birth cohort effects on adolescent alcohol use: The influence of social norms from 1976–2007. *Archives of General Psychiatry, 69*(12), 1304–1313.

Kiesner, J., Poulin, F., & Dishion, T. J. (2010). Adolescent substance use with friends: Moderating and mediating effects of parental monitoring and peer activity contexts. *Merrill-Palmer Quarterly, 56*(4), 529–556.

Larson, R. W., Richards, M. H., Moneta, G., Holmbeck, G., & Duckett, E. (1996). Changes in adolescents' daily interactions with their families from ages 10 to 18: Disengagement and transformation. *Developmental Psychology, 32,* 744–754.

Laursen, B., & Collins, W. A. (2009). Parent–child relationships during adolescence. In R. M. Lerner & L. Steinberg (Eds.), *Handbook of adolescent psychology* (3rd ed.). Hoboken, NJ: Wiley.

Lerner, R. M. (2006). Developmental science, developmental systems, and contemporary theories of human development. In W. Damon & R. M. Lerner (Eds.), *Theoretical models of human development. Volume 1 of the Handbook of child psychology* (6th ed.). Hoboken, NJ: Wiley.

Lewis, M. (1999). Contextualism and the issue of continuity. *Infant Behavior and Development, 22,* 431–444.

Li, Y., & Lerner, R. M. (2011). Trajectories of school engagement during adolescence: Implications for grades, depression, delinquency, and substance use. *Developmental Psychology, 47,* 233–247.

Low, S., Shortt, J. W., & Snyder, J. (2012). Sibling influences on adolescent substance use: The role of modeling, collusion, and conflict. *Development and Psychopathology, 24*(1), 287–300.

Maggs, J. L., Almeida, D. M., & Galambos, N. L. (1995). Risky business: The paradoxical meaning of problem behavior for young adolescents. *Journal of Early Adolescence, 15*, 339–357.

Maggs, J. L., & Schulenberg, J. E. (2005a). Initiation and course of alcohol consumption among adolescents and young adults. In M. Galanter (Ed.), *Recent developments in alcoholism* (Alcohol problems in adolescents and young adults, Vol. 17, pp. 29–47). New York, NY: Kluwer Academic/Plenum Publishers.

Maggs, J. L., & Schulenberg, J. E. (2005b). Trajectories of alcohol use during the transition to adulthood. *Alcohol Research and Health, 28*, 195–211.

Maggs, J., Schulenberg, J., & Hurrelmann, K. (1997). Developmental transitions during adolescence: Health promotion implications. In J. Schulenberg, J. Maggs, & K. Hurrelmann (Eds.), *Health risks and developmental transitions during adolescence* (pp. 522–546). New York, NY: Cambridge University Press.

Marcia, J. (1994). Identity and psychotherapy. In S. L. Archer (Ed.), *Interventions for adolescent identity development* (pp. 29–46). Thousand Oaks, CA: Sage.

Maslowsky, J., Buvinger, E., Keating, D., Steinberg, L., & Cauffman, E. (2011). Cost-benefit analysis mediation of the relationship between sensation seeking and risk behavior. *Personality and Individual Differences, 51*, 802–806.

Maslowsky, J., Keating, D., Monk, C., & Schulenberg, J. E. (2011). Planned versus unplanned risks: Neurocognitive predictors of subtypes of adolescents' risk behavior. *International Journal of Behavioral Development, 35*, 152–160.

Maslowsky, J., & Schulenberg, J.E. (2013). Interaction matters: Quantifying conduct problem by depressive symptoms interaction and its association with adolescent alcohol, cigarette, and marijuana use in a national sample. *Development and Psychopathology, 25*(4), 1029–1043.

Masten, A. S. (2001). Ordinary magic: Resilience processes in development. *American Psychologist, 56*, 227–238.

Masten, A. S., Faden, V. B., Zucker, R. A., & Spear, L. P. (2008). Underage drinking: A developmental framework. *Pediatrics, 121*, S235–S251.

McCaffery, J. M., Papandonatos, G. D., Stanton, C., Lloyd-Richardson, E. E., & Niaura, R. (2008). Depressive symptoms and cigarette smoking in twins from the National Longitudinal Study of Adolescent Health. *Health Psychology, 27*(S3), S207–215.

McCluskey, C. P., Krohn, M. D., Lizotte, A. J., & Rodriguez, M. L. (2002). Early substance use and school achievement: An examination of Latino, White, and African American youth. *Journal of Drug Issues, 32*, 921–943.

McGue, M., & Sharma, A. (1995). Parent and sibling influences on adolescent alcohol use and misuse: Evidence from a U.S. adoption cohort. *Journal of Studies on Alcohol, 57*, 8–18.

Mendle, J., & Ferrero, J. (2012). Detrimental psychological outcomes associated with pubertal timing in adolescent boys. *Developmental Review, 32*, 49–65.

Mercken, L., Candel, M., Willems, P., & de Vries, H. (2007). Disentangling social selection and social influence effects on adolescent smoking: The importance of reciprocity in friendships. *Addiction, 102*, 1483–1492.

Moffitt, T. E., & Caspi, A. (2001). Childhood predictors differentiate life-course persistent and adolescent-limited antisocial pathways among males and females. *Development and Psychopathology, 13*, 355–375.

Monahan, K. C., Lee, J. M., & Steinberg, L. D. (2011). Revisiting the impact of part-time work on adolescent adjustment: Distinguishing between selection and socialization using propensity score matching. *Child Development, 82*, 96–112.

Mortimer, J. T. (2003). *Working and growing up in America*. Cambridge, MA: Harvard University Press.

National Institute on Drug Abuse. (2003). *Drug use among racial/ethnic minorities, revised* (NIH Publication No. 03–3888). Bethesda, MD: National Institutes of Health.

National Institute on Drug Abuse. (2012). *Health effects of commonly abused drugs*. Available from http://www.drugabuse.gov/drugs-abuse/commonly-abused-drugs/health-effects

Negriff, S., & Trickett, P. K. (2012). Peer substance use as a mediator between early pubertal timing and adolescent substance use: Longitudinal associations and moderating effect of maltreatment. *Drug and Alcohol Dependence, 126*, 95–101.

O'Brien, L., Albert, D., Chein, J., & Steinberg, L. (2011). Adolescents prefer more immediate rewards when in the presence of their peers. *Journal of Research on Adolescence, 21*(4), 747–753.

O'Neil, K. A., Conner, B. T., & Kendall, P. C. (2011). Internalizing disorders and substance use disorders in youth: Comorbidity, risk, temporal order, and implications for intervention. *Clinical Psychology Review, 31*(1), 104–112.

Olds, R. S., & Thombs, D. L. (2001). The relationship of adolescent perceptions of peer norms and parent involvement to cigarette and alcohol use. *Journal of School Health, 71*, 223–228.

Osgood, D. W., Wilson, J. K., O'Malley, P. M., Bachman, J. G., & Johnston, L. D. (1996). Routine activities and individual deviant behaviors. *American Sociological Review, 61*, 635–655.

Patrick, M. E., & Schulenberg, J. E. (2010). Alcohol use and heavy episodic drinking prevalence and predictors among national samples of American 8th and 10th grade students. *Journal of Studies on Alcohol and Drugs, 71*, 41–45.

Patrick, M. E., & Schulenberg, J. E. (2011). How trajectories of reasons for alcohol use relate to trajectories of binge drinking: National panel data spanning late adolescence to early adulthood. *Developmental Psychology, 47*, 311–317.

Patrick, M. E., & Schulenberg, J. E. (2014). Prevalence and predictors of adolescent alcohol use and binge drinking in the United States. *Alcohol Research: Current Reviews, 35*(2), 193–200.

Patrick, M. E., Schulenberg, J. E., Maggs, J. L., & Maslowsky, J. (in press). Substance use and peers during adolescence and emerging/early adulthood: Socialization, selection, and developmental transitions. In K. Sher (Ed.), *Handbook of substance use disorders*. Oxford: Oxford University Press.

Patrick, M. E., Schulenberg, J. E., O'Malley, P. M., Johnston, L., & Bachman, J. (2011). Adolescents' reported reasons for alcohol and marijuana use as predictors of substance use and problems in adulthood. *Journal of Studies on Alcohol and Drugs, 72*, 106–116.

Patterson, G. R., Dishion, T. J., & Yoerger, K. (2000). Adolescent growth in new forms of problem behavior: Macro- and micro-peer dynamics. *Prevention Science, 1*(1), 3–13.

Petraitis, J., Flay, B. R., & Miller, T. Q. (1995). Reviewing theories of adolescent substance use: Organizing pieces of the puzzle. *Psychological Bulletin, 11*, 67–86.

Pilgrim, C. C., Schulenberg, J. E., O'Malley, P. M., Bachman, J. G., & Johnston, L. D. (2006). Mediators and moderators of parental involvement on substance use: A national study of adolescents. *Prevention Science, 10*, 1–15.

Prinstein, M. J., & Dodge, K. A. (2008). Current issues in peer influence research. In M. J. Prinstein & K. A. Dodge (Eds.), *Understanding peer influence in children and adolescents* (pp. 3–13). New York, NY: The Guilford Press.

Rankin, B. H., & Quane, J. M. (2002). Social contexts and urban adolescent outcomes: The interrelated effects of neighborhoods, families, and peers on African-American youth. *Social Problems, 49*(1), 79–100.

Reardon, S. F., & Buka, S. L. (2002). Differences in onset and persistence of substance abuse and dependence among whites, blacks, and Hispanics. *Public Health Reports, 117*(Suppl. 1), S51–S59.

Reboussin, B. A., Hubbard, S., & Ialongo, N. S. (2007). Marijuana use patterns among African-American middle-school students: A longitudinal latent class regression analysis. *Drug and Alcohol Dependence, 90*(1), 12–24.

Reyna, V. F., & Farley, F. (2006). Risk and rationality in adolescent decision making: Implications for theory, practice, and public policy. *Psychological Science in the Public Interest, 7*, 1–44.

Romer, D., & Jamieson, P. (2001). Do adolescents appreciate the risks of smoking? Evidence from a national survey. *Journal of Adolescent Health, 29*, 12–21.

Rudolph, K. D., & Troop-Gordon, W. (2010). Personal-accentuation and contextual-amplification models of pubertal timing: Predicting youth depression. *Development and Psychopathology, 22*, 433–451.

Rutter, M. (1996). Transitions and turning points in developmental psychopathology: As applied to the age span between childhood and mid-adulthood. *International Journal of Behavioral Development, 19*, 603–626.

Samek, D. R., & Rueter, M. A. (2011). Considerations of elder sibling closeness in predicting younger sibling substance use: Social learning versus social bonding explanations. *Journal of Family Psychology, 25*(6), 931–941.

Sameroff, A. (2010). A unified theory of development: A dialectic integration of nature and nurture. *Child Development, 81*, 6–22.

Schulenberg, J. E., & Maggs, J. L. (2002). A developmental perspective on alcohol use and heavy drinking during adolescence and the transition to young adulthood. *Journal of Studies on Alcohol. Supplement, 14*, 54–70.

Schulenberg, J., Maggs, J. L., Dielman, T. E., Leech, S. L., Kloska, D. D., Shope, J. T., et al. (1999). On peer influences to get drunk: A panel study of young adolescents. *Merrill-Palmer Quarterly, 45*, 108–142.

Schulenberg, J., Maggs, J., & Hurrelmann, K. (Eds.). (1997). *Health risks and developmental transitions during adolescence*. New York, NY: Cambridge University Press.

Schulenberg, J. E., Maggs, J. M., & O'Malley, P. M. (2003). How and why the understanding of developmental continuity and discontinuity is important: The sample case of long-term consequences of adolescent substance use. In J. T. Mortimer & M. J. Shanahan (Eds.), *Handbook of the life course* (pp. 413–436). New York, NY: Plenum Publishers.

Schulenberg, J. E., & Maslowsky, J. (2009). Taking substance use and development seriously: Developmentally distal and proximal influences on adolescent drug use. *Monographs of the Society for Research in Child Development, 74*, 121–130.

Schulenberg, J. E., & Patrick, M. E. (2012). Historical and developmental patterns of alcohol and drug use among college students: Framing the problem. In H. R. White & D. Rabiner (Eds.), *College drinking and drug use* (pp. 13–35). New York, NY: Guilford Press.

Schulenberg, J. E., Sameroff, A. J., & Cicchetti, D. (2004). Editorial: The transition to adulthood as a critical juncture in the course of psychopathology and mental health. *Development and Psychopathology, 16*, 799–806.

Schulenberg, J., Wadsworth, K. N., O'Malley, P. M., Bachman, J. G., & Johnston, L. D. (1996). Adolescent risk factors for binge drinking during the transition to young adulthood: Variable- and pattern-centered approaches to change. *Developmental Psychology, 32*, 659–674.

Schulenberg, J. E., & Zarrett, N. R. (2006). Mental health during emerging adulthood: Continuity and discontinuity in courses, causes, and functions. In J. J. Arnett & J. L. Tanner (Eds.), *Emerging adults in America: Coming of age in the 21st century* (pp. 135–172). Washington, DC: American Psychological Association.

Simons, J., Correia, C. J., & Carey, K. B. (2000). A comparison of motives for marijuana and alcohol use among experienced users. *Addictive Behaviors, 25*, 153–160.

Spear, L. (2007). The developing brain and adolescent-typical behavior patterns: An evolutionary approach. In D. Romer & E. F. Walker (Eds.), *Adolescent psychopathology and the developing brain: Integrating brain and prevention science* (pp. 9–30). New York, NY: Oxford University Press.

Staff, J., Messersmith, J., & Schulenberg, J. E. (2009). Adolescents and the world of work. In R. M. Lerner & L. Steinberg (Eds.), *Handbook of adolescent psychology* (3rd ed.). Hoboken, NJ: Wiley.

Steinberg, L., Albert, D., Cauffman, E., Banich, M., Graham, S., & Woolard, J. (2008). Age differences in sensation seeking and impulsivity as indexed by behavior and self-report: Evidence for a dual systems model. *Developmental Psychology, 44*, 1764–1778.

Steinberg, L., & Monahan, K. C. (2007). Age differences in resistance to peer influence. *Developmental Psychology, 43*, 1531–1543.

Stice, E., Burton, E. M., & Shaw, H. (2004). Prospective relations between bulimic pathology, depression, and substance abuse: Unpacking comorbidity in adolescent girls. *Journal of Consulting and Clinical Psychology, 72*, 62–71.

Sturman, D. A., & Moghaddam, B. (2011). The neurobiology of adolescence: Changes in brain architecture, functional dynamics, and behavioral tendencies. *Neuroscience and Biobehavioral Reviews, 35*(8), 1704–1712.

Susman, E. J., & Dorn, L. D. (2009). Puberty: Its role in development. In R. M. Lerner & L. Steinberg (Eds.), *Handbook of adolescent psychology* (3rd ed.). Hoboken, NJ: Wiley.

Tauras, J. A., O'Malley, P. M., & Johnston, L. D. (2001). *Effects of price and access laws on teenage smoking initiation: A national longitudinal analysis* (ImpacTeen/Youth, Education, and Society Research Paper No. 1). Chicago, IL: University of Illinois at Chicago.

Urberg, K. A., Luo, Q., Pilgrim, C., & Degirmencioglu, S. M. (2003). A two-stage model of peer influence in adolescent substance use: Individual and relationship-specific differences in susceptibility to influence. *Addictive Behaviors, 28*(7), 1243–1256.

Wallace, J. M., Jr., Bachman, J. G., O'Malley, P. M., Schulenberg, J. E., Cooper, S. M., & Johnston, L. D. (2003). Gender and ethnic differences in smoking, drinking, and illicit drug use among American 8th, 10th and 12th grade students, 1976–2000. *Addiction, 98*, 225–234.

Wallace, J. M., Jr., Yamaguchi, R., Bachman, J. G., O'Malley, P. M., Schulenberg, J. E., & Johnston, L. D. (2007). Religiosity and adolescent substance use: The role of individual and contextual influences. *Social Problems, 54*(2), 308–327.

Werner, H. (1957). The concept of development from a comparative and organismic point of view. In D. B. Harris (Ed.), *The concept of development: An issue in the study of human behavior* (pp. 125–148). Minneapolis, MN: University of Minnesota Press.

White, H. R., McMorris, B. J., Catalano, R. F., Fleming, C. B., Haggerty, K. P., & Abbott, R. D. (2006). Increases in alcohol and marijuana use during the transition out of high school into emerging adulthood: The effects of leaving home, going to college, and high school protective factors. *Journal of Studies on Alcohol, 67*, 810–822.

Windle, M., Spear, L. P., Fuligni, A. J., Angold, A., Brown, J. D., Pine, D., et al. (2008). Transitions into underage and problem drinking: Developmental processes and mechanisms between 10 and 15 years of age. *Pediatrics, 121*, S273–S289.

Wood, M. D., Read, J. P., Mitchell, R. E., & Brand, N. H. (2004). Do parents still matter? Parent and peer influences on alcohol involvement among recent high school graduates. *Psychology of Addictive Behaviors, 18*, 19–30.

Zucker, R. A., Donovan, J. E., Masten, A. S., Mattson, M. E., & Moss, H. B. (2008). Early developmental processes and the continuity of risk for underage drinking and problem drinking. *Pediatrics, 121*(Suppl. 4), S252–S272.

Zuckerman, M. (1979). *Sensation seeking: Beyond the optimal level of arousal*. Hillsdale, NJ: Erlbaum.

Developmental Trajectories of Disordered Eating: Genetic and Biological Risk During Puberty

Kelly L. Klump

Eating disorders [i.e., anorexia nervosa (AN), bulimia nervosa (BN)] and disordered eating symptoms (e.g., body dissatisfaction, weight concerns, dieting, binge eating) have traditionally been viewed as developmental clinical conditions. They have a stereotypic adolescent age of onset and rarely begin after mid-adulthood (American Psychiatric Association, 2013). These trajectories of onset/offset have led many researchers to study specific developmental factors and periods that might contribute to developmental patterns of risk. The most frequently studied factor in this regard is puberty. This focus is understandable given the significant psychological, psychosocial, and biological changes of puberty and the fact that most eating disorders do not begin until during/after puberty (American Psychiatric Association, 2013; Bulik, 2002; Favaro, Caregaro, Tenconi, Bosello, & Santonastaso, 2009; Favaro, Ferrara, & Santonastaso, 2003; Klump, 2013).

This chapter will review evidence in support of puberty as a critical risk period for eating disorders. The chapter begins with basic definitions of eating disorders and the disordered eating phenotypes that have been the focus of most investigations. Data supporting a role for puberty in the development of disordered eating phenotypes will then be reviewed, with a particular emphasis on differentiating pubertal status (i.e., pubertal stage at a given point in time) from pubertal timing (i.e., onset of puberty relative to peers, including early, on-time, and late onset). Evidence from studies examining mechanisms of puberty's effects will then be discussed. An emphasis will be placed on emerging data highlighting genetic and biological mechanisms during puberty, as these data are contributing important new insights into the nature of puberty's effects on eating disorder risk. Given the significant sex difference in eating disorders (female to male ratio = 4:1 to 10:1) (American Psychiatric Association, 2013; Hudson, Hiripi, Pope, & Kessler, 2007), most studies have focused on females rather than males, although studies examining both sexes are reviewed below.

Definitions of Eating Disorders and the Symptoms

In brief, AN is characterized by a refusal to maintain a minimally healthy body weight (e.g., ≥85 % of ideal for age and height) coupled with intense fears of becoming fat and a self-evaluation significantly influenced by body weight and shape (American Psychiatric Association, 2013). Individuals with AN may restrict their food intake only, although most go on to develop binge eating and/or purging behaviors over the course of their illness (Eddy et al., 2007). By contrast, BN sufferers are of at least normal weight and

K.L. Klump, Ph.D. (✉)
Department of Psychology, Michigan State University,
316 Physics Rd – Room 107B, East Lansing,
MI 48824-1116, USA
e-mail: klump@msu.edu

M. Lewis and K.D. Rudolph (eds.), *Handbook of Developmental Psychopathology*,
DOI 10.1007/978-1-4614-9608-3_31, © Springer Science+Business Media New York 2014

engage in recurrent (i.e., ≥1×/week) binge eating episodes (i.e., the consumption of an unusually large amount of food within a discrete period and a loss of control over eating during the episode) as well as inappropriate compensatory behaviors, including purging behaviors (self-induced vomiting, misuse of laxatives, diuretics, or enemas) and non-purging behaviors (fasting, excessive exercise) (American Psychiatric Association, 2013). Similar to individuals with AN, individuals with BN experience undue influence of weight/shape on self-evaluation (American Psychiatric Association, 2013).

Although AN and BN are relatively rare (~0.5–3 % of females) (American Psychiatric Association, 2013), related otherwise specified feeding and eating disorders (OSFED) more common (~10 % of young adult females) (Fairburn & Bohn, 2005). These OSFED represent clinically significant disorders of eating that do not meet the specific criteria for an eating disorder. The fact that OSFED diagnoses are the most frequently encountered eating disorders in clinical (Thomas, Vartanian, & Brownell, 2009) and community (Machado, Machado, Goncalves, & Hoek, 2007) samples led the DSM-5 Workgroup to broaden the criteria for AN and BN to capture these more commonly encountered cases (Walsh, 2009). It also led to a push for dimensional rather than categorical models of eating disorders and other forms of psychopathology (Cuthbert, 2005; Krueger & Markon, 2011). Fortunately, because of the rarity of AN and BN, particularly before puberty, studies of pubertal risk have focused on dimensional measures of disordered eating symptoms (e.g., the tendency to binge eat, have concerns about body weight/shape, be dissatisfied with the size/shape of body parts— see Table 31.1) that are known to predate the onset of the full disorders (Jacobi, Hayward, de Zwaan, Kraemer, & Agras, 2004) and cut across diagnostic boundaries of AN and BN.

Phenotypic Associations Between Puberty and Disordered Eating

As discussed extensively by Klump (2013), studies of pubertal risk have examined pubertal status (e.g., prepuberty vs. postpuberty) as well as

Table 31.1 Definitions of eating disorder symptoms that have been examined in studies of puberty

Symptoms	Definition
Body dissatisfaction, weight/shape concerns	Dissatisfaction with the size/shape of one's body or body parts, and/or preoccupation with weight and a desire to lose weight
Dieting/weight management	Behavioral attempts to restrict food intake and/or engage in other behaviors to lose weight (e.g., exercise)
Dietary restraint	A cognitive intent to diet (i.e., desire to lose weight, plans to restrict food intake) as well as actual attempts to lose weight through dieting, avoidance of high-fat foods, and/or fasting
Binge eating	The consumption of a large amount of food in a short period of time (i.e., 2 h) with a loss of control over the binge episode
Purging behaviors	The use of inappropriate compensatory behaviors including purging (i.e., self-induced vomiting, or abuse of laxatives, diuretics, or enemas) and non-purging (e.g., excessive exercise, fasting) behaviors

pubertal timing (i.e., early, on-time, vs. late maturers). Most studies have examined how pubertal status and/or timing at one point in time are associated with concurrent eating disorders and their symptoms. Although cross-sectional studies are important for understanding *proximal correlates* of the disorder, longitudinal/prospective studies are needed to ensure that pubertal status and timing are *risk factors* for eating disorders even after all girls "catch up" and have completed their pubertal development. Persistence of pubertal status and timing effects can be examined via (1) longitudinal/prospective studies that examine whether pubertal status/timing effects at time 1 predict later risk at time 2, particularly when time 2 occurs in postpuberty and/or (2) retrospective studies that assess whether recalled markers of pubertal development (e.g., menarche) occurred earlier or later than peers and/or population norms. The latter studies are obviously less rigorous, as they rely on retrospective reports that are prone to memory biases (Coughlin, 1989).

Nonetheless, rare syndromes like eating disorders can be difficult to investigate in prospective studies due to the small number of expected cases, and so most studies of clinical eating disorders rely on retrospective reports.

Findings in Girls

Overall, data from cross-sectional and longitudinal studies are remarkably consistent in suggesting that pubertal status and timing are associated with a significantly increased risk of developing eating disorders and their component symptoms in girls (Klump, 2013). Studies consistently show that prepubertal onset of AN, BN, and OSFED is rare (Bulik, 2002), as mean ages of onset for the disorders (i.e., 15–19 years for AN and BN) (American Psychiatric Association, 2013; Favaro et al., 2003, 2009) reflect a postpubertal bias. Girls who are at more advanced stages of pubertal development have increased rates of BN and OSFED, and with few exceptions, a higher percentage of early maturers are among those diagnosed with BN as compared to females without eating disorders (for a review, see Klump, 2013). Importantly, although two prospective studies failed to find an effect of pubertal status (Killen et al., 1994) or timing (Stice, Presnell, & Bearman, 2001) on risk for BN, findings from retrospective studies clearly show that the effects of early pubertal timing on BN persist across late adolescence (Biederman et al., 2007; Graber, Lewinsohn, Seeley, & Brooks-Gunn, 1997; Kaltiala-Heino, Marttunen, Rantanen, & Rimpela, 2003; Kaltiala-Heino, Rimpela, Rissanen, & Rantanen, 2001; Ruuska, Kaltiala-Heino, Koivisto, & Rantanen, 2003) into young (Corcos et al., 2000; Fairburn, Welch, Doll, Davies, & O'Connor, 1997; Romans, Gendall, Martin, & Mullen, 2001) and middle (Romans et al., 2001) adulthood. Discrepant results between study types could be due to the small number of prospective studies conducted (i.e., only two) and/or to the low base rate of BN (1–3 %); this low base rate can make it difficult to detect prospective associations between pubertal status/timing and the disorder in small to moderately sized ($N=939$ and 496, respectively;

Killen et al., 1994; Stice et al., 2001) community samples. By contrast, associations are easier to detect in retrospective studies that include a larger number of BN cases and then "look back" at the presence of early pubertal timing. Results for AN have been even more mixed than those for BN (see Klump, 2013); although some studies find that early maturing girls are at increased risk (Crisp, 1970; Nicholls & Viner, 2009), no studies have examined differential rates of AN across pubertal status.

Findings for individual disordered eating symptoms corroborate those of clinical disorders by showing higher levels of all of the symptoms in Table 31.1 in girls who are at more advanced stages of pubertal development (Klump, 2013). Pubertal timing results largely replicate these findings where the highest rates of eating disorder symptoms are found in early maturing as compared to on-time and late-maturing girls (Klump, 2013). Findings have been particularly robust for body dissatisfaction and weight/shape concerns (Klump, 2013), and most results have been confirmed via prospective and/or retrospective studies. For example, several prospective studies found that pubertal status and timing effects persisted several years (range = 8 months to 30 years) after the initial assessment (Klump 2013).

Findings in Boys

Far fewer studies have examined the effects of puberty on eating disorder symptoms in males, and to date, findings are quite mixed. Similar to results in girls, several studies found that early maturing boys and/or those at advanced stages of puberty had higher rates of AN, BN, and eating disorder symptoms (Klump, 2013). However, an equal number of studies failed to find significant effects of pubertal status/timing on BN or disordered eating symptoms (Klump, 2013). When significant effects were observed, they typically were for the body dissatisfaction and weight/shape concerns that are associated with puberty in girls, although even these studies were mixed in their reports of significant versus null associations (Klump, 2013).

Summary

Overall, results are relatively consistent in showing significant effects of both pubertal status and timing on most eating disorder phenotypes in girls. Findings for boys have been much less consistent, suggesting that puberty is likely to play a much larger role in eating disorder risk in girls than boys and that sex-specific processes during puberty may differentially contribute to eating disorder risk across the sexes. These sex-specific processes highlight both psychosocial and genetic/biological factors that could serve as mechanisms of puberty's effects on eating disorders and their symptoms.

Mechanisms Underlying Puberty's Effects

Psychosocial Theories

Prevailing theories of risk have posited that significant pubertal status and timing effects in girls are due to the physical changes of puberty and their effects on body satisfaction, self-esteem, and mood (Bulik, 2002; Fornari & Dancyger, 2003). These theories emphasize the role of body dissatisfaction in causing increased dieting, which then leads to AN and BN. Early maturers are thought to be at particular risk given that they experience these physical changes earlier than their peers and may therefore experience even more body dissatisfaction than their developmentally on-time counterparts. Girls are believed to be at increased risk relative to boys given that pubertal physical changes in girls (i.e., increased adiposity) move them away from beauty ideals, while physical changes in boys (i.e., increased muscle mass) move them closer to their beauty ideals (Bulik, 2002; Fornari & Dancyger, 2003).

Although data testing the full psychosocial model are relatively sparse, some studies have supported its major tenants, at least in regard to the association between pubertal status, body dissatisfaction, and dieting (Attie & Brooks-Gunn, 1989; Bulik, 2002; Gralen, Levine, Smolak, & Murnen, 1990). However, no studies have examined whether these processes ultimately lead to the development of AN or BN, and given the individual association of each of these risk factors with puberty and disordered eating (see review above), the temporal ordering of the risk process (i.e., increased body fat leading to body dissatisfaction, which then leads to dieting and then to eating disorders) has not been established.

Genetic and Biological Theories

The pubertal activation of ovarian hormones and their substantial role in sex-differentiated behaviors have made this system a prime candidate in the hunt for biological factors underlying pubertal risk. Emerging data from human and animal studies provide support for these hypotheses. For example, twin studies of adolescent female twins found significant increases in genetic influences on disordered eating symptoms across adolescence, where there was essentially no genetic influence (i.e., 0 % heritability) in preadolescent female twins (age 11), but significant genetic effects ($\geq$50 % heritability) in twins during mid- (age 14) and late (age 17 or 18) adolescence (Klump, Burt, McGue, & Iacono, 2007; Klump, Burt, McGue, Iacono, & Wade, 2010). Developmental differences were observed in both cross-sectional (Klump, Burt, et al., 2010; Klump, McGue, & Iacono, 2000) and longitudinal (Klump, Burt, et al., 2007) studies, suggesting that the effects were robust and reflected within-twin pair shifts in etiologic influences across adolescence.

Given that puberty typically begins between preadolescence and middle adolescence in girls, puberty was an obvious candidate for studies examining mechanisms underlying age differences in genetic risk. Twin studies subsequently examined differences in genetic risk across puberty by comparing heritability across female twins who varied in their pubertal status and/or timing. In terms of pubertal status, several studies found substantial differences in genetic effects, such that genes accounted for 0 % of the variance in disordered eating symptoms in pre-early puberty, but ~50 % of the variance during mid-puberty and beyond (Culbert, Burt, McGue, Iacono, & Klump, 2009; Klump, McGue, & Iacono, 2003; Klump, Perkins, Burt, McGue, & Iacono, 2007). Twin studies of pubertal timing extended these findings by showing that associations between early pubertal timing and disordered eating symptoms (e.g., dieting, body dissatisfaction, drive for thinness, binge eating) were due to a shared set of genetic risk factors contributing to both phenotypes (Baker, Thornton, Bulik, Kendler, & Lichtenstein, 2012; Harden, Mendle, & Kretsch, 2012). Importantly, after controlling for these shared genetic risk factors, phenotypic associations between early pubertal timing and dieting were eliminated, suggesting that genetic risk factors (rather than environmental influences) entirely account for the co-occurrence of early menarche and dieting in girls (Harden et al., 2012).

Overall, data from twin studies provide strong support for puberty as a period of significant genetic risk for eating disorders in girls. These results have led to an increased interest in examining biological factors that may account for increased genetic effects across puberty. Thus far, theories and studies have focused on the ovarian hormones (estrogen, in particular) that become activated during puberty as potential mechanisms underlying puberty's effects. This focus is predicated on the fact that one of the primary functions of estrogen is to regulate gene transcription, and thereby protein synthesis, within the central nervous system (Ostlund, Keller, & Hurd, 2003; Wilson, Foster, Kronenberg, & Larsen, 1998). Some of the genes regulated by estrogen have been found to be significantly associated with eating disorders, particularly those in the serotonin system (Hildebrandt, Alfano, Tricamo, & Pfaff, 2010; Ostlund et al., 2003) and those associated with brain-derived neurotrophic factor (BDNF) (Klump & Culbert, 2007). Researchers have proposed (Klump & Culbert, 2007; Klump, Keel, Sisk, & Burt, 2010) that increases in estrogen during puberty may contribute to genetic risk via the hormone's effects on the production of these important neurotransmitters/neurotrophins, their receptors, and/or their signal transduction mechanisms.

To date, only one pilot study has investigated these possibilities, and it did so indirectly using a twin study design. Klump, Keel et al. (2010) compared the magnitude of genetic effects on disordered eating in twins with high (i.e., above the median value) versus low (i.e., below the median value) estradiol levels during puberty. Results suggested significant differences in genetic influences on overall eating disorder symptoms by estradiol levels, with no genetic influence in twins with low estradiol levels, but significant genetic effects in twins with high estradiol levels. Findings remained unchanged after controlling for age, BMI, and the physical changes of puberty (e.g., breast development), suggesting direct effects of estrogen on genetic risk for eating disorders during puberty in girls.

Clearly, additional research is needed to replicate these results, particularly given the small sample size ($N=99$ twin pairs) for this pilot project. However, corroborating data come from twin studies of males examining the effects of puberty on genetic risk for disordered eating (Klump et al., 2012). Boys do not experience increases in estrogen during puberty, as their pubertal development is driven primarily by increases in testosterone. If pubertal increases in genetic effects are present in boys, then factors other than (or in addition to) estrogen may drive increases in genetic effects in girls. In contrast to findings in girls, results showed no changes in genetic effects on overall levels of disordered eating in male twins across pre-early puberty, mid-late puberty, or young adulthood. The heritability remained constant at ~50 % of the variance in all groups (Klump et al., 2012). These findings suggest that pubertal increases in genetic influences are specific to girls and may be related to the estrogen effects described above.

Conclusions and Future Directions

In summary, data are clear in showing that both advanced pubertal status and early pubertal timing significantly increase risk for eating disorders and their symptoms in girls. Findings further suggest that these effects are at least partially genetically mediated, as dramatic increases in genetic effects have been observed across adolescence that appear to be due to estrogen activation during puberty. These changes are not uniformly present in boys, providing further indirect support for pubertal hormone influences on risk for eating disorders in girls. Finally, emerging data confirm that associations between early pubertal timing and key disordered eating symptoms (i.e., dieting) are due to genetic (rather than environmental) risk factors.

Although these studies do not rule out psychosocial explanations for pubertal risk, they call into question the predominance of these factors in etiologic models. Harden et al. (2012) showed rather convincingly that phenotypic associations between early pubertal timing and dieting are eliminated when within-family, genetic risk factors are controlled. Likewise, twin studies of puberty that control for age and BMI, and the twin study of estrogen that controlled for age, BMI, and the physical changes of puberty, suggest direct effects of puberty and estrogen on genetic and phenotypic risk. Recent studies in animals corroborate these impressions. Using a rodent model of binge eating, Klump, Suisman, Culbert, Kashy, and Sisk (2011) showed that binge eating proneness, or the tendency to consistently consume large amounts of palatable food (i.e., food that is high in fat and/or sugar) in a short period of time, emerged during puberty in female rats. In prepuberty, there were no significant differences in palatable food intake between binge eating prone and binge eating resistant (i.e., the tendency to consistently consume small amounts of palatable food) rats, but significant differences emerged during mid-late puberty and persisted into adulthood (Klump et al., 2011). Importantly, the two groups did not differ in their chow intake or body weight at any stage of development, suggesting that the pubertal effects were specific to palatable food intake and binge eating phenotypes. Notably, these findings in rats are unlikely to be due to environmental or psychosocial influences, as female rats do not experience key psychosocial/psychological risk factors (i.e., increased body dissatisfaction) that are present in humans.

Future Directions

Studies of puberty have made great strides in confirming the importance of this developmental period for phenotypic, genetic, and biological risk for eating disorders. They have also highlighted several areas in need of future research. On the phenotypic side, more studies are needed examining pubertal risk for clinical eating disorders, most notably AN, binge eating disorder (BED), and OSFED. Studies of AN have been fewer in number and much more mixed in their findings than studies of BN. BED is a new disorder in DSM-5, and OSFED diagnoses are of significant interest due to their increased prevalence in the population (relative to AN and BN). To some extent, the dimensional approach of most studies ameliorates concerns about the lack of data for these disorders, as their key symptoms (e.g., binge eating, dieting) show the pubertal phenotypic and genetic effects described herein. Nonetheless, future phenotypic and genetic studies should examine puberty's effects on AN, BED, and OSFED to determine the role of puberty in their development.

With regard to genetic and hormonal mechanisms, more twin studies of estrogen are clearly needed to replicate initial pilot data and confirm a role for estrogen in pubertal emergence of phenotypic and genetic risk for eating disorders. Longitudinal studies would go a long way in determining whether *within-person changes* in phenotypic and genetic risk across puberty are due to estrogen activation. It would be helpful for these studies to examine other phenotypes that are comorbid with eating disorders and have been linked to pubertal processes (e.g., depression, anxiety, substance use). Some developmental twin studies show that changes in genetic risk for disordered eating are independent of mood (e.g., (Klump, Burt, et al., 2007), but most studies have not examined comorbid psychiatric traits. These studies should also aim to integrate psychosocial risk factors into studies of biological/genetic risk. As an example of this type of integration, in the Harden et al. (2012) twin study discussed above, subjectively rated pubertal timing (i.e., whether the twin thought her development was earlier than her peers) was environmentally associated with increased risk for dieting in girls. This was in stark contrast to the findings for objectively measured pubertal timing (i.e., comparison of the twin's actual pubertal development to population norms) that was associated with increased dieting through genetic factors. The possibility that pubertal timing may be differentially associated with eating disorder risk depending upon the measurement/perspective underscores the strong need for multi-method, multilevel studies that examine biological and psychosocial risk factors and their interplay in the progression of eating disorder symptoms across development.

Finally, additional studies also are needed to identify the specific genes and neurobiological systems that may be activated by hormones during puberty. Emerging data show strong phenotypic and genetic effects of estrogen on the pattern and timing of changes in brain structure and function during puberty (Ahmed et al., 2008; Nunez, Sodhi, & Juraska, 2002; Peper, Brouwer, et al., 2009; Peper, Schnack, et al., 2009; Primus & Kellogg, 1991; Spear, 2000; Zehr, Todd, Schulz, McCarthy, & Sisk, 2006). Yet, none of these studies have linked these changes to eating disorders or their symptoms. Several of the neurobiological systems that are regulated by estrogen and have been implicated in the etiology of eating disorders (e.g., serotonin, neurotrophic factors, dopamine) would be ideal targets for such investigations (Hildebrandt et al., 2010; Ostlund et al., 2003; Young, 2010). Notably, many of these systems show significant changes/maturation during the pubertal period (Becker, 2009; Friemel, Spanagel, & Schneider, 2010; Iughetti, Casarosa, Predieri, Patianna, & Luisi, 2011) that may be linked to estrogen (Becker, 2009) and may contribute to increases in pubertal risk. Human and animal studies examining whether estrogen regulation of these systems accounts for increased risk are needed to confirm a role for estrogen in pubertal increases in eating disorders.

Acknowledgements Work on this chapter was supported by a grant from the National Institute of Mental Health awarded to Dr. Klump (MH 070542). The content is solely the responsibility of the author and does not necessarily represent the official views of the NIMH.

References

Ahmed, E. I., Zehr, J. L., Schulz, K. M., Lorenz, B. I. Doncarlos, L. L., & Sisk, C. L. (2008). Pubertal hormones modulate the addition of new cells to sexually dimorphic brain regions. *Nature Neuroscience, 11*, 995–997.

American Psychiatric Association. (2013). *Diagnostic and statistical manual of mental disorders, Fifth edition (DSM-5)*. Washington, DC: American Psychiatric Association.

Attie, I., & Brooks-Gunn, J. (1989). Development of eating problems in adolescent girls: A longitudinal study. *Developmental Psychology, 25*(1), 70–79.

Baker, J. H., Thornton, L. M., Bulik, C. M., Kendler, K. S., & Lichtenstein, P. (2012). Shared genetic effects between age at menarche and disordered eating. *Journal of Adolescent Health, 51*(5), 491–496.

Becker, J. B. (2009). Sexual differentiation of motivation: A novel mechanism? *Hormones and Behavior, 55*(5), 646–654.

Biederman, J., Ball, S. W., Monuteaux, M. C., Surman, C. B., Johnson, J. L., & Zeitlin, S. (2007). Are girls with ADHD at risk for eating disorders? Results from a controlled, five-year prospective study. *International Journal of Eating Disorders, 40*(3), 232–240.

Bulik, C. M. (2002). Eating disorders in adolescents and young adults. *Child and Adolescent Psychiatric Clinics of North America, 11*, 201–218.

Corcos, M., Flament, M. F., Giraud, M. J., Paterniti, S., Ledoux, S., Atger, F., et al. (2000). Early psychopathological signs in bulimia nervosa. A retrospective comparison of the period of puberty in bulimic and control girls. *European Child and Adolescent Psychiatry, 9*(2), 115–121.

Coughlin, S. S. (1989). Recall bias in epidemiologic studies. *Journal of Clinical Epidemiology, 43*(1), 87–91.

Crisp, A. H. (1970). Reported birth weights and growth rates in a group of patients with primary anorexia nervosa (weight phobia). *Journal of Psychosomatic Research, 14*(1), 23–50.

Culbert, K. M., Burt, S. A., McGue, M., Iacono, W. G., & Klump, K. L. (2009). Puberty and the genetic diathesis of disordered eating attitudes and behaviors. *Journal of Abnormal Psychology, 118*(4), 788–796.

Cuthbert, B. N. (2005). Dimensional models of psychopathology: Research agenda and clinical utility. *Journal of Abnormal Psychology, 114*(4), 565–569.

Eddy, K. T., Dorer, D. J., Franko, D. L., Tahilani, K., Thompson-Brenner, H., & Herzog, D. B. (2007). Should bulimia nervosa be subtyped by history of anorexia nervosa? A longitudinal validation. *International Journal of Eating Disorders, 40*, S67–S71.

Fairburn, C. G., & Bohn, K. (2005). Eating disorder NOS (EDNOS): An example of the troublesome "Not Otherwise Specified" (NOS) category in DSM-IV. *Behaviour Research and Therapy, 43*, 691–701.

Fairburn, C. G., Welch, S. L., Doll, H. A., Davies, B. A., & O'Connor, M. E. (1997). Risk factors for bulimia nervosa: A community-based case–control study. *Archives of General Psychiatry, 54*(6), 509–517.

Favaro, A., Caregaro, L., Tenconi, E., Bosello, R., & Santonastaso, P. (2009). Time trends in age at onset of anorexia nervosa and bulimia nervosa. *Journal of Clinical Psychiatry, 70*(12), 1715–1721.

Favaro, A., Ferrara, S., & Santonastaso, P. (2003). The spectrum of eating disorders in young women: A prevalence study in a general population sample. *Psychosomatic Medicine, 65*(4), 701–708.

Fornari, V., & Dancyger, I. F. (2003). Psychosexual development and eating disorders. *Adolescent Medicine, 14*(1), 61–75.

Friemel, C. M., Spanagel, R., & Schneider, M. (2010). Reward sensitivity for a palatable food reward peaks during pubertal developmental in rats. *Frontiers in Behavioral Neuroscience, 4*(39), 1–10.

Graber, J. A., Lewinsohn, P. M., Seeley, J. R., & Brooks-Gunn, J. (1997). Is psychopathology associated with the timing of pubertal development? *Journal of the American Academy of Child and Adolescent Psychiatry, 36*(12), 1768–1776.

Gralen, S. J., Levine, M. P., Smolak, L., & Murnen, S. K. (1990). Dieting and disordered eating during early and middle adolescence: Do the influences remain the same? *International Journal of Eating Disorders, 9*(5), 501–512.

Harden, K. P., Mendle, J., & Kretsch, N. (2012). Environmental and genetic pathways between early pubertal timing and dieting in adolescence: Distinguishing between objective and subjective timing. *Psychological Medicine, 42*(1), 183–193.

Hildebrandt, T., Alfano, L., Tricamo, M., & Pfaff, D. W. (2010). Conceptualizing the role of estrogens and serotonin in the development and maintenance of bulimia nervosa. *Clinical Psychology Review, 30*(6), 655–668.

Hudson, J. I., Hiripi, E., Pope, H. G., & Kessler, R. C. (2007). The prevalence and correlates of eating disorders in the National Comorbidity Survey Replication. *Biological Psychiatry, 61*(3), 348–358.

Iughetti, L., Casarosa, E., Predieri, B., Patianna, V., & Luisi, S. (2011). Plasma brain-derived neurotrophic factors in children and adolescents. *Neuropeptides, 45*, 205–211.

Jacobi, C., Hayward, C., de Zwaan, M., Kraemer, H. C., & Agras, W. S. (2004). Coming to terms with risk factors for eating disorders: Application of risk terminology and suggestions for a general taxonomy. *Psychological Bulletin, 130*(1), 19–65.

Kaltiala-Heino, R., Marttunen, M., Rantanen, P., & Rimpela, M. (2003). Early puberty is associated with mental health problems in middle adolescence. *Social Science and Medicine, 57*, 1055–1064.

Kaltiala-Heino, R., Rimpela, M., Rissanen, A., & Rantanen, P. (2001). Early puberty and early sexual activity are associated with bulimic-type eating pathology in middle adolescence. *Journal of Adolescent Health, 28*, 346–352.

Killen, J. D., Taylor, C. B., Wilson, D. M., Haydel, K. F., Hammer, L. D., Simmonds, B., et al. (1994). Pursuit of thinness and onset of eating disorder symptoms in a community sample of adolescent girls: A three-year prospective analysis. *International Journal of Eating Disorders, 16*(3), 227–238.

Klump, K. L. (2013). Puberty as a critical risk period for eating disorders: A review of human and animal studies. *Hormones and Behavior, 64*, 399–410.

Klump, K. L., Burt, S. A., McGue, M., & Iacono, W. G. (2007). Changes in genetic and environmental influences on disordered eating across adolescence: A longitudinal twin study. *Archives of General Psychiatry, 64*(12), 1409–1415.

Klump, K. L., Burt, S. A., McGue, M., Iacono, W. G., & Wade, T. M. (2010). Age differences in genetic and environmental influences on weight and shape concerns. *International Journal of Eating Disorders, 43*(8), 679–688.

Klump, K. L., & Culbert, K. M. (2007). Molecular genetic studies of eating disorders: Current status and future directions. *Current Directions in Psychological Science, 16*(1), 37–41.

Klump, K. L., Culbert, K. M., Slane, J. D., Burt, S. A., Sisk, C. L., & Nigg, J. T. (2012). The effects of puberty on genetic risk for disordered eating: Evidence for sex difference. *Psychological Medicine, 42*(3), 627–638.

Klump, K. L., Keel, P. K., Sisk, C. L., & Burt, S. A. (2010). Preliminary evidence that estradiol moderates genetic influences on disordered eating attitudes and behaviors during puberty. *Psychological Medicine, 40*(10), 1745–1753.

Klump, K. L., McGue, M., & Iacono, W. G. (2000). Age differences in genetic and environmental influences on eating attitudes and behaviors in female adolescent twins. *Journal of Abnormal Psychology, 109*(2), 239–251.

Klump, K. L., McGue, M., & Iacono, W. G. (2003). Differential heritability of eating attitudes and behaviors in prepubertal versus pubertal twins. *International Journal of Eating Disorders, 33*(3), 287–292.

Klump, K. L., Perkins, P., Burt, S. A., McGue, M., & Iacono, W. G. (2007). Puberty moderates genetic influences on disordered eating. *Psychological Medicine, 37*(5), 627–634.

Klump, K. L., Suisman, J. L., Culbert, K. M., Kashy, D. A., & Sisk, C. L. (2011). Binge eating proneness emerges during puberty in female rats: A longitudinal study. *Journal of Abnormal Psychology, 120*(4), 948–955.

Krueger, R. F., & Markon, K. E. (2011). A dimensional-spectrum model of psychopathology: Progress and opportunities. *Archives of General Psychiatry, 68*(1), 10–11.

Machado, P. P., Machado, B. C., Goncalves, S., & Hoek, H. W. (2007). The prevalence of eating disorders not otherwise specified. *International Journal of Eating Disorders, 40*(3), 212–217.

Nicholls, D. E., & Viner, R. M. (2009). Childhood risk factors for lifetime anorexia nervosa by age 30 years in a national birth cohort. *Journal of the American Academy of Child and Adolescent Psychiatry, 48*(8), 791–799.

Nunez, J. L., Sodhi, J., & Juraska, J. M. (2002). Ovarian hormones after postnatal day 20 reduce neuron number in the rat primary visual cortex. *Journal of Neurobiology, 52*(4), 312–321.

Ostlund, H., Keller, E., & Hurd, Y. L. (2003). Estrogen receptor gene expression in relation to neuropsychiatric disorders. *Annals of the New York Academy of Sciences, 1007*, 54–63.

Peper, J. S., Brouwer, R. M., Schnack, H. G., van Baal, G. C., van Leeuwen, M., van den Berg, S. M., et al. (2009). Sex steroids and brain structure in pubertal boys and girls. *Psychoneuroendocrinology, 34*(3), 332–342.

Peper, J. S., Schnack, H. G., Brouwer, R. M., Van Baal, G. C., Pjetri, E., Szekely, E., et al. (2009). Heritability of regional and global brain structure at the onset of puberty: A magnetic resonance imaging study in 9-year-old twin pairs. *Human Brain Mapping, 30*(7), 2184–2196.

Primus, R. J., & Kellogg, C. K. (1991). Gonadal status and pubertal age influence the responsiveness of the benzodiazepine/GABA receptor complex to environmental challenge in male rats. *Brain Research, 561*(2), 299–306.

Romans, S. E., Gendall, K. A., Martin, J. L., & Mullen, P. E. (2001). Child sexual abuse and later disordered eating: A New Zealand epidemiological study. *International Journal of Eating Disorders, 29*(4), 380–392.

Ruuska, J., Kaltiala-Heino, R., Koivisto, A. M., & Rantanen, P. (2003). Puberty, sexual development and eating disorders in adolescent outpatients. *European Child and Adolescent Psychiatry, 12*(5), 214–220.

Spear, L. P. (2000). The adolescent brain and age-related behavioral manifestations. *Neuroscience and Biobehavioral Reviews, 24*(4), 417–463.

Stice, E., Presnell, K., & Bearman, S. K. (2001). Relation of early menarche to depression, eating disorders, substance abuse, and comorbid psychopathology among adolescent girls. *Developmental Psychology, 37*(5), 608–619.

Thomas, J. J., Vartanian, L. R., & Brownell, K. D. (2009). The relationship between eating disorder not otherwise specified (EDNOS) and officially recognized eating disorders: Meta-analysis and implications for DSM. *Psychological Bulletin, 135*(3), 407–433.

Walsh, B. T. (2009). Eating disorders in DSM-V: Review of existing literature (Part 1). *International Journal of Eating Disorders, 42*(7), 579–580.

Wilson, J. D., Foster, D. W., Kronenberg, H. M., & Larsen, P. R. (1998). *Williams textbook of endocrinology* (9th ed.). Philadelphia, PA: W.B. Saunders Company.

Young, J. K. (2010). Anorexia nervosa and estrogen: Current status of the hypothesis. *Neuroscience and Biobehavioral Reviews, 34*(8), 1195–1200.

Zehr, J. L., Todd, B. J., Schulz, K. M., McCarthy, M. M., & Sisk, C. L. (2006). Dendritic pruning of the medial amygdala during pubertal development of the male Syrian hamster. *Journal of Neurobiology, 66*(6), 578–590.

Enuresis and Encopresis: The Elimination Disorders

Janet E. Fischel and Kate E. Wallis

The childhood elimination disorders have been written about extensively in the psychological, medical, child developmental, urological, and pediatrics literature. In fact, the Winter 1976 issue of the *Journal of Pediatric Psychology* was entirely devoted to this topic. Nearly four decades later, there is still abundant ongoing research addressing etiological frameworks as well as risk factors, comorbidities, and treatment strategies.

Toilet training has as its goal the individual's continence of urine and feces, with elimination occurring in socially acceptable places. None of us began life with this skill in place; instead we learned it with the help of parents and other adults who taught us when to eliminate and when to withhold urine and feces. In their classic study of 22 cultures, Whiting and Child (1953) described that achieving continence is among the most basic and universal targets of socialization everywhere. Furthermore, virtually every culture appears to succeed in toilet training between 80 and 90 % of its new members within the expected time limit. The few who remain untrained, or who do train and then relapse, are said to have an elimination disorder.

J.E. Fischel, Ph.D. (✉)
Division Chief for Developmental and Behavioral Pediatrics, Department of Pediatrics, Stony Brook University and Stony Brook Long Island Children's Hospital, Stony Brook, NY 11794, USA
e-mail: janet.fischel@stonybrookmedicine.edu

K.E. Wallis, M.D., M.P.H.
Department of Pediatrics, New York University School of Medicine, New York, NY 10016, USA

Our goal in this chapter is to summarize what is known about the etiology, diagnosis, and treatment of elimination disorders in children who do not achieve continence at the culturally expected time or who revert to incontinence after a period of continence has been achieved. We rely on the diverse current literature as well as clinical experience to gain a comprehensive understanding of these important childhood disorders.

Physiology of Urination and Defecation

The Physiology of Urination

The human bladder is a hollow organ made up of an inner epithelial layer (uroepithelium), a muscular layer (detrusor vesicae), and connective tissue. Urine is continuously collected as the ureters allow the passage of urine from the kidneys into the posterior portion of the bladder. As urine accumulates, the bladder stretches while the detrusor muscle relaxes, and the bladder neck and sphincter muscle contract to prevent the passage of urine into the urethra. As this occurs, an initial urge to urinate must be voluntarily suppressed until reaching a toilet.

Casey (2011) provides an excellent review of both healthy and atypical bladder function. The bladder has input from three different nervous system pathways: somatic, parasympathetic, and sympathetic. When controlling the urge to urinate, the somatic nervous system pathway is

M. Lewis and K.D. Rudolph (eds.), *Handbook of Developmental Psychopathology*,
DOI 10.1007/978-1-4614-9608-3_32, © Springer Science+Business Media New York 2014

stimulated, leading to contraction of the sphincter muscle to maintain continence. During this filling phase, the sympathetic nervous system assists by causing active relaxation of the detrusor muscle. Through this mechanism, the bladder can increase its volume without increasing its pressure.

When a conscious decision to urinate is made, or when the bladder reaches its capacity, the somatic pathway is inhibited, leading to sphincter relaxation. The parasympathetic nervous system pathway overcomes the sympathetic signals, causing contraction of the detrusor muscle. This increases the pressure within the bladder to exceed the pressure of the bladder outlet, allowing urination to occur (Casey, 2011).

Bladder control relies on careful coordination of the various neurological inputs. To achieve successful toilet training, a child must be trained to sense bladder filling, to coordinate the suppression of urination, and to release urine upon reaching a toilet. The inability to reach this developmental milestone is known as *urine incontinence* or, also termed, *enuresis*. Successful toilet training is presumed to involve increasing the individual's sensitivity to appropriate body signals and/or increasing voluntary control over the relevant muscles.

The Physiology of Defecation

The digestive tract is a long, hollow tube, with the colon (large intestines) and rectum at the distal end. After food is digested in the stomach and small intestine, the remaining waste products move through the colon and gradually shift from a liquid state to a semisolid state as water is reabsorbed. When sufficient waste accumulates, muscle contractions move that waste down the colon and into the rectum. The resultant stretching of the walls of the rectum leads to the urge to defecate, prompting the automatic relaxation of the internal anal sphincter. If convenient, voluntary actions allow for defecation to take place by relaxing the external anal sphincter and the puborectalis muscle. As this occurs, diaphragmatic contraction raises the intra-abdominal pressure to allow for the passage of stool

(Bharucha, 2008). The urge to defecate can be controlled until a toilet is available by the voluntary contraction of the external anal sphincter and the levator ani muscles. Alternately, the inability to exhibit control over these mechanisms is known as encopresis, defined as passing feces anywhere but into a toilet.

Developmental Considerations

Readiness in Typically Developing Children

Most parents in the USA focus on the task of toilet training between 2 and 3 years of age, and most children complete toilet training before their fourth birthdays. In other cultures, the timing of this active training phase may be older or indeed younger. Societal expectations about continence and parental methods to achieve that goal differ widely as well (Whiting & Child, 1953). In western cultures, where the active phase of toilet training typically occurs between 2 and 3 years of age, there are "readiness" skills that afford caregivers the opportunity to lay the groundwork for training. Usually, parents or caregivers recognize a child's adoption of regular routines for feeding and sleeping and note that the child has the communication skills and motivation to step up to the active training phase.

There are several important skills children need to acquire in order to succeed in toilet training. These can be framed in five domains: communication skills, social and emotional skills, fine motor skills, gross motor skills, and cognitive skills. In the communication realm, a child needs to convey to caretakers that the need to eliminate is imminent. The child's social-emotional development must be at a level to understand the parental or caretaker expectations of appropriate toilet use. Fine motor skills are required to manipulate such items as clothing or toilet paper, while gross motor skills are necessary to achieve the posture/positions for defecation and urination into a toilet. The cognitive requirements in toilet learning are several. Cognitive monitoring is required in the form of planfulness, self-control, and understanding the meaning of relevant bodily sensations. Parents and caretakers are helpful in this regard during the active training period, engaging in frequent prompting, inviting, reminding, or other close monitoring, and these efforts afford the child guidance to facilitate success.

Transient Regression

Once toilet learning is achieved, parental prompting generally continues for several months more, focused mostly on high-risk times when the child's motivation or attention might be challenged (e.g., before attending a birthday party and before car, train, or airplane journeys). Events involving major changes, whether stressful or joyous, such as moving to a new family home or the birth of a sibling, should be viewed as risks for relapse or regression with newly acquired toileting skills. Such regression is typically transient if managed appropriately and promptly, helping the child return to continent status. Importantly, these relapses, if short lived, do not merit a diagnosis of an elimination disorder.

Challenges in Children with Developmental Atypicalities

Children with developmental delays or atypicalities that impact communication skills, social and emotional development, fine or gross motor abilities, or more global cognitive skills face unusual challenges in toilet learning. For some, delaying toilet training affords the child more time to mature in developmental areas called into play in the training process. For others, modifications in communication, such as employing nonverbal signals or signs or training programs that enhance motivation to use the toilet or careful attention to clothing that does not require the more complex fine motor skills of unbuttoning or unzipping, may help to structure successful toilet learning. For others, parents and caretakers

might shift to time training, a method of scheduled toilet visits, often after meals or snacks, or perhaps even hourly, in lieu of the more typical combination of parental prompts and child recognition of bodily cues.

The challenges for children with significant developmental difficulties are several. Among them are managing such problems as fear of toilets, "pot phobia," poor engagement with parental/societal expectations, difficulty in identifying appropriate motivators or small rewards to strengthen appropriate behaviors in child training, or poor generalization of training success from one toilet or locale to others. Of note, quality of life for children with significant developmental disabilities and their families is certainly enhanced if continence can be achieved. Such children can participate in school excursions and a wider range of activities and will likely have more social options than children who remain untrained and require diaper changes and caretakers willing to attend to their cleanliness.

Nomenclature

Terminology

The terminology to define variations in types of childhood elimination disorders has not enjoyed firm standardization. In fact, the nomenclature of these disorders is frequently difficult or elusive, with terms that are seemingly interchangeable and with conditions that can be both a symptom and a disorder. Diagnosis is, in part, dependent on age or developmental status and impacted by functional or organic factors, further complicating the diagnostic schema. In this section, terminology is offered according to current literature preferences, and those labels will be used throughout this work as consistently as possible. Figures 32.1 and 32.2 reflect current terminology and distinctions of importance in urinary incontinence (continuous vs. intermittent, daytime vs. nocturnal) and fecal incontinence or encopresis.

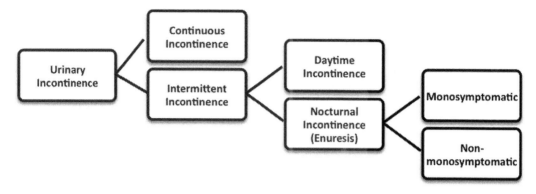

Fig. 32.1 Graphic representation of nomenclature of urinary incontinence

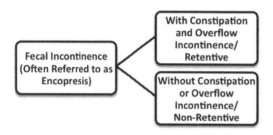

Fig. 32.2 Graphic representation of nomenclature of fecal incontinence

Important Dichotomies

Primary vs. Secondary Incontinence. Primary incontinence refers to a child of at least 5 years of age (for urinary incontinence) and 4 years of age (for fecal incontinence) who has never achieved continence. Secondary incontinence can only be diagnosed in a child who has become incontinent after achieving continence for at least 6 months.

The Functional-Organic Distinction. A fundamental distinction is made between elimination disorders thought to be of organic etiology and those that are functional. In the organic category are those disorders based on physical illness or structural abnormality with accompanying aberration of the workings of those structures. The functional disorders have no identifiable physical basis to explain their occurrence. This diagnosis of exclusion should not be made by casual judgment; although organically caused elimination disorders are rare, they can be extremely serious.

It is important to have any child with an elimination disorder checked by a physician to evaluate for possible organic contributions.

Urinary Incontinence

Work done in the fields of urology, general pediatrics, gastroenterology, and neurology sometimes utilizes nomenclature different from the Diagnostic and Statistical Manual of Mental Disorders (DSM-5). One such classification system that has been discussed and adopted in several research protocols is that proposed by the International Children's Continence Society in 2006 (Nevéus et al., 2006). Researchers had advocated for its inclusion (von Gontard, 2011), but this nomenclature was not adopted in DSM-5. Nonetheless, the terminology is utilized below because it provides for important clinical distinctions.

Continuous Incontinence vs. Intermittent Incontinence. Continuous incontinence means constant urine leakage and is associated with anatomic abnormalities. Intermittent incontinence is urine leakage that occurs in discrete amounts alternating with maintenance of urinary continence (Nevéus et al., 2006).

Nocturnal vs. Daytime Incontinence. The 2006 recommendations differentiate nocturnal incontinence, defined as enuresis, from daytime incontinence. Children who wet themselves during both the day- and nighttime have dual diagnoses, both daytime incontinence and enuresis. Daytime incontinence is characterized based on the frequency of incontinence, the voiding frequency in a 24-h period, voided volumes, and fluid intake. Children who suffer from urinary urgency are considered to have an overactive bladder (Nevéus et al., 2006).

Of note, the American Sleep Disorders Association has its own Classification Manual that describes the diagnostic criteria for "Sleep Enuresis," which is "characterized by recurrent involuntary micturition that occurs during sleep" (Diagnostic Classification Steering Committee, 1991, p. 101).

Monosymptomatic vs. Nonmonosymptomatic Enuresis. Children who present with enuresis (nighttime incontinence) alone without bladder dysfunction are considered to have monosymptomatic enuresis. Children with enuresis and other lower urinary tract symptoms are considered to have nonmonosymptomatic enuresis. These additional symptoms can include abnormal voiding frequency (considered fewer than or equal to three voids or more than or equal to eight voids daily), daytime incontinence, urgency, hesitancy at initiation of micturition, pain, or abnormal urine stream (including a weak stream, intermittency, or straining) (Nevéus et al., 2006).

Fecal Incontinence

Retentive vs. Nonretentive Encopresis The Diagnostic and Statistical Manual of Mental Disorders, 5th Edition, makes a distinction between encopresis with constipation and overflow incontinence and encopresis without these features (American Psychiatric Association, 2013). Fecal incontinence in children with evidence of constipation on physical exam or by history occurs as a result of leakage of generally poorly formed stool. This more common cause of encopresis is referred to as retentive constipation and overflow incontinence. In fact, Loening-Baucke (2007) reports that among a cohort of children with constipation, 18.3 % had functional fecal incontinence, but among children without constipation, only 0.3 % had functional fecal incontinence.

Retentive encopresis can become a vicious cycle. In its normal state, the rectal vault is empty. However, when a person withholds stool voluntarily, the rectum and lower colon become filled with fecal material. If withholding continues, a large quantity of stool will accumulate, and, as a result, the lower colon will become very distended. Concurrently, the body will absorb almost all of the water from the fecal mass, leaving hard, impacted stool. In this condition, passing stool is extremely painful or impossible, compounding the problem and causing the child to withhold to avoid the pain. The urge and ability to defecate are therefore significantly reduced. Fluid-containing stool from the upper colon now can no longer be passed due to obstruction of the rectum. But liquid stool will almost invariably leak around the impacted fecal mass, producing soiled underwear.

Accompanying the retentive pattern may also be inappropriate closure of the external anal sphincter precisely at times when its relaxation is necessary for proper defecation. This "paradoxical constriction" of the sphincter can delay defecation or truncate the experience, yielding only partial defecation, further compounding the child's constipation. It is therefore not surprising that a history of painful and effortful defecation is present in the majority of children who suffer from fecal soiling (Partin, Hamill, Fischel, & Partin, 1992). Children who suffer from encopresis without constipation or overflow incontinence tend to have encopretic feces that are "of normal form and consistency" (American Psychiatric Association, 2013, p. 358).

These distinctions are adopted into the literature using the following terms: retentive encopresis to describe fecal incontinence with constipation and nonretentive encopresis to describe fecal incontinence without constipation. Literature in the last decade, however, sometimes refers to *soiling* and *overflow soiling* to describe the retentive pattern more specifically (Dobson & Rogers, 2009; Murphy & Carney, 2004), while researchers and practitioners also utilize the term *soiling* as a simple descriptor of fecal incontinence.

Prevalence

The prevalence of the childhood elimination disorders is difficult to quantify, both because of the various methodologies used to estimate prevalence and the definitional issues described above that have been modified over time. It is clear that prevalence estimates for both urinary and fecal incontinence decrease with increasing age, and the prevalence of urinary incontinence outweighs that of fecal incontinence by a factor of about three or more. Approximately 5–10 % of 5-year-olds, 3–5 % of 10-year-olds, and about 1 % of 15-year-olds or beyond meet the definition for urinary incontinence (American Psychiatric Association, 2013). Some authors have found substantially higher prevalence rates, especially when looking at enuresis alone (Joinson et al., 2007; von Gontard, Heron, & Joinson, 2011). The prevalence of fecal incontinence at age 5 years has been estimated at 1–2.2 % (American Psychiatric Association, 2013; Bellman, 1966) and at age 6 years at 1.4–1.9 % (Bellman, 1966; von Gontard, Moritz, Thome-Granz, & Freitag, 2011).

Etiological Considerations

A number of broad models have been put forth as general explanations of functional (nonorganic) elimination disorders. These may be structured along parallel paths for enuresis and encopresis. Additionally, two models have emerged with a focus on the etiology of nocturnal enuresis, or monosymptomatic nocturnal enuresis, the most prevalent of the elimination disorders. One provides a predominantly physiologically based conceptual framework, and one highlights potential neurodevelopmental underpinnings of the disorder. While there are variations within each of the following approaches, no causal model of the elimination disorders is complete without acknowledgment of the familial nature of the disorders, that is, the disorders tend to run in families (Bellman, 1966; von Gontard, Heron, et al., 2011). Evidence to that effect suggests that a genetic etiological picture deserves continued exploration.

The Psychodynamic Model

According to a psychodynamic formulation, toilet training reflects a psychological conflict between child and parents, one that must be resolved in the child's psyche before full continence is attained. In this perspective, achievement of bladder and bowel control occurs during the anal stage of psychosexual development. Inspired by psychodynamic views that parent–child conflict or poor parent–child dynamics may be characteristic of the family with an incontinent child (e.g., Stein, 1998), one might interpret the correlation between parent–child conflict and elimination disorders by assuming that the interpersonal conflicts cause the elimination disorders. In contrast, such conflicts are interpretable as the effects rather than the cause of incontinence (Vivian, Fischel, & Liebert, 1986). In their discussion of enuresis from a biopsychosocial perspective, Bischof and Benson (2004) provide an interesting discussion of family characteristics, acknowledging the difficulty in determining causal pathways of impact.

The Learning or Skills Deficit Model

According to the learning/skills deficit model, individuals with elimination disorders have not received the amount or kind of training necessary to become continent. A child's failure to become continent may occur because caregivers or parents used inadequate teaching methods or perhaps because the child was an unusually slow learner or learned faulty elimination skills. In sum, the child is presumed to have not yet learned to attend and respond appropriately to bodily cues indicating the need to eliminate.

When applied to the case of nocturnal enuresis, the learning or skills deficit model might suggest that the child has not developed adequate learned arousal from sleep in response to cues of a full bladder (Moffatt, 1997). When applied to retentive encopresis, the learning or skills deficit model might be exemplified by escape and avoidance learning. Whether initial toilet training was "complete" or not, a child who experiences highly effortful or uncomfortable stool passage gradually learns to avoid defecating. Whatever the cause of painful defecation may have been initially, the acquired tendency to inappropriately suppress the urge to defecate by stopping the necessary sphincter relaxation eventually leads to stool retention, overdistention of the rectal vault, and inordinately hard and large fecal matter retained instead of released. Subsequent attempts to defecate will prove uncomfortable, which the child avoids or escapes by further stool retention, compounding the problem.

The Improper Diet Hypothesis

A third etiological model of elimination disorders is the improper diet hypothesis. According to this view, dietary excesses or deficits cause problems with voiding or defecating. In the case of retentive encopresis, diets with inadequate roughage are considered to potentiate constipation and effortful, painful stools with the eventual development of withholding. In parallel fashion, enuresis is sometimes blamed on excess fluid intake during the hours just before bedtime.

Neurodevelopmental Immaturity or Delay

Bed-wetting beyond the age of 5 years and without other clear organic or pathological findings is the most prevalent of the elimination disorders and has spawned interest in etiological considerations. Subtle developmental delay, subtle maturational delay, or difficult temperament are raised in considerations of etiological or concomitant factors associated with bed-wetting, day wetting, or soiling problems (Joinson, Heron, Butler, & von Gontard, 2006; Joinson et al., 2008; Sethi, Bhargava, & Shipra, 2005). Speculation of neurodevelopmental atypicalities or immaturity, sometimes focused on bladder control, but more recently viewed in a broader

framework, has received research attention in a number of studies. For example, an increased frequency of bed-wetting in children with, compared to children without, minor neurological dysfunction has been noted (Lunsing, Hadders-Algra, Touwen, & Huisjes, 1991). Further support for maturational deficits in motor performance is found in work focusing on the brain stem in an extensive assessment of the motor function of children with, and comparison children without, nocturnal enuresis (Freitag, Rohling, Seifen, Pukrop, & von Gontard, 2006). These studies suggest that maturational deficits in motor cortex circuitry may play a role in the development of enuresis (von Gontard, Freitag, Seifen, Pukrop, & Rohling, 2006). Support for a neurodevelopmental model can be found in the expectation that prevalence rates of intermittent urinary incontinence diminish with age.

A Three-Systems View of Enuresis

Butler and Holland (2000) and Butler (2004) have proposed a "three systems" model of children's nocturnal enuresis, with supporting evidence from the literature to assert that one or more physiologic/biochemical/psychologic systems is functioning inadequately in enuretic children. The model includes (a) excessive nocturnal urine production (because of a lack of circadian rhythmicity and inadequate production of vasopressin during sleep), (b) bladder overactivity, and (c) the inability to awaken from sleep when the bladder is full. Importantly, the model does not implicate "deep sleep," as enuresis appears to be uncorrelated with sleep stage, but rather the inability to arouse in response to important bladder capacity cues. The model provides guidance for considering treatment options such as the urine alarm and anticholinergic medication (Butler, 2004) or perhaps the use of focused training exercises such as the holding exercise (Van Hoeck et al., 2007) by identifying the probable etiologic cause among the three described above and selecting a therapy considered to be most appropriate for that causal pathway.

Risk Factors and Concomitant Problems

A number of concomitant conditions have been considered as contributors to, correlates of, or risk factors for the elimination disorders. Several of these are reviewed here. Note, however, that consensus is missing on four key issues: (1) prioritizing the relative importance of each, (2) careful attention to the prevalence of each, (3) evidence base for a singular or unique model of contribution vs. a multifaceted one, and (4) evidence for causal vs. correlative relationships between elimination disorders and concomitant conditions.

Concomitant Problems with Affective, Behavioral, and Social Characteristics

Psychological and behavioral problems often co-occur with elimination disorders. Understanding these relationships is challenging, but the co-occurrence affirms the importance of appropriate screening for affective, behavioral, academic, or social concerns. Further, treatment success may be impacted by concomitant difficulties (Stark, Spirito, Lewis, & Hart, 1990), whether eventually viewed as causal or correlated characteristics.

Enuresis and Self-Esteem, Attachment, and Prosocial Skills. Studies with relatively small samples have explored the psychological correlates of enuresis from a variety of perspectives. For example, a Brazilian study embedded in the Rorschach method found that a sample of children with enuresis (not of organic origin, predominantly primary enuretics) demonstrated characteristics of lower self-esteem than controls (Semer & Yezigi, 2009). An Italian study in which enuretics and nonenuretics were matched on gender and age also found significantly lower self-esteem, as well as lower incidence of secure attachment, and higher rates of behavioral difficulties for the enuretic sample, with no differences in six dimensions of temperament studied between

groups. Of note, the behavior difficulties spanned a wide range of characteristics, including conduct and emotional problems, hyperactivity, diminished prosocial behaviors, and difficulty with peers (Coppola, Costantini, et al. 2011). Zink, Freitag and von Gontard (2008) reported that in their sample of children between 5 and 16 years of age with day and night wetting disorders referred to a tertiary care center for evaluation of behavioral concerns, the Achenbach Child Behavior Checklist (CBCL) completed by parents demonstrated that externalizing disorders were more than twice as likely to be present than internalizing disorders. Within the subset of children with monosymptomatic nocturnal enuresis, both internalizing disorders and the frequency of occurrence of at least one ICD-10 psychiatric diagnosis were diminished compared with children for whom nonmonosymptomatic nocturnal enuresis or urge incontinence or voiding postponement were diagnosed. Again employing the parent completed CBCL in an evaluation of over 300 5- to 7-year-olds in Istanbul, Erdogan et al. (2008) found that children with enuresis had elevated total problem scores and elevated social problem scale scores compared with nonenuretics, but the percentage of children with elevated scores that reached the clinically significant range of the CBCL did not differ between the two groups.

Enuresis and Attentional Problems. Particular focus has been given to the prevalence of attention-deficit/hyperactivity disorder (ADHD) as an associated finding for children with enuresis. This is an interesting association, as ADHD is among the most prevalent of childhood psychological problems and the co-occurrence of ADHD and elimination disorders stimulate consideration of immaturity or delays in central nervous system function in the context of etiological hypotheses (Shreeram, He, Kalaydjian, Brothers, & Merikangas, 2009). von Gontard, Moritz, and colleagues (2011) identified an association between attention-deficit/hyperactivity disorder and enuresis, particularly *daytime* urinary incontinence. Baeyens et al. (2004) found an impressively increased occurrence of attention-deficit/

hyperactivity disorder associated with enuresis (based on a mostly nonmonosymptomatic nocturnal enuretic sample) in their university hospital setting in Belgium. And their 2-year follow-up study suggested that the presence of ADHD increased the probability of continuing with difficult-to-cure enuresis. Specifically, enuretics with ADHD were over three times more likely to have continued enuresis than children without ADHD (Baeyens et al., 2005). The authors provided a further 4-year follow-up report, in which 64 % of the baseline attention-deficit/hyperactivity disorder diagnoses were reconfirmed. At that end point, the continued occurrence of enuresis had declined and did not differ between children with and children without an initial or a 4-year follow-up point diagnosis of attention-deficit/hyperactivity disorder (Baeyens, Roeyers, Van Erdeghem, Hoebeke, & Vande Walle, 2007). In other words, the early trajectory of the co-occurrence of the two disorders suggests delayed achievement of continence, while 4-year outcomes do not appear to differ between children with or without ADHD.

In a nationally representative sample of US children aged 8–11 years, attention-deficit/hyperactivity disorder was highly associated with nocturnal incontinence (Shreeram et al., 2009). As Shreeram et al. (2009) and others point out, it is clearly important to further disentangle subcategories of attentional disorders, elimination disorders, and the outcomes of interest in these data, when treatment is ongoing for enuresis, attention-deficit/hyperactivity disorder, or both.

Encopresis and Anxiety, Depression, and Attentional, School-Related and Disruptive, and Oppositional Problems. The associated behavioral problems and lower self-esteem suggested in studies of childhood enuresis are echoed in investigations of the concomitant difficulties of children with encopretic problems. However, there appears to be less specificity in identifying any one or set of consistent problems concomitant with fecal incontinence (von Gontard, Baeyens, Van Hoecke, Warzak, & Bachmann, 2011). Joinson and colleagues (2006) reported that a large population-based sample of children

aged 7–8 years with soiling problems experienced significantly higher rates of anxiety disorders, depressive disorders, and attentional and oppositional disorders, with rates of most of these disorders increasing as a function of frequency of soiling. Cox, Morris, Borowitz, and Sutphen (2002) utilized an extensive set of psychometric evaluations to investigate differences between children with and without chronic encopresis. They found substantial evidence for the more likely presence of school achievement problems, anxiety and depressive symptoms, family environment difficulties, more attentional problems, social problems, and increased disruptive behavior for children with encopresis compared with those without the difficulty. Interestingly, the lower self-esteem sometimes reported as characteristic of these children did not reach significance in this sample.

While there remain a number of nuanced and perhaps tangled findings in our understanding of the possible affective, behavioral, and social problems associated with the elimination disorders, it is clear that psychological issues occur at disproportionately higher rates in children with vs. without elimination difficulties. Such considerations make the comprehensiveness of evaluation as well as the careful consideration of treatment of clinical symptoms beyond the elimination disorder all the more important in the effort to enhance both treatment adherence and success (von Gontard, Baeyens, et al., 2011).

Concomitant Problems with Biophysical Characteristics

Several variables have been explored from a biophysical context in the search for correlates or causes of the functional elimination disorders. For example, smaller bladder capacity, hormonal variations, or circadian rhythm disturbances have been explored in the study of urinary incontinence (Jackson, 2007; Van Hoeck et al., 2007) and hormonal variations, as well as motility issues have been explored in the study of fecal incontinence (e.g., Raghunath et al., 2011; Stern et al., 1995).

Sleep Apnea/Sleep Disturbances. Recent studies have documented a relationship between enuresis and sleep disordered breathing or obstructive sleep apnea (OSA). For example, Barone et al. (2009) found that 80 % of children with mono-symptomatic nocturnal enuresis had OSA, compared with 45.1 % without monosymptomatic nocturnal enuresis. Bascom et al. (2011) found a statistically significant difference in sleep disordered breathing among children with enuresis and daytime incontinence compared to children with monosymptomatic enuresis alone.

The etiological mechanism thought to be responsible for this relationship is related to the increases in intrathoracic pressure from apneic episodes. In turn, this increased pressure transmitted to the right atrium of the heart may result in the release of natriuretic peptides, increasing the excretion of sodium and water, thus increasing urine volume. Therefore, a plausible biological mechanism may link the presence of OSA to the development of enuresis through the production of large urine volumes (Su et al., 2011).

Other studies have been unable to find a uniform association between OSA symptoms and the prevalence of enuresis. For example, Su et al. (2011) found that among males, there was no correlation between OSA and the enuresis prevalence. But among females, the prevalence of nocturnal enuresis increased with increasing severity of OSA symptoms as assessed by a sleep questionnaire. Utilizing home sleep studies, Bader, Nevéus, Kruse, and Sillen (2002) found minor differences in the sleep of children with and without enuresis, namely, an increased number of shorter sleep cycles during the night in enuretic children, but their results lacked a correlation between OSA and enuresis. In conclusion, while sleep disordered breathing and OSA may provide a plausible biological mechanism for explaining enuresis, current data do not consistently demonstrate a relationship.

Breast-Feeding. Enuresis is thought to be related to developmental delay, and breast-feeding is thought to be a protective factor against developmental delay. Therefore, researchers have attempted to analyze the relationship between enuresis and breast-feeding. A study of 55 cases and 117 controls suggests that breast-feeding is protective against enuresis (Barone et al., 2006). While this single study suggests a correlation, the protective effects of breast-feeding on the development of enuresis must be confirmed.

Genetic Factors. Although specific genetic factors have not been fully elucidated, there is a clear family history associated with enuresis. It is estimated that about 75 % of children with primary nocturnal enuresis (in other terminology, this is monosymptomatic primary enuresis) have a first-degree relative who also had the condition (Bayoumi et al., 2006). A family history of bedwetting was associated more commonly with cases of enuretic children than nonenuretic controls (Barone et al., 2006). Results from twin studies provide further evidence of heritability; for example, in a large Finnish twin cohort, the concordance of enuresis was higher among monozygotic (identical) than dizygotic (fraternal) twins (Hublin, Kaprio, Partinen, & Koskenvuo, 1998). Because monozygotic twins share more genetic material than dizygotic twins, this lends further weight to the genetic implications of the development of enuresis. Specific genes have been investigated among families with multiple cases of enuresis (e.g., Bayoumi et al., 2006). However, clear linkage patterns have not been consistently observed across multiple populations, suggesting the need for additional research to find the genes responsible for the observed hereditary phenomena.

Hypercalciuria. It has been suggested that increased urinary calcium excretion, known as *hypercalciuria*, is related to nocturnal enuresis. Researchers have found that hypercalciuria is more common among children with nocturnal enuresis than among continent children (Raes et al., 2010). For example, when 24-h urine calcium was measured (a more accurate measurement technique than a random urine calcium level) in a study of 122 enuretic children and 110 continent children, 21.3 % of the enuretic children had hypercalciuria compared with 4.5 % of children without enuresis (Valavi, Ahmadzadeh, Hooman, & Aminzadeh, 2011).

Nocturnal hypercalciuria (higher quantities of calcium excreted at night in urine) has been identified as significantly more common in children with nocturnal enuresis than in children without nocturnal enuresis (Aceto et al., 2003). This suggests that the nighttime excretion of calcium in urine may create nocturnal diuresis of large urinary volumes, perhaps potentiating the development of enuresis.

Demographic Variables. Prevalence estimates of the elimination disorders vary markedly. In a population-based sample with a mean age of 7.3 years, the prevalence of daytime urinary incontinence among boys is 13.7 % and among girls, 21.5 %, when children with mild, moderate, and severe incontinence were included (Sureshkumar, Jones, Cumming, & Craig, 2009). Additional data support the near equality of prevalence of daytime wetting at 8 years of age (7 and 8.7 %, respectively, for boys and girls) (Joinson et al., 2007), while other research suggests a male predominance, with 4.1 % of males and 3.0 % of females in a geographically defined sample of children with mean age of 6.22 years suffering from daytime incontinence (von Gontard, Moritz, et al., 2011).

For nocturnal enuresis, there is a male predominance (Sureshkumar, Jones, Caldwell, & Craig, 2009). At age 8, 21 % of males and 10.8 % of females were bed wetters (Joinson et al., 2007), and at age 7, the difference was 12.9 vs. 6.4 %, respectively (von Gontard, Moritz, et al., 2011).

More males than females suffer from encopresis, in a ratio of approximately 3–6 boys for every girl affected (Bellman, 1966; Har & Croffie, 2010). Loening-Baucke (2007) cites a prevalence of fecal incontinence among boys at 7.3 and 1.3 % among girls. Others find a less disparate ratio among 8-year-olds, with 8.8 % males and 4.8 % of females affected with soiling (Joinson et al., 2007), and still others find no difference in prevalence between boys and girls at age 7 (von Gontard, Moritz, et al., 2011). Of note, researchers

have found no relationship between encopresis and socioeconomic status, family size, birth order, or parental age.

Evaluation

Criteria for Diagnosis

The diagnosis of each elimination disorder should emerge from a careful interview of parent(s) and, as appropriate, the child. It is our preference to use a highly structured initial consultation, including a thorough toileting history and a determination of whether parents or other family members have experienced similar problems. Clear information must be gathered about the age of onset, to help determine primary or secondary status; correlates of onset (e.g., important family changes, start of school); current frequency of wetting or soiling; and social, behavioral, or cognitive symptoms that might impact the problem or its treatment. Especially important to learn is whether the problem has been brought to the attention of a physician. A physical examination is always requested if the child has not had one recently that included discussion of this concern. It is also essential to learn what the family is doing about the problem right now and require discontinuation of treatments or practices that seem inappropriate.

Key to accurate diagnosis is the guideline provided by DSM criteria. For encopresis, DSM guidelines require a chronological or developmental level of 4 years and passage of feces into inappropriate places, whether involuntary or intentional, at least once monthly for at least 3 months, and not attributable to other medical conditions except the involvement of constipation (American Psychiatric Association, 2013, p. 357). For enuresis, DSM guidelines require that the child be voiding into the bed or clothing, whether involuntarily or intentionally, at least twice weekly for at least 3 consecutive months or must cause significant distress or impairment; the child must achieve a chronological or developmental age of 5 years (American Psychiatric Association, 2013, p. 355).

Treatment Considerations

A variety of treatment approaches to the elimination disorders have emerged from the work of researchers and clinicians in the several disciplines interested in these problems. There is no singular standard treatment for either the voiding or the defecation disorders. There is consensus, however, that a careful medical review of the child's symptoms is warranted and that careful classification of the problem as primary vs. secondary may be important to illuminate fuller concern for organic problems or psychological considerations that deserve prompt attention (see McGrath, Mellon, and Murphy (2000) and Mellon and McGrath (2000) for a discussion of the importance of both medical and psychological assessment before intervention). In this section we will focus on what is known about management approaches for the elimination disorders.

Treatment for Monosymptomatic Primary Enuresis

Historical Treatments. Several writers have described cruel and barbarous methods of managing enuresis from ancient times to only hundreds of years ago. Mattresses with protruding metal spikes, penile tourniquets, and electrical currents are among the practices once touted as treatments (Bloom, 1993; Mishne, 1993).

Current Treatment Approaches. Present-day treatments range from pharmaceutical to behavioral methods, with exercises to alter bladder capacity and tone, and a number of combination strategies to address what is appreciated to be a challenging problem. The preponderance of behavioral methods includes a urine alarm as a key component of treatment, although verbal psychotherapies, counseling, simple reward programs, fluid restriction before bedtime, and hypnosis have been utilized. The urine alarm method, initially popularized by Mowrer and Mowrer (1938), relies on the initial drops of urine to initiate the alarm, expose the child to the alarm's sound, and awaken the sleeping bed wetter.

Sometimes the alarm is enhanced by adding an open intercom to the parental bedroom so that an adult can join and guide the child appropriately to address the supposed deep sleep characteristic of bed wetters. Eventually, with nightly use over several weeks, one learns to "avoid" being startled by the alarm by maintaining continence or awakening before the alarm signals in response to cues of bladder fullness so that voiding urine can occur into the toilet.

In the past several decades, urine alarm training has been combined with a number of other methods in the effort to enhance or speed its success and to diminish relapse once initial arrest of bed-wetting has been accomplished. The resulting "packages" of procedures and behavioral contingencies are favored by researchers (see Houts, Berman, & Abramson, 1994), although it is unclear whether or which additional procedures might enhance success rates, produce more rapid continence, or diminish relapse. Nonetheless, training times are generally at least 8 weeks, and relapse remains a concern of behavioral packages and pharmacological strategies alike.

Among the first such behavioral packages to be described was full-spectrum home training (FSHT) (Houts & Liebert, 1984; Houts, Liebert, & Padawer, 1983). An updated description of FSHT can be found in Houts (2003) which details the several components of the program: (1) urine alarm treatment; (2) a carefully executed family support agreement, with specific responsibilities for parent(s) and child; (3) a daily record to monitor wet and dry nights; (4) a daytime bladder training exercise initially described by Kimmel and Kimmel (1970), now known as retention control training, with the goal of expanding the child's ability to hold urine comfortably; (5) overlearning, an adjunctive procedure pioneered by Young and Morgan (1972) to prevent relapse; and (6) an optional waking component based on the work of Azrin, Sneed, and Foxx (1974) to facilitate achieving the initial goal of 14 consecutive dry nights.

Houts et al. (1994) provide an extensive and rigorous evaluation of the two current broad approaches to treatment, psychological and pharmacological interventions, as well as evaluation of placebo or no-treatment controls. Their review examined 78 published reports in which data met specific criteria for inclusion in their effectiveness analysis. Among the most pertinent findings was the fact that cessation of bed-wetting at posttreatment favored children who received treatment—either psychological or pharmacological—over those receiving placebos or no treatment. This finding provides support for the view that recommending treatment is a prudent step, in contrast with a "wait and see" approach where the delay might impact social and affective spheres adversely (Houts et al., 1994). At follow-up in their review, Houts et al. found that children receiving psychological treatment modalities continued to show superior outcomes to controls, while those receiving pharmacological interventions no longer differed significantly from controls. In further analyses, which included a covariate marker of investigator "allegiance" to one method or another, two treatments, the alarm and desmopressin, had stronger outcomes by the end of treatment than three other treatment categories (psychological therapy without urine alarm, tricyclics, or other medications). And at follow-up, those utilizing the urine alarm in psychological treatment had more favorable outcomes than all other treatments.

Daytime Incontinence and Secondary Incontinence. Daytime intermittent incontinence and the onset of either day or night incontinence after a substantial period of continence has been achieved are much less frequent than monosymptomatic primary enuresis. These conditions have not received nearly as much research attention as the nighttime problem. Such conditions deserve careful medical review for infection, significant constipation, or other organic concerns and relevant psychological review for behavioral concerns and for significant stressors impacting the child's health. Additionally, a careful inquiry into the child's access to comfortable and clean school bathrooms or scheduled access to the nursing office bathroom may be warranted. Interestingly, a prospective investigation of the age of initiation of toilet training within the Avon Longitudinal Study of Parents and Children provides suggestive data

on subsequent diurnal wetting difficulties when training has been delayed until after 2 years of age (Joinson et al., 2009). Treatments including timed voiding (Allen, Austin, Boyt, Hawtrey, & Cooper, 2007) have improved daytime incontinence, and the utilization of systematic retention control training as a bladder-toning exercise has sometimes joined into our treatment package as well.

Treatment for Encopresis with Constipation or History of Constipation

A number of different treatments have been tried for encopresis. For review of the treatment spectrum, from psychotherapy and play therapy to hypnosis; biofeedback; holistic, integrative, or complementary/alternative medicine; Internet-enhanced intervention; and behavioral interventions, see Brooks et al. (2000), Culbert and Banez (2007), Howe and Walker (1992), McGrath et al. (2000), and Ritterband et al. (2008). Few treatments have been evaluated in rigorous and controlled methodological comparison studies, and samples in such research tend to be relatively small. Of additional concern to practitioners and researchers alike is the fact that sample selection is often of the convenience sort, with subjects who have failed medical management and recommended for psychological intervention (e.g., Stark, 2000); treatment components are often described without sufficient detail or fidelity evaluation (McGrath et al., 2000); varying procedures for initial constipation treatment and cleanout have not been rigorously compared; and outcomes of "improvement" are not provided in a consistent metric across studies (Brooks et al., 2000). Despite these methodological considerations, there is reasonable consensus that the most successful efforts to treat encopresis appear to be founded on behavioral management principles used in conjunction with laxative or stool softener and dietary prescriptions (e.g., Weissman & Bridgemohan, 2009). These are often referred to as mixed medical-behavioral (Brooks et al., 2000), combination, or package treatments. Such joint management approaches appear to receive optimal attention in the recent literature, with behavioral management addressing a broad spectrum of skills, a training structure, schedules for toilet sitting, techniques for handling toilet refusal, and carefully planned positive reinforcement and with medical management addressing initial medical evaluation, pharmacologic aids, and dietary recommendations (Reimers, 1996; Weissman & Bridgemohan, 2009).

Treatment for the child with encopresis and current constipation or significant holding behavior usually includes (1) medical cleanout plan followed by the ongoing use of a stool softener or laxative under physician supervision; (2) a prescribed toilet-sitting schedule as a behavioral technique and as a caregiver-guided adjunct to medical management; (3) a dietary program to enhance fiber and assure adequate water intake; (4) education about the disorder and its management steps and expectations; and (5) behavioral management strategies to increase stooling frequency, increase toilet use, and decrease soiling. The behavioral strategies will be addressed more fully below.

While detailed training protocols may be found in the literature (e.g., Friman, Hofstadter, & Jones, 2006), studies on treatment often lack data on dosage of the intervention(s) and on their families' fidelity to the intervention techniques (see McGrath et al., 2000). Further, we find that some degree of custom tailoring is often required for each family, because families have often tried, in sequential fashion, several strategies with varying consistency before seeking consultation, and every child has his or her individual training needs. For example, the child who is reluctant to toilet sit poses a challenge to the scheduled toilet-sitting requirement. This deserves evaluation to ascertain whether the interpersonal dynamics of caregiver and child are significantly problematic, whether the child is displaying pot phobic characteristics, or if the child is showing expected levels of anxiety or toilet refusal, perhaps related to earlier constipation and pain on stool passage. Caregivers need help in accomplishing toilet sitting when the child is somewhat oppositional or fearful. Some children are responsive to being "paid back" if cooperative, and we recommend payback in the form of time (minutes) back for the

time spent on the toilet, often easing toilet-sitting struggles substantially.

Behavioral management strategies aimed at enhancing soft stools and regular defecation differ from one another in their particulars, but all seem to include a set of key components, namely, record keeping; scheduled toilet sitting; structured toilet-skills training with systematic reinforcement of appropriate behaviors; family education about the problem; and laxative, stool softener, and/or dietary intervention.

Ensuring Soft and Frequent Stool Passage

For children with retentive encopresis, the first goal is to clear the rectal vault, using enemas, suppositories, stool softeners, or laxatives per pediatrician or pediatric gastroenterologist advice. (Montgomery and Navarro (2008) and Weissman and Bridgemohan (2009) offer tables of the most common choices.) Stool passage in a timely manner is important, as it precludes the moisture reabsorption that would otherwise result in hard stools and painful defecation, and it better controls excessively large stools; timely stool passage also diminishes the need for behaviors and postures that exercise the child's skills in holding back.

Record Keeping

Record keeping is instituted to help monitor the frequency of occurrence and the time of day of soiling incidents as well as the occurrence of successful toilet use, both prompted and spontaneous. Records are helpful to the clinician in reviewing frequency of stooling and in identifying times of day or days of the week that might be "high risk" for soiling incidents. With that knowledge, one might modify the toilet-sitting plan accordingly to be preventive. One expects prompted or scheduled toilet visits to be predominant at the start of training, but recognition of the bodily need and spontaneous toilet approach is essential to the eventual independence of successful toileting.

Scheduled Toilet Sitting

It is useful to establish a daily schedule of toilet-sitting times for the child or appropriate prompting to visit the toilet (Kuhn, Marcus, & Pitner, 1999;

Levine & Bakow, 1976). Attention should be paid to relevant aspects of the child's routine and the timing of medication in selecting toilet-sitting times, as well as an opportunity to sit after meals or snacks to work with the gastrocolic reflex. The use of adaptor seats, potty-training chairs, or the standard toilet should be dependent on the child's age, preference, and convenience.

Systematic Reinforcement

A central behavioral technique for controlling encopresis and motivating proper toilet use is systematic reinforcement of appropriate behaviors. An important reward is immediate social praise, which is always given for successful stool passage on the toilet and for appropriate toilet sitting, including both scheduled and spontaneous sits. Along with social reward, small immediate rewards for defecation in the toilet can be helpful for younger children as a motivator both to work on this skill and perform at the toilet. For nonretentive encopretic children, days of "no soiling" deserve reward, but care must be taken not to reward "no soiling" without some link to proper defecation in the toilet, as retentive behavior might inadvertently be strengthened.

The initial goal for severely retentive young children with a history of fear or pain on defecation is to bring them to the status of soft, frequent stool, even when the toilet is not used and a diaper is used instead. Social praise and small rewards can be helpful in that regard. Once stooling is repeatedly experienced as both appropriately frequent and without pain, fear, or emotionality, the more active phase of toilet training may be started, with systematic reinforcement, record keeping, and scheduled toilet sits.

Helpful Additions to Management

It can be useful to end a day in which soiling has occurred with a warm bath, because soiling often signals incomplete evacuation of feces. A bath affords a young child a context of relaxation or play that might facilitate stool passage.

Parents should guide children's skill development in cleanliness training and appropriate removal of soiled undergarments. These skills are dependent upon the child's age, but the eventual goal of self-cleaning needs to be incorporated into the training plans as appropriate, so that the ultimate outcome is a child with healthy and relatively independent toileting skills.

There is often a dramatic initial reduction in soiling behavior in the early weeks after combination training for encopresis is initiated with the multiple components described above. This initial arrest has reasonable probability to be sustained when careful and continued monitoring for adherence to the plan's several components is a priority. Caregivers sometimes take initial improvement over a first few weeks as a signal to pull away from close monitoring; this is not recommended because the self-regulation required of the child may be inadequately established early on, and the supports of a multipronged behavioral management plan are important to shifting the child's stooling interest, skills, and habits. Treatment failure and relapse are difficult realities deserving of best efforts to identify and rectify whatever the problematic issues may be.

Treatment Challenges

Secondary Disorders. The most encouraging fact about the functional elimination disorders is that successful treatments exist for the most common forms, especially those that fit one of the specific learning models. Of concern and deserving of very careful evaluation and review are cases involving the functional enuretic or encopretic disorders *after* initial continence has been achieved for several months or years or those that appear to be unresponsive to reasonable treatment modalities and excellent family adherence.

Children with Special Needs. Children with a variety of developmental disorders can bring challenging variations in motivation; behavioral repertoire; fine and gross motor coordination; and intellectual, language, and social interactional skills to the development of their self-help skills. Even typical toilet training, whether initiated at the typical age range for training or somewhat later, might require modifications for children with specific developmental problems.

Identifying developmental readiness in the child with a developmental disability can be problematic and sometimes requires explicit training of language or gestures to cue or announce toileting needs. For some, readiness skills or motivation may be lacking, but frequent toilet visits can be an optimal way to achieve continence in between toilet visits, or skills may best be introduced and discretely taught in small steps (Weissman & Bridgemohan, 2009). Appropriate rewards need to be identified carefully if they are to serve, in fact, as positive reinforcers of the toileting behaviors being trained. Achieving reliable toileting skill is an important, albeit challenging goal for those guiding the educational, social, recreational, and family participations of children with developmental problems.

In Sum

The elimination disorders are a set of prominent and important childhood disorders that enjoy active theorizing about etiologies with abundant research on correlates and comorbidities as well as strong research interest in the effectiveness of a variety of treatment approaches. Nonetheless, there are important gaps in our understanding of these disorders and in the evidence base for their optimal management. Developing the toileting skills to achieve reliable continence is a significant milestone of early childhood. Disorders of elimination that delay, challenge, or interfere with this accomplishment deserve careful and timely professional evaluation and prudent management so that a repertoire of skills supporting a healthy elimination pattern can be achieved.

References

Aceto, G., Penza, R., Coccioli, M. S., Palumbo, F., Cresta, L., Cimador, M., et al. (2003). Enuresis subtypes based on nocturnal hypercalciuria: A multicenter study. *Journal of Urology, 170*(4 Pt 2), 1670–1673.

Allen, H. A., Austin, J. C., Boyt, M. A., Hawtrey, C. E., & Cooper, C. S. (2007). Initial trial of timed voiding is warranted for all children with daytime incontinence. *Urology, 69*(5), 962–965.

American Psychiatric Association. (2013). *Diagnostic and statistical manual of mental disorders* (5th ed.), Arlington, VA: American Psychiatric Association.

Azrin, N. H., Sneed, T. J., & Foxx, R. M. (1974). Dry-bed training: Rapid elimination of childhood enuresis. *Behaviour Research and Therapy, 12*(3), 147–156.

Bader, G., Nevéus, T., Kruse, S., & Sillen, U. (2002). Sleep of primary enuretic children and controls. *Sleep, 25*(5), 579–583.

Baeyens, D., Roeyers, H., Demeyere, I., Verte, S., Hoebeke, P., & Vande Walle, J. (2005). Attention-deficit/hyperactivity disorder (ADHD) as a risk factor for persistent nocturnal enuresis in children: A two-year follow-up study. *Acta Paediatrica, 94*(11), 1619–1625.

Baeyens, D., Roeyers, H., Hoebeke, P., Verte, S., Van Hoecke, E., & Vande Walle, J. (2004). Attention deficit/hyperactivity disorder in children with nocturnal enuresis. *Journal of Urology, 171*(6 Pt 2), 2576–2579.

Baeyens, D., Roeyers, H., Van Erdeghem, S., Hoebeke, P., & Vande Walle, J. (2007). The prevalence of attention deficit-hyperactivity disorder in children with non-monosymptomatic nocturnal enuresis: A 4-year followup study. *Journal of Urology, 178*(6), 2616–2620.

Barone, J. G., Hanson, C., DaJusta, D. G., Gioia, K., England, S. J., & Schneider, D. (2009). Nocturnal enuresis and overweight are associated with obstructive sleep apnea. *Pediatrics, 124*(1), e53–e59.

Barone, J. G., Ramasamy, R., Farkas, A., Lerner, E., Creenan, E., Salmon, D., et al. (2006). Breastfeeding during infancy may protect against bed-wetting during childhood. *Pediatrics, 118*(1), 254–259.

Bascom, A., Penney, T., Metcalfe, M., Knox, A., Witmans, M., Uweira, T., et al. (2011). High risk of sleep disordered breathing in the enuresis population. *Journal of Urology, 186*(4 Suppl), 1710–1714.

Bayoumi, R. A., Eapen, V., Al-Yahyaee, S., Al Barwani, H. S., Hill, R. S., & Al Gazali, L. (2006). The genetic basis of inherited primary nocturnal enuresis: A UAE study. *Journal of Psychosomatic Research, 61*(3), 317–320.

Bellman, M. (1966). Studies on encopresis. *Acta paediatrica Scandinavica*, Suppl 170:171+.

Bharucha, A. E. (2008). Lower gastrointestinal functions. *Neurogastroenterology and Motility, 20*(Suppl 1), 103–113.

Bischof, G. H., & Benson, B. M. (2004). Childhood enuresis: A biopsychosocial systems approach. *Journal of Family Psychotherapy, 15*(3), 1–17.

Bloom, D. A. (1993). The American experience with desmopressin. *Clinical pediatrics (Phila),* Spec No:28–31.

Brooks, R. C., Copen, R. M., Cox, D. J., Morris, J., Borowitz, S., & Sutphen, J. (2000). Review of the treatment literature for encopresis, functional constipation, and stool-toileting refusal. *Annals of Behavioral Medicine, 22*(3), 260–267.

Butler, R. J. (2004). Childhood nocturnal enuresis: Developing a conceptual framework. *Clinical Psychology Review, 24*(8), 909–931.

Butler, R. J., & Holland, P. (2000). The three systems: A conceptual way of understanding nocturnal enuresis. *Scandinavian Journal of Urology and Nephrology, 34*(4), 270–277.

Casey, G. (2011). Incontinence and retention – How the bladder misfunctions. *Nursing New Zealand, 17*(7), 26–31.

Coppola, G., Costantini, A., Gaita, M., & Saraulli, D. (2011). Psychological correlates of enuresis: a case-control study on an Italian sample. Pediatric Nephrology, *26*(10), 1829–1836.

Cox, D. J., Morris, J. B., Jr., Borowitz, S. M., & Sutphen, J. L. (2002). Psychological differences between children with and without chronic encopresis. *Journal of Pediatric Psychology, 27*(7), 585–591.

Culbert, T. P., & Banez, G. A. (2007). Integrative approaches to childhood constipation and encopresis. *Pediatric Clinics of North America, 54*(6), 927–947. xi.

Diagnostic Classification Steering Committee, A. S. D. A. (1991). *International classification of sleep disorders: Diagnostic and coding manual.* Rochester, MN: American Sleep Disorders Association.

Dobson, P., & Rogers, J. (2009). Assessing and treating faecal incontinence in children. *Nursing Standard, 24*(2), 49–56. quiz 58, 60.

Erdogan, A., Akkurt, H., Boettjer, N. K., Yurtseven, E., Can, G., & Kiran, S. (2008). Prevalence and behavioural correlates of enuresis in young children. *Journal of Paediatrics and Child Health, 44*(5), 297–301.

Freitag, C. M., Rohling, D., Seifen, S., Pukrop, R., & von Gontard, A. (2006). Neurophysiology of nocturnal enuresis: Evoked potentials and prepulse inhibition of the startle reflex. *Developmental Medicine and Child Neurology, 48*(4), 278–284.

Friman, P. C., Hofstadter, K. L., & Jones, K. M. (2006). A biobehavioral approach to the treatment of functional encopresis in children. *Journal of Early and Intensive Behavior Intervention, 3*(3), 263–272.

Har, A. F., & Croffie, J. M. (2010). Encopresis. *Pediatrics in Review, 31*(9), 368–374. quiz 374.

Houts, A. C. (2003). Behavioral treatment for enuresis. In E. Kazdin & J. R. Weisz (Eds.), *Evidence-based psychotherapies for children and adolescents* (pp. 389–406). New York, NY: Guilford.

Houts, A. C., Berman, J. S., & Abramson, H. (1994). Effectiveness of psychological and pharmacological treatments for nocturnal enuresis. *Journal of Consulting and Clinical Psychology, 62*(4), 737–745.

Houts, A. C., & Liebert, R. M. (1984). *Bedwetting: A guide for parents and children.* Springfield, IL: Charles C. Thomas.

Houts, A. C., Liebert, R. M., & Padawer, W. (1983). A delivery system for the treatment of primary enuresis. *Journal of Abnormal Child Psychology, 11*(4), 513–519.

Howe, A. C., & Walker, C. E. (1992). Behavioral management of toilet training, enuresis, and encopresis. *Pediatric Clinics of North America, 39*(3), 413–432.

Hublin, C., Kaprio, J., Partinen, M., & Koskenvuo, M. (1998). Nocturnal enuresis in a nationwide twin cohort. *Sleep, 21*(6), 579–585.

Jackson, E. C. (2007). Is lack of bladder inhibition during sleep a mechanism of nocturnal enuresis? *The Journal of pediatrics, 151*(6), 559–560.

Joinson, C., Heron, J., Butler, U., & von Gontard, A. (2006). Psychological differences between children with and without soiling problems. *Pediatrics, 117*(5), 1575–1584.

Joinson, C., Heron, J., Butler, R., Von Gontard, A., Butler, U., Emond, A., et al. (2007). A United Kingdom population-based study of intellectual capacities in children with and without soiling, daytime wetting, and bed-wetting. *Pediatrics, 120*(2), e308–e316.

Joinson, C., Heron, J., Von Gontard, A., Butler, U., Emond, A., & Golding, J. (2009). A prospective study of age at initiation of toilet training and subsequent daytime bladder control in school-age children. *Journal of Developmental and Behavioral Pediatrics, 30*(5), 385–393.

Joinson, C., Heron, J., von Gontard, A., Butler, U., Golding, J., & Emond, A. (2008). Early childhood risk factors associated with daytime wetting and soiling in school-age children. *Journal of Pediatric Psychology, 33*(7), 739–750.

Kimmel, H. D., & Kimmel, E. (1970). An instrumental conditioning method for the treatment of enuresis. *Journal of Behavior Therapy and Experimental Psychiatry, 1*, 121–123.

Kuhn, B. R., Marcus, B. A., & Pitner, S. L. (1999). Treatment guidelines for primary nonretentive encopresis and stool toileting refusal. *American Family Physician, 59*(8), 2171–2178.

Levine, M. D., & Bakow, H. (1976). Children with encopresis: A study of treatment outcome. *Pediatrics, 58*(6), 845–852.

Loening-Baucke, V. (2007). Prevalence rates for constipation and faecal and urinary incontinence. *Archives of Disease in Childhood, 92*(6), 486–489.

Lunsing, R. J., Hadders-Algra, M., Touwen, B. C., & Huisjes, H. J. (1991). Nocturnal enuresis and minor neurological dysfunction at 12 years: A follow-up study. *Developmental Medicine and Child Neurology, 33*(5), 439–445.

McGrath, M. L., Mellon, M. W., & Murphy, L. (2000). Empirically supported treatments in pediatric psychology: Constipation and encopresis. *Journal of Pediatric Psychology, 25*(4), 225–254. discussion 255–256.

Mellon, M. W., & McGrath, M. L. (2000). Empirically supported treatments in pediatric psychology: Nocturnal enuresis. *Journal of Pediatric Psychology, 25*(4), 193–214. discussion 215-198, 219–124.

Mishne, J. M. (1993). Primary nocturnal enuresis: A psychodynamic clinical perspective. *Child and Adolescent Social Work Journal, 10*, 469–495.

Moffatt, M. E. (1997). Nocturnal enuresis: A review of the efficacy of treatments and practical advice for clinicians. *Journal of Developmental and Behavioral Pediatrics, 18*(1), 49–56.

Montgomery, D. F., & Navarro, F. (2008). Management of constipation and encopresis in children. *Journal of Pediatric Health Care, 22*(3), 199–204.

Mowrer, O. H., & Mowrer, W. M. (1938). Enuresis: A method for its study and treatment. *American Journal of Orthopsychiatry, 8*, 436–459.

Murphy, S., & Carney, T. (2004). The classification of soiling and encopresis and a possible treatment protocol. *Child and Adolescent Mental Health, 9*(3), 125–129.

Nevéus, T., von Gontard, A., Hoebeke, P., Hjalmas, K., Bauer, S., Bower, W., et al. (2006). The standardization of terminology of lower urinary tract function in children and adolescents: Report from the Standardisation Committee of the International Children's Continence Society. *Journal of Urology, 176*(1), 314–324.

Partin, J. C., Hamill, S. K., Fischel, J. E., & Partin, J. S. (1992). Painful defecation and fecal soiling in children. *Pediatrics, 89*(6 Pt 1), 1007–1009.

Raes, A., Dossche, L., Hertegonne, N., Nuytemans, L., Hoebeke, P., Van Laecke, E., et al. (2010). Hypercalciuria is related to osmolar excretion in children with nocturnal enuresis. *Journal of Urology, 183*(1), 297–301.

Raghunath, N., Glassman, M. S., Halata, M. S., Berezin, S. H., Stewart, J. M., & Medow, M. S. (2011). Anorectal motility abnormalities in children with encopresis and chronic constipation. *Journal of Pediatrics, 158*(2), 293–296.

Reimers, T. M. (1996). A biobehavioral approach toward managing encopresis. *Behavior Modification, 20*(4), 469–479.

Ritterband, L. M., Ardalan, K., Thorndike, F. P., Magee, J. C., Saylor, D. K., Cox, D. J., et al. (2008). Real world use of an Internet intervention for pediatric encopresis. *Journal of Medical Internet Research, 10*(2), e16.

Semer, N. L., & Yezigi, L. (2009). The Rorschach and the body: The study of self-esteem in enuretic children through the Rorschach method. *Rorschachiana, 30*(1), 3–25.

Sethi, S., Bhargava, S., & Shipra, M. P. (2005). Nocturnal enuresis: A review. *Journal of Pediatric Neurology, 3*, 11–18.

Shreeram, S., He, J. P., Kalaydjian, A., Brothers, S., & Merikangas, K. R. (2009). Prevalence of enuresis and its association with attention-deficit/hyperactivity disorder among U.S. children: Results from a nationally representative study. *Journal of the American Academy of Child and Adolescent Psychiatry, 48*(1), 35–41.

Stark, L. J. (2000). Commentary: Treatment of encopresis: Where do we go from here? *Journal of Pediatric Psychology, 25*(4), 255–256.

Stark, L. J., Spirito, A., Lewis, A. V., & Hart, K. J. (1990). Encopresis: Behavioral parameters associated with children who fail medical management. *Child Psychiatry and Human Development, 20*(3), 169–179.

Stein, S. M. (1998). Enuresis, early attachment and intimacy. *British Journal of Psychotherapy, 15*(2), 167–176.

Stern, H. P., Stroh, S. E., Fiedorek, S. C., Kelleher, K., Mellon, M. W., Pope, S. K., et al. (1995). Increased plasma levels of pancreatic polypeptide and decreased plasma levels of motilin in encopretic children. *Pediatrics, 96*(1), 111–117.

Su, M. S., Li, A. M., So, H. K., Au, C. T., Ho, C., & Wing, Y. K. (2011). Nocturnal enuresis in children: Prevalence, correlates, and relationship with obstructive sleep apnea. *Journal of Pediatrics, 159*(2), 238.e1–242.e1.

Sureshkumar, P., Jones, M., Caldwell, P. H., & Craig, J. C. (2009). Risk factors for nocturnal enuresis in school-age children. *Journal of Urology, 182*(6), 2893–2899.

Sureshkumar, P., Jones, M., Cumming, R., & Craig, J. (2009). A population based study of 2,856 school-age children with urinary incontinence. *Journal of Urology, 181*(2), 808–815. discussion 815-806.

Valavi, E., Ahmadzadeh, A., Hooman, N., & Aminzadeh, M. (2011). Clinical correlation between hypercalciuria and nocturnal enuresis. *Saudi Journal of Kidney Diseases and Transplantation, 22*(5), 976–981.

Van Hoeck, K., Bael, A., Lax, H., Hirche, H., Van Dessel, E., Van Renthergem, D., et al. (2007). Urine output rate and maximum volume voided in school-age children with and without nocturnal enuresis. *Journal of Pediatrics, 151*(6), 575–580.

Vivian, D., Fischel, J. E., & Liebert, R. M. (1986). Effect of "wet nights" on daytime behavior during concurrent treatment of enuresis and conduct problems. *Journal of Behavior Therapy and Experimental Psychiatry, 17*(4), 301–303.

von Gontard, A. (2011). Elimination disorders: A critical comment on DSM-5 proposals. *European Child and Adolescent Psychiatry, 20*(2), 83–88.

von Gontard, A., Baeyens, D., Van Hoecke, E., Warzak, W. J., & Bachmann, C. (2011). Psychological and psychiatric issues in urinary and fecal incontinence. *Journal of Urology, 185*(4), 1432–1436.

von Gontard, A., Freitag, C. M., Seifen, S., Pukrop, R., & Rohling, D. (2006). Neuromotor development in nocturnal enuresis. *Developmental Medicine and Child Neurology, 48*(9), 744–750.

von Gontard, A., Heron, J., & Joinson, C. (2011). Family history of nocturnal enuresis and urinary incontinence: Results from a large epidemiological study. *Journal of Urology, 185*(6), 2303–2306.

von Gontard, A., Moritz, A. M., Thome-Granz, S., & Freitag, C. (2011). Association of attention deficit and elimination disorders at school entry: A population based study. *Journal of Urology, 186*(5), 2027–2032.

Weissman, L., & Bridgemohan, C. (2009). Bowel function, toileting, and encopresis. In W. B. Carey, A. C. Crocker, W. L. Coleman, E. Roy Elias, & H. M. Feldman (Eds.), *Developmental-behavioral pediatrics* (4th ed.). Philadelphia, PA: Saunders Elsevier.

Whiting, J. W. M., & Child, I. L. (1953). *Child training and personality: A cross-cultural study*. New Haven, CT: Yale University Press.

Young, G. C., & Morgan, R. T. (1972). Overlearning in the conditioning treatment of enuresis. *Behaviour Research and Therapy, 10*(2), 147–151.

Zink, S., Freitag, C. M., & von Gontard, A. (2008). Behavioral comorbidity differs in subtypes of enuresis and urinary incontinence. *Journal of Urology, 179*(1), 295–298. discussion 298.

Part VIII

Chronic Developmental Disorders

Helen Tager-Flusberg

Introduction

Over the past decade, there have been exponential changes in perspectives on autism spectrum disorder (ASD), which includes classic autism, pervasive developmental disorder not otherwise specified (PDD-NOS), and Asperger syndrome (APA, 1994). Perhaps the most striking changes are in the prevalence rates for this group of disorders (now generally referred to with the umbrella term ASD; APA, 2013), not only in the USA but in all countries where epidemiological studies have been conducted. The latest statistics from the Centers for Disease Control estimate that 1 in 88 children in the USA has an ASD and an even more alarming figure of 1 in 54 boys (ADDM, 2012). These soaring rates, which still seem to be rising, have led to growing public awareness about ASD coupled with serious fears and concerns as some media reports refer to a new epidemic of this once rare neurodevelopmental disorder.

These changes have led to increased attention to the need for more funding and scientific research into the causes, pathophysiology, and treatments for ASD. Contemporary research on ASD has built on the important advances that have been made in recent years in the fields of genetics, genomics, neuroscience, and cognitive science, and clearly substantial progress has been made. This chapter summarizes the history and current knowledge about ASD, surveys what is known about the etiology of the disorder, and then provides a review of early development in infants and children with ASD framed within a conceptual model that underscores the significance of developmental processes in our understanding of this complex disorder.

History of ASD

Kanner and Asperger

In the midst of the Second World War, two important papers were published introducing the construct of a developmental disorder that involved fundamental disturbances in social behavior (Asperger, 1944; Kanner 1943). The case histories of the children documented by both Kanner and Asperger are easily recognized today as examples of ASD, and despite the significant heterogeneity in the presentation of these children's problems, the common features of impaired *social affective communication* led to the introduction of a new diagnostic category. Importantly,

H. Tager-Flusberg, Ph.D. (✉)
Department of Psychology, Boston University, Boston, MA 02215, USA

Departments of Anatomy & Neurobiology and Pediatrics, Boston University School of Medicine, Boston, MA 02215, USA
e-mail: htagerf@bu.edu

M. Lewis and K.D. Rudolph (eds.), *Handbook of Developmental Psychopathology*,
DOI 10.1007/978-1-4614-9608-3_33, © Springer Science+Business Media New York 2014

Kanner and Asperger both noted that their patients were predominantly boys, though why this should be so was not understood. Although it would take many years for Asperger's work to be recognized (Wing, 1981) and for autism to make its way into the DSM (APA, 1980), clinical studies began to appear in the literature soon after Kanner's seminal paper was published.

Early Theories

Throughout its relatively brief history, the dominant views about ASD reflected the conceptual frameworks that prevailed in all areas of psychopathology. Thus, during the 1950s and 1960s, psychoanalytic explanations of the core impairments in ASD focused on the mother: her cold "refrigerator" style of parenting was to blame for the child's withdrawal from the social world. Beginning in the 1970s, cognitive and neurobiological approaches gradually came to replace psychoanalysis, and ASD was now understood as a disorder of the brain that was manifest in impaired cognition and observable behavioral symptoms (Hermelin & O'Connor, 1970; Rimland, 1964). Environmental theories were gradually replaced by biological theories, and evidence began to emerge that ASD ran in families and therefore was rooted largely in genetics (Folstein & Rutter, 1977).

Research on ASD steadily accumulated over the next two decades, particularly within psychology where the emphasis lay on finding a unitary cognitive explanation for the range of behavioral symptoms that defined the disorder. During this period little attention was paid to the significant heterogeneity that would challenge any simple view of ASD, and few developmental studies were undertaken that might also challenge the popular view of ASD as a static disorder. Still, considerable progress was made in research that focused not only on the deficits (e.g., theory of mind, face processing, executive functions) but also on some of the cognitive strengths that could be found in people with ASD (e.g., savant skills, visual search speed).

Current Perspectives

In the past decade, new views of ASD have emerged emphasizing the view that ASD is a *complex* disorder. This complexity is manifest at every level of analysis, from genetics to neurobiology to behavioral symptoms. Thus, while earlier genetic studies were interpreted as suggesting that only a handful of genes were associated with ASD, current research has implicated hundreds of risk genes, the majority of which are involved in critical brain developmental processes and that vary considerably within the population (State & Sestan, 2012). At the neurobiological level, system-level developmental explanations (e.g., altered balance between excitatory and inhibitory synaptic processes) are replacing theories about localized lesions. Earlier claims that a single cognitive deficit could explain all the symptoms of ASD are no longer viewed as tenable; instead, researchers are now embracing a broader approach that includes several core cognitive deficits that emerge over time (Charman et al., 2011). And at the behavioral level, heterogeneity particularly in associated symptoms (e.g., IQ, language, psychopathology, medical conditions) and comorbidity with other disorders is now understood as the norm rather than as exceptions that are not relevant to the definition of ASD. Future advances will depend on researchers embracing this view of ASD as a complex and developmental disorder.

Defining ASD

DSM IV Criteria

Classifications of ASD (APA, 1994) focused on three core symptom domains: social reciprocity, language and communication, and repetitive behaviors and restricted interests. Deficits in all three domains define classic autism; for Asperger syndrome no deficits in communication are included, and delays in language development or cognitive impairment are exclusionary criteria; PDD-NOS is diagnosed when a child fails to meet full criteria for autism. It is generally accepted that symptoms emerge before the pre-school years, though may go unrecognized until children are four or five years old. For nearly two decades, these subtypes of pervasive developmental disorder were the basis of both clinical and research practice, and objective diagnostic instruments were developed to aid in consensus views of who would be classified with ASD (Lord, Rutter, & LeCouteur, 1994; Lord, Rutter, DiLavore, & Risi, 1999).

The DSM IV (and ICD-10) definitions of ASD were a significant advance over previous classification systems, and their criteria have been used over the past two decades in the vast majority of clinical studies spanning genetics to treatment. At the same time as these new definitions appeared, the prevalence rates began to rise. At least some of this rise can be attributed to the broadening of criteria for diagnosing ASD, particularly at the higher end of the spectrum, including children with less intellectual disability and more advanced language skills. The increase in the number of children with ASD also reflects greater awareness in the community and better detection in younger children, at least in some geographical regions (ADDM, 2012).

In recognition of the phenotypic heterogeneity of ASD, many studies explored the possibility of defining meaningful subtypes, beginning with the obvious distinctions embodied within DSM IV between autism, Asperger syndrome, and PDD-NOS. Recent reviews of these studies have concluded that the distinctions between these subtypes have not proven useful either for research purposes or in clinical practice (e.g., Huerta, Bishop, Duncan, Hus, & Lord, 2012; Ozonoff, 2012), though comorbid features (e.g., developmental language delay) are a more promising route to creating useful genetic and behavioral subtypes.

DSM 5

In part as a response to research findings based on DSM IV, the newly proposed DSM 5 classification collapsed the three subtypes into a single disorder: autism spectrum disorder (http://www.dsm5.org). The new diagnostic criteria also comprise two domains instead of three: (1) deficits in social/communication and (2) fixated interests and repetitive behaviors, in recognition of factor analytic studies that demonstrate the commonalities among symptoms of social and communication impairment (e.g., Frazier, Youngstrom, Kubu, Sinclair, & Rezai, 2008). Not surprisingly, these changes have generated controversy, particularly over concerns that the new narrower definition will exclude many individuals from receiving a diagnosis that is the gateway to services and intervention (e.g., Ghaziuddin, 2011; McPartland, Reichow, & Volkmar, 2012). Nevertheless, systematic comparisons of the old and new criteria using large samples of participants suggest that overall, the new criteria will not lead to a significant reduction in the numbers of diagnosed individuals (Huerta et al., 2012).

Another important change in DSM 5 is the introduction of severity levels. A person receiving an ASD diagnosis will now also be rated for the severity of their symptoms; these ratings are important for clinical planning and provide explicit recognition of the quantitative variability found in the population. In addition, comorbid conditions will need to be documented including intellectual disability, language impairment, and other psychiatric conditions that are commonly found in people with ASD, such as mood disorders, sleep disturbance, or attention deficit disorder. All these changes reflect current understanding of the major defining characteristics of children and adults with ASD.

Etiology of ASD

Genetic Studies

The first twin study, which included a small sample of participants, found that concordance rates for monozygotic twins were significantly higher than for dizygotic twins, establishing a relatively high heritability estimate for ASD (Folstein & Rutter, 1977). These findings were replicated in later studies, culminating in estimates of over 90 % heritability (Bailey, Phillips, & Rutter, 1996). But these studies were all carried out at a time when ASD was relatively rare, and they relied on earlier narrower definitions of the disorder. One recent study, which included almost 200 twin pairs and used more rigorous diagnostic measures, found a much more modest heritability estimate (about 37 %), reflecting lower concordance for MZ twins and much higher concordance for DZ twins compared to the earlier studies (Hallmayer et al., 2011). The findings suggested a more significant influence of shared environmental factors (55 %–58 %), which the authors speculate would need to be operating primarily during the prenatal or early postnatal period.

In addition to twin studies, there have been numerous studies of recurrence rates among siblings and other relatives, as well as research on what has come to be called the "broader autism phenotype" – the presence of milder subclinical phenotypic traits in first-degree relatives. The risk recurrence rate among siblings is now estimated at just under 20 %, based on prospective studies of infants who have older diagnosed siblings; this compares to estimates of 3 %–6 % found in studies conducted almost 30 years ago (Ozonoff, Young, Carter, et al., 2011; see also Constantino, Zhang, Frazier, Abbacchi, & Law, 2010). Broader autism phenotype characteristics have been documented in almost half the parents or siblings enrolled in recent behavioral, cognitive, and neuroimaging studies of social, language, or personality characteristics (Gerdts & Bernier, 2011). These more recent twin and family-based studies reveal different findings than earlier behavior genetic studies on ASD. In part, these differences may reflect more rigorous methodology, but it is also likely that the differences reflect changes in the mix of genetic and nongenetic factors associated with ASD that parallel the rising prevalence rates and perhaps also cohort effects (Szatmari, 2011).

Toward the end of the twentieth century, at a time when ASD was still viewed as relatively uncommon, there was an informal consensus among researchers that ASD was largely inherited

and that while there were methodological hurdles to surmount, it should not take long to identify the relatively small number of genes responsible (e.g., Bailey et al., 1995; Rutter, 1996). Less than two decades later, the landscape has changed considerably. While advances have been made in identifying genes and gene variants associated with ASD, progress has been slower than the optimists had hoped for and no major gene or gene locus has emerged from genome-wide association studies that would account for the majority of cases, reflecting the same pattern found in studies of other complex medical and psychiatric disorders (State & Levitt, 2011; Sullivan, Daly, & O'Donovan, 2012). It now seems that non-inherited *de novo* genetic factors, for example, copy number variants (CNVs) and point mutations, account for significantly more ASD cases than had previously been thought, but each specific genomic variant accounts for fewer than 1 % of cases (Sebat et al., 2007; State & Sestan, 2012). Moreover, some of these recently identified CNVs are associated not only with ASD but also with other neurodevelopmental disorders including, for example, schizophrenia or language impairment (Shen et al., 2011; Vernes et al., 2008).

Nongenetic Factors

In recognition of the fact that inherited genes cannot fully explain the etiology of ASD, a fact that is underscored by the newer twin studies, scientists have turned their attention to a wide range of alternative risk factors. The now discredited hypothesis that autism was caused by the measles–mumps–rubella vaccine, traditionally administered at around 18 months of age, led to a storm of controversy that has still not completely disappeared (Bearman, 2010; Wakefield et al., 1998). Other researchers are investigating the possibility of other environmental toxins, though to date, no strong contenders have emerged (Newschaffer et al., 2012). More promising findings have been obtained in epidemiological studies of demographic factors including parental, particularly fathers', age; close spacing of births; multiple births; low birth weight; and prematurity; and there is some evidence that the maternal–fetal environment, including drugs, maternal infection, and maternal–fetal immune reactivity, may all contribute to the etiology of ASD, particularly as these factors interact with familial-genetic and epigenetic risk (Szatmari, 2011). Changes over the past two decades in all these factors may also be contributing to the rise in prevalence rates. As with all complex disorders, it will take significant time and effort to understand the interactions between genetic and nongenetic risk contributions to ASD, and we are still a long way from having a complete picture of what causes this neurodevelopmental disorder.

Developmental Model of ASD

Risk and Outcome

The most comprehensive model of ASD has been proposed by Dawson and her colleagues within a developmental framework (Dawson, 2008; Dawson, Sterling, & Faja, 2009). In this model, there is a set of *risk indices*, including susceptibility genes, environmental risk factors, and neurobehavioral or phenotypic risk indices (e.g., reduced social interest, atypical brain organization for language or face perception). These risk indices influence a range of *risk processes* that include atypical behavioral and brain development and lead to altered interactions of infants with their social environment. Most importantly, these risk processes involve children's reciprocal social interactions with primary caregivers, which in turn lead to alterations in their social, language, and cognitive development. On this model, optimal social engagement in infancy is the key to later development across multiple domains (cf. Kuhl, 2007). Together, risk indices and risk processes lead to ASD *outcomes* that emerge typically during the second year of life. Within this model behavioral intervention directly influences risk processes and in turn can mediate outcomes in children that are at high risk for ASD or who are in the early developmental stages of the full-blown disorder.

Early Identification and Treatment

Dawson's model integrates research on etiology, developmental processes, and treatment of ASD with a view to understanding the enormous heterogeneity in the outcomes of children with ASD. There is significant heterogeneity in the genetic risk indices and, though less clearly understood, presumably in other risk indices and processes. Dawson's model clearly advocates for the early identification of ASD risk indices in the expectation that children identified as high risk should have access to intervention that will mediate their eventual outcomes, including the possibility of preventing the onset of ASD. The efficacy of early intensive behavioral intervention for children with ASD has now been well documented in rigorous research studies, including randomized control trials (Dawson & Burner, 2011). In particular, developmentally based behavioral interventions that are conducted in structured one-to-one interactions produce optimal outcomes, especially if implemented in the toddler and preschool years (e.g., Dawson et al., 2010; Kasari, Gulsrud, Wong, Kwon, & Locke, 2010). Recent findings showing that the earlier interventions are implemented the better the outcomes will be for young children at risk for ASD (cf. Rogers et al., 2012) underscore the significance of brain and behavioral plasticity during the early years in mediating the processes that shape the developmental trajectory for ASD.

The Development of Young Children with ASD

Early Development in Infants at Risk for ASD

As we have seen, Dawson's model places significant emphasis on the role of developmental processes in both brain and behavior in determining the outcomes of children with ASD, and effective interventions are based within a developmental framework. In recent years researchers have paid close attention to investigating development in ASD using longitudinal research designs.

Perhaps the most important studies that are now emerging in the literature focus on longitudinal studies of infants at risk for ASD, following these infants long before the emergence of symptoms and diagnosis (Zwaigenbaum et al., 2007). In most of these studies, risk is defined genetically, based on the presence of an older sibling that is diagnosed with ASD; as noted earlier, prevalence rate for these high-risk infants is now estimated at almost 20 % (Ozonoff et al., 2011). Prospective longitudinal studies replace earlier reliance on either parental retrospective recall, which is notoriously susceptible to bias, or home video analyses of infants later diagnosed with ASD (e.g., Osterling & Dawson, 1994) that had revealed important quantitative differences in social responsiveness by 12 months.

There are now more than 20 different research groups from around the world who are engaged in studying infants at risk for ASD (http://www.autismspeaks.org/science/initiatives/high-risk-baby-sibs). Their research has yielded important findings about the earliest signs of ASD in this population (which may not be representative of all children with ASD) that can be found in the first two years of life.

The First Twelve Months

Despite parental reports to the contrary, studies of high-risk infants have not identified any clear behavioral signs of the core symptoms of the disorder before the age of 12 months. On the contrary, at 6 months these babies are socially engaged, smile at their caregivers, and respond to social bids, just like typically developing infants (Zwaigenbaum et al., 2005). At 10–12 months of age, differences can be assessed in infants who later receive an ASD diagnosis. Their vocalization and nonverbal communication are less frequent, they are less responsive to their name being called, and they exhibit other signs of lower social engagement and unusual motor and attention problems (see Rogers, 2009; Tager-Flusberg, 2010 for reviews). There is considerable variability in the specific behavioral features seen in each

high-risk baby, but together these signs all bear close similarity to the full-blown symptoms that are used in diagnosing older children with ASD. Interestingly, there is preliminary evidence that during the first year of life, subtle, nonspecific secondary features may distinguish high-risk infants who are later diagnosed with ASD, including temperamental characteristics (Garon et al., 2009) or developmental delay in motor control (Flanagan, Landa, Bhat, & Bauman, 2012).

Studies of brain structure and function in infants later diagnosed with ASD have revealed differences that emerge before overt behavioral signs. While these findings await replication, they offer the promise that this line of research might lead to even earlier diagnosis, at least of significantly high risk if not full-blown ASD, using a mix of bio- and behavioral markers. Using diffusion tensor imaging to investigate the development of the organization of white matter fiber tracts, Wolff and his colleagues found that at 6 months, fractional anisotropy (FA) values, a measure of white matter development, were higher in the infants who met criteria for ASD at 24 months of age. Moreover, the developmental trajectories of FA were slower in these infants between 6 and 24 months compared to those high-risk infants who did not have an ASD outcome (Wolff et al., 2012). In another study, Elsabbagh and her colleagues collected event-related potentials (ERP) from infants at 6–10 months of age, while they were looking at dynamic faces directed toward or away from the infants (Elsabbagh et al., 2012). The infants later diagnosed with ASD at 36 months did not show the expected differences in ERP response to the dynamic gaze shifts.

Several other studies have found that as a group, high-risk infants, regardless of their outcome, differ significantly from low-risk controls who have no family history of ASD. These studies highlight the significance of endophenotypes for ASD that can be detected in the first year of life, which, in Dawson's model, would be termed phenotypic risk indices. Examples of such endophenotypes include lower power measured in electroencephalogram (EEG) recordings at 6 months (Tierney, Gabard-Durnam, Vogel-Farley, Tager-Flusberg, & Nelson, 2012), reduced entropy in EEG at 9 months (Bosl, Tierney, Tager-Flusberg, & Nelson, 2011), differences in neural markers of attention to faces at 12 months (Luyster, Wagner, Vogel-Farley, Tager-Flusberg, & Nelson, 2011), and ERP latency to familiar and unfamiliar faces (Key & Stone, 2012). As with the studies finding early markers that distinguish infants later diagnosed with ASD, several of these studies found differences in the developmental trajectories of these endophenotypes over the first 2 or 3 years of life suggesting that it is important to take a dynamic view of development and not simply investigate infants at one point in time.

This is a very active area of current research, and future investigations will need to follow up on these findings to see whether there are subtle differences in the endophenotypes seen in high-risk infants based on their long-term developmental outcomes. At the same time, these are early days for research on identifying early risk signs for ASD. So far few of the findings in the literature have been replicated in independent studies. More importantly perhaps, because none of the published studies have compared infants at risk for ASD to infants at risk for other neurodevelopmental disorders, we do not know whether the putative risk signs or endophenotypes are specific to ASD or whether they may be shared by infants who are genetic risk for other complex disorders (e.g., language impairment or ADHD) that have overlapping etiology and some shared behavioral characteristics.

Another key issue, not directly addressed in Dawson's model, is whether there are protective factors that may be identified in infancy or toddlerhood that might explain why the majority of high-risk infants do not go on to meet criteria for ASD, even though they have many of the same risk indices (from genetics to phenotypes) as infants who do go on to have ASD. So far, no published studies have directly addressed this issue. Protective factors could include genetic, neurocognitive, or environmental factors, which may influence the child's developmental trajectory toward a more normative outcome. Understanding

what protective factors might be operating within a broader framework of developmental psychopathology for ASD will undoubtedly lead to new ways of conceptualizing notions of risk and resilience within this population and may lead to novel methods for behavioral interventions.

The Toddler Years

In the majority of cases, ASD is a disorder that emerges gradually during the second or third year of life. The precise timing differs across infants, but the general pattern found across high-risk infants who are later diagnosed with ASD is that their behavioral developmental trajectory goes awry at some point between 12 and 36 months. During this period of onset, there are significant declines in social engagement (including smiling, eye contact, and vocalizations directed toward others) and slowed or absent growth in language and nonverbal cognition (Ozonoff et al., 2010). In some children, usually those who had already begun speaking by 12 months, there may be a complete loss of language (Pickles et al., 2009). This atypical pattern of loss is referred to as "regression." While earlier studies focused only on regression in language skills, it is now clear that social communication behaviors also show a pattern of regression or decline in frequency and that this regression may be a defining feature of ASD (Ozonoff, Hueng & Thompson, 2011).

As in older children with ASD, toddlers vary widely in the presentation of their symptoms, but the core features of deficits in social reciprocity, language and communication, and repetitive behaviors and restricted interests are present at this early age. Social impairments are strikingly evident in abnormal eye contact, absent or very limited joint attention behaviors, imitation, and functional or pretend play. Coupled with these reductions in social interest and motivation are deficits in language and communication. Toddlers with ASD rarely communicate even using nonverbal gestures. Their language development is often quite delayed, and even when they begin to speak, they vocalize very little and seldom initiate conversation, limiting their language to simple requests and responses (Tager-Flusberg, Edelson, & Luyster, 2011). Sensitivity to a variety of sensory stimuli emerges during this time in many toddlers which may take the form of unusual reactions to touch, sounds, sights, or tastes (Ben-Sasson et al., 2007). They show an increased and sometimes quite focused interest in objects, often developing a significant attachment to particular objects or parts of objects (Zwaigenbaum et al., 2009).

The striking imbalance between their lack of engagement with people and enhanced engagement with things is at the heart of what differentiates toddlers with ASD from both typically developing toddlers and toddlers with other neurodevelopmental disorders. This imbalance also disrupts developmental processes, with potentially cascading effects on language and cognitive development, depending on the severity of the symptoms (Jones & Klin, 2009). The normally close and natural interchanges that take place between child and caregiver during mealtimes, play, and other activities are no longer possible when the child ignores or even avoids all social approaches, and this has significant consequences for development. ASD highlights the deeply intertwined connections between social, cognitive, and language development that is evident across all children; these interconnections are even more disturbed when the child with ASD also has comorbid intellectual disability.

What theories have been proposed to explain the cognitive mechanisms that may underlie these interconnections between the developmental domains that are at the core of ASD? The most widely investigated proposal is that ASD is characterized by impairments in theory of mind, the ability to interpret and predict behavior in terms of mental states (Baron-Cohen, Tager-Flusberg, & Cohen, 1993; Baron-Cohen, Tager-Flusberg, & Cohen, 2000). While early studies investigated the understanding (or failure to understand) of false belief and related mental states in older children with ASD, which is achieved at around the age of four or five, later research focused on the developmental precursors of classic theory of mind, including shared gaze, intentionality, and joint

attention skills which emerge in the first year of life and more advanced imitation, symbolic play, and self-/other understanding that emerge during the second and third years of life, the period when ASD symptoms begin to appear. Michael Lewis and his colleagues have argued that in typically developing toddlers, self-representation develops at around the age of 18 months, as evidenced by the closely related developments in visual self-recognition, the use of personal pronouns such as "me" and "mine," and engaging in self and other pretense play (Lewis & Ramsay, 2004). Self-representation is the foundation for the development of empathy and for emotions such as pride, embarrassment, and guilt. These core social affective communicative skills are significantly impaired in older children with ASD, and Carmody and Lewis (2012) recently demonstrated that preschoolers with ASD also show deficits in self-representation, which were particularly severe in children with autistic disorder.

The acquisition of language is often viewed as the single most important factor predicting long-term outcomes for children with ASD (Tager-Flusberg, Paul, & Lord, 2005). Early language milestones, such as canonical babbling, first words, and phrases, are usually delayed; however, some children with ASD, particularly those receiving early intervention, can make rapid progress and may catch up with their peers by the time they start school. Nevertheless, there is enormous heterogeneity in the success of children with ASD in developing spoken language, with over one-quarter of the population remaining nonverbal. A number of prelinguistic factors are important precursors for language in typically developing children, and studies have found that the same precursors predict language acquisition in children with ASD (Luyster, Kadlec, Connolly, Carter, & Tager-Flusberg, 2008). These factors include joint attention, imitation, nonverbal cognition, motor, gesture, and symbolic development as indexed by level of play skills. Gestural communication is the single most significant predictor of later language for children with ASD, perhaps because it encompasses joint attention, imitation, cognition, and motor components while serving core communication functions (Luyster et al., 2011). It is still not known why some children with ASD fail to acquire language despite years of intense intervention, and because these children have not been included in most research studies, very little is known about them (Tager-Flusberg & Kasari, 2013).

For typically developing children, parental behavior is an additional important predictor of language development. The quantity and quality of parents' gestural and linguistic input significantly influences the rate of early language development and is particularly important in determining the growth of children's vocabulary (Gathercole & Hoff, 2007; Rowe & Goldin-Meadow, 2009). Recent research found that comparable relationships were seen among mothers and their high-risk infants and that these mothers consistently provided high-quality communicative input to their children, and even higher rates of gesturing were found for mothers of infants who were not later diagnosed with ASD (Talbott, Nelson, & Tager-Flusberg, 2013). Siller and Sigman (2002) had earlier reported that caregivers of children with ASD were, as a group, similar to caregivers of both typically developing children and children with developmental delay in the ways they offered optimal input to their children during free play by synchronizing their behaviors to the focus of their children's attention and activity. Importantly, this synchronous behavior, demonstrating the caregiver's sensitivity to their child's behavior, predicted later long-term gains in joint attention skills and language development. These studies provide an important foundation for the development of parent-based interventions that can be implemented early in life with high-risk infants suggesting ways in which protective processes, grounded in high-quality parent–child interactions, might operate to reduce the likelihood of the onset or severity of ASD in the toddler years (Rogers et al., 2012).

While the majority of studies on brain structure and function in ASD using magnetic resonance imaging (MRI) have been carried out in older, mostly high functioning individuals, in recent years several studies of brain development in young children with ASD have been conducted that have demonstrated the early emergence of an atypical developmental trajectory in brain size and organization, which parallels the emergence of core symptoms. Courchesne and his colleagues have focused on the changes in brain growth that begin toward the end of the first year of life: a proportion of children with ASD show accelerated brain enlargement (as evidenced by changes in head circumference and in MRI studies) that plateaus in the preschool years (Redcay & Courchesne, 2005). This abnormal growth trajectory is most evident in frontal and temporal brain regions, affecting both grey and white matter (Courchesne, Redcay, & Kennedy, 2004; Hazlett et al., 2011). In addition, older children and adolescents with ASD show atypical asymmetry patterns in brain development with reduced left hemisphere asymmetry evident in both structural and functional brain organization (see Courchesne et al., 2007 for review). Recent work suggests that these atypical patterns emerge early, at the time when symptoms of ASD are first observed. For example, one small-scale study found white matter enlargement in frontal areas, but reduced white matter in the left temporal–parietal junction, in preschoolers with ASD (Carmody & Lewis, 2010). Those children with more severe social communication symptoms showed more significant differences in left hemisphere white matter in frontal and temporal brain regions. In another study, Redcay and Courchesne (2008) found that toddlers with ASD showed greater activation in the right hemisphere when listening to speech. Together, these studies show that there is close timing in the emergence of behavioral symptoms of ASD and abnormalities in brain development that are most evident in those neural systems that are associated with social and communicative functioning.

The research summarized here underscores the importance of earlier identification of ASD, or even risk for ASD before the full-blown onset of the disorder, and this is reflected in widespread calls for screening among primary care physicians (e.g., http://www.medicalhomeinfo.org/downloads/pdfs/AutismAlarm.pdf). Today, many experienced clinicians feel more comfortable diagnosing ASD by the age of 2 or 3, in large part because only with a diagnosis will a child be eligible for early intervention and other services that are available in many regions. Nevertheless in the majority of places around the world, and in rural areas or among minorities in the USA, diagnosis may be delayed for several years (Mandell et al., 2009). These delays have an enormous impact on the long-term outcomes of these children, who lack access to treatment, and to their families.

Beyond the Toddler Years

It is generally accepted that ASD is a lifelong disorder. Longitudinal studies have found that symptoms peak during the preschool years, a time when most children are diagnosed (Lord, Luyster, Guthrie, & Pickles, 2012). Although far less emphasis has been on understanding the course of development into adulthood, one important study found that over time, there is a general reduction in symptom severity for the majority of older adolescents and adults (Seltzer et al., 2011). Exactly what drives these changes is not known, though it is likely to be a combination of the natural course of development coupled with experiences that promote greater social engagement over time, including perhaps continued access to structured interventions and education.

Fein and her colleagues have investigated a group of children who had been diagnosed with ASD when they were toddlers but who had lost the diagnosis by the time they were preschoolers (Fein et al., 2013; Sutera et al., 2007). The single most important predictor of which toddlers would achieve this optimal outcome was motor skills and less severe social deficits. By the time the toddlers were retested after they no longer met criteria for an ASD diagnosis, they had made very significant gains in both IQ and language skills, which may be attributed in part to the intensive behavioral interventions they all had received. Although these children were able to move into regular school settings, some subtle deficits in pragmatic language skills remained

suggesting that there are residual effects of ASD that are not completely eliminated or outgrown (Kelley, Paul, Fein, & Naigles, 2006).

Summary and Future Directions

Because of the alarming rise in prevalence rates, there is now far greater awareness and interest in ASD. We now recognize that this is a complex disorder with multiple etiologies and heterogeneity in the phenotypes, which change over time. Dawson's developmental model of ASD highlights the role of risk indices and risk processes as central to our understanding of the unfolding trajectory that leads to the emergence of ASD symptoms during the second and third years of life. In recent years we have begun to make inroads in what is known about not only these risk profiles but also of potential protective factors that may prevent onset or reduce the severity of ASD in later years.

Studies of high-risk infants have allowed us to observe the full range of developmental pathways for infants who are genetically vulnerable, with about one-fifth eventually having an ASD outcome. At the same time, when compared to infants later diagnosed with ASD, the majority of high-risk infants may share similar atypical brain and behavioral patterns but do not meet criteria for ASD in later years, and in some cases, toddlers who are diagnosed with ASD can fall "off the spectrum" by the time they reach kindergarten. The key to understanding what may protect these children comes from taking a *developmental* perspective. The same processes are critical for social, cognitive, and language development in both typically developing children and those at risk for or with ASD. Interestingly, some studies suggest that motor skills may be the single best child-related factor that predicts eventual outcomes for this population. It may be that motor development is a sensitive marker for cortical maturation and development. Future studies should address this issue and explore additional potential child-related protective processes such as emotional regulation and other executive functions.

Behavioral interventions that encompass these developmental processes and are presented in an intense and highly structured setting can significantly improve a child's cognitive and language skills and may lead to optimal outcomes. Parent–child interactions are also important influences on children with ASD: it may be even more essential to synchronize with the attentional focus and activities of a child at risk for ASD, even though these may be somewhat unusual in content and focus.

Despite all these advances in our understanding of ASD, the rates are still rising and there is much work to be done. How are we to understand the exponential increase in the numbers of children diagnosed with ASD? In addition to the focus on potential risk indices, more research is needed on the role of risk processes and potential protective factors. Advances in our understanding of the developmental processes will lay a foundation for enhanced early detection and diagnosis of ASD and lead to even more targeted interventions that can be implemented by parents and professionals. Finally, we need a concerted effort to bring what we have already learned to the many areas of the world where there are still almost no resources available for children and adults with ASD and their families.

Acknowledgments The preparation of this chapter was supported by grants from NIH (RO1 DC 10290; RO1 DC 11339; P50 DC 13027) and the Simons Foundation.

References

American Psychiatric Association. (1980). *Diagnostic and statistical manual of mental disorders* (3rd ed.). Washington, DC: Author.

American Psychiatric Association. (1994). *Diagnostic and statistical manual of mental disorders* (4th ed.). Washington, D.C.: Author.

American Psychiatric Association. (2013). *Diagnostic and statistical manual of mental disorders* (5th ed.). Arlington, VA: American Psychiatric Publishing.

Asperger, H. (1944/1991). 'Autistic psychopathy' in childhood. In U. Frith (Ed.), *Autism and Asperger syndrome* (pp. 37–91). Cambridge: Cambridge University Press.

Autism and Developmental Disabilities Monitoring Network (2012). Prevalence of autism spectrum disorder – Autism and Developmental Disabilities Monitoring Network, United States, 2008. *MMWR Surveillance Summary, 61*, 1–19.

Bailey, A., Le Couteur, A., Gottesman, I., Bolton, P., Simonoff, E., Yuzda, E., et al. (1995). Autism as a strongly genetic disorder: Evidence from a British twin study. *Psychological medicine, 25*, 63–77.

Bailey, A., Phillips, W., & Rutter, M. (1996). Autism: Towards an integration of clinical, genetic, neuropsychological and neurobiological perspectives. *Journal of Child Psychology and Psychiatry, 37*, 89–126.

Baron-Cohen, S., Tager-Flusberg, H., & Cohen, D. J. (Eds.). (1993). *Understanding other minds: Perspectives from autism.* Oxford: Oxford University Press.

Baron-Cohen, S., Tager-Flusberg, H., & Cohen, D. J. (Eds.). (2000). *Understanding other minds: Perspectives from developmental cognitive neuroscience* (2nd ed.). Oxford: Oxford University Press.

Ben-Sasson, A., Cermak, S., Orsmond, G., Tager-Flusberg, H., Carter, A. S., Kadlec, M. B., et al. (2007). Extreme sensory modulation behaviors in toddlers with autism spectrum disorders. *American Journal of Occupational Therapy, 61*, 584–592.

Bosl, W., Tierney, A., Tager-Flusberg, H., & Nelson, C. A. (2011). EEG complexity as a biomarker for autism spectrum disorder risk. *BMC Medicine, 9*, 1–18.

Bearman, P. (2010). Just-so stories: Autism, and the single-bullet disorder. *Social Psychology Quarterly, 20*, 1–4.

Carmody, D., & Lewis, M. (2010). Regional white matter development in children with autism spectrum disorders. *Developmental Psychobiology, 52*, 755–763.

Carmody, D., & Lewis, M. (2012). Self representation in children with and without autism spectrum disorders. *Child Psychiatry and Human Development, 43*, 227–237.

Charman, T., Jones, C., Pickles, A., Simonoff, E., Baird, G., & Happé, F. (2011). Defining the cognitive phenotype of autism. *Brain Research, 1380*, 10–21.

Constantino, J., Zhang, Y., Frazier, T., Abbacchi, A., & Law, P. (2010). Sibling recurrence and the genetic epidemiology of autism. *American Journal of Psychiatry, 167*, 1349–1356.

Courchesne, E., Redcay, E., & Kennedy, D. (2004). The autistic brain: Birth through adulthood. *Current Opinion in Neurobiology, 17*, 489–496.

Courchesne, E., Pierce, K., Schumann, C., Redcay, E., Buckwalter, J., Kennedy, D., et al. (2007). Mapping early brain development in autism. *Neuron, 56*, 399–413.

Dawson, G. (2008). Early behavioral intervention, brain plasticity, and the prevention of autism spectrum disorder. *Development and Psychopathology, 20*, 775–803.

Dawson, G., Rogers, S., Munson, J., Smith, M., Winter, J., Greenson, J., et al. (2010). Randomized controlled trial of an intervention for toddlers with autism: The Early Start Denver Model. *Pediatrics, 125*, 17–23.

Dawson, G., & Burner, K. (2011). Behavioral interventions in children and adolescents with autism spectrum disorder: A review of recent findings. *Current Opinion in Pediatrics, 23*, 616–620.

Dawson, G., Sterling, L., & Faja, S. (2009). Autism: Risk factors, risk processes and outcome. In M. de Haan & M. R. Gunnar (Eds.), *Handbook of developmental social neuroscience* (pp. 435–458). New York: Guilford Press.

Elsabbagh, M., Mercure, E., Hudry, K., Chandler, S., Pasco, G., Charman, T., et al. (2012). Infant neural sensitivity to dynamic eye gaze is associated with later emerging autism. *Current Biology, 22*, 1–5.

Fein, D., Barton, M., Eigsti, I.-M., Kelley, E., Naigles, L., Schultz, R., et al. (2013). Optimal outcome in individuals with a history of autism. *Journal of Child Psychology and Psychiatry, 54*, 195–205.

Flanagan, J., Landa, R., Bhat, A., & Bauman, M. (2012). Head lag in infants at risk for autism: A preliminary study. *American Journal of Occupational Therapy, 66*, 577–585.

Folstein, S., & Rutter, M. (1977). Infantile autism: A genetic study of 21 twin pairs. *Journal of Child Psychology and Psychiatry, 18*, 297–321.

Frazier, T., Youngstrom, E., Kubu, C., Sinclair, L., & Rezai, A. (2008). Exploratory and confirmatory factor analysis of the autism diagnostic interview-revised. *Journal of Autism and Developmental Disorders, 38*, 474–480.

Garon, N., Bryson, S., Zwaigenbaum, L., Smith, I., Brian, J., Roberts, W., et al. (2009). Temperament and its relationship to autism symptoms in a high-risk infant sib cohort. *Journal of Abnormal Child Psychology, 37*, 59–78.

Gathercole, V. C. M., & Hoff, E. (2007). Input and the acquisition of language: Three questions. In E. Hoff & M. Shatz (Eds.), *Blackwell handbook of language development* (pp. 107–127). Oxford: Blackwell.

Gerdts, J., & Bernier, R. (2011). The broader autism phenotype and its implications on the etiology and treatments of autism spectrum disorders. *Autism Research and Treatment*. Article ID 545901.

Ghaziuddin, M. (2011). Asperger disorder in the DSM-V: Sacrificing utility for validity. *Journal of the American Academy of Child and Adolescent Psychiatry, 50*, 192–193.

Hallmayer, J., Cleveland, S., Torres, A., Philips, J., Cohen, B., Torigoe, T., et al. (2011). Genetic heritability and shared environmental factors among twin pairs with autism. *Archives of General Psychiatry, 68*, 1095–1102.

Hazlett, H., Poe, M., Gerig, G., Styner, M., Chappell, C., Smith, R., et al. (2011). Early brain overgrowth in autism associated with an increase in cortical surface area before age 2 years. *Archives of General Psychiatry, 68*, 467–476.

Hermelin, B., & O'Connor, N. (1970). *Psychological experiments with autistic children*. Oxford: Pergamon Press.

Huerta, M., Bishop, S., Duncan, A., Hus, V., & Lord, C. (2012). Application of DSM-5 criteria for autism spectrum disorder to three samples of children with DSM-IV diagnoses of pervasive developmental disorders. *American Journal of Psychiatry, 169*, 1056–1064.

Jones, W., & Klin, A. (2009). Heterogeneity and homogeneity across the autism spectrum: The role of development. *Journal of the American Academy of Child and Adolescent Psychiatry, 48*, 471–473.

Kanner, L. (1943). Autistic disturbance of affective contact. *Nervous Child, 2*, 217–250.

Kasari, C., Gulsrud, A., Wong, C., Kwon, S., & Locke, J. (2010). Randomized controlled caregiver mediated joint engagement intervention for toddlers with autism. *Journal of Autism and Developmental Disorders, 40*, 1045–1056.

Kelley, E., Paul, J., Fein, D., & Naigles, L. (2006). Residual language deficits in optimal outcome children with a history of autism. *Journal of Autism and Developmental Disorders, 36*, 807–828.

Key, A., & Stone, W. (2012). Processing of novel and familiar faces in infants at average and high risk for autism. *Developmental Cognitive Neuroscience, 2*, 244–255.

Kuhl, P. (2007). Is speech learning 'gated' by the social brain? *Developmental Science, 10*, 110–120.

Lewis, M., & Ramsay, D. (2004). Development of self-recognition, personal pronoun use, and pretend play during the 2nd year. *Child Development, 75*, 1821–1931.

Lord, C., Rutter, M., & LeCouteur, A. (1994). Autism diagnostic interview-revised: A revised version of a diagnostic interview for caregivers of individuals with possible pervasive developmental disorders. *Journal of Autism and Developmental Disorders, 24*, 659–685.

Lord, C., Rutter, M., DiLavore, P., & Risi, S. (1999). *Autism Diagnostic Observation Schedule (ADOS)*. Los Angeles, CA: Western Psychological Services.

Lord, C., Luyster, R., Guthrie, W., & Pickles, A. (2012). Patterns of developmental trajectories in toddlers with autism spectrum disorder. *Journal of Consulting and Clinical Psychology, 80*, 477–489.

Luyster, R., Kadlec, M. B., Connolly, C., Carter, A., & Tager-Flusberg, H. (2008). Language assessment and development in toddlers with autism spectrum disorders. *Journal of Autism and Developmental Disorders, 38*, 1426–1438.

Luyster, R., Wagner, J. B., Vogel-Farley, V., Tager-Flusberg, H., & Nelson, C. A. (2011). Neural correlates of familiar and unfamiliar face processing in infants at risk for autism. *Brain Topography, 24*, 220–228.

Luyster, R., Seery, A.M., Thompson, M.R., & Tager-Flusberg, H. (2011). Identifying early risk markers and developmental trajectories for language impairment in neurodevelopmental disorders. *Developmental Disabilities Research Review, 17*, 151–159.

Mandell, D., Wiggins, L., Carpenter, L., Daniels, J., DiGuiseppi, C., Durkin, M., et al. (2009). Racial/ethnic disparities in the identification of children with autism spectrum disorders. *American Journal of Public Health, 99*, 493–498.

McPartland, J., Reichow, B., & Volkmar, F. (2012). Sensitivity and specificity of proposed DSM-5 diagnostic criteria for autism spectrum disorder. *Journal of the American Academy of Child and Adolescent Psychiatry, 51*, 368–383.

Newschaffer, C., Croen, L., Fallin, M., Hertz-Picciotto, I., Nguyen, D., Lee, N., et al. (2012). Infant siblings and the investigation of autism risk factors. *Journal of Neurodevelopmental Disorders, 4*, 7.

Osterling, J., & Dawson, G. (1994). Early recognition of children with autism: A study of first birthday home videotapes. *Journal of Autism and Developmental Disorders, 24*, 247–257.

Ozonoff, S. (2012). Editorial perspective: Autism spectrum disorders in DSM-5 – An historical perspective and the need for change. *Journal of Child Psychology and Psychiatry, 53*, 1092–1094.

Ozonoff, S., Iosif, A.-M., Baguio, F., Cook, I., Hill, M., Hutman, T., et al. (2010). A prospective study of the emergence of early behavioral signs of autism. *Journal of the American Academy of Child and Adolescent Psychiatry, 49*, 256–266.

Ozonoff, S., Hueng, K., & Thompson, M. (2011). Regression and other patterns of onset. In D. G. Amaral, G. Dawson, & D. Geschwind (Eds.), *Autism spectrum disorders*. New York: Oxford University Press.

Ozonoff, S., Young, G., Carter, A., Messinger, D., Yirmiya, N., Zwaigenbaum, L., et al. (2011). Recurrence risk for autism spectrum disorders: A baby siblings research consortium study. *Pediatrics, 128*, 488–495.

Pickles, A., Simonoff, E., Conti-Ramsden, G., Falcaro, M., Simkin, Z., Charman, T., et al. (2009). Loss of language in early development of autism and specific language impairment. *Journal of Child Psychology and Psychiatry, 50*, 843–852.

Redcay, E., & Courchesne, E. (2005). When is the brain enlarged in autism? A meta-analysis of all brain size reports. *Biological Psychiatry, 58*, 1–9.

Redcay, E., & Courchesne, E. (2008). Deviant functional magnetic resonance imaging patterns of brain activity to speech in 2-3-year-old children with autism spectrum disorder. *Biological Psychiatry, 64*, 589–598.

Rimland, B. (1964). *Infantile autism: The syndrome and its implications for a neural theory of behavior*. New York: Prentice-Hall.

Rogers, S. (2009). What are infant siblings teaching us about autism in infancy? *Autism Research, 2*, 125–137.

Rogers, S., Estes, A., Lord, C., Vismara, L., Winter, J., Fitzpatrick, A., et al. (2012). Effects of a brief Early Start Denver Model (ESDM)-based parent intervention on toddlers at risk for autism spectrum disorders: A randomized controlled trial. *Journal of the American Academy of Child and Adolescent Psychiatry, 51*, 1052–1065.

Rowe, M. L., & Goldin-Meadow, S. (2009). Early gesture selectively predicts later language learning. *Developmental Science, 12*, 182–187.

Rutter, M. (1996). Autism research: Prospects and priorities. *Journal of Autism and Developmental Disorders, 26*, 257–275.

Sebat, J., Lakshmi, B., Malhotra, D., Troge, J., Lese-Martin, C., Walsh, T., et al. (2007). Strong association of de novo copy number mutations with autism. *Science, 316*, 445–449.

Seltzer, M. M., Greenberg, J. S., Taylor, J. L., Smith, L., Orsmond, G. I., Esbensen, A., et al. (2011). Adolescents and adults with autism spectrum disorders. In D. G. Amaral, G. Dawson, & D. Geschwind (Eds.), *Autism spectrum disorders*. New York: Oxford University Press.

Shen, Y., Chen, X., Wang, L., Guo, J., Shen, J., An, Y., et al. (2011). Intra-family phenotypic heterogeneity of 16p11.2 deletion carriers in a three-generation Chinese family. *American Journal of Medical Genetics B: Neuropsychiatric Genetics, 156*, 225–232.

Siller, M., & Sigman, M. (2002). The behaviors of parents of children with autism predict the subsequent development of their children's communication. *Journal of Autism and Developmental Disorders, 32*, 77–89.

State, M., & Levitt, P. (2011). The conundrum of understanding genetic risks for autism spectrum disorders. *Nature Neuroscience, 14*, 1499–1506.

State, M., & Sestan, N. (2012). The emerging biology of autism spectrum disorders. *Science, 337*, 1301–1303.

Sullivan, P., Daly, M., & O'Donovan, M. (2012). Genetic architectures of psychiatric disorders: The emerging picture and its implications. *Nature Reviews. Genetics, 13*, 537–551.

Sutera, S., Pandey, J., Esser, E., Rosenthal, M., Wilson, L., Barton, M., et al. (2007). Predictors of optimal outcome in toddlers diagnosed with autism spectrum disorders. *Journal of Autism and Developmental Disorders, 37*, 98–107.

Szatmari, P. (2011). Is autism, at least in part, a disorder of fetal programming? *Archives of General Psychiatry, 68*, 1091–1092.

Tager-Flusberg, H. (2010). The origins of social impairments in autism spectrum disorder: Studies of infants at risk. *Neural Networks, 23*, 1072–1076.

Tager-Flusberg, H., Paul, R., & Lord, C. E. (2005). Language and communication in autism. In F. Volkmar, R. Paul, A. Klin, & D. J. Cohen (Eds.), *Handbook of autism and pervasive developmental disorder* (3rd ed., Vol. 1, pp. 335–364). New York: Wiley.

Tager-Flusberg, H., Edelson, L., & Luyster, R. (2011). Language and communication in autism spectrum disorders. In D. Amaral, G. Dawson, & D. Geschwind (Eds.), *Autism spectrum disorders*. Oxford: Oxford University Press.

Tager-Flusberg, H., & Kasari, C. (2013). Minimally verbal school-aged children with autism spectrum disorder: The neglected end of the spectrum. *Autism Research*. Oct 7. doi: 10.1002/aur.1329.

Talbott, M.R., Nelson, C.A., & Tager-Flusberg, H. (2013). Maternal gesture use and language development in infant siblings of children with autism spectrum disorder. *Journal of Autism and Developmental Disorders.* Apr 13. PMCID:PMC3823696.

Tierney, A., Gabard-Durnam, L., Vogel-Farley, V., Tager-Flusberg, H., & Nelson, C. A. (2012). Developmental trajectories of resting EEG power: An endophenotype of autism spectrum disorder. *PLOS One, 7.*

Vernes, S., Newbury, D., Abrahams, B., Winchester, L., Groszer, M., Alarcho, M., et al. (2008). A functional genetic link between distinct developmental language disorders. *New England Journal of Medicine, 359,* 2337–2345.

Wakefield, A. J., Murch, S. H., Anthony, A., Linnell, J., Casson, D. M., Malik, M., et al. (1998). Ileal lymphoid nodular hyperplasia, non-specific colitis, and pervasive developmental disorder in children. *Lancet, 35,* 637–41 [retracted].

Wing, L. (1981). Asperger's syndrome: A clinical account. *Psychological Medicine, 11,* 115–129.

Woolf, J., Gu, H., Gerig, G., Elison, J., Styner, M., Gouttard, S., et al. (2012). Differences in white matter fiber tract development present from 6 to 24 months in infants with autism. *American Journal of Psychiatry, 169,* 589–600.

Zwaigenbaum, L., Bryson, S., Rogers, T., Roberts, W., Brian, J., & Szatmari, P. (2005). Behavioral manifestations of autism in the first year of life. *International Journal of Developmental Neuroscience, 23,* 143–152.

Zwaigenbaum, L., Thurm, A., Stone, W., Baranek, G., Bryson, S., Iverson, J. et al. (2007). Studying the emergence of autism spectrum disorders in high-risk infants: Methodological and practical issues. *Journal of Autism and Developmental Disorders, 37,* 466–480.

Zwaigenbaum, L., Bryson, S., Lord, C., Rogers, S., Carter, A., Carver, L., et al. (2009). Clinical assessment and management of toddlers with suspected autism spectrum disorder: Insights from studies of high-risk infants. *Pediatrics, 123,* 1383–1391.

Intellectual Disability

34

Barbara Tylenda, Rowland P. Barrett, and Henry T. Sachs, III

Introduction

Change in Terminology

Intellectual disability has been recognized perhaps longer than anything else we currently study in psychiatry and psychology (Berkson, 2004; Tylenda, Hooper, & Barrett, 1987). However, the term intellectual disability (ID) is relatively new. It replaces the previous and long-used term mental retardation (MR).

In 2007, the American Association on Mental Retardation (AAMR) successfully voted to rename its organization the American Association on Intellectual and Developmental Disabilities (AAIDD). At that time, the organization also put forth the formal diagnostic name change from MR to ID (Schalock et al., 2007).

According to the AAIDD, the diagnostic term ID is preferred over the term MR because it reflects a changed construct of disability (AAMR, 2002; Buntinx, 2006; World Health Organization, 2001). Specifically, the construct changes from disability as a problem residing within a person to understanding disability as residing at least partly in the gap between a person's capacities and the demands of typical contexts or environments

B. Tylenda, Ph.D., A.B.P.P. (✉) • R.P. Barrett, Ph.D.
H.T. Sachs, III, M.D.
Alpert Medical School of Brown University,
Providence, RI 02912, USA
e-mail: BTylenda@Lifespan.org

(AAIDD, 2012). Further, the construct changes from a static, unchanging condition to a condition that can change over time (Harris, 2006).

The AAIDD was clear to stipulate that "… anyone eligible in the past for a diagnosis of MR is now considered eligible for a diagnosis of ID. The term ID covers the same population of individuals previously diagnosed with MR in number, kind, level, type and duration, and the need for services and supports; and every individual who is or was eligible for a diagnosis of mental retardation is eligible for a diagnosis of ID" (AAIDD, 2010, p. xvi).

Overview

ID is a categorization for a heterogeneous group of individuals with deficits in cognitive and adaptive behavior functioning manifest prior to their 18th birthday. Those presenting with ID display individual patterns of strengths and weaknesses across academic, language, social, emotional, and physical skill performances. The developmental course for individuals with ID is not as inflexible as once thought (AAIDD, 2012). Multiple, unique developmental challenges face these children and their caregivers alike. How these challenges are resolved contributes significantly to the eventual developmental outcomes of children with ID.

ID is not a medical disorder, although it may be coded in a medical classification of diseases. Further, despite its inclusion in all the editions of the APA's *Diagnostic and Statistical Manual of Mental Disorders* (*DSM*) (American Psychiatric Association, 1952, 1968, 1980, 1987, 1994, 2000), ID is not a mental disorder. Rather, it is a deviation in development that can increase the risk of mental disorder. In general, the definition and severity of ID refers to a level of behavioral performance without reference to etiology.

Until recently, ID was wrongly viewed as a protective or exclusionary factor in mental disorders. "Diagnostic overshadowing" (Reiss, Levitan, & Szyszko, 1982) attributed most behavioral and emotional abnormalities in those with ID to their cognitive limitations or underlying medical condition. However, it is now clear that individuals with ID have three to four times the general population risk for the full range of psychiatric disorders (cf. Matson & Barrett, 1993). This is not surprising when one considers the factors contributing to developmental psychopathology: biology, learned behavior, psychodynamic issues, social factors, family systems functioning, and cognitive abilities. ID and its various etiologies are likely to impact on most or all of these components. In this regard, individuals with ID and psychiatric disorder represent a unique population requiring the integration of numerous treatment modalities.

Diagnosis of ID

Diagnostic Criteria

While there are several different diagnostic criteria for ID (e.g., WHO, 2008), the authoritative definition of ID is that of the AAIDD (Harris, 2006). The 2010 definition in 11th edition of the *Manual* is essentially the same definition as that from its 2002 *Manual* with the minor edit that substitutes the term ID for MR: "ID is characterized by significant limitations both in intellectual functioning and in adaptive behavior as expressed in conceptual, social, and practical adaptive skills. This disability originates before age 18" (p. 1).

The 2010 *Manual* also provides the listing of five *assumptions* that are now *an explicit part* of

the definition because they clarify the context from which the definition arises and indicate how the definition must be applied (AAIDD, 2010). The five AAIDD definition *assumptions* are as follows: "(*1*) Limitations in present functioning must be considered within the context of community environments typical of the individual's age peers and culture; (*2*) Valid assessment considers cultural and linguistic diversity as well as differences in communication, sensory, motor, and behavioral factors; (*3*) Within an individual, limitations often coexist with strengths; (*4*) An important purpose of describing limitations is to develop a profile of needed supports; and (*5*) With appropriate supports over a sustained period, the life functioning of the person with ID generally will improve" (p. 1).

Since 2002, the AAIDD definition no longer includes a classification system based on degrees of severity of ID. This came about from the AAIDD's position of incorporating measured intelligence only in the initial diagnosis. The AAIDD definition emphasizes identification of an individual's specific areas of "ability" rather than "disability" and then classifies the intensity of needed support services in various cognitive and adaptive behavior domains. The intent has been to drive recognition of the relative strengths of individuals with ID and create awareness among service providers, researchers, and policymakers that the population is vastly heterogeneous, even within sets of individuals possessing a common IQ.

Review of APA's *Diagnostic and Statistical Manual of Mental Disorders, Fifth Edition* (*DSM-5*) (American Psychiatric Association, 2013), reveals a significant shift of definitional criteria for ID by APA. The APA definition of ID is now quite consistent with the AAIDD definition. The APA *DSM-5* definition for ID (referred to as "Intellectual Disability (Intellectual Developmental Disorder")) is as follows:

"Intellectual Disability (Intellectual Developmental Disorder) is a disorder with onset during the developmental period that includes both intellectual and adaptive functioning deficits in conceptual, social, and practical domains. The following three criteria must be met:

A. Deficits in intellectual functions, such as reasoning, problem solving, planning, abstract thinking, judgment, academic learning, and learning from experience, confirmed by both clinical assessment and individualized, standardized intelligence testing.

AND

B. Deficits in adaptive functioning that result in failure to meet developmental and sociocultural standards for personal independence and social responsibility. Without ongoing support, the adaptive deficits limit functioning in one or more activities of daily life, such as communication, social participation, and independent living, across multiple environments, such as home, school, work, and community.

AND

C. Onset of intellectual and adaptive deficits during the developmental period." (p. 33)

In doing so, *DSM-5* (American Psychiatric Association, 2013) has not only eliminated the terminology MR to be consistent with AAIDD practices and international opinion, it also has added rigor to wording regarding cultural sensitivity and adaptive behavior functioning.

Clinical Profile of ID Severity Level

While the AAIDD and APA have eliminated ID IQ subtypes from definitional criteria for diagnostic purposes, general clinical profiles are associated with respective identified ranges of cognitive functioning. These profiles of severity levels have been the way that educators, psychologists, adult service providers, and researchers have identified the ID population and are considered to have continued qualitative value (McMillan, Gresham, & Siperstein, 1993, 1995).

Individuals with IQ scores falling in the range of 2 to 3 SD below the mean comprise approximately 85 % of all persons diagnosed with ID (APA, 2000). Comparable limitations with regard to adaptive functioning also are present.

Individuals in this range of functioning often are not identified as having ID until they enter school (Grossman, 1983; Tylenda, Beckett, &

Barrett, 2007). Parents of these children, however, frequently report that their child displayed delays in acquisition of developmental speech and motor milestones. Children with cognitive functioning in this range may have a history of referral for speech and occupational therapy services in early childhood. Once identified as having ID, these children become eligible for special education services to aid acquisition of academic, vocational, and life skills. Individuals with cognitive functioning in this range typically develop social and communication skills by age 4 and achieve academic skills approximating the sixth-grade level by their late teenage years. For many children in this range of functioning, cognitive deficits will be misinterpreted as decreased motivation, an oppositional response style, or attention deficits, and appropriate special education interventions will not be sought.

Beyond the school-age years, individuals with cognitive functioning in this range develop sufficient social and vocational abilities to live and work independently without coming to the attention of the professional service community. Some may need assistance when facing unusual personal, economic, or social stressors. Some also will require ongoing vocational, social, and self-care support.

Individuals with IQ scores falling in the range of more than 3 SD below the mean make up the remaining 15 % of all individuals diagnosed with ID (APA, 2000). Comparable limitations with regard to adaptive functioning also are present.

Individuals whose eventual IQ scores fall between 3 and 4 SD below the mean usually are first identified during infancy or early childhood secondary to displaying delays in attaining developmental milestones (Tylenda, Beckett, & Barrett, 2007). Individuals functioning in this range usually develop communication skills in early childhood. With the support of special education services, these individuals may acquire academic skills similar to a second- to fourth-grade student, usually by the period of late adolescence. They usually will be able to interpret social cues but may have difficulty organizing a timely and appropriate response to social interactions. Even as adults, these individuals will likely require increased support, supervision, and/or assistance in most areas of vocational and daily living in comparison to their mildly affected counterparts. These individuals make up approximately 10 % of the ID population (Harris, 2006).

Individuals whose eventual IQ scores fall 4 to 5 SD below the mean commonly are identified as needing supports/services in infancy as they manifest delays in acquiring motor and language skills (Tylenda et al., 2007). Physical abnormalities are not unusual, and they often have concurrent medical problems. These individuals develop very limited language. While they acquire some basic self-help skills, they cannot function independently and usually require significant daily support and professional supervision throughout their entire lives. This group constitutes 3 to 4 % of those diagnosed with ID (Harris, 2006).

Individuals whose eventual IQ scores fall more than 5 SD below the mean are typically identified as needing supports/services at birth or soon thereafter (Tylenda et al., 2007). Early identification is usually secondary to their apparent physical abnormalities and/or compromise. Such may hinder or preclude the ability to ambulate or speak. Neurological impairments are most common in this group. Skills for simple tasks, such as basic communication, may be learned with frequent repetition and dedicated individual attention. Others will have to take on responsibility for all basic care and activities of daily living for individuals in this range of functioning. This level of care will be lifelong. This group makes up 1 % to 2 % of persons with ID (Harris, 2006).

Epidemiology

The statistical component of the definition of ID would presume a population prevalence of approximately 3 % (2 SD below the mean in a normal distribution of intelligence). An early study by Heber (1961) put the prevalence of ID in the United States at 3 %, a very significant number. A very well-conducted population study of the Isle of Wight by Rutter, Tizard, and Whitmore (1970) confirmed these findings. However, more recent studies (cf. Murphy, Boyle, Schendel, Decoufle, & Yeargin-Allsopp, 1998) have repeatedly demonstrated a prevalence rate equal to or less than 1 % (Baird & Sadovnick, 1985) with males being 50 % more likely to have ID. Males also are at greater risk of genetic abnormality (McLaren & Bryson, 1987) and are more likely to come to professional attention for psychiatric (i.e., aggressive, disruptive behaviors) disorders. Approximately 2.5 million individuals in the United States have ID (Centers for Disease Control, 1996; Committee on Disability Determination for Mental Retardation, 2002), which is identified as the largest categorical disability among children. The prevalence rate of ID in children between the ages of 6 and 17 is 11.4/1,000.

The reasons for the apparent overestimation of ID prevalence are probably multifactorial. The mortality rate for those with moderate-profound ID is elevated (McLaren & Bryson, 1987). Genetic counseling and prenatal testing have decreased the likelihood of children with chromosomal abnormalities. Abortion service for high-risk pregnancies also is a factor. Improved obstetrical techniques have lowered the incidence of brain damage at birth (Harris, 2006). Newborn screening (e.g., PKU), hormone replacement, vaccination, and immunotherapy have nearly eliminated some causes of ID (Alexander, 1998). Finally, the reduction in poverty and improvements in early childhood nutrition and education (e.g., lead exposure) have decreased the rate of mild ID, the classification most likely impacted by environmental variables associated with poverty (Thompson & Hupp, 1992).

Undiagnosed ID also plays a role in suppressing prevalence rates. As individuals become adults and function independently in society, many no longer meet the adaptive impairment criteria of ID.

Etiology

Overall, the potential etiologies for ID are as diverse as they are numerous (Accardo & Capute,

1998). Such reflect the interaction of genetics and environmental factors and can occur prenatally, perinatally, or postnatally during the developmental period (AAMR, 2002). Chromosomal abnormalities, deficits of metabolism, intrauterine infections, and toxic exposure or brain developmental errors are among the prenatal causes of ID (Bale, 2002; Burd, Cotsonas-Hassler, Martsolf, & Kerbeshian, 2003; Jones, Lopez, & Wilson, 2003; Mochida & Walsh, 2004; Rhead & Irons, 2004; Rovet, 2002). Normally developed fetuses may experience perinatal insult. Toxemia, obstetrical trauma, intracranial hemorrhage, hydrocephalus, seizures, and infections may create permanent deficits (Vannucci, 1990). Throughout the child's development, head injuries, infections, seizure disorders, genetic disorders, toxic exposures, and/or environmental deprivation may contribute to a presentation consistent with ID (Matson & Barrett, 1993).

The roles of deprivation and cultural and familial factors have been cited as dominant etiologically for individuals where the degree of ID is less severe. Specifically, low socioeconomic status, maternal education, positive family histories of ID, consanguinity, child abuse, and child neglect have been identified as risk factors for individuals with less severe ID (Zigler, 1967).

However, advances in biomedical technology have enabled identification of a neurobiological etiology for an increasing number of ID syndromes (Harris, 2006). A cause can be confirmed for approximately 80 % of individuals presenting with ID in the more severe forms. Neurobiological factors are also being found to play a significant etiological role in milder ID—where a variety of biomedical abnormalities may be responsible for 30 % to 45 % of cases of milder ID (Lamont and Dennis, 1988). These results have led to a reexamination of the causative role of psychosocial disadvantage and polygenic inheritance in those presenting with ID in the milder form of severity level. Current evidence does not support the existence of the etiological distinction between "organic ID" and "cultural/familiar ID" as newer knowledge about brain functioning and behavior becomes available (Rutter, Simonoff, & Plomin, 1996).

Disabilities Frequently Associated with ID

In comparison to the general population, individuals with ID are more likely to have significant disabilities (Frazier, Barrett, Feinstein, & Walters, 1997). The frequency of associated physical disabilities increases in proportion to the level of cognitive and adaptive delay. Blindness and hearing impairment occur at 20 to 30 times the rate of the general population, respectively (Baroff, 1986), in those with the most severe degree of ID. Cerebral palsy, scoliosis, kyphosis, and other impairments of motor functioning are much more frequent. Even constipation, enuresis, and encopresis have significant impacts on social and life skill development in those with ID (Matson, Anderson, & Bamburg, 2000).

Comorbid psychopathology also is present in the ID population. Rutter et al. (1970) in their study of the Isle of Wight showed that mental illness occurred about five times as often among individuals with ID compared to the non-ID population. Menolascino (1970) published a compendium on psychiatric approaches to ID and coined the term "dual diagnosis" to designate people who have both ID and mental illness simultaneously. A more complete discussion of comorbid psychopathology among individuals with ID can be found later in this chapter.

Finally, difficult behaviors expressed by individuals with ID also are not uncommon. Unfortunately, these difficult behaviors often grab unwanted attention by the public or can create feelings of apprehension and/or danger for family members, professionals, or direct care staff. For individuals with ID who are nonverbal, behavioral disruption may indicate a very mild annoyance to a serious medical or mental condition (Lowe et al., 2007). For example, some of the causative sources for difficult behavior could include internal triggers (e.g., pain, seizure, sensory, fear, psychosis), external triggers (e.g., threats, environmental cues, lack of safety), trauma (e.g., physical, sexual, posttraumatic, stress), limited range of expression (e.g., through illness, disability, or habit, different emotions are expressed in few visible expressive behaviors), and differentiation from mental illness diagnoses (e.g., overlap of conditions and behaviors which could include behavioral syndromes, learned behaviors, mannerisms, or manifestations of other disease processes such as change in arousal secondary to toxic effects of medication). Each of these categories requires assessment for potential causes, and they are not mutually exclusive of another category. The task for the evaluator is to assess the likely reasons for the disruptive behavior and to address individual and environmental contributions to the situation in which it arose.

Differentiating Children with ID from Children with Other Handicaps

In general, diagnostic issues with individuals who may be presenting with an ID may not be as straightforward as one would think. It is possible that an individual is presenting with an ID, is manifesting dual diagnosis, or is presenting with another disability altogether. Thus, psychiatrists, psychologists, and other evaluators who will be specializing in the diagnosis of ID would be well served to understand the unique concerns that present when undertaking such an evaluation.

It is possible that young children, particularly those of preschool age, who are referred for a first time developmental/cognitive evaluation for clarification of a diagnosis of ID are actually manifesting either (1) a diagnosis other than ID or (2) one or more additional diagnoses concomitant with the diagnosis of ID. Consequently, an evaluator who will be specializing in the evaluation and diagnosis of ID should be well versed in the presenting features and profiles for a range of other disorders and problems frequently diagnosed in the preschool and school-age population. Table 34.1 lists a range of these disorders and problems.

Table 34.1 List of disorders and problems to consider when a child is referred for a diagnostic evaluation to "rule in/rule out" intellectual disability

When conducting an assessment with a child for a possible diagnosis of intellectual disability (ID), the evaluator needs to consider the following range of disorders or problems as possible alternative or additional diagnoses/conditions:

1. Developmental delay
2. The "umbrella of neurological impairment" which includes:
   (a) Autism spectrum disorder[a]
   (b) Childhood disintegrative disorder
   (c) Neurological inefficiency/nonverbal learning disability
   (d) Attention deficit/hyperactivity disorder
3. Language/communication disorder
4. Hearing impairment
5. Visual impairment
6. Cerebral palsy
7. Rett's syndrome
8. Motor coordination disorder
9. Regulatory disorder
10. Reactive attachment disorder
11. Elective mutism
12. Psychosocial deprivation
13. Other psychiatric condition
14. Some form of a behavioral disorder
15. Dyadic problem between caretaker and child
16. Challenging temperament and/or inconsistency of temperament between caretaker and child

[a]Childhood disorders subsumed under "autism spectrum disorder" in *DSM-5* include (1) pervasive developmental disorder, not otherwise specified; (2) high-functioning autism; and (3) Asperger's disorder

Components of a Comprehensive Evaluation

The determination of ID is rarely a simple matter. While assessment of an individual's cognitive and adaptive behavior functioning during the developmental period is the core criteria for diagnosis of ID, a comprehensive evaluation for ID typically goes beyond this. A comprehensive evaluation includes consideration of genetic and nongenetic etiologies and assessment of cognitive and adaptive behavior functioning. Associated medical conditions (e.g., cerebral palsy or a seizure disorder) and mental, emotional, and behavioral problems should also be closely reviewed as they may influence cognitive functioning. A comprehensive evaluation may involve several assessment visits over time and, for a younger child, may occur within the context of a multidisciplinary treatment team.

Determining the etiology of ID can be critical. If a genetic disorder is suspected, genetic testing may be used to confirm a diagnosis. Confirmation of a genetic disorder also may lead to uncovering other associated medical and behavioral features requiring attention. Information on the etiology of ID may impact trajectory as some developmental disorders can be arrested or sometimes prevented through early detection and treatment. Knowledge of etiology can inform for the future of the individual with ID or other family members as they consider their own family planning. Finally, etiological clarification can identify an appropriate support group and, in certain cases, facilitate funding for special services.

A full medical history and a thorough physical examination are first steps to deciphering the etiology of ID. Following these events, laboratory and diagnostic studies are chosen based on the clinical findings. Formal evaluation of cognitive and adaptive behavior functioning is also completed along with evaluation of comorbid emotional and/or behavioral problems. A comprehensive treatment plan is created based on all evaluation findings which may include medical, psycho-educational, genetic, and/or behavioral counseling and family support services.

Not all evaluations will result in a clear etiology or a diagnosed condition. The cause for ID can be identified in 40 % to 60 % of those undergoing an evaluation (Curry et al., 1997). Diagnostic accuracy is gradually increasing with improved neuroimaging techniques and cytogenetic techniques (Harris, 2006).

Harris (2006) has provided a comprehensive review of guidelines for a medical and genetic evaluation of an individual with ID. Tylenda et al. (2007) have provided an extensive examination of various standardized verbal and nonverbal intelligence tests useful in assessing for ID in individuals across the age range (and who

may present with various forms of concomitant challenge). They review in detail the history, conceptual bases, method of test construction, psychometric properties, testing procedures, scoring protocols, and examiner qualifications, as well as indications and contraindications for the use of each test. They also walk professionals through the intricacies of accurate intelligence testing and reporting of results for children and adolescents with ID. A companion review for the assessment of adaptive behavior functioning can be found in Dixon (2007). Aman has (1991a, 1991b) reviewed instruments for assessing emotional and behavioral disorders in individuals at all levels of ID.

Developmental Challenges for Individuals with ID

Development is a complex process of growth and change through which children acquire a variety of skills and abilities that allow them to understand and function in their world. The normal trajectory of development enables a child to progress from complete dependency on others to near- or complete independency for his/her needs and well-being. Although there is great variability in development, there are earlier and later limits to what is considered "normal/typical" development. Statistically, children with ID are those who develop at a rate significantly below average—the lowest 3 % on the normal, bell-shaped curve distribution—indicating why ID is called a "developmental disability."

These children make progress at a rate that is significantly slower than is expected of children their age. However, just as the development of children who do not have ID varies, so does the development of children with ID. Further, for any child with ID, the development for different areas (i.e., cognitive abilities, language and speech skills, gross motor skills, fine motor skills, social-emotional skills, and play skills) may proceed at different rates, on different timelines, and in different orders. As a result, the timetable for achievement of developmental milestones for a child with ID can be difficult to predict as well as eventual developmental trajectories. However, over time, such trajectories become more predictable based on the child's prior rates and breadth of performance. Variables key to the eventual developmental progression for any child with ID will include the following: (1) the child's inborn biological and neurological capacity (which set the general limits for the rate and eventual endpoints of development), (2) the ongoing environmental factors to which the child is exposed (e.g., type and amount of stimulation), (3) any associated disabilities or medical problems of the child, and (4) the child's support network's ability to assist him/her in addressing these challenges.

Disruption of Mastery of Developmental Skills Specific to Developmental Periods

The mastery of developmental "skills" specifically associated to each developmental period can present unique challenges for a child or adolescent with ID. A disruption in the mastery of specific developmental skills also can present unique challenges for the child or adolescent's caregivers and family, in how they initiate as well as respond to the child.

Infancy

Infancy is characterized by the development of attachment, self-regulation, and environmental awareness and exploration (Lieberman & Pawl, 1988). ID and associated disorders may disrupt mastery in each of these areas. Many developmental processes in infancy focus on strengthening attachment. Eye contact, a social smile, and cooing and other vocalizations often are delayed or nonexistent in children with ID. For infants with significant neurological or physical disabilities, uncertainty about their survival or prognosis, long-term postnatal hospitalization, or prolonged intrusive medical interventions also inhibit normal attachment.

Families often experience anger, denial, sorrow, and a prolonged grieving process (Lewis & MacLean, 1982) in response to having a child with ID. This also may interfere with the attachment process. In children with more subtle delays, the inability to achieve milestones at expected intervals may lead to misgivings about parental skills and increasing frustration. Autism spectrum disorders (American Psychiatric Association, 2013), often associated with ID, create further obstacles to attachment.

Delays in motor coordination and exploration of the environment often create a greater dependence on caregivers that is a harbinger of future interactive patterns. This may be enhanced by comorbid medical disorders, such as seizures, that enhance parental vigilance. Conversely, social withdrawal and isolation are frequent presentations.

Early Childhood

Many children's ID and associated delays are identified during this period. Parental response, both emotionally and in terms of expectations, impacts on this period of personal mastery. Maintaining unrealistic expectations of trying to "prove the experts wrong" leads to increasing frustration and tension in the parent–child relationship. Conversely, removing or minimizing expectations may inhibit the development of many key skills. This may create an environment of overprotection or chronic parental apathy that squelches individual initiative.

Language development is usually delayed in persons with ID. Mild delays are often overlooked or misinterpreted. Early intervention, which can be very helpful, is often unintentionally delayed. Deficits in language and communication development are some of the best predictors of behavioral difficulties in children with developmental disabilities (Carr & Durand, 1985). Frustration at not being able to communicate needs or desires may lead to disruptive, aggressive, or self-injurious behavior. Social failures are often the result of an inability to follow the flow of communication and basic interpersonal cues. Isolation or increased reliance on selected caregivers may be inadvertently reinforced. In this regard, it is important to recognize that children with specific language disorders may develop effective alternative communication systems to express their needs (Bondy & Frost, 1994).

Self-care skills are frequently delayed. Associated fine and gross motor delays may prevent children from successfully dressing, going to the toilet, or feeding themselves. Children with less severe delays may express the desire to perform these tasks without the requisite skills. This may lead to increasing conflict with caregivers. For those with a more severe form of ID, there is often a lifelong inability to contribute effectively to activities of daily living. Opportunities for child care may be greatly reduced by the child's lack of self-care skills. Unfortunately, it is just those parents who must continue providing their children with intensive assistance who would benefit most from more readily available child care.

Spontaneous, meaningful play may be delayed or missing. Children with a more severe form of ID may engage in seemingly undirected or self-stimulatory behavior instead of appropriate play. Children with lesser delays may only develop some symbolic play as they are about to enter school. Isolated or parallel play may predominate, especially when communicative skills are significantly impaired.

As with all children, many factors during this formative period contribute to personality development. The challenges of skill mastery, communication, emotional and physiological self-regulation, and how caregivers address these issues have significant implications. For children with milder severity ID, self-esteem, trust, and perceived competence form the basis of interpersonal relationships and a sense of self in the world. For those with more severe delays, the caregiver's ability to assist the child effectively in regulating responses to internal and environmental stimuli helps create a lifelong style of behavior.

Childhood

For many children with ID, beginning school is the first exposure to a large number of children without disabilities. It may be the first time descriptors such as "intellectually disabled," "slow learner," or other pejorative terms are encountered. This may be particularly challenging to children with mild ID. While increased academic mainstreaming has elevated the awareness of many typical children regarding disabilities, children with ID often still are perceived as different and are the target of peer taunting and rejection. As important, they perceive themselves as different. This becomes particularly challenging in the later elementary grades as peers become less tolerant of anyone seen as different. It is also a time when children with mild to moderate severity ID become increasingly aware of their limitations. Social withdrawal, isolation, and depression often manifest during this period. Some children display externalizing or acting-out behavior as an increasing desperation to be socially accepted coincides with peers increased willingness to use them as foils.

Participation in extracurricular and community activities is a hallmark of this age. Athletics may be inaccessible for some with significant associated physical handicaps. The nationwide Special Olympics initiative and greater understanding and support from many school districts have increased the participation rate of children with ID and other developmental delays in athletics. Group activities such as scouting have created subgroups that are more geared toward children with special needs but may isolate them from the mainstream, increasing their awareness of perceived differences. Dance and martial arts classes are often very well received by parents and children alike.

Most children with ID need support in the classroom in terms of either special resource support or placement in a self-contained special education classroom. As peers tackle more demanding language and abstract concepts, children with mild ID increasingly struggle to keep up. Academic failures are common. For children with more severe delays, the goals of education often change from preparation for higher education to life skills and vocational activities, further differentiating them from peers. The rigid demands of an academic schedule may be very different from the previous flexibility of home. Children with ID will have greater difficulty adapting to this change. This difficulty often will be expressed behaviorally as they are unable to convey via communicative skills the ensuing frustration and confusion. The subtleties of communication and behavioral routines, well learned by families, may be lost on teachers caring for numerous children with varying special needs.

Adolescence

Adolescence is a challenging period for every teen as well as for those living and working with them. Physical changes, striving for greater independence, and social acceptance are even more difficult for teens presenting with cognitive and adaptive skill deficits.

Increasing sensitivity of the erogenous zones may lead to inappropriate touching in children unable to master social rules. Some females with more severe levels of ID may be unable to understand the physical sensation of menstruation. Physical discomfort may lead to increased irritability, self-injury, and aggression (Kaminer, Feinstein, Barrett, Tylenda, & Hole, 1988). Personal hygiene also may be a problem.

The commonly held prejudice that those with ID are likely perpetrators of sexual assaults belies the reality that they more likely may be victims of sexual mistreatment or abuse (Ammerman, Hersen, van Hasselt, Lubetsky, & Sieck, 1994). Adolescence is a particularly risky period. Many children at this age are living in institutional settings, such as residential group homes, which may further increase the risk of abuse.

Deficits in social skills are particularly debilitating during this period (Borden, Walters, & Barrett, 1995). Complex social interactions, rapidly changing trends, and group cohesiveness are the norm. It is very challenging for adolescents with mild ID to keep up with their developmentally intact age-mates. Friendships with nondelayed peers, which may have flourished for years, are strained as these peers begin dating, working, and expressing their own independence. Children with ID may have the same dreams and expectations as their peers. Status symbols such as driving or a "cool" job may be out of reach. Medical or neurological conditions may contribute to physical abnormalities at an age when personal appearance has heightened significance. Depression and withdrawal are common as social failures accumulate. Suicidal ideation is not unusual (Walters, Barrett, Knapp, & Borden, 1995). Relationships with adults are often more rewarding. Somatization or creative storytelling may increase as a means of soliciting professional help or to otherwise fill the void of loneliness.

Academic challenges often change during this period. Vocational skill development predominates. Those with more severe levels of ID will frequently be taught repetitive "prevocational" tasks that are often minimally rewarding. For adolescents with milder delays, attending vocational classes may be stigmatizing and a source of shame (Lewis, 1998). Self-worth may diminish rapidly as teens with ID come to blame themselves for having a developmental disability.

Families face different stressors. Parents are aging and may feel increasingly overwhelmed by the demands of a teenager with ID. The normal developmental trajectory of increasing child independence may be disrupted, forcing families to face issues that have previously been avoided. For example, the opportunity for increased freedom for parents as their children leave the nest may prove illusory. In addition, issues of long-term care may arise when parents are no longer able to support more seriously delayed children. This is frequently a period when professional agencies become involved in the child's life to plan vocational, social, and residential opportunities. However, many families find it stressful to relinquish some or all of the care of their children to others. Brothers and sisters may be overprotective or resentful of a sibling with special needs and find that the changes of adolescence have a greater impact on family functioning.

Adulthood

As individuals with mild forms of ID reach adulthood, some might no longer be considered intellectually disabled. Relieved of the imposed structure of academics, some individuals with ID find appropriate jobs and housing arrangements that allow them to live independently. Unfortunately, stressors around child rearing, occupational or financial matters, and social relationships may lead to minor or major regression that requires additional family or professional support. Others with milder severity levels of ID receive support around occupational, residential, and social issues, as needed. Self-motivation and time management may be a challenge when rewards (i.e., a paycheck) are not immediate. In less supported worksites, relationships with coworkers can be challenging. Being criticized or taken advantage of is common.

Managing home finances, food shopping, laundry, and other life skills may be daunting tasks for individuals with milder severity levels of ID (Antonello, 1996). Those individuals are more at risk for con artists and "scams." Some engage in inappropriate or illegal activities without understanding the full import of their actions. Many have legal guardians. Sometimes, individuals and guardians disagree on issues, which may lead to tension and frustration. All of these factors may contribute to greater dependence on others than the individual desires.

Those with ID may have physical handicaps, limited mobility, or limited access to transportation. This enhances difficulties in keeping appointments and job expectations and creates further isolation. Individuals with more severe levels of ID in adulthood often work in a very structured and supportive environment. Behavioral issues such as aggression, self-injury, compulsions, and opposition are common and limit productivity. Ongoing assistance around self-care skills requires close supervision by family or agencies.

Family Stress

Having a child with ID can change family life in many ways, impacting on the family's time, finances, and physical and emotional energy. Krantz (1993) extensively reviewed the many facets of family life that can be affected while raising a child with ID.

Family stress is often significantly increased while parents care for a child with ID. These children will often have coexisting conditions requiring frequent medical involvement (Knoll, 1992). The paroxysmal nature of seizures, loss of functioning in numerous associated degenerative genetic disorders, and monitoring of multiple medications and their potential side effects contribute to heightened parental vigilance and a perception of greater fragility in the child.

The normal maturation of the family is inhibited or may even regress as the child fails to meet developmental milestones. Constant advocacy for special education and support services diverts energy from other family responsibilities. Parental career progress may be impacted. Siblings often feel ignored or overburdened and may exhibit problematic behaviors (Lobato, 1990; Stoneman & Berman, 1993). The family's sense of loss and guilt in not having the anticipated "perfect child" cannot be overlooked (Lewis, 1998). "Managing" extended family dynamics also can be extremely challenging when, for example, grandparents consistently respond that there is nothing wrong with their grandchild and that the child's parents are "reading too much into things" when developmental progression begins to fall behind or goes awry.

Parents may have to master many skills unique to their situation (Baker, 1989). More intensive behavioral management techniques or medical care interventions may be needed. Up to 80 % of children with developmental delays have significant sleep difficulties (Quine, 1986). This may lead to pervasive family sleep deprivation that further increases household stress and limited adaptability. There is also an increased incidence of ID and illiteracy in family members of probands with ID. This may impact on a family's coping ability in the face of the unique demands associated with raising a child with ID (Knoll, 1992).

Finally, children and adolescents with ID have three to four times the general population risk for the full range of psychiatric disorders (cf. Matson & Barrett, 1993). This can lead to a family becoming totally overwhelmed (Dykens, 2000), particularly if periods of inpatient psychiatric hospitalization are required. Sometimes, hospitalization of the child requires the temporary domestic relocation of a family member near to where the child is hospitalized, given the limited number of inpatient facilities that treat children and adolescents with ID and comorbid psychopathology. Understanding of the various psychotropic medications used for children and adolescents with ID and a coexisting psychiatric condition may be unfamiliar territory for the family. Equally unfamiliar may be the necessity of treating the child's psychiatric condition via multiple medication trials, various behavioral intervention strategies, and ongoing data collection. Such also requires the close co-collaboration and development of trust with the hospital clinical team which can become a long-standing relationship as the child may move between inpatient, day treatment, outpatient, and/or residential care.

Comorbid Psychopathology for Individuals with ID

The incidence of psychopathology in those with ID is elevated above the rate observed in non-ID individuals (Dekker & Koot, 2003; Reiss, 1990). One study (Einfield & Tonge, 1996) found that 20 % of children with an IQ less than 70 had severe emotional or behavioral disorders, and only 1 in 10 of these children and adolescents with major psychiatric disorders had received specialized psychiatric care. Individual and family stress, neurological impairment, sensory deficits, and limited adaptive skills increase the risk of developing psychopathology.

Controversy persists as to the efficacy of *DSM* diagnoses in those with greater severity of ID. It is not clear if abnormal behaviors seen in this population meet the specific criteria for psychiatric disorders. However, in those with milder severity ID, presentations meeting *DSM* diagnostic criteria are readily apparent (Dekker & Koot; 2003; Harden & Sahl, 1997; Szymanski, 1994).

Abnormal behaviors are often the presenting complaint of dually diagnosed children and adolescents. More often than not, a functional analysis of behaviors, including review of antecedent issues and behavioral consequences, is a necessary first step to better understand the etiology of a given behavior. More recently, professionals in the field have been able to supplement these behavioral analyses with the development of many new diagnostic scales specific to the ID population across a variety of psychiatric disorders. Matson (2007) has extensively reviewed this body of assessment materials with thoughtful commentary regarding diagnostic efficacy with regard to this population for the following areas: self-injurious behavior, aggressive behavior, feeding disorders, pain, and depression, anxiety, and related disorders.

Self-Injurious Behavior

Self-injurious behavior (SIB) is common in persons with ID, occurring in 16 % of the population (cf. Barrett, 2008). Prevalence rates vary in accordance with the level of severity of ID. Self-injury is rare (1 %) in children with mild ID, but more common in children with moderate ID (9 %), severe ID (16 %), and profound ID (27 %). Self-injurious responses may range from skin picking and head-banging to severe self-mutilation. There is an inverse correlation between the amount and severity of SIB and expressive language and cognitive development (Schroeder, Schroeder, Smith, & Dalldorf, 1978). Self-injury may be a final common pathway for several psychiatric and behavioral phenomena (Schroeder, Oster-Granite, & Thompson, 2002). Identifying specific etiologies will presumably dictate appropriate treatment interventions.

Inadvertently reinforced self-injury may occur in children with limited communication skills or sensory deficits (Barrett, 2008). These children appear to learn rapidly that engaging in self-mutilating behaviors commands instant and close attention from caregivers. Often, these behavioral patterns arise from periods of physical discomfort such as headaches, earaches, dental pain, menstrual periods, constipation, or eczema. The child's inability to describe discomfort leads to physical expression of pain and frustration.

For some children, self-injury appears to be internally reinforced by the release of endogenous opiates (Barrett, Feinstein, & Hole, 1989). Repeated self-injury apparently induces endorphin release and a temporarily favorable sensory consequence. In these situations, medications that inhibit the effectiveness of endogenous opiates effectively extinguish the drive to self-injury (Sandman et al., 1998).

Some SIBs suggest an underlying affective disorder or obsessive–compulsive disorder (Matson, 1986). Cyclic presentations, co-occurring vegetative symptoms, and associated affective changes may indicate a mood disorder. In milder severity ID, a child or adolescent will often be able to describe depressed mood, anhedonia, or even manic symptoms. The apparent ego-dystonic nature of self-injury and the desire for imposed physical restraint to prevent the acts in some are consistent with a compulsive drive. This may be difficult to differentiate from stereotypical behaviors often seen in individuals with severe developmental delays. Interestingly, medications that address mood disorders and obsessive–compulsive behaviors have diminished SIB in some individuals (Cook, Rowlett, Jaselskis, & Leventhal, 1992; Kastrom, Finesmith, & Walsh, 1993; King, 2000). Mental disorders such as Lesch–Nyhan syndrome, and chromosomal abnormalities such as Cornelia de Lange syndrome (Opitz, 1985), have phenotypic presentations that include severe self-injury.

Abnormal Movements

Individuals with ID and associated neurological impairments are at increased risk for movement disorders. Motor tics and Tourette's syndrome are common in this population. Differentiating motor tics from stereotypies and vocal tics from echolalia is challenging and impacts treatment recommendations. Vocal and complex motor tics often are misdiagnosed as oppositional, aggressive, and disruptive behaviors.

Many adolescents and young adults with ID have been on neuroleptics for extended periods, targeting aggression or disruptive behavior. Comorbid neurological abnormalities increase the risk of tardive dyskinesia, involuntary muscle movements often centering on the oral musculature. The use of neuroleptics also may increase a sense of restlessness, known as akathisia. This may present as hyperactivity, irritability, or

dysphoria and, if not properly diagnosed, could lead to a cascade of inappropriate psychopharmacological and behavioral interventions (Wilson, Lott, & Tsai, 1998).

Aggressive/Destructive Behaviors

Aggressive behaviors appear in approximately 25 % of the community sample of children and adolescents with developmental disabilities (Emerson, 2003). These behaviors contribute significantly to the social isolation and institutional placement of this population (Hill & Bruininks, 1981). Frustration stemming from communication deficits is a common source of aggressive and destructive behavior. Adjustment difficulties created by environmental changes may be expressed aggressively. Disruption in living arrangements, support staff, or routine that is not understood or explained can lead to significant outbursts. If these outbursts lead to the reinstatement of the status quo, such behavioral patterns are strongly reinforced.

Mood disorders, both major depression (Dosen, 1984) and mania (Sovner, 1989), may present as disruptive behavior. This is especially challenging to diagnose in nonverbal children. Associated changes in sleep, appetite, and energy patterns are frequently seen. There is also often an ebb and flow to the presenting symptoms.

Previous traumatic events including abuse and neglect may create a long-standing pattern of disruptive behaviors in an attempt at self-protection. Withdrawal and social isolation often may be seen in these situations. The interictal, or between-seizure, phase in some seizure disorders may increase aggressive tendencies. Comorbid schizophrenia or substance abuse may lead to increased confusion and poor impulse control, exacerbating aggressive tendencies.

Attention and Motivational Deficits

Attention difficulties and motivational difficulties are found as common presentations for numerous disorders, including attention deficit/hyperactivity disorder (ADHD), depression, mania, anxiety, and hyperthyroidism. Differentiation of these disorders in cognitively limited and often medically complicated populations is particularly challenging but important. There is evidence that treatments helpful to otherwise intact children with ADHD are useful for ID children with a diagnosis of ADHD, but their rate of beneficial response appears to be well under that found for those children in the normal IQ range, and their response to treatment shows great variability (Aman, Buican, & Arnold, 2003). The symptom presentation in these individuals may represent underlying neurocognitive deficits in attention and arousal, or other psychiatric disorders, and not ADHD per se. Medications for seizures or other medical conditions as well as sensory deficits also may diminish attention (cf. Aman & Singh, 1988; Reiss & Aman, 1998).

Anxiety, Mood Disorders, and Related Disorders

Rates of significant anxiety symptoms appear to be much higher in children with ID, approximately 25 % (Benson, 1985), than the general population estimate of 2–5 % (Clum & Pickett, 1984). The typical predominance of females is not seen. There is an increased prevalence for anxiety disorders in specific neurogenetic syndromes (Dykens, 2003). It remains unclear if an individual's level of cognitive delay contributes to the severity and frequency of anxiety disorders.

Mood disorders (e.g., major depression, bipolar disorder, and dysthymia) occur commonly in individuals with ID. Approximately 2 % to 10 % of individuals with ID manifest major affective disorders, and approximately 25 % suffer from dysthymia (Cooper, Melville, & Einfeld, 2003). Cain et al. (2003) reported that bipolar disorder can be distinguished from behavioral and psychiatric diagnoses in adults with ID. Specifically, those with clinical symptoms of bipolar disorder had significantly more mood-related and non-mood-related symptoms and greater functional impairment than those with major depression.

The inability of many with developmental delays to describe internal states accurately is particularly problematic around anxiety disorders and mood disorders. Careful observation is often the most helpful diagnostic tool. One must differentiate general anxiety, avoidance, panic, posttraumatic stress, and obsessive–compulsive behaviors from several other diagnoses. This list should include mania, ADHD, stereotypical movements, akathisia, hyperthyroidism, and seizures.

Limited adaptability, sensory deficits, concrete thought processes, and increased family stress also may contribute to an increased rate of anxiety symptoms in this population. If identified, these symptoms are frequently responsive to typical interventions (cf. Barlow, 1993; Reiss & Aman, 1998; Werry & Aman, 1993).

Adjustment Disorders

Those with ID often thrive and rely on consistency in routine. Even minor changes in the environment can have a disproportionately significant impact on behavior and mood. Careful analysis of recent changes in living situation, education, or caretaker interaction is necessary when sudden changes in behavior are seen. The *DSM* criterion of resolution of symptoms in 6 months is not always relevant in this population. It is not unusual for children with ID to be excluded from full or partial explanations for the sudden disappearance of a relative from death or moving. Entering the school situation where one is teased or ignored can lead to withdrawal or provocative behaviors across settings. Entering or leaving institutions may create changes in mood or behavior as long-standing routines are disrupted. Understanding underlying issues is essential for efficacious treatment.

Conclusion

The societal perception of individuals with ID and, consequently, their social acceptance has changed dramatically over the past 40 years. The results of parent advocacy, deinstitutionalization, academic and vocational mainstreaming, increased respect for individual rights, increased interdisciplinary collegiality between various professional groups, and the de-emphasis of chemical restraint have caused an enormous shift in paradigms for treatment and support. While challenges remain for individuals with ID and their families, advances in understanding and treating children with ID, while still evolving, have resulted in marked improvements in the quality of life.

References

Accardo, P. J., & Capute, A. J. (1998). Mental retardation. *Mental Retardation and Developmental Disabilities Research Reviews, 4*, 2–5.

Alexander, D. (1998). Prevention of mental retardation: Four decades of research. *Mental Retardation and Developmental Disabilities Research Reviews, 4*, 50–58.

Aman, M. G. (1991a). *Assessing psychopathology and behavioral problems in persons with mental retardation: A review of available instruments*. Rockville, MD: S. Department of Health and Human Services (DHHS) (DHHS Publication No. [ADM] 91-1712.).

Aman, M. G. (1991b). Review and evaluation of instruments for assessing emotional and behavioral disorders. *Australia and New Zealand Journal of Developmental Disabilities, 17*, 127–145.

Aman, M. G., Buican, B., & Arnold, L. E. (2003). Methylphenidate treatment in children with borderline IQ and mental retardation: Analysis of three aggregated studies. *Journal of Child and Adolescent Psychopharmacology, 13*, 29–40.

Aman, M. G., & Singh, N. N. (Eds.). (1988). *Psychopharmacology of the developmental disabilities*. New York: Springer.

American Association on Intellectual and Developmental Disabilities (AAIDD). (2010). *Intellectual disability: Definition, classification, and systems of support* (11th ed.). Washington, DC: Author.

American Association on Intellectual and Developmental Disabilities (AAIDD). (2012). *User's guide—To accompany the 11th edition of intellectual disability: Definition, classification, and systems of support*. Washington, DC: Author.

American Association on Mental Retardation (AAMR). (2002). *Mental retardation: Definition, classification, and systems of support* (10th ed.). Washington, DC: Author.

American Psychiatric Association. (1952). *Diagnostic and statistical manual of mental disorders* (1st ed.). Washington, DC: Author.

American Psychiatric Association. (1968). *Diagnostic and statistical manual of mental disorders* (2nd ed.). Washington, DC: Author.

American Psychiatric Association. (1980). *Diagnostic and statistical manual of mental disorders* (3rd ed.). Washington, DC: Author.

American Psychiatric Association. (1987). *Diagnostic and statistical manual of mental disorders* (3rd ed., revised). Washington, DC: Author.

American Psychiatric Association. (1994). *Diagnostic and statistical manual of mental disorders* (4th ed.). Washington, DC: Author.

American Psychiatric Association. (2000). *Diagnostic and statistical manual of mental disorders* (4th ed., text revision). Washington, DC: Author.

American Psychiatric Association. (2013). *Diagnostic and statistical manual of mental disorders* (5th ed.). Washington, DC: Author.

Ammerman, R. T., Hersen, M., van Hasselt, V., Lubetsky, M. J., & Sieck, W. R. (1994). Maltreatment in psychiatrically hospitalized children and adolescents with developmental disabilities: Prevalence and correlates. *Journal of the American Academy of Child and Adolescent Psychiatry, 33*, 567–576.

Antonello, S. J. (1996). *Social skills development. Practical strategies for adolescents and adults with developmental disabilities*. Boston, MA: Allyn & Bacon.

Baird, P. A., & Sadovnick, A. D. (1985). Mental retardation in over half a million consecutive live births: An epidemiologic study. *American Journal of Mental Deficiency, 89*, 323.

Baker, B. L. (1989). *Parent training and developmental disabilities*. Washington, DC: American Association on Mental Retardation.

Bale, J. F. (2002). Congenital infections. *Neurology Clinics, 20*, 1039–1060.

Barlow, D. (Ed.). (1993). *Clinical handbook of psychological disorders* (2nd ed.). New York: Guilford Press.

Baroff, G. S. (1986). *Mental retardation: Nature, causes, and management* (2nd ed.). Washington, DC: Hemisphere.

Barrett, R. P. (2008). Atypical behavior: Self-injury and pica. In M. L. Wolraich, D. D. Drotar, P. H. Dworkin, & E. C. Perrin (Eds.), *Developmental-behavioral pediatrics: Evidence and practice* (pp. 871–885). Philadelphia, PA: Mosby Elsevier.

Barrett, R. P., Feinstein, C., & Hole, W. (1989). Effects of naloxone and naltrexone on self-injury in autism: A double blind, placebo controlled analysis. *American Journal on Mental Retardation, 93*, 644–651.

Benson, B. A. (1985). Behavioral disorders in mental retardation: Association with age, sex, and level of functioning in an outpatient clinic sample. *Applied Research in Mental Retardation, 6*, 79–85.

Berkson, G. (2004). Intellectual and physical disabilities in prehistory and early civilization. *Mental Retardation, 42*, 195–208.

Bondy, A. S., & Frost, L. A. (1994). The picture exchange communication system. *Focus on Autistic Behavior, 9*, 1–19.

Borden, M. C., Walters, A. S., & Barrett, R. P. (1995). Mental retardation and developmental disabilities. In V. van Hasselt & M. Herson (Eds.), *Handbook of adolescent psychopathology: A guide to diagnosis and treatment* (pp. 497–524). New York: Lexington Books.

Buntinx, W. H. E. (2006). The relationship between WHO-ICF and the AAMR-2002 system. In H. Switzky & S. Greenspan (Eds.), *What is mental retardation? Ideas for an evolving disability in the 21st century* (pp. 303–323). Washington, DC: American Association on Mental Retardation.

Burd, L., Cotsonas-Hassler, T. M., Martsolf, J. T., & Kerbeshian, J. (2003). Recognition and management of fetal alcohol syndrome. *Neurotoxicology and Teratology, 25*, 681–688.

Cain, N. N., Davidson, P. W., Burhan, A. M., Andolsek, M. E., Baxter, J. T., Sullivan, L., et al. (2003). Identifying bipolar disorders in individuals with intellectual disability. *Journal of Intellectual Disability Research, 47*, 31–38.

Carr, E. G., & Durand, V. M. (1985). Reducing behavior problems through functional communication. *Journal of Applied Behavior Analysis, 18*, 111–126.

Centers for Disease Control. (1996). State-specific rates of mental retardation—United States. 1993. *Morbidity Mortality Weekly Reports, 45*, 61–65.

Clum, G. A., & Pickett, L. (1984). Panic disorder and generalized anxiety disorders. In P. B. Sutkon & H. Adams (Eds.), *Comprehensive handbook of psychopathology* (pp. 123–146). New York: Plenum Press.

Committee on Disability Determination for Mental Retardation. (2002). Introduction. In D. J. Reschly, T. G. Myers, & C. R. Hartel (Eds.), *Mental retardation: Determining eligibility for social security benefits* (pp. 15–37). Washington, DC: National Academy Press.

Cook, E. H., Rowlett, R., Jaselskis, C., & Leventhal, B. L. (1992). Fluoxetine treatment of children and adults with autistic disorder and mental retardation. *Journal of the American Academy of Child and Adolescent Psychiatry, 31*, 739–745.

Cooper, S. A., Melville, C. A., & Einfeld, S. L. (2003). Psychiatric diagnosis, intellectual disabilities, and diagnostic criteria for psychiatric disorders for use with adults with learning disabilities/mental retardation (DC-LD). *Journal of Intellectual Disability Research, 47*(suppl. 1), 3–15.

Curry, C. J., Stevenson, R. E., Aughton, D., Byrnes, J., Carey, J. C., Cassidy, S., et al. (1997). Evaluation of mental retardation: Recommendations of a consensus conference: American College of Medical Genetics. *American Journal of Medical Genetics, 72*, 468–477.

Dekker, M. C., & Koot, H. M. (2003). DSM-IV disorders in children with borderline to moderate intellectual disability. II: Child and family predictors. *Journal of the American Academy of Child and Adolescent Psychiatry, 42*, 923–931.

Dixon, D. R. (2007). Adaptive behavior scale. In J. L. Matson (Vol. Ed.), *International review of research in mental retardation: Vol. 34. Handbook of assessment*

in persons with intellectual disability (pp. 99–140). San Diego, CA: Elsevier.

Dosen, A. (1984). Depressing conditions in mentally handicapped children. *Acta Paedopsychiatrica, 50*, 29–40.

Dykens, E. M. (2000). Psychopathology in children with intellectual disability. *Journal of Child Psychology and Psychiatry, 41*, 407–417.

Dykens, E. M. (2003). Anxiety, fears, and phobias in persons with Williams syndrome. *Developmental Neuropsychology, 23*, 291–316.

Einfield, S. L., & Tonge, B. J. (1996). Population prevalence of psychopathology in children and adolescents with intellectual disability: II. Epidemiological findings. *Journal of Intellectual Disabilities Research, 40*, 99–109.

Emerson, E. (2003). Prevalence of psychiatric disorders in children and adolescents with and without intellectual disability. *Journal of Intellectual Disability Research, 47*, 51–58.

Frazier, J., Barrett, R. P., Feinstein, C. B., & Walters, A. S. (1997). Moderate to profound mental retardation. In J. Noshpitz (Ed.), *Handbook of child and adolescent psychiatry* (Vol. 4, pp. 397–408). New York: Wiley.

Grossman, H. J. (1983). *Classification in mental retardation*. Washington, DC: American Association on Mental Deficiency.

Harden, A., & Sahl, R. (1997). Psychopathology in children and adolescents with developmental disorders. *Research in Developmental Disabilities, 18*, 369–382.

Harris, J. C. (2006). *Intellectual disability: Understanding its development, causes, classification, evaluation, and treatment*. New York: Oxford University Press.

Heber, R. (1961). *Epidemiology of mental retardation*. Springfield, IL: Charles C. Thomas.

Hill, B. K., & Bruininks, R. H. (1981). *Physical and behavioral characteristics and maladaptive behavior of mentally retarded individuals in residential facilities*. Minneapolis: University of Minnesota, Department of Psychoeducational Studies.

Jones, J., Lopez, A., & Wilson, M. (2003). Congenital toxoplasmosis. *American Family Physicians, 67*, 2131–2138.

Kaminer, Y., Feinstein, C., Barrett, R. P., Tylenda, B., & Hole, W. (1988). Menstrually related mood disorders in developmentally disabled adolescents: Review and current status. *Child Psychiatry and Human Development, 18*, 239–249.

Kastrom, T., Finesmith, R., & Walsh, K. (1993). Long-term administration of valproic acid in the treatment of affective symptoms in people with mental retardation. *Journal of Clinical Psychopharmacology, 15*, 448–451.

King, B. H. (2000). Pharmacological treatment of mood disturbance, aggression, and self-injury in persons with developmental disabilities. *Journal of Autism & Developmental Disabilities, 30*, 439–445.

Knoll, J. (1992). Being a family: The experience of raising a child with a disability or chronic illness. In V. J. Bradley, J. Knoll, & J. M. Agosta (Eds.), *Emerging issues in family support* (pp. 9–56). Washington, DC: American Association on Mental Retardation.

Krantz, J. Z. (1993). Family and community life. In R. Smith (Ed.), *Children with mental retardation* (pp. 259–301). Bethesda, MD: Woodbine House.

Lamont, M. A., & Dennis, N. R. (1988). Aetiology of mild mental retardation. *Archives of Diseases of Children, 63*, 1032–1038.

Lewis, M. (1998). Shame and stigma. In P. Gilbert & B. Andrews (Eds.), *Shame: Interpersonal behavior, psychopathology, and culture* (pp. 126–140). New York: Oxford University Press.

Lewis, M. H., & MacLean, W. E., Jr. (1982). Issues in treating emotional disorders of the mentally retarded. In J. L. Matson & R. P. Barrett (Eds.), *Psychopathology in the mentally retarded* (pp. 1–36). New York: Grune & Stratton.

Lieberman, A. F., & Pawl, J. H. (1988). Clinical applications of attachment theory. In M. Greenberg (Ed.), *Attachment beyond infancy* (pp. 327–351). Chicago: University of Chicago Press.

Lobato, D. J. (1990). *Brothers, sisters, and special needs: Information and activities for helping young siblings of children with chronic illnesses and developmental disabilities*. Baltimore: Paul H. Brooks.

Lowe, K., Allen, D., Jones, E., Brophy, S., Moore, K., & Jones, W. (2007). Challenging behaviors: Prevalence and topographies. *Journal of Intellectual Disability Research, 51*, 625–636.

Matson, J. L. (1986). Self-injury and its relationship to diagnostic schemes in psychopathology. *Applied Research in Mental Retardation, 7*, 223–227.

Matson, J. L. (Vol. Ed.). (2007). *International review of research in mental retardation: Vol. 34. Handbook of assessment in persons with intellectual disability*. San Diego, CA: Elsevier.

Matson, J. L., Anderson, S. J., & Bamburg, J. W. (2000). The relationship of social skills to psychopathology for individuals with mild and moderate mental retardation. *The British Journal of Developmental Disabilities, 46*, 15–22.

Matson, J. L., & Barrett, R. P. (Eds.). (1993). *Psychopathology in the mentally retarded* (2nd ed.). Boston, MA: Allyn & Bacon.

McLaren, J., & Bryson, S. E. (1987). Review of recent epidemiological studies of mental retardation: Prevalence associated disorders and etiology. *American Journal of Mental Retardation, 92*(5), 243–254.

McMillan, D. L., Gresham, F. M., & Siperstein, G. N. (1993). Conceptual and psychological concerns about the 1992 AAMR definition of mental retardation. *American Journal of Mental Retardation, 98*, 325–335.

McMillan, D. L., Gresham, F. M., & Siperstein, G. N. (1995). Heightened concerns over the 1992 AAMR definition: Advocacy versus precision. *American Journal on Mental Retardation, 100*, 87–97.

Menolascino, F. J. (Ed.). (1970). *Psychiatric approaches to mental retardation*. New York, NY: Basic Books.

Mochida, G. H., & Walsh, C. A. (2004). Genetic basis of developmental malformations of the cerebral cortex. *Archives of Neurology, 61*, 637–640.

Murphy, C. C., Boyle, C., Schendel, D., Decoufle, P., & Yeargin-Allsopp, M. (1998). Epidemiology of mental retardation in children. *Mental Retardation and Developmental Disabilities Research Reviews, 4*, 6–13.

Opitz, J. M. (1985). The Brachmann-de Lange syndrome. *American Journal of Medical Genetics, 22*, 761–767.

Quine, L. (1986). Behavior problems in severely mentally handicapped children. *Psychological Medicine, 16*, 761–767.

Reiss, S. (1990). Prevalence of dual diagnosis in community-based day programs in the Chicago metropolitan area. *American Journal of Mental Retardation, 94*, 578–585.

Reiss, S., & Aman, M. G. (Eds.). (1998). *Psychotropic medications and developmental disabilities*. Columbus: Ohio State University Press.

Reiss, S., Levitan, G. W., & Szyszko, J. (1982). Emotional disturbance and mental retardation: Diagnostic overshadowing. *American Journal of Mental Deficiency, 86*, 567–574.

Rhead, M. J., & Irons, M. (2004). The call from the newborn screening laboratory. *Pediatric Clinics of North America, 51*, 803–818.

Rovet, J. F. (2002). Congenital hypothyroidism: An analysis of persisting deficits and associated factors. *Neuropsychology, Development and Cognition, Section C, Child Neuropsychology, 8*, 150–162.

Rutter, M., Simonoff, E., & Plomin, R. (1996). Genetic influences on mild mental retardation: Concepts, findings, and research implications. *Journal of Biosocial Science, 28*, 509–526.

Rutter, M., Tizard, J., & Whitmore, K. (1970). *Education, health, and behavior*. New York: Wiley.

Sandman, C. A., Thompson, T. T., Barrett, R. P., Verhoeven, W. M., McCubbin, J. A., Schroeder, S. R., et al. (1998). Opiate blockers. In S. Reiss & M. G. Aman (Eds.), *Psychotropic medications and developmental disabilities* (pp. 291–302). Columbus: Ohio State University Press.

Schalock, R. L., Luckasson, R. A., Shogren, K. A., Borthwick-Duffy, S., Bradley, V., Buntinx, W. H. E., et al. (2007). The renaming of mental retardation: Understanding the change to the term intellectual disability. *Intellectual and Developmental Disabilities, 45*, 116–124.

Schroeder, S. R., Oster-Granite, M. L., & Thompson, T. (2002). *Self-injurious behavior: Gene-brain-behavior relationships*. Washington, DC: American Psychological Association.

Schroeder, S. R., Schroeder, C. S., Smith, B., & Dalldorf, J. (1978). Prevalence of self- injurious behaviors in a large state facility for the retarded: A three year follow-up study. *Journal of Autism and Childhood Schizophrenia, 8*, 261–269.

Sovner, R. (1989). The use of valproate in the treatment of mentally retarded persons with typical and atypical bipolar disorders. *Journal of Clinical Psychiatry, 50*, 40–43.

Stoneman, Z., & Berman, P. W. (Eds.). (1993). *The effects of mental retardation, disability, and illnesses on sibling relationships: Research issues and challenges.* Baltimore: Paul H. Brookes.

Szymanski, L. S. (1994). Mental retardation and mental health: Concepts, etiology, and incidence. In N. Bouras (Ed.), *Mental health in mental retardation: Recent advances and practices* (pp. 19–33). Cambridge: Cambridge University Press.

Thompson, T., & Hupp, S. C. (Eds.). (1992). *Saving children at risk: Poverty and disabilities.* London: Sage.

Tylenda, B., Beckett, J., & Barrett, R. P. (2007). Assessing mental retardation using standardized intelligence tests. In J. L. Matson (Vol. Ed.), *International review of research in mental retardation: Vol. 34. Handbook of assessment in persons with intellectual disability* (pp. 27–97). San Diego, CA: Elsevier.

Tylenda, B., Hooper, S. R., & Barrett, R. P. (1987). Developmental learning disorders. In C. L. Frame & J. L. Matson (Eds.), *Handbook of assessment in child psychopathology: Applied issues in differential diagnosis and treatment evaluation* (pp. 187–217). New York: Plenum Press.

Vannucci, R. C. (1990). Experimental biology of cerebral hypoxia-ischemia: Relation to perinatal brain damage. *Pediatric Research, 27,* 317–326.

Walters, A. S., Barrett, R. P., Knapp, L., & Borden, M. C. (1995). Suicidal behavior in children and adolescents with mental retardation. *Research in Developmental Disabilities, 16,* 85–96.

Werry, J. S., & Aman, M. G. (Eds.). (1993). *Practitioner's guide to psychoactive drugs for children and adolescents.* New York: Plenum Press.

Wilson, J. G., Lott, R. S., & Tsai, L. (1998). Side effects: Recognition and management. In S. Reiss & M. G. Aman (Eds.), *Psychotropic medications and developmental disabilities* (pp. 95–114). Columbus: Ohio State University Press.

World Health Organization. (2001). *International classification of functioning, disability, and health (ICF).* Geneva: Author.

World Health Organization. (2008). *Revision of the international classification of diseases (ICD).* Available at http://www.who.int/classifications/icd/ICDRevision/en/index.html

Zigler, E. (1967). Familial mental retardation: A continuing dilemma. *Science, 155,* 292–298.

Gender Dysphoria

Kenneth J. Zucker

Since the second edition of the *Handbook of Developmental Psychopathology* was published 14 years ago (Sameroff, Lewis, & Miller, 2000), there has been a remarkable increase in clinical, research, and media attention afforded to children and adolescents who meet the DSM-IV-TR (American Psychiatric Association, 2000) diagnostic criteria for Gender Identity Disorder (GID), which, as I will note in more detail below, has been somewhat reconceptualized and renamed as gender dysphoria (GD) in the DSM-5 (American Psychiatric Association, 2013). In this chapter, I will provide an update on the GD diagnosis, drawing on new data sets that have become available since the prior volume of this handbook (Zucker, 2000). I will also consider new lines of research that have considered the interface between what we know about typical and atypical gender development.

Phenomenology

Children and adolescents with GD show an array of sex-typed behaviors that suggest a strong identification with the opposite sex. In many

K.J. Zucker, Ph.D. (✉)
Gender Identity Service, Child, Youth,
and Family Services, Centre for Addiction and
Mental Health, Intergenerational Wellness Centre,
Beamish Family Wing, 80 Workman Way, Toronto,
ON, Canada M6J 1H4
e-mail: Ken.Zucker@camh.ca

respects, GD is a deeply phenomenological and subjective condition. Children and adolescents match their felt gender identity in a sociocultural context in which they have the opportunity to observe and learn how boys and girls/men and women are categorized and behave (Fausto-Sterling, Garcia Coll, & Lamarre, 2012; Martin, Ruble, & Szkrybalo, 2002; Owen Blakemore, Berenbaum, & Liben, 2009; Ruble, Martin, & Berenbaum, 2006). The surface expression of GD can be constructed only in relation to what is normatively sex dimorphic in a particular culture and in a particular historical time period. Since GID was first described in the DSM-III (American Psychiatric Association, 1980) 30+ years ago, its surface manifestations in children have been characterized by several parameters: toy and activity interests, peer affiliation preferences, roles in fantasy and pretend play, and in cross-dressing. There is also a marked rejection or avoidance of behaviors typically associated with one's natal sex. In addition, both children and adolescents express a strong desire to be of the other gender (or some alternative gender that departs from one's assigned gender at birth). Some children go beyond the mere desire to be of the other gender: they declare that they "are" the other gender. In some children and almost always in adolescents, there is an accompanying desire to be rid of the sex-related somatic features associated with the natal sex and the desire to change one's body to match that of the desired gender. Two examples illustrate this phenomenology:

Case Example 1

Frank is a 4-year-old natal male who was referred by his parents because of concerns that he was unhappy as a boy. At the age of 2, he became quite interested, if not preoccupied, with female characters that he saw in films, such as Ariel from *The Little Mermaid*. In his mother's words, he became "obsessed" with long hair and would spend hours creating long hair using string, which he would attach to popsicle sticks or pencils. He would "beg" his mother to allow him to brush and stroke her hair during the day and at bedtime. He often would put long towels on his head to simulate long hair. By age 3, he was primarily interested in stereotypical feminine objects and activities, such as Barbie dolls, and adopted female roles in fantasy play (he would enact being his mother or one of his three nannies). He preferred to play with girls and complained that boys were too rough and vile ("They say bad words, mommy"). By age 4, Frank began to verbalize the desire to be a girl or that he "was" a girl. He has not verbalized any negative feelings about his sexual anatomy. At first, Frank's parents thought that his behavior was a phase because he was surrounded by females (his mother, the three female nannies, and the daughters of mother's female friends) and that his father was much less salient because of work commitments, which led him to be away from home in total for 3 months of each calendar year. Because Frank was now entering preschool, the parents were worried that his marked cross-gender identification would lead to social ostracism within the peer group. The parents sought out advice as to how to best deal with Frank's apparent rejection of himself as a boy and his desire to be a girl.

Case Example 2

Diane is a 14-year-old natal female who was referred by a school social worker. Diane had been truant from school for weeks on end. When seen by the social worker, Diane presented phenotypically as an adolescent boy, based on hairstyle and clothing style. Diane self-identified as "trans," had adopted the given name of James, and asked that the social worker use male pronouns in talking to the teachers and principal about "her." As a child, Diane had stereotypical masculine interests and activity choices. Diane always enacted male roles in fantasy play. By age 5, Diane refused to wear stereotypical girls' clothing. Diane had her hair cut short and was often perceived by strangers and new peers to be a boy. However, through the elementary school years, the teachers would ask Diane to "line up" with the girls when gender segregation activities were required (e.g., attending gym class), and this led, in part, to a lot of social ostracism. Diane was referred to as a "boy-girl" or as an "in-between." During childhood, Diane never verbalized the desire to be a boy, and her mother, with whom she lived, commented that she simply thought that her daughter was a "tomboy." By late childhood, Diane had become quite oppositional and, in adolescence, was often depressed. Frequent self-harm (cutting to the forearms) led to several emergency room visits. With the development of secondary sex characteristics at puberty (e.g., breast development) and the onset of menses, Diane became more distraught. She would conceal her breasts by wearing layers of t-shirts and would avoid going outside during the summer months. According to her mother, Diane's reaction to menarche was "dreadful." At the time of assessment, James indicated a strong desire for male sex hormones (testosterone) and asked about the possibility of surgery to remove her breasts. James reported a sexual attraction to females. James self-identified as "straight" because "I have the mind of a boy." The idea of adopting a lesbian sexual identity was abhorrent ("I got nothing against lesbians, but I'm not one of those").

Referral Rates, Diagnosis, and Assessment

Referral Rates

The epidemiology of GD is still quite uncertain other than the fact that it is a relatively uncommon psychiatric diagnosis compared to many other diagnoses that can be applied to children and adolescents. We do know somewhat more about sex differences in referral rates and recent changes in the number of referred children and adolescents to specialized gender identity clinics (as summarized in Wood et al., 2013). Three facts will be noted here: first, among children (12 years of age and younger), the sex ratio favors boys. In our clinic for children and youth, for the years 1975–2011, the sex ratio for children was 4.49:1 of boys to girls ($N = 577$), which was significantly larger than the 2.02:1 sex ratio of boys to girls ($N = 468$) from the Amsterdam clinic in the Netherlands. Second, for our adolescent cases, the sex ratio was near parity, at 1:04:1 of boys to girls ($N = 253$), quite comparable to the Dutch sex ratio of 1.01:1 ($N = 393$). Third, the number of referred adolescent cases has increased dramatically over the past 8 years, with an almost fivefold increase in annual referrals from prior years.

The sex difference in child referrals likely reflects the greater tolerance for gender-variant behavior in natal females compared to natal males. Thus, the threshold for referrals seems to be higher for girls, and, indeed, some studies have shown that GD girls display more marked cross-gender behavior than GD boys (Cohen-Kettenis, Owen, Kaijser, Bradley, & Zucker, 2003; Wallien et al., 2009; Zucker, Bradley, & Sanikhani, 1997a). By adolescence, however, the sex ratio is likely reduced because both natal males and females show comparable intensity levels of GD. As noted above, the Toronto clinic has a higher proportion of referred boys than the Amsterdam clinic. Two factors may account for this finding. First, the threshold for referral appears to be higher in the Netherlands than it is in Toronto, in the sense that the Dutch children appear to show more extreme gender-variant behaviors than the Toronto children (e.g., Cohen-Kettenis et al., 2006; Steensma, Zucker, Kreukels et al., 2013; Wallien et al., 2009). Second, in the Netherlands, it is quite rare for a child to be referred at the age of 5 years or younger, whereas in the Toronto clinic the percentage is much higher (2.3 % vs. 22.6 %) (Cohen-Kettenis et al., 2003). This is important because, among children 5 years of age or younger in the Toronto clinic, the sex ratio is highly skewed (e.g., among 3–4-year-olds, the sex ratio was an astonishing 33:1 of boys to girls).

Diagnosis

In Zucker (2000), I summarized the changes in the GID diagnostic criteria for children that appeared in the DSM-IV, compared to the DSM-III and the DSM-III-R. Here, I will summarize six substantive changes in the DSM-5 criteria compared to the DSM-IV. Table 35.1 shows the diagnostic criteria for gender dysphoria in the DSM-5.

1. The first change pertains to a relabeling of the diagnostic label: Gender Dysphoria instead of Gender Identity Disorder. There were a few reasons for this. Some critics argued that it is not gender identity that is "disordered" per se, but that it is the distress that accompanies the incongruence between one's assigned gender at birth (almost always in synchrony with one's presumed natal sex: boy = male; girl = female). Initially, the Gender Identity Disorders subworkgroup, which was part of the DSM-5 Work Group on Sexual and Gender Identity Disorders, had proposed the term Gender Incongruence as an alternative label, but some critics felt that this was a bit too vague (De Cuypere, Knudson, & Bockting, 2010). Thus, the Gender Identity Disorders subworkgroup proposed a second alternative—Gender Dysphoria. This proposed relabeling received a fair amount of positive support during the second and third phases in which professionals and the general public could provide feedback on the DSM-5 website. The term gender dysphoria has a long history in clinical sexology (e.g., Fisk, 1973) and was thus deemed to be one that would be familiar to specialists.[1]

---

[1] I was the Chair of the DSM-5 Work Group on Sexual and Gender Identity Disorders. Peggy T. Cohen-Kettenis was the Chair of the subworkgroup on Gender Identity Disorders.

Table 35.1 DSM-5 diagnostic criteria for gender dysphoria

A. A marked incongruence between one's experienced/
   expressed gender and assigned gender, of at least 6
   months duration, as manifested by at least six of the
   following (one of which must be Criterion A1):

1. A strong desire to be of the other gender or an
   insistence that one is the other gender (or some
   alternative gender different from one's assigned
   gender).

2. In boys (assigned gender), a strong preference for
   cross-dressing or simulating female attire; or in
   girls (assigned gender), a strong preference for
   wearing only typical masculine clothing and a
   strong resistance to the wearing of typical
   feminine clothing.

3. A strong preference for cross-gender roles in
   make-believe play or fantasy play.

4. A strong preference for the toys, games, or
   activities stereotypically used or engaged in by
   the other gender.

5. A strong preference for playmates of the other
   gender.

6. In boys (assigned gender), a strong rejection of
   typically masculine toys, games, and activities
   and a strong avoidance of rough-and-tumble play;
   or in girls (assigned gender), a strong rejection of
   typically feminine toys, games, and activities

7. A strong dislike of one's sexual anatomy.

8. A strong desire for the primary and/or secondary
   sex characteristics that match one's experienced
   gender.

B. The condition is associated with clinically significant
   distress or impairment in social, school, or other
   important areas of functioning.

Specify if:

With a disorder of sex development (e.g., a congenital
adrenogenital disorder such as… congenital adrenal
hyperplasia or…androgen insensitivity syndrome).

Note: Reprinted with the permission of the American
Psychiatric Association.

2. In DSM-5, the proposed introductory
   descriptor reads as follows: "A marked incongruence between one's experienced/expressed
   gender and assigned gender, of at least 6
   months' duration, as manifested by at least…"
   In the DSM-IV-TR, the introductory descriptor read as follows: "A strong and persistent
   cross-gender identification…"

   The reasons for the proposed changes were
   as follows: (1) the use of the term "incongruence" is a descriptive one that better reflects
   the core of the problem, namely, on the one
   hand, an incongruence between the identity

that one experiences and expresses and, on the
other hand, how one is expected to live based
on one's assigned gender (usually at birth)
(Meyer-Bahlburg, 2010). This was deemed
preferable to the term "cross-gender identification" in that a strictly binary gender identity
concept is no longer in line with the spectrum
of gender identity variations that one sees
clinically. (2) The term "sex" has been
replaced by assigned "gender" in order to
make the criteria applicable to individuals
with a disorder of sex development (DSD)
(see below) (Meyer-Bahlburg, 2009, 2010).
During the course of physical sex differentiation, some aspects of biological sex (e.g., 46,
XY genes) may be incongruent with other
aspects (e.g., the external genitalia); thus,
using the term "sex" would be confusing.

3. The third change pertains to the collapsing of
   the Point A ("A strong and persistent cross-
   gender identification…") and Point B
   ("Persistent discomfort with his or her sex, or
   a sense of inappropriateness in the gender role
   of that sex") criteria for GID that were present
   in the DSM-IV. Although the DSM-IV
   Subcommittee on Gender Identity Disorders
   (Bradley et al., 1991) had already recommended this change, this suggestion was not
   implemented. The DSM-5 Gender Identity
   Disorders subworkgroup persisted in recommending this change: the distinction between
   the Point A and B criteria is not supported by
   factor analytic studies suggesting that the concept of GD was best captured by one underlying dimension (e.g., Deogracias et al., 2007;
   Johnson et al., 2004; Singh et al., 2010;
   Steensma et al., in press; Zucker et al., 1998)
   as well as Mokken scale analysis for the ado-
   lescent/adult symptoms (Paap et al., 2011).

4. The fourth change pertains to a tightening of
   the threshold for diagnosis in children. In
   DSM-IV and DSM-IV-TR, it was possible to
   receive a diagnosis of GID in the absence of an
   expressed desire to be of the other gender and/
   or in the absence of an expressed discomfort
   with one's sexual anatomy. In this situation, a
   child could receive the diagnosis if he or she
   manifested all of the other symptoms, which
   were all markers of a strong cross-gender

identification and a rejection of behaviors associated with one's natal gender. The reasoning behind this decision was that some clinicians felt that there were a small number of children who likely had a GID, but did not express it, perhaps because of a sense of social inhibition or opprobrium (Bradley et al., 1991).

Since the DSM-IV (American Psychiatric Association, 1994) was published, some critics expressed concern that this diagnostic algorithm might not accurately distinguish between children with a bona fide GID and children with marked gender-variant behavior who did not experience any discomfort with their gender identity (for review, see Zucker, 2010). In an analysis of secondary data sets, Zucker (2010) showed that there was a reliable association between the degree to which mothers indicated that their child expressed the wish to be of the other gender and the degree to which their child manifested surface indicators of cross-gender behavior and also the degree to which the child indicated the desire to be of the other gender (and other indicators of gender dysphoria) on a structured diagnostic interview. In part because of these supporting data sets, the DSM-5 criteria require that the "strong desire" to be of the other gender or the insistence that one is of the other gender is a necessary, but not sufficient, criterion for the diagnosis to be made. This change will likely make the threshold for the diagnosis somewhat more conservative and should, in theory, reduce the stigmatization of gender nonconforming children who do not experience gender dysphoria.

5. For the adolescent/adult criteria, the diagnostic criteria are more nuanced than they were in the DSM-IV and, unlike the DSM-IV criteria, are represented in a polythetic format.

Based on secondary data analysis, it was proposed that the presence of at least two indicators (out of 6) would be required to meet the diagnostic criteria for GD. This was based on an analysis of 154 adolescent and adult patients with GID compared to 684 controls (Deogracias et al., 2007; Singh et al., 2010). From a 27-item dimensional measure of gender dysphoria, the Gender Identity/Gender Dysphoria Questionnaire for Adolescents and Adults (GIDYQ), five items were extracted that corresponded to the A2–A6 indicators (we could not extract a corresponding item for A1). Each item was rated on a 5-point response scale, ranging from never to always, with the past 12 months as the time frame. In this analysis, a symptom was coded as present if the participant endorsed one of the two most extreme response options (frequently or always) and as absent if the participant endorsed one of the three other options (never, rarely, sometimes). This yielded a true positive rate of 94.2 % and a false-positive rate of 0.7 %. These findings suggest that the proposed diagnostic criteria will have a very high true positive rate and a very low false-positive rate.

6. In DSM-III, the presence of a physical intersex condition (now termed a DSD) was not an exclusionary criterion for GID, but it became one in DSM-IV (see Meyer-Bahlburg, 1994). Over the past 20 years, considerable additional evidence has accumulated that some individuals with a DSD experience GD and may wish to change their assigned gender; the percentage of such individuals who experience GD is syndrome dependent (see, e.g., Meyer-Bahlburg, 1994, 2005, 2009, 2010; Pasterski et al., 2013). From a phenomenological perspective, DSD individuals with GD have both similarities and differences to individuals with GD with no known DSD (Meyer-Bahlburg, 1994, 2009; Richter-Appelt & Sandberg, 2010). Developmental trajectories also show similarities and differences. In DSM-5, the presence of a DSD is coded as a subtype. Its presence is suggestive of a specific causal mechanism that may not be present in individuals without a diagnosable DSD.

Assessment

Biomedical Tests

Because GD is overrepresented among specific DSDs, including congenital adrenal hyperplasia (CAH) in genetic females, in various androgen-resistant conditions in genetic males (e.g., partial androgen insensitivity syndrome) who are assigned to the female gender at, or shortly after, birth, in genetic males with penile agenesis or cloacal exstrophy who are assigned to the female gender (also at birth or shortly thereafter), it is important to inquire about any physical signs of these conditions; however, it is rare that these conditions have not already been diagnosed prior to a clinical assessment for GD. An exception to this might be instances of adolescent-onset DSDs, such as nonclassical (late-onset) CAH, or an endocrine condition called polycystic ovary syndrome, with its consequent androgenization effects. In the latter condition, some studies have found an elevated percentage of GD patients, but other studies have not (e.g., Baba et al., 2011; Mueller et al., 2008). In the absence of a known DSD, karyotyping of the sex chromosomes is invariably congruent with the assigned gender at birth (Inoubli et al., 2011).

Psychological Testing

Over the past 30+ years, there have been many psychometrically sound measures developed to complement the clinical diagnosis of GD (for reviews, see Zucker, 2005; Zucker & Wood, 2011). These include parent-report questionnaires, self-report questionnaires (for adolescents), play assessments, structured tasks, projective tests, and gender identity interview schedules. Most of these measures show very good discriminant validity (with various comparisons groups as controls, such as siblings, clinically referred children, and nonclinically referred children), with very low rates of false-positives using sensitivity and specificity procedures. Moreover, within samples of gender-referred children, these measures have also reliably discriminated children threshold vs. subthreshold for the GID diagnosis. As noted in the section on Developmental Trajectories, some of these measures have also shown evidence of predictive validity.

Associated Features

Apart from the behavioral characteristics that define the GD diagnostic criteria, these children have other sex-dimorphic characteristics that distinguish them from comparison children. For example, masked adult raters judged photographs of boys with GD to have a physical appearance that was more stereotypically feminine (e.g., "beautiful," "pretty") and less stereotypically masculine (e.g., "all-boy," "rugged") than same-sex controls, whereas the converse was found for girls with GD (e.g., less "beautiful," "pretty," but more "masculine," "tomboyish") (Fridell, Zucker, Bradley, & Maing, 1996; McDermid, Zucker, Bradley, & Maing, 1998; Zucker, Wild, Bradley, & Lowry, 1993). Other research showed that boys with GID were perceived by their parents as having been particularly "beautiful" and "feminine" during their infancy compared to control boys (Green, 1987). Boys with GD have a lower parent-rated activity level than same-sex controls, whereas girls with GD have a higher activity level than same-sex controls. Indeed, boys with GD have a lower activity level than girls with GD (Zucker & Bradley, 1995), the inverse from what is found in samples of boys and girls unselected for any other particular attribute of sex-typed behavior (Eaton & Enns, 1986).

General Behavior Problems

Since the last edition of this volume, a considerable amount of new data has accrued, which shows that, on average, both children and adolescents have more general behavior problems than their siblings and non-referred controls. Much of these data comes from analyses of the Child Behavior Checklist (CBCL), the Teacher's Self-Report Form, and the Youth Self-Report Form, which are now part of a family of forms known as the Achenbach System of Empirically Based Assessment (ASEBA) (Achenbach & Rescorla, 2001). In general, children and adolescents with GD have behavior problems that approximate what is seen in other children and adolescents referred for other reasons although there is some variation depending on the metric, the age group (children vs. adolescents), and the clinic site (Cohen-Kettenis et al., 2003; de Vries, Doreleijers, Steensma, & Cohen-Kettenis, 2011; Steensma et al., 2013; Wallien, Swaab, & Cohen-Kettenis,

2007; Zucker & Bradley, 1995; Zucker, Wood, Singh, & Bradley, 2012; for a detailed review, see Zucker, Wood, & VanderLaan, 2014).

In recent years, there has also been an emerging interest in the possible co-occurrence of GD with autism spectrum disorders (ASD), as reviewed in de Vries, Noens, Cohen-Kettenis, van Berckelaer-Onnes, and Doreleijers (2010). A number of clinician have reported on an apparent increase in the number of GD children and adolescents who appear to meet criteria for a high-functioning ASD, such as Asperger's Disorder or Pervasive Developmental Disorder Not Otherwise Specified. One explanation for a possible linkage between GD and ASD is the intense focus/obsessional interest in specific activities (e.g., Baron-Cohen & Wheelwright, 1999; Klin, Danovitch, Merz, & Volkmar, 2007). These children and adolescents appear to develop a fixation on gender, in much the same way that they develop other types of intense/obsessional/ restricted interests (e.g., in street routes, in makes of dishwashers, etc.).

To address the idea of focused and obsessional interests, VanderLaan et al. (2014) examined two items from the CBCL: Item 9 ("Can't get his/her mind off certain thoughts; obsessions") and Item 66 ("Repeats certain acts over and over; compulsions") in a sample of 534 GD children (439 boys, 95 girls) and 419 siblings (241 boys, 178 girls), who ranged in age from 3 to 12 years. As for all CBCL items, ratings were on a 0–2-point scale. The mother–father correlation was 0.50 for Item 9 and 0.39 for Item 66.

Item 9 was endorsed more frequently for the GD children than for the siblings (for males, 61.5 % vs. 27.3 %; for females, 66.7 % vs. 15.4 %), as was Item 66 (for males, 26.2 % vs. 10.5 %; for females, 21.5 % vs. 5.1 %). For Item 9, the percentage was even higher than for referred children in the standardization sample (for males, 49 %; for females, 47 %) and considerably higher than for non-referred children (for males, 24 %; for females, 20 %). For Item 66, the percentage was comparable to the referred children in the standardization sample (for males, 26 %; for females, 24 %) and considerably higher than for non-referred children (for males, 5 %; for females, 6 %).

Thematic analysis for Item 9 indicated that gender-related content was significantly more common for the GD boys than for their male siblings (54.6 % vs. 13.0 %), but the difference between GD girls and their female siblings was not significant (40.9 % vs. 26.3 %). For Item 66, gender-related content was not more prevalent among the GD children than among their siblings.

In a second study, Wood (2011) administered the Social Responsiveness Scale (SRS) (Constantino & Gruber, 2005) to the mothers of 38 GD children. The SRS is a 65-item parent-report questionnaire, with response options ranging from 1 (not true) to 4 (almost always true). The SRS has five factors: Social Awareness, Social Cognition, Social Communication, Social Motivation, and Autistic Mannerisms. The last factor contains items that correspond to the construct of focused/intense interests (e.g., "Has an unusually narrow range of interests").

Wood (2011) found that 60.5 % of the sample had a T score ≥ 60 (indicating a clinical range score) on the Autistic Mannerisms factor. The corresponding percentages for the other factors were 39.5 %, 39.5 %, 47.4 %, and 44.7 %, respectively. For the total score, 55.3 % of the sample met criterion for caseness. Although these findings are suggestive of an elevation of ASD traits, much additional work is required; for example, it is not yet clear if these elevated traits of ASD in GD children will prove to be diagnostic specific—it is possible that they are characteristic of clinical populations in general (see, e.g., Pine, Guyer, Goldwin, Towbin, & Leibenluft, 2008).

From a conceptual perspective, the key issue is how to best account for the presence of associated behavior problems in both children and adolescents with GD: (1) Is it caused by an inherent stress or distress that co-occurs with GD? (2) Is it secondary to other forms of psychopathology, which, in turn, "cause" the GD to develop? (3) Is it caused by the social ostracism or rejection (e.g., from peers and parents) that can be elicited by the marked gender-variant behavior that expresses the underlying GD? (4) Is it unrelated to GD per se, but related to generic risk factors within the family for the expression of psychopathology (e.g., biological factors, parental psychopathology, familial adversity)?

To date, two lines of research have provided clear empirical support for two of these hypothesized pathways: the social ostracism model and the generic risk factor model. Several studies have shown that social ostracism by the peer group (which, most likely, results in poor peer relations) is a very strong predictor of general behavior problems in both GD children and adolescents. Other research has shown that composite measures of maternal psychopathology also predict general behavior problems (for review, see Zucker et al., 2014). Considerably less work has attempted to examine if self-reported stress or distress surrounding the GD can be linked to general measures of behavior problems and psychodynamic models which posit that other psychopathology induces the GD have not been formally tested by temporal methods (see Coates & Person, 1985).

Understanding the empirical evidence that supports or contests these different pathways is extremely important with regard to clinical management policies and decisions. For example, if the model of social ostracism is correct, one therapeutic approach would be to reduce the child's expression of gender-variant behavior. If these children became more gender typical, it would eliminate the surface behaviors that elicit the social ostracism. An alternative therapeutic approach would be to provide the child a safer social environment (e.g., attendance at schools in which gender nonconforming behavior is better tolerated, if not embraced, or to work with parents around "accepting" their child's gender-variant behavior). If the model of generic risk factors is correct, then the focus of treatment would be to alleviate, where possible, the activating effects of such factors (e.g., reduction of concurrent parental psychopathology, pharmacological treatment of the child when they have disorders that might be related to an underlying biological diathesis, etc.). If the association with an ASD is correct, then one therapeutic approach would be to help a child think more flexibly regarding gender, to move the child away from the intense/restricted focus on gender, etc. Finally, if GD is an inherent source of distress, then treatment designed to eliminate the GD (whether by psychotherapeutic methods or biomedical treatments) should reduce the associated psychopathology.

Developmental Trajectories

When a child presents to a clinician with a behavior pattern that corresponds to the DSM-5 diagnosis of GD, many parents want information about long-term developmental trajectories. Will their child continue to feel gender dysphoric and, eventually, seek out biomedical treatment (hormonal treatment and genital reassignment surgery) and "formally" transition to living in the desired gender? Will their child's GD "desist" and thus become more comfortable with a gender identity that matches their birth sex? Regardless of their child's long-term gender identity, how will their sexual orientation differentiate? Will their child be sexually attracted to males, to females, to both, or to neither? In this section, I will provide a summary of the current database that has accumulated with regard to long-term developmental trajectories.

At the time of the 2000 volume, the most extensive long-term follow-up of boys with GD had been reported on by Green (1987) (for other follow-up studies available at that time, see the summary in Zucker & Bradley (1995), pp. 283–290). Green's study contained 66 feminine boys and 56 control boys assessed initially at a mean age of 7.1 years (range, 4–12). At the time of follow-up (M age, 18.9 years; range, 14–24), data were available for 44 of the feminine boys and 30 of the control boys. At follow-up, gender identity was assessed via a clinical interview, and sexual orientation was assessed by means of a semi-structured interview, in which Kinsey ratings, on a 7-point scale, were made for fantasy and behavior, ranging from exclusive heterosexuality (gynephilia) to exclusive homosexuality (androphilia) in relation to the participant's birth sex.

In Green's follow-up study, there was virtually no evidence for the persistence of GD: only 1 (2.2 %) of the 44 feminine boys was considered to be gender dysphoric at the time of follow-up.

Table 35.2 Summary of three new follow-up studies of children with gender dysphoria

Study	N/sex	Age at assessment (in years)		Age at follow-up (in years)		Gender dysphoric (%)	Bisexual/homosexual in fantasy (%)	Bisexual/homosexual in behavior (%)
		M	SD	M	SD			
Wallien and Cohen-Kettenis (2008)	59/M	8.3	2.0	19.4	3.4	20.3	81/68[a]	79[b]
	18/F	8.6	1.5	18.7	2.7	50.0	70/100[a]	60[b]
Drummond et al. (2008)	25/F	8.8	3.1	23.2	5.8	12.0	32[c]	24[c]
Singh (2012)	139/M	7.4	2.6	20.5	5.2	12.2	63.6[d]	47.2[d]

Note: M = natal male; F = natal female

[a]The first value was based on a question pertaining to "fantasy" and the second value was based on a question pertaining to "attraction" (see the supplemental material for the article at http://www.jaacap.com). For the male participants, the N was 21 for fantasy and 37 for attraction; for the female participants, the N was 3 for fantasy and 10 for attraction

[b]For the male participants, N = 19; for the female participants, N = 5 (see Wallien & Cohen-Kettenis, 2008, Table 5)

[c]For fantasy, the denominator included 1 participant who did not report any sexual fantasies; for behavior, the denominator included 8 participants who had not engaged in sexual behavior (see Drummond et al., 2008, Table 3)

[d]For fantasy, N = 129, including 4 participants who did not report any sexual fantasies; for behavior, N = 108, including 28 participants who did not report any sexual behavior (see Singh, 2012, Tables 9 and 10)

The remainder appeared to be comfortable with a male gender identity. Regarding sexual orientation, 75–80 % of the feminine boys were classified as either bisexual or homosexual at follow-up compared to 0–4 % of the comparison boys in fantasy or behavior.

Three new follow-up studies now provide a basis for comparison to Green: Drummond, Bradley, Peterson-Badali, and Zucker (2008), Wallien and Cohen-Kettenis (2008), and Singh (2012). Two of these studies were from my own clinic, and the third study was conducted at the sole gender identity clinic for children in the Netherlands. Table 35.2 provides a summary of these three studies with regard to gender identity and sexual orientation at the time of follow-up.

From Table 35.2, it can be seen that the rate of persistent GD was higher in these three new follow-up studies, with a range of 12–50 %, when compared to Green's persistence rate of 2.2 %. The most notable variation was between the two follow-up samples of girls (12 % vs. 50 %), but the sample sizes were sufficiently small that it would be imprudent to over-interpret the meaning of this variation. Regarding sexual orientation, for the males, a substantial majority were homosexual/bisexual (androphilic/biphilic) in fantasy and at least half were homosexual or bisexual in behavior. For the females, one-third

to one-quarter of the participants in Drummond et al. were homosexual or bisexual, which was notably lower than the percentage in Wallien and Cohen-Kettenis, but their study had only a maximum of 10 participants for these ratings.

From these new follow-up studies, I think that several provisional conclusions can be made: (1) with the exception of the female data from Wallien and Cohen-Kettenis, the percentage of children where the GD persists into late adolescence or early adulthood is on the low side. The persistence rate is certainly much lower than what one finds in GD patients who are evaluated for the first time in adolescence (not childhood) (for review, see Zucker et al., 2011). (2) For the male children, the new studies certainly confirm Green's finding that marked feminine behaviors in boys are reliably associated with either a bisexual or a homosexual sexual orientation in adolescence/adulthood, at rates that are dramatically higher than the base rate of androphilia in males that one can discern from epidemiological studies (perhaps around 2–3 % using rigorous assessment methods and no more than 10 % using much looser metrics). In itself, this has important implications for theory regarding causal mechanisms that posit an intersection between gender identity and sexual orientation (see below). (3) For females, the numbers for follow-up are still pitifully small, but even the percentage from the Drummond et al. (2008) study certainly suggests a much higher rate of a bisexual/homosexual sexual orientation than one would predict based on epidemiological research.

Predictors of Long-Term Gender Identity

When one asks adolescents or adults with GD about their recollections of sex-typed behavior in childhood, for those who have a sexual orientation directed to members of their birth sex, it is almost universal to find a childhood history of marked gender-variant or cross-gender behavior (Deogracias et al., 2007).[2] Thus, there appears to be evidence for retrospective continuity between an early cross-gender identification that persists into later phases of the life course. In contrast, the prospective data summarized above show much less continuity between cross-gender identification in childhood and at follow-up. A key challenge, then, for developmental theories of psychosexual differentiation is to account for the disjunction between retrospective and prospective data with regard to GD persistence.

Regarding children with GD, then, we need to understand why, for the majority, gender dysphoria appears to remit by adolescence, if not earlier. One possible explanation concerns referral bias. Green (1974) argued that children with GD who are referred for clinical assessment (and then, in some cases, therapy) may come from families in which there is more concern than is the case for adolescents and adults, the majority of whom did not receive a clinical evaluation and treatment

during childhood. Thus, a clinical evaluation and subsequent therapeutic intervention during childhood may alter the natural history of GD. Of course, this is only one account of the disjunction, and there may well be additional factors that might distinguish those children who are more likely to persist than those who do not.

One such explanation pertains to the concepts of developmental malleability and plasticity. It is possible, for example, that gender identity shows relative malleability during childhood, with a gradual narrowing of plasticity as the gendered sense of self consolidates as one approaches adolescence. As noted above, some support for this idea comes from follow-up studies of adolescents with GD, who appear to show a much higher rate of GD persistence as they are followed into young adulthood.

One contextual issue is that the vast majority of these samples entered these clinic-based prospective studies during historical periods when the predominant therapeutic guidelines were to somehow try and help a child feel more comfortable with a gender identity that matched his or her birth sex or to at least not "encourage" a cross-gender identity (Zucker et al., 2012). This has changed rather dramatically in the past few years. For example, there is now what I would call an early gender transition movement or subculture (see, e.g., http://www.transkidspurplerainbow.org/) in which some clinicians and some parents view a child's early cross-gender identification as a fixed, unalterable, and essential part of the child's sense of self. Accordingly, some clinicians recommend that a young child begin a social transition to the desired gender long before puberty—in some cases, as early as the preschool years (e.g., Brown, 2006; Byne et al., 2012; Padawar, 2012; Rosin, 2008; Saeger, 2006; Santiago, 2006; Schwartzapfel, 2013; Vanderburgh, 2009) and some parents implement this approach on their own.

In some respects, this approach to clinical management can be conceptualized as an alternative treatment to the more traditional "treatment-as-usual" (TAU) approaches which likely shared an underlying goal of reducing, not "supporting," the child's intense desire to be of the other gender.

---

[2] For GD adolescents and adults who have a sexual orientation predominantly directed to members of the opposite sex (relative to their own natal sex), it is much less common to recall a childhood history of cross-sex-typed behavior (Zucker et al., 2012). In these individuals, it is common for the GD to be overtly expressed only at the time of puberty or long after. In the literature, this is often referred to as "late-onset" GD. It is beyond the scope of this chapter to describe in detail this form of GD. A useful overview of late-onset GD in natal males can be found in Lawrence (2013).

One could even go so far as to posit that this contemporary approach is akin to a social experiment of nurture. Thus, it can be asked if the rate of persistent GD will be higher among those children who make an early social transition to the desired gender when compared to the TAU approaches.

Steensma, McGuire, Kreukels, Beekman, and Cohen-Kettenis (2013) have provided the first empirical evidence that this appears to be the case–at least for natal males. Steensma et al. followed up 127 children (79 natal boys, 48 natal girls) (M age at assessment, 9.1 years; range, 6–12) at a mean age of 16.1 years (range, 15–19). At the time of the childhood assessment, Steensma et al. classified 12 (15.1 %) of the natal boys and 27 (56.2 %) of the natal girls as having already made either a "partial" or a "complete" social transition to living in the cross-gender role. At follow-up, the participants were classified as either "persisters" or "desisters." Of the 79 natal boys, 29 % were classified as persisters and, of the 48 natal girls, 50 % were classified as persisters. Of the 79 natal boys, a greater percentage of persisters had made a social transition in childhood compared to the desisters (43.4 % vs. 3.6 %); the corresponding figures for the girls were 58.4 % vs. 45.8 %, respectively. In logistic regression for natal males, early gender transition independently predicted persistence, but this was not the case for the natal females. At least for natal boys, then, it could be argued that the "act" of early gender social transition had some type of feedback effect in contributing to the persistence of GD. For natal girls, however, early gender social transition did not appear to have the same effect (see below). It is possible that the reason for the sex difference pertains to the complexity in defining what exactly constitutes a gender social transition. For many GD boys, they might well go to school wearing gender-typical clothing and thus are perceived to be boys, whereas many more GD girls, if they wear boy's clothes and have very short haircuts, may well be perceived as boys; thus, at least in part, natal boys might have to do more to be classified as social transitioners than are natal girls. Indeed, in Steensma et al., the percentage of natal boys classified as social transitioners was much lower than that of the natal girls (15.1 % vs. 52.0 %).

From the new follow-up studies, there was sufficient variability in gender identity outcome to analyze various predictors. In all three follow-up studies, dimensional measures of cross-gender identity and cross-gender role behavior in childhood predicted GD persistence. Children whose cross-gender identity and behavior were more extreme were more likely to be persisters than desisters. Thus, even within samples of children with marked gender-variant behavior, the extremeness of the phenotype could predict gender identity outcome. In Singh (2012), an older age at assessment in childhood marginally predicted persistence (at $p = 0.09$), and a lower social class background significantly predicted persistence ($p < 0.001$), independently of a dimensional composite of cross-gender behavior.

Why, one might ask, would a lower socioeconomic (SES) background predict persistence within a sample of GD children? An early study in the normative gender developmental literature reported that children from "working-class" backgrounds had an earlier awareness of "sex-appropriate" behavior than children from middle-class backgrounds (Rabban, 1950) and a subsequent study found that boys from lower SES backgrounds had more traditional patterns of sex-typed behavior than upper SES boys (Hall & Keith, 1964), but there was no significant social class effect for girls (for a similar null finding for girls, see Hines et al., 2002). Other studies hint at social class differences in parenting style that are related to gender socialization (greater egalitarianism in middle-class families) (Shinn & O'Brien, 2008).

In Singh (2012), it was speculated that the GD boys from lower SES families had more "rigid" notions of within-sex variation in sex-typed behavior and that, later on, the acceptability of a homosexual sexual orientation (without "becoming" a female to "normalize" such attractions) perhaps intensified the desire to be of the other gender. Thus, between-social class variation in the acceptability of homosexuality was posited as a potential mediator variable. On this point, there is some interesting evidence to suggest that gay men from higher social class backgrounds are more likely to show behavioral defeminization over the life course than are gay men from lower social class backgrounds (Harry, 1985). It has been argued that, within gay male subculture, extreme effeminate behavior is appraised negatively. It is possible, therefore, that males with persistent cross-gender behaviors would be subject to rejection by potential sexual partners (see Taywadietop, 2001). Consistent rejections may predispose some of these individuals to consider transitioning to the female gender role as an alternative to living as a homosexual man.

Causal Mechanisms

In my view, understanding the genesis of GD requires that we understand the mechanisms that explain the development of normative sex differences in sex-dimorphic behavior (including gender identity, gender role, and sexual orientation). In this respect, I endorse the long-established tradition that emphasizes the importance of understanding the interplay between normative and atypical development and the idea that, in many instances, the underlying mechanisms regarding the latter are inversions of the underlying mechanisms of the former.

The field of psychosexual differentiation has relied on at least two theoretical models: one model asks what is known about the factors that contribute to normative between-sex differences in sex-dimorphic behavior (the between-sex model); the second model asks what is known about the factors that contribute to normative within-sex differences in sex-dimorphic behavior (the within-sex model).

As an example of the first model, it has long been theorized that the well-established between-sex difference in prenatal exposure to androgen accounts, at least in part, for normative sex differences in sex-dimorphic behavior (Berenbaum, Owen Blakemore, & Bletz, 2011; Hines, 2011). Let us suppose that it does. Then, one could ask if within-sex variation in prenatal androgen exposure would also account for within-sex variation

in sex-dimorphic behavior. Affirmative support for this question comes from numerous studies of genetic females with CAH, who are exposed to high levels of prenatal testosterone as a result of this endocrine abnormality and who also show, on a number of sex-dimorphic measures, masculinized (or defeminized) behavior (Hines, 2004). In unaffected boys and girls, Auyeung et al. (2009) showed that within-sex variation in fetal testosterone, as assayed from amniotic fluid, was related to within-sex variation in parent-reported sex-typed behavior at a mean age of 8.5 years: within-sex analyses showed that both boys and girls with higher levels of prenatal testosterone had more male-typical behavior (for a similar study that assayed testosterone in infancy, see Lamminmäki et al., 2012).

As an example of the second model, numerous studies have now documented that gay men come from sibships with an excess of older brothers when compared to heterosexual men (known as the fraternal birth order effect). In contrast, there is no evidence to indicate that there is an analogous effect associated with within-sex variation in sexual orientation among women. Thus, the fraternal birth order effect in males requires some kind of within-sex explanation. Blanchard (2001) and Blanchard and Klassen (1997) theorized that maternal immune reaction during pregnancy is one candidate explanation. Because the male fetus is experienced by the mother as more "foreign" (antigenic) than the female fetus, it was argued that the production of maternal antibodies has the (inadvertent) consequence of demasculinizing or feminizing the male fetus. Because the mother's antigenicity increases with each successive male pregnancy, the model predicts that males born later in a sibline would be more affected and thus this is why the odds of male homosexuality increase with the number of older brothers. Bogaert (2006) provided some further support for this theory by showing that only biological older brothers, but not any other sibling characteristics, including nonbiological older brothers, predicted within-sex variation in sexual orientation in men.

In this section, I will provide a selective summary of "causal" research on GD that has, at least in part, relied on these theoretical models (for a more detailed overview, see Zucker & Bradley, 1995).

Biological Influences

Genetics

Candidate gene studies have yielded mixed results in adult males and females with GD, including high rates of "false-positives" in control groups and failures to replicate (Ngun, Ghahramani, Sánchez, Bocklandt, & Vilain, 2011). Similar studies have not been conducted on either children or adolescents with GD. As this is a very new line of research, it is premature to draw any definitive conclusions. However, there is some supportive behavior genetic evidence: in clinical samples, identical twins are more likely to be concordant for GD than nonidentical twins (Heylens et al., 2012; for a nonclinical sample, see Coolidge, Thede, & Young, 2002). Moreover, in the general population, twin studies have shown that the liability for cross-gender behavior has a strong heritable component (Alanko et al., 2010; Burri, Cherkas, Spector, & Rahman, 2011; van Beijsterveldt, Hudziak, & Boomsma, 2006). Other studies, however, have also identified strong shared and non-shared environmental influences (Iervolino, Hines, Golombok, Rust, & Plomin, 2005; Knafo, Iervolino, & Plomin, 2005). Such environmental influences could, of course, pertain to nongenetic biological factors but could also involve postnatal psychosocial factors. In any case, it should be recognized that these studies have not identified the specific genetic and environmental factors, or the gene × environmental interactions, underlying the liability to cross-gender behavior. That genetic factors do not account for all of the variance in the liability to cross-gender behavior is demonstrated quite clearly from clinical case reports of identical twins discordant for GD (Heylens et al., 2012).

Prenatal Sex Hormones

It has long been noted that classical prenatal hormone theory does not easily account for GD since the vast majority have a grossly phenotype (e.g., normal externa there is little reason to believe hormonal milieu was grossly it is conceivable that more subtl ... terns of prenatal sex hormone secretion play a predisposing role. For example, in experimental studies of female rhesus monkey offspring, it has been possible, by varying the timing of exogenous administration of hormones during the pregnancy, to alter the normal patterning of sex-dimorphic behavior but to keep normal genital differentiation intact (Goy, Bercovitch, & McBrair, 1988) (for an analogous model in male nonhuman primates, see Herman & Wallen, 2007). This animal model, which shows a dissociation between sex-dimorphic behavioral differentiation and genital differentiation, has the most direct relevance for explaining the marked cross-gender behavior of GD children and adolescents. The Auyeung et al. (2009) finding noted above suggests that subtle within-sex variation in prenatal testosterone might well apply to children with GD, but it would be difficult to test this possibility except by locating children who eventually developed a GD and who happened to be part of a sample in which prenatal testosterone had been assayed.

Because of this sampling obstacle, some studies have used biophysical markers that might be related, at least in theory, with variation in prenatal androgen exposure. An example of this is the measurement of the length of the second and fourth digits and their corresponding ratio (2D:4D). It is now well established that there is a normative sex difference in 2D:4D, with males having, on average, a longer fourth digit than second digit than females (for a meta-analytic summary, see Grimbos, Dawood, Burris, Zucker, & Puts, 2010). Although some studies on GD adults have shown evidence for an altered within-sex difference in 2D:4D, the one study on 2D:4D in children with GD did not detect any significant difference from same-sex controls (Wallien, Zucker, Steensma, & Cohen-Kettenis, 2008).

Fraternal Birth Order Effect

As noted above, a fraternal birth order effect has been established as a correlate of within-sex

.ariation in sexual orientation. The fraternal birth order effect has also been documented in several independent samples of boys with GD (assessed either in childhood or in adolescence) (Blanchard, Zucker, Bradley, & Hume, 1995; Schagen, Delemarre-van de Waal, Blanchard, & Cohen-Kettenis, 2012; VanderLaan, Blanchard, Wood, & Zucker, in press; Zucker et al., 1997b). If the maternal immune hypothesis is correct, it could be the case that the demasculinizing or feminizing effect also extends to gender identity, which, of course, in GD males is shifted in a female-typical direction.

Psychosocial Influences

To merit truly causal status, psychosocial factors should be able to account for the emergence of marked cross-gender behavior in GD children in the first few years of life, when its behavioral expressions are first manifested. Otherwise, psychosocial factors would be better conceptualized as having a perpetuating role.

Maternal Prenatal Sex Preference

One early hypothesis was rather simple: mothers of boys with GD were more likely to have desired a daughter during the pregnancy than control mothers. This prenatal gender preference was hypothesized to have influenced the mother's subsequent gender socialization of the GD boy (e.g., by subtly encouraging or fostering feminine behavior). Zucker et al. (1994), however, found no evidence that mothers of GD boys were more likely to recall a prenatal preference for a daughter than mothers of same-sex controls. However, Zucker et al. did find that mothers of GD boys who only had older sons were more likely to have wanted a daughter during the pregnancy than mothers of GD boys from other classes of sibships; however, the same pattern was detected in the mothers of control boys. Thus, there was no support for the hypothesis.

Social Reinforcement

Parental tolerance or encouragement of the early cross-gender behavior of GD children has been reported on by clinicians of diverse theoretical persuasions and has also marshaled some degree of empirical support (Green, 1987; Zucker & Bradley, 1995).

The reasons why parents might tolerate, if not encourage, early cross-gender behaviors appear to be quite diverse, suggesting that the antecedents to this "end state" are multiple in origin. For example, if one listens to the reports by contemporary parents of children who have made an early gender social transition, a common narrative is that the parents are simply "supporting" what they view as their child's essential "nature" (cf. Smiler & Gelman, 2008). Such parents would argue that the direction of effect is from child to parent, not the other way around or even some kind of interactive, iterative transactional process (for an important study implicating transactional processes in the sex-typed play behavior of girls with CAH, see Wong, Pasterski, Hindmarsh, Geffner, & Hines, 2013).

In an earlier generation of parents of GD children, parents reported being influenced by ideas regarding nonsexist child-rearing and thus were as likely to encourage cross-gender behavior as same-gender behavior. In other parents, the antecedents seem to be rooted in pervasive conflict that revolved around gender issues. For example, I coined the term *pathological gender mourning* to describe a small subgroup of mothers who had a strong desire for a girl (after having giving birth only to older sons), and they seemed quite troubled by the fact that they had given birth to another son (Zucker, 1996). This was expressed in various ways: marked jealousy of friends with daughters, assignment of a gender-ambiguous or gender-neutral given name, delayed naming of the newborn, severe postpartum depression, replacement and adoption fantasies, recurrent night dreams about being pregnant with a girl, and active cross-dressing of the boy during infancy and toddlerhood.

In the normative developmental literature, the role of parental reinforcement efforts in inducing sex-typed behavioral sex differences was studied extensively between the 1970s and early 1990s. Lytton and Romney's (1991) meta-analysis concluded that, with one exception, there was "little differential socialization for social behavior or abilities" (p. 267). The exception was in the domain of "encouragement of sex-typed activities and perceptions of sex-stereotyped characteristics" (p. 283), for which the mean effect sizes for mothers, fathers, and parents combined were 0.34, 0.49, and 0.43, respectively. Although Lytton and Romney's overall conclusion minimized the influence of parental socialization on sex-dimorphic behavior, the domain for which clear parental gender socialization effects were found is precisely the domain that encompasses many of the initial behavioral features of GD (for further discussion, see Zucker & Bradley, 1995, pp. 222–226).

Cognitive-Developmental Factors

Over the past couple of decades, cognitive-developmental models have come to play a much more central role in the normative literature regarding gender development (see, e.g., Martin et al., 2002; Tobin et al., 2010), building on the seminal theoretical work from the 1960s to 1980s, and its emphasis on "self-socialization." Two elements of this complex work will be discussed here. First, there is the literature on how early gender self-labeling as a boy or as a girl organizes the child's search for gender-related information in the social environment. Several empirical studies have shown that sex-typed behavior increases following the toddler's or young child's ability to self-label correctly as a boy or as a girl, an early phase in the development of mature cognitive gender constancy.

Studies of children with GD have shown that they are more likely than control children to mislabel themselves as of the other gender and to also show a "developmental lag" in cognitive gender constancy (e.g., Wallien et al., 2009; Zucker et al., 1999). Perhaps this early cognitive mislabeling of gender contributes to their cross-gender identification although the reasons why such mislabeling occurs are unclear. It could, for example, be argued that there is some kind of interactive effect between gender cognitions and the strong interest in cross-gender behavior.

A second aspect of the cognitive-developmental literature pertains to the observation that young children have rather rigid, if not obsessional, interests in engaging in sex-typed behavior: for girls, Halim et al. (2013) dubbed this the "pink frilly dress" phenomenon. Halim et al. argued that this gender rigidity was part of the young child's effort to master gender categories and to securely (affectively) place oneself in the "right" category. Parents of such children do not particularly encourage the rigidity, but they also do not discourage it, and there is the assumption that such rigidity will wane over developmental time and that there will be a concomitant increase in gender flexibility.

Halim et al.'s (2013) observations jibe rather nicely with empirical data suggesting that many children with GD show very focused and intense cross-gender interests (VanderLaan et al., 2014). If these early cross-gender intense interests are reinforced rather than ignored or compensated for by efforts to increase gender-flexible thinking and behavior, perhaps this contributes to their continuation and an increase in the likelihood that a cross-gender identity will persist.

Clinical Management: Is There a Best Practice?

For the practicing developmental clinician, it will be readily apparent from a perusal of the treatment guideline literature that there are some therapeutic approaches for which there is reasonable consensus—especially for adolescents—but for other approaches much is "up in the air," especially for children.

For probably the majority of adolescents with GD, there is now a reasonable consensus that psychological interventions designed to reduce the gender dysphoria are relatively ineffective and most adolescents with GD are not "interested" in such an approach anyways. Because the desire to be of the other gender has, more or less, become part of the youth's gendered sense of self, the most common therapeutic approach has been to support a social gender transition (if it has not already occurred) and to support the initiation of biomedical treatments that permit an approximation of the phenotype of the desired gender. Thus, in adolescents, it has become a more standard practice to recommend the institution of hormonal treatment to delay or suppress somatic puberty via the use of gonadotropin-releasing hormone analogues prior to the age of 16 years, followed by the institution of contra-sex hormonal therapy at 16+ years, and then sex-reassignment surgery at 18+ years. For carefully evaluated adolescents, this therapeutic approach reduces the GD and appears to contribute to better psychosocial functioning in general (see, e.g., Cohen-Kettenis, Steensma, & de Vries, 2011; Coleman et al., 2011). It should, however, also be recognized that not all adolescents with GD are immediate candidates for this treatment approach: there are some adolescents who report being "confused" about their gender identity, some wonder if their gender dysphoria is related to adverse psychosocial experiences, and others are in a phase of exploring how their felt gender identity relates to their emerging sexual orientation. For these adolescents, it is more appropriate to begin treatment with a trial of psychosocial therapy to help them sort out these issues, prior to consideration of the utility of biomedical treatments (Smith, van Goozen, & Cohen-Kettenis, 2001; Zucker et al., 2011).

For children, the contemporary therapeutic literature is hampered by the relative, if not complete, absence of well-designed comparative treatment approaches (Zucker, 2008). Therapeutic goals need to be clearly articulated and agreed upon in a collaborative manner with parents. The clinician needs to be well versed in the conceptual and philosophical discourse about what constitutes "best practice" in order to contextualize the therapeutic needs of individual children (Drescher & Byne, 2012). The clinician will also need to be quite mindful of the different philosophies, values, and "ideologies" that parents bring to the consulting room. Some parents very much want their child to feel comfortable with a gender identity that matches their birth sex, others are more comfortable with their child expressing a cross-gender identity, and still others simply don't know what to think and, therefore, look to the clinician for expert guidance.

My own view is that, for young children with GD, gender identity differentiation is far from fixed, as suggested by the long-term follow-up data reviewed above. Thus, a therapeutic approach that attempts to reduce the GD via psychosocial treatments is likely to be successful.

If this conjecture is correct, then the clinician must contemplate a myriad of value judgments, such as whether or not it is easier for the child to grow up with a gender identity that matches his or her birth sex vs. a gender identity that is incongruent with the birth sex, and does the former result in a better life-course psychosocial adaptation? On this point, much remains unknown.

We are currently in an era in which some parents and some clinicians have adopted a very different course of therapeutics, as I outlined earlier in describing the early gender transition social movement. It is my own view that this therapeutic approach will result in a much higher rate of children persisting in their desire to change genders and to pursue the biomedical treatments that become available at the time of adolescence. As more data become available that track the psychosocial adjustment of these youngsters, we will be in a better empirical position to draw conclusions about best practice. For the time being, the contemporary developmental clinician will have to tolerate the ambiguity of the gaps in the literature on what is not known.

Summary

In this chapter, I have reviewed aspects of the core phenomenology, diagnosis and assessment, associated features, developmental trajectories, and selected causal mechanisms pertaining to GD in children and adolescents. Given the recent increase in clinical referrals of children and adolescents in the GD spectrum that has been reported internationally, it is important that practitioners be aware of the various methods that are available for a comprehensive diagnostic assessment, to have information on the common associated problems seen in this population, and to be aware of the follow-up data on known developmental trajectories. Much empirical work remains to be done in identifying what is clearly a complex biopsychosocial pathway that leads to this relatively uncommon, but fascinating, psychiatric condition.

References

Achenbach, T. M., & Rescorla, L. A. (2001). *Manual for the ASEBA school-age forms & profiles*. Burlington, VT: University of Vermont, Research Center for Children, Youth, & Families.

Alanko, K., Santtila, P., Harlaar, N., Witting, K., Varjonen, M., Jern, P., et al. (2010). Common genetic effects of gender atypical behavior in childhood and sexual orientation in adulthood: A study of Finnish twins. *Archives of Sexual Behavior, 39*, 81–92.

American Psychiatric Association. (1980). *Diagnostic and statistical manual of mental disorders* (3rd ed.). Washington, DC: Author.

American Psychiatric Association. (1994). *Diagnostic and statistical manual of mental disorders* (4th ed.). Washington, DC: Author.

American Psychiatric Association. (2000). *Diagnostic and statistical manual of mental disorders* (4th ed., text rev.). Washington, DC: Author.

American Psychiatric Association. (2013). *Diagnostic and statistical manual of mental disorders* (5th ed.). Arlington, VA: Author.

Auyeung, B., Baron-Cohen, S., Ashwin, E., Knickmeyer, R., Taylor, K., & Hines, M. (2009). Fetal testosterone predicts sexually differentiated childhood behavior in boys and girls. *Psychological Science, 20*, 144–148.

Baba, T., Endo, T., Ikeda, K., Shimizu, A., Honnma, H., Ikeda, H., et al. (2011). Distinctive features of female-to-male transsexualism and prevalence of gender identity disorder in Japan. *Journal of Sexual Medicine, 8*, 1686–1693.

Baron-Cohen, S., & Wheelwright, S. (1999). 'Obsessions' in children with autism or Asperger syndrome: Content analysis in terms of core domains of cognition. *British Journal of Psychiatry, 175*, 484–490.

Berenbaum, S. A., Owen Blakemore, J. E., & Beltz, A. M. (2011). A role for biology in gender-related behavior. *Sex Roles, 64*, 804–825.

Blanchard, R. (2001). Fraternal birth order and the maternal immune hypothesis of male homosexuality. *Hormones and Behavior, 40*, 105–114.

Blanchard, R., & Klassen, P. (1997). H-Y antigen and homosexuality in men. *Journal of Theoretical Biology, 185*, 373–378.

Blanchard, R., Zucker, K. J., Bradley, S. J., & Hume, C. S. (1995). Birth order and sibling sex ratio in homosexual male adolescents and probably prehomosexual feminine boys. *Developmental Psychology, 31*, 22–30.

Bogaert, A. F. (2006). Biological versus nonbiological older brothers and men's sexual orientation. *Proceedings of the National Academy of Sciences of the United States of America, 103*, 10771–10774.

Bradley, S. J., Blanchard, R., Coates, S., Green, R., Levine, S. B., Meyer-Bahlburg, H. F. L., et al. (1991). Interim report of the DSM-IV subcommittee on gender identity disorders. *Archives of Sexual Behavior, 20*, 333–343.

Brown, P. L. (2006, December 2). Supporting boys or girls when the line isn't clear. *New York Times*, pp. A1, A11.

Burri, A., Cherkas, L., Spector, T., & Rahman, Q. (2011). Genetic and environmental influences on female sexual orientation, childhood gender typicality and adult gender identity. *PLoS ONE, 6*(7), e21982. doi:10.1371/journal.pone.0021982.

Byne, W., Bradley, S. J., Coleman, E., Eyler, A. E., Green, R., Menvielle, E. J., et al. (2012). Report of the American Psychiatric Association Task Force on treatment of gender identity disorder. *Archives of Sexual Behavior, 41*, 759–796.

Coates, S., & Person, E. S. (1985). Extreme boyhood femininity: Isolated behavior or pervasive disorder? *Journal of the American Academy of Child Psychiatry, 24*, 702–709.

Cohen-Kettenis, P. T., Owen, A., Kaijser, V. G., Bradley, S. J., & Zucker, K. J. (2003). Demographic characteristics, social competence, and behavior problems in children with gender identity disorder: A cross-national, cross-clinic comparative analysis. *Journal of Abnormal Child Psychology, 31*, 41–53.

Cohen-Kettenis, P. T., Steensma, T. D., & de Vries, A. L. C. (2011). Treatment of adolescents with gender dysphoria in the Netherlands. *Child and Adolescent Psychiatric Clinics of North America, 20*, 689–700.

Cohen-Kettenis, P. T., Wallien, M., Johnson, L. L., Owen-Anderson, A. F. H., Bradley, S. J., & Zucker, K. J. (2006). A parent-report gender identity questionnaire for children: A cross-national, cross-clinic comparative analysis. *Clinical Child Psychology and Psychiatry, 11*, 397–405.

Coleman, E., Bockting, W., Botzer, M., Cohen-Kettenis, P., DeCuypere, G., ... Zucker, K. (2011). Standards of care for the health of transsexual, transgender, and gender-nonconforming people, Version 7. *International Journal of Transgenderism, 13*, 165–232.

Constantino, J. N., & Gruber, C. P. (2005). *Social responsiveness scale*. Los Angeles, CA: Western Psychological Services.

Coolidge, F. L., Thede, L. L., & Young, S. E. (2002). The heritability of gender identity disorder in a child and adolescent twin sample. *Behavior Genetics, 32*, 251–257.

De Cuypere, G., Knudson, G., & Bockting, W. (2010). Response of the World Professional Association for transgender health to the proposed *dsm 5* criteria for gender incongruence. *International Journal of Transgenderism, 12*, 119–123.

de Vries, A. L. C., Doreleijers, T. A. H., Steensma, T. D., & Cohen-Kettenis, P. T. (2011). Psychiatric comorbidity in gender dysphoric adolescents. *Journal of Child Psychiatry and Psychiatry, 52*, 1195–1202.

de Vries, A. L. C., Noens, I. L., Cohen-Kettenis, P. T., van Berckelaer-Onnes, I. A., & Doreleijers, T. A. H. (2010). Autism spectrum disorders in gender dysphoric children and adolescents. *Journal of Autism and Developmental Disorders, 40*, 930–936.

Deogracias, J. J., Johnson, L. L., Meyer-Bahlburg, H. F. L., Kessler, S. J., Schober, J. M., & Zucker, K. J. (2007). The gender identity/gender dysphoria questionnaire for adolescents and adults. *Journal of Sex Research, 44*, 370–379.

Drescher, J., & Byne, W. (2012). Introduction to the special issue on "The Treatment of Gender Dysphoric/Gender Variant Children and Adolescents". *Journal of Homosexuality, 59*, 295–300.

Drummond, K. D., Bradley, S. J., Badali-Peterson, M., & Zucker, K. J. (2008). A follow-up study of girls with gender identity disorder. *Developmental Psychology, 44*, 34–45.

Eaton, W. O., & Enns, L. R. (1986). Sex differences in human motor activity level. *Psychological Bulletin, 100*, 19–28.

Fausto-Sterling, A., Garcia Coll, C., & Lamarre, M. (2012). Sexing the baby: Part 2–applying dynamic systems theory to the emergences of sex-related differences in infants and toddlers. *Social Science & Medicine, 74*, 1693–1702.

Fisk, N. (1973). Gender dysphoria syndrome (the how, what, and why of a disease). In D. Laub & P. Gandy (Eds.), *Proceedings of the second interdisciplinary symposium on gender dysphoria syndrome* (pp. 7–14). Palo Alto, CA: Stanford University Press.

Fridell, S. R., Zucker, K. J., Bradley, S. J., & Maing, D. M. (1996). Physical attractiveness of girls with gender identity disorder. *Archives of Sexual Behavior, 25*, 17–31.

Goy, R. W., Bercovitch, F. B., & McBrair, M. C. (1988). Behavioral masculinization is independent of genital masculinization in prenatally androgenized female rhesus macaques. *Hormones and Behavior, 22*, 552–571.

Green, R. (1974). *Sexual identity conflict in children and adults*. New York: Basic Books.

Green, R. (1987). *The "sissy boy syndrome" and the development of homosexuality*. New Haven, CT: Yale University Press.

Grimbos, T., Dawood, K., Burris, R., Zucker, K. J., & Puts, D. A. (2010). Sexual orientation and the second to fourth finger length ratio: A meta-analysis in men and women. *Behavioral Neuroscience, 124*, 278–287.

Halim, M. L., Ruble, D. N., Tamis-Lemonda, C. S., Zosuls, K. M., Lurye, L. E., & Greulich, F. K. (2013). The case of the pink frilly dress and the avoidance of all things "girly": Children's appearance rigidity and cognitive theories of gender development. *Developmental Psychology*, doi:10.1037/a0034906.

Hall, M., & Keith, R. A. (1964). Sex-role preferences among children of upper- and lower social class. *Journal of Social Psychology, 62*, 101–110.

Harry, J. (1985). Defeminization and social class. *Archives of Sexual Behavior, 14*, 1–12.

Herman, R. A., & Wallen, K. (2007). Cognitive performance in rhesus monkeys varies by sex and prenatal androgen exposure. *Hormones and Behavior, 51*, 496–507.

Heylens, G., De Cuypere, G., Zucker, K. J., Schelfaut, C., Elaut, E., Vanden Bossche, H., et al. (2012). Gender identity disorder in twins: A review of the literature. *Journal of Sexual Medicine, 9*, 751–757.

Hines, M. (2004). *Brain gender*. New York: Oxford University Press.

Hines, M. (2011). Prenatal endocrine influences on sexual orientation and on sexually differentiated childhood behavior. *Frontiers in Neuroendocrinology, 32*, 170–182.

Hines, M., Golombok, S., Rust, J., Johnston, K. J., Golding, J., & the Avon Longitudinal Study of Parents and Children Study Team. (2002). Testosterone during pregnancy and gender role behavior of preschool children: A longitudinal, population study. *Child Development, 73*, 1678–1687.

Iervolino, A. C., Hines, M., Golombok, S. E., Rust, J., & Plomin, R. (2005). Genetic and environmental influences on sex-typed behavior during the preschool years. *Child Development, 76*, 826–840.

Inoubli, A., De Cuypere, G., Rubens, R., Heylens, G., Elaut, E., Van Caenegem, E., et al. (2011). Karyotyping, is it worthwhile in transsexualism? *Journal of Sexual Medicine, 8*, 475–478.

Johnson, L. L., Bradley, S. J., Birkenfeld-Adams, A. S., Radzins Kuksis, M. A., Maing, D. M., & Zucker, K. J. (2004). A parent-report gender identity questionnaire for children. *Archives of Sexual Behavior, 33*, 105–116.

Klin, A., Danovitch, J. H., Merz, A. B., & Volkmar, F. R. (2007). Circumscribed interests in higher functioning individuals with autism spectrum disorders: An exploratory study. *Research & Practice for Persons with Severe Disabilities, 32*, 89–100.

Knafo, A., Iervolino, A. C., & Plomin, R. (2005). Masculine girls and feminine boys: Genetic and environmental contributions to atypical gender development in early childhood. *Journal of Personality and Social Psychology, 88*, 400–412.

Lamminmäki, A., Hines, M., Kuriri-Hänninen, T., Kilpeläinen, L., Dunkel, L., & Sankilampi, U. (2012). Testosterone measured in infancy predicts subsequent sex-typed behavior in boys and in girls. *Hormones and Behavior, 61*, 611–616.

Lawrence, A. A. (2013). *Men trapped in men's bodies: Narratives of autogynephilic transsexualism*. New York: Springer.

Lytton, H., & Romney, D. M. (1991). Parents' differential socialization of boys and girls: A meta- analysis. *Psychological Bulletin, 109*, 267–296.

Martin, C. L., Ruble, D. N., & Szkrybalo, J. (2002). Cognitive theories of early gender development. *Psychological Bulletin, 128*, 903–933.

McDermid, S. A., Zucker, K. J., Bradley, S. J., & Maing, D. M. (1998). Effects of physical appearance on masculine trait ratings of boys and girls with gender identity disorder. *Archives of Sexual Behavior, 27*, 253–267.

Meyer-Bahlburg, H. F. L. (1994). Intersexuality and the diagnosis of gender identity disorder. *Archives of Sexual Behavior, 23*, 21–40.

Meyer-Bahlburg, H. F. L. (2005). Gender identity outcome in female-raised 46, XY persons with penile agenesis, cloacal exstrophy of the bladder, or penile ablation. *Archives of Sexual Behavior, 34*, 423–438.

Meyer-Bahlburg, H. F. L. (2009). Variants of gender differentiation in somatic disorders of sex development: Recommendations for Version 7 of the World Professional Association for Transgendered Health's Standards of Care. *International Journal of Transgenderism, 11*, 226–237.

Meyer-Bahlburg, H. F. L. (2010). From mental disorder to iatrogenic hypogonadism: Dilemmas in conceptualizing gender identity variants as psychiatric conditions. *Archives of Sexual Behavior, 39*, 461–476.

Mueller, A., Gooren, L. J., Naton-Schöotz, S., Cupisti, S., Beckmann, M., & Dittrich, R. (2008). Prevalence of polycystic ovary syndrome and hyperandrogenemia in female-to-male transsexuals. *Journal of Clinical Endocrinology and Metabolism, 93*, 1408–1411.

Ngun, T. C., Ghahramani, N., Sánchez, F. J., Bocklandt, S., & Vilain, E. (2011). The genetics of sex differences in brain and behavior. *Frontiers in Neuroendocrinology, 32*, 227–246.

Owen Blakemore, J. E., Berenbaum, S. A., & Liben, L. S. (2009). *Gender development*. New York: Psychology Press/Taylor & Francis Group.

Paap, M. C., Kreukels, B. P., Cohen-Kettenis, P. T., Richter-Appelt, H., de Cuypere, G., & Haraldsen, I. R. (2011). Assessing the utility of diagnostic criteria: A multisite study on gender identity disorder. *Journal of Sexual Medicine, 8*, 180–190.

Padawar, R. (2012, August 12). Boygirl. *New York Times Magazine*, pp. 18–23, 36, 46.

Pasterski, V., Zucker, K. J., Hindmarsh, P. C., Hughes, I. A., Acerini, C., Spencer, D., et al. (2013). *Increased gender dysphoria in girls with congenital adrenal hyperplasia*. Manuscript submitted for publication.

Pine, D. S., Guyer, A. E., Goldwin, M., Towbin, K. A., & Leibenluft, E. (2008). Autism spectrum disorder scale scores in pediatric mood and anxiety disorders. *Journal of the American Academy of Child and Adolescent Psychiatry, 47*, 652–661.

Rabban, M. (1950). Sex-role identification in young children from two diverse social groups. *Genetic Psychology Monographs, 42*, 81–158.

Richter-Appelt, H., & Sandberg, D. E. (2010). Should disorders of sex development be an exclusion criterion for gender identity disorder in DSM 5? *International Journal of Transgenderism, 12*, 94–99.

Rosin, H. (2008, November). A boy's life. *The Atlantic*, 56–71.

Ruble, D. N., Martin, C. L., & Berenbaum, S. A. (2006). Gender development. In W. Damon & R. M. Lerner (Series Ed.) and N. Eisenberg (Vol. Ed.), *Handbook of child psychology* (6th ed.). *Vol. 3: Social, emotional, and personality development* (pp. 858–932). New York: Wiley.

Saeger, K. (2006). Finding our way: Guiding a young transgender child. *Journal of GLBT Family Studies, 2*(3/4), 207–245.

Sameroff, A. J., Lewis, M., & Miller, S. M. (Eds.). (2000). *Handbook of developmental psychopathology* (2nd ed.). New York: Kluwer Academic/Plenum.

Santiago, R. (2006). 5-year-old 'girl' starting school is really a boy. *The Miami Herald*. Retrieved from http://www.miami.com/mld/miamiherald/living/education/15003026.htm

Schagen, S. E., Delemarre-van de Waal, H. A., Blanchard, R., & Cohen-Kettenis, P. T. (2012). Sibling sex ratio and birth order in early-onset gender dysphoric adolescents. *Archives of Sexual Behavior, 41*, 541–549.

Schwartzapfel, B. (2013, March). Born this way? *The American Prospect*. Retrieved from http://prospect.org/article/born-way

Shinn, L. K., & O'Brien, M. (2008). Parent–child conversational styles in middle childhood: Gender and social class differences. *Sex Roles, 59*, 61–67.

Singh, D. (2012). *A follow-up study of boys with gender identity disorder*. Unpublished doctoral dissertation, University of Toronto.

Singh, D., Deogracias, J. J., Johnson, L. L., Bradley, S. J., Kibblewhite, S. J., Owen-Anderson, A., et al. (2010). The gender identity/gender dysphoria questionnaire for adolescents and adults: Further validity evidence. *Journal of Sex Research, 47*, 49–58.

Smiler, A. P., & Gelman, S. A. (2008). Determinants of gender essentialism in college students. *Sex Roles, 58*, 864–874.

Smith, Y. L. S., van Goozen, S. H. M., & Cohen-Kettenis, P. T. (2001). Adolescents with gender identity disorder who were accepted or rejected for sex reassignment surgery: A prospective follow-up study. *Journal of the American Academy of Child and Adolescent Psychiatry, 40*, 472–481.

Steensma, T. D., Kreukels, B., Jürgensen, M., Thyen, U., de Vries, A., & Cohen-Kettenis, P. T. (in press). The Utrecht Gender Dysphoria Scale: A validation study. *Archives of Sexual Behavior*.

Steensma, T. D., McGuire, J. K., Kreukels, B. P. C., Beekman, A. J., & Cohen-Kettenis, P. T. (2013). Factors associated with desistence and persistence of childhood gender dysphoria: A quantitative follow-up study. *Journal of the American Academy of Child and Adolescent Psychiatry, 52*, 582–590.

Steensma, T. D., Zucker, K. J., Kreukels, B. P. C., VanderLaan, D. P., Wood, H., Fuentes, A., & Cohen-Kettenis, P. T. (2013). Behavioral and emotional problems on the Teacher's Report Form: A cross-national, cross-clinic comparative analysis of gender dysphoric children and adolescents. *Journal of Abnormal Child Psychology*, doi:10.1007/s10802-013-9802-2.

Taywaditep, K. J. (2001). Marginalization among the marginalized: Gay men's anti-effeminacy attitudes. *Journal of Homosexuality, 42*(1), 1–28.

Tobin, D. D., Menon, M., Menon, M., Spatta, B. C., Hodges, E. V. E., & Perry, D. G. (2010). The intrapsychics of gender: A model of self-socialization. *Psychological Review, 117*, 601–622.

van Beijsterveldt, C. E. M., Hudziak, J. J., & Boomsma, D. I. (2006). Genetic and environmental influences on cross-gender behavior and relations to psychopathology: A study of Dutch twins at ages 7 and 10 years. *Archives of Sexual Behavior, 35*, 647–658.

Vanderburgh, R. (2009). Appropriate therapeutic care for families with pre-pubescent transgender/gender-dissonant children. *Child and Adolescent Social Work Journal, 26*, 135–154.

VanderLaan, D. P., Blanchard, R., Wood, H., & Zucker, K. J. (in press). Birth order and sibling sex ratio of children and adolescents referred to a Gender Identity Service. *PLOS ONE*.

Vanderlaan, D. P., Postema, L., Wood, H., Singh, D., Fantus, S., Hyun, J., ... and Zucker, K. J. (2014). Do children with gender dysphoria have intense/obsessional interests? *Journal of Sex Research*, doi: 10.1080/00224499.2013.860073

Wallien, M. S. C., & Cohen-Kettenis, P. T. (2008). Psychosexual outcome of gender dysphoric children. *Journal of the American Academy of Child and Adolescent Psychiatry, 47*, 1413–1423.

Wallien, M. S. C., Quilty, L. C., Steensma, T. D., Singh, D., Lambert, S. L., Leroux, A., et al. (2009). Cross-national replication of the gender identity interview for children. *Journal of Personality Assessment, 91*, 545–552.

Wallien, M. S. C., Swaab, H., & Cohen-Kettenis, P. T. (2007). Psychiatric comorbidity among children with gender identity disorder. *Journal of the American Academy of Child and Adolescent Psychiatry, 46*, 1307–1314.

Wallien, M. S. C., Zucker, K. J., Steensma, T. D., & Cohen-Kettenis, P. T. (2008). 2D:4D finger-length ratios in children and adults with gender identity disorder. *Hormones and Behavior, 54*, 450–454.

Wong, W. I., Pasterski, V., Hindmarsh, P. C., Geffner, M. E., & Hines, M. (2013). Are there parental socialization effects on the sex-typed behavior of individuals with congenital adrenal hyperplasia? *Archives of Sexual Behavior, 42*, 381–391.

Wood, H. (2011, October). The relationship between gender identity disorder and autism spectrum disorder. In K. J. Zucker (Chair), *Gender identity disorder in children and adolescents: Theoretical and empirical advances*. Symposium presented at the meeting of the joint meeting of the American Academy of Child and Adolescent Psychiatry and the Canadian Academy of Child and Adolescent Psychiatry, Toronto.

Wood, H., Sasaki, S., Bradley, S. J., Singh, D., Fantus, S., Owen-Anderson, A., et al. (2013). Patterns of referral to a gender identity service for children and adolescents (1976–2011): Age, sex ratio, and sexual orientation [Letter to the Editor]. *Journal of Sex & Marital Therapy, 39*, 1–6.

Zucker, K. J. (1996, March). *Pathological gender mourning in mothers of boys with gender identity disorder: Clinical evidence and some psychocultural hypotheses*. Paper presented at the meeting of the Society for Sex Therapy and Research, Miami Beach, FL.

Zucker, K. J. (2000). Gender identity disorder. In A. J. Sameroff, M. Lewis, & S. M. Miller (Eds.), *Handbook of developmental psychopathology* (2nd ed., pp. 671–686). New York: Kluwer Academic/Plenum.

Zucker, K. J. (2005). Measurement of psychosexual differentiation. *Archives of Sexual Behavior, 34*, 375–388.

Zucker, K. J. (2008). Children with gender identity disorder: Is there a best practice? [Enfants avec troubles de l'identité sexuée: y-a-t-il une pratique la meilleure?]. *Neuropsychiatrie de l'Enfance et de l'Adolescence, 56*, 358–364.

Zucker, K. J. (2010). The DSM diagnostic criteria for gender identity disorder in children. *Archives of Sexual Behavior, 39*, 477–498.

Zucker, K. J., & Bradley, S. J. (1995). *Gender identity disorder and psychosexual problems in children and adolescents*. New York: Guilford Press.

Zucker, K. J., Bradley, S. J., Kuksis, M., Pecore, K., Birkenfeld-Adams, A., Doering, R. W., et al. (1999). Gender constancy judgments in children with gender identity disorder: Evidence for a developmental lag. *Archives of Sexual Behavior, 28*, 475–502.

Zucker, K. J., Bradley, S. J., Owen-Anderson, A., Kibblewhite, S. J., Wood, H., Singh, D., et al. (2012). Demographics, behavior problems, and psychosexual characteristics of adolescents with gender identity disorder or transvestic fetishism. *Journal of Sex & Marital Therapy, 38*, 151–189.

Zucker, K. J., Bradley, S. J., Owen-Anderson, A., Singh, D., Blanchard, R., & Bain, J. (2011). Puberty-blocking hormonal therapy for adolescents with gender identity disorder: A descriptive clinical study. *Journal of Gay & Lesbian Mental Health, 15*, 58–82.

Zucker, K. J., Bradley, S. J., & Sanikhani, M. (1997a). Sex differences in referral rates of children with gender identity disorder: Some hypotheses. *Journal of Abnormal Child Psychology, 25*, 217–227.

Zucker, K. J., Green, R., Coates, S., Zuger, B., Cohen-Kettenis, P. T., Zecca, G. M., et al. (1997b). Sibling sex ratio of boys with gender identity disorder. *Journal of Child Psychology and Psychiatry, 38*, 543–551.

Zucker, K. J., Green, R., Bradley, S. J., Williams, K., Rebach, H. M., & Hood, J. E. (1998). Gender identity disorder of childhood: Diagnostic issues. In T. A. Widiger, A. J. Frances, H. A. Pincus, R. Ross, M. B. First, W. Davis, & M. Kline (Eds.), *DSM-IV sourcebook* (Vol. 4, pp. 503–512). Washington, DC: American Psychiatric Association.

Zucker, K. J., Green, R., Garofano, C., Bradley, S. J., Williams, K., Rebach, H. M., et al. (1994). Prenatal gender preference of mothers of feminine and masculine boys: Relation to sibling sex composition and birth order. *Journal of Abnormal Child Psychology, 22*, 1–13.

Zucker, K. J., Wild, J., Bradley, S. J., & Lowry, C. B. (1993). Physical attractiveness of boys with gender identity disorder. *Archives of Sexual Behavior, 22*, 23–36.

Zucker, K. J., & Wood, H. (2011). Assessment of gender variance in children. *Child and Adolescent Psychiatric Clinics of North America, 20*, 665–680.

Zucker, K. J., Wood, H., Singh, D., & Bradley, S. J. (2012). A developmental, biopsychosocial model for the treatment of children with gender identity disorder. *Journal of Homosexuality, 59*, 369–397.

Zucker, K. J., Wood, H., & VanderLaan, D. P. (2014). Models of psychopathology in children and adolescents with gender dysphoria. In B. P. C. Kreukels, T. D. Steensma, & A. L. C. de Vries (Eds.), *Gender dysphoria and disorders of sex development: Progress in care and knowledge* (pp. 171–192). New York: Springer.

Daniel N. Klein, Sara J. Bufferd, Margaret W. Dyson,
and Allison P. Danzig

In this chapter, we begin by outlining the classification of personality disorders (PDs) in the *Diagnostic and Statistical Manual of Mental Disorders*, 4th edition (*DSM-IV*; American Psychiatric Association, 2000) and 5th edition (*DSM-5*; American Psychiatric Association, 2012), and the alternative hybrid dimensional-categorical system that appears in Section III (Emerging Measures and Models) of *DSM-5*. The rest of the chapter is organized around the three main elements of the newly proposed hybrid dimensional-categorical classification. Specifically, we consider the development of (1) the proposed core impairments in personality functioning; (2) specific PD diagnoses, focusing on borderline PD (BPD) and antisocial PD (ASPD); and (3) normal and pathological personality traits. We will focus on personality pathology in youth, although there also is a growing literature on PD in older adults (Tackett, Balsis, Oltmanns, & Krueger, 2009).

D.N. Klein, Ph.D. (✉) • A.P. Danzig, M.A.
Department of Psychology, Stony Brook University,
Stony Brook, NY 11794, USA
e-mail: Daniel.Klein@stonybrook.edu

S.J. Bufferd, Ph.D.
Department of Psychology, California State
University San Marcos, San Marcos, CA 92096, USA

M.W. Dyson, Ph.D.
Child and Adolescent Services Research Center,
University of California – San Diego,
La Jolla, CA 92093, USA

Classification of Personality Disorder

DSM-IV and DSM-5

The *DSM-IV* classification of PDs was carried over unchanged into *DSM-5*, with two significant exceptions that will be discussed below: the elimination of *DSM-IV*'s multiaxial classification and the addition of an alternative hybrid dimensional-categorical classification of PDs as a model requiring further study. In both editions, there are 10 specific PD categories, which are diagnosed using polythetic criteria sets (i.e., the presence of a minimum number from a larger set of features). Of all the sections in *DSM-IV*, the PDs evoked the greatest controversy (Clark, 2007; Widiger & Trull, 2007). Criticisms included the general definition of PD, the distinction between Axis I (major syndromes) and Axis II (PDs) in the multiaxial system, the use of categorical diagnoses, the fact that the PDs were derived from clinical experience without attention to the overall structure of the PD domain, and the use of polythetic criteria.

The *DSM-IV* and *DSM-5* defines PD as enduring and pervasive, with an onset by adolescence or early adulthood. Unfortunately, this definition is quite broad and is not explicitly included in the criteria for specific PDs and is therefore typically ignored. The *DSM*s also make assumptions about the age of onset and development of PDs that have been called into question by clinical and

M. Lewis and K.D. Rudolph (eds.), *Handbook of Developmental Psychopathology*,
DOI 10.1007/978-1-4614-9608-3_36, © Springer Science+Business Media New York 2014

epidemiological research. With the exception of antisocial PD (ASPD), which cannot be diagnosed before age 18, PDs can be diagnosed in children and adolescents. However, due to concerns about distinguishing PDs from transient developmental disturbances and other mental disorders, the DSMs discourage making these diagnoses in children and adolescents. Contrary to the DSM perspective, however, there is growing evidence that PDs (1) can be identified in adolescents (Westen & Chang, 2000), (2) are at least as common in adolescents as in adults (Johnson, Bromley, Bornstein, & Sneed, 2006), and (3) are largely similar in adolescence and adulthood with respect to structure (Westen, Shedler, Durrett, Glass, & Martens, 2003) and stability over time (Chanen et al., 2004; Grilo, Becker, Edell, & McGlashan, 2001; Johnson et al., 2000).

DSM-IV distinguished PDs from other mental disorders by placing them on separate axes to encourage clinicians to pay greater attention to personality pathology. However, the conceptual basis for this distinction was problematic (Krueger, 2005; Widiger, 2003). Many Axis I disorders also have an adolescent or early adult onset, chronic course, and pervasive effects on functioning. In addition, at least several PDs have etiological influences that overlap with Axis I disorders and can be conceptualized as lying on a spectrum that cuts across the Axis I–Axis II boundary (e.g., schizotypal personality disorder and schizophrenia, avoidant personality disorder, and generalized social phobia). From a developmental psychopathology perspective, this reflects the significant heterotypic continuity that exists between PDs and Axis I disorders (Beauchaine, Klein, Crowell, Derbidge, & Gatzke-Kopp, 2009). Partly as a result of these problems, DSM-5 eliminated the multiaxial system and classifies PDs on the same axis as the major clinical syndromes.

Perhaps the strongest criticism of the *DSM-IV DSM-5* classification of PDs concerns its categorical format (Clark, 2007; Widiger & Trull, 2007). As the DSM itself suggests, most PDs are probably the extreme end of a continuum of normally distributed personality traits. Hence, selecting a boundary between normal and pathological is somewhat arbitrary. Moreover, small changes in the criteria sets and/or cutoffs can have dramatic effects on prevalence rates. In addition, it is unclear whether the specific criteria and cutoffs are appropriate across developmental periods. For example, although there is evidence for continuity between PDs in adolescents and adults, there may be some age-related differences in their manifestations (Becker, Grilo, Edell, & McGlashan, 2001; Durrett & Westen, 2005; Westen et al., 2003). Finally, dichotomizing a continuous variable reduces the amount of information in that variable, attenuating reliability. Indeed, when the DSM PDs are treated as continuous variables by summing criteria, increases are observed in interrater reliability (Zimmerman, 1994), agreement between self- and informant-reports (Riso, Klein, Anderson, Crosby Ouimette, & Lizardi, 1994), and stability over time (Durbin & Klein, 2006; Sanislow et al., 2009).

The existing PDs are based largely on clinical observations, without systematic attention to the overall structure of the PD domain (Skodol et al., 2011). In particular, many criteria (and the traits they represent) overlap across PDs (e.g., inappropriate, intense anger or difficulty controlling anger in BPD and irritability and aggressiveness in ASPD), contributing to high rates of comorbidity. Indeed, among individuals with a PD diagnosis, over 50 % meet criteria for multiple PDs (Zimmerman, Rothschild, & Chelminski, 2005), and PD comorbidity may be even greater among adolescents (Becker, Grilo, Edell, & McGlashan, 2000).

Finally, the polythetic criteria are problematic in several respects. First, they contribute to high within-category heterogeneity, as individuals with the same diagnosis may have few or no features in common. Second, the criteria sets for different PDs vary in breadth and complexity (e.g., the features of some PDs, such as paranoid and dependent, are variations on a single trait, whereas other PDs are multidimensional). Finally, many of the criteria sets are a combination of stable traits (e.g., for BPD, chronic dysphoria, intolerance of being alone) and acute symptoms (self-injurious behavior, quasi-psychotic thinking) that may contribute to the modest stability of the PDs (Clark, 2007).

Alternative DSM-5 Model for PDs Classification for DSM-5

In an effort to address these problems, the *DSM-5* Personality Disorders Work Group proposed a hybrid dimensional-categorical system (Skodol et al., 2011) that was included as an alternative model in Section III (Emerging Measures and Models). First, unlike *DSM-IV*, where the definition of PD could be ignored in formulating specific diagnoses and to recognize the commonalities that cut across specific PDs, the alternative *DSM-5* model requires at least two core elements for the diagnosis of all forms of PD: impairment in self and interpersonal functioning.

Second, the alternative *DSM-5* model proposes a "hybrid" dimensional-categorical structure (Skodol et al., 2011). Over the past decade, a number of dimensional classification systems of PDs have been proposed, many of which are variants of the Five-Factor Model (FFM) of general personality dimensions: extraversion, neuroticism, agreeableness, conscientiousness versus impulsivity, and openness to experience (Widiger & Simonsen, 2005; Widiger & Trull, 2007). These dimensions map the structure of normal personality in a systematic and an efficient manner, and apart from openness, each of these dimensions has meaningful associations with PDs (Samuel & Widiger, 2008). Importantly, the associations between these trait dimensions and measures of PDs in adolescents are similar to those observed in adults (DeClercq & DeFruyt, 2007; Tackett et al., 2009), suggesting that there is substantial homotypic continuity in the traits that comprise PDs from youth through adulthood.

Drawing on this literature, the alternative *DSM-5* model includes a set of five higher order personality trait dimensions, each of which is comprised of lower order specific traits (facets). The five higher order traits are negative affectivity (neuroticism), detachment (low extraversion or positive affectivity), antagonism (low agreeableness), disinhibition (vs. compulsivity), and psychoticism (replacing openness and capturing an important aspect of PD that is not included in most models of normal personality structure) (Krueger et al., 2011).

Finally, the alternative *DSM-5* model reduces the number of specific PD categories from 10 to 6 (borderline, obsessive–compulsive, avoidant, schizotypal, antisocial, narcissistic), and replaces the mixed symptom/trait criteria used in *DSM-IV* with traits from the five domains and their facets described above. For example, BPD is characterized by negative affectivity (specifically, the facets emotional lability, anxiousness, separation insecurity, depressivity, and hostility) and disinhibition (impulsivity and risk-taking). The traits characterizing each PD were selected by matching them to the *DSM-IV* PD criteria.

Individuals who meet the general diagnostic criteria for PD, but whose trait profiles do not match those of any of the six PD types specified in *DSM-5*, meet the criteria for PD-Trait Specified (PD-TS). This also provides a means of classifying PDs that are not specifically included in the alternative *DSM-5* model. For example, the definition and criteria of *DSM-IV* paranoid PD map closely onto the *DSM-5* trait facet of suspiciousness, and those of *DSM-IV* dependent PD map onto the facets of separation insecurity and submissiveness.

Given the likely influence of the alternative *DSM-5* hybrid dimensional-categorical model in the future, in the next three sections we will address the development of core impairments in personality functioning; the specific PDs, with a focus on BPD and ASPD, two of the most studied and impairing PD types; and the proposed *DSM-5* trait domains.

Core Impairments in Personality Functioning

The proposed initial requirement for diagnosing PD in the alternative *DSM-5* model is the presence of impairment in two core areas of personality functioning: self and interpersonal (American Psychiatric Association, 2012). Each of these areas, which are conceptually independent of specific PDs and trait dimensions, includes two subdomains. The "self" domain includes the subdomains of identity and self-direction. Identity encompasses accurate self-perception, setting appropriate boundaries with others, exhibiting a stable sense of self-esteem, and experiencing and regulating a range of emotional experiences. Self-direction includes the ability to set and pursue appropriate goals, both short and long term, and the capacity to learn from experience and apply this knowledge to subsequent behavior.

The "interpersonal" domain also includes two subdomains: empathy and intimacy. Empathy refers to the ability to understand and appreciate others' perspectives and motivations in a tolerant and respectful way, as well as the ability to understand the effects of one's behaviors, both positive and negative, on others' feelings. Intimacy encompasses the ability to form and maintain stable, close, and long-lasting positive relationships with others that is reflected in shared respect and regard.

These four subdomains were selected based on conceptual work from multiple theoretical perspectives suggesting that they reflect core aspects of personality pathology and empirical research indicating that general severity of personality pathology is the best predictor of later functional impairment (Bender, Morey, & Skodol, 2011). A dimension encompassing each of these elements discriminated patients with and without PDs with moderate sensitivity and specificity (Morey et al., 2011). However, it remains to be demonstrated that these core impairments are *more* characteristic of PDs than other mental disorders.

Instability in self-identity is a well-established feature in the adult personality pathology literature, particularly in BPD (Wilkinson-Ryan & Westen, 2000). Low self-esteem is also associated with numerous Axes I and II disorders. For example, Watson (1998) reported that self-esteem was associated with dimensional measures of almost all PDs, and particularly with avoidant, borderline, dependent, and obsessive–compulsive PDs. Emotion dysregulation is a core feature of BPD (Putnam & Silk, 2005), as well as a number of Axis I (Kring & Sloan, 2010) and other Axis II disorders (Bender et al., 2011). Finally, almost all PDs are associated with low self-directedness (Mulder, Joyce, Sullivan, Bulik, & Carter, 1999; Svrakic, Whitehead, Przybeck, & Cloninger, 1993), although dimin-

ished self-directedness is also evident in many Axis I disorders (e.g., Klein, Durbin, & Shankman, 2009).

PDs are also characterized by a variety of interpersonal deficits, including problems with empathy and intimacy (e.g., Benjamin, 2003; Blatt, 2008). For example, lack of empathy is a hallmark of antisocial and narcissistic PDs (Ritter et al., 2011). Failure of mentalization, the capacity to recognize one's own and others' intentions and feelings, is common in BPD (Gunderson, 2007). Most PDs are also characterized by problems with intimate relationships, such as exploitiveness in antisocial and narcissistic PD, disinterest in schizotypal PD, and intense, unstable relationships characterized by idealization and devaluation and fear of abandonment in BPD (Bender et al., 2011; Gunderson, 2007).

The four subdomains of functioning constructs in the alternative *DSM-5* model overlap with important developmental milestones for children and adolescents and are important components of healthy development. Problems in these areas may indicate, serve as precursors of, or predispose to PD.

The ability to self-regulate in emotionally arousing situations develops rapidly in childhood, paralleling increases in cognitive control (e.g., executive attention improves around 30 months of age; task-shifting ability improves from middle childhood to early adolescence). The development of emotion regulation continues at a slower pace through adolescence and early adulthood (Crick, Murray-Close, & Woods, 2005; Eisenberg, Spinrad, & Eggum, 2010).

Children develop a realistic self-concept during the preadolescent period (Thomaes, Bushman, Stegge, & Olthof, 2008). Children's self-esteem tends to be unrealistically high in early childhood, decreases in middle childhood, and exhibits an even steeper decline during adolescence, before rising over the course of adulthood (Robins & Trzesniewski, 2005).

Finally, there are multiple shifts in children's self-directedness over the course of development. The initial stirrings of autonomy arise in toddlerhood when young children begin asserting the desire for independence. Autonomy continues to increase over childhood and into adolescence, particularly after puberty. Child adjustment is positively associated with parents who gradually begin to grant greater autonomy around entry into middle school (Grolnick, Kurowski, Dunlap, & Hevey, 2000).

Interactive play increases dramatically during the preschool period, moving from nonsocial activity to parallel play, before shifting to associative and cooperative play. Specific peer groups begin to form in middle childhood (Rubin, Bukowski, & Parker, 2006), with friendship groups initially comprised of same-sex pairs before changing to include opposite-sex pairs around mid-adolescence. The development of peer functioning in childhood and adolescence is closely linked to the child's growing desire for autonomy from their family of origin, as time spent with the peer group substantially increases around the onset of puberty (Parker, Rubin, Erath, Wojslawowicz, & Buskirk, 2006). Romantic intimacy also increases over adolescence, with roughly half of 15–16-year-olds reporting a current romantic relationship (Feiring, 1996).

Empathy, an important component of interpersonal relationships, begins developing in toddlerhood (e.g., giving comforting hugs) and into preschool (e.g., using comforting words) and continues to develop through middle childhood as children become better at understanding emotions (Hoffman, 2000). Children who display higher levels of empathy are better liked and more likely to be popular among classmates (Cillessen & Bellmore, 2004). The theory of mind, which refers to understanding that others have beliefs, desires, and intentions that may differ from one's own, begins developing around 2 years of age, with steep increases in middle childhood (Carpendale & Chandler, 1996) and in adolescence (Kuhn & Dean, 2004). Finally, social communication, a construct that includes linguistic complexity and pragmatic advances (e.g., taking pauses, turn-taking in conversation), improves substantially in middle childhood when children begin to express themselves more articulately and understand the distinction between what people say and what they mean (Lee, Torrance, & Olson, 2001). The development of complex social communication continues in adolescence (e.g., increased use of sarcasm and irony; Winner, 1988).

There are bidirectional influences between the development of self- and interpersonal functioning. For example, adolescents who rated themselves as higher on self-esteem are more popular among their peers (Glendinning & Inglis, 1999), and having at least one close friend increases self-esteem (Bishop & Inderbitzen, 1995). The attachment literature has demonstrated that a healthy parent–child relationship serves an emotion-regulatory function for young children (Morris, Silk, Steinberg, Myers, & Robinson, 2007), and research on adolescent peer functioning indicates that same- and opposite-sex peer relationships in mid-adolescence predict less emotional volatility in later adolescence (Hay & Ashman, 2003).

Disruptions in the development of stable identity, self-direction, intimacy, and empathy may predispose to future PD. Self-esteem is relatively stable over the course of development (Robins & Trzesniewski, 2005), suggesting that it could precede the onset of personality pathology. Indeed, Orth, Robins, and Widaman (2011) reported that self-esteem predicted a number of later life outcomes (e.g., relationship satisfaction, psychological health, and physical health), rather than merely being a correlate or consequence. However, research is needed to test whether self-esteem predicts the subsequent emergence of personality pathology.

Individual differences in emotion regulation are also relatively stable (Eisenberg et al., 2010), and problems with emotion regulation predict subsequent internalizing and externalizing psychopathology (McLaughlin, Hatzenbuehler, Mennin, & Nolen-Hoeksema, 2011). Cross-sectional and prospective longitudinal studies indicate that individuals who fail to develop appropriate empathy are at risk for ASPD and psychopathy, and possibly BPD and narcissistic PD (Frick & Viding, 2009; Mullins-Nelson, Salekin, & Leistico, 2006). In addition, children who have difficulty developing and maintaining interpersonal relationships due to deficits in social competence are at risk for later Axis I (Parker & Asher, 1987) and Axis II (Kupersmidt,

Coie, & Dodge, 1990) disorders as adults. Taken together, these data suggest that it is reasonable to hypothesize that maladaptive child development across the "self" and "interpersonal" domains play an important role in the genesis of later personality pathology.

Personality Disorder Diagnoses

There has been increasing interest in understanding the complex, dynamic processes that contribute to personality pathology (Tackett et al., 2009). Although assessment is complicated by possible discontinuity between phenotypes of childhood, adolescent, and adult features, the etiology of symptoms may be continuous across development (Cicchetti & Crick, 2009). Longitudinal research on both normative and pathological processes is necessary to identify antecedents of personality disorders and refine our understanding of the course and presentations of such pathology (Shiner, 2009).

In the few studies have that examined the prevalence of PDs in youth, rates have ranged from 6 to 17 % based on direct and informant interviews and self-report measures in community and primary care samples of adolescents (Johnson et al., 2006). These studies raise the intriguing possibility that PDs may be more prevalent in early and middle adolescence than in later adolescence, when the rates tend to be similar to those found in adults (approximately 10 %). DSM-IV Cluster B diagnoses (antisocial, borderline, histrionic, narcissistic) appear to be the most common PDs in youth (Johnson et al., 2000). Similar to findings in adults, the stability of PD diagnoses range from low to moderate in adolescents (Chanen et al., 2004), but are higher for PD trait dimensions (Grilo et al., 2001). There are virtually no data on the prevalence or stability of prepubertal PD.

There are several non-mutually exclusive explanations of why rates of PDs may decline during adolescence. First, even in adults, PDs are not as stable as has typically been assumed. Thus, several studies of large samples of adults with PDs have reported surprisingly high remission rates (Sanislow et al., 2009; Zanarini, Frankenburg, Reich, & Fitzmaurice, 2012). Second, as discussed below, mean levels of personality traits change over the course of development, often in the direction of greater adjustment and maturity (Roberts, Walton, & Viechtbauer, 2006). In particular, some of the normative developmental changes in adolescence (e.g., greater emotional reactivity and risk-taking, exploration of identity, experimentation with roles) may be difficult to distinguish from PD features. Thus, if one views PDs as stable conditions, this suggests that the more transient cases of adolescent PD are "false positives" that may be better conceptualized in other ways (e.g., adjustment disorder or a V code). Finally, Tackett et al. (2009) have suggested that at least some of the differences in levels of PD traits between adolescents and adults may reflect age-related measurement biases.

In this next section, we focus on BPD and ASPD. These are the two best-researched PDs and have high prevalence rates in inpatient and corrections facilities, respectively. Both have substantial personal and societal costs and are associated with an increased risk for depression and suicide (Beauchaine et al., 2009).

Borderline Personality Disorder

BPD is characterized by dysregulation in emotional, behavioral, interpersonal, and cognitive functioning, including unstable and intense negative affect, impulsivity and suicidal behavior, volatile interpersonal relationships and efforts to avoid abandonment, and a poorly integrated sense of self. The diagnosis of BPD in youth can be challenging, as many symptoms mirror developmentally normative behaviors. In addition, diagnosing BPD in youth may seem inconsistent with the notion that personality is still evolving and that PD reflects enduring and pervasive patterns of behavior. However, the limited available data suggest that, at least by adolescence, BPD can be diagnosed reliably, is characterized by similar clinical features and comorbidity as adults, and is associated with significant functional impairment

(Becker et al., 2000; Grilo et al., 2001; Miller, Muehlenkamp, & Jacobson, 2008). The few studies examining the stability of BPD diagnoses over time in adolescents have found that it is fairly low but similar to the stability of BPD in adults (Miller et al., 2008). However, some youth continue to meet full criteria for BPD in adulthood, and many exhibit persistent subclinical features (Crawford, Cohen, & Brook, 2001; Miller et al., 2008). Thus, from a dimensional perspective, mean levels of BPD features decrease over time [Bornovalova, Hicks, Iacono, & McGue (2009); but see discussion above] yet still maintain moderate rank-order stability (Chanen et al., 2004).

Within the past decade or so, there has been increasing theoretical and empirical attention to the early manifestations of BPD (Belsky et al., 2012; Bornovalova et al., 2009; Crowell, Beauchaine, & Linehan, 2009). These studies suggest that characteristics related to BPD can be identified in childhood and early adolescence.

Early biological deficits in affect regulation and impulsivity appear to render individuals vulnerable to environmental challenges such as life stressors, traumatic events, and problematic familial and interpersonal processes that, together, increase risk for BPD. The biological factors associated with BPD and BPD-related behaviors include genetic influences (Bornovalova et al., 2009; Torgersen et al., 2000); dysfunction across several neurotransmitter systems (Gurvits, Koenigsberg, & Siever, 2000), including deficits in the central serotonin system (Goodman & New, 2000); and abnormalities in frontolimbic circuitry (Brendel, Stern, & Silbersweig, 2005). In addition, BPD is associated with the early emerging, biologically based temperament traits of negative affectivity and impulsivity (Crowell et al., 2009). However, with rare exceptions (e.g., Bornovalova et al., 2009), these studies have focused on adults; prospective studies in youth are needed to identify neurodevelopmental processes in BPD.

Research has implicated a range of psychosocial variables in the development of BPD, including an invalidating and/or abusive rearing environment, disrupted attachment, and familial psychopathology. A harsh, invalidating rearing environment has been identified as an influential predictor of BPD, particularly in the context of the biological and temperamental vulnerabilities described above (Linehan, 1993). This type of environment can include caregiver behaviors such as minimizing or denying children's emotions and punishing affective expression, which convey to the child that her emotions are unacceptable, while also neglecting to teach skills to manage feelings. Additionally, physical, sexual, and emotional abuse and neglect are implicated as common risk factors for BPD in numerous retrospective studies in adults (e.g., Zanarini, 2000), as well as in prospective studies following children into young adulthood (e.g., Widom, Czajia, & Paris, 2009). Harsh treatment has also been identified as a possible antecedent of borderline pathology in youth in prospective studies (Belsky et al., 2012; Carlson, Egeland, & Sroufe, 2009; Winsper, Zanarini, & Wolke, 2012).

Disrupted and insecure attachment to caregivers is also linked to risk for BPD (Levy, 2005), possibly due to limited opportunities to develop self-control and emotion regulation skills via this relationship (Fonagy & Bateman, 2008). Specifically, unresolved, preoccupied, and fearful attachment patterns have been associated with BPD in adults (Agrawal, Gunderson, Holmes, & Lyons-Ruth, 2004). A history of disrupted attachment was associated with BPD in a clinical sample of adolescent girls (Ludolph et al., 1990). In prospective studies, early attachment disruption or disorganization have predicted later BPD symptoms (Carlson et al., 2009; Crawford, Cohen, Chen, Anglin, & Ehrensaft, 2009). It is likely that these attachment problems are related to the pervasive interpersonal problems associated with BPD. Some have suggested that a temperamental style reflecting high stress reactivity may evoke problematic attachment, perhaps by increasing the likelihood of negative parenting and further interfering with the development of self-regulation and social interaction (Gunderson & Lyons-Ruth, 2008).

Finally, familial psychopathology also confers risk for BPD, likely through both biological and social processes. Impulse control disorders, including BPD, and, to a lesser extent, mood disorders, have been found to aggregate in relatives of individuals with BPD (White, Gunderson, Zanarini, & Hudson, 2003). In a clinical sample of children, those with BPD symptoms were more likely to have parents with substance use disorders than a comparison group with similarly poor functioning (Guzder, Paris, Zelkowitz, & Marchessault, 1996).

Antisocial Personality Disorder

ASPD is characterized by a marked indifference to social norms and the rights of others, deceitfulness, impulsivity, irritability, aggressiveness, and lack of remorse. ASPD is the only PD that requires evidence of pathology prior to adulthood. Thus, the pattern of antisocial behavior must be pervasive since at least age 15, with evidence of conduct problems earlier in life. The developmental trajectory of most adults with ASPD includes early hyperactivity, impulsivity, and oppositionality, preadolescent conduct problems, and substance use problems in adolescence and adulthood (Beauchaine et al., 2009; Dishion & Patterson, 2006). An early age of onset of conduct disorder, versus onset in adolescence, is associated with a higher risk of persistent ASPD in adulthood (Moffitt, 2003). Similar to the antecedents of BPD, both biological and environmental vulnerabilities appear to render individuals susceptible to developing ASPD. Research in this area has included antisocial behaviors, as well as related constructs such as aggression and criminality. In addition, much of this work focuses on psychopathy, a construct that overlaps with ASPD but is defined more by psychological deficits (e.g., lack of anxiety, remorse, and loyalty) than by behavioral deviance.

There are broad genetic influences on externalizing problems, including antisocial behavior, aggression, and substance misuse (Krueger et al., 2002). However, genetic and environmental influences also vary as a function of both the type of antisocial behavior and developmental stage. For example, there is a particularly strong genetic influence among antisocial children with a callous-unemotional interpersonal style, which is thought to be a precursor of psychopathy (Viding, Blair, Moffitt, & Plomin, 2005). In addition, in a multivariate twin analysis, Silberg, Rutter, Tracy, Maes, and Eaves (2007) found evidence for a single genetic factor influencing antisocial behavior from childhood through young adulthood, a genetic influence that was specific to adult antisocial behavior, and a shared environmental effect beginning in adolescence. There was also a transient, there was a transient genetic effect at puberty that may reflect pubertal timing, which could influence the expression of high-risk behaviors (e.g., reward-seeking, risk-taking) and exposure to environmental risk factors (e.g., deviant peers).

Children with behavior problems associated with risk for ASPD exhibit fearless and impulsive/bold temperament styles (Lahey & Waldman, 2003). Each of these styles may reflect a distinct developmental pathway to adult antisocial behavior (Fowles & Dindo, 2009). Both low fearfulness/high disinhibition and high sociability/sensation seeking at age 3 predicted self-reported psychopathic features at age 28 (Glenn, Raine, Venables, & Mednick, 2007). Consistent with a transactional framework, such temperament styles may respond differently to different types of parental behavior (Fowles & Dindo, 2009) and evoke negative treatment from significant adults (e.g., harsh parenting) (Larsson, Viding, Rijsdijk, & Plomin, 2008).

A number of social and contextual variables, such as ineffective parenting, conflictive parent–child relationships, a history of abuse, academic failure, limited access to resources, and exposure to violence in the community, predict the development of antisocial and related behaviors (Lynam, Loeber, & Stouthamer-Loeber, 2008; Murray & Farrington, 2010). Moreover, the presence of both biological and social risk factors greatly increases the risk for antisocial behavior (Raine, 2008). For example, Caspi et al. (2002) reported that a genetic polymorphism in the monoamine oxidase A gene, which encodes an enzyme central to the metabolism of serotonin and dopamine, was highly predictive of antisocial behavior in adolescence and adulthood but only in the context of childhood maltreatment.

The neurotransmitters modulated by this polymorphism may influence key neural circuitry that includes the medial prefrontal cortex, rostral cingulate, and amygdala, which have been implicated in antisocial behavior. This, in turn, is likely to influence reactivity to social and affective information and potentiate the effects of early environmental risks (see Buckholtz & Meyer-Lindenberg, 2008). Research in this area suggests that the effects of biological and social vulnerabilities may be synergistic, rather than additive (Beauchaine et al., 2009).

Overlapping Etiological Features of BPD and ASPD

As our discussion above suggests, ASPD and BPD have a number of risk factors in common. Indeed, twin studies indicate that the PDs have shared genetic and environmental influences (Torgersen et al., 2008). Much of the shared vulnerability is likely to reflect trait impulsivity stemming from dysregulation of serotonergic and dopaminergic functioning (Beauchaine et al., 2009). High-risk family environments, characterized by coercive and conflictual relationships, render impulsive individuals vulnerable to PD due to their limited emotion regulation skills. Sex appears to moderate these "multifinal" genetic and environmental risk processes, as females are more likely to develop BPD and males are more likely to develop ASPD (Beauchaine et al., 2009). It is not currently known, however, whether this reflects sex-specific genetic influences or socialization processes that channel shared vulnerabilities in a more externalizing or internalizing direction.

Personality Trait Dimensions

Research on the relationship between child and adolescent personality traits and PD is limited (Widiger, De Clercq, & De Fruyt, 2009). However, growing evidence regarding the heritability of PDs (e.g., Livesley & Jang, 2008), the applicability of the FFM of adult personality to youth (e.g., Lamb, Chung, Wessels, Broberg, & Hwang, 2002), and trait research supporting the stability of personality from childhood to adulthood (e.g., Caspi, 2000; Shiner, Masten, & Roberts, 2003) has encouraged developmental researchers to more systematically examine traits as developmental antecedents and early manifestations of PD.

Individual differences in emotional reactivity and regulation in youth have traditionally been characterized as temperament, whereas in adults these differences are described as personality. Temperament is often defined (and distinguished from personality) as the narrower attentional, activational, and affective core of the broader construct of personality, which is typically described as individual differences in thinking, feeling, and behaving (Shiner, 2009; Tackett, 2006). Thus, it is assumed that temperament traits are most evident and relevant in infancy/toddlerhood and early childhood, and as children mature, are exposed to a wider range of experiences, and develop new skills, competencies, and ways to regulate their emotions, temperament traits evolve into the broader, more cognitively complex, domain of personality (Shiner, 2009; Tackett, 2006).

Nonetheless, there are close relationships between the major dimensions included in the most common models of child temperament and adult personality (Caspi, Roberts, & Shiner, 2005; Tackett et al., 2009). Most models in both domains include constructs related to neuroticism/negative affectivity and extraversion/positive affectivity/surgency. In addition, the temperament dimension of effortful control encompasses most aspects of the personality dimensions of conscientiousness versus impulsivity and agreeableness.

The close link between temperament and personality is further supported by evidence of the stability of individual differences in traits over the life course. In a comprehensive meta-analysis examining the rank-order stability of traits from infancy to late adulthood, Roberts and DelVecchio (2000) combined stability coefficients for a variety of temperament and personality traits. Rank-order stability was modest prior to age 3 but increased to a moderate level by ages 3–6, where it remained fairly consistent through the college years, and then slowly increased again before plateauing in middle age. Roberts et al. (2006) subsequently used meta-analysis to examine mean-level change in personality over the lifespan. They found that the mean level of neuroticism peaked, and conscientiousness and agreeableness were lowest, in adolescence. As these are common features of PD, this is consistent with suggestions, noted above, that rates of PDs decline slightly after adolescence (Johnson et al., 2006; Shiner, 2009).

Inspired by studies investigating the utility of the FFM to describe maladaptive personality in adulthood, developmental researchers have become increasingly interested in using the FFM and related models to identify childhood and adolescent antecedents and manifestations of PD (Shiner, 2009; Widiger et al., 2009). For instance, De Clercq and De Fruyt (2003) employed a top-down approach (i.e., using adult personality measures to examine traits in younger age groups) to test the association of self-reported PDs with the FFM, assessed with the widely used NEO Personality Inventory (NEO-PI-R; Costa & McCrae, 1992), in a non-clinical sample of 419 adolescents. The pattern of correlations of the NEO factors with PDs was highly consistent with the results in adult samples (e.g., Samuel & Widiger, 2008). Thus, these findings indicate that the relation between the FFM traits and PD extend across developmental periods.

Despite these and related findings, instruments initially developed for adults may not be optimal for assessing individual differences in children and adolescents (De Clercq, De Fruyt, & Van Leeuwen, 2004). In an attempt to create an age-specific and comprehensive instrument of adaptive personality for younger age groups, Mervielde and De Fruyt (1999) employed a bottom-up approach to develop the Hierarchical Personality Inventory for Children (HiPIC). This lexically based instrument was constructed by examining the structure of a large pool of parents' free descriptions of individual differences in youth ranging from 6 to 13 years. The HiPIC factor structure consists of the traits of extraversion, emotional instability/neuroticism, benevolence, conscientiousness, and imagination and, with a few exceptions, is highly similar to the FFM (Mervielde & De Fruyt, 2002; Widiger et al., 2009). De Clercq and colleagues (2004) have also used the HiPIC to examine the relationship between personality traits and PDs in youth. Using a sample of 454 non-clinical adolescents, they found that the patterns of associations of the HiPIC and NEO with PD features were very similar to the results reported in adults, although the HiPIC accounted for somewhat greater variance in PD than the NEO.

Despite the close associations between adaptive and maladaptive personality, the two domains do not map completely onto one another (Krueger et al., 2011). For example, as noted above, the FFM dimension of openness does not have a counterpart in the PD domain, and the FFM does not include important aspects of personality pathology, such as quasi-psychotic experiences and intentional self-injury. There have been several attempts to develop instruments and models for maladaptive personality in youth. Westen and colleagues developed one of the first empirically grounded classification systems of personality pathology for adolescents (i.e., the Shedler-Westen Assessment Procedure-200 for Adolescents [SWAP-200-A]) (Westen et al., 2003). This Q-sort measure was constructed based on ratings of *DSM-IV* PD features in adolescents by 296 randomly selected clinicians. Results supported the validity and clinical utility of the measure, suggesting that personality pathology in adolescents is similar to that in adults (Westen et al., 2003). The development of the SWAP-200-A involved a top-down approach, in which adult PD features were adapted for a younger age group. Thus, similar to the application of the NEO-PI-R to youth, this may not be the optimal approach for examining the early manifestations and developmental antecedents of PDs in youth (De Clercq, De Fruyt, Van Leeuwen, & Mervielde, 2006). Rather, a bottom-up approach beginning with a comprehensive set of traits exhibited in youth may provide a better approach to investigating personality pathology in younger age groups.

Utilizing a bottom-up approach, De Clercq and colleagues (2006) developed an age-appropriate, dimensional taxonomy of trait-related PD features in youth. The Dimensional Personality Symptom Item Pool (DIPSI) is a 172-item scale that can be rated by caregivers or by youth. It includes 27 lower order facets which are subsumed by four higher order dimensions: disagreeableness (which consists of low-end variants of benevolence, such as egocentrism/dominance), emotional instability (which includes both anxious and depressed traits and dependency), compulsivity (which consists of high-end variants of conscientiousness such as perfectionism), and introversion (which includes of low-end variants of extraversion, including shyness and withdrawal). Consistent with the adult literature (Widiger & Simonsen, 2005), the DIPSI does not include a fifth dimension reflecting openness to experience.

The four DIPSI dimensions exhibited significant associations with the corresponding higher order factors of the HiPIC (De Clercq et al., 2006). In addition they showed high levels of structural and rank-order stability over a 2-year period (De Clercq, Van Leeuwen, Van den Norortgate, De Bolle, & De Fruyt, 2009).

The structure of the DIPSI is similar to recent taxonomies of adult personality pathology (e.g., Schedule for Nonadaptive and Adaptive Personality [Clark, 1990]) and Dimensional Assessment of Personality Pathology—Basic Questionnaire [Livesley, Jackson, & Schroeder, 1992]) and to Widiger and Simonsen's (2005) consensus model, which provided a foundation for the alternative *DSM-5* model trait criteria discussed earlier. This similarity in maladaptive personality structure in childhood and adulthood underscores the relevance of personality pathology in youth and its continuity across development.

Conclusions

Although *DSM-5* adopted the *DSM-IV* PD section without change, in response to the many criticisms of the *DSM-IV* approach to classifying

PD, *DSM-5* included an alternative model for PDs in section III (Emerging Measures and Models). The alternative model adds general criteria for PD and introduces a hybrid dimensional-categorical system with six specific PDs that are defined by five dimensional trait domains, each with a number of lower order facets. This model is likely to attract considerable attention in the coming years.

The general criteria for PD include impairment in identity and interpersonal functioning. As there is a substantial literature on the development of these domains in typical youth, this offers an exciting opportunity to use developmental science to elucidate the genesis of personality pathology. Precisely because these functions develop over time, however, this also raises challenging questions about distinguishing typical from atypical manifestations at different ages. Creating developmentally sensitive measures to assess impairments in these core areas should be a priority. In addition, many mental disorders other than PDs are associated with disturbances in self and interpersonal functioning; hence, it will be important to demonstrate the discriminant validity of the general definition of PD.

The alternative *DSM-5* model for PDs retained six of the 10 specific PD categories. As discussed above, there is growing evidence that PDs can be diagnosed in adolescence and have comparable validity to adult PDs. However, the challenge of distinguishing normative from pathological manifestations of personality in youth persists, and it will be important for future versions of the *DSM-5* to provide some guidance. Moreover, the question of whether PDs can be validly diagnosed in childhood remains unclear.

There are only a few prospective studies of development of PDs (e.g., Cohen, Crawford, Johnson, & Kasen, 2005; Widom et al., 2009). Longitudinal studies are essential to distinguish behaviors that are normative at some stages of development but problematic at different ages (e.g., oppositionality, fear of strangers). In addition, there may be heterotypic continuity in that some problems which appear to have resolved take different forms at later ages (e.g., conduct problems in girls becoming BPD in women).

Moreover, some of what may appear to be personality pathology may be context-dependent and resolve when contexts change (Tackett et al., 2009). Hence, identifying predictors of transient versus stable personality pathology is a critical task.

The growing evidence of continuity between child temperament and adult personality is now at the point that some are questioning the meaningfulness of the temperament-personality distinction (Shiner, 2009). Moreover, the close links that have been demonstrated between the major domains of adult personality and PD are also evident between temperament and personality pathology in youth. These data suggest that the *DSM-5* alternative trait-based taxonomy may be useful in children and adolescents. However, facet-level traits play a critical role in defining PDs in *DSM-5*. In both the adult and child literatures, there is still no consensus on the number, nature, and structural relations of constructs at the facet level. In addition, more psychometric work is needed on developmental differences in trait expression [for a good example using item-response theory, see Tackett et al. (2009)].

In future work, it will be important to distinguish between the antecedents and the early manifestations of PDs. This is a challenging conceptual distinction that hinges on the difference between extreme and maladaptive traits. Extreme traits are not necessarily maladaptive, but may become so in the future, hence may be antecedents of PD. The alternative *DSM-5* model distinguishes extreme trait levels from impairments in self and interpersonal function. This may help sharpen conceptualizations of, and research on, antecedents and early manifestations of PD.

In addition, it is critical to elucidate the processes through which extreme traits confer risk for personality pathology. For example, do traits intensify over time as a function of increasingly demanding developmental contexts and life stress? In addition, to what extent do traits influence the contexts and stressors that, in turn, exacerbate them (Klein, Bufferd, Ro, & Clark, in press)? Finally, it is important to delineate the relationships between personality traits and core impairments in self and interpersonal functioning.

It is reasonable to posit that extreme traits adversely influence self- and interpersonal functioning. On the other hand, drawing on McAdams and Pals (2006), Shiner (2009) has hypothesized that "characteristic adaptations" such as mental representations, coping styles, and personal narratives, all of which are related to the alternative *DSM-5* PD model core impairments, moderate early temperament and determine whether extreme traits develop into personality pathology.

Increased identification of antecedents and early manifestations of PD, and elucidation of the processes associated with their development should facilitate prevention and early intervention efforts targeting vulnerable children in at-risk families and communities (Belsky et al., 2012). Hopefully, such interventions will shift developmental trajectories away from more severe personality pathology and reduce the considerable personal and societal costs of PD throughout the life course (Beauchaine et al., 2009).

References

Agrawal, H. R., Gunderson, J., Holmes, B. M., & Lyons-Ruth, K. (2004). Attachment studies with borderline patients: A review. *Harvard Review of Psychiatry, 12*, 94–104.

American Psychiatric Association. (2000). *Diagnostic and statistical manual of mental disorders: Fourth edition text revision*. Washington, DC: American Psychiatric Press.

American Psychiatric Association. (2012). *DSM-5 development*. Retrieved from http://www.dsm5.org/Pages/Default.aspx.

Becker, D. F., Grilo, C. M., Edell, W. S., & McGlashan, T. H. (2000). Comorbidity of borderline personality disorder with other personality disorders in hospitalized adolescents and adults. *American Journal of Psychiatry, 157*, 2011–2016.

Becker, D. F., Grilo, C. M., Edell, W. S., & McGlashan, T. H. (2001). Applicability of personality disorder criteria in late adolescence: Internal consistency and criterion overlap 2 years after psychiatric hospitalization. *Journal of Personality Disorders, 15*, 255–262.

Beauchaine, T. P., Klein, D. N., Crowell, S. E., Derbidge, C., & Gatzke-Kopp, L. (2009). Multifinality in the development of personality disorders: A Biology × Sex × Environment interaction model of antisocial and borderline traits. *Development and Psychopathology, 21*, 735–770.

Belsky, D. W., Caspi, A., Arseneault, L., Bleidorn, W., Fonagy, P., Goodman, M., et al. (2012). Etiological features of borderline personality related characteristics in a birth cohort of 12-year-old children. *Development and Psychopathology, 24*, 251–265.

Bender, D. S., Morey, L. C., & Skodol, A. E. (2011). Toward a model for assessing level of personality functioning in DSM-5, Part I: a review of theory and methods. *Journal of Personality Assessment, 93*, 332–346.

Benjamin, L. S. (2003). *Interpersonal diagnosis and treatment of personality disorders* (2nd ed.). New York: Guilford Press.

Bishop, J. A., & Inderbitzen, H. M. (1995). Peer acceptance and friendship: An investigation of their relation to self-esteem. *The Journal of Early Adolescence, 15*(4), 476–489.

Blatt, S. J. (2008). *Polarities of Experience: Relatedness and Self-Definition in Personality Development, Psychopathology, and the Therapeutic Process.* Washington, DC: American Psychological Association.

Bornovalova, M. A., Hicks, B. M., Iacono, W. G., & McGue, M. (2009). Stability, change, and heritability of borderline personality disorder traits from adolescence to adulthood: A longitudinal twin study. *Development and Psychopathology, 21*, 1335–1353.

Brendel, G. R., Stern, E., & Silbersweig, D. (2005). Defining the neurocircuitry of borderline personality disorder: Functional neuroimaging approaches. *Development and Psychopathology, 17*, 1197–1206.

Buckholtz, J. W., & Meyer-Lindenberg, A. (2008). MAOA and the neurogenetic architecture of human aggression. *Trends in Neurosciences, 31*, 120–129.

Carlson, E. A., Egeland, B., & Sroufe, L. A. (2009). A prospective investigation of the development of borderline personality symptoms. *Development and Psychopathology, 21*, 1311–1334.

Carpendale, J. I., & Chandler, M. J. (1996). On the distinction between false belief understanding and subscribing to an interpretive theory of mind. *Child Development, 67*, 1686–1706.

Caspi, A. (2000). The child is farther of the man: Personality continuities from childhood to adulthood. *Journal of Personality and Social Psychology, 78*, 158–172.

Caspi, A., McClay, J., Moffitt, T. E., Mill, J., Martin, J., Craig, I. W., et al. (2002). Role of genotype in the cycle of violence in maltreated children. *Science, 297*, 851–854.

Caspi, A., Roberts, B. W., & Shiner, R. L. (2005). Personality development: Stability and change. *Annual Review of Psychology, 56*, 453–484.

Chanen, A. M., Jackson, H. J., McGorry, P. D., Allot, K. A., Clarkson, V., & Yuen, H. P. (2004). Two-year stability of personality disorder in older adolescent outpatients. *Journal of Personality Disorders, 18*, 526–541.

Cicchetti, D., & Crick, N. R. (2009). Precursors and diverse pathways to personality disorder in children and adolescents. *Development and Psychopathology, 21*, 683–685.

Cillessen, A. H. N., & Bellmore, A. D. (2004). Social skills and interpersonal perception in early and middle childhood. In P. K. Smith & C. H. Hart (Eds.), *Blackwell handbook of childhood social development* (pp. 355–374). Malden, MA: Blackwell.

Clark, L. A. (1990). Toward a consensual set of symptom clusters for assessment of personality disorder. In J. Butcher & C. Spielberger (Eds.), *Advances in Personality Assessment* (Vol. 8, pp. 243–266). Hillsdale, NJ: Lawrence A Erlbaum Associates.

Clark, L. A. (2007). Assessment and diagnosis of personality disorder: Perennial issues and an emerging reconceptualization. *Annual Review of Psychology, 58*, 227–257.

Cohen, P., Crawford, T. N., Johnson, J. G., & Kasen, S. (2005). The children in the community study of developmental course of personality disorder. *Journal of Personality Disorders, 19*, 466–486.

Costa, P. T., Jr., & McCrae, R. R. (1992). *Revised NEO Personality Inventory (NEO-PI-R) and NEO Five-Factor Inventory (NEO-FFI) professional manual.* Odessa, FL: Psychological Assessment Resources.

Crawford, T. N., Cohen, P., & Brook, J. S. (2001). Dramatic–erratic personality disorder symptoms: I. *Continuity from early adolescence into adulthood.* *Journal of Personality Disorders, 15*, 319–335.

Crawford, T. N., Cohen, P. R., Chen, H. N. A., Anglin, D. M., & Ehrensaft, M. (2009). Early maternal separation and the trajectory of borderline personality disorder symptoms. *Development and Psychopathology, 21*, 1013–1030.

Crick, N. R., Murray-Close, D., & Woods, K. (2005). Borderline personality features in childhood: A short-term longitudinal study. *Development and Psychopathology, 17*(4), 1051–1070.

Crowell, S. E., Beauchaine, T. P., & Linehan, M. (2009). The development of borderline personality: Extending Linehan's model. *Psychological Bulletin, 135*, 495–510.

De Clercq, B., & De Fruyt, F. (2003). Personality disorder symptoms in adolescence: A five-factor model perspective. *Journal of Personality Disorders, 17*, 269–292.

DeClercq, B., & DeFruyt, F. (2007). Childhood antecedents of personality disorder. *Current Opinion in Psychiatry, 20*, 57–61.

De Clercq, B., De Fruyt, F., & Van Leeuwen, K. (2004). A "little five" lexically based perspective on personality disorder symptoms in adolescence. *Journal of Personality Disorders, 18*, 479–499.

De Clercq, B., De Fruyt, F., Van Leeuwen, K., & Mervielde, I. (2006). The structure of maladaptive personality traits in childhood: A step toward an Integrative developmental perspective for the DSM-V. *Journal of Abnormal Psychology, 115*, 639–657.

De Clercq, B., Van Leeuwen, K., Van den Norortgate, W., De Bolle, M., & De Fruyt, F. (2009). Childhood personality pathology: Dimensional stability and change. *Developmental and Psychopathology, 21*, 853–869.

Dishion, T., & Patterson, G. (2006). The development and ecology of antisocial behavior in children and adolescents. In D. Cicchetti & D. J. Cohen (Eds.), *Developmental psychopathology: Vol. 3. Risk, disorder, and adaptation* (2nd ed., pp. 503–541). Hoboken, NJ: Wiley.

Durbin, C. E., & Klein, D. N. (2006). Ten-year stability of personality disorders among outpatients with mood disorders. *Journal of Abnormal Psychology, 115*, 75–84.

Durrett, C., & Westen, D. (2005). The structure of Axis II disorders in adolescents: A cluster- and factor-analytic investigation of DSM-IV categories and criteria. *Journal of Personality Disorders, 19*, 440–461.

Eisenberg, N., Spinrad, T. L., & Eggum, N. D. (2010). Emotion-related self-regulation and its relation to children's maladjustment. *Annual Review of Clinical Psychology, 6*, 495–525.

Feiring, C. (1996). Lovers as friends: Developing conscious views of romance in adolescence. *Journal of Research on Adolescence, 7*, 214–224.

Fonagy, P., & Bateman, A. (2008). The development of borderline personality disorder—A mentalizing model. *Journal of Personality Disorders, 22*, 4–21.

Fowles, D. C., & Dindo, L. (2009). Temperament and psychopathy: A dual-pathway model. *Current Directions in Psychological Science, 18*, 179–183.

Frick, P. J., & Viding, E. (2009). Antisocial behavior from a developmental psychopathology perspective. *Development & Psychopathology, 21*, 1111–1131.

Glendinning, A., & Inglis, D. (1999). Smoking behavior in youth: The problem of low self-esteem? *Journal of Adolescence, 22*, 673–682.

Glenn, A. L., Raine, A., Venables, P. H., & Mednick, S. A. (2007). Early temperamental and psychophysiological precursors of adult psychopathic personality. *Journal of Abnormal Psychology, 116*, 508–518.

Goodman, M., & New, A. (2000). Impulsive aggression in borderline personality disorder. *Current Psychiatry Reports, 2*, 56–61.

Grilo, C. M., Becker, D. F., Edell, W. S., & McGlashan, T. H. (2001). Stability and change of DSM-III-R personality disorder dimensions in adolescents followed up 2 years after psychiatric hospitalization. *Comprehensive Psychiatry, 42*, 364–368.

Grolnick, W. S., Kurowski, C. O., Dunlap, K. G., & Hevey, C. (2000). Parental resources and the transition to junior high. *Journal of Research on Adolescence, 10*, 466–488.

Gunderson, J. G. (2007). Disturbed relationships as a phenotype for borderline personality disorder. *American Journal of Psychiatry, 164*, 1637–1640.

Gunderson, J. G., & Lyons-Ruth, K. (2008). Borderline personality disorder's interpersonal hypersensitivity phenotype: A gene–environment–developmental model. *Journal of Personality Disorders, 22*, 22–41.

Gurvits, I. G., Koenigsberg, H. W., & Siever, L. (2000). Neurotransmitter dysfunction in patients with borderline personality disorder. *Psychiatric Clinics of North America, 23*, 27–40.

Guzder, J., Paris, J., Zelkowitz, P., & Marchessault, K. (1996). Risk factors for borderline pathology in children. *Journal of the American Academy of Child and Adolescent Psychiatry, 35*, 26–33.

Hay, I., & Ashman, A. F. (2003). The development of adolescents' emotional stability and general self-concept: The interplay of parents, peers, and gender. *International Journal of Disability, Development and Education, 50*, 77–91.

Hoffman, M. L. (2000). *Empathy and moral development*. New York: Cambridge University Press.

Johnson, J. G., Bromley, E., Bornstein, R. F., & Sneed, J. R. (2006). *Adolescent personality disorders. In D.A.Wolfe & E.J. Mash (Eds.), Behavioral and emotional disorders in children and adolescents: Nature, assessment, and treatment (pp. 463–484)*. New York: Guilford Press.

Johnson, J. G., Cohen, P., Kasen, S., Skodol, A., Hamagami, F., & Brook, J. (2000). Age-related change in personality disorder traits levels between early adolescence and adulthood: A community-based longitudinal investigation. *Acta Psychiatrica Scandinavica, 102*, 265–275.

Klein, D. N., Bufferd, S. J., Ro, E., & Clark, L. A. (in press). Depression and comorbidity: Personality disorders. In C. S. Richards & M. W. O'Hara (Eds.), *The Oxford handbook of depression and comorbidity*. New York, NY: Oxford University Press.

Klein, D. N., Durbin, C. E., & Shankman, S. A. (2009). Personality and mood disorders. In I. H. Gotlib & C. L. Hammen (Eds.), *Handbook of Depression and Its Treatment* (Vol. 2, pp. 93–112). New York: Guilford Press.

Kring, A. M., & Sloan, D. M. (2010). *Emotion regulation and psychopathology: A transdiagnostic perspective*. New York: Guilford Press.

Krueger, R. F. (2005). Continuity of Axes I and II: Toward a unified model of personality, personality disorders, and clinical disorders. *Journal of Personality Disorders, 19*, 233–261.

Krueger, R. F., Eaton, N. B., Clark, L. A., Watson, D., Markon, K. E., Derringer, J., et al. (2011). Deriving an empirical structure of personality pathology for DSM-5. *Journal of Personality Disorders, 25*, 170–191.

Krueger, R. F., Hicks, B. M., Patrick, C. J., Carlson, S. R., Iacono, W. G., & McGue, M. (2002). Etiologic connections among substance dependence, antisocial behavior, and personality: Modeling the externalizing spectrum. *Journal of Abnormal Psychology, 111*, 411–424.

Kuhn, D., & Dean, D. (2004). Connecting scientific reasoning and causal inference. *Journal of Cognition and Development, 5*, 261–288.

Kupersmidt, J. B., Coie, J. D., & Dodge, K. A. (1990). The role of poor peer relationships in the development of disorder. In S. R. Asher & J. D. Coie (Eds.), *Peer Rejection in Childhood* (pp. 274–308). New York: Cambridge University Press.

Lahey, B. B., & Waldman, I. D. (2003). A developmental propensity model of the origins of conduct problems during childhood and adolescence. In B. B. Lahey, T. E. Moffitt, & A. Caspi (Eds.), *Causes of conduct disorder and juvenile delinquency* (pp. 76–117). New York: Guilford.

Lamb, M. E., Chung, S. S., Wessels, H., Broberg, A. G., & Hwang, C. P. (2002). Emergence and construct validation of the big five factors in early childhood: A longitudinal analysis of their ontogeny in Sweden. *Child Development, 73*, 1517–152.

Larsson, H., Viding, E., Rijsdijk, F., & Plomin, R. (2008). Relationships between a parental negativity and childhood antisocial behavior over time: A bidirectional effect model in a longitudinal genetically informative design. *Journal of Abnormal Child Psychology, 36*, 633–645.

Lee, E. A., Torrance, N., & Olson, D. R. (2001). Young children and the say/mean distinction: Verbatim and paraphrase recognition in narrative and nursery rhyme contexts. *Journal of Child Language, 28*, 531–543.

Levy, K. L. (2005). The implications of attachment theory and research for understanding borderline personality disorder. *Development and Psychopathology, 17*, 959–986.

Linehan, M. (1993). *Cognitive– behavioral treatment of borderline personality disorder*. New York: Guilford Press.

Livesley, W. J., Jackson, D. N., & Schroeder, M. L. (1992). Factorial structure of traits delineating personality disorders in clinical and general population samples. *Journal of Abnormal Psychology, 101*, 432–440.

Livesley, W. J., & Jang, K. L. (2008). The behavioral genetics of personality disorder. *Annual Review of Clinical Psychology, 4*, 247–274.

Ludolph, P. S., Westen, D., Misle, B., Jackson, A., Wixom, J., & Wiss, F. C. (1990). The borderline diagnosis in adolescents: Symptoms and developmental history. *American Journal of Psychiatry, 147*, 470–476.

Lynam, D. R., Loeber, R., & Stouthamer-Loeber, M. (2008). The stability of psychopathy from adolescence into adulthood: The search for moderators. *Criminal Justice and Behavior, 35*, 228–243.

McAdams, D. P., & Pals, J. L. (2006). The new Big Five: Fundamental principles for an integrative science of personality. *American Psychologist, 61*, 204–217.

McLaughlin, K. A., Hatzenbuehler, M. L., Mennin, D. S., & Nolen-Hoeksema, S. (2011). Emotion dysregulation and adolescent psychopathology: A prospective study. *Behaviour Research and Therapy, 49*, 544–554.

Mervielde, I., & De Fruyt, F. (1999). Construction of the Hierarchical Personality Inventory for Children (HiPIC). In I. Mervielde, I. Deary, F. De Fruyt, & F. Ostendorf (Eds.), *Personality psychology in Europe* (pp. 107–127). Tilburg: Tilburg University Press.

Mervielde, I., & De Fruyt, F. (2002). Assessing children's traits with the Hierarchical Personality Inventory for Children. In B. De Raad & M. Perugini (Eds.), *Big Five Assessment* (pp. 129–146). Seattle, WA: Hogrefe and Huber.

Miller, A. L., Muehlenkamp, J. J., & Jacobson, C. M. (2008). Fact or fiction: Diagnosing borderline personality disorder in adolescents. *Clinical Psychology Review, 28*, 969–981.

Moffitt, T. E. (2003). Life-course-persistent and adolescent-limited antisocial behavior: A 10-year research review and a research agenda. In B. Lahey, T. E. Moffitt, & A. Caspi (Eds.), *Causes of conduct disorder and juvenile delinquency* (pp. 49–75). New York: Guilford Press.

Morey, L. C., Berghuis, H., Bender, D. S., Verheul, R., Krueger, R. F., & Skodol, A. E. (2011). Toward a model for assessing level of personality functioning in DSM-5, Part III: Empirical articulation of a core dimension of personality pathology. *Journal of Personality Assessment, 93*, 347–353.

Morris, A. S., Silk, J. S., Steinberg, L., Myers, S. S., & Robinson, L. R. (2007). The role of the family context in the development of emotion regulation. *Social Development, 16*, 361–388.

Mulder, R. T., Joyce, P. R., Sullivan, P. F., Bulik, C. M., & Carter, F. A. (1999). The relationship among three models of personality psychopathology: DSM-III-R personality disorder, TCI scores and DSQ defences. *Psychological Medicine, 29*, 943–951.

Mullins-Nelson, J. L., Salekin, R. T., & Leistico, A.-M. R. (2006). Psychopathy, empathy, and perspective-taking ability in a community sample: Implications for the successful psychopathy concept. *The International Journal of Forensic Mental Health, 5*, 133–149.

Murray, J., & Farrington, D. P. (2010). Risk factors for conduct disorder and delinquency: Key findings from longitudinal studies. *Canadian Journal of Psychiatry, 55*, 633–642.

Orth, U., Robins, R. W., & Widaman, K. F. (2011). Life-span development of self-esteem and its effects on important life outcomes. *Journal of Personality and Social Psychology, 101*, 607–619.

Parker, J. G., & Asher, S. R. (1987). Peer relations and later personal adjustment: Are low-accepted children at risk? *Psychological Bulletin, 102*, 357–389.

Parker, J. G., Rubin, K. H., Erath, S. A., Wojslawowicz, J. C., & Buskirk, A. A. (2006). Peer relationships, child development, and adjustment: A developmental psychopathology perspective. In D. Cicchetti & D. J. Cohen (Eds.), *Developmental psychopathology, Vol. One: Theory and method* (2nd ed., pp. 419–493). Hoboken, NJ: Wiley.

Putnam, K. M., & Silk, K. R. (2005). Emotion dysregulation and the development of borderline personality disorder. *Development and Psychopathology, 17*, 899–925.

Raine, A. (2008). From genes to brain to antisocial behavior. *Current Directions in Psychological Science, 17*, 323–328.

Riso, L. P., Klein, D. N., Anderson, R. L., Crosby Ouimette, P., & Lizardi, H. (1994). Concordance between patients and informants on the Personality Disorder Examination. *American Journal of Psychiatry, 151*, 568–573.

Ritter, K., Dziobek, I., Preissler, S., Ruter, A., Vater, A., Fydrich, T., et al. (2011). Lack of empathy in patients with narcissistic personality disorder. *Psychiatry Research, 187*, 241–247.

Roberts, B. W., & DelVecchio, W. F. (2000). The rank-order consistency of personality traits from childhood old age: A quantitative review of longitudinal studies. *Psychological Bulletin, 126*, 3–25.

Roberts, B.W., Walton, K.E., & Viechtbauer, W. (2006). Patterns of mean-level change in personality traits across the life course: A meta-analysis of longitudinal studies. *Psychological Bulletin, 132*, 1–25.

Robins, R. W., & Trzesniewski, K. H. (2005). Self-esteem development across the lifespan. *Current Directions in Psychological Science, 14*, 158–162.

Rubin, K. H., Bukowski, W. M., & Parker, J. G. (2006). Peer interactions, relationships, and groups. In N. Eisenberg (Ed.), *Handbook of child psychology: Vol. 3. Social, emotional, and personality development* (pp. 571–645). Hoboken, NJ: Wiley.

Samuel, D. B., & Widiger, T. A. (2008). A meta-analytic review of the relationships between the five-factor model and DSM-IV-TR personality disorders: A facet-level analysis. *Clinical Psychology Review, 28*, 1326–1342.

Sanislow, C. A., Little, T. D., Grilo, C. M., Daversa, M., Markowitz, J. C., Pinto, A., et al. (2009). Ten-year stability and latent structure of the DSM-IV schizotypal, borderline, avoidant, and obsessive-compulsive personality disorders. *Journal of Abnormal Psychology, 118*, 507–519.

Shiner, R. L., Masten, A. S., & Roberts, J. M. (2003). Childhood personality foreshadows adult personality and life outcomes two decades later. *Journal of Personality, 71*, 1145–1170.

Shiner, R. L. (2009). The development of personality disorders: Perspectives from normal personality development in childhood and adolescence. *Development and Psychopathology, 21*, 715–734.

Silberg, J. L., Rutter, M., Tracy, K., Maes, H. H., & Eaves, L. (2007). Etiological heterogeneity in the development of antisocial behavior: The Virginia Twin Study of Adolescent Behavioral Development and the Young Adult Follow-Up. *Psychological Medicine, 37*, 1193–1202.

Skodol, A. E., Clark, L. C., Bender, D. S., Krueger, R. F., Morey, L. C., Verheul, R., et al. (2011). Proposed changes in personality and personality disorder assessment and diagnosis for DSM-5 Part I: Description and rationale. *Personality Disorders: Theory, Research, and Treatment, 2*, 4–22.

Svrakic, D. M., Whitehead, C., Przybeck, T. R., & Cloninger, C. R. (1993). Differential diagnosis of personality disorder by the seven factor model of temperament and character. *Archives of General Psychiatry, 50*, 991–999.

Tackett, J. L. (2006). Evaluating models of the personality—psychopathology relationship in children and adolescents. *Clinical Psychology Review, 26*, 584–599.

Tackett, J. L., Balsis, S., Oltmanns, T. F., & Krueger, R. F. (2009). A unifying perspective on personality pathology across the life span: Developmental considerations for the fifth edition of the Diagnostic and Statistical Manual of Mental Disorders. *Development and Psychopathology, 21*, 687–713.

Thomaes, S., Bushman, B. J., Stegge, H., & Olthof, T. (2008). Trumping shame by blasts of noise: Narcissism, self-esteem, shame, and aggression in young adolescents. *Child Development, 79*, 1792–1801.

Torgersen, S., Lygren, S., Oien, P. A., Skre, I., Onstad, S., Edvardsen, J., et al. (2000). A twin study of personality disorders. *Comprehensive Psychiatry, 41*, 416–425.

Torgersen, S., Czajkowski, N., Jacobson, K., Reichborn-Kjennerud, T., Røysamb, E., Neale, M. C., et al. (2008). Dimensional representations of DSM-IV cluster B personality disorders in a population-based sample of Norwegian twins: A multivariate study. *Psychological Medicine, 38*, 1–9.

Viding, E., Blair, R. J. R., Moffitt, T. E., & Plomin, R. (2005). Evidence for substantial genetic risk for psychopathy in 7-year-olds. *Journal of Child Psychology and Psychiatry, 46*, 592–597.

Watson, D. C. (1998). The relationship of self-esteem, locus of control, and dimensional models to personality disorders. *Journal of Social Behavior & Personality, 13*, 399–420.

Westen, D., & Chang, C. (2000). Personality pathology in adolescence: A review. *Adolescent Psychiatry, 25*, 61–100.

Westen, D., Shedler, J., Durrett, C., Glass, S., & Martens, A. (2003). Personality diagnoses in adolescence: DSM-IV Axis II diagnoses and an empirically derived alternative. *American Journal of Psychiatry, 160*, 952–966.

White, C. N., Gunderson, J. G., Zanarini, M. C., & Hudson, J. I. (2003). Family studies of borderline personality disorder: A review. *Harvard Review of Psychiatry, 11*, 8–19.

Widiger, T. A. (2003). Personality disorder and Axis I psychopathology: The problematic boundary of Axis I and Axis II. *Journal of Personality Disorders, 17*, 90–108.

Widiger, T. A., De Clercq, B., & De Fruyt, F. (2009). Childhood antecedents of personality disorder: An alternative. *Development and Psychopathology, 21*, 771–791.

Widiger, T. A., & Simonsen, E. (2005). Alternative dimensional models of personality disorder: Finding common ground. *Journal of Personality Disorders, 19*, 110–130.

Widiger, T. A., & Trull, T. J. (2007). Plate tectonics in the classification of personality disorders: Shifting to a dimensional model. *American Psychologist, 62*, 71–83.

Widom, C. S., Czajia, S. J., & Paris, J. (2009). A prospective investigation of borderline personality disorder in abused and neglected children followed up into adulthood. *Journal of Personality Disorders, 23*, 433–446.

Wilkinson-Ryan, T., & Westen, D. (2000). Identity disturbance in borderline personality disorder: An empirical investigation. *American Journal of Psychiatry, 157*, 528–541.

Winner, E. (1988). *The point of words: Children's understanding of metaphor and irony*. Cambridge, MA: Harvard University Press.

Winsper, C., Zanarini, M., & Wolke, D. (2012). Prospective study of family adversity and maladaptive parenting in childhood and borderline personality disorder symptoms in a non-clinical population at 11 years. *Psychological Medicine, 42*(11), 2405–2420.

Zanarini, M. C. (2000). Childhood experiences associated with the development of borderline personality disorder. *Psychiatric Clinics of North America, 23*, 89–101.

Zanarini, M. C., Frankenburg, F. R., Reich, D. B., & Fitzmaurice, G. (2012). Attainment and stability of sustained symptomatic remission and recovery among patients with Borderline Personality Disorder and Axis II comparison subjects: A 16-year prospective follow-up study. *American Journal of Psychiatry, 169*, 476–483.

Zimmerman, M. (1994). Diagnosing personality disorders: A review of issues and research models. *Archives of General Psychiatry, 51*, 225–245.

Zimmerman, M., Rothschild, L., & Chelminski, I. (2005). The prevalence of DSM-IV personality disorders in psychiatric outpatients. *American Journal of Psychiatry, 162*, 1911–1918.

Part IX

Trauma Disorders

A Developmental Psychopathology Perspective on Child Maltreatment

37

Dante Cicchetti and Adrienne Banny

Introduction

Child maltreatment exemplifies a pathogenic relational environment that confers considerable risk for maladaptation across diverse psychological and biological domains of development. Deprived of many of the experiences believed to promote adaptive functioning across the life span, maltreated children traverse a probabilistic pathway characterized by an increased likelihood for compromised resolution of stage-salient developmental tasks. Because the maltreating home represents such a dramatic violation of the average expectable environment, research on child maltreatment informs developmental theory by elucidating the conditions necessary for normal development and healthy adaptation. Moreover, research on child maltreatment enhances clinical, legal, and policy decisions aimed to promote children's safety and well-being.

D. Cicchetti, Ph.D. (✉)
Institute of Child Development,
University of Minnesota, 51 E River Rd,
Minneapolis, MN 55455, USA

Mt. Hope Family Center, University of Rochester,
500 Wilson Blvd, Rochester, NY 14608, USA
e-mail: cicchett@umn.edu

A. Banny, M.A.
Institute of Child Development,
University of Minnesota, 51 E River Rd,
Minneapolis, MN 55455, USA

The goal of this chapter is to provide a selective review of research in the area of child maltreatment, updating the chapter from the prior edition of this volume (Cicchetti, Toth, & Maughan, 2000). Therefore, we will be largely focusing on developments in the field since 2000, with a particular emphasis on the growing contribution of genetic and neurobiological research. We begin by addressing definitional, epidemiological, and etiological aspects of child maltreatment. Guided by a developmental psychopathology perspective and organizational view of development, we describe the psychological and neurobiological sequelae of child maltreatment, in addition to a discussion of resilience. Finally, we address recent advances in intervention and prevention.

Definitional and Epidemiological Issues

Definitional and epidemiological issues in the area of child maltreatment are integrally related, as definitional decisions directly affect subsequent estimates of incidence and prevalence. Despite widespread consensus that child maltreatment is a serious societal problem, there exists a long history of discordance among researchers, lawmakers, and clinicians with regard to what exactly constitutes child maltreatment. Disagreement partially stems from the fact that these professional domains are motivated by different goals in their operationalization of child

M. Lewis and K.D. Rudolph (eds.), *Handbook of Developmental Psychopathology*,
DOI 10.1007/978-1-4614-9608-3_37, © Springer Science+Business Media New York 2014

maltreatment. For example, a medical-diagnostic definition focuses on the individual abuser and overt signs of maltreatment. Although this definition effectively informs medical practice, it tends to overlook more subtle, psychological effects. A legal definition, on the other hand, emphasizes demonstratable physical and emotional harm, with the purpose of garnering information that would be useful as evidence for prosecution. Also contributing to the controversy surrounding the definition of child maltreatment are cultural and historical variations in what is deemed to be acceptable versus maltreating parenting (Barnett, Manly, & Cicchetti, 1993).

Due to methodological advances in the operationalization of child maltreatment, four general categories of child maltreatment have emerged and appear to be widely accepted: (1) *physical abuse*, which involves the nonaccidental infliction of physical injury on the child; (2) *sexual abuse*, which includes attempted or actual sexual contact between the child and a family member or person caring for the child for purposes of that person's sexual satisfaction or financial benefit; (3) *neglect*, which pertains to failure to provide for the child's basic physical needs for adequate food, clothing, shelter, and medical treatment; and (4) *emotional maltreatment*, which involves extreme thwarting of children's basic emotional needs for psychological safety and security, acceptance and self-esteem, and age-appropriate autonomy.

In order to address more detailed definitional considerations, Barnett, Manly, and Cicchetti developed the Maltreatment Classification System (MCS; Barnett et al., 1993), a multidimensional nosology for categorizing and quantifying maltreatment experiences. The MCS codes official substantiated records of child abuse and assesses many salient features of maltreatment including the subtype, severity, onset, frequency, chronicity, and identity of the perpetrators. The MCS also specifies the developmental period during which each subtype occurred. By providing a comprehensive account of maltreatment history, the MCS allows researchers to ascertain how various aspects of child maltreatment influence development. Moreover, the utilization of

an objective classification system like the MCS facilitates the comparison of research findings from different laboratories.

Keeping in mind the complexities associated with defining maltreatment, it is possible to evaluate incidence and prevalence, while also remaining cognizant of the limitations inherent in such estimates. According to recently published US government statistics (U.S. Department of Health and Human Services, 2010), an estimated 3.3 million referrals concerning approximately 5.9 million children were received by Child Protective Services (CPS) agencies in 2010. Of these, 60.7 %, or nearly two million referrals, were screened in for a CPS response. The majority of screened in reports (i.e., 90.3 %) received an investigation response, resulting in 436,321 substantiated cases of child maltreatment. The rate of victimization per 1,000 children in the national population is 9.2, with children in the age group comprising birth to 1 year having the highest rates of victimization—20.6 per 1,000 children. Furthermore, 1,560 children died from abuse and neglect, and nearly 80 % of all child fatalities were younger than 4 years old.

Even in the case of unsubstantiated reports, significant psychosocial maladjustment occurs (Kohl, Jonson-Reid, & Drake, 2009). Moreover, "unsubstantiated" does not necessarily mean that maltreatment did not occur. In fact, research suggests that substantiated and unsubstantiated cases may not vary significantly in terms of existing risk factors or future risk (Kohl et al., 2009).

In addition to including children who were investigated by CPS agencies, the National Incidence Studies (NIS) obtains data on other maltreated children who were not reported to CPS or who were screened out by CPS. These additional children were identified by community professionals (e.g., physicians, social workers, teachers, day care providers). The NIS reports use two definitions of child maltreatment: the Harm Standard, which requires demonstratable harm (e.g., bruises, abrasions, cuts, burns, fractures), and the less stringent Endangerment Standard, which includes maltreated children who are at risk for demonstratable harm. Perhaps most notably, NIS has consistently found that

CPS agencies investigate only a minority of children identified by NIS. The most recently published NIS-4 (Sedlak et al., 2010) verified this result, finding that CPS investigated the maltreatment of only 32 % of children who experienced the Harm Standard and 43 % of those under the Endangerment Standard. Moreover, NIS-4 found that if all maltreated children identified by NIS were reported to CPS, more than 80 % would have received CPS investigation if current CPS screening policies were followed. Such evidence of low CPS investigation rates highlights the likelihood that official statistics underestimate the actual prevalence of child maltreatment.

The impact of child maltreatment is profound, affecting individual victims and their families, as well as society more broadly. A 2007 study conducted by Prevent Child Abuse America estimated that the total cost (i.e., direct and indirect costs) of child abuse and neglect in the United States is $103.8 billion per year (Wang & Holton, 2007). Annual direct costs, estimated at $33,101,302,133, reflect costs associated with meeting the immediate needs of the child, such as hospitalization, mental health care, child welfare services, and law enforcement. Yearly indirect costs, estimated at $70,652,715,359, include special education, juvenile delinquency, mental and physical health care, criminality, and lost productivity to society. Furthermore, a recent study by the Centers for Disease Control and Prevention (CDC) estimated the total lifetime economic burden resulting from child maltreatment in the United States to be as large as $585 billion (Fang, Brown, Florence, & Mercy, 2012).

Etiology

With respect to etiology, years of research have eventuated in the conclusion that no single risk factor can account for the occurrence of child maltreatment. Although factors such as poverty, parental psychopathology, and a history of maltreatment in one's own childhood have emerged as robust predictors, none act as a necessary or sufficient cause of child maltreatment. Thus, a number of etiological models have evolved that

focus on multiple transacting levels of the ecology (Belsky, 1980; Cicchetti & Lynch, 1993; Cicchetti & Rizley, 1981).

The ecological-transactional model developed by Cicchetti and Lynch (1993) explains how cultural, community, and family factors, in concert with characteristics of the individual, mutually interact to determine the likelihood of child maltreatment, as well as the course of subsequent development. According to this model, risk and protective factors can exist at every level of the ecology (i.e., micro-, meso-, macro-, and exosystem). Potentiating factors increase the probability of maltreatment (e.g., community violence, low SES, job loss, mental illness), whereas compensatory factors reduce the likelihood that child maltreatment will occur (e.g., parent's own history of good parenting, marital harmony, improvement in financial conditions). Potentiating and compensatory factors at any given level of the ecology can affect processes and outcomes in surrounding levels of the environment. For example, in addition to increasing the ultimate risk of child maltreatment, potentiating factors at more distal levels (e.g., community, culture) affect processes and outcomes that occur in more proximal levels of the ecology (e.g., family). Overall, the balance of potentiating and compensatory factors that are present in the various ecological levels determines the absence or presence of child maltreatment.

An Organizational Perspective on Development

We approach the current review of the consequences of child maltreatment within an organizational framework that examines the resolution of stage-salient developmental tasks. According to this perspective, development may be conceptualized as a series of reorganizations, whereby previously developed structures become incorporated into subsequently emerging ones via a process of hierarchical integration (Sroufe & Rutter, 1984). In this way, competence at one stage prepares a child for adaptive functioning at the next stage. Conversely, maladaptation may be carried forward, disrupting the development of later competencies. Consistent with this perspective, maltreatment is viewed as placing children on a probabilistic pathway marked by compromised resolution of stage-salient developmental tasks. As negative transactions between the child and the environment continue, risk for repeated developmental failures and the emergence of psychopathology increases. Although a comprehensive review of the sequelae of child maltreatment is beyond the scope of the present chapter, we cover developmental issues that forebode later maladaptation in the absence of proper intervention.

Despite the broad profile of risk associated with the experience of child maltreatment, not all abused and neglected children are destined to follow a trajectory of developmental deviation and disruption. Therefore, we invoke the concepts of equifinality and multifinality in order to stress diversity in process and outcome (Cicchetti & Rogosch, 1996). Equifinality refers to the observation that numerous pathways to the same outcome are possible. Consequently, a variety of processes may culminate in the same disorder. The principal of multifinality asserts that a particular risk or protective factor may result in a variety of outcomes. Therefore, numerous outcomes are possible for maltreated children, including healthy adaptation.

Affect Differentiation and Modulation of Attention and Arousal

An early stage-salient developmental task in infancy involves the ability to regulate and differentiate emotions. Defined as the monitoring, evaluating, and modifying of emotional reactions for the purpose of achieving individual goals, emotion regulation optimizes one's adaptive engagement with the environment (Thompson, Lewis, & Calkins, 2008). Because the ability to autonomously regulate one's emotions is believed to emerge from early parent–child interactions, maltreatment poses a serious risk to children's affective development. In fact,

maltreated children demonstrate numerous disturbances in the expression, recognition, and regulation of emotions.

Maltreated children are exposed to an atypical emotional environment, characterized by less positive emotion (Bugental, Blue, & Lewis, 1990) and more negative emotion (Herrenkohl, Herrenkohl, Egolf, & Wu, 1991) in comparison to that expressed in nonmaltreating homes. Among maltreating families, physically abusive parents are more negative than neglecting parents and engage in higher rates of aggression directed toward their children. Neglected children experience an impoverished emotional environment, marked by infrequent affective exchanges with their caregivers (Crittenden, 1981). Ultimately, it is believed that these aberrant emotional experiences eventuate in neuropathological connections that undermine effective emotion regulation capabilities.

Deviations in the development of emotional expression among maltreated children have been noted as early as 3 months of age. Maltreated children exhibit distortions in affect differentiation, manifested as either excessive negative affect or blunted patterns of affect (Gaensbauer & Hiatt, 1984). Moreover, negative emotions, such as fear, anger, and sadness, have been observed in physically abused infants long before they occur in normal development (Gaensbauer, 1980).

Child maltreatment also affects the development of emotion recognition abilities. Neglected children have difficulties discriminating emotional expressions in general, whereas physically abused children demonstrate a response bias for angry facial expressions (Pollak, Cicchetti, Hornung, & Reed, 2000). Research shows that physically abused children display differential processing of emotion that appears to be specific to anger. In a study that required participants to distinguish faces along a continuum varying in signal intensity, physically abused children demonstrated a broader category boundary for angry faces compared to nonabused children (Pollak & Kistler, 2002). Similarly, Pollak and Sinha (2002) utilized a sequence of affective stimuli that presented the image structure in increasing increments. Physically abused children accurately identified anger based on less perceptual information than nonmaltreated children (Pollak & Sinha, 2002). In order to approximate more naturalistic emotional input, Pollak, Messner, and Kistler (2009) presented children with a series of images that showed the unfolding of various emotional expressions. Relative to non-maltreated comparisons, physically abused children accurately recognized anger earlier in the formation of the facial expression, when less cues were available (Pollak, Messner, Kistler, & Cohn, 2009). Moreover, research indicates that once oriented to cues of anger, maltreated children may have difficulty disengaging their attention (Pollak & Tolley-Schell, 2003).

Psychophysiological studies also provide evidence that maltreated children allocate more attentional resources to the detection of anger (Pollak, Klorman, Thatcher, & Cicchetti, 2001). In particular, measurement of cognitive event-related brain potentials (ERP) indicates that school-age maltreated children display larger P3b amplitude when their attention is directed toward angry, as opposed to happy, targets (Pollak et al., 2001; Pollak & Tolley-Schell, 2003; Shackman, Shackman, & Pollak, 2007). Moreover, this pattern of response appears to be specific to anger, rather than to negative emotions in general (Pollak et al., 2001). Similar findings indicate that maltreated children exhibit brain-based abnormalities in the processing of facial affect as early as 30–42 months of age (Cicchetti & Curtis, 2005; Curtis & Cicchetti, 2011). Together, these results suggest more efficient cognitive organization and processing of anger among abused children.

Behavioral and psychophysiological evidence of maltreated children's differential processing of affective information suggests that early experience influences subsequent emotional development and shapes implicated brain circuitry. The effects observed among maltreated children may reflect experience-dependent processes that involve the fine-tuning of attention, learning, perceptual, and memory systems that facilitate the rapid identification of anger (Pollak, 2009). Enhanced sensitivity to anger may provide a behavioral advantage in maltreating homes where anger may be a particularly salient cue of imminent harm. However, the failure of regulatory capacities that enable flexibility and control makes what is adaptive in the maltreating home maladaptive when generalized to more normative social contexts (Pollak, 2009).

Development of Attachment Relationships

The formation of attachment relationships represents a primary developmental task during the first year of life. Securely attached infants derive a sense of security from their primary caregiver and can use their attachment figure as a secure base from which to explore the environment (Bowlby, 1969). Within the context of the parent–child relationship, children develop attitudes and expectations regarding the self and others, which are subsequently applied to later social interactions (Sroufe & Fleeson, 1986). Exposed to insensitive and pathological care, maltreated children may develop negative expectations regarding the availability and trustworthiness of others, as well as mental representations of the self as incompetent and unworthy.

Maltreated children are especially at risk for developing disorganized attachments (i.e., Type D) with their primary caregiver (see Cyr, Euser, Bakermans-Kranenburg, & Van Ijzendoorn, 2010, for meta-analysis). Estimates of the manifestation of disorganized attachment among maltreated children range from 80 to over 90 % (Cyr et al., 2010). In the Strange Situation paradigm, Type D infants demonstrate inconsistent and disorganized strategies for coping with separation from and reunion with the caregiver (Hesse & Main, 2006). In addition, these infants display bizarre behaviors such as freezing, stilling, and stereotypies, as well as contradictory behavior directed toward the attachment figure (e.g., approach parent with head averted; Hesse & Main, 2006).

Several explanations have been proposed to account for the preponderance of disorganized attachment relationships between maltreated children and their primary caregivers. Because inconsistent care is a hallmark of maltreating families, some have hypothesized that a combination of insensitive overstimulation and insensitive understimulation may lead to the contradictory behaviors observed among maltreated infants classified as Type D (Crittenden, 1985). According to Hesse and Main (2006), attachment disorganization is caused by frightened and frightening (FR) parental behavior, which is believed to have its origins in unresolved parental trauma. Maltreating behaviors are arguably among the most frightening parenting behaviors, placing children in an irresolvable paradox in which their attachment figure is simultaneously their source of safety and their source of fear (Hesse & Main, 2006).

Genetic variation has also been explored as a contributor to the development of disorganized attachment; however, little consistent evidence has emerged for a candidate gene main effect on attachment disorganization (see Luijk et al., 2011). Among maltreated children, Cicchetti, Rogosch, and Toth (2011) found that neither the serotonin transporter gene (5-HTT) nor the dopamine receptor D4 gene (DRD4) were associated with disorganized attachment. They concluded that the anomalous aspects of maltreating parenting may be so robust that they overpower the potential effect of genetic variation in the etiological pathway to attachment disorganization (Cicchetti, Rogosch, & Toth, 2011).

Although attachment is conceptualized as an important stage-salient developmental task during the first year of life, attachment security continues to exert its influence on development across the life span. First, substantial stability in insecure and disorganized patterns of attachment has been observed among maltreated children (Barnett, Ganiban, & Cicchetti, 1999). Additionally, disorganized attachment initiates a maladaptive trajectory that heightens risk for future relational dysfunction, as well as various forms of psychopathology (Hesse & Main, 2006).

Development of the Self-System

The development of an integrated sense of self typically occurs in the toddler and preschool years, arising from the successful resolution of previous stage-salient tasks, such as the formation of a secure attachment relationship (Cicchetti, 1991). Early caregiving experiences serve as the basis for the development of representational models of the attachment figure, as well as corresponding and coherent representational models of the self and of the self in relation to others (Sroufe & Fleeson, 1986). As discussed above, many maltreated infants fail to develop an organized pattern of attachment, increasing the probability of subsequent perturbations in representational development (Cicchetti, 1991). Indeed, maltreated children show disruptions in many aspects of the self-system.

Aberrations in self-development have been observed as early as 18 months of age, as demonstrated by investigations of visual self-recognition. On the mirror-rouge paradigm, an assessment of the presence of a cognitive self, maltreated and nonmaltreated children are comparable in their capacity to recognize themselves; however, differences emerge with respect to their affective responses (Schneider-Rosen & Cicchetti, 1991). Specifically, maltreated toddlers are more likely than nonmaltreated comparison children to display neutral or negative emotions upon seeing their images in a mirror, which may be interpreted as reflecting negative feelings about the self.

At 30 months of age, maltreated children demonstrate disruptions in their development of an internal-state lexicon. Even after controlling for receptive vocabulary, maltreated toddlers produce proportionately fewer internal-state words, show less differentiation in their attributional focus, and are more context-bound in their use of internal-state language than nonmaltreated comparisons (Beeghly & Cicchetti, 1994).

Negative self-system processes continue to be evident in the preschool period. Maltreated children's narrative representations of parents and of self are more negative than those of nonmaltreated children (Toth, Cicchetti, Macfie, Maughan, & Vanmeenen, 2000). With respect to subtype, neglected children have been found to tell narratives containing more negative self-representations compared to nonmaltreated children, whereas physically abused children possess more grandiose self-representations.

These variations by subtype may reflect differences in maltreating experiences. For example, grandiose self-representations may reflect a coping process to maintain personal control in an adverse and threatening home environment, while negative self-representations may develop from the chronic absence of attention and validation in a neglecting home (Toth, Cicchetti, Macfie, Rogosch, & Maughan, 2000).

Research among school-age maltreated children provides further evidence of self-system deviation. Relative to teacher ratings, younger maltreated children overestimate their own sense of social competence and peer acceptance (Vondra, Barnett, & Cicchetti, 1989). These children may be engaging in defensive processing in order to increase their sense of competence. In fact, research indicates that the development of a grandiose self, as reflected by inflated social self-efficacy, may serve as a protective factor in the link between maltreatment and internalizing symptomatology (Kim & Cicchetti, 2003). However, as maltreated children mature, they tend to underestimate their competence and are rated by teachers as having lower self-esteem (Vondra et al., 1989).

Finally, maltreated children are at risk for developing dissociative features and disorder, perhaps the most severe deficit in the integration of the self (Macfie, Cicchetti, & Toth, 2001a, 2001b; Valentino, Cicchetti, Rogosch, & Toth, 2008b). The link between maltreatment and dissociation has been observed across a wide age range, from preschoolers to adults. Among preschoolers, physical and sexual abuse appear to be most robustly related to dissociative features, with physical abuse emerging as particularly salient for the development of dissociation at clinical levels. Furthermore, longitudinal research indicates that, among maltreated preschoolers, the self becomes more fragmented over time.

Peer Relations

Consistent with an organizational perspective on development, it has been theorized that the negative relational patterns acquired in a maltreating environment become incorporated into the structures that are pertinent for successful peer relations. Within the context of their early caregiving experiences, maltreated children may develop negative expectations regarding the self and others, as well as a concept of relationships as involving victimization and coercion. These internalizations lead to the selection and structuring of later social interactions, such that familiar relationship patterns are recreated and validated (Sroufe & Fleeson, 1986). Research supports this conceptualization of continuity in relational functioning, as maltreated children have been shown to exhibit a broad range of difficulties in the peer domain.

With regard to peer relations, maltreated children appear to traverse one of two general developmental pathways: (1) withdrawal from peer interactions or (2) heightened aggression toward peers. The link between maltreatment and aggressive behavior is particularly robust (e.g., Cullerton-Sen et al., 2008; Shields & Cicchetti, 2001; Teisl & Cicchetti, 2008). Moreover, aggression appears to largely account for the association between maltreatment and peer rejection (Bolger & Patterson, 2001). Emphasizing a gender-informed approach to the study of maltreatment and aggression, Cullerton-Sen and colleagues (2008) showed that maltreatment was associated with physical aggression for boys and relational aggression for girls. Sexual abuse emerged as a particularly salient predictor of relational aggression among girls. Findings suggest that boys and girls may internalize the experience of maltreatment in different ways, initiating gender-specific pathways to the expression of externalizing behaviors. For example, maltreated girls may learn from their early parent–child interactions that love and affection can be withdrawn as punishment. When confronted with conflict in the peer group, maltreated girls may draw upon what they have learned in the home, such that they use the relationship as a vehicle of harm against their peers (i.e., relational aggression; Cullerton-Sen et al., 2008).

Maltreatment also places children at risk for being victimized by their peers. Schwartz, Dodge, Pettit, and Bates (1997) demonstrated that abusive family treatment predicted boys' status as aggressive victims. In an investigation of bullying and peer victimization that included both boys and girls, Shields and Cicchetti (2001) found that maltreated children were more likely than nonmaltreated children to bully other children and more likely to be victimized by their peers. Gender did not act as a moderator, suggesting that maltreated boys and girls are at comparable risk for bullying and victimization (Shields & Cicchetti, 2001).

The effects of maltreatment on disrupted peer group functioning may be explained by perturbations in cognitive and emotional processes. With regard to social information processing, physically abused children make errors in encoding social cues, exhibit biases toward attributing hostile intent, generate more aggressive responses, and positively evaluate aggression as an appropriate response (Teisl & Cicchetti, 2008). These deficits, in turn, mediate the association between physical abuse and aggression in the peer context (Teisl & Cicchetti, 2008). Whereas maladaptive social cognition emerges as a salient explanatory factor for physically abused children, emotion dysregulation appears to play an integral role in the link between maltreatment and aggression for all maltreated groups (Shields & Cicchetti, 2001; Teisl & Cicchetti, 2008). Poor emotion regulation also mediates the association between maltreatment and victimization by peers (Shields & Cicchetti, 2001).

In addition to their difficulties in the larger peer group, maltreated children demonstrate weaknesses in developing and maintaining friendships (Howe & Parke, 2001; Parker & Herrera, 1996). Maltreated children report less caring and validation and more conflict and betrayal in their friendships compared to nonmaltreated children (Howe & Parke, 2001). In an observational setting, Parker and Herrera (1996) found that friendship dyads containing a physically abused adolescent displayed more conflict and less intimacy than dyads without an abused adolescent. Alternatively, having friends may serve as an important buffer for maltreated children against feelings of loneliness, low self-esteem, and victimization by the larger peer group (Bolger, Patterson, & Kupersmidt, 1998; Schwartz, Dodge, Pettit, & Bates, 2000).

Memory

Research investigating the effects of maltreatment on memory is only recently emerging. There are a number of reasons why maltreatment might be expected to alter basic memory processes (Howe, Cicchetti, & Toth, 2006). For example, the experience of stress associated with living in a maltreating home may potentiate neurological changes in the structures implicated in encoding and storing information. Observed delays in intellectual functioning, executive functioning, and language may also be implicated in potential memory deficits. Furthermore, maltreated children are at risk for the development of posttraumatic stress disorder (PTSD) and dissociation, both of which have been linked to memory distortion among adults.

For the most part, hypothesized adverse effects of maltreatment on memory have not been empirically supported. Although the field is still in its infancy, many studies show no differences between maltreated and nonmaltreated children in terms of basic memory processes. Maltreated children are comparable to their nonmaltreated peers with respect to basic recall and recognition, as well as in their degree of suggestibility to misinformation (Cicchetti, Rogosch, Howe, & Toth, 2010; Eisen, Goodman, Qin, Davis, & Crayton, 2007; Howe, Cicchetti, Toth, & Cerrito, 2004; Porter, Lawson, & Bigler, 2005). Moreover, Beers and DeBellis (2002) did not find any differences in basic memory processes between maltreated children with PTSD and normative comparison youth. Similarity in memory functioning is evident in studies involving both neutral and emotionally laden stimuli (Howe et al., 2004; Howe, Toth, & Cicchetti, 2011). In addition, differences in memory processes fail to emerge with respect to ecologically valid and stressful information (Eisen et al., 2007). For example, Eisen and colleagues (2007), tested memory for an anogenital exam that occurred in the context of an inpatient abuse assessment. Memory accuracy and suggestibility did not vary by abuse status.

Although no between-group differences have been discovered, within-group investigations suggest variation in basic memory processes as a function of maltreatment subtype. For example, in a depth-of-processing incidental recall task of self-referent information, neglected children demonstrated a greater proportion of negative false recall and less positive false recall than did the abused children, suggesting greater memory inaccuracy among neglected children (Valentino, Cicchetti, Rogosch, & Toth, 2008b). In another study by Valentino, Cicchetti, Rogosch, and Toth (2008a), subtype differences emerged for memory of maternal-referent information, such that abused children exhibited lower recall compared to neglected children. Findings are suggestive of defensive processing of information that activates the attachment system as a protective mechanism among abused children. Finally, Cicchetti, Rogosch, Howe, and Toth (2010) showed that children with a history of neglect and/or emotional maltreatment and low cortisol evinced increased levels of memory inaccuracy.

In addition to subtype differences in basic memory processes, Valentino, Toth, and Cicchetti (2009) revealed subtype-specific variation in autobiographical memory for nontraumatic events. Abused children's memories were more overgeneral compared to the memories of neglected and nonmaltreated children. Retrieving memory in generic form may reflect a strategy for avoiding negative affect associated with painful memories. Consistent with a dynamic skills framework, defensive, traumatogenic responses become more habitual and generalized over time, resulting in less integration of memories (Ayoub et al., 2006).

Overall, given the extensive policy implications for legal contexts involving child testimony, further translational research on the effects of maltreatment on memory is warranted.

Maltreatment and Psychopathology

As we have illustrated, the experience of child maltreatment places children on a probabilistic pathway characterized by compromised resolution of stage-salient developmental tasks. Failure to meet the demands of a particular stage undermines the development of subsequently emerging capacities. These cascading effects, in turn, heighten the risk for maladaptation and the emergence of psychopathology. Indeed, consistent with the concept of multifinality (Cicchetti & Rogosch, 1996), maltreated children develop a broad range of psychopathological outcomes (Keyes et al., 2012; Scott, Smith, & Ellis, 2010).

In general, the literature indicates that exposure to child maltreatment increases the risk for greater lifetime prevalence of many psychiatric symptoms and diagnoses. These include mood and anxiety disorders (Kim & Cicchetti, 2006; Widom, DuMont, & Czaja, 2007), dissociation and suicidal behavior (Yates, Carlson, & Egeland, 2008), substance use disorders (Rogosch, Oshri, & Cicchetti, 2010; Widom, Marmorstein, & White, 2006), disruptive and antisocial behaviors (Egeland, Yates, Appleyard, & van Dulmen, 2002; Widom & Maxfield, 2001), and psychosis (Arseneault et al., 2011). Longitudinal research by Kaplow and Widom (2007) suggests that the age of onset of maltreatment may be an important factor in differentiating the effects of maltreatment on later mental health outcomes. In particular, individuals who were maltreated earlier in life (i.e., before the age of six and/or during the infancy or preschool years) evinced higher levels of internalizing problems as adults, whereas those who were older at the time of maltreatment went on to develop more externalizing outcomes in adulthood. The preschool years emerged as a potential sensitive period during which maltreatment may have an especially robust effect, potentiating the development of both internalizing and externalizing disorders (i.e., anxiety, depression, antisocial personality disorder).

Maltreatment has also been implicated in the etiology of personality disorders. Given that personality disorders do not emerge spontaneously at the age of 18, some researchers have adopted a developmental psychopathology approach by seeking to identify early precursors and processes that confer vulnerability to later personality pathology. Consistent with this approach, Rogosch and Cicchetti (2005) found that maltreated children exhibit higher mean levels of potential precursors to borderline personality disorder (e.g., emotional lability, conflictual relationships with adults and peers, relational aggression, self-harm) than do nonmaltreated comparisons. An examination of early risk factors for paranoid personality identified a history of child maltreatment as a predictor, alongside significant behavioral disturbances and negative peer relationships (Natsuaki, Cicchetti, & Rogosch, 2009). In a prospective investigation of personality organization, Rogosch and Cicchetti (2004) found that 6-year-old maltreated children exhibited lower agreeableness, conscientiousness, and openness to experiences, as well as higher neuroticism, than did nonmaltreated children. Analysis of personality clusters revealed that the majority of nonmaltreated children were represented in the adaptive Gregarious and Reserved personality clusters, whereas maltreated children largely accounted for the makeup of less adaptive personality profiles (i.e., Undercontroller, Overcontroller, and Dysphoric). Furthermore, longitudinal stabilities were observed across ages seven, eight, and nine, suggesting continuity in maltreated children's personality liabilities.

Recent research in molecular genetics suggests that maltreated children's risk for psychopathology is not inevitable. In a landmark epidemiological study, Caspi and colleagues (2002) followed a large sample of male children from birth to adulthood to ascertain why some maltreated children grow up to develop antisocial personality disorder, whereas others do not. Results revealed that a functional polymorphism in the promoter of the monoamine oxidase A (MAOA) gene moderated the effect of child maltreatment. The MAOA gene is located on the X chromosome and encodes the MAOA enzyme, which metabolizes neurotransmitters such as norepinephrine, serotonin, and dopamine, rendering them inactive. Maltreated children with the genotype conferring high MAOA activity were significantly less likely to develop antisocial behavior problems compared to maltreated children with the low MAOA activity genotype. In addition, maltreatment groups did not differ on MAOA activity, suggesting a lack of an evocative gene-environment correlation as an explanation

for maltreatment. Subsequent research has been successful in replicating Caspi's original findings and in extending them to samples of children and adolescents (Cicchetti, Rogosch, & Thibodeau, 2012; Foley et al., 2004; Kim-Cohen et al., 2006; Widom & Brzustowicz, 2006).

With respect to the link between maltreatment and depression, Caspi et al. (2003) found that genetic variation in a functional polymorphism (5-HTTLPR) in the promoter region of the serotonin transporter gene (5-HTT) plays a moderating role. Specifically, adults carrying the s allele exhibited more depressive symptoms, diagnosable depression, and suicidality in response to stressful life events than individuals homozygous for the l allele. In addition, an examination of early life stress showed that a history of child maltreatment longitudinally predicted depression in adulthood, but only among s carriers.

Although not all studies have confirmed the findings of Caspi et al. (2003), efforts at replication have demonstrated that the 5-HTTLPR by maltreatment interaction effect may be generalized to child and adolescent populations (Åslund et al., 2009; Cicchetti, Rogosch, & Oshri, 2011; Cicchetti, Rogosch, & Sturge-Apple, 2007; Kaufman et al., 2004, 2006). In the first of such investigations, Kaufman et al. (2004) found that maltreated children with the s/s genotype evinced depression scores that were almost twice as high as the depression scores of maltreated children with the s/l and l/l genotypes. Kaufman et al. (2006) replicated these findings in a subsequent study, the results of which revealed a significant three-way interaction between BDNF genotype, 5-HTTLPR, and maltreatment in predicting heightened levels of depression. In another instance of G X G X E, Cicchetti and colleagues (2007) found that adolescents with a history of sexual abuse who carried both the s/s genotype and the low MAOA activity genotype evinced higher levels of depression symptomatology compared to sexually abused adolescents with alternative combinations of the variants of the 5-HTT and MAOA genes. Åslund et al. (2009) also demonstrated a positive maltreatment X 5-HTTLPR effect for depression among adolescents; however, results were only significant for females. Furthermore, recent research indicates that 5-HTTLPR appears to have a moderating effect within the context of a process model linking child maltreatment to depression via peer victimization (Banny, Cicchetti, Rogosch, Oshri, & Crick, 2013).

A haplotype in the corticotropin-releasing hormone receptor 1 gene (CRHR1) also has been shown to moderate the effect of child maltreatment on the development of depression in adulthood (Bradley et al., 2008; Polanczyk et al., 2009). The CRHR1 gene plays a key role in the regulation of the hypothalamic-pituitary-adrenal (HPA) axis in response to stress, making it an important candidate gene for depression. In a study by Bradley et al. (2008), the TAT haplotype was found to exert a protective effect, such that individuals exposed to moderate to severe child abuse showed diminished depression symptoms compared to those with a history of maltreatment in other genotype groups. Polanczyk et al. (2009) replicated these findings among women in the E-Risk Study who were exposed to severe child maltreatment. Similarly, DeYoung, Cicchetti, and Rogosch (2011) found that having two copies of the CRHR1 gene exerted a protective effect against neuroticism among children who had experienced three to four subtypes of maltreatment, but not among those who had experienced one to two subtypes. The CRHR1 gene has also been implicated in G X G X E interactions, such that maltreated children with two copies of the TAT haplotype of CRHR1 and the *l/l* genotype of 5-HTTLPR exhibit higher levels of internalizing symptoms than nonmaltreated children with the same combination of gene variants (Cicchetti, Rogosch, & Oshri, 2011).

Maltreatment and Allostatic Load

In addition to the socioemotional and psychological consequences of child maltreatment, child abuse and neglect appear to be implicated in the disruption of diverse biological systems. The concepts of allostasis and allostatic load (AL) provide an integrative framework for understanding how exposure to chronic stress, such as child maltreatment, potentiates long-term liabilities for

physical and mental health (Rogosch, Dackis, & Cicchetti, 2011). Allostasis is a process that involves the activation of multiple interactive physiological systems (e.g., HPA and sympathetic-adrenal-medullary axes and cardiovascular, immune, and metabolic systems). In the short term, mobilization of these systems exerts a protective effect on the body and promotes an adaptive response to stress; however, with chronic activation, physiological reactions to stress become less efficient in protecting the individual. Ensuing damage to the body results in allostatic overload, which in turn contributes to changes in the brain and the development of various disease states.

Research by Cicchetti and Rogosch (2001a) investigated the extent to which maltreated children vary with respect to cortisol regulation, a biomarker of AL. Although no differences in cortisol regulation were found between the maltreated and nonmaltreated groups, findings revealed significant within-group variation as a function of maltreatment subtype. In particular, children who had experienced both physical and sexual abuse, in combination with neglect or emotional maltreatment, exhibited substantial elevations in morning cortisol levels (i.e., hypercortisolism). In addition, a subgroup of physically abused children showed a trend toward lower morning cortisol relative to nonmaltreated children (i.e., hypocortisolism). Furthermore, the neglected and emotionally maltreated groups did not differ from nonmaltreated children in terms of cortisol regulation. These differential outcomes are illustrative of the systems concept of multifinality. Specifically, the experience of child maltreatment does not uniformly affect the neuroendocrine functioning of all victims, but rather eventuates in a diversity of outcomes.

Longitudinal analysis of the developmental course of cortisol dysregulation accommodates findings of both hyper- and hypocortisolism among maltreated children. Trickett, Noll, Susman, Shenk, and Putnam (2010) measured cortisol activity at six time points spanning across childhood, adolescence, and young adulthood to determine the effects of maltreatment on cortisol regulation. Although the cortisol levels of sexually abused females were initially higher compared to nonabused females, their levels were lower by early adulthood. Results support an attenuation hypothesis, whereby the HPA axis adapts to hypersecretion by downregulating its response to stress, eventually resulting in hyposecretion (Trickett et al., 2010).

Research has also examined whether cortisol differentially relates to social and psychological functioning based on maltreatment status. This research is driven by two hypotheses, the first of which posits that the association between HPA axis dysregulation and social/psychological problems is stronger for maltreated children. This hypothesis was supported by the findings of Cicchetti and Rogosch (2001b), which indicated that depressed maltreated children exhibited a pattern of cortisol dysregulation that was not evident among depressed nonmaltreated children. Similarly, in a later study by Cicchetti, Rogosch, Gunnar, and Toth (2010), children who had experienced early sexual and/or physical abuse in the first 5 years of life and who also had high internalizing symptoms uniquely exhibited an attenuated diurnal decrease in cortisol, whereas nonmaltreated children with high internalizing symptomatology did not evince neuroendocrine dysregulation. Parallel findings have been demonstrated by Heim, Mletzko, Purselle, Musselman, and Nemeroff (2008) who found that abused, but not nonabused, men showed HPA hyperactivity. A second hypothesis predicts that these associations will be more pronounced among nonmaltreated children (i.e., social push perspective; Raine, 2002). Consistent with this perspective, research by Murray-Close, Han, Cicchetti, Crick, and Rogosch (2008) demonstrated that physical and relational aggression were associated with greater cortisol dysregulation in nonmaltreated children than in maltreated children. Overall, these findings highlight equifinality, such that two phenotypically similar children may have biologically distinct characteristics (Cicchetti & Rogosch, 1996).

In addition to cortisol dysregulation, maltreatment appears to be associated with other adverse health outcomes that may be implicated in the development of allostatic overload. For example, maltreatment predicts increased risk for hospital-based treatment of asthma, cardiorespiratory, and infectious disease in childhood (Lanier, Johnson-Reid, Stahlschmidt, Drake, & Constantino, 2010). Early child abuse has been linked to more health-related symptoms (e.g., sleep, eating, general health status), higher body mass index (BMI), and compromised immune system functioning in adolescence (Clark, Thatcher, & Martin, 2010; Shirtcliff, Coe, & Pollak, 2009; Shin & Miller, 2012). In addition, evidence suggests that maltreatment is related to structural and functional abnormalities in the brain (Hart & Rubia, 2012). Furthermore, health liabilities extend into adulthood, as child maltreatment has been found to predict adult cardiovascular disease, elevated inflammation levels, type II diabetes, and self-reported physical symptoms across a range of organ systems (Batten, Aslan, Maciejewski, & Mazure, 2004; Danese et al., 2008; Rich-Edwards et al., 2010; Springer, Sheridan, Kuo, & Carnes, 2007).

Consistent with the concept of AL, Rogosch et al. (2011) conducted a multi-domain assessment of stress-sensitive systems among low-income maltreated and nonmaltreated comparison children. An AL composite was created from measurements of salivary cortisol and dehydroepiandrosterone, BMI, waist-hip ratio, and blood pressure. Results indicated that maltreatment and AL independently predicted psychopathology and health difficulties (i.e., parent report of child's physical health status and utilization of health-care system). As AL increased, the level of child health and psychological problems increased for all low-income children. Child maltreatment had an additive effect, contributing to the degree of physical and mental health problems beyond that accounted for by the AL composite. Therefore, children with both high AL and a history of maltreatment had the most health problems.

Resilience

Despite their heightened risk for maladaptation and psychopathology, not all maltreated children follow negative developmental trajectories.

Maltreated children also demonstrate the capacity for resilience, a dynamic process involving the attainment of positive adaptation within the context of significant adversity (Luthar, Cicchetti, & Becker, 2000). The study of resilience among maltreated children has traditionally examined psychosocial predictors of competent functioning. Among them include neighborhood characteristics, secure attachment relationships, mother–child relationship quality, regulatory skills, and supportive peer relationships (Alink, Cicchetti, Kim, & Rogosch, 2009; Haskett, Nears, Ward, & McPherson, 2006). Personality characteristics and self-processes, such as high self-esteem and perceived self-efficacy, have also emerged as significant predictors of resilience in maltreated children (Cicchetti & Rogosch, 2007; Kim & Cicchetti, 2003).

Advances in technology have allowed for the expansion of research on resilience to include biological mechanisms. In the first of such investigations, Curtis and Cicchetti (2007) measured EEG asymmetry and emotion regulation as predictors of resilient functioning. They were particularly interested in the degree of left frontal EEG activity, which has been consistently linked to positive emotions/approach behavior. Findings indicated that maltreated children with left hemispheric activation asymmetry were functioning resiliently based on a competence composite index (e.g., good peer relations, successful school adaptation, low internalizing and externalizing symptoms). Moreover, adult observational ratings of emotion regulation made a unique contribution to resilience.

A second multilevel investigation conducted by Cicchetti and Rogosch (2007) found that personality characteristics (i.e., ego control, ego resiliency) and adrenal steroid hormones (i.e., cortisol, DHEA) independently contributed to resilience and that these predictors functioned differentially for maltreated and nonmaltreated children. For example, lower morning cortisol was related to higher resilient functioning for nonmaltreated children, whereas high morning cortisol was associated with higher resilient functioning for physically abused children. Furthermore, maltreated children with high

resilience showed an atypical rise in DHEA from morning to afternoon.

Finally, with advances in molecular genetics, knowledge that particular genotypes confer protection to vulnerable children has motivated researchers to examine potential genetic mechanisms involved in resilience (Kim-Cohen & Gold, 2009). In a study by Cicchetti and Rogosch (2012), genetic variation had more of an impact on the resilient functioning of nonmaltreated children, with little to no influence on the resilience of maltreated children. It is possible that the experience of maltreatment is so significant that it overpowers potential genetic effects. However, future research that incorporates multiple levels of analysis is needed to determine whether other genes or biological factors may be at play. Such research will be critical in the development of prevention and intervention programs aimed at promoting adaptive functioning in the face of adversity.

Prevention and Intervention

As reviewed in the current chapter, years of empirical research indicate that child maltreatment initiates a probabilistic pathway marked by heightened risk for maladaptation across a broad range of psychological and biological domains. Moreover, child maltreatment exerts a considerable toll on society at large. Systematic observation of such wide-reaching effects emphasizes the urgency of translating basic research into the development of evidence-based prevention and intervention programs for maltreated children and their families.

Findings regarding the extensive influence of child maltreatment stress the criticality of preventing maltreatment before it occurs. Emerging evidence suggests that maltreatment can be prevented. Two programs, the Chicago Parenting Center (CPC) and the Nurse Family Partnership (NFP), have been identified as the most successful in the reduction of maltreatment (Reynolds, Mathieson, & Topitzes, 2009). CPC adopts a school-based approach, providing high-quality preschool education, while NFP implements an intensive home visitation model. Although they differ with regard to service implementation, both programs are ecologically based and deliver comprehensive family support services, highlighting the utility of a multisystemic approach to the prevention of maltreatment. Participation in CPC and NFP has been linked to an average reduction in the occurrence of maltreatment that is more than double that of other prevention programs (Reynolds et al., 2009).

Ultimately, a review of the empirical support for maltreatment prevention programs indicates that the evidence base remains relatively weak (Reynolds et al., 2009); therefore, the development of intervention programs remains a priority. Interventions informed by an organizational perspective seek to effect change in the course of development by promoting the successful resolution of stage-salient developmental tasks. Inherent in this approach is an emphasis on early intervention, before the initiation of negative developmental cascades. Consistent with organizational theory, a number of attachment-informed interventions have been developed and evaluated in abused and neglected populations. Among them include child–parent psychotherapy (CPP), the goal of which is to improve mother–child attachment relationships by modifying mothers' internal working models. Cicchetti, Rogosch, and Toth (2006) compared the effectiveness of CPP with a psychoeducational parenting intervention (PPI) and with the community standard (CS). At the conclusion of the intervention approximately 1 year later, infants in the CPP and PPI groups evidenced a significant change in their attachment security, such that their attachment security no longer differed from that of the infants in the nonmaltreated comparison group. Furthermore, for maltreated children in the CPP and PPI groups, HPA axis functioning was normalized (Cicchetti, Rogosch, Toth, & Sturge-Apple, 2011). In contrast, infants in the CS group did not show any improvements in their attachment security, and their trajectories of cortisol regulation became more divergent over time (Cicchetti et al., 2006; Cicchetti, Rogosch, Toth, & Sturge-Apple, 2011). Results demonstrate that behavioral interventions may positively alter psychological and neurobiological processes that have long-term implications for development.

Utilizing a similar treatment design, Toth, Maughan, Manly, Spagnola, and Cicchetti (2002) demonstrated the efficacy of CPP for preschool-aged children, compared to PPI and CS. In this study, only CPP had significant treatment effects. Specifically, preschoolers in the CPP intervention showed a greater decline in maladaptive maternal representations, a greater decrease in negative self-representations, and more positive mother–child relationship expectations over the course of treatment compared to the PPI and CS groups. This pattern of results suggests that as self-system development progresses and becomes more consolidated, an attachment-based intervention (i.e., CPP) may be more effective at improving representations of the self and of others, compared to a didactic parenting intervention (i.e., PPI).

Conclusions

In this chapter, we have adopted an organizational approach to development in order to provide a framework for understanding the extensive consequences of child maltreatment. Our review conveys the negative and often lifelong effects of child maltreatment on diverse psychological and biological systems. The experience of child maltreatment potentiates a pathway marked by repeated developmental failures, wherein unsuccessful resolution of stage-salient issues initiates a cascade of sequelae that compromises the development of later competencies.

Longitudinal studies that incorporate multiple levels of analysis will contribute to the creation of prevention and intervention programs aimed at mitigating the impact of early life stress and promoting adaptive functioning at multiple levels of influence. By elucidating the various pathways by which maltreated children develop or avert maladaptation, basic research can inform translational efforts that have the potential to reduce the burden of mental illness on individuals, families, and society. It is possible that theoretically informed early interventions that target multiple systems may prevent developmental cascades leading to costlier interventions.

Acknowledgments Our work on this chapter was supported by grants from the National Institute of Drug Abuse (R01 DA017741), the National Institute of Mental Health (R01 MH083979, R01 MH091070, R01 MH054643), and the Spunk Fund, Inc.

References

Alink, L. R. A., Cicchetti, D., Kim, J., & Rogosch, F. A. (2009). Mediating and moderating processes in the relation between maltreatment and psychopathology: Mother-child relationship quality and emotion regulation. *Journal of Abnormal Child Psychology, 37*, 831–843.

Arseneault, L., Cannon, M., Fisher, H. L., Polanczyk, G., Moffitt, T. E., & Caspi, A. (2011). Childhood trauma and children's emerging psychotic symptoms: A genetically sensitive longitudinal cohort study. *American Journal of Psychiatry, 168*, 65–72.

Åslund, C., Leppert, J., Comasco, E., Nordquist, N., Oreland, L., & Nilsson, K. W. (2009). Impact of the interaction between the 5HTTLPR polymorphism and maltreatment on adolescent depression: A population-based study. *Behavior Genetics, 39*, 524–531.

Ayoub, C. C., O'Connor, E., Rappolt-Schlichtmann, G., Fischer, K. W., Rogosch, F. A., Toth, S. L., et al. (2006). Cognitive and emotional differences in young maltreated children: A translational application of dynamic skill theory. *Development and Psychopathology, 3*, 679–706.

Banny, A. M., Cicchetti, D., Rogosch, F. A., Oshri, A., & Crick, N. R. (2013). Pathways to depression: A moderated mediation model of the roles of child maltreatment, peer victimization, and genetic variation among children from low-SES backgrounds. *Development and Psychopathology, 25*, 599–614.

Barnett, D., Ganiban, J., & Cicchetti, D. (1999). Maltreatment, negative expressivity, and the development of Type D attachments from 12- to 24-months of age. *Society for Research in Child Development Monograph, 64*, 97–118.

Barnett, D., Manly, J. T., & Cicchetti, D. (1993). Defining child maltreatment: The interface between policy and research. In D. Cicchetti & S. L. Toth (Eds.), *Child abuse, child development, and social policy* (pp. 7–73). Norwood, NJ: Ablex.

Batten, S. V., Aslan, M., Maciejewski, P. K., & Mazure, C. M. (2004). Childhood maltreatment as a risk factor for adult cardiovascular disease and depression. *Journal of Clinical Psychiatry, 65*, 245–254.

Beeghly, M., & Cicchetti, D. (1994). Child maltreatment, attachment, and the self system: Emergence of an internal state lexicon in toddlers at high social risk. *Development and Psychopathology, 6*, 5–30.

Beers, S. R., & DeBellis, M. D. (2002). Neuropsychological function in children with related posttraumatic stress disorder. *American Journal of Psychiatry, 159*, 483–486.

Belsky, J. (1980). Child maltreatment: An ecological integration. *American Psychologist, 35*, 320–335.

Bolger, K. E., & Patterson, C. J. (2001). Developmental pathways from child maltreatment to peer rejection. *Child Development, 72*, 549–568.

Bolger, K. E., Patterson, C. J., & Kupersmidt, J. B. (1998). Peer relationships and self-esteem among children who have been maltreated. *Child Development, 69*, 1171–1197.

Bowlby, J. (1969). *Attachment and Loss* (Vol. I). New York: Basic Books.

Bradley, R. G., Binder, E. B., Epstein, M. P., Tang, Y., Nair, H. P., Liu, W., et al. (2008). Influence of child abuse on adult depression: Moderation by the corticotropin-releasing hormone receptor gene. *Archives of General Psychiatry, 65*, 190–200.

Bugental, D. B., Blue, J., & Lewis, J. (1990). Caregiver beliefs and dysphoric affect directed to difficult children. *Developmental Psychology, 26*, 631–638.

Caspi, A., McClay, J., Moffitt, T., Mill, J., Martin, J., Craig, I. W., et al. (2002). Role of genotype in the cycle of violence in maltreated children. *Science, 297*, 851–854.

Caspi, A., Sugden, K., Moffitt, T. E., Taylor, A., Craig, I. W., Harrington, H. L., et al. (2003). Influence of life stress on depression: Moderation by a polymorphism in the 5-HTT gene. *Science, 301*, 386–389.

Cicchetti, D. (1991). Fractures in the crystal: Developmental psychopathology and the emergence of the self. *Developmental Review, 11*, 271–287.

Cicchetti, D., & Curtis, W. J. (2005). An event-related potential (ERP) study of processing of affective facial expressions in young children who have experienced maltreatment during the first year of life. *Development and Psychopathology, 17*(3), 641–677.

Cicchetti, D., & Lynch, M. (1993). Toward an ecological/transactional model of community violence and child maltreatment: Consequences for children's development. *Psychiatry, 56*, 96–118.

Cicchetti, D., & Rizley, R. (1981). Developmental perspectives on the etiology, intergenerational transmission and sequelae of child maltreatment. *New Directions for Child Development, 11*, 31–55.

Cicchetti, D., & Rogosch, F. A. (1996). Equifinality and multifinality in developmental psychopathology. *Development and Psychopathology, 8*, 597–600.

Cicchetti, D., & Rogosch, F. A. (2001a). Diverse patterns of neuroendocrine activity in maltreated children. *Development and Psychopathology, 13*, 677–693.

Cicchetti, D., & Rogosch, F. A. (2001b). The impact of child maltreatment and psychopathology on neuroendocrine functioning. *Development and Psychopathology, 13*, 783–804.

Cicchetti, D., & Rogosch, F. A. (2007). Personality, adrenal steroid hormones, and resilience in maltreated children: A multi-level perspective. *Development and Psychopathology, 19*, 787–809.

Cicchetti, D., & Rogosch, F. A. (2012). Gene by environment interaction and resilience: Effects of child maltreatment and serotonin, corticotropin releasing hormone, dopamine, and oxytocin genes. *Development and Psychopathology, 24*, 411–427.

Cicchetti, D., Rogosch, F. A., Gunnar, M. R., & Toth, S. L. (2010). The differential impacts of early abuse on internalizing problems and diurnal cortisol activity in school-aged children. *Child Development, 25*, 252–269.

Cicchetti, D., Rogosch, F. A., Howe, M. L., & Toth, S. L. (2010). The effects of maltreatment on neuroendocrine regulation and memory performance. *Child Development, 81*, 1504–1519.

Cicchetti, D., Rogosch, F. A., & Oshri, A. (2011). Interactive effects of corticotrophin releasing hormone receptor 1, serotonin transporter linked polymorphic region, and child maltreatment on diurnal cortisol regulation and internalizing symptomatology. *Development and Psychopathology, 23*, 1125–1138.

Cicchetti, D., Rogosch, F. A., & Sturge-Apple, M. (2007). Interactions of child maltreatment and serotonin transporter and monoamine oxidase A polymorphisms: Depressive symptomatology among adolescents from low socioeconomic status backgrounds. *Development and Psychopathology, 19*, 1161–1180.

Cicchetti, D., Rogosch, F. A., & Thibodeau, E. L. (2012). The effects of child maltreatment on early signs of antisocial behavior: Genetic moderation by Tryptophan Hydroxylase, Serotonin Transporter, and Monoamine Oxidase-A-Genes. *Development and Psychopathology, 24*, 907–928.

Cicchetti, D., Rogosch, F. A., & Toth, S. L. (2006). Fostering secure attachment in infants in maltreating families through preventive interventions. *Development and Psychopathology, 18*, 623–650.

Cicchetti, D., Rogosch, F. A., & Toth, S. L. (2011). The effects of child maltreatment and polymorphisms of the serotonin transporter and dopamine D4 receptor genes on infant attachment and intervention efficacy. *Development and Psychopathology, 23*, 357–372.

Cicchetti, D., Rogosch, F. A., Toth, S. L., & Sturge-Apple, M. L. (2011). Normalizing the development of cortisol regulation in maltreated infants through preventive interventions. *Development and Psychopathology, 23*, 789–800.

Cicchetti, D., Toth, S. L., & Maughan, A. (2000). An ecological-transactional model of child maltreatment. In A. J. Sameroff, M. Lewis, & S. M. Miller (Eds.), *Handbook of developmental psychopathology* (2nd ed., pp. 689–722). New York: Plenum.

Clark, D. B., Thatcher, D. L., & Martin, C. S. (2010). Child abuse and other traumatic experiences, alcohol use disorders, and health problems in adolescence and young adulthood. *Journal of Pediatric Psychology, 35*, 499–510.

Crittenden, P. M. (1981). Abusing, neglecting, problematic, and adequate dyads: Differentiating by patterns of interaction. *Merrill-Palmer Quarterly, 27*, 201–218.

Crittenden, P. M. (1985). Social networks, quality of child-rearing, and child development. *Child Development, 56*, 1299–1313.

Cullerton-Sen, C., Cassidy, A. R., Murray-Close, D., Cicchetti, D., Crick, N. R., & Rogosch, F. A. (2008). Childhood maltreatment and the development of relational and physical aggression: The importance of a gender-informed approach. *Child Development, 79*(6), 1736–1751.

Curtis, W. J., & Cicchetti, D. (2007). Emotion and resilience: A multi-level investigation of hemispheric electroencephalogram asymmetry and emotion regulation in maltreated and non-maltreated children. *Development and Psychopathology, 19*, 811–840.

Curtis, W. J., & Cicchetti, D. (2011). Affective facial expression processing in young children who have experienced maltreatment during the first year of life: An event-related potential (ERP) study. *Development and Psychopathology, 23*, 373–395.

Cyr, C., Euser, E. M., Bakermans-Kranenburg, M. J., & Van Ijzendoorn, M. H. (2010). Attachment security and disorganization in maltreating and high-risk families: A series of meta-analyses. *Development and Psychopathology, 22*, 87–108.

Danese, A., Moffitt, T. E., Pariante, C. M., Ambler, A., Poulton, R., & Caspi, A. (2008). Elevated inflammation levels in depressed adults with a history of childhood maltreatment. *Archives of General Psychiatry, 65*, 409–415.

DeYoung, C. G., Cicchetti, D., & Rogosch, F. A. (2011). Moderation of the association between childhood maltreatment and neuroticism by the corticotrophin-releasing hormone receptor 1 gene. *Journal of Child Psychology and Psychiatry, 52*, 898–906.

Egeland, B., Yates, T., Appleyard, K., & van Dulmen, M. (2002). The long-term consequences of maltreatment in the early years: A developmental pathway model to antisocial behavior. *Children's Services: Social Policy, Research, and Practice, 5*, 249–260.

Eisen, M. L., Goodman, G. S., Qin, J., Davis, S., & Crayton, J. (2007). Maltreated children's memory: Accuracy, suggestibility, and psychopathology. *Developmental Psychology, 43*, 1275–1294.

Fang, X., Brown, D. S., Florence, C. S., & Mercy, J. A. (2012). The economic burden of child maltreatment in the United States and implications for prevention. *Child Abuse & Neglect, 36*, 156–165.

Foley, D. L., Eaves, L. J., Wormley, B., Silberg, J. L., Maes, H. H., Kuhn, J., et al. (2004). Childhood adversity, monoamine oxidase A genotype, and risk for conduct disorder. *Archives of General Psychiatry, 61*, 738–744.

Gaensbauer, T. (1980). Anaclitic depression in a three-and-one-half-month-old-child. *American Journal of Psychiatry, 137*, 841–842.

Gaensbauer, T., & Hiatt, S. (1984). Facial communication of emotion in early infancy. In N. A. Fox & R. J. Davidson (Eds.), *The psychobiology of affective development* (pp. 207–230). Hillsdale, NJ: Erlbaum.

Hart, H., & Rubia, K. (2012). Neuroimaging of child abuse: A critical review. *Frontiers in Human Neuroscience, 6*, 1–24.

Haskett, M. E., Nears, K., Ward, C. S., & McPherson, A. V. (2006). Diversity in adjustment of maltreated children: Factors associated with resilient functioning. *Clinical Psychology Review, 26*, 796–812.

Heim, C., Mletzko, T., Purselle, D., Musselman, D. L., & Nemeroff, C. B. (2008). The dexamethasone/corticotropin-releasing factor test in men with major depression: Role of childhood trauma. *Biological Psychiatry, 63*, 398–405.

Herrenkohl, R. C., Herrenkohl, E. C., Egolf, B. P., & Wu, P. (1991). The developmental consequences of child abuse: The Lehigh longitudinal study. In R. H. Starr & D. A. Wolfe (Eds.), *The effects of child abuse and neglect* (pp. 57–81). New York: Guilford Press.

Hesse, E., & Main, M. (2006). Frightened, threatening, and dissociative parental behavior in low-risk samples: Description, discussion, and interpretations. *Development and Psychopathology, 18*, 309–344.

Howe, M. L., Cicchetti, D., & Toth, S. L. (2006). Children's basic memory processes, stress, and maltreatment. *Development and Psychopathology, 18*, 759–769.

Howe, M. L., Cicchetti, D., Toth, S. L., & Cerrito, B. M. (2004). True and false memories in maltreated children. *Child Development, 75*, 1402–1417.

Howe, T. R., & Parke, R. D. (2001). Friendship quality and sociometric status: Between-group differences and links to loneliness in severely abused and nonabused children. *Child Abuse & Neglect, 25*, 585–606.

Howe, M. L., Toth, S. L., & Cicchetti, D. (2011). Can maltreated children suppress true and false memories for emotional information? *Child Development, 82*, 967–981.

Kaplow, J. B., & Widom, C. S. (2007). Age of onset of child maltreatment predicts long-term mental health outcomes. *Journal of Abnormal Psychology, 116*, 176–187.

Kaufman, J., Yang, B., Douglas-Palumberi, H., Grasso, D., Lipschitz, D., Houshyar, S., et al. (2006). Brain-derived neurotrophic factor—5-HTTLPR gene interactions and environmental modifiers of depression. *Biological Psychiatry, 59*, 673–680.

Kaufman, J., Yang, B., Douglas-Palumberi, H., Houshyar, S., Lipschitz, D., Krystal, J. H., et al. (2004). Social supports and serotonin transporter gene moderate depression in maltreated children. *Proceedings of the National Academy of Sciences of the United States of America, 101*, 17316–17321.

Keyes, K. M., Eaton, N. R., Krueger, R. F., McLaughlin, K. A., Wall, M. M., Grant, B. F., et al. (2012). Childhood maltreatment and the structure of common psychiatric disorders. *British Journal of Psychiatry, 200*, 107–115.

Kim, J. E., & Cicchetti, D. (2003). Social self-efficacy and behavior problems in maltreated and nonmaltreated children. *Journal of Clinical Child and Adolescent Psychology, 32*, 106–117.

Kim, J. E., & Cicchetti, D. (2006). Longitudinal trajectories of self-system processes and depressive symptoms among maltreated and nonmaltreated children. *Child Development, 77*, 624–639.

Kim-Cohen, J., Caspi, A., Taylor, A., Williams, B., Newcombe, R., Craig, I. W., et al. (2006). MAOA, maltreatment, and gene–environment interaction predicting children's mental health: New evidence and a meta-analysis. *Molecular Psychiatry, 11*, 903–913.

Kim-Cohen, J., & Gold, A. L. (2009). Measuring gene-environment interactions and mechanisms promoting resilient development. *Current Directions in Psychological Science, 18*, 138–142.

Kohl, P. L., Jonson-Reid, M., & Drake, B. (2009). Time to leave substantiation behind: Findings from a national probability study. *Child Maltreatment, 14*, 17–26.

Lanier, P., Johnson-Reid, M., Stahlschmidt, M. J., Drake, B., & Constantino, J. (2010). Child maltreatment and pediatric health outcomes: A longitudinal study of low-income children. *Journal of Pediatric Psychology, 35*, 511–522.

Luijk, M. P., Roisman, G. I., Haltigan, J. D., Tiemeier, H., Booth-LaForce, C., van IJzendoorn, M. H., et al. (2011). Dopaminergic, serotonergic, oxytonergic candidate genes associated with infant attachment security and disorganization? In search of main and interaction effects. *Journal of Child Psychology and Psychiatry, 52*, 1295–1307.

Luthar, S. S., Cicchetti, D., & Becker, B. (2000). The construct of resilience: A critical evaluation and guidelines for future work. *Child Development, 71*, 543–562.

Macfie, J., Cicchetti, D., & Toth, S. L. (2001a). Dissociation in maltreated versus nonmaltreated preschool-aged children. *Child Abuse and Neglect, 25*, 1253–1267.

Macfie, J., Cicchetti, D., & Toth, S. L. (2001b). The development of dissociation in maltreated preschool-aged children. *Development and Psychopathology, 13*, 233–254.

Murray-Close, D., Han, G., Cicchetti, D., Crick, N. R., & Rogosch, F. A. (2008). Neuroendocrine regulation and aggression: The moderating roles of physical and relational aggression and child maltreatment. *Developmental Psychology, 44*, 1160–1176.

Natsuaki, M., Cicchetti, D., & Rogosch, F. A. (2009). Examining the developmental history of child maltreatment, peer relations, and externalizing problems among adolescents with symptoms of paranoid personality disorder. *Development and Psychopathology, 21*, 1181–1193.

Parker, J. G., & Herrera, C. (1996). Interpersonal processes in friendship: A comparison of abused and nonabused children's experiences. *Developmental Psychology, 32*, 1025–1038.

Polanczyk, G., Caspi, A., Williams, B., Price, T. S., Danese, A., Sugden, K., et al. (2009). Protective effect of CRHR1 gene variants on the development of adult depression following childhood maltreatment. *Archives of General Psychiatry, 66*, 978–985.

Pollak, S. D. (2009). Mechanisms linking early experience and the emergence of emotions: Illustrations from the study of maltreated children. *Current Directions in Psychological Science, 17*, 370–375.

Pollak, S. D., Cicchetti, D., Hornung, K., & Reed, A. (2000). Recognizing emotion in faces: Developmental effects of child abuse and neglect. *Developmental Psychology, 36*, 679–688.

Pollak, S. D., & Kistler, D. J. (2002). Early experience is associated with the development of categorical representations for facial expressions of emotion. *Proceedings of the National Academy of Sciences of the United States of America, 99*, 9072–9076.

Pollak, S. D., Klorman, R., Thatcher, J. E., & Cicchetti, D. (2001). P3b reflects maltreated children's reactions to facial displays of emotion. *Psychophysiology, 38*, 267–274.

Pollak, S. D., Messner, M., Kistler, D. J., & Cohn, J.F. (2009). Development of perceptual expertise in emotion recognition. *Cognition, 110*, 242–247.

Pollak, S. D., & Sinha, P. (2002). Effects of early experience on children's recognition of facial displays of emotion. *Developmental Psychology, 38*, 784–791.

Pollak, S. D., & Tolley-Schell, S. A. (2003). Selective attention to facial emotion in physically abused children. *Journal of Abnormal Psychology, 112*, 323–338.

Porter, C., Lawson, J. S., & Bigler, E. D. (2005). Neurobehavioral sequelae of child abuse. *Child Neuropsychology, 11*, 203–220.

Raine, A. (2002). Biosocial studies of antisocial and violent behavior in children and adults: A review. *Journal of Abnormal Child Psychology, 30*, 311–326.

Reynolds, A. J., Mathieson, L. C., & Topitzes, J. W. (2009). Do early childhood interventions prevent child maltreatment? A review of research. *Child Maltreatment, 14*, 182–206.

Rich-Edwards, J. W., Spiegelman, D., Hibert, E. N. L., Jun, H., Todd, T. J., Kawachi, I., et al. (2010). Abuse in childhood and adolescence as a predictor of type 2 diabetes in adult women. *American Journal of Preventive Medicine, 39*, 529–536.

Rogosch, F. A., & Cicchetti, D. (2004). Child maltreatment and emergent personality organization: Perspectives from the Five-Factor model. *Journal of Abnormal Child Psychology, 32*, 123–145.

Rogosch, F. A., & Cicchetti, D. (2005). Child maltreatment, attention networks, and potential precursors to borderline personality disorder. *Development and Psychopathology, 17*(4), 1071–1089.

Rogosch, F. A., Dackis, M. N., & Cicchetti, D. (2011). Child maltreatment and allostatic load: Consequences for physical and mental health in children from low-income families. *Development and Psychopathology, 23*, 1107–1124.

Rogosch, F. A., Oshri, A., & Cicchetti, D. (2010). From child maltreatment to adolescent cannabis abuse and dependence: A developmental cascade model. *Development and Psychopathology, 22*, 883–897.

Schneider-Rosen, K., & Cicchetti, D. (1991). Early self-knowledge and emotional development: Visual self-recognition and affective reactions to mirror self-image in maltreated and nonmaltreated toddlers. *Developmental Psychology, 27*, 481–488.

Schwartz, D., Dodge, K. A., Pettit, G. S., & Bates, J. E. (1997). The early socialization of aggressive victims of bullying. *Developmental Psychology, 68*, 665–675.

Schwartz, D., Dodge, K. A., Pettit, G. S., & Bates, J. E. (2000). Friendship as a moderating factor in the pathway between early harsh home environment and later victimization in the peer group. *Developmental Psychology, 36*, 646–662.

Scott, K. M., Smith, D. R., & Ellis, P. M. (2010). Prospectively ascertained child maltreatment and its association with DSM-IV mental disorders in young adults. *Archives of General Psychiatry, 67*, 712–719.

Sedlak, A., Mettenburg, J., Basena, M., Petta, I., McPherson, K., Greene, A., et al. (2010). *Fourth national incidence study of child abuse and neglect (NIS-4): Report to congress*. Washington, DC: Department of Health and Human Services.

Shackman, J. E., Shackman, A. J., & Pollak, S. D. (2007). Physical abuse amplifies attention to threat and increases anxiety in children. *Emotion, 7*, 838–852.

Shields, A., & Cicchetti, D. (2001). Parental maltreatment and emotion dysregulation as risk factors for bullying and victimization in middle childhood. *Journal of Clinical Child Psychology, 30*, 349–363.

Shin, S. H., & Miller, D. P. (2012). A longitudinal examination of childhood maltreatment and adolescent obesity: Results from the National Longitudinal Study of Adolescent Health (AddHealth) Study. *Child Abuse & Neglect, 36*, 84–94.

Shirtcliff, E. A., Coe, C. L., & Pollak, S. D. (2009). Early childhood stress is associated with elevated antibody levels to herpes simplex virus type 1. *Proceedings of the National Academy of Sciences of the United States of America, 106*, 2963–2967.

Springer, K. W., Sheridan, J., Kuo, D., & Carnes, M. (2007). Long-term physical and mental health consequences of childhood physical abuse: Results from a large population-based sample of men and women. *Child Abuse & Neglect, 31*, 517–530.

Sroufe, L. A., & Fleeson, J. (1986). Attachment and the construction of relationships. In W. Hartup & Z. Rubin (Eds.), *Relationships and development* (pp. 51–71). Hillsdale, NJ: Erlbaum.

Sroufe, L. A., & Rutter, M. (1984). The domain of developmental psychopathology. *Child Development, 55*, 17–29.

Teisl, M., & Cicchetti, D. (2008). Physical abuse, cognitive and emotional processes, and aggressive/disruptive behavior problems. *Social Development, 16*(1), 1–23.

Thompson, R. A., Lewis, M. D., & Calkins, S. D. (2008). Reassessing emotion regulation. *Child Development Perspectives, 2*, 124–131.

Toth, S. L., Cicchetti, D., Macfie, J., Maughan, A, & Vanmeenen, K. (2000). Narrative representations of caregivers and self in maltreated preschoolers. *Attachment & Human Development, 2*, 271–305.

Toth, S. L., Cicchetti, D., Macfie, J., Rogosch, F. A., & Maughan, A. (2000). Narrative representations of moral-affiliative and conflictual themes and behavioral problems in maltreated preschoolers. *Journal of Clinical Child Psychology, 29*(3), 307–318.

Toth, S. L., Maughan, A., Manly, J. T., Spagnola, M., & Cicchetti, D. (2002). The relative efficacy of two interventions in altering maltreated preschool children's representational models: Implications for attachment theory. *Development and Psychopathology, 14*, 777–808.

Trickett, P. K., Noll, J. G., Susman, E. J., Shenk, C. E., & Putnam, F. W. (2010). Attenuation of cortisol across development for victims of sexual abuse. *Development and Psychopathology, 22*, 165–175.

U.S. Department of Health and Human Services, Administration for Children and Families, Administration on Children, Youth and Families, Children's Bureau. (2011). *Child maltreatment 2010.* Available from http://www.scf.hhs.gov/programs/cb/stats_research/index.htm#can

Valentino, K., Cicchetti, D., Rogosch, F. A., & Toth, S. L. (2008a). Memory, maternal representations and internalizing symptomatology among abused, neglected and nonmaltreated children. *Child Development, 79*, 705–719.

Valentino, K, Cicchetti, D., Rogosch, F.A., & Toth, S.L. (2008b). True and false recall and dissociation among maltreated children: The role of self-schema. *Development and Psychopathology, 20*, 213–232.

Valentino, K., Toth, S. L., & Cicchetti, D. (2009). Autobiographical memory functioning among abused, neglected and nonmaltreated children: The overgeneral memory effect. *Journal of Child Psychology and Psychiatry, 79*, 1029–1038.

Vondra, J., Barnett, D., & Cicchetti, D. (1989). Perceived and actual competence among maltreated and comparison school children. *Development and Psychopathology, 1*, 237–255.

Wang, C., & Holton, J. (2007). *Total estimated cost of child abuse and neglect in the United States. Prevent child abuse America.* Available at http://member.preventchildabuse.org/site/DocServer/cost_analysis.pdf?docID=144

Widom, D. S., & Brzustowicz, L. M. (2006). MAOA and the "cycle of violence": Childhood abuse and neglect, MAOA genotype, and risk for violent and antisocial behavior. *Biological Psychiatry, 60*(7), 684–689.

Widom, C. S., DuMont, K., & Czaja, S. J. (2007). A prospective investigation of major depressive disorder and comorbidity in abused and neglected children grown up. *Archives of General Psychiatry, 64*, 49–56.

Widom, C. S., Marmorstein, N. R., & White, H. R. (2006). Childhood victimization and illicit drug use in middle adulthood. *Psychology of Addictive Behaviors, 20*, 394–403.

Widom, C. S., & Maxfield, M. G. (2001). *An update on the "cycle of violence".* Washington, DC: U.S. Department of Justice, Office of Justice Programs, National Institute of Justice.

Yates, T. M., Carlson, E. A., & Egeland, B. (2008). A prospective study of child maltreatment and self-injurious behavior in community sample. *Development and Psychopathology, 20*, 651–671.

Posttraumatic Stress Disorder in Children and Adolescents

38

Stephanie M. Keller and Norah C. Feeny

Epidemiology

Children experience traumatic events at rates similar to those of adults (Boney-McCoy & Finkelhor, 1995; Copeland, Keeler, Angold, & Costello, 2007; Kilpatrick et al., 2003). In contrast to the considerable literature on trauma exposure as well as the development, maintenance, and treatment of PTSD in adults, relatively little is known about the onset and course of this disorder in children and adolescents. In a large longitudinal study, about two-thirds (67.8 %) of children reported experiencing a traumatic event by the age of 16, and over 13 % of these children reported some posttraumatic stress symptoms (Copeland et al., 2007). Moreover, over half of the trauma-exposed children reported exposure to 2 or more traumatic events (Copeland et al., 2007). Hearing about or being confronted with traumatic news, witnessing a traumatic event (e.g., witnessing parental violence), and experiencing violence (e.g., physical abuse) appear to be the most common traumatic events reported by children and adolescents (e.g., Copeland et al., 2007; Luthra et al., 2009). Childhood sexual abuse appears to be less common, with a national survey estimate suggesting

that 13.5 % of females and 2.5 % of males report being sexually abused before the age of 18 (Molnar, Buka, & Kessler, 2001). Despite high rates of trauma exposure, in a national sample of children and adolescents aged 12–17 years old, 3.7 % of males and 6.3 % of females met criteria for a DSM-IV diagnosis of PTSD (Kilpatrick et al., 2003). Thus, trauma exposure, often exposure to multiple events, is common among individuals of all ages, and a small subset of these individuals develops PTSD.

Similar to the pattern in adults (e.g., Charuvastra & Cloitre, 2008; Resnick, Kilpatrick, Dansky, Saunders, & Best, 1993), among children and adolescents, exposure to violent and interpersonal traumas (e.g., witnessing a murder, sexual abuse) appears be associated with greater risk for developing PTSD than exposure to nonviolent traumas, such as natural disasters (Copeland et al., 2007; Garrison et al., 1995; Horowitz, McKay, & Marshall, 2005; Luthra et al., 2009). Also similar to findings in adults, (e.g., Breslau, 2001), among children and adolescents, males are more likely to experience traumatic events, but higher rates of PTSD are seen in females (e.g., Foster, Kuperminc, & Price, 2004; Osofksy, Osofksy, Kroenenberg, Brennan, & Hansel, 2009; Schwab-Stone et al., 1995; Thabet, Abu Tawahina, El Sarraj, & Vostanis, 2008; Vernberg, Silverman, La Greca, & Prinstein, 1996). In addition to gender, age may be a factor associated with the development of PTSD symptoms in children and adolescents. It appears that younger children are more likely than adolescents

S.M. Keller, M.A. (✉) • N.C. Feeny, Ph.D.
Case Western Reserve University, Cleveland, OH, USA
e-mail: smp28@case.edu; ncf2@case.edu;
norah.feeny@case.edu

M. Lewis and K.D. Rudolph (eds.), *Handbook of Developmental Psychopathology*,
DOI 10.1007/978-1-4614-9608-3_38, © Springer Science+Business Media New York 2014

to develop PTSD following trauma exposure (e.g., Chen, Lin, Tseng, & Wu, 2002; Green et al., 1991), although others have found no effect of age (e.g., Hunt, Martens, & Belcher, 2011; Thabet et al., 2008).

In both genders and across age ranges, trauma exposure during childhood is associated with increased risk for a number of psychological difficulties including depression, anxiety, and PTSD (e.g., Saywitz, Mannarino, Berliner, & Cohen, 2000). Children who have been traumatized also tend to display social and emotional difficulties during adulthood (Brent et al., 2002; Nelson et al., 2002). For example, childhood sexual abuse is associated with increased risk for anxiety, depression, and substance use disorders during adulthood (Nelson et al., 2002). Moreover, children who experience sexual abuse are at increased risk of being sexually abused as adults. In general, trauma exposure during childhood and adolescence can lead to a number of long-lasting negative outcomes, particularly PTSD.

PTSD in children and adolescents is often chronic and unremitting if left untreated (Meiser-Stedman, Smith, Glucksman, Yule, & Dalgleish, 2008; Scheeringa, Zeanah, Myers, & Putnam, 2005; Shaw, Applegate, & Schorr, 1996). Shaw and colleagues (1996) followed a group of children aged 6–11 years for 21 months after exposure to Hurricane Andrew. Even after 21 months, 70 % of children reported moderate to severe levels of PTSD symptoms. Interestingly, PTSD symptoms decreased more over the 21-month period for males than for females (Shaw et al., 1996).

Overall, it appears that trauma exposure is common among children and adolescents. Given that many children experience trauma and most do not develop PTSD (Kendall-Tackett, Williams, & Finkelhor, 1993), understanding factors that contribute to the development and maintenance of PTSD is vital. This chapter will provide an outline of factors that contribute to the development of PTSD in children in adolescents. Second, the chapter will provide an overview on PTSD diagnosis and treatment in this population. Third, the chapter will briefly examine neurobiological correlates of PTSD in children and adolescents. Finally, conclusions and future directions will be discussed.

Risk and Resiliency Factors

A child's resiliency or vulnerability to psychopathology following exposure to trauma is determined by a multitude of factors, including both personal and social components. Overall, risk or resiliency following trauma involves complex interactions between the child's intrinsic (e.g., temperament) and extrinsic (e.g., family support) environment (e.g., Pynoos, Steinberg, & Piacentini, 1999; Vernberg, 1999). Findings from a recent meta-analysis examining 64 studies that assessed risk factors associated with PTSD development in children (Trickey, Siddaway, Meiser-Stedman, Serpell, & Field, 2012) suggest that subjective factors relating to the traumatic event (e.g., subjective threat to life) and posttrauma variables (e.g., social support) have a stronger relationship to PTSD development than pretrauma, demographic variables such as age and gender. Specifically, we will examine three sets of risk and resiliency factors including pretrauma, trauma-related, and posttrauma factors that contribute to PTSD development.

Pretrauma Factors. Pretrauma factors are defined as characteristics of the child or the child's environment that existed or originated prior to the traumatic event (e.g., demographic variables, family history of psychopathology, temperament). These factors have produced somewhat inconsistent findings and appear to be less related to PTSD development than trauma-related and post-event variables (Trickey et al., 2012). First, as previously discussed, children who are younger appear to be more likely to develop PTSD (Chen et al., 2002; Green et al., 1991; Trickey et al., 2012). Some researchers have suggested that younger children may be more susceptible to PTSD due to a lack of cognitive resources, including a limited understanding of the world, fewer coping skills, and fewer opportunities to rely on community support (e.g., Vernberg, 1999). Bokszczanin (2007) provided some support for this theory, suggesting that older adolescent boys, as compared to adolescent females and younger females and males, reported the lowest level of distress following a Poland flood and participated the most in post-disaster community repair. However, others have found that following trauma exposure, older children and adolescents are more likely to develop PTSD (Copeland et al., 2007; Khamis, 2005). For example, following exposure to various types of traumatic events, adolescents aged 14–16 years displayed higher levels of posttraumatic stress symptoms than children aged 9–13 years (Copeland et al., 2007). Overall, recent meta-analytic findings suggest that age plays a small role in PTSD development (Trickey et al., 2012). Some researchers have suggested that developmental stage and emotional or cognitive maturity may have more of an impact on PTSD development than actual child age (Khamis, 2005; Margolin & Vickerman, 2007). Thus, in order to deepen our knowledge of the role of age in predicting PTSD development, future researchers may benefit from examining the child's developmental stage rather than chronological age. For example, clinicians and researchers may want to consider a child's level of cognitive, language, emotional, and social development as well as the achievement of developmental skills and milestones when assessing trauma-related symptoms (Chu & Lieberman, 2010).

Second, similar to findings in adults (e.g., Foa & Tolin, 2008), female gender appears to be associated with PTSD development (e.g., Foster et al., 2004; Osofsky et al., 2009; Schwab-Stone et al., 1995; Thabet et al., 2008; Walker, Carey, Mohr, Stein, & Seedat, 2004) but the effect is small (Trickey et al., 2012). Generally, some have suggested that female children are more likely to develop internalizing symptoms (e.g., anxiety/distress) following trauma exposure, whereas boys report higher levels of externalizing symptoms, such as anger (e.g., Cummings, Iannotti, & Zahn-Waxler, 1985). Given that a number of PTSD symptoms are internalizing in nature (e.g., reexperiencing symptoms such as repeatedly thinking about the event), this may partially explain the link between higher rates of PTSD in females. Furthermore, recent evidence suggests that male and female children may respond differently when exposed to similar traumas, which may partially account for the

observed higher rates of PTSD among females. For example, in a sample of inner-city youth aged 11–16 years old, girls responded with distress both when they were victims of violence and when witnessing violence (Foster et al., 2004). However, boys were more likely to develop psychological symptoms from being victimized than from witnessing violence (Foster et al., 2004). Thus, trauma-related symptoms, such as PTSD, are likely determined by a number of interacting factors such as gender and trauma type.

Third, pretrauma child characteristics (e.g., temperament, psychopathology) have been linked to risk for PTSD development. For example, children with a history of pretrauma psychopathology appear to have a higher likelihood of developing PTSD following trauma exposure (Copeland et al., 2007; La Greca, Silverman, & Wasserstein, 1998; Lengua, Long, Smith, & Meltzoff, 2005; Paradise, Rose, Sleeper, & Nathanson, 1994). Both internalizing problems such as anxiety and externalizing problems have been shown to increase risk for PTSD development following exposure to multiple types of trauma, such as a natural disaster (La Greca et al., 1998). Among children exposed to the September 11, 2001, terrorist attacks, higher pretrauma depression, more externalizing problems, and low self-esteem were related to a higher number of PTSD symptoms postexposure to September 11, 2001, attacks (Lengua et al., 2005). Moreover, Paradise and colleagues (1994), in a review of medical records, found that children receiving treatment for sexual abuse were more likely to have been previously (i.e., pretrauma) treated by a psychiatrist (for non-abuse-related reasons) than children admitted to the hospital for other reasons (e.g., injury, illness). Additionally, there is a small but growing body of evidence to suggest that temperament may play an important role in posttraumatic stress reactions following trauma exposure (Werner & Smith, 1982; Wertlieb, Weigel, Springer, & Feldstein, 1987). Temperament is broadly defined as an emotional and behavioral style that is consistent across time and situations (Derryberry & Rothbart, 1988). Negative emotionality and poor effortful control (e.g., attention regulation, inhibitory skills) have been suggested as possible dispositional characteristics that may lead to increased risk for PTSD in children following potentially traumatic events (e.g., Lengua et al., 2005; Salmon & Bryant, 2002; Wilson, Lengua, Meltzoff, & Smith, 2010). Overall, child temperament and/or pretrauma psychopathology appears to influence risk for PTSD in children and adolescents.

Fourth, an adverse family environment appears to influence posttrauma psychopathology, including PTSD (Copeland et al., 2007; De Bellis, Hooper, Woolly, & Shenk, 2010; Ostrowski, Christopher, & Delahanty, 2007). For example, among children aged 8–18 years old, lower family income was significantly associated with higher levels of PTSD symptoms following exposure to a pediatric injury (Ostrowski et al., 2007). Some have suggested (e.g., Desjarlais, Eisenberg, Good, & Kleinman, 1995; Khamis, 2005) that living in a poor environment may hinder individuals from accessing resources that are necessary (e.g., health services, community support) to ward off the impact of traumatic stress.

Finally, there is limited research examining the impact of culture and ethnicity on trauma exposure and PTSD development. Rates of some types of trauma exposure such as homicide (Centers for Disease Control and Prevention, 2010) and maltreatment (Sedlak et al., 2010) are reportedly higher among African American children and adolescents than other ethnic groups. After exposure to a hurricane, African American children reported higher levels of PTSD symptoms than Caucasian children or other minority children (e.g., Shannon, Lonigan, Finch, & Taylor, 1994). However, others have not found ethnic differences in rates of PTSD (e.g., Russoniello et al., 2002; Vernberg, 1999). Overall, research on cultural and ethnic factors associated with trauma exposure and PTSD development among children and adolescents is limited.

Pretrauma factors such as demographic variables and pretrauma psychopathology appear to influence PTSD development following trauma exposure, although the effects are generally in the small range. These variables are likely to interact and be influenced by other subsequent factors such as the nature of the trauma exposure and posttrauma events such as family support and coping strategies.

Trauma-Related Factors. There are a number of variables associated with the traumatic event itself that influence PTSD development (e.g., severity of trauma, subjective perception of threat of danger). A recent meta-analysis (Trickey et al., 2012) suggests that subjective trauma-related variables such as perception of threat may be more influential in predicting PTSD development in children than objective trauma characteristics (e.g., duration or severity of event).

Interpersonal traumas (e.g., physical or sexual abuse) appear to be related to higher rates of PTSD than non-interpersonal traumas (e.g., serious accident) (e.g., Copeland et al., 2007; Lonigan, Shannon, Taylor, Finch, & Sallee, 1994; Rossman, Hughes, & Rosenberg, 2000). For example, rates of PTSD following serious pediatric injury range from about 5 to 16 % (Landolt, Vollrath, Ribi, Gnehm, & Sennhauser, 2003), whereas rates of PTSD following exposure to interparental abuse range from 13 to 50 % (Rossman et al., 2000). Generally, among adults, it appears that interpersonal trauma creates an ongoing sense of fear and threat (Forbes et al., 2012), leading to an increased risk of PTSD. Further research in children and adolescent populations is needed to understand factors that contribute to an increased risk of PTSD following interpersonal trauma.

Second, exposure to multiple traumatic events increases the odds of developing PTSD among children and adolescents (Jaffee, Caspi, Moffitt, Polo-Tomas, & Taylor, 2007; Grych, Jouriles, Swank, McDonald, & Norwood, 2000; Thabet et al., 2008; Copeland et al., 2007). Children who are victims of dual violence (e.g., interparental violence and parent–child violence) tend to report higher levels of psychological distress than children exposed to only one type of violence (Grych et al., 2000; Jaffee et al., 2007). It appears that experiencing one type of violence in the home increases a child's risk for experiencing additional trauma. For example, child abuse is 18 times more likely to occur in families where interparental violence is present (Straus & Smith, 1990). Margolin and Vickerman (2007) suggest that child abuse and dual violence may lead to a child developing a low self-esteem due to a lack of family cohesion and low familial social support. Similarly, low self-esteem may result from other factors such as self-blame. Often, children may develop a sense of self-blame, believing that they should have done more to stop or prevent the violence (Silvern, Karyl, & Landis, 1995). Others suggest that the accumulation of stress from multiple traumatic experiences places children on a risk trajectory for developing psychopathology, including PTSD (Jaffee et al., 2007; Margolin & Vickerman, 2007). For example, children in an environment filled with chronic trauma exposure may feel a sense of constant danger or threat of danger, even when the traumatic event is not being witnessed or experienced (Kaysen, Resick, & Wise, 2003). Overall, exposure to multiple traumatic events places children at an increased risk of developing PTSD.

Finally, traumatic events with a high likelihood of "secondary stressors" (Shaw et al., 1996) are associated with an increased risk for both developing and maintaining PTSD. Children living in a war zone experience high rates of PTSD, which may partially be due to the fact that additional stressors are likely to occur. Such secondary stressors may include being exiled, separation from family members, damage to property, or experiencing a loss of belongings (e.g., Ajdukovic, 1998; Kuterovac, Dyregrov, & Stuvland, 1994; Thabet et al., 2008). For example, among 45 adolescents aged 14–19 exposed to the war in the Republic of Croatia, posttrauma psychopathology was associated with exposure to a higher number of stressful events (Ajdukovic, 1998). Exposure to natural disasters, such as a hurricane, may also lead to high levels of experience of secondary stressors. For example, high rates of PTSD (85 %) were exhibited among children 8 weeks after exposure to Hurricane Andrew, which was likely due to the experience of secondary stressors such as parental unemployment, loss of home or belongings, and school disruption (Shaw et al., 1995).

Trauma-related factors impact posttrauma distress including PTSD development. Generally, factors such as trauma type and severity appear influential in PTSD development. Yet, these factors likely interact with pre- and posttrauma variables to determine risk or resiliency following trauma exposure.

Posttrauma Factors. Variables that occur or are present after the traumatic event (e.g., family response, coping strategies) are determined to be posttrauma factors. Among adults, lack of social support appears to be one of the strongest risk factors for PTSD development (Brewin, Andrews, & Valentine, 2000; Ozer, Best, & Lipsey, 2003). There is accumulating evidence to suggest a similar pattern in children and adolescents (Pine & Cohen, 2002; Valentino, Berkowitz, & Stover, 2010; Vernberg et al., 1996). Overall, it appears that positive support is a protective factor following trauma exposure (e.g., Thabet et al., 2008), whereas hostile support (Valentino et al., 2010) or a lack of support is a risk factor for PTSD development.

Generally, researchers suggest that in the aftermath of a traumatic event, multiple sources of support (e.g., peer, family, parental) are beneficial (Vernberg et al., 1996). Yet, parental support seems to be the most influential or primary source of support (Masten, 2001; Thabet et al., 2008; Valentino et al., 2010; Vernberg et al., 1996) determining risk or resiliency following trauma. In a generalized trauma sample of youth between 7 and 17 years old, youth report of hostile and coercive parenting was significantly associated with higher levels of PTSD symptoms (Valentino et al., 2010). Although parents may be the primary source of support, additional sources of support are important as well. In the aftermath of community trauma (e.g., natural disaster), teachers may also provide a sense of support for children by providing factual information about the event and resuming normal, pretrauma scheduling and routines (Vernberg et al., 1996; Vernberg & Vogel, 1993). In some cultures, such as the African American community, relationships with extended family in particular are related to better psychological adjustment (Taylor, Seaton, &

Dominguez, 2008). Thus, for some cultures, extended family relationships may be linked to resiliency following trauma. Generally, social support from multiple sources following child and adolescent trauma exposure appears to play a salient role in recovery.

Many theorists have highlighted the role of cognitions in the development and continuation of PTSD in adults (e.g., Ehlers & Clark, 2000). Evidence for the role of trauma-related cognitions in PTSD among adults suggests that negative beliefs about the self (i.e., self as incompetent) and the world (i.e., the world is dangerous) are associated with PTSD development (e.g., O'Donnell, Elliott, Wolfgang, & Creamer, 2007). There is a growing body of evidence to suggest that cognitive attributions and strategies following trauma exposure affect PTSD development in children and adolescents as well (Durakovic-Belko, 2003; Ehlers, Mayou, & Bryant, 2003; Kolko, Brown, & Berliner, 2002; Meiser-Stedman, Dalgleish, Glucksman, Yule, & Smith, 2009; Silvern et al., 1995). In particular, it appears that a negative posttrauma worldview, such as a pessimistic view of the future, has been associated with PTSD severity in children (e.g., Schwarzwald, Weisenberg, Solomon, & Waysman, 1997). Stallard and Smith (2007) examined 75 children and adolescents between the ages of 7 and 18 years who were involved in motor vehicle accidents and found that a sense of alienation from others, future danger, and negative permanent change were associated with higher levels of PTSD symptoms. Similarly, negative attributional styles and negative self-views (i.e., shame) following trauma, such as abuse, are related to poorer adjustment and increased risk of PTSD (e.g., Feiring, Taska, & Lewis, 2002; Lewis, 1992). For example, in a sample of 137 sexually abused children and adolescents, abuse-specific internal attributions (i.e., blaming self for the abuse) and shame were associated with higher levels of psychopathology, including PTSD (Feiring, Taska, & Chen, 2002). Generally, negative trauma-related beliefs about the self and world appear to impact PTSD development.

Finally, parental distress following child trauma exposure appears to be related to PTSD development (McFarlane, 1987; Ostrowski et al., 2007; Trickey et al., 2012). Some have theorized that parental avoidance in particular may be related to PTSD symptoms in children (McFarlane, 1987). Adults may aim to protect their children from additional emotional distress by not discussing the traumatic event (Steward, O'Connor, Adredolo, & Steward, 1996). Yet, although parents may believe they are shielding their children from distress, parental hesitation to confront or discuss emotional difficulties may hinder the child's ability to express or resolve their own psychological distress (McFarlane, 1987). Ostrowski and colleagues (2007) examined both maternal and child PTSD symptoms (e.g., reexperiencing, avoidance, and hyperarousal) among 41 children and adolescents aged 8–18 years following a pediatric injury. Findings suggested that maternal symptoms, particularly avoidance, were associated with more posttraumatic stress symptoms in children (Ostrowski et al., 2007). Thus, it appears that parental distress may influence their child's reaction following trauma exposure.

Overall, determining vulnerability or resiliency following trauma among children and adolescents is complex and determined by multiple factors. Meta-analytic findings suggest that posttrauma variables (e.g., social support) appear to be the most strongly associated with PTSD development among both children and adolescents as well as adults (e.g., Ozer et al., 2003; Trickey et al., 2012). It is likely that risk factors and protective factors interact with one another. Many have suggested (e.g., Vogt, King, & King, 2007) that pathways leading to PTSD development are multi-determined and considering multiple risk factors is important.

Diagnosis and Phenomenology

Historically, the criteria for a diagnosis of PTSD in both children and adolescents have been similar to that in adults and guided by the Diagnostic and Statistical Manual for Mental Disorders (DSM). In order to be diagnosed with PTSD, based on DSM-V (APA, 2013) criteria, a child must be exposed to a traumatic event. A traumatic event may include directly experiencing a trauma (e.g., experiencing sexual abuse, serious injury, etc.), witnessing a traumatic event (e.g., witnessing a murder), learning about a traumatic event that occurred to a close family member or friend (e.g., learned about a parental trauma), or experiencing repeated or extreme exposure to aversive details of a traumatic event (not through media such as movies) (APA, 2013). In addition to the exposure to a traumatic event, the child or adolescent must experience symptoms in four different clusters including re-experiencing (e.g., upset by trauma reminders), avoidance (e.g., pushing away trauma-related thoughts or feelings), negative cognitions and mood (e.g., self-blame), and arousal (e.g., hypervigilance) in order to be diagnosed with PTSD (APA, 2013).

Previous versions of the DSM acknowledged that children may display some of these symptoms differently than adults. Researchers and clinicians have suggested that these criteria were not developmentally appropriate or sensitive (e.g., Aaron, Zaglul, & Emery, 1999; Carrion, Weems, Ray, & Reiss, 2002; Levendosky, Huthbocks, Semel, & Shapiro, 2002; Scheeringa, Zeanah, & Cohen, 2011). For example, a large portion of trauma-exposed children and adolescents failed to meet the threshold for a DSM-IV (APA, 1994) PTSD diagnosis, yet report similar levels of impairment as those who meet diagnostic criteria (e.g., Aaron et al., 1999; Carrion et al., 2002). Examining 59 trauma-exposed children aged 7-14 years, Carrion and colleagues (2002) found that individuals meeting the criteria for all three DSM-IV symptom clusters of PTSD (e.g., at least 1 re-experiencing, 3 avoidance, and 2 hyperarousal symptoms) did not significantly differ from individuals meeting criteria for only two symptom clusters of PTSD (e.g., 1 re-experiencing, 1 avoidance, and 2 hyperarousal symptoms) on levels of impairment or emotional distress. The DSM-V (APA, 2013) now includes a developmental subtype for PTSD in pre-school aged children, which includes children less than 6 years of age, in order to account for developmental considerations. These revised criteria include a reduction in the number of avoidance symptoms required for a PTSD diagnosis.

Childhood and adolescence are times of critical physical, emotional, psychological, and social growth and development (Davis & Siegel, 2000). Thus, the expression of PTSD symptoms may vary widely depending on the developmental age of the child. Young children often display PTSD symptoms in more behavioral and limited ways, such as play (Perrin, Smith, & Yule, 2000) or regressive behaviors such as enuresis or thumb-sucking (Armsworth & Holaday, 1993). Language development may partially account for this symptom presentation. For example, preschool-age children who have been sexually abused often do not possess the proper grammar, vocabulary, or language skills necessary to describe the details of the sexual event (Poole & Lamb, 1998).

Scheeringa, Zeanah, & Cohen (2011) advocated altering the DSM criteria for a PTSD diagnosis in young children (i.e., preschool age), by placing more emphasis on behavioral manifestations of symptoms. For example, many young children fail to meet the 3-symptom threshold for the avoidance/numbing symptom cluster of PTSD (Scheeringa, Peebles, Cook, & Zeanah, 2001). Many of the avoidance symptoms of PTSD (e.g., avoidance of thoughts or feelings associated with the traumatic event) require a high level of cognitive and abstract reasoning. Older children are able to avoid thinking about traumatic reminders or distressing thoughts by shifting their attention to happier or more pleasing thoughts (Harris, 1994). However, these are skills that young children have likely not yet developed (Scheeringa, Zeanah, & Cohen, 2011).

Overall, it is important to create developmentally sensitive criteria for a diagnosis of PTSD in children and adolescents in order to ensure proper assessment and treatment. Missed or improper diagnosis may lead to inappropriate treatment plans or lack of intervention. Given that PTSD in youth appears to be chronic and unremitting if left untreated (e.g., Meiser-Stedman et al., 2008; Scheeringa et al., 2005), a proper diagnosis is the first step in providing adequate clinical care to reduce the potentially long-lasting emotional distress and psychosocial impairment of these children.

PTSD Treatment in Children and Adolescents

In contrast to the large literature examining treatment for PTSD in adults, there is relatively limited data examining effective treatment options for youth. Generally, relatively few randomized controlled treatment trials have been conducted in youth samples (Stallard, 2006). Psychotherapy, particularly trauma-focused therapy, has demonstrated effectiveness in the treatment of PTSD for children and adolescents (Cohen et al., 2010; Silverman et al., 2008). The National Child Traumatic Stress Network (NCTSN) has been integral in disseminating the information and training in evidence-based treatment for youth with PTSD (Pynoos et al., 2008). Pharmacotherapy has been less examined, and the evidence for the use of medication to treat PTSD in youth is limited (Huemer, Erhart, & Steiner, 2010). However, evidence is growing for the use of selective serotonin reuptake inhibitors (SSRIs; Seedat, Lockhat, Kaminer, Zungu-Dirwayi, & Stein, 2001) in this population.

Psychotherapy. There has recently been an increased focus on evaluating the efficacy of psychotherapy for children and adolescents with PTSD (e.g., Feeny, Foa, Treadwell, & March, 2004). The recent guidelines for the assessment and treatment of PTSD in youth, put forth by the *American Academy of Child and Adolescent Psychiatry* (Cohen et al., 2010), state that trauma-focused therapy, as opposed to other treatments (e.g., nondirective psychotherapy or pharmacotherapy), should be considered as the first-line treatment for PTSD in youth. There is evidence for both trauma-focused psychoanalytic (Trowell et al., 2002) and cognitive behavioral therapy for PTSD (e.g., Silverman et al., 2008). However, only one randomized controlled trial has been conducted on psychoanalytic therapy for children with PTSD (Trowell et al., 2002), and all participants had sexual abuse-related PTSD. Thus, more evidence with diverse samples is needed to explore the generalizability of these findings.

Trauma-focused cognitive behavioral therapy (TF-CBT; Cohen, Mannarino, & Deblinger, 2006) has received the most empirical support for the treatment of PTSD in youth (Feeny et al., 2004; Kowalik, Weller, Venter, & Drachman, 2011; Silverman et al., 2008). There are a growing number of well-controlled, randomized clinical trials supporting TF-CBT's effectiveness in children and adolescents (e.g., Cohen, Deblinger, Mannarino, & Steer, 2004; Cohen & Mannarino, 1996; Deblinger, Lippman, & Steer, 1996). Recent evidence suggests that TF-CBT can be effective for children as young as 3 years old (Scheeringa, Weems, Cohen, Amaya-Jackson, & Guthrie, 2011). TF-CBT is a brief cognitive behavioral therapy, often lasting for approximately 12–18 sessions, and involves both the child and a non-offending parent (Cohen et al., 2006). In general, children are taught behavioral and cognitive strategies in order to express their emotions effectively, challenge and change unhelpful thought patterns, and reduce their overall distress (Cohen et al., 2006). The parental component involves teaching the parent helpful ways to respond to their child's trauma, discussing effective parent–child communication strategies, and encouraging the parent to support their child in practicing the skills they learn in therapy (Cohen et al., 2006).

In many trials, TF-CBT has provided greater PTSD symptom reduction than other treatments including individual nondirective supportive therapy (Cohen & Mannarino, 1996) and client-centered therapy (Cohen et al., 2004). For example, in a large, randomized trial of 229 sexually abused children aged 8–14 years old, TF-CBT provided greater symptom reduction than client-centered therapy. In addition, TF-CBT provided more symptom reduction in other areas of functioning including depression and externalizing problems (Cohen et al., 2004). Despite TF-CBT's overall effectiveness, 21 % of children who received TF-CBT retained their PTSD diagnosis at posttreatment. Thus, future research should explore potential mechanisms and processes of change that occur during TF-CBT in order to highlight for whom and under what conditions treatment works best for children with PTSD.

Overall, trauma-focused treatment appears to be effective in the treatment of PTSD for children and adolescents. Given that there are still some children who do not significantly benefit from the current evidence-based psychotherapy options, there has been a growing interest in exploring other treatment modalities, such as pharmacotherapy, for the treatment of PTSD in this population.

Pharmacotherapy. The evidence for the use of medication to treat PTSD in youth is limited, and no medications are FDA approved for PTSD in children. There are few well-conducted, randomized controlled trials of medication treatments for PTSD in this population. Despite limited data to support the use of medication for PTSD in children and adolescents, a high proportion of child psychiatrists report prescribing medication for the treatment of PTSD in this population (Cohen, Mannarino, & Rogal, 2001). In fact, in a survey of child psychiatrists, 95 % reported using pharmacotherapy to treat PTSD in children and adolescents (Cohen et al., 2001). In this survey, child psychiatrists reported prescribing antidepressants, anticonvulsants, antipsychotics, and alpha- and beta-adrenergic blocking agents to treat PTSD in children (Cohen et al., 2001).

Among adults with PTSD, effective pharmacotherapy treatment options exist, particularly SSRIs. Recently, researchers have begun to examine the efficacy of SSRI treatment for PTSD in children and adolescents (Cohen, Mannarino, Perel, & Staron, 2007; Robb, Cueva, Sporn, Yang, & Vanderburg, 2010; Seedat et al., 2001, 2002; Yorbik, Akbiyik, Kirmizigul, & Söhmen, 2004). However, some caution that the effectiveness of this medication in adults may not be applicable to children due to differences in neurobiological functioning and structures (Cohen, 2001; Pervanidou, 2008). For example, neurological, biological, and cognitive changes occur during development, and therefore there may be differences in the effectiveness of medications between adults and children.

There is tentative evidence to suggest that SSRIs are effective in reducing PTSD symptoms (e.g., Seedat et al., 2001). Yet, most studies to date examining the efficacy of SSRIs in children have been characterized by small sample sizes, lack of control groups, no randomization to treatment conditions, and only short-term follow-up. Moreover, in a recent randomized controlled trial comparing the effectiveness of sertraline, an SSRI, to placebo in 131 children aged 6–17 years old with PTSD, both placebo and sertraline produced similar reductions in PTSD (Robb et al., 2010). Thus, at this point in time, most have concluded that there is limited support for the efficacy of pharmacotherapy treatment in children and adolescents (Huemer et al., 2010; Nikulina et al., 2008; Wethington et al., 2008).

Some have suggested that pharmacotherapy, such as an SSRI, may be useful as an add-on treatment to psychotherapy for children with PTSD (Cohen et al., 2007).

In a recent small trial, Cohen and colleagues (2007) examined the efficacy of adding an SSRI to TF-CBT. A group of 24 sexually abused children and adolescents between the ages of 10 and 17 years old were randomly assigned TF-CBT, TF-CBT plus sertraline, or TF-CBT plus placebo for 12 weeks (Cohen et al., 2007). Results indicated that both groups experienced similar reductions in PTSD symptoms. Based on these findings, the authors suggest an initial trial of psychotherapy prior to adding medication for children with PTSD. Importantly, one-third of participants referred to complete this study refused participation due to concerns related to administering medication (Cohen et al., 2007). Thus, it appears that many parents do not want their children to receive medication for trauma-related symptoms.

Overall, there has been an increase in research examining the effectiveness of pharmacotherapy for child and adolescent PTSD. Given the small number of trials examining the efficacy of medication, the evidence for the effectiveness of this treatment modality is limited. The recent guidelines for treatment of PTSD in children and adolescents (Cohen et al., 2010) suggest that combination treatment (i.e., adding a medication to psychotherapy) may be helpful when a child has severe PTSD, a co-occurring psychological disorder that also requires treatment, or a poor response to psychotherapy.

Neurobiological Correlates of PTSD

Trauma exposure and PTSD development affect multiple facets of a child's development including emotional, cognitive, behavioral, and physiological functioning. Recent research has begun to shed light on the neurobiological impact of trauma exposure and PTSD development (e.g., De Bellis et al., 2010; Jackowski, Araujo, de Lacerda, Jesus Mari, & Kaufman, 2009; van der Kolk, 2003). Yet, there is still a great deal of information to be explored in this area. Analyzing the neurobiology of PTSD has the potential to improve our understanding of the pathways leading to PTSD development and inform treatment options.

PTSD appears to produce alterations in biological systems that regulate stress response (De Bellis, Baum, Birmaher, Keshavan, & Ryan, 1999; van der Kolk, 2003). A number of neural systems seem to be altered by trauma exposure, particularly those involved in memory formation and emotional responsivity (e.g., van der Kolk, 2003). Theoretically, researchers have proposed that PTSD influences neurobiological functioning in three primary ways (van der Kolk, 2003). First, PTSD affects the maturational processes of the structures of the brain. Second, PTSD affects neuroendocrine and chemical release (van der Kolk, 2003). Finally, PTSD influences the interactions among biological, cognitive, affective, and behavioral functioning (Pechtel & Pizzagalli, 2011; van der Kolk, 2003). Generally, it appears that neurodevelopment may be particularly impacted by chronic long-term trauma (e.g., De Bellis et al., 1999).

Many brain structures have been investigated as playing a role in PTSD development including the amygdala (e.g., Carrion et al., 2001; De Bellis, Hall, Boring, Frustaci, & Moritz, 2001; Karl et al., 2006; Woon & Hedges, 2008), hippocampus (e.g., De Bellis et al., 2010), and prefrontal cortex (e.g., Richert, Carrion, Karchemskiy, & Reiss, 2006). However, findings have generally been inconclusive. The amygdala, which plays a role in threat assessment and emotional responses (Shin, Rauch, & Pitman, 2006), has been found to have a reduced volume in adults with PTSD

(e.g., Karl et al., 2006). However, results have been mixed among children and adolescents, with some suggesting no differences in amygdala volume between PTSD and control groups (e.g., De Bellis et al., 2001) and others finding a reduction in amygdala volume in children with PTSD (e.g., Carrion et al., 2001). The prefrontal cortex, which serves a variety of neurocognitive functions including regulating (e.g., activating or inhibiting) the activity in other brain structures such as the amygdala and hippocampus (Shimamura, 2000), has also been an area of interest (e.g., Richert et al., 2006).

The hippocampus, a brain structure involved in learning and memory, is the structure which has received the most empirical attention. In particular, the hippocampus plays a critical role in the ability to consciously recall previous life events (Fanselow, 2000). Generally, adults with child abuse-related PTSD appear to have a smaller hippocampal volume than both non-PTSD trauma-exposed adults and healthy controls (e.g., Bremner et al., 1997; Stein, Koverola, Hanna, Torchia, & McClarty, 1997). However, these findings have not been well replicated in child and adolescent samples (e.g., De Bellis et al., 2001, 2010). For example, De Bellis and colleagues (2010) examined neurobiological correlates of PTSD in three groups of children: children with a maltreatment history, children with a maltreatment history and PTSD, and children with no maltreatment. Overall, no significant difference in hippocampal volume emerged (De Bellis et al., 2010). However, PTSD was associated with lower visual memory. These findings suggest that although children with PTSD may not have structural hippocampal abnormalities, hippocampal dysfunction may still be present.

Overall, childhood and adolescence are periods of rapid and discontinuous brain development. Trauma exposure during these critical periods may have a particularly detrimental effect on both structural and functional development (Schwartz & Perry, 1994). The increasing technology and accessibility to neuroimaging techniques continues to provide powerful tools for the examination of neural disruptions associated with PTSD in youth. Future research is needed to more clearly examine the impact of trauma on neural development. In general, the majority of neurobiological research has been limited to child abuse survivors. Thus, less is known regarding the impact of other traumas (e.g., natural disaster) on long-term neural dysregulation. In addition, age of trauma may be a critical factor in predicting neurobiological disruptions, given that development occurs discontinuously (e.g., van der Kolk, 2003).

Conclusions and Future Directions

Trauma exposure during childhood and adolescence is common, with approximately two-thirds of children reporting exposure to a traumatic event by the age of 16 (Copeland et al., 2007). Although trauma is common, PTSD develops in only a small subset of children and adolescents. A recent meta-analysis suggests that subjective experiences of the traumatic event itself, as well as posttrauma variables, such as family support, appear to be the strongest predictors of PTSD development in children and adolescence (Trickey et al., 2012). Pretrauma or demographic variables have only a small impact on PTSD development. This is encouraging, given that posttrauma variables are potentially modifiable. Social support appears to be particularly influential in predicting PTSD development in children and adolescents. Clinicians can work with children and their primary support network (e.g., parents) to provide stable, supportive environments to effectively recover from a traumatic experience. Clinicians and researchers should also consider cultural factors when working with children with PTSD. With regard to social support, it appears that some cultures may benefit from utilizing support from their extended family (e.g., Taylor et al., 2008). For other children, it may be that parental support is particularly influential. Overall, ethnic and cultural variables associated with PTSD development and treatment in youth have been underexamined. However, among all cultures, following trauma exposure, activating and utilizing one's social support network is important for recovery.

Given that childhood and adolescence encompass such a broad age range, it will be important for future research to take into account the developmental stage and maturity of a child during trauma exposure when examining risk for PTSD. Research on PTSD in youth has encompassed a wide age range and various types of trauma exposure. Given the rapid pace of cognitive, affective, and behavioral advances that occur throughout childhood, it may be beneficial to examine subgroups of children to examine differential effects of trauma exposure.

Recently, in order to examine the validity and efficacy of the previous DSM-IV criteria for a PTSD diagnosis, researchers have begun to examine the usefulness of the diagnostic criteria among very young children (e.g., ages 3–6; Cohen & Mannarino, 1996; Scheeringa, Zeanah, & Cohen, 2011). These findings have helped to provide guidelines to clinicians and researchers regarding potential differences in symptom presentation of PTSD among specific age groups and have been influential in shaping the PTSD criteria for preschool age children in the current version of the DSM, the DSM-V (APA, 2013). For example, young children may be more likely to display behavioral, as opposed to verbal, symptoms. In addition, findings regarding the neurobiological impact of trauma have been somewhat inconclusive. Given that children develop at different rates, it may be important for researchers to examine not only the effects of chronological age but also the impact of developmental age on the neural effects of PTSD. Overall, taking into account developmental stage when examining the effects of trauma on youth will be beneficial for advancing our current understanding.

PTSD was not introduced into the DSM until 1980. Thus, the disorder is relatively new. Developmental considerations and diagnostic algorithms for PTSD are still being refined for children and adolescents (e.g., Scheeringa, Zeanah, & Cohen, 2011) and are now incorporated into the DSM-V. The continued effort in refining the diagnosis will be helpful in guiding the successful treatment of PTSD. Currently, trauma-focused therapy is suggested as the first-line treatment for youth with PTSD (Cohen et al.,

2010). Medication, particularly SSRIs, has shown some promise in the treatment of PTSD, but evidence is limited. Future research with large, diverse samples and randomized assignment to treatment groups will help to expand our understanding of efficacy of pharmacotherapy for youth with PTSD. In addition to efficacy of a particular treatment, clinicians and researchers should examine parent and child treatment preference. For example, Cohen and colleagues (2007) reported that a large portion of their referrals refused to participate in their treatment trial comparing TF-CBT vs. TF-CBT plus medication, due to concerns with medication. In addition, there are no published studies to date comparing the efficacy of the first-line psychotherapy for PTSD in youth to medication. Therefore, evidence for the use of medication in this population is limited.

Overall, there has been a recent growth of empirical literature examining PTSD diagnosis and treatment among youth. Given the high rates of trauma exposure and resulting symptoms in this population, future research is needed to refine the PTSD diagnosis and enhance the delivery of treatment for children and adolescents.

References

Aaron, J., Zaglul, H., & Emery, R. E. (1999). Posttraumatic stress in children following acute physical injury. *Journal of Pediatric Psychology, 24*, 335–343.

Ajdukovic, M. D. (1998). Displaced adolescents in Croatia: A source of stress and post-traumatic stress reaction. *Adolescence, 33*, 209–217.

American Psychiatric Association. (1994). *Diagnostic and statistical manual of mental disorders* (4th ed.). Washington, DC: American Psychiatric Association.

Armsworth, M. W., & Holaday, M. (1993). The effects of psychological trauma on children and adolescents. *Journal of Counseling and Development, 72*(1), 49–56.

Bokszczanin, A. (2007). PTSD symptoms in children and adolescents 28 months after a flood: Age and gender differences. *Journal of Traumatic Stress, 20*, 347–351.

Boney-McCoy, S., & Finkelhor, D. (1995). Psychosocial sequelae of violent victimization in a national youth sample. *Journal of Consulting and Clinical Psychology, 63*, 726–736.

Bremner, J. D., Randall, P., Vermetten, E., Staib, L., Bronen, R. A., Mazure, C., et al. (1997). Magnetic resonance imaging-based measurement of hippocampal volume in posttraumatic stress disorder related to childhood physical and sexual abuse- A preliminary report. *Biological Psychiatry, 41*(1), 23–32.

Brent, D. A., Oquenda, M., Birmaher, B., Greenhill, L., Kolko, D., Stanley, B., et al. (2002). Familial pathways to early-onset suicide attempt. *Archives of General Psychiatry, 59*, 801–807.

Breslau, N. (2001). The epidemiology of posttraumatic stress disorder: What is the extent of the problem? *Journal of Clinical Psychiatry, 62*(17), 16–22.

Brewin, C. R., Andrews, B., & Valentine, J. D. (2000). Meta-analysis risk factors for posttraumatic stress disorder in trauma-exposed adults. *Journal of Consulting and Clinical Psychology, 68*, 748–766.

Carrion, V. G., Weems, C. F., Eliez, S., Patwardhan, A., Brown, W., Ray, R. D., et al. (2001). Attenuation of frontal asymmetry in pediatric posttraumatic stress disorder. *Biological Psychiatry, 50*, 943–951.

Carrion, V. G., Weems, C. F., Ray, R., & Reiss, A. L. (2002). Toward an empirical definition of pediatric posttraumatic stress disorder: The phenomenology of posttraumatic stress disorder symptoms in youth. *Journal of the American Academy of Child and Adolescent Psychiatry, 41*, 166–173.

Centers for Disease Control and Prevention. (2010). *Centers for Disease Control and Prevention: Youth violence: Facts at a glance.* Retrieved from http://www.cdc.gov/ViolencePrevention/youthviolence/index.html

Charuvastra, A., & Cloitre, M. (2008). Social bonds and posttraumatic stress disorder. *Annual Review of Psychology, 59*, 301–328.

Chen, S. H., Lin, Y. H., Tseng, H. M., & Wu, Y. C. (2002). Post-traumatic stress reactions in children and adolescents one year after the 1999 Taiwan Chi-Chi earthquake. *Journal of the Chinese Institute of Engineers, 25*(5), 597–608.

Chu, A. T., & Lieberman, A. F. (2010). Clinical implications of traumatic stress from birth to age five. *Annual Review of Clinical Psychology, 6*, 469–494.

Cohen, J. A. (2001). Pharmacologic treatment of children. *Trauma, Violence & Abuse, 2*(2), 155–171.

Cohen, J. A., Bukstein, O., Walter, H., Benson, S., Chrisman, A., Farchione, T. R., et al. (2010). Practice parameter for the assessment and treatment of children and adolescents with posttraumatic stress disorder. *Journal of the American Academy of Child and Adolescent Psychiatry, 49*(4), 414–430.

Cohen, J. A., Deblinger, E., Mannarino, A. P., & Steer, R. A. (2004). A multisite, randomized controlled trial for children with sexual abuse-related PTSD symptoms. *Journal of the American Academy of Child and Adolescent Psychiatry, 43*, 393–402.

Cohen, J., & Mannarino, A. (1996). A treatment outcome study for sexually abused preschool children: Initial findings. *Journal of the American Academy of Child and Adolescent Psychiatry, 35*, 42–50.

Cohen, J. A., Mannarino, A. P., & Deblinger, E. (2006). *Treating trauma and traumatic grief in children and adolescents.* New York: Guilford Press.

Cohen, J. A., Mannarino, A. P., Perel, J. M., & Staron, V. (2007). A pilot randomized controlled trial of combined trauma-focused CBT and sertraline for childhood PTSD symptoms. *Journal of the American Academy of Child and Adolescent Psychiatry, 46*, 811–819.

Cohen, J. A., Mannarino, A. P., & Rogal, S. (2001). Treatment practices for childhood posttraumatic stress disorder. *Child Abuse and Neglect, 25*, 123–135.

Copeland, W. E., Keeler, G., Angold, A., & Costello, J. (2007). Traumatic events and posttraumatic stress in childhood. *Archives of General Psychiatry, 64*, 577–584.

Cummings, E. M., Iannotti, R. J., & Zahn-Waxler, C. (1985). Influence of conflict between adults on the emotions and aggression of young children. *Developmental Psychology, 21*(3), 495–507.

Davis, L., & Siegel, L. (2000). Posttraumatic stress disorder in children and adolescents: A review and analysis. *Clinical Child and Family Psychology Review, 3*(3), 135–154.

De Bellis, M. D., Baum, A., Birmaher, B., Keshavan, M. S., & Ryan, N. D. (1999). Developmental traumatology part I: Biological stress systems. *Biological Psychiatry, 45*, 1259–1270.

De Bellis, M. D., Hall, J., Boring, A. M., Frustaci, K., & Moritz, G. (2001). A pilot longitudinal study of hippocampal volumes in pediatric maltreatment-related posttraumatic stress disorder. *Biological Psychiatry, 50*, 305–309.

De Bellis, M. D., Hooper, S. R., Woolly, D. P., & Shenk, C. E. (2010). Demographic, maltreatment, and neurobiological correlates of PTSD symptoms in children and adolescents. *Journal of Pediatric Psychology, 35*(5), 570–577.

Deblinger, E., Lippman, J., & Steer, R. A. (1996). Sexually abused children suffering posttraumatic stress symptoms: Initial treatment outcome findings. *Child Maltreatment, 1*, 310–321.

Derryberry, D., & Rothbart, M. K. (1988). Arousal, affect, and attention as components of temperament. *Journal of Personality and Social Psychology, 55*, 958–966.

Desjarlais, R., Eisenberg, L., Good, B., & Kleinman, A. (1995). *World mental health: Problems and priorities in low-income countries*. New York: Oxford University Press.

Durakovic-Belko, E. (2003). Determinants of posttraumatic adjustment in adolescents from Sarajevo who experienced war. *Journal of Clinical Psychology, 59*(1), 27–40.

Ehlers, A., & Clark, D. M. (2000). A cognitive model of posttraumatic stress disorder. *Behaviour Research and Therapy, 38*, 319–345.

Ehlers, A., Mayou, R. A., & Bryant, B. (2003). Cognitive Predictors of posttraumatic stress disorder in children: Results of a prospective longitudinal study. *Behaviour Research and Therapy, 41*, 1–10.

Fanselow, M. S. (2000). Contextual fear, gestalt memories, and the hippocampus. *Behavioural Brain Research, 110*(1–2), 73–81.

Feeny, N. C., Foa, E. B., Treadwell, K. R., & March, J. (2004). Posttraumatic stress disorder in youth: A critical review of the cognitive and behavioral treatment outcome literature. *Professional Psychology: Research and Practice, 35*, 466–476.

Feiring, C., Taska, L., & Chen, K. (2002). Trying to understand why horrible things happen: Attribution, shame, and symptom development following sexual abuse. *Child Maltreatment, 7*(1), 26–41.

Feiring, C., Taska, L., & Lewis, M. (2002). Adjustment following sexual abuse discovery: The role of shame and attributional style. *Developmental Psychology, 38*(1), 79–92.

Foa, E. B., & Tolin, D. F. (2008). Sex differences in trauma and posttraumatic stress disorder: A quantitative review of 25 years of research. *Psychological Bulletin, 132*(6), 959–992.

Forbes, D., Fletcher, S., Parslow, R., Phelps, A., O'Donnell, M., Bryant, R. A., et al. (2012). Trauma at the hands of another: Longitudinal study of differences in the posttraumatic stress disorder symptom profile following interpersonal compared with noninterpersonal trauma. *The Journal of Clinical Psychiatry, 73*(3), 372–376.

Foster, J. D., Kuperminc, G. P., & Price, A. W. (2004). Gender differences in posttraumatic stress and related symptoms among inner-city minority youth exposed to community violence. *Journal of Youth and Adolescence, 33*(1), 59–69.

Garrison, C. Z., Bryant, E. S., Addy, C. L., Spurier, P. G., Freedy, J. R., & Kilpatrick, D. G. (1995). Posttraumatic stress disorder in adolescents after Hurricane Andrew. *Journal of the American Academy of Child and Adolescent Psychiatry, 34*(9), 1193–1201.

Green, B. L., Korol, M., Grace, M. C., Vary, M. G., Leonard, A., Gleser, G. C., et al. (1991). Children and disaster: Age, gender, and parental effects on PTSD symptoms. *Journal of the American Academy of Child and Adolescent Psychiatry, 30*(6), 945–951.

Grych, J. H., Jouriles, E. N., Swank, P. R., McDonald, R., & Norwood, W. D. (2000). Patterns of adjustment among children of battered women. *Journal of Consulting and Clinical Psychology, 68*, 84–94.

Harris, P. L. (1994). The child's understanding of emotion: Developmental change and the family environment. *Journal of Child Psychology and Psychiatry, and Allied Disciplines, 35*, 3–28.

Horowitz, K., McKay, M., & Marshall, R. (2005). Community violence and urban families: Experiences, effects, and directions for intervention. *American Journal of Orthopsychiatry, 75*(3), 356–368.

Huemer, J., Erhart, F., & Steiner, H. (2010). Posttraumatic stress disorder in children and adolescents: A review of psychopharmacological treatment. *Child Psychiatry and Human Development, 41*, 624–640.

Hunt, K. L., Martens, P. M., & Belcher, H. M. E. (2011). Risky business: Trauma exposure and rate of posttraumatic stress disorder in African American children and adolescents. *Journal of Traumatic Stress, 24*(3), 365–369.

Jackowski, A., Araujo, C., de Lacerda, A., Jesus Mari, J., & Kaufman, J. (2009). Neurostructural imaging findings in children with post-traumatic stress disorder. *Psychiatry and Clinical Neurosciences, 63*, 1–8.

Jaffee, S., Caspi, A., Moffitt, T. E., Polo-Tomas, M., & Taylor, A. (2007). Individual, family, and neighborhood factors predict children's resilience to maltreatment: A cumulative stressors model. *Child Abuse and Neglect, 31*, 231–253.

Karl, A., Schaefer, M., Malta, L. S., Dorfel, D., Rohleder, N., & Werner, A. (2006). A meta-analysis of structural brain abnormalities in PTSD. *Neuroscience and Biobehavioral Reviews, 30*, 1004–1031.

Kaysen, D., Resick, P., & Wise, D. (2003). Living in danger: The impact of chronic traumatization and the traumatic context on posttraumatic stress disorder. *Trauma, Violence & Abuse, 4*(3), 247–264.

Kendall-Tackett, K. A., Williams, L. M., & Finkelhor, D. (1993). Impact of sexual abuse on children: A review and synthesis of recent empirical studies. *Psychological Bulletin, 113*, 164–180.

Khamis, V. (2005). Post-traumatic stress disorder among school age Palestinian children. *Child Abuse and Neglect, 29*, 81–95.

Kilpatrick, D. G., Ruggiero, K. J., Acierno, R., Saunders, B. E., Resnick, H. S., Best, C. L., et al. (2003). Violence and risk of PTSD, major depression, substance abuse/dependence, and comorbidity: Results from the national survey of adolescents. *Journal of Consulting and Clinical Psychology, 71*(4), 692–700.

Kolko, D. J., Brown, E. J., & Berliner, L. (2002). Children's perceptions of their abusive experiences: Measurement and preliminary findings. *Child Maltreatment, 7*, 42–55.

Kowalik, J., Weller, J., Venter, J., & Drachman, D. (2011). Cognitive behavioral therapy for the treatment of pediatric posttraumatic stress disorder: A review and meta-analysis. *Journal of Behavior Therapy and Experimental Psychiatry, 42*, 405–413.

Kuterovac, G., Dyregrov, A., & Stuvland, R. (1994). Children in war: A silent majority under stress. *British Journal of Medical Psychology, 67*, 363–375.

La Greca, A. M., Silverman, W. K., & Wasserstein, S. B. (1998). Children's predisaster functioning as a predictor of posttraumatic stress following Hurricane Andrew. *Journal of Consulting and Clinical Psychology, 66*, 883–892.

Landolt, M. A., Vollrath, M., Ribi, K., Gnehm, H. E., & Sennhauser, F. H. (2003). Incidence and associations of parental and child posttraumatic stress symptoms in pediatric patients. *Journal of Child Psychology and Psychiatry, and Allied Disciplines, 44*, 1199–1207.

Lengua, L. J., Long, A. C., Smith, K. A., & Meltzoff, A. N. (2005). Pre-attack symptomatology and temperament as predictors of children's response to the September 11th terrorist attacks. *Journal of Child Psychology and Psychiatry, 46*, 631–645.

Levendosky, A., Huth-bocks, A., Semel, M., & Shapiro, D. (2002). Trauma symptoms in preschool-age children exposed to domestic violence. *Journal of Interpersonal Violence, 17*(2), 150–164.

Lewis, M. (1992). *Shame, the exposed self*. New York: The Free Press.

Lonigan, C. J., Shannon, M. P., Taylor, C. M., Finch, A. J., & Sallee, F. R. (1994). Children exposed to disaster: Risk factors for the development of posttraumatic symptomatology. *Journal of the American Academy of Child and Adolescent Psychiatry, 33*, 94–105.

Luthra, R., Abramovitz, R., Greenberg, R., Schoor, A., Newcorn, J., Schmeidler, J., et al. (2009). Relationship between type of trauma exposure and posttraumatic stress disorder among urban children and adolescents. *Journal of Interpersonal Violence, 24*(11), 1919–1927.

Margolin, G., & Vickerman, A. (2007). Posttraumatic stress in children and adolescents exposed to family violence: I. Overview and issues. *Professional Psychology: Research and Practice, 38*(6), 613–619.

Masten, A. S. (2001). Ordinary magic: Resilience processes in development. *American Psychologist, 56*, 227–238.

McFarlane, A. C. (1987). Posttraumatic phenomena in a longitudinal study of children following a natural disaster. *Journal of the American Academy of Child and Adolescent Psychiatry, 26*, 764–769.

Meiser-Stedman, R., Dalgleish, T., Glucksman, E., Yule, W., & Smith, P. (2009). Maladaptive cognitive appraisals mediate the evolution of posttraumatic stress reactions: A 6-month follow-up of child and adolescent assault and motor vehicle accident survivors. *Journal of Abnormal Psychology, 118*(4), 778–787.

Meiser-Stedman, R., Smith, P., Glucksman, E., Yule, W., & Dalgleish, T. (2008). The Posttraumatic stress disorder diagnosis in preschool- and elementary school-age children exposed to motor vehicle accidents. *American Journal of Psychiatry, 165*, 1326–1337.

Molnar, B. E., Buka, S. L., & Kessler, R. C. (2001). Child sexual abuse and subsequent psychopathology: Results from the National Comorbidity Survey. *American Journal of Public Health, 91*(5), 753–760.

Nelson, E. C., Heath, A. C., Madden, P. A. F., Cooper, M. L., Dinwiddie, S. H., et al. (2002). Association between self-reported childhood sexual abuse and adverse psychosocial outcomes. *Archives of General Psychiatry, 59*, 139–145.

Nikulina, V., Hergenrother, J. M., Brown, E. J., Doyle, M. E., Filton, B. J., Carson, G. S., et al. (2008). From efficacy to effectiveness: The trajectory of the treatment literature for children with PTSD. *Expert Review of Neurotherapeutics, 8*(8), 1233–1246.

O'Donnell, M. L., Elliott, P., Wolfgang, B. J., & Creamer, M. (2007). Posttraumatic appraisals in the development and persistence of posttraumatic stress symptoms. *Journal of Traumatic Stress, 20*(2), 173–182.

Osofsky, H. J., Osofsky, J. D., Kroenenberg, M., Brennan, A., & Hansel, T. C. (2009). Posttraumatic stress symptoms in children after Hurricane Katrina: Predicting the need for mental health services. *American Journal of Orthopsychiatry, 79*(2), 212–220.

Ostrowski, S. A., Christopher, N. C., & Delahanty, D. L. (2007). The impact of maternal posttraumatic stress disorder symptoms and child gender on risk for persistent posttraumatic stress disorder symptoms in child trauma victims. *Journal of Pediatric Psychology, 32*, 338–342.

Ozer, E. J., Best, S. R., & Lipsey, T. L. (2003). Predictors of posttraumatic stress disorder and symptoms in adults: A meta-analysis. *Psychological Bulletin, 129*, 52–73.

Paradise, J., Rose, L., Sleeper, L., & Nathanson, M. (1994). Behavior, family function, school performance, and predictors of persistent disturbance in sexually abused children. *Pediatrics, 93*, 452–459.

Pechtel, P., & Pizzagalli, D. A. (2011). Effects of early life stress on cognitive and affective function: An integrated review of human literature. *Psychopharmacology, 214*, 55–70.

Perrin, S., Smith, P., & Yule, W. (2000). Practitioner review: The assessment of post-traumatic stress disorder in children and adolescents. *Journal of Child Psychology and Psychiatry, 41*(3), 277–289.

Pervanidou, P. (2008). Biology of post-traumatic stress disorder in childhood and adolescence. *Journal of Neuroendocrinology, 20*, 632–638.

Pine, D. S., & Cohen, J. A. (2002). Trauma in children and adolescents: Risk and treatment of psychiatric sequelae. *Biological Psychiatry, 51*, 519–531.

Poole, D. A., & Lamb, M. (1998). Investigative Interviewing of children: A guide for professionals. Washington DC: American Psychological Association.

Pynoos, R. S., Fairbank, J. A., Steinberg, A. M., Amaya-Jackson, L., Gerrity, E., & Mount, M. L. (2008). The National Child Traumatic Stress Network: Collaborating to improve the standard of care. *Professional Psychology: Research and Practice, 39*, 389–395.

Pynoos, R. S., Steinberg, A. M., & Piacentini, J. C. (1999). A developmental psychopathology model of childhood traumatic stress and intersection with anxiety disorders. *Biological Psychiatry, 46*, 1542–1554.

Resnick, H. S., Kilpatrick, D. G., Dansky, B. S., Saunders, B. E., & Best, C. L. (1993). Prevalence of civilian trauma and posttraumatic stress disorder in a representative national sample of women. *Journal of Consulting and Clinical Psychology, 61*(6), 984–991.

Richert, K. A., Carrion, V. G., Karchemskiy, A., & Reiss, A. L. (2006). Regional differences of the prefrontal cortex in pediatric PTSD: An MRI study. *Depression and Anxiety, 23*, 17–25.

Robb, A. S., Cueva, J. E., Sporn, J., Yang, R., & Vanderburg, D. G. (2010). Sertraline treatment of children and adolescents with posttraumatic stress disorder: A double-blind, placebo-controlled trial. *Journal of Child and Adolescent Psychopharmacology, 20*(6), 463–471.

Rossman, B. B. R., Hughes, H. M., & Rosenberg, M. S. (2000). *Children and interparental violence: The impact of exposure*. Philadelphia, PA: Taylor and Francis.

Russoniello, C. V., Skalko, T. K., O'Brien, K., McGhee, S. A., Bingham-Alexander, D., & Beatley, J. (2002). Childhood posttraumatic stress disorder and efforts to cope after Hurricane Floyd. *Behavioral Medicine, 28*, 61–71.

Salmon, K., & Bryant, R. A. (2002). Posttraumatic stress disorder in children: The influence of developmental factors. *Clinical Psychology Review, 22*, 163–188.

Saywitz, K. J., Mannarino, A. P., Berliner, L., & Cohen, J. A. (2000). Treatment for sexually abused children and adolescents. *American Psychologist, 55*, 1040–1049.

Scheeringa, M. S., Peebles, C. D., Cook, C. A., & Zeanah, C. H. (2001). Toward establishing procedural, criterion, and discriminant validity for PTSD in early childhood. *Journal of the American Academy of Child and Adolescent Psychiatry, 40*, 52–60.

Scheeringa, M. S., Weems, C. F., Cohen, J. A., Amaya-Jackson, L., & Guthrie, D. (2011). Trauma-focused cognitive-behavioral therapy for posttraumatic stress disorder in three-through six year-old children: A randomized clinical trial. *Journal of Child Psychology and Psychiatry, 52*(8), 853–860.

Scheeringa, M. S., Zeanah, C. H., & Cohen, J. A. (2011). PTSD in children and adolescents: Toward an empirically based algorithm. *Depression and Anxiety, 28*, 770–782.

Scheeringa, M. S., Zeanah, C. H., Myers, L., & Putnam, F. W. (2005). Predictive validity in a prospective follow-up of PTSD in preschool children. *Journal of the American Academy of Child and Adolescent Psychiatry, 44*(9), 899–906.

Schwab-Stone, M., Ayers, T., Kasprow, W., Voyce, C., Barone, C., Shriver, T., et al. (1995). No safe haven: A study of violence exposure in an urban community. *Journal of the American Academy of Child and Adolescent Psychiatry, 34*, 1343–1352.

Schwarz, E. D., & Perry, B. D. (1994). The post-traumatic response in children and adolescents. *Psychiatric Clinics of North America, 17*, 311–326.

Schwarzwald, J., Weisenberg, M., Solomon, Z., & Waysman, M. (1997). What will the future bring? Thoughts of children after missile bombardment. *Anxiety, Stress and Coping: An International Journal, 10*(3), 257–267.

Sedlak, A. J., Mettenburg, J., Basena, M., Petta, I., McPherson, K., Greene, A., et al. (2010). *Fourth national incidence study of child abuse and neglect (NIS–4): Report to congress*. Washington, DC: U.S. Department of Health and Human Services, Administration for Children and Families.

Seedat, S., Lockhat, R., Kaminer, D., Zungu-Dirwayi, N., & Stein, D. J. (2001). An open trial of citalopram in adolescents with post-traumatic stress disorder. *International Clinical Psychopharmacology, 16*(1), 21–25.

Seedat, S., Stein, D. J., Ziervogel, C., Middleton, T., Kaminer, D., Emsley, R. A., et al. (2002). Comparison of response to a selective serotonin reuptake inhibitor in children, adolescents, and adults with posttraumatic stress disorder. *Journal of Child and Adolescent Psychopharmacology, 12*, 37–46.

Shannon, M. P., Lonigan, C. J., Finch, A. J., & Taylor, C. M. (1994). Children exposed to disaster: I: Epidemiology of post-traumatic symptoms and symptom profiles. *Journal of the American Academy of Child and Adolescent Psychiatry, 33,* 80–93.

Shaw, J. A., Applegate, B., & Schorr, C. (1996). Twenty-one-month follow-up study of school-age children exposed to Hurricane Andrew. *Journal of the American Academy of Child and Adolescent Psychiatry, 35*(3), 359–364.

Shaw, J. A., Applegate, B., Tanner, S., Perez, D., Rothe, E., et al. (1995). Psychological effects of Hurricane Andrew on an elementary school population. *Journal of The American Academy of Child and Adolescent Psychiatry, 34*(9), 1185–1192.

Shimamura, A. P. (2000). The role of the prefrontal cortex in dynamic filtering. *Psychobiology, 28,* 207–218.

Shin, L. M., Rauch, S. L., & Pitman, R. K. (2006). Amygdala, medial prefrontal cortex, and hippocampal function in PTSD. *Annals of the New York Academy of Sciences, 1071,* 67–79.

Silverman, W. K., Ortiz, C. D., Viswesvaran, C., Burns, B. J., Kolko, D. J., Putnam, F. W., et al. (2008). Evidence-based psychosocial treatments for children and adolescents exposed to traumatic events. *Journal of Clinical Child and Adolescent Psychology, 37,* 156–183.

Silvern, L., Karyl, J., & Landis, T. Y. (1995). Individual psychotherapy for the traumatized children of abused women. In E. Peled & P. G. Jaffe (Eds.), *Ending the cycle of violence* (pp. 43–76). Thousand Oaks, CA: Sage.

Stallard, P. (2006). Psychological interventions for post-traumatic reactions in children and young people: A review of randomised controlled trials. *Clinical Psychology Review, 26*(7), 895–911.

Stallard, P., & Smith, E. (2007). Appraisals and cognitive coping styles associated with chronic post-traumatic symptoms in child road traffic accident survivors. *Journal of Child Psychology and Psychiatry, 48,* 194–201.

Stein, M. B., Koverola, C., Hanna, C., Torchia, M. G., & McClarty, B. (1997). Hippocampal volume in women victimized by childhood sexual abuse. *Psychological Medicine, 27*(4), 951–959.

Steward, M. S., O'Connor, J., Adredolo, C., & Steward, D. S. (1996). The trauma and memory of cancer treatment in children. In M. H. Bornstein & J. L. Genevro (Eds.), *Child development and behavioral pediatrics* (pp. 105–128). Mahwah, NJ: Lawrence Erlbaum and Associates.

Straus, M. A., & Smith, C. (1990). Family patterns and child abuse. In M. A. Straus & R. J. Gelles (Eds.), *Physical violence in American families: Risk factors and adaptations to violence in 8,145 families* (pp. 507–525). New Brunswick, NJ: Transaction Publishing.

Taylor, R. D., Seaton, E., & Dominguez, A. (2008). Kinship support, family relations and psychological adjustment among low-income African-American mothers and adolescents. *Journal of Research on Adolescence, 18,* 1–22.

Thabet, A. A., Abu Tawahina, A., El Sarraj, E., & Vostanis, P. (2008). Exposure to war trauma and PTSD among parents and children in the Gaza strip. *European Child and Adolescent Psychiatry, 17*(4), 191–199.

Trickey, D., Siddaway, A. P., Meiser-Stedman, R., Serpell, L., & Field, A. (2012). A meta-analysis of risk factors for post-traumatic stress disorder in children and adolescents. *Clinical Psychology Review, 32,* 122–138.

Trowell, J., Kolvin, I., Weeramanthri, T., Sadowski, H., Berelowitz, M., Galsser, D., et al. (2002). Psychotherapy for sexually abused girls: Psychopathological outcome findings and patterns of change. *British Journal of Psychiatry, 180,* 234–247.

Valentino, K., Berkowitz, S., & Smith Stover, C. (2010). Parenting behaviors and posttraumatic symptoms in relation to children's symptomatology following a traumatic event. *Journal of Traumatic Stress, 23*(3), 403-407.

van der Kolk, B. A. (2003). The neurobiology of childhood trauma. *Child and Adolescent Psychiatric Clinics of North America, 21*(1), 293–317.

Vernberg, E. M. (1999). Children responses to disaster: Family and system approaches. In R. Gist & B. Lubin (Eds.), *Response to disaster: Psychological, community and ecological approaches* (pp. 193–209). Washington, DC: Taylor & Francis.

Vernberg, E. M., Silverman, W. K., La Greca, A. M., & Prinstein, M. J. (1996). Prediction of posttraumatic stress symptoms in children after hurricane Andrew. *Journal of Abnormal Psychology, 105,* 237–248.

Vernberg, E. M., & Vogel, J. (1993). Interventions with children following disasters. *Journal of Clinical Child Psychology, 22,* 485–498.

Vogt, D. S., King, D. W., & King, D. W. (2007). Risk pathways for PTSD: Making sense of the literature. In M. J. Friedman, T. M. Keane, & P. A. Resick (Eds.), *Chapter 6: Handbook of PTSD Science and Practice.* New York: Guilford Press.

Walker, J. L., Carey, P. D., Mohr, N., Stein, D. J., & Seedat, S. (2004). Gender differences in the prevalence of childhood sexual abuse and in the development of pediatric PTSD. *Archives of Women's Mental Health, 7*(2), 111–121.

Werner, E. E., & Smith, R. S. (1982). *Vulnerable but invincible: A longitudinal study of resilient children and youth.* New York: McGraw-Hill.

Wertlieb, D., Weigel, C., Springer, T., & Feldstein, M. (1987). Temperament as a moderator of children's stressful experiences. *American Journal of Orthopsychiatry, 57,* 234–245.

Wethington, H. R., Hahn, R. A., Fuqua-Whitley, D. S., Sipe, T. A., Crosby, A. E., Johnson, R. L., et al. (2008). The effectiveness of interventions to reduce psychological harm from traumatic events among children and adolescents: A systematic review. *American Journal of Preventive Medicine, 35*(3), 287–313.

Wilson, A. C., Lengua, L. J., Meltzoff, A. N., & Smith, K. A. (2010). Parenting and temperament prior to

September 11, 2001 and parenting specific to 9/11 as predictors of children's post-traumatic stress symptoms following 9/11. *Journal of Clinical Child & Adolescent Psychology, 39*(4), 445–459.

Woon, F. L., & Hedges, D. W. (2008). Hippocampal and amygdala volumes in children and adults with childhood maltreatment-related posttraumatic stress disorder: A meta-analysis. *Hippocampus, 18*, 729–736.

Yorbik, O., Akbiyik, D. I., Kirmizigul, P., & Söhmen, T. (2004). Post-traumatic stress disorder symptoms in children after the 1999 Marmara earthquake in Turkey. *International Journal of Mental Health, 33*, 46–58.

Dissociative Disorders in Children and Adolescents

39

Joyanna L. Silberg

There is a widespread national and international interest in the neurophysiological and psychological effects of trauma on youth. This interest has been sparked in part by recent scientific developments in the field of neuroscience documenting that clear-cut brain abnormalities result from children's early exposure to domestic violence, verbal abuse, physical abuse, sexual abuse, and neglect (Teicher, Samson, Polcari, & McGreenery, 2006). There have been a record number of natural disasters worldwide in the last fifteen years with increased professional awareness of the enduring effect on the children exposed to these, as well as increasing documentation of the effects on children of terrorism, displacement, and ongoing armed warfare (Brom, Pat-Horenczyk, & Ford, 2008).

Parallel to this developing professional interest in childhood trauma, there has been increased attention to dissociation, a psychological process associated with trauma that presents in traumatized children with dazed states, confusion in identity, and dysregulations in behavior, mood, cognitions, somatic experiences, and relationships. Dissociation in children and adolescents has been increasingly documented by a variety of researchers and clinicians who have found that

dissociative symptoms are often associated with histories of severe trauma.

The field of dissociative disorders in adults underwent a significant resurgence in the early 1980s with a variety of books (i.e., Kluft, 1985a, 1985b; Putnam, 1989; Ross, 1989) and a major NIMH-funded research study (Putnam, Guroff, Silberman, Barban, & Post, 1986) showing that adults diagnosed with multiple personality disorder (MPD, now renamed dissociative identity disorder, DID) had documented histories of severe sexual and physical abuse in childhood. The contemporary identification of children and adolescents with dissociative disorders began in the early 1980s when Fagan and McMahon (1984) discussed four cases of children and young adolescents who presented with marked shifts in identity, severe self-destructive behaviors, and loss of memory for recent events and noted these children had a clear history of trauma including sexual and physical abuse. Fagan and McMahon described treating these children fairly rapidly compared to their adult counterparts and suggested that the early manifestations of dissociation in children be called "incipient multiple personality disorder." Kluft (1984, 1985a, 1985b) described the use of hypnotherapy techniques with several cases of children with early signs of multiple personality disorder, some of whom also had parents with the disorder.

By the late 1980s and early 1990s, additional case histories and larger case series of dissociative children began to appear in the literature (Albini & Pease, 1989; Coons, 1996; Dell &

J.L. Silberg, Ph.D. (✉)
The Sheppard Pratt Health System, Baltimore, MD 21285, USA
e-mail: jsilberg@sheppardpratt.org; jlsilberg@aol.com

M. Lewis and K.D. Rudolph (eds.), *Handbook of Developmental Psychopathology*, DOI 10.1007/978-1-4614-9608-3_39, © Springer Science+Business Media New York 2014

Eisenhower, 1990; Hornstein & Tyson, 1991; Klein, 1985; Riley & Mead, 1988) and single case reports (Jacobsen, 1995; Laporta, 1992; Peterson, 1991; Snow, White, Pilkington, & Beckman, 1995). Hornstein and Putnam (1992) collected the largest series of patients from two sites and describe 64 children showing amnesia, trance states, self-destructive behavior, profound fluctuations, a sense of divided identity, hallucinations, and an array of posttraumatic and other comorbid symptoms.

As research has proliferated, researchers have documented a strong association between a history of sexual abuse in children and adolescents and dissociative symptoms (Bonanno, Noll, Putnam, O'Neill, & Trickett, 2003; Collin-Vézina & Hébert, 2005; Macfie, Cicchetti, & Toth, 2001). Dissociative symptoms in sexual abused children correlate to early onset of sexual abuse and multiple perpetrators (Trickett, Noll, & Putnam, 2011) and are associated with risk-taking behaviors (Kisiel & Lyons, 2001). Sexual abuse from caregivers may be one of the most confusing forms of maltreatment which may set the stage for dissociation in children and adolescents. Forced to engage with caregivers in this invasive and intimate way, multiple sets of confusing and competing feelings may be aroused at the same time—pleasure and pain, dependency and fear, love and rage, shame and intimacy, and the feelings of betrayal aroused when a caregiver is also an abuser may contribute powerfully to dissociative processes (Freyd, 1998). Dividing their awareness may help children cope with this array of contradictory feelings. Some research has found that physical abuse may produce even higher levels of dissociation in young children (Hulette, Freyd, & Fisher, 2011; Macfie et al., 2001).

Impaired caregiving is also associated with higher levels of dissociation. For example, research has found correlations between dissociation and parents who are psychologically insensitive and avoidant (Dutra, Bureau, Holmes, Lyubchik, & Lyons-Ruth, 2009), neglectful (Ogawa, Sroufe, Weinfield, Carlson, & Egeland, 1997), inconsistent and rejecting (Mann & Sanders, 1994), and punitive (Kim, Trickett, & Putnam, 2010). High levels of dissociation and

dissociative disorders have also been found in children following war trauma (Cagiada, Camaido, & Pennan, 1997) and medical trauma (Diseth, 2006; Silberg, 2011; Stolbach, 2005). Children's experience of multiple types of trauma are associated with the highest levels of dissociation (Hulette et al., 2011; Hulette, Fisher, Kim, Ganger, & Landsverk, 2008; Teicher et al., 2006).

Dissociative symptoms are more frequently found in girls and tend to worsen with age becoming more similar to adult presentations (Putnam, Hornstein, & Peterson, 1996). Significant levels of dissociation have been found in a variety of populations of children and adolescents receiving psychiatric care including delinquent adolescents (Carrion & Steiner, 2000), adolescents with sexual behavior problems (Friedrich et al., 2001; Leibowitz, Laser, & Burton, 2011), adolescents who engage in risk-taking behaviors (Kisiel & Lyons, 2001), and general psychiatric inpatients (Brunner, Parzer, Schuld, & Resch, 2000; Goffinet, 2005).

While research continues to document the prevalence of dissociation as a measurable symptom in a variety of clinical populations, research on treatment of dissociation in children has lagged behind that of dissociation in adults. In 1996, the first book on childhood dissociation treatment appeared (Shirar, 1996), closely followed by my own edited volume *The Dissociative Child* (Silberg, 1996/1998). Frank Putnam's (1997) book made significant advances in our understanding of dissociation in children by providing theoretical underpinnings for understanding dissociative phenomena in children. The International Society for the Study of Trauma and Dissociation (ISST-D, formerly known as the International Society for the Study of Dissociation or ISSD) published guidelines for the treatment of children and adolescents in 2003 (ISSD, 2003). These guidelines were developed by expert clinicians from around the world and were developed for children with a variety of diagnoses who manifest dissociative symptoms, rather than being confined only to children who show the most severe dissociative symptoms. As chair of that guideline task force, I worked with my colleagues to comb and organize the existing literature and integrate it with the results of our developing expertise. A recent book contains contributions by many of the guideline task force members and has added significantly to the treatment literature. The book, *Dissociation in Traumatized Children and Adolescents*, provides a collection of international case studies and details the step-by-step treatment of dissociative children and adolescents across the age span (Wieland, 2011). A treatment model for the comprehensive care of dissociative children and teens has recently been published (Silberg, 2013) which outlines a treatment approach which moves methodically from psychoeducation through affect regulation techniques into trauma processing and resolution. A main feature of this approach includes helping the dissociative child or teen accept and embrace dissociated material so that gaps in awareness are minimized.

Although professional interest in dissociation in children and adolescents has expanded in the last decade, evaluation and treatment of dissociative children and adolescents is still relatively unfamiliar to clinicians. Recognition of dissociative symptoms and disorders in children is important as many dissociative symptoms can be mistaken for other childhood psychiatric problems for which the treatment approach differs markedly. For example, the dazed states of dissociative children may be confused with symptoms of attention deficit, and the voices many dissociative children hear internally may be confused with signs of a psychotic process. These misdiagnoses can lead to the misuse of medications which may have no effect on dissociative symptoms or may lead to clinicians missing some subtle signs of abuse. On the other hand, careful attention to dissociative processes among clinical providers will lead to significant benefits to children in their care, as recent clinical reports indicate that these conditions are fairly treatable with early intervention averting the extreme and morbid course of the disorder in adulthood (Silberg, 2013; Wieland, 2011; Wieland & Silberg, 2013).

Currently, there is increasing recognition of dissociative symptoms and disorders in children and adolescents, with recent books (Silberg, 2013; Wieland, 2011), chapters in textbooks (Silberg, 2001a; Silberg & Dallam, 2009; Waters, 2012; Wieland & Silberg, 2013), and journal articles researching how dissociation correlates with a variety of other symptoms and trauma-related variables as described above. Yet there remains an absence of agreed-upon protocols for symptom assessment, and so large cohorts of uniformly diagnosed dissociative youngsters have not yet been carefully studied (Boysen, 2011).

Theoretical Overview

One of the leading theories explaining dissociation is the structural dissociation model developed by Van der hart, Nijenhuis, and Steele (2006). According to this model, the brain's adaptive system involved in daily activities and the defensive system involved in fear reactions and self-defense become disconnected from each other during trauma. According to the structural dissociation model, further trauma can divide the split parts of the personality into further fragments, what is called secondary and then tertiary dissociation. Van der Hart and colleagues advocate a therapeutic approach that builds attachment and security of the adaptive part of the personality, simultaneously reducing the fear and avoidance of the emotional part of the personality.

Child clinicians familiar with the concepts of developmental psychopathology often find this model too mechanistic to explain the development of dissociation in children and adolescents whose dissociative fragmentation is best viewed as a developmental lack of integration, rather than a "splitting." As pointed out by Michael Lewis (1992), the notion of the unitary self may be a late developing Western idea, as other cultures see the self as multifaceted, dual, or heavily linked with social roles or group identity. Dissociative manifestations may be one cultural bound way that children with disruptions in the development of a unified self may present. According to Lewis, a developing child confronted with experiences of sexual abuse may be overwhelmed by the affect shame and to avoid the overwhelming pain of this experience may disconnect from the shame-filled self, adopting a self-conception that allows avoidance of this affect state. Separated self-conceptions may manifest in dissociative identity states. Kluft (2007), a key theorist and innovator in the field of adult dissociative disorders, has also emphasized that the affect of shame underlies severe dissociative pathology.

Feiring, Taska, and Lewis (1996) suggest that the shame after sexual abuse stems from the experience of stigmatization and the negative attributions about the self associated with these stigmatizing experiences. The absence of support enhances these shame-based conceptions of self that result from sexual abuse. In fact, research has found that feelings of shame as measured by cognitions such as feeling exposed, dirty, and wanting to hide are associated with increased posttraumatic stress symptomatology in sexually abused children (Feiring & Taska, 2005; Feiring, Taska, & Lewis, 2002).

Putnam's discrete behavioral states model of dissociation (Putnam, 1997) also views the phenomenon from a more developmentally sensitive viewpoint. Putnam based his theories on observations from the infant observation studies of Peter Wolff (1987) who identified the basic states of infants observed throughout the day—deep sleep, to REM sleep, to crying, to fussy, to alert. As the babies developed, Wolff observed increasing flexibility between states. In contrast, Putnam theorized that a rigidity and impermeability between fear-based states characterized the chronically traumatized child. According to Putnam, normal development involves a process of alternating and shifting states, and flexibility and freedom to move within states is a hallmark of health and normal development. Putnam further theorizes that attentive responses of a loving caregiver promote the independent self-regulation that is characteristic of the emotionally healthy child. On the other hand, the chronically traumatized child has rigid and impermeable states that are resistant to self-regulation as they are triggered automatically by traumatic environmental cues.

Important theoretical advances to our understanding of dissociation have been offered by the attachment literature as disorganized attachment provides an early prototype of the blank looks, avoidant eye gaze, and shifting affect of children exposed to inconsistent and abusive caregivers (Lyons-Ruth, Dutra, Schuder, & Bianchi, 2006). As described by Liotti (2009), a child lacking consistent caregiving may develop contrasting internal working models, or expectation of caregiver response, and alternate in their responses, trying to make internal sense of the shifting and inconsistent environment to which they are exposed. In fact, longitudinal research has found that disorganized attachment styles can predict dissociation in teenagers, lending strong support to the theoretical association between disorganized attachment and dissociation (Ogawa et al., 1997).

My own, affect avoidance theory of dissociation (Silberg, 2013), relies on Putnam's insights, the insights from attachment theories, as well as Tomkins' affect theory to explain the automatic shifts in state seen in dissociative children and adolescents. According to Tomkins (1962), "affect scripts" are collections of learned associations between affect, what stimulated them, and behaviors that provide useful responses to these affects. Practiced scripts can begin to take on a life of their own and are increasingly relied on for dealing with affect in rote and automatic ways. For example, the affect of shame, associated with sexual abuse and other emotionally painful affective memories of abusive interactions with caregivers, can become particularly acute over time. Avoidance of this affect through practiced behavioral scripts of attack provides a successful method for learning to deal with the pain associated with shame. According to affect avoidance theory, new scripts evolve to develop avoidance to the arousal of affects associated with trauma— terror, humiliation, disgust—and these painful affects are soon mistaken for the sources of trauma themselves and thus in turn provoke avoidance scripts of their own. The traumatized child engages in practiced, automatic behavioral scripts evoked by multiple triggers in the environment. As the process of affective awareness becomes disrupted in traumatized children, these children miss out on the basic building blocks of identity and consciousness. Affect, which normally helps to integrate a developing sense of self by connecting similar experiences and promoting self-awareness, becomes instead a signal of avoidance, memory loss, initiation of nonconscious action plans, and disorganization.

In this model, dissociation is the activation of automatic thoughts, behaviors, identities, or affect scripts which become increasingly autonomous and outside the child's or teen's awareness. This model points the way to a clear approach to treatment—the dissociative child in treatment must focus on the transitional moments that trigger these automatic programs of response and learn to identify, express, and regulate the affective responses that they are avoiding. A key treatment intervention is also the detoxification of shame-based self-conceptions so that the self that experiences the shamed affect can find a way to be tolerated within the entire self-conception of the child.

Some children may have inborn predispositions to cope with trauma with dissociative strategies, perhaps due to fantasy-proneness, hypnotizability, or interpersonal sensitivity (Silberg, 2013), and some research suggests a possible genetic component of dissociative traits (Jang, Paris, Zweig-Frank, & Livelsey, 1998).

Assessing Dissociation in Children and Adolescents

The current DSM 5 contains four categories of dissociative disorders. The most severe disorder is dissociative identity disorder (DID), which is characterized by marked discontinuity in a sense of identity and gaps in autobiographical memory. Children with significant dissociative symptoms may be better characterized as having other specified dissociative disorder (OSDD), as the alterations in identity may not be as marked as seen in adults and the gaps in memory may be more amenable to rapid intervention. The other categories of dissociative amnesia, characterized by global memory loss for autobiographical details of one's life, or depersonalization/derealization disorder are less common in the pediatric population.

Assessment may be aided by a variety of assessment tools that have been developed to identify dissociative symptoms in children and adolescents. Frank Putnam's 20-question parent report screening instrument, the Child Dissociative Checklist (CDC), asks parents or observers to rate from 0 to 2 how often a child evidences behaviors such as rapid regressions, fluctuation states, vivid imaginary friends, disavowed behaviors, sleep disruptions, and sexual precocity (Putnam, Helmers, & Trickett, 1993). Stolbach's, Children's Dissociative Experience Scale and Traumatic Stress Inventory (Silberg, 2013; Stolbach, 1997) asks latency age children to rate how alike or different they are to children with described dissociative and posttraumatic traits. In 1997, Armstrong and colleagues introduced the Adolescent Dissociative Experiences Scale (A-DES) that allows adolescents to rate how frequently they experience a variety of dissociative symptoms including amnesia, passive influence, depersonalization, and fantasy involvement, through the contexts of school, family, and friends (Armstrong, Putnam, Carlson, Libero, & Smith, 1997; Smith & Carlson, 1996). This measure has been translated to a variety of languages and culturally appropriate norms developed (Nilsson & Svedin, 2006; Shin, Jeong, & Chung, 2009; Soukup, Papežová, Kuběna, & Mikolajová, 2010; Zoroglu, Sar, Tuzun, Tutkun, & Savas, 2002). Silberg developed an Imaginary Friends Questionnaire based on research comparing hospitalized children with normal preschoolers (Silberg, 1998a, 2013) and also found that dissociative children showed unique behaviors on standard psychological testing and showed dissociative themes in their projective stories (Silberg, 1998b). The Multidimensional Inventory of Dissociation (Dell, 2006) is an inventory that taps phenomenological aspects of dissociation and covers 23 symptoms. An adolescent version has undergone preliminary testing in the United States (Ruths, Silberg, Dell, & Jenkins, 2002) and Belgium (Goffinet, 2005), and the symptom picture pattern in adolescent with dissociative pathology closely mirrors adult symptomatology. Briere's Trauma Symptom Checklist for Children (1996) and Briere's Trauma Symptom Checklist for Young Children (2005) include scales that assess dissociation. Researchers have developed a posttraumatic stress disorder and dissociation scale from a composite of items in the commonly used Child Behavior Checklist (Achenbach, 1991; Sim et al., 2005).

While these screening measures are helpful as an initial tool, it is through the clinical interview that the clinician will gain entrance into the phenomenological world of the child with dissociative symptoms or disorders. Questionnaires and screening tools serve a useful functioning in steering the evaluator regarding what to inquire about in more detail.

Sometimes clinicians are caught off guard by dramatic dissociative presentations, with children or adolescents changing their voices, carriage, and manner and identifying themselves with different names. Even the most skeptical clinician witnessing these dramatic presentations will soon come to appreciate the complexity and intransigence of dissociative processes. These cases, where clients perceptibly shift identities and amnesia is displayed, are best diagnosed as dissociative identity disorder. However, it is more common for the child or adolescent client to present with more subtle symptomatology, best diagnosed as other specified dissociative disorder not otherwise specified, and a careful clinical interview that covers several major symptoms areas may uncover these hidden dissociative processes. Table 39.1 summarizes the key symptoms that children and teens with dissociative symptoms may display which covers five important categories—perplexing shifts in consciousness; hallucinatory phenomena; fluctuations in behavior, affects, and skills; difficulties with memory; and unusual somatic manifestations.

Perplexing Shifts in Consciousness

Children with dissociative symptoms and disorders may have unusual lapses in attention and focus. Some parents and teachers describe that they may have a blank look on their face "as if no one is home." These episodes may appear seizure-like, but on careful interview the child may be able to tell you that he/she was in an imaginary world or hearing the sound of an imaginary friend talking to them. Unlike many children with

Table 39.1 Five classes of symptoms related to dissociation

1. Perplexing shifts in consciousness
   Momentary lapses in consciousness or shutdown states that could last for hours
   Entry into flashback states where present and past are confused
   Sleep anomalies including sleepwalking, difficulty being aroused, sleeplessness, or having personality changes upon afwakening from deep sleeps
   Feeling in a fog, or not in one's own body, depersonalization
   Feeling that one's sense of self shifts markedly

2. Vivid hallucinatory experiences
   Hearing voices
   Seeing ghosts or other imaginary entities that interact with them
   Vivid imaginary friends and belief that these can "take over" or influence behavior
   Feeling younger or markedly older than one's chronological age

3. Marked fluctuations in knowledge, moods, or patterns of behavior and relating
   Feeling one's moods have a "mind of their own"
   Extreme changes in relationships with family members
   Skills and abilities are inconsistent
   Sense of one's self as divided
   Extreme behaviors that seem uncharacteristic—sexual promiscuity, extreme aggression

4. Perplexing memory lapses for one's own behavior or recently experienced events
   Cannot remember what happened during an angry episode
   Cannot remember whole months or years of life (after age 4 or 5)
   Cannot remember assignments that one has completed
   Cannot remember experiences with friends or family that others report

5. Abnormal somatic experiences
   Shifting somatic complaints
   Self-harming behaviors
   Conversion symptoms, pseudoseizures
   Pain insensitivity
   Bowel or bladder incontinence

Reprinted with permission of author from *The Child Survivor: Healing Developmental Trauma and Dissociation*, Routledge, 2013

attention deficit disorders, they may not appear distractible or impulsive when not paying attention, but internally focused, as if in a trance.

Sometimes these profound changes in awareness may be severe and last for several hours. The child or teen seems lost in a trance and not easily aroused. Perry (2002) has recommended use of naltrexone to reverse these severe states that may follow overwhelming trauma and understands these kinds of episodes as sensitization and dysregulation of the central nervous system opioid systems which have been repeatedly activated due to extreme stress (Perry, Pollard, Blakely, Baker, & Vigilante, 1995). Some children, no longer exposed to severe trauma, may enter these profound states of dissociative shutdown at seemingly minor provocation, when stimuli reminiscent of the trauma are aroused (Silberg, 2013). Many of these children are worked up for seizure disorders by neurologists and ultimately are diagnosed with PNES (psychogenic nonepileptic seizures) as no EEG findings are found. Sometimes these states will include flashback reenactments where children or teens seem caught in a bad dream with shouts of "no" and body movements that may simulate a violent assault. These psychogenic episodes tend to last longer than neurological seizures and when the patients awaken they are more clearheaded, not showing the lethargy and confusion that follows EEG-documented seizures (Luther, McNamara, Carwile, Miller, & Hope, 1982). Some dissociative clients may have particular difficulty upon awakening from sleep, may show aggressive behavior with little awareness, enter regressed states, or be difficult to arouse.

Clinicians observing these profound changes in consciousness may feel out of their element, but it is important to remember that these states involve a component of self-hypnosis, so that suggestive comments by the clinician, soothing talk, and a calming therapeutic presence of a clinician may play a large role in helping restore the child to a state of wakefulness and awareness.

Children and teens may also complain of changes in their sense of identity—feeling like when they are angry or upset, it is not really them. Sometimes they have colorful ways of describing these changes in identity, as one 14-year-old sexual abuse victim stated, "Adrenalin Man takes over when I get angry." Some adopted children may believe that a part of themselves retains the name they had in a pre-adoptive home, and it is important to inquire about nicknames, previous names, or what various people call the child to further assess this subjective sense of identity

shift. Case histories have documented that children may be called different names as they move between households of divorcing families, which may lead to a disjointed sense of self and divided identity particularly if one of the homes is a source of trauma (Baita, 2011).

Depersonalization experience, seeing oneself as if through a fog or through a camera lens as if in a movie, is a common perception of teens with significant dissociative symptoms. Sometimes they will feel like their own body does not belong to them or feel a sense that it is not really them when they look in a mirror. When this is the primary symptom, teens may qualify for the diagnosis of depersonalization disorder/derealization disorder. It is important to differentiate these symptoms from the effects of chronic use of drugs such as marijuana which can also produce symptoms of depersonalization in young people. The onset of depersonalization/derealization disorder tends to be around the age of 16, and it is associated with a history of emotional abuse. This disorder is particularly difficult to treat both in teenagers and adults (Simeon, Guralnik, Schmeidler, Sirof, & Knutelska, 2001; Simeon, Knutelska, Nelson, & Guralnik, 2003).

Hallucinatory Experiences

Hallucinatory phenomenon are commonly found in dissociative clients, but clinicians should be aware that hearing voices is increasingly recognized as a more common problem among child and adolescent clients than once thought (Altman, Collins, & Mundy, 1997) and can be associated with a history of traumatic events (Arseneault et al., 2011). When asking children or adolescents if they hear voices, clinicians should find other ways to inquire as children identify "hearing voices" with automatic hospitalization and will deny this rather than acknowledge something that they believe will be interpreted as very serious. Instead, clinicians can ask, "Do you sometimes hear the sound of people who you used to know talking to you?" and "Do you hear pretend friends in your mind talking to you or giving you advice?" The most difficult voice that dissociative children cope with is the harassing sound of past perpetrators of abuse that they may hear in their mind often commanding them to act out in the abusive ways they themselves have experienced. When responding to these internal harassing voices, children may become extremely aggressive, agitated, or speak in an uncharacteristically gruff voice, with inappropriate language apparently mirroring an abuser's behavior.

When young children describe hearing the sound of imaginary friends in their mind, it is often difficult to distinguish these from the developmentally normative experiences of many young children. About 28 % of normal children may have imaginary friends (Taylor, 1999) and these imaginary creations serve normal developmental functions, assisting with role development, working out internal conflicts, and providing a form of stimulating fantasy play. The voices or imaginary friends of dissociative children can be distinguished from these normal phenomena by their often malevolent influence on the child's behavior, the lack of memory the child might have for behavior performed under the influence of these voices, and the child's belief that these imaginary phenomena are "real" (Mclewin & Muller, 2006; Silberg, 2013; Trujillo, Lewis, Yeager, & Gidlow, 1996). Unlike dissociative children, normal children have no problem identifying their imaginary friends as fantasy creations, under their own control. Normal children usually dispense with their imaginary friends by the age of 8, whereas dissociative children may describe having their imaginary friends way into their teens. A series of questions that may assist with uncovering these processes in teenagers are to ask, "Did you ever have imaginary friends when you were younger? Do you sometimes think they are still there?" Once the clinician finds out about these imaginary friends, questions about their roles, their feelings, and how they influence behavior can follow.

Younger children may also see the imaginary friends, pointing to where they have entered the room through a window or door and can describe them sitting on a couch. These vivid perceptions are common with children with dissociative features and do not in themselves indicate a psychotic process.

Fluctuations

The rapid fluctuations seen in dissociative children are confusing to caregivers and teachers who often pereceive that these changes are not precipitated. Generally, an internal or external stimulus associated with a traumatic reminder may instigate these rapid changes. For example, a teenage girl hid under her desk and began sucking her thumb while watching a movie with her high school class. Later, she revealed that a scene in the movie of a large open meadow looked like the site of a violent rape she had experienced and triggered this regressive behavior. Other dramatic changes in behavior may be more concerning, as children may engage in dangerous self-destructive behavior, engage in risky sexual encounters or sexualized behaviors (Grimminck, 2011), or use illicit substances. In a large data sample of children in the welfare system, dissociation was the symptom that most readily predicted the need for rapid hospitalization (Kisiel & Mcllelland, 2012, data in preparation, personal communication, March 28, 2012).

The fluctuations in mood that these youth experience feel foreign and illogical to them. They may describe their moods as unpredictable like the weather, often descending on them without warning and without the normal cause and effect relationship between events and moods that most children can describe. Particularly disconcerting to caregivers is the rapid shifts in relationship to caregivers, from loving, solicitous, and affectionate to hostile and aggressive in rapid succession. Some clinicians have also documented wildly fluctuating variations in cognitive skill level from time to time, which can become very frustrating in school settings where the behavior may be interpreted as willful or avoidant.

Perplexing Memory Lapses

Unusual memory lapses may be difficult to assess in children and teenagers as saying "I forgot" is a common distraction technique that young people use to avoid confrontation and accountability. Nonetheless, asking young people about their own concerns about memory, rather than confronting them on things they claim to have forgotten, may help with the clinical assessment of amnesia. Dissociative children and adults have particular difficulty remembering what they did when in rageful states. Sometimes children in regressed states will have trouble recognizing their caregivers (Waters, 2005a). When assessing for difficulties in memory, it is best to focus on areas in which the child or teen has motivation to remember like forgetting planned excursions with friends or school work that they turned in but don't remember doing. Recent research suggests that motivation may play a key role in memory (Anderson & Huddleston, 2012) and that many children dealing with a history of traumatic events may practice avoidance so that they no longer can access troubling and traumatic information (Kenardy et al., 2007). While uncovering hidden traumatic memories is not appropriate during an initial interview, having memory for one's own recent autobiographical history is very important for successful functioning, and lack of autobiographical memory can lead to havoc in peer relationships, at home, and at school. It is important that a child or teen's environment holds them gently accountable for behavior even if it is executed outside of their awareness, as central consciousness is built through this kind of accountability (Silberg, 2013; Waters & Silberg, 1998). When global forgetfulness about life events is the primary symptom, a diagnosis of dissociative amnesia may be most appropriate. Unusual cases of dissociative amnesia, where teens forget their names or life circumstances, may be associated with a sudden onset of a traumatic event (Waters, 2005b).

Abnormal Somatic Experiences

Children with dissociative symptoms and disorders may have shifting areas of the body with heightened sensitivity or diminished sensitivity, and conversion symptoms are common in this population (Bowman, 2006). Young people may complain of pain at the site of previous caregiver-inflicted injuries or complain of lack of sensitivity

to pain or normal bodily sensations like defecation and urination. Many of these children may have daytime or nighttime enuresis or encopresis, as repeated stimulation of the anogenital areas during sexual abuse may lead to conditioned avoidance responses to any sensation in these areas (Silberg, 2013; Waters, 2011). Fear may also lead to loss of sphincter control which can lead to these accidents. Work in conjunction with a pediatric specialist may be important in these cases.

Self-injury in these children or teenagers may serve a variety of functions such as identifying with abusive caregivers, punishing the self for the trauma endured, calling attention to their pain, or releasing internal opioids (Ferentz, 2012; Yates, 2004). Sometimes children engage in repetitive self-harming such as headbanging to silence the internal voices of harassing perpetrators. In assessing children with trauma histories, a careful inquiry into the methods and intended purpose of self-harming behaviors may yield important information that can be addressed in therapy.

Treatment

Empirically validated approaches to the treatment of trauma-based disorders have proliferated with the work of the National Child Traumatic Stress Network (NCTSN). One of these techniques includes trauma-focused cognitive behavioral therapy (Cohen, Deblinger, Mannarino, & Steer, 2004; Cohen, Mannarino, & Deblinger, 2006). Developing trauma narratives, a key component of this approach, is a well-validated technique that should be incorporated in any trauma-based intervention. However, the disabling symptoms of rage, self-destruction, and extreme mood variability may make this cognitively based approach unrealistic for children with dissociative symptoms and disorders.

Another empirically validated practice supported through the NCTSN is Child–Parent Psychotherapy (Busch & Lieberman, 2007; Lieberman & Van Horn, 2005; Lieberman, Van Horn, & Ghosh-Ippen, 2005). Child–Parent Psychotherapy emphasizes the important role that parents play in facilitating a joint language that diffuses any secrecy about the trauma. However, a traumatized child with dissociative states may block from awareness his or her parents' attempts to support the child's growth and recovery post trauma so these techniques need to be augmented with directly addressing the dissociation which blocks the child's awareness. Blaustein and Kinniburgh (2010) developed the ARC approach to therapy which emphasizes attachment, self-regulation, and competency, which has received some initial validation in preliminary research (Arvidson et al., 2011). Effective approaches for dissociative symptoms and disorders similarly need to emphasize affect- and self-regulation, building relationships and mastery, and the analysis of triggers for trauma processing which is emphasized in this approach.

Another theorist and clinician who influenced our view of dissociation and the treatment of childhood trauma is Bruce Perry. Perry's (2009) Neurosequential Model of Therapeutics emphasizes the hierarchical nature of the brain which organizes itself from the "bottom up" starting with the primitive brainstem and moving up to the middle and upper brain centers such as the diencephalon, limbic system, and cortex. According to Perry's theory, dissociation is viewed as a "brain habit" or "trait" that must be reversed on a neurological level. Perry emphasizes that remediation for trauma involves restructuring the impaired neural networks with repetitive and organized stimulation geared to the brain structure that was affected during the time of trauma.

Successful remediation for dissociation involves incorporating many of these accepted methods of treatment such as building a trauma narrative, working with the parents to validate experiences, encouraging affect regulation skills, and appealing to the child on a somatosensory level (Marks, 2011; Waters, 2011; Wieland, 2011; Wieland & Silberg, 2013). In addition, therapy must focus specifically on the onset of dissociative episodes and the traumatic triggers of these episodes so that the child or teen can learn new ways to respond to traumatic reminders and interrupt these conditioned, automatic processes (Blaustein & Kinniburgh, 2010; Johnson,

2003; Silberg, 2013). Therapy must emphasize building bridges between the rejected and sequestered parts of the self contained in voices, imaginary friends, or dissociated identities with an attitude of acceptance modeled by the therapist and eventually embraced by the child or teen (Wieland, 2011; Wieland & Silberg, 2013).

Cognitive interventions which help to address shame-based cognitions such as "I am dirty" or "This happened to me because I am a bad person" can be helpful (Silberg, 2013), particularly when identity states which harbor these negative attributions about the self are accessed for the therapeutic work. Family work is extremely important as an accompaniment to treatment as parents can serve as ancillary therapists helping to provide predictability and structure at home and serving as witnesses when traumatic material is processed (Marks, 2011; Silberg, 1999, 2004, 2013; Waters, 1998; Wieland, 2011). Parents may require their own therapy as issues of loss and trauma in their own early history can directly affect parenting (Hesse, Main, Abrams, & Rifkin, 2003). A variety of stabilization techniques have been described using safe-place imagery, suggestions to contain overwhelming traumatic content in imaginary vaults, or imagining the self with heroic or special powers which harness the dissociative child's capacity for fantasy in positive ways (Silberg, 2013; Wieland, 1998; Williams & Velazquez, 1996). Creative interventions such as art therapy may be particularly helpful with this population (Sobol & Schneider, 1998). The accepted treatment guidelines of the ISST-D incorporate all of these features and emphasize that a child or teen's physical and emotional safety must be assured before any successful treatment interventions can occur (ISSD, 2003). There are no psychopharmacological interventions that target dissociation per se, but medication may be used for reducing anxiety, depression, attentional difficulties, or other comorbid symptoms.

I have introduced a treatment model of Dissociation-Focused Interventions (DFI) which follow a sequential path organized into the acronym EDUCATE (Silberg, 2013). These steps begin with psychoeducation about trauma and dissociation (E: Education) and assessing the child's motivations to hold on to their dissociation (D: Dissociation motivation). The next group of interventions assists the child in (U) understanding the hidden parts of the self and (C) claiming and embracing the affective experiences and memories associated with these dissociated states. Their rage, for example, may be sequestered and inaccessible, harbored in a part of the self that they call "bad Joey," and their fears may be projected into childlike states. Healing involves self-acceptance of all of the feelings associated with these different self-conceptions.

The A in EDUCATE stands for regulation of Arousal, Affect, and Attachment. Hyperaroused children may see danger everywhere and their neurological system may act as if the trauma is still ongoing. Hyperarousal can be calmed through empathic connection, sensory-motor interventions, and teaching children to use imagery for self-soothing.

The crux of treatment is learning affect regulation techniques which are best reinforced in the context of relationships with attachment figures. These important skills are based on helping the child to identify affects, understand the purpose of affects, express and tolerate them, and ultimately learning to interact with the world in a more effective way. Through empathic connection with the child's whole self, the loving caregiver can be guided in family therapy sessions to provide the "glue" that reinforces the young person's unified sense of self.

Traumatic processing and understanding triggers is the "T" in the EDUCATE model. Processing traumatic events involves attending to the content of early trauma and its meaning to the child. Full processing includes uncovering the affects that were aroused at the time of trauma and analyzing the triggers that stimulate those feelings anew. The therapist must help create mastery experiences that help counter the child's feelings of powerlessness in the context of a validating relationship. The focus of E (Ending Stage of Therapy) is embracing new developmental challenges as the child or teen with dissociative symptoms and disorders learns to fully accept the self and appreciate the ways their new life differs from the traumatic past.

Clinicians interested in learning to work with children or teens with these severe clinical presentations can find continuing education available at the meetings of international trauma societies, such as the International Society for the Study of Trauma and Dissociation (http://www.ISST-D.org) or the International Society for the Study of Traumatic Stress (http://www.ISTSS.org). There is emerging evidence that when therapist with specialized training in dissociation treats adults, there is significant reduction in symptoms, and the younger clients respond even more quickly (Brand et al., 2009, 2012; Myrick et al., 2012). Specialized techniques for working with trauma and dissociation using bilateral stimulation to achieve more rapid processing are also taught by EMDR (Eye Movement Desensitization and Reprocessing) practitioners (Adler-Tapia & Settle, 2008; Gomez, 2012; see EMDRIA.org).

While clinicians faced with their first dissociative child clients may find the work overwhelming and unfamiliar, clinical case reports and follow-up suggest that early intervention can remediate dissociative symptoms (Silberg, 2001b, 2013, Silberg & Waters, 1998; Wieland, 2011) which can progress to increasingly intransigent presentations in adulthood. Early intervention for these severe trauma-based disorders may return children to a normal life trajectory and even interrupt the intergenerational transmission of maltreatment in families.

References

Achenbach, T. M. (1991). *Manual for the child behavior checklist*. Burlington, VT: University of Vermont Department of Psychiatry.

Adler-Tapia, R., & Settle, C. (2008). *EMDR and the art of psychotherapy with children*. New York: Springer.

Albini, T. K., & Pease, T. E. (1989). Normal and pathological dissociations of early childhood. *Dissociation, 2*, 144–150.

Altman, H., Collins, M., & Mundy, P. (1997). Subclinical hallucinations and delusions in nonpsychotic adolescents. *Journal of Child Psychology and Psychiatry, 38*, 413–420.

Anderson, M. C., & Huddleston, E. (2012). Towards a cognitive and neurobiological model of motivated forgetting. In R. F. Belli (Ed.), *True and false recovered memories: Toward a reconciliation of the debate*

(Nebraska symposium on motivation, Vol. 58, pp. 53–120). New York: Springer.

Armstrong, J., Putnam, F. W., Carlson, E., Libero, D., & Smith, S. (1997). Development and validation of a measure of adolescent dissociation: The adolescent dissociative experience scale. *Journal of Nervous and Mental Disease, 185*, 491–497.

Arseneault, L., Cannon, M., Fisher, H. L., Polanczyk, G., Moffitt, T. E., & Caspi, A. (2011). Childhood trauma and children's emerging psychotic symptoms: A genetically sensitive longitudinal cohort study. *American Journal of Psychiatry, 168*, 65–72.

Arvidson, J., Kinniburgh, K., Howard, K., Spinazzola, J., Strothers, H., Evans, M., et al. (2011). Treatment of complex trauma in young children: Developmental and cultural considerations in application of the ARC Intervention Model. *Journal of Child and Adolescent Trauma, 4*(1), 34–51.

Baita, S. (2011). Dalma (4 to 7 years old) – "I've got all my sisters with me": Treatment of dissociative identity disorder in a sexually abused young child. In S. Wieland (Ed.), *Dissociation in traumatized children and adolescents: Theory and clinical interventions* (pp. 29–74). New York: Routledge.

Blaustein, M. E., & Kinniburgh, K. M. (2010). *Treating traumatic stress in children and adolescents: How to foster resilience through attachment, self-regulation, and competency*. New York: Guilford Press.

Bonanno, G. A., Noll, J. G., Putnam, F. W., O'Neill, M., & Trickett, P. K. (2003). Predicting the willingness to disclose childhood sexual abuse from measures of repressive coping and dissociative tendencies. *Child Maltreatment, 8*, 302–318.

Bowman, E. S. (2006). Why conversion seizures should be classified as a dissociative disorder. *Psychiatric Clinics of North America, 29*, 185–211.

Boysen, G. A. (2011). The scientific status of childhood dissociative identity disorder: A review of published research. *Psychotherapy and Psychosomatics, 80*, 329–334.

Brand, B. L., Classen, C. C., Lanius, R., Loewenstein, R., McNary, S., Pain, C., et al. (2009). A naturalistic study of dissociative identity disorder and dissociative disorder not otherwise specified patients treated by community clinicians. *Psychological Trauma: Theory, Research, Practice, and Policy, 1*(2), 153–171.

Brand, B. L., McNary, S. W., Myrick, A. C., Loewenstein, R. J., Classen, C. C., Lanius, R. A., Pain, C. & Putnam, F. W. (2012). A longitudinal, naturalistic study of dissociative disorder patients treated by community clinicians. *Psychological Trauma: Theory, Research, Practice, and Policy*. Advance On-Line Publication. doi:10.1037/a0027654

Briere, J. (1996). *Trauma symptom checklist for children*. Lutz, FL: Psychological Assessment Resources.

Briere, J. (2005). *Trauma symptom checklist for young children*. Lutz, FL: Psychological Assessment Resources.

Brom, D., Pat-Horenczyk, R., & Ford, J. D. (Eds.). (2008). *Treating traumatized children: Risk, resilience and recovery* (pp. 225–239). London: Routledge.

Brunner, R., Parzer, P., Schuld, V., & Resch, F. (2000). Dissociative symptomatology and traumatogenic factors in adolescent psychiatric patients. *Journal of Nervous and Mental Disease, 188*, 71–77.

Busch, A. L., & Lieberman, A. F. (2007). Attachment and trauma: An integrated approach to treating young children exposed to family violence. In D. O. Oppenheim & D. F. Goldsmith (Eds.), *Attachment theory in clinical work with children* (pp. 139–171). New York: Guilford Press.

Cagiada, S., Camaido, L., & Pennan, A. (1997). Successful integrated hypnotic and psychopharmacological treatment of a war-related post-traumatic psychological and somatoform dissociative disorder of two years duration (psychogenic coma). *Dissociation, 10*, 182–189.

Carrion, V. G., & Steiner, H. (2000). Trauma and dissociation in delinquent adolescents. *Journal of the American Academy of Child & Adolescent Psychiatry, 39*, 353–359.

Cohen, J. A., Deblinger, E., Mannarino, A. P., & Steer, R. A. (2004). A multisite, randomized controlled trial for children with sexual abuse-related PTSD symptoms. *Journal of the American Academy of Child and Adolescent Psychiatry, 43*, 393–402.

Cohen, J. A., Mannarino, A. P., & Deblinger, E. (2006). *Treating trauma and traumatic grief in children and adolescents*. New York: Guilford Press.

Collin-Vézina, D., & Hébert, M. (2005). Comparing dissociation and PTSD in sexually abused school-aged girls. *Journal of Nervous and Mental Disease, 93*, 47–52.

Coons, P. M. (1996). Clinical phenomenology of 25 children and adolescents with dissociative disorders. *Child and Adolescent Psychiatric Clinics of North America, 5*, 361–374.

Dell, P. F. (2006). The multidimensional inventory of dissociation (MID): A comprehensive measure of pathological dissociation. *The Journal of Trauma and Dissociation, 7*(2), 77–106.

Dell, P. F., & Eisenhower, J. W. (1990). Adolescent multiple personality disorder: A preliminary study of eleven cases. *Journal of the American Academy of Child and Adolescent Psychiatry, 29*, 359–366.

Diseth, T. (2006). Dissociation following traumatic medical procedures in childhood: A longitudinal follow-up. *Development and Psychopathology, 18*, 233–251.

Dutra, L., Bureau, J., Holmes, B., Lyubchik, A., & Lyons-Ruth, K. (2009). Quality of early care and childhood trauma: A prospective study of developmental pathways to dissociation. *Journal of Nervous and Mental Disease, 197*(6), 383–390.

Fagan, J., & McMahon, P. P. (1984). Incipient multiple personality in children. *Journal of Nervous and Mental Disease, 172*, 26–36.

Feiring, C., & Taska, L. (2005). The persistence of shame following sexual abuse: A longitudinal look at risk and recovery. *Child Maltreatment, 10*(4), 337–349.

Feiring, C., Taska, L., & Lewis, M. (1996). A process model for understanding adaptation to sexual abuse: The role of shame in defining stigmatization. *Child Abuse and Neglect, 20*(8), 767–792.

Feiring, C., Taska, L., & Lewis, M. (2002). Adjustment following sexual abuse discovery: The role of shame and attributional style. *Developmental Psychology, 38*(1), 79–92.

Ferentz, L. (2012). *Treating self-destructive behaviors in trauma survivors*. New York: Routledge.

Freyd, J. (1998). *Betrayal trauma: The logic of forgetting childhood abuse*. Boston: Harvard University Press.

Friedrich, W. N., Gerber, P. N., Koplin, B., Davis, M., Giese, J., Mykelbust, C., et al. (2001). Multimodal assessment of dissociation in adolescents: Inpatients and juvenile sex offenders. *Sexual Abuse, 13*, 167–177.

Goffinet, S. (2005, November). *The prevalence of dissociative disorders in adolescent inpatients*. Paper presented at 22nd international conference, International Society for the Study of Dissociation, Toronto, Canada.

Gomez, A. (2012). *EMDR therapy and adjunct approaches with children: Complex trauma, attachment, and dissociation*. New York: Springer Publishing.

Grimminck, E. (2011). Emma (6 to 9 years old)–From kid actress to healthy child: Treatment of the early sexual abuse led to integration. In S. Wieland (Ed.), *Dissociation in traumatized children and adolescents: Theory and clinical interventions* (pp. 75–96). New York: Routledge.

Hesse, E., Main, M., Abrams, K. Y., & Rifkin, A. (2003). Unresolved states regarding loss or abuse can have "second-generation" effects: Disorganized, role-inversion and frightening ideation in the offspring of traumatized non-maltreating parents. In D. J. Siegel & M. F. Solomon (Eds.), *Healing trauma: Attachment, mind body and brain* (pp. 57–106). New York: Norton.

Hornstein, N. L., & Putnam, F. W. (1992). Clinical phenomenology of child and adolescent dissociative disorders. *Journal of the American Academy of Child and Adolescent Psychiatry, 31*, 1077–1085.

Hornstein, N. L., & Tyson, S. (1991). Inpatient treatment of children with multiple personality/dissociation and their families. *Psychiatric Clinics of North America, 4*, 631–648.

Hulette, A. C., Fisher, P. A., Kim, H. K., Ganger, W., & Landsverk, J. L. (2008). Dissociation in foster preschoolers: A replication and assessment study. *Journal of Trauma and Dissociation, 9*, 173–190.

Hulette, A. C., Freyd, J. J., & Fisher, P. A. (2011). Dissociation in middle childhood among foster children with early Maltreatment experiences. *Child Abuse and Neglect, 35*, 123–126.

International Society for the Study of Dissociation. (2003). Guidelines for the evaluation and treatment of dissociative symptoms in children and adolescents. *Journal of Trauma and Dissociation, 5*(3), 119–149.

Jacobsen, T. (1995). Case study: Is selective mutism a manifestation of dissociative identity disorder? *Journal of American Academy of Child and Adolescent Psychiatry, 31*, 1077–1085.

Jang, K. L., Paris, J., Zweig-Frank, H., & Livelsey, W. J. (1998). Twin study of dissociative experience. *Journal of Nervous and Mental Disease, 186*, 345–351.

Johnson, T. C. (2003). Some considerations about sexual abuse and children with sexual behavior problems. *Journal of Trauma and Dissociation, 3*(4), 83–105.

Kenardy, J., Smith, A., Spence, S. H., Lilley, P. R., Newcombe, P., Dob, R., et al. (2007). Dissociation in children's trauma narratives: An exploratory investigation. *Journal of Anxiety Disorders, 21*, 456–466.

Kim, K., Trickett, P. K., & Putnam, F. W. (2010). Childhood experiences of sexual abuse and later parenting practices among non-offending mothers of sexually abused and comparison girls. *Child Abuse and Neglect, 34*, 610–622.

Kisiel, C., & Lyons, J. S. (2001). Dissociation as a mediator of psychopathology among sexually abused children and adolescents. *American Journal of Psychiatry, 158*, 1034–1039.

Klein, B. R. (1985). A child's imaginary companion: A transitional self. *Clinical Social Work, 13*, 272–282.

Kluft, R. P. (1984). MPD in childhood. *Psychiatric Clinics of North America, 7*, 9–29.

Kluft, R. P. (1985a). Childhood Multiple Personality Disorder: Predictors, clinical findings and treatment results. In R. P. Kluft (Ed.), *Childhood antecedents of multiple personality disorder* (pp. 168–196). Washington, DC: American Psychiatric Press.

Kluft, R. P. (Ed.). (1985b). *Childhood antecedents of multiple personality disorder* (pp. 168–196). Washington, DC: American Psychiatric Press.

Kluft, R. P. (2007). Applications of innate affect theory to the understanding and treatment of Dissociative Identity Disorder. In E. Vermetten, M. J. Dorahy, & D. Spiegel (Eds.), *Traumatic dissociation: Neurobiology and treatment* (pp. 301–316). Washington, DC: American Psychiatric Publishing.

Laporta, L. D. (1992). Childhood trauma and multiple personality disorder: The case of a 9-year-old girl. *Child Abuse and Neglect, 16*, 615–620.

Leibowitz, G. S., Laser, J. A., & Burton, D. L. (2011). Exploring the relationships between dissociation, victimization, and juvenile sexual offending. *Journal of Trauma and Dissociation, 12*(1), 38–52.

Lewis, M. (1992). *Shame: The exposed self*. New York: The Free Press.

Lieberman, A. F., & Van Horn, P. (2005). *"Don't hit my mommy!": A manual for child-, parent psychotherapy with young witnesses of family violence*. Washington, DC: Zero to Three Press.

Lieberman, A. F., Van Horn, P., & Ghosh-Ippen, C. (2005). Toward evidence-based treatment: Child–parent psychotherapy with preschoolers exposed to marital violence. *Journal of the American Academy of Child and Adolescent Psychiatry, 44*, 1241–1248.

Liotti, G. (2009). Attachment and dissociation. In P. Dell & J. O'Neil (Eds.), *Dissociation and the dissociative disorders: DSM V and beyond* (pp. 53–65). New York: Routledge.

Luther, J. S., McNamara, J. O., Carwile, S., Miller, P., & Hope, V. (1982). Pseudoepileptic seizures: Methods and video analysis to aid diagnosis. *Annals of Neurology, 12*, 458–462.

Lyons-Ruth, K., Dutra, L., Schuder, M. R., & Bianchi, I. (2006). From infant attachment disorganization to adult dissociation: Relational adaptations or traumatic experiences? *Psychiatric Clinics of North America, 29*, 63–86.

Macfie, J., Cicchetti, D., & Toth, S. L. (2001). The development of dissociation in maltreated preschool-aged children. *Development and Psychopathology, 13*, 233–254.

Mann, B. J., & Sanders, S. (1994). Child dissociation and the family context. *Journal of Abnormal Child Psychology, 22*, 373–388.

Marks, R. P. (2011). Jason (7 years old)–Expressing past neglect and abuse: Two-week intensive therapy for an adopted child with dissociation. In S. Wieland (Ed.), *Dissociation in traumatized children and adolescents: Theory and clinical interventions* (pp. 97–140). New York: Routledge.

Mclewin, L. A., & Muller, R. T. (2006). Childhood trauma, imaginary companions and the development of pathological dissociation. *Aggression and Violent Behavior, 11*, 531–545.

Myrick, A. C., Brand, B. L., McNary, S. W., Loewenstein, R. J., Classen, C. C., Lanius, R. A., et al. (2012). An exploration of young adults' progress in treatment for dissociative disorder. *Journal of Trauma and Dissociation, 13*(5), 582–595.

Nilsson, D., & Svedin, C. G. (2006). Dissociation among Swedish adolescents and the connection to trauma: An evaluation of the Swedish version of adolescent dissociative experience scale. *Journal of Nervous and Mental Disease, 194*, 684–689.

Ogawa, J. R., Sroufe, L. A., Weinfield, N. S., Carlson, E. A., & Egeland, B. (1997). Development and the fragmented self: Longitudinal study of dissociative symptomatology in a nonclinical sample. *Developmental Psychopathology, 9*, 855–979.

Perry, B. D. (2002). *Adaptive responses to childhood trauma*. Retrieved from http://74.52.31.127/~oldnew/fasa/FASA%20PDF/For%20Professionals/Neurodevelopment%20&%20Trauma.pdf

Perry, B. D. (2009). Examining child maltreatment through a neurodevelopmental lens: Clinical application of the neurosequential model of therapeutics. *Journal of Loss and Trauma, 14*, 240–255.

Perry, B. D., Pollard, R., Blakely, T., Baker, W., & Vigilante, D. (1995). Childhood trauma, the neurobiology of adaptation and use-dependent development of the brain: How states become traits. *Infant Mental Health Journal, 16*, 271–291.

Peterson, G. (1991). Children coping with trauma: Diagnosis of dissociation identity disorder. *Dissociation, 4*, 152–164.

Putnam, F. W. (1989). *Diagnosis and treatment of multiple personality disorder*. New York: Guilford Press.

Putnam, F. W. (1997). *Dissociation in children and adolescents: A developmental approach*. New York: Guilford.

Putnam, F. W., Guroff, J. J., Silberman, E. K., Barban, L., & Post, R. M. (1986). The clinical phenomenology of multiple personality disorder: Review of 100 recent cases. *Journal of Clinical Psychiatry, 47*, 285–293.

Putnam, F. W., Helmers, K., & Trickett, P. K. (1993). Development, reliability, and validity of a child dissociation scale. *Child Abuse and Neglect, 17*, 731–741.

Putnam, F. W., Hornstein, N., & Peterson, G. (1996). Clinical phenomenology of child and adolescent dissociative disorders: Gender and age effects. *Child and Adolescent Psychiatric Clinics of North America, 5*, 303–442.

Riley, R. L., & Mead, J. (1988). The development of symptoms of multiple personality in a child of three. *Dissociation, 1*, 41–46.

Ross, C. (1989). *Multiple personality: Diagnosis, clinical features, and treatment*. New York: Wiley.

Ruths, S., Silberg, J. L., Dell, P. F., & Jenkins, C. (2002, November). *Adolescent DID: An elucidation of symptomatology and validation of the MID*. Paper presented at the 19th meeting of the International Society for the Study of Dissociation, Baltimore, MD.

Shin, J. U., Jeong, S. H., & Chung, U. S. (2009). The Korean version of the adolescent dissociative experience scale: Psychometric properties and the connection to trauma among Korean adolescents. *Psychiatry Investigation, 6*(3), 163–172.

Shirar, L. (1996). *Dissociative children: Bridging the inner and outer worlds*. New York: W. W. Norton.

Silberg, J. L. (Ed.). (1996/1998). *The dissociative child: Diagnosis, treatment and management*. Lutherville, MD: Sidran Press.

Silberg, J. L. (1998a). Interviewing strategies for assessing dissociative disorders in children and adolescents. In J. L. Silberg (Ed.), *The dissociative child: Diagnosis, treatment and management* (2nd ed., pp. 47–68). Lutherville, MD: Sidran Press.

Silberg, J. L. (1998b). Dissociative symptomatology in children and adolescents as displayed on psychological testing. *Journal of Personality Assessment, 71*, 421–439.

Silberg, S. L. (1999). Parenting the dissociative child. *Many Voices, 11*(1), 6–7.

Silberg, J. L. (2001a). Treating maladaptive dissociation in a young teenage girl. In H. Orvaschel, J. Faust, & M. Hersen (Eds.), *Handbook of conceptualization and treatment of child psychopathology* (pp. 449–474). Oxford, UK: Elsevier Science.

Silberg, J. L. (2001b). An optimistic look at childhood dissociation. *ISSD NEWS, 19*(2), 1.

Silberg, J. L. (2004). Treatment of dissociation in sexually abused children: A family/attachment perspective. *Psychotherapy: Theory, Research, Practice and Training, 41*, 487–496.

Silberg, J. L. (2011). Angela (14 to 16 years old) - Finding words for pain: Treatment of a dissociative teen presenting with medical trauma. In S. Wieland (Ed.), *Dissociation in children and adolescents: Clinical case studies* (pp. 263–284). New York: Routledge Press.

Silberg, J. L. (2013). *The child survivor: Healing developmental trauma and dissociation*. New York: Routledge.

Silberg, J. L., & Dallam, S. (2009). Dissociation in children and adolescents: At the crossroads. In P. F. Dell & J. O'Neill (Eds.), *Dissociation: DSM-V and beyond* (pp. 67–81). New York: Routledge Press.

Silberg, J. L., & Waters, F. W. (1998). Factors associated with positive therapeutic outcome. In J. L. Silberg (Ed.), *The dissociative child: Diagnosis, treatment and management* (2nd ed., pp. 105–112). Lutherville, MD: Sidran Press.

Sim, L., Friedrich, W. N., Davies, W. H., Trentaham, B., Lengua, L., & Pithers, W. (2005). The child behavior checklist as an indicator of posttraumatic stress disorder and dissociation in normative, psychiatric, and sexually abused children. *Journal of Traumatic Stress, 18*(6), 697–705.

Simeon, D., Guralnik, O., Schmeidler, J., Sirof, B., & Knutelska, M. (2001). The role of childhood interpersonal trauma in depersonalization disorder. *American Journal of Psychiatry, 58*(7), 1027–1033.

Simeon, D., Knutelska, M., Nelson, D., & Guralnik, O. (2003). Feeling unreal; a depersonalization update on 117 cases. *Journal of Clinical Psychiatry, 64*(9), 990–997.

Smith, S. R., & Carlson, E. B. (1996). Reliability and validity of the adolescent dissociative experiences scale. *Dissociation, 9*, 125–129.

Snow, M. S., White, J., Pilkington, L., & Beckman, D. (1995). Dissociative identity disorder revealed through play therapy: A case study of a four year old. *Dissociation, 8*, 120–123.

Sobol, B., & Schneider, K. (1998). Art as an adjunctive therapy in the treatment of children who dissociate. In J. L. Silberg (Ed.), *The dissociative child: Diagnosis, treatment and management* (2nd ed., pp. 219–230). Lutherville, MD: Sidran Press.

Soukup, J., Papežová, H., Kuběna, A. A., & Mikolajová, V. (2010). Dissociation in non-clinical and clinical sample of Czech adolescents. Reliability and validity of the Czech version of the Adolescent Dissociative Experiences Scale. *European Psychiatry, 25*, 390–395.

Stolbach, B. C. (1997). The children's dissociative experiences scale and posttraumatic symptom inventory: Rationale, development, and validation of a self-report measure. *Dissertation Abstracts International, 58*(03), 1548B.

Stolbach, B. C. (2005). Psychotherapy of a dissociative 8-year-old boy burned at age 3. *Psychiatric Annals, 35*, 685–694.

Taylor, M. (1999). *Imaginary companions and the children who create them*. New York: Oxford University Press.

Teicher, M., Samson, J. A., Polcari, A., & McGreenery, C. E. (2006). Sticks and stones and hurtful words. Relative effects of various form of childhood maltreatment. *American Journal of Psychiatry, 163*, 993–1000.

Tomkins, S. S. (1962). *Affect imagery consciousness – volume 1: The positive affects*. New York: Springer Publishing Co.

Trickett, P. K., Noll, J. G., & Putnam, F. W. (2011). The impact of sexual abuse on female development:

Lessons from a multi-generational, longitudinal study. *Development and Psychopathology, 23*, 453–476.

Trujillo, K., Lewis, D. O., Yeager, C. A., & Gidlow, B. (1996). Imaginary companions of school boys and boys with dissociative identity disorder/multiple personality disorder: A normal to pathological continuum. *Child and Adolescent Psychiatric Clinics of North America, 5*, 375–391.

Van der hart, O., Nijenhuis, E. R. S., & Steele, K. (2006). *The haunted self: Structural dissociation and the treatment of chronic traumatization*. New York: W. W. Norton.

Waters, F. S. (1998). Parents as partners in the treatment of dissociative children. In J. L. Silberg (Ed.), *The dissociative child: Diagnosis, treatment and management* (2nd ed., pp. 273–296). Lutherville, MD: Sidran Press.

Waters, F. S. (2005a). Recognizing dissociation in preschool children. *ISSTD News, 23*, 4.

Waters, F. S. (2005b). Atypical DID adolescent case. *ISSTD News, 23*(3), 1–2. 4–5.

Waters, F. S. (2011). Ryan (8 to 10 years old) – Connecting with the body: Treatment of somatoform dissociation (encopresis and multiple physical complaints) in a young boy. In S. Wieland (Ed.), *Dissociation in traumatized children and adolescents: Theory and clinical interventions* (pp. 141–186). New York: Routledge.

Waters, F. S. (2012). Assessing and diagnosing dissociation in children: Beginning the recovery. In A. Gomez (Ed.), *EMDR therapy and adjunct approaches with children: Complex trauma, attachment and dissociation*. New York: Springer.

Waters, F. S., & Silberg, J. L. (1998). Therapeutic phases in the treatment of dissociative children. In J. L. Silberg (Ed.), *The dissociative child: Diagnosis, treatment and management* (2nd ed., pp. 135–156). Lutherville, MD: Sidran Press.

Wieland, S. (1998). *Techniques and issues in abuse-focused therapy*. Thousand Oaks, CA: Sage.

Wieland, S. (Ed.). (2011). *Dissociation in traumatized children and adolescents: Theory and clinical interventions*. New York: Routledge.

Wieland, S., & Silberg, J. S. (2013). Dissociation focused therapy in children and adolescents. In J. Ford & C. Courtois (Eds.), *The treatment of complex trauma in children and adolescents*. New York: Guilford Press.

Williams, D. T., & Velazquez, L. (1996). The use of hypnosis in children with dissociative disorders. *Child and Adolescent Psychiatric Clinics of North America, 5*, 495–508.

Wolff, P. H. (1987). *The development of behavioral states and the expression of emotions in early infancy*. Chicago: University of Chicago Press.

Yates, T. M. (2004). The developmental psychopathology of self-injurious behavior: Compensatory regulation in posttraumatic adaptation. *Clinical Psychology Review, 24*, 35–74.

Zoroglu, S. S., Sar, V., Tuzun, U., Tutkun, H., & Savas, H. A. (2002). Reliability and validity of the Turkish version of the adolescent dissociative experiences scale. *Psychiatry and Clinical Neurosciences, 56*, 551–556.

About the Editors

Michael Lewis Ph.D. is University Distinguished Professor of Pediatrics and Psychiatry and Director of the Institute for the Study of Child Development at Rutgers Robert Wood Johnson Medical School. He is also Professor of Psychology, Education, and Biomedical Engineering and currently serves as Founding Director of Rutgers Robert Wood Johnson Medical School's Autism Center. He has been the recipient of the Urie Bronfenbrenner Award for Lifetime Contribution to Developmental Psychology in the Service of Science and Society from the American Psychological Association, the Hedi Levenback Pioneer Award from the New York Zero-to-Three Network, and the award for Distinguished Scientific Contributions to Child Development from the Society for Research in Child Development. He is also the author of *Shame: The Exposed Self, Altering Fate: Why the Past Does Not Predict the Future*, and the recently published *The Rise of Consciousness and the Development of Emotional Life*.

Karen D. Rudolph Ph.D. is a professor at the University of Illinois, Urbana-Champaign. She received her doctorate in clinical psychology at the University of California, Los Angeles, and completed a clinical internship at the Neuropsychiatric Institute and Hospital at UCLA. She has been a recipient of a William T. Grant Foundation Faculty Scholars Award and a James McKeen Cattell Sabbatical Award and has served as a PI and co-PI on several large-scale longitudinal studies funded by the National Institute of Mental Health. She serves on the editorial boards of *Development and Psychopathology* and the *Journal of Abnormal Child Psychology* and is an associate editor for the *Journal of Clinical Child and Adolescent Psychology*. Her research focuses on person-by-environment interactions that predict the emergence and continuity of depressive disorders, with a focus on developmental transitions (e.g., puberty, school transitions) that create a context of risk for the onset or exacerbation of psychopathology.

M. Lewis and K.D. Rudolph (eds.), *Handbook of Developmental Psychopathology*,
DOI 10.1007/978-1-4614-9608-3, © Springer Science+Business Media New York 2014

Author Index

A

Aarnoudse-Moens, C.S., 395
Aaron, J., 749
Aase, H., 532
Abaied, J.L., 210, 504
Abbacchi, A., 654
Abbott, R.D., 174
Abela, J.R.Z., 495, 500, 501, 504, 505
Abela, J.Z., 194, 209, 215
Aber, J.L., 173, 213
Abidin, R., 574
Abramowitz, J.S., 563, 572
Abrams, K.Y., 770
Abramson, H., 642
Abramson, L.Y., 113, 331, 493, 500, 501, 506
Abu Tawahina, A., 743
Accardo, P.J., 668–669
Acebo, C., 414, 415
Aceto, G., 641
Achenbach, T.M., 16–18, 67–82, 216, 319, 544, 688, 766
Achermann, P., 410
Ackerman, B.P., 147
Adam, E.K., 205–218
Adams, P., 505
Adelman, H., 163, 165, 170, 171
Adler, A., 278
Adler, N.E., 209, 215, 287, 288, 290, 292, 296
Adler-Tapia, R., 771
Adolphs, R., 266, 269
Adredolo, C., 748
Adrien, J., 496
Afifi, T.O., 129
Afrank, J., 475
Agerbo, E., 104
Ageton, S.S., 31
Aggen, S., 110
Agras, W.S., 622
Agrawal, H.R., 709
Ahlqvist-Bjorkroth, S., 394
Ahmadzadeh, A., 641
Ahmed, E.I., 627
Ahmed, S., 97
Ahnlide, J.-A., 533
Aiken, L.S., 114, 115, 131, 213
Aikins, J.W., 189, 505
Ainsworth, M.D.S., 7, 150, 315, 358

Ainsworth, M.S., 150, 452
Aisenberg, E., 130
Aitken, D.H., 289
Aitken, M.E., 171
Ajayi, C.A., 133
Ajdukovic, M.D., 747
Akande, A., 543
Akbiyik, D.I., 751
Akerman, A., 300
Akiba, M., 172
Akinbami, L.J., 165
Akiskal, H.S., 506
Akiva, T., 173
Aksan, N., 319
Alanko, K., 695
Albano, A.M., 207
Albert, D., 609
Albin, G.R., 171
Albini, T.K., 761
Albus, K.E., 251, 366
Alcorn, K.L., 392
Alegría, M., 227
Alexander, D., 668
Alexander, K.L., 172
Alfano, L., 625
Alfredsson, L., 57
Algoe, S.B., 134
Alink, L.A., 210
Alink, L.R.A., 735
Alkon, A., 292, 297
Alkon–Leonard, A., 296
Allan, N.P., 319, 550
Allebeck, P., 56
Allen, E.C., 394
Allen, H.A., 643
Allen, J.P., 127, 188, 606, 611
Allen, L., 213
Allen, M., 169
Allen, N.B., 506
Allen, T.D., 171
Allen, V.L., 336
Alloy, L.B., 113, 500, 504
Allport, F.H., 8
Allport, G.W., 8
Almas, A.N., 311
Almeida, D.M., 147, 601

Almqvist, F., 74
Alpern, L., 476
Alpert, A., 504
Alsaker, F.D., 336, 339, 345
al-Shabbout, M., 497
Alsobrook, J.I., 562
Alsobrook, J.P., 564
Alsobrook, K., 567
Altemeier, W.A., 397
Altham, P.M., 497
Altman, H., 767
Aman, M.G., 671, 678
Amato, P.R., 145
Amato, R., 57
Amatya, K., 190
Amaya-Jackson, L., 750
Ames, E.W., 374, 380
Ames, L., 567
Aminzadeh, M., 641
Amir, N., 554, 563, 570, 572
Ammerman, R.T., 674
Amronmin, J., 165
Anand, A., 498
Anand, K.J., 434
Anastopoulos, A.D., 440
Anderman, E.M., 168
Anderman, L.H., 168
Anders, T.F., 410
Andersen, S.L., 295
Anderson, C.A., 478
Anderson, J., 91, 472
Anderson, L.W., 178
Anderson, M.C., 769
Anderson, R.L., 704
Anderson, S.E., 393
Anderson, S.J., 669
Anderson, W.M., 419
Andersson, T., 339, 340, 347
Andreasson, S., 56
Andrews, B., 747
Andrews, D.W., 451, 459, 612
Andrews, J.A., 342, 494, 504
Andrews, M.H., 503
Aneshensel, C.S., 95, 96, 206, 338
Angermeyer, M.C., 571
Angleitner, A., 167
Anglin, D.M., 709
Angold, A., 33, 65, 87, 88, 91, 110–112, 165, 333,
        337–339, 428–432, 491–494, 546–548, 566, 589,
        610, 743, 745, 746, 753
Anisman, H., 289
Ankerst, D.P., 498
Ann Wright, P., 213
Ansorge, M.S., 273
Ansseau, M., 533
Anthony, E.J., 4, 125, 126
Antle, M.C., 410
Antonello, S.J., 675
Applegate, B., 428, 744

Appleyard, K., 592, 731
Arango, V., 533
Araujo, C., 752
Archer, J., 470, 471
Archer, M., 362
Arcus, D., 132, 321, 568
Ardic, U.A., 572
Arel, S., 173
Arend, R.A., 504
Arendt, J., 416
Ariagno, R.L., 410
Armer, M., 234
Armitage, R., 496
Armstrong, J., 765
Armstrong, T.D., 588
Armsworth, M.W., 749
Arnds, K., 454
Arndt, S., 536
Arnett, J.J., 457
Arnold, L.E., 678
Arnold, P.D., 548, 549
Arnsten, A.F., 436
Aron, A., 135, 312
Aron, E.N., 312, 317
Aronson, J., 168
Arseneault, L., 56, 731, 767
Arvidson, J., 770
Arvidsson, T., 505
Asarnow, J.R., 504
Asendorpf, J.B., 167, 234
Asher, S.R., 707
Ashman, A.F., 707
Ashwin, C., 268
Aslan, M., 734
Åslund, C., 732
Asparouhov, T., 112
Asperger, H., 651
Assel, M.A., 393
Astor, R.A., 177
Atkins, M.S., 131
Atlas-Corbett, A., 365
Attar-Schwartz, S., 209
Attie, I., 624
Aud, S., 163–165
Audenaert, K., 533
Auerbach, J.E., 430
Auerbach, J.G., 427
Auerbach, R., 209, 213
Auerbach, S.H., 418
Aunola, K., 166, 194
Aupperle, R.L., 278
Aurora, R.N., 418
Austin, A.A., 228
Austin, J.C., 643
Austin, M.P., 503
Auyeung, B., 694, 695
Avenevoli, S., 88, 103, 490, 492, 493
Axelson, D., 492
Ayduk, O., 169

Ayhan, Y., 57
Aylward, E., 532
Aylward, G.P., 391
Ayoub, C.C., 731
Azrin, N.H., 642

B
Baack, M.L., 391
Baba, T., 688
Babor, T.F., 585
Babson, K.A., 341
Bacallao, M., 211
Bachman, J.G., 602, 604, 605, 610–614
Bachmann, C., 639
Bacon, A., 495
Badali-Peterson, M., 691
Bader, G., 640
Baer, P.E., 611
Baeyens, D., 638, 639
Bagot, R.C., 253, 272, 494, 495
Bagwell, C.L., 193
Bailey, A., 654
Baird, P.A., 668
Baita, S., 767
Baker, B.L., 675
Baker, J.H., 50, 625
Baker, J.P., 391
Baker, L., 531
Baker, W., 767
Bakermans-Kranenburg, M.J., 38, 48, 54, 55, 155, 248,
        252, 255, 270–272, 275, 296, 297, 322, 357, 358,
        361, 363, 364, 366, 374, 379, 552, 727
Bakker, M.P., 210
Bakow, H., 645
Baldasaro, R.E., 110
Baldwin, A.L., 28, 33, 165
Baldwin, C.A., 28, 33, 165
Bale, J.F., 669
Bale, T.L., 47, 258
Balentine, A., 428
Ball, J.E., 553
Ballabh, P., 390
Balsis, S., 703
Balster, R.L., 455
Balthazor, M., 505
Bamburg, J.W., 669
Ban, M., 495, 496
Bancila, D., 212
Bandalos, D., 119
Bandura, A., 10, 168
Banerjee, R., 554
Banez, G.A., 643
Bannon, K., 437
Banny, A.M., 723–736
Baptista, J., 365
Baram, T.Z., 373
Barban, L., 761
Barbas, H., 266

Barber, B.K., 144, 145, 504
Barber, B.L., 331
Bardin, C., 393
Bar-Haim, Y., 270, 554, 555
Barker, E.D., 114
Barker, R., 177
Barkin, S.H., 130
Barkley, R.A., 68, 291, 312, 316, 317, 323, 427–433
Barlow, D.H., 110, 207, 229, 554, 678
Barnes, A.R., 250
Barnes, G.M., 611
Barnett, D., 724, 728, 729
Barnett, J.H., 171
Barnett, M.A., 130
Barocas, R., 33
Baroff, G.S., 669
Baron, I.S., 392
Baron, R., 209, 210
Baron-Cohen, S., 268, 658, 689
Barone, J.G., 640
Barr, C.S., 53, 290, 293
Barrett, L.C., 37
Barrett, P.M., 551–552, 569, 571–573
Barrett, R.P., 665–679
Barrett, S., 291
Barrocas, A.L., 555
Barron, K., 115
Barros, A.J., 397
Barros, F.C., 397
Barrueco, S., 128
Barry, R.A., 255, 256, 322, 361
Barry, R.J., 377
Barry, T.D., 456
Bartels, M., 72, 494
Bartko, W.T., 33, 34
Bartram, A.F., 392
Bascoe, S.M., 153
Bascom, A., 640
Baskin, C.H., 17
Bateman, A., 709
Bates, B., 251, 366
Bates, J.E., 155, 156, 187, 188, 227, 250, 297, 311–325,
        430, 478, 499, 502, 729, 730
Battaglia, M., 273, 549
Batten, S.V., 734
Batty, M.J., 436
Bauchner, H., 396
Baucom, D.H., 589
Bauer, D.J., 110, 113–116, 119, 208
Bauer, P.M., 377, 382
Baum, A., 752
Bauman, M., 656
Baumeister, R.F., 135
Baumrind, D., 601
Bayles, K., 317, 318
Bayoumi, R.A., 640
Bazinet, A., 320
Beach, S.R.H., 48, 49, 257, 274, 275
Beam, M., 230

Bean, R.A., 197
Beard, J., 114
Beardslee, W.R., 127, 130
Bearman, P., 654
Bearman, S.K., 338, 623
Beauchaine, T.P., 154, 297, 429, 471–474, 521–538, 704, 708–711, 714
Beautrais, A., 92
Beaver, K.M., 55
Bechara, A., 594
Beck, A.T., 212, 500, 506
Becker, B.E., 127, 155, 167, 213, 735
Becker, D.F., 704, 709
Becker, J.B., 333, 339, 627
Becker, K., 435
Beckett, C., 357, 376, 385
Beckett, J., 667
Beckman, D., 762
Bédard, A.C.V., 427
Beeghly, M., 728
Beekman, A.J., 693
Beers, J., 173
Beers, S.R., 730
Behen, M.E., 382
Behre, W.J., 177
Behrman, R.E., 390
Beirens, K., 229
Belay, H., 53
Belcher, H.M.E., 744
Beldavs, Z.G., 152
Belden, A.C., 503
Belizán, J.M., 391
Bell, R.Q., 18, 249, 312, 322
Bell, S.R., 172
Bellanti, C.J., 146
Bellin, H., 6
Bellis, M.A., 608
Bellivier, F., 533
Bellman, M., 341, 636
Bellmore, A.D., 192, 707
Bellodi, L., 566
Belsky, D.W., 535, 709, 714
Belsky, J., 38, 54, 55, 149, 155, 175, 248, 257, 271, 296, 302, 321, 322, 347, 358, 366, 393, 450, 725
Beltran, I., 601
Beltz, A.M., 694
Bem, D.J., 235
Bem, S.L., 5
Ben Amor, L., 434
Benca, R., 165
Bender, D.S., 706
Benedict, R., 225, 226
Ben-Efraim, Y.J., 55
Benjamin, L.S., 706
Benjet, C., 212, 336, 338
Benn, R., 173
Benner, A.D., 178
Bennett, A.J., 53
Bennett, D.S., 440
Benning, S.D., 334

Benoit, D., 393
Benoit, M.Z., 228
Bensadoun, J., 288
Ben-Sasson, A., 658
Benson, B.A., 678
Benson, B.M., 636
Benson, P., 249
Bercovitch, F.B., 695
Berenbaum, S.A., 683, 694
Berenson, K., 169
Berg, C.Z., 563
Bergen, S.E., 590, 593
Berger, L.M., 129
Bergeron, N., 230
Bergman, L.R., 110, 114, 115, 188, 571
Berkman, L.F., 97, 397
Berkowitz, S., 747
Berkson, G., 27, 665
Berliner, L., 744, 748
Berman, A.L., 522, 525
Berman, J.S., 642
Berman, P.W., 675
Bermant, G., 136
Bernard, K., 291
Bernard, R.S., 392
Bernburg, J., 233
Berndt, T.J., 193
Bernier, R., 654
Bernstein, A., 543, 544, 556, 609
Bernstein, I.H., 73
Berntson, G.G., 291
Berridge, K.C., 532, 594
Bérubé, R.L., 74
Berument, S.K., 378
Berwick, D.M., 396
Berwid, O.G., 431
Bessler, A., 428
Best, C.L., 743
Best, K.M., 504
Best, S.R., 747
Beyers, W., 551
Bhargava, S., 637
Bharucha, A.E., 632
Bhat, A., 656
Bhatnagar, S., 289
Bhutta, A.T., 434
Bianchi, I., 764
Bidesi, A.P., 498
Biederman, J., 68, 431, 623
Biehl, M.C., 338, 341
Bienvenu, O.J., 566
Bierman, K.L., 146, 188, 467–482
Bifulco, A.T., 505
Bigbee, M.A., 191
Bigda-Peyton, J.S., 209
Biggar, H., 93
Biggs, J., 168
Biglan, A., 449, 450, 452
Bigler, E.D., 730
Bilenberg, N., 74

Billet, E.A., 568
Binet, A., 69
Bingham, C.R., 591, 592
Birch, D., 401
Birch, H.G., 311
Birch, L.L., 401
Birmaher, B., 468, 491, 492, 497, 752
Biro, F.M., 332, 333, 345
Bischof, G.H., 636
Bishop, J.A., 707
Bishop, J.L., 475
Bishop, S., 653
Biswal, B., 280
Biswas-Diener, R., 135
Bithoney, W.G., 401
Bizot, J.C., 533
Blachman, D.R., 193
Black, M.M., 397, 398, 402
Blackford, J.U., 319
Blackwell, L.S., 168
Blair, C., 165, 167, 476
Blair, P.S., 396, 397, 399
Blair, R.J.R., 710
Blakely, R.D., 271
Blakely, T., 767
Blakemore, S.J., 608
Blanchard, R., 694, 696
Bland, R.C., 531
Blanton, H., 195
Blatt, S.J., 706
Blaustein, M.E., 770
Blehar, M.C., 150, 315, 358
Blenner, S., 389–402
Blijlevens, P., 323
Block, J., 4
Block, J.H., 127, 167
Block, R.W., 398
Block, T.H., 4
Block-Lerner, J., 173
Bloom, D.A., 642
Blöte, A.W., 554
Blue, J., 726
Blumenthal, H., 341
Blumenthal, S.J., 530
Blyth, D.A., 334, 336
Bocklandt, S., 695
Bockting, W., 685
Boden, J.M., 54, 258
Boeding, S., 589
Boergers, J., 191, 536
Bogaert, A.F., 694
Bogdan, R., 46, 265, 293, 296, 301
Bögels, S.M., 152, 169, 175, 545
Boggs, S.R., 479
Bogle, M., 399
Bohn, K., 622
Bohon, C., 209, 501
Boislard, P., 233
Boivin, M., 192, 196, 479
Bokhorst, C.L., 251

Bokszczanin, A., 744
Bolger, K.E., 729, 730
Bolhofner, K., 491
Bollen, K.A., 110, 112, 119
Bolt, D., 392
Bolton, D., 563, 564
Bonanno, G.A., 762
Bond, J., 94
Bondy, A.S., 672
Bonefant, E., 585
Boney-McCoy, S., 743
Bongar, B., 526
Bonner, M.J., 571
Bonn-Miller, M.O., 609
Boodoosingh, L., 17
Bookman, E.B., 258
Boomsma, D.I., 72, 494, 593, 695
Booth, A., 291
Booth-LaForce, C., 149
Bootzin, R.R., 413
Bor, W., 212
Borbély, A.A., 410
Borden, M.C., 674
Borduin, C.M., 481
Borelli, J.L., 189, 193, 194, 505
Borges, G., 212, 583
Borghini, A., 393
Borghol, N., 294
Boring, A.M., 752
Borkenau, P., 167
Borkowski, J.G., 144
Borman-Spurrell, E., 397
Bornovalova, M.A., 709
Bornstein, M.H., 37
Bornstein, R.F., 704
Borodkin, K., 416
Borowitz, S.M., 639
Borowsky, I.W., 504
Borry, P., 522
Bos, A.F., 395
Bos, K.J., 377, 381
Bosello, R., 621
Bosker, F.J., 532, 533
Bosl, W., 657
Bosmans, G., 543–556
Bosquet Enlow, M., 393
Bosquet, M., 555
Botteron, K.N., 497
Botvin, G.J., 339
Bouchard, T.J. Jr., 248
Boulton, M.J., 190, 554
Bowker, J., 234
Bowlby, J., 7, 149, 358–360, 364–367, 373, 504, 552, 727
Bowman, E.S., 769
Boxer, A.M., 335, 338
Boxer, P., 234
Boxmeyer, C.L., 456
Boyce, W.T., 11, 16, 38, 54, 155, 209, 271,
       287–302, 322, 348
Boyle, C., 668

Boyle, M.H., 395, 467, 493
Boysen, G.A., 763
Boyt, M.A., 643
Bradley, R.G., 733
Bradley, S.J., 319, 685–691, 695–697
Bradshaw, M., 249
Brady, S.S., 291
Braet, C., 491, 551, 552
Brand, B.L., 771
Brand, N.H., 611
Branje, S.J.T., 146
Bransford, J., 175
Bratslavsky, E., 135
Brauner, J., 478
Braungart, J.M., 51
Braveman, P., 287
Bray, J.H., 611
Brechwald, W.A., 188, 194
Bredenkamp, D., 380
Bredy, T.W., 293, 299
Bremner, J.D., 752
Brendel, G.R., 709
Brendgen, M., 192, 194, 196, 472, 473, 500, 505
Brener, N.D., 171
Brennan, A., 743
Brennan, J., 478
Brennan, L.M., 454
Brennan, P.A., 110, 209–212, 493, 495, 504
Brennan, R.T., 341
Brenner, A.B., 131
Brenner, J., 186
Brenner, S.L., 297, 537
Brenning, K., 552
Brent, D.A., 533, 744
Breslau, J., 392
Breslau, N., 743
Brewin, C.R., 747
Brezo, J., 533
Bridgemohan, C., 643, 644, 646
Brigidi, B.D., 563
Brinkmeyer, M.Y., 480
Brisch, K., 357
Bristol-Power, M., 144
Britner, P.A., 380
Britton, J.C., 268, 550
Broberg, A.G., 505, 711
Brock, S.E., 171
Broderick, P.C., 173
Brodsky, N.L., 171
Brody, G.H., 48, 49, 129, 132, 257, 274, 339, 341, 449, 611
Broeren, S., 556
Broidy, L.M., 454, 457, 468, 470
Brom, D., 761
Bromet, E.J., 88
Bromley, E., 704
Bronfenbrenner, U., 10, 30, 32, 225, 449, 602, 606, 614
Brook, D.W., 610
Brook, J.S., 565, 610, 709
Brooks, R.C., 643

Brooks-Gunn, J., 92, 96, 127, 129, 172, 209, 332–334,
    336–339, 341–343, 345, 346, 375, 392, 623, 624
Brophy, K., 433
Brothers, S., 638
Brouwer, R.M., 627
Brown, A.C., 129
Brown, B.B., 611, 612
Brown, C.H., 589
Brown, D.S., 725
Brown, E.J., 748
Brown, G.W., 206, 207, 503, 528
Brown, J.L., 173
Brown, K.J., 133
Brown, L., 440
Brown, M.Z., 522
Brown, N.L., 188
Brown, P.J., 127–130, 133, 135
Brown, P.L., 692
Brown, R.T., 440
Brown, S.A., 601, 608
Brown, S.M., 56, 273
Brown, T., 110
Brown, T.L., 605
Brown, T.N., 614
Browne, C.B., 187
Brownell, K.D., 622
Broyd, S.J, 437
Brozina, K., 215
Brubakk, A.M., 395
Bruce, A.E., 503
Bruce, J., 375, 376, 378, 380
Bruce, M.L., 103
Bruininks, R.H., 677
Brumariu, L.E., 504, 551, 552
Brumbach, B.H., 450
Brune, C.W., 271
Brunner, R., 762
Bruno, R., 567, 573
Brunwasser, S.M., 135
Bryant, A., 613
Bryant, B., 748
Bryant, F.B., 211, 333
Bryant, R.A., 746
Bryson, S.E., 668
Brzustowicz, L.M., 54, 732
Buchanan, A., 209
Buchanan, C.M., 333, 339
Buchanan, N.R., 186
Buchanan, R.L., 211
Buchmayer, S., 395
Bucholz, K.K., 494
Buehler, C., 147, 213
Bufferd, S.J., 492, 499, 703–714
Bugental, D.B., 316, 726
Buican, B., 678
Buitelaar, J.K., 433, 436, 468
Buka, S.L., 126, 503, 605, 743
Bukowski, W.M., 192, 194, 505, 707

Bukstein, O.G., 432
Bulik, C.M., 621, 623–625, 706
Bullmore, E.T., 268, 436
Bullock, B.M., 195, 457
Bunaciu, L., 341
Bunge, S.A., 437
Bunting, J., 527
Buntinx, W.H.E., 665
Burchinal, M., 113
Burd, L., 669
Bureau, J., 762
Burge, D., 193, 501, 504
Burgess, K.B., 321
Burghy, C.A., 301
Burk, W.J., 194, 196, 339
Burke, H.M., 290
Burke, J.D., 95, 313, 468–470
Burke, K.C., 95
Burks, V., 189
Burmeister, M., 49, 258, 533
Burner, K., 655
Burns, B.J., 98
Burraston, B.O., 300
Burrell, N.A., 169
Burri, A., 695
Burris, R., 695
Burt, K.B., 129
Burt, S.A., 249–251, 624–626
Burton, C., 505
Burton, D.L., 762
Burton, E.M., 209, 501, 610
Bus, A.G., 48
Busatto, G.F., 565
Busby, K.A., 496
Busch, A.L., 769
Bush, G., 436
Bush, N.R., 16, 209, 287–302, 321, 476
Bushley, T., 392
Bushman, B.J., 478, 706
Buskirk, A.A., 707
Buss, K.A., 314, 315, 317, 320, 323, 324, 554
Butler, A.S., 390
Butler, M.J., 210–211
Butler, R.J., 637
Butler, S.M., 114
Butler, U., 637
Button, T.M.M., 590
Buu, A., 592, 593
Buvinger, E., 608
Byne, W., 692, 698
Bynum, M.S., 132
Byrd, A.L., 468
Byrnes, H.F., 131

C
Cacioppo, J.T., 291
Cadaveira, F., 594
Cadoret, R.J., 250, 536
Cagiada, S., 762

Cain, C.A., 250
Cain, D.P., 299
Cain, N.N., 678
Cairns, B.D., 10, 166, 475
Cairns, R.B., 10, 114, 166, 167, 172, 605, 608, 612
Calder, Y.M., 155
Calderon, M., 164
Caldwell, P.H., 641
Caldwell, T., 235
Calkins, S.D., 193, 430, 431, 726
Calvocoressi, L., 569, 574
Camaido, L., 762
Cameron, R.P., 493
Campbell, K.D.M., 228
Campbell, S.B., 427–442, 498
Candel, M., 611
Canino, G., 227, 492
Canli, T., 274
Cannell, C.F., 103
Canning, R.D., 188
Cantwell, D.P., 338, 504
Capaldi, D., 188, 451, 505
Capitman, J., 610
Caplan, M.Z., 186
Cappuccio, F.P., 409, 413
Capute, A.J., 668–669
Carbone, M.A., 255
Carbonneau, R., 114
Card, N.A., 192
Cardoos, S.L., 192
Caregaro, L., 621
Carey, K.B., 609
Carey, P.D., 745
Carey, W.B., 410
Carleton, R.A., 205–218
Carlson, E.A., 7, 9, 37, 150, 317, 359, 360, 709, 731, 762, 765
Carlson, G.A., 492
Carlson, M., 290
Carlson, W., 194
Carmody, D.P., 269, 658, 659
Carmona, S., 436
Carnes, M., 734
Carney, T., 635
Carpendale, J.I., 707
Carpenter, T.P., 209
Carpenter, W.B., 585
Carr, E.G., 672
Carrasco, M., 269
Carrillo, N., 172
Carrion, V.G., 749, 752, 762
Carroll, A.E., 176
Carskadon, M.A., 174, 175, 413–415, 496
Carson, C., 391
Carter, A.S., 561–575, 658
Carter, F.A., 706
Carter, J.D., 392
Carter, J.S., 205–218, 501, 503, 504
Carter, M.C., 380
Carter, R., 338

Caruthers, A.S., 457
Carver, C.S., 502
Carwile, S., 767
Casadio, P., 57
Casarosa, E., 627
Casey, B.J., 268, 609
Casey, G., 631, 632
Casey, P.H., 399, 402, 434
Casiglia, A.C., 233
Caspers, K., 275
Caspi, A., 38, 46, 49, 52–57, 93, 94, 131, 167, 250, 256,
        272, 311, 334, 335, 338–342, 435, 449, 470, 474,
        499, 503, 506, 526, 533, 535, 589, 606, 607, 613,
        710, 711, 732, 746
Cassidy, J., 3, 150, 153, 552
Castellanos, F.X., 436, 437
Castelli, K.L., 430
Castle, D.J., 565
Castle, J., 357, 376
Catalano, R.F., 115, 164, 174, 176, 589
Cauffman, E., 608
Cavanagh, S.E., 145
Caverzasi, E., 498, 499
Cedeno, L.A., 130
Celimli, S., 378
Cen, G., 228
Cerdá, M., 603
Cerrito, B.M., 730
Céspedes, Y.M., 228
Chabane, N., 562
Chaffin, M., 364
Chagnon, N.A., 233
Chaiyasit, W., 225
Chamberlain, P., 480
Chambers, P.L., 394
Chambless, D.L., 573
Champagne, F.A., 252, 312
Champoux, M., 53, 554
Chan, K.P., 252
Chan, W., 376
Chandler, A.L., 147
Chandler, M.J., 6, 28, 38, 707
Chandra, A., 97
Chanen, A.M., 704, 708, 709
Chang, C., 704
Chao, R.K., 228
Charman, T., 652
Charness, N., 30
Charney, D., 496, 499
Charnov, E., 7
Charpak, N., 391
Charpak, Y., 391
Charuvastra, A., 743
Chase-Lansdale, P.L., 96
Chassin, L., 211, 589, 601, 608, 609
Chatoor, I., 397, 398, 400, 401
Chattarji, S., 382
Chau, C., 190
Cheah, C.L., 189, 192
Cheah, C.S.L., 505

Cheely, C., 212
Chein, J., 609
Chelminski, I., 704
Chemineau, P., 416
Chen, C.H., 230, 233–236, 278
Chen, E., 205–218, 287, 289–291, 375
Chen, H.N.A., 232, 235, 236, 709
Chen, K., 748
Chen, L.A., 497–499
Chen, M.C., 495
Chen, S.H., 744
Chen, W.J., 213
Chen, X., 197, 225–237
Chen, Y.F., 49, 257
Cheng, H., 230
Cherkas, L., 695
Cheslow, D., 567
Chesney, M., 296
Chess, S., 6, 14, 311, 499
Chesson, A.L. Jr., 419
Chetty, R., 175
Cheung, R.Y.M., 236
Chhangur, R., 48, 49
Chiao, J.Y., 302
Child, I.L., 631, 632
Childs, C.P., 226
Chisholm, K., 374, 380
Chiu, W.T., 562
Chiu, Y.J., 213
Chmielewski, M., 70, 110
Cho, E., 291
Choi, H., 228
Chomsky, N., 6
Chong, R., 229
Chorpita, B.F., 207, 228, 554
Choukas-Bradley, S.C., 185–198
Chow, S.-M., 134, 315
Christakis, D.A., 299
Christener, R.W., 163
Christoforidou, A., 229
Christopher, N.C., 746
Chu, A.T., 745
Chu, B.C., 130
Chugani, H.T., 381, 382
Chung, B., 277
Chung, I.-J., 115
Chung, J., 197, 228
Chung, K.F., 229
Chung, S.S., 711
Chung, U.S., 765
Cicchetti, D., 11, 27, 40, 49, 90, 119, 127–130, 135, 146,
        154, 155, 195, 210, 213, 256, 258, 265, 290, 300,
        302, 312, 313, 317, 331, 340, 342, 366, 377–378,
        474, 476, 492, 494, 537, 605, 606, 614, 708,
        723–736, 762
Cicirelli, V.G., 146
Ciesla, J.A., 209, 501, 504
Cillessen, A.H.N., 187, 190, 505, 707
Cillessen, A.N., 187, 190
Cirulli, E.T., 253, 254

Claes, M., 457
Claessens, A., 324
Clark, A.G., 494, 505
Clark, C., 235
Clark, D.A., 563
Clark, D.B., 734
Clark, D.M., 414, 748
Clark, K.E., 145
Clark, L.A., 499, 550, 703, 704, 713, 714
Clark, R., 390
Clarke, A.R., 377
Clarke, G., 496, 499
Clausen, J.S., 612
Clauss, J.A., 319
Clayton, R.R., 605
Clemans, K.H., 341
Clements, M., 394
Cleves, M.A., 434
Cloitre, M., 743
Cloninger, C.R., 583, 706
Clum, G.A., 678
Coates, S., 690
Cobb, J.A., 451
Cobb, N., 171
Coccia, M.A., 173
Cochran, S.D., 92
Coe, C.L., 734
Coffino, B., 7
Coghill, D., 427–429, 433
Cohen, D.J., 268, 331, 340, 342, 658
Cohen, G.L., 176, 195
Cohen, J.A., 75, 744, 747, 749–751, 753–754, 769
Cohen, J.D., 594
Cohen, M.A., 467
Cohen, P.R., 88, 89, 565, 610, 709, 713
Cohen, S., 206, 214, 287, 289, 290
Cohen-Almagor, R., 522
Cohen-Kettenis, P.T., 685, 688–689, 691, 693, 695, 696, 698
Cohn, J., 502, 727
Coie, J.D., 185, 187–189, 235, 315, 456, 475, 707–708
Colaizy, T., 391
Colbus, D., 18
Colder, C.R., 321
Cole, D.A., 210, 211, 213, 320, 490, 494, 501, 504
Cole, D.J., 197
Cole, H.E., 150
Cole, P.M., 154, 230, 232
Cole, R., 34
Cole, S.W., 186, 252
Cole, S.Z., 396
Coleman, C.C., 190
Coleman, E., 698
Coleman, J.C., 607, 608
Coleman, R.W., 396
Coles, M.E., 168
Coley, R.L., 129
Colin, V., 398
Collins, F.S., 254, 257
Collins, L.M., 111, 607

Collins, M., 767
Collins, W.A., 9, 37, 150, 610
Collin-Vézina, D., 762
Collishaw, S., 132
Colonnesi, C., 552
Colvert, E., 378
Coman, D.C., 271
Comeau, C.A., 129
Compas, B.E., 30, 205, 207, 208, 499–502, 506
Compian, L., 336
Compton, S.N., 91, 97
Compton, W.M., 584, 585
Comtois, K.A., 522
Conde-Agudelo, A., 391
Conger, R.D., 130, 147, 156, 337–339, 341, 346, 503, 504, 554, 611
Conley, C.S., 333, 336–338, 340, 341, 343, 345, 493, 500–501, 505
Connell, A.M., 113, 115, 461, 505
Conner, B.T., 610
Conners, C.K., 70, 72
Connolly, C., 658
Connolly, J., 336, 337
Connolly, N.P., 211
Connor, C.M., 37
Connor-Smith, J.K., 499, 501
Constantine, N.A., 393
Constantino, J.N., 654, 689, 734
Conti, G., 293
Conway, C.C., 110, 194, 495
Cook, C.A., 749
Cook, E.H., 677
Cook, K.V., 4
Cook, T.D., 26, 178
Cooley, M.R., 228
Coolidge, F.L., 695
Cooney, R.E., 501
Coons, P.M., 761
Cooper, C.S., 643
Cooper, K., 402
Cooper, M.L., 569, 609
Cooper, P.J., 550, 551
Cooper, S.A., 678
Cope, J., 373
Copeland, W.E., 165, 491, 493, 546, 743, 745, 746, 753
Coplan, J.D., 497
Coplan, R.J., 234
Coppola, G., 638
Corcos, M., 623
Corfas, G., 292
Corno, L., 167
Corr, P.J., 533
Corral, M.M., 594
Correia, C.J., 609
Correnti, R., 175
Corteses, S., 419
Cortesi, F., 414
Costa, P.T. Jr., 712
Costantini, A., 638
Costanzo, P.R., 493

Costello, E.J., 33, 65, 87–91, 95, 97, 102, 103, 110, 111, 119, 165, 333, 337, 339, 492, 493, 546–548, 566, 588, 589, 610

Costello, J., 111, 429, 491, 743, 745, 746, 753

Cote, J.E., 609

Cothern, L., 231

Cotsonas-Hassler, T.M., 669

Cottrell, D., 402

Couchoud, E.A., 186

Coughlin, S.S., 622

Coulton, C.J., 96

Courchesne, E., 269, 659

Courtney, M., 112

Coury, D.L., 401

Coussons-Read, M.E., 390

Cowan, R.L., 319

Cowen, P.J., 278

Cox, C., 338

Cox, D.J., 639

Cox, M.J., 144, 146–148, 152, 255, 316

Coyne, J.C., 504, 506

Craddock, M.M., 434

Craig, J.C., 641

Craig, W.M., 336, 337

Cramer, A., 475

Crampton, D.S., 96

Craney, J.L., 491

Crawford, T.N., 709, 713

Crayton, J., 730

Creamer, M., 748

Creedy, D., 392

Cregger, B., 573

Creswell, C., 550, 551, 555

Crick, N.R., 188, 190, 191, 236, 706, 708, 733, 734

Crisp, A.H., 623

Crittenden, P.M., 726, 728

Crockett, L., 338

Croen, L.A., 103

Croffie, J.M., 641

Croft, C.M., 251

Cronbach, L.J., 318

Crone, E.A., 609, 614

Crosby, L., 459

Crosby Ouimette, P., 704

Crosnoe, R., 33, 177, 601, 604, 607, 612

Crossman, E.J., 125–136, 296

Croudace, T., 495, 496

Crouter, A.C., 10, 146

Crowe, R.R., 250

Crowell, S.E., 522, 524, 526, 529, 530, 532–538, 704, 709

Crowley, S.J., 413, 415

Crozier, M., 547

Csepe, V., 118–119

Csikszentmihalyi, C., 132

Csikszentmihalyi, M., 135

Cudeck, R., 114

Cuellar, D., 164

Cueva, J.E., 751

Cui, M., 147, 156

Cukor, D., 505

Culbert, J.P., 413

Culbert, K.M., 625, 626

Culbert, T.P., 643

Cullen, K.R., 498

Cullerton-Sen, C., 729

Culley, B.S., 394

Cumming, R., 641

Cummings, E.M., 11, 145–148, 150, 153, 156, 297, 315, 427, 477, 745

Cummings, J., 131

Curchack-Lichtin, J.T., 427

Curran, M., 148

Curran, P.J., 112–116, 119, 208, 502, 548, 589

Currie, C., 336

Currier, D., 532

Curry, C.J., 671

Curry, J.F., 574

Curtis, D., 440

Curtis, W.J., 727, 735

Cusi, A.M., 498

Cusick, G., 112

Cuskelly, M., 395

Cuthbert, B.N., 622

Cutts, D., 402

Cutuli, J.J., 317

Cyr, C., 727

Cyranowski, J.M., 493, 545

Cytryn, L., 31

Czaja, S.J., 731

Czajia, S.J., 709

Czeisler, C.A., 415

D

Dackis, M.N., 129, 733

Dadds, M.R., 478, 548, 550–552, 553, 555

Dagan, Y., 416

Dahl, R., 409

Dahl, R.A., 332, 333, 345

Dahl, R.E., 174, 333, 334, 343, 349, 496, 497, 609, 614

Daleiden, E.L., 268

Dalen, L., 431

Daley, D., 427, 431

Daley, S.E., 211, 331, 503–505

Dalgleish, T., 744, 748

Dallaire, D.H., 552

Dallam, S., 763

Dalldorf, J., 676

Dalton, K.M., 268, 269, 277

Daly, M., 654

D'Amato, F.R., 56

D'Amico, E.J., 611

Dancyger, I.F., 624

Danese, A., 734

D'Angelo, E.J., 531

D'Angiulli, A., 130, 292

Daniels, D., 248.250

Dannefer, D., 607

Danovitch, J.H., 689

Dansky, B.S., 743

Danzig, A.P., 703–714
Darling-Hammond, L., 175
Darlow, B.A., 392
Darwin, C., 18
Datar, A., 165
Davey, G.C.L., 553
David, C.F., 228
Davidov, M., 149
Davidson, R.J., 377, 497, 535
Davies, B.A., 623
Davies, M., 536, 546, 563
Davies, P.T., 143–157, 427
Davila, D., 419
Davila, J., 112, 504
Davis, B., 504
Davis, E.L., 323
Davis, L., 391, 392, 749
Davis, N.S., 410
Davis, R.L., 565
Davis, S.K., 115, 212, 730
Dawood, K., 695
Daws, L.C., 270, 271, 273
Dawson, D.A., 589
Dawson, G., 265, 268, 494, 497, 537, 614, 655, 656
Day, N.E., 252
De Bellis, M.D., 382, 746, 752
De Bolle, M., 713
De Clercq, B.J., 499, 711–713
De Curtis, M., 398
De Cuypere, G., 685
de Figueroa, C.Z., 391
De Fruyt, F., 499, 705, 711–713
de Groat, C., 215
de Haan, M., 291
de Kloet, E.R., 289
de Lacerda, A., 752
De Los Reyes, A., 191
De Meyer, T., 294
De Ocampo, A.C., 394
De Pauw, S.S.W., 311, 319
De Schipper, J.C., 291, 366
De Vocht, F., 57
de Vries, A.L.C., 688, 689, 698
de Vries, H., 611
De Wilde, A., 551
de Winter, A.F., 395, 500
de Zwaan, M., 622
Deacon, B.J., 572
Deale, A., 565
Dean, D., 707
Deater-Deckard, K., 49, 113, 247–249, 478, 534
DeBaryshe, B.D., 534
DeBellis, M.D., 730
Deblinger, E., 750, 769
Deblois, T., 392
DeCarlo, C.A., 156
DeClercq, B., 705
Decoufle, P., 668
DeFries, J.C., 48, 51, 249, 250
DeGarmo, D.S., 152

Degirmencioglu, S.M., 611
Degnan, K.A., 311, 431, 550, 555
Dekker, M.C., 676
Del Giudice, M., 208, 211, 297
Delahanty, D.L., 746
DelBello, M.P., 278
Delemarre-van de Waal, H.A., 696
Delgado, P., 564
DelGiudice, M., 349
Dell, P.F., 761–762, 765
DeLoache, J.S., 555
Delorme, R., 564, 565
DeLucia, C., 589
Delva, J., 605
DelVecchio, W.F., 711
Demaree, H.A., 431
DeMaso, D.R., 531
Dement, W.C., 496
DeMier, R.L., 392
Demirakca, T., 498
Denckla, M.B., 436
Denham, S.A., 186
Denissen, J.J.A., 234
Dennis, C.L., 392
Dennis, N.R., 669
Denny, G.S., 171
Deogracias, J.J., 686, 687, 692
Derbidge, C.M., 521–538, 704
Derks, L.M., 72
DeRose, L.M., 346
DeRosier, M.E., 236
Derryberry, D., 745
DeSantis, A.S., 290
Desjarlais, R., 746
DeSouza, A., 232
D'Esposito, M., 11, 293
Dettling, A.C., 291, 312
Dettmer, A.M., 289, 293, 299, 301
Devaud, L.L., 590
Dever, B.V., 609, 611
Devilly, G.J., 392
Dewald, J.F., 175, 409
DeYoung, C.G., 733
Di Forti, M., 56, 57
Diaferia, G., 566
Diamantopoulou, S., 72
Diamond, A., 165, 167
Diaz, R.M., 92, 536
Diaz-Rossello, J., 391
Dichter, G.S., 497
Dick, D.M., 341, 590, 591, 593
Dick, R., 171
Dickstein, S.G., 437
Diener, E., 135
Dienstbier, R.A., 290
Dierickx, K., 522
Dierker, L., 525
Dietrich, S., 571
Diez Roux, A.V., 95, 97
Digdon, N.L., 413

DiLavore, P., 653
Dimas, J., 215
Dinan, T.G., 497
Dindo, L., 710
Ding, B., 57
Dintcheff, B.A., 611
Diorio, J., 252
DiRago, A.C., 592
Diseth, T., 762
Dishion, T.J., 113, 131, 188, 189, 191, 194, 195, 233,
        234, 313, 449–462, 471, 475, 476, 505, 536, 611,
        612, 710
Dixon, D.R., 671
Doan, S.N., 210
Dobscha, S.K., 522
Dobson, P., 635
Dodge, K.A., 40, 89, 119, 130, 153, 156, 166,
        187–189, 195, 235, 236, 250, 297, 312,
        313, 315, 316, 318, 322–324, 450, 452,
        456, 461, 471, 478, 601, 606, 608, 610,
        611, 613, 707–708, 729, 730
Doering, L.V., 392
Doernberger, C.H., 126
Dohrenwend, B., 206, 207, 214, 215
Dolan, C.V., 72
Dolan, L., 215
Dolan, R.J., 273, 382
Doll, H.A., 623
Domenech, J.M., 494
Domes, G., 277
Domingues, M.R., 397
Dominguez, A., 747–748
Dong, Q., 230, 232, 233, 543
Donnellan, M.B., 147
D'Onofrio, B.M., 54, 250
Donovan, J.E., 601
Donzella, B., 291
Doreleijers, T.A.H., 688, 689
Doremus-Fitzwater, T.L., 608, 609
Dorn, L.D., 331–333, 338–340, 342, 345, 346, 348, 608
Dornbusch, S.M., 145
Dosen, A., 677
Dougherty, L.R., 112, 492
Downey, G., 169
Downing, J., 608
Dowsett, C., 324
Doyle, A.E., 427, 431
Dozier, M., 251, 290, 291, 300, 366
Drabant, E.M., 53
Drabick, D.G., 211
Drachman, D., 750
Dracup, K., 392
Drake, B., 724, 734
Draper, P., 347, 450
Dreger, R.M., 70
Drescher, J., 698
Drevets, W.C., 266, 497, 498
Drewett, R.F., 396, 402
Driscoll, A.K., 338
Driscoll, K., 499
Drotar, D., 402

Drummond, K.D., 691, 692
Drury, S.S., 294, 295, 299, 376
Dryfoos, J.G., 171
Duarte, C.S., 131
Dubas, J.S., 333, 336
DuBois, D.L., 131, 171, 192, 214
Dubowitz, H., 402
Ducci, F., 589
Duckett, E., 610
Dudbridge, F., 496
Dudukovic, N.M., 437
Duffy, S.N., 214
Duggal, S., 215
Duhig, A.M., 69
Dumas, J.E., 231
Dumenci, L., 69, 74
Dumitrescu, A., 365
DuMont, K., 731
Duncan, A., 653
Duncan, G.J., 92, 96, 163–165, 172, 324
Duncan, L.E., 57
Duncan, S.C., 118, 611
Duncan, T.E., 118, 454, 611
Dunger, D.B., 397
Dunlap, K.G., 707
Dunlop, L.C., 339, 340, 346
Dunn, E., 171, 503
Dunn, J., 146, 150, 250
Dunn, V., 491
DuPaul, G.J., 431–433, 440
Durakovic-Belko, E., 748
Durand, V.M., 418, 672
Durbin, C.E., 499, 500, 704, 706
Durkheim, E., 521, 523, 525, 528, 536
Durlak, J.A., 172
Durrant, C., 258
Durrett, C., 110, 704
Dusick, A.M., 398
Dutra, L., 762, 764
Dweck, C.S., 165, 168, 169
Dyck, R.J., 531
Dyer-Friedman, J., 573
Dykens, E.M., 675, 678
Dymnicki, A.B., 172
Dyregrov, A., 747
Dyson, M.W., 311, 499, 703–714
Dziobek, I., 268, 269

E
Eagle, M.N., 3
Earls, F., 96, 290, 341
Earls, M., 440
East, P.L., 611
Easteal, S., 54
Easterlin, R.A., 528, 529
Eaton, W.O., 688
Eaton, W.W., 547
Eaves, L.J., 48, 51, 246, 249–251, 347, 493, 494, 710
Eberhart, N.K., 209, 211, 493
Ebersöhn, L., 130

Ebstein, R.P., 272, 297
Eby, J., 505
Eby, L.T., 171
Eccles, J.S., 26, 34, 40, 131, 163–179, 331, 333, 339, 612
Eckenrode, J.E., 536
Eddy, J.M., 454
Eddy, K.T., 621
Eddy, M.J., 194
Edelbrock, C., 70, 71, 431
Edell, W.S., 704
Edelson, L., 658
Eder, D., 189
Edinger, J.D., 414
Edwards, A.C., 341
Edwards, C.P., 228
Edwards, D.M., 395
Edwards, H., 391
Edwards, M.C., 112
Edwards, M.E., 119
Edwards, P., 153, 453
Egan, S.K., 192
Egeland, B., 9, 37, 90, 126, 150, 317, 359, 555, 592, 709, 731, 762
Egerter, S., 287
Egger, H.L., 87, 111–112, 430–432, 492, 546, 547, 566
Eggleston, E.P., 114
Eggum, N.D., 457, 501–502, 706
Egolf, B.P., 726
Ehlers, A., 748
Ehrenkranz, R.A., 398
Ehrenreich, S.E., 198
Ehrensaft, M., 709
Ehrman, K., 269
Einfield, S.L., 676, 678
Eisen, J.L., 568, 571
Eisen, M.L., 730
Eisenberg, L., 746
Eisenberg, N., 128, 132, 232, 236, 315, 323, 457, 501–502, 706, 707
Eisenhower, A., 505
Eisenhower, J.W., 761–762
Eklund, K., 115
El Sarraj, E., 743
Elder, G.H. Jr., 19, 26, 33, 177, 337, 338, 346, 347, 503, 554, 605, 607
Eldredge, N., 18, 38
Eley, T.C., 211, 256, 494, 501, 548, 549, 552
El-Faddagh, M., 435
Elias, M.J., 130
Elkind, D., 608
Elkins, I., 589
Ellickson, S.L., 610
Elliott, D.S., 31
Elliott, P., 748
Elliott, R., 382
Ellis, B.B., 77
Ellis, B.J., 54, 155, 208, 271, 296, 297, 322, 347–349, 450, 459, 460, 504
Ellis, J.E., 38
Ellis, L.K., 452

Ellis, P.M., 731
Ellis, T.A., 525
Ellison, C.G., 249
Ellison-Wright, I., 436
Ellison-Wright, Z., 436
Elnour, A.A., 527
Elsabbagh, M., 656
Else-Quest, N., 493
El-Sheikh, M., 297, 319, 472, 477, 478
Eluvathingal, T.J., 382
Emde, R.N., 36
Emerson, E., 677
Emery, R.E., 156, 196, 332, 749
Emmett, P.M., 396
Emond, A.M., 396
Emslie, G.J., 491, 496
Ende, G., 498
Endo, T., 276
Engel, M., 324
Engels, R.C.M.E., 339
Engert, V., 298
England, S.J., 419
Englund, M.M., 317
Enns, L.R., 688
Enoch, M.A., 258
Ensminger, M.E., 589
Ensor, R., 146
Entringer, S., 294
Entwisle, D.R., 172
Epel, E.S., 294, 295
Epps, A., 208
Epstein, M.K., 69
Erath, S.A., 297, 472, 477, 478, 707
Ercan, E.S., 572
Erdogan, A., 638
Erhart, F., 750
Erhart, M., 74
Ericsson, K.A., 30
Erikson, E.H., 360, 609
Eriksson, M., 392
Erkanli, A., 65, 88, 95, 111, 333, 492, 493, 546, 589, 610
Erklani, A., 429
Ernst, M., 498
Eron, L.D., 152
Escobar, J.I., 229
Esparza, N.P., 210
Espelage, D.L., 166, 236
Espie, C.A., 414
Espinoza, G., 198
Esposito, E.A., 348, 349, 371–385
Esposito, L., 118
Essau, C.A., 493
Esser, G., 435
Essex, M.J., 252, 291, 293, 296, 297, 503
Estell, D.B., 475
Estes, D., 11
Estrada, G., 56
Esveldt-Dawson, I., 17
Etkin, A., 268
Ettelt, S., 569
Etter, E.M., 209

Euser, E.M., 727
Evans, D.W., 565, 567
Evans, G.W., 210, 290, 291, 295
Evans, J., 56
Evans, S.C., 171
Evans, S.W., 171
Evenden, J.L., 533
Evindar, A., 393
Ewing, L.J., 431
Ey, S., 208
Eyberg, S.M., 479, 480
Eyer, J., 295
Eysenck, H.J., 313, 499
Eysenck, M.W., 499
Ezpeleta, L., 494

F
Fabbri, C., 252
Fabbri, M., 414
Fabes, R.A., 198, 475
Faden, V.B., 601, 602
Fagan, J., 761
Fagg, J., 528
Fagot, B.I., 4, 454
Fairburn, C.G., 397, 622, 623
Fairchild, G., 372, 436
Faja, S., 655
Fan, X., 498
Fang, X., 725
Fanselow, M.S., 752
Farah, M.J., 292
Farahmand, F.K., 214
Faraone, S.V., 429, 431, 433, 434, 436
Farber, E.A., 126
Farberow, N.L., 522
Farberow, R., 524
Fargeon, S., 432
Farley, F., 608, 609
Farmer, T.W., 233, 475
Farrell, A., 118
Farrell, L.J., 563, 568, 572–574
Farrell, M.P., 611
Farrington, D.P., 457, 470, 471, 710
Farris, A.M., 147
Farver, J., 230
Fask, D., 250
Fast, D.K., 416
Faturi, C.B., 373
Fausto-Sterling, A., 683
Favaro, A., 621, 623
Fearon, P., 252
Fearon, R.M.P., 149, 393
Fearon, R.P., 357, 358, 360, 361, 552
Federman, E., 589
Feehan, M., 91
Feeley, N., 394
Feeny, N.C., 743–754
Feifel, J., 192
Fein, D., 660

Fein, G.G., 186
Feinstein, C.B., 669, 674, 676
Feiring, C., 4, 6, 9, 358, 707, 748, 764
Feldman, H.M., 440
Feldman, R., 394
Feldman, S., 188
Feldstein, M., 745
Fenton, M., 585
Ferber, R., 410, 411, 417, 418
Ferdinand, R.F., 72
Ferentz, L., 769
Ferenz-Gillies, R., 150
Fergusson, D.M., 54, 56, 58, 92, 93, 146, 235, 258, 491, 495, 499
Fernald, L.C., 290
Fernandes, C., 57
Fernández-Navarro, P., 533
Ferrara, S., 621
Ferreira, R., 130
Ferrero, J., 334, 337, 338, 347, 348, 608
Fetrow, R., 454
Fiedler, F.E., 131
Field, A.P., 543, 551, 553–555, 744
Field, T.A., 392, 393
Fiese, B.H., 35, 38, 393
Figueredo, A.J., 450
Finch, A.J., 17, 746
Fincham, F.D., 133, 145, 147, 150
Findenauer, C., 135
Findlay, R., 147
Fine, S., 17
Finesmith, R., 677
Finkelhor, D., 743, 744
Fischel, J.E., 631–346
Fischer, M., 428, 429, 431, 432
Fischman, A.I., 436
Fish, L., 366
Fisher, L., 374, 378
Fisher, P.A., 290, 291, 300, 302, 380, 762
Fisk, N., 685
Fiske, A., 529
Fiske, S.T., 169
Fitzgerald, H.E., 591, 592
Fitzgerald, M., 433
Fitzmaurice, G.M., 114, 119, 492, 503, 708
Fivaz-Depeursinge, E., 146
Flament, M.F., 562, 563, 567
Flanagan, J., 656
Flannery, D.J., 114, 339
Flay, B.R., 115, 607
Fleeson, J., 727–729
Fleischmann, R.L., 564
Fleitlich-Bilyk, B., 73
Fleiz, C., 212
Fleming, J., 493
Fleming, W.S., 150
Flemings, C.B., 164
Flemming, J.E., 31
Fletcher, K., 428, 432
Flint, J., 46, 258

Flook, L., 173
Florence, C.S., 725
Flores, E., 215
Flores, G., 165
Flory, K., 605
Flouri, E., 209, 210
Flynn, C., 501, 504
Flynn, M., 212, 213, 215, 348, 502–504
Foa, E.B., 563, 570–572, 745, 750
Foley, D.L., 54, 87, 492, 732
Folkman, S., 206
Folstein, S., 652, 653
Fonagy, P., 549, 709
Fonseca, A.C., 546, 548
Fontaine, J., 229
Fontaine, N.M.G., 114, 479
Fontaine, R.G., 166, 477
Fonzi, A., 233
Forbes, D., 746
Forbes, E.E., 343, 498, 502
Forcada-Guex, M., 393, 394
Ford, J.D., 151, 761
Forehand, R.L., 93, 480, 505
Forgatch, M.S., 152, 451, 456
Formoso, D., 213
Fornari, V., 624
Forston, J.L., 173
Fosco, G.M., 457
Foster, C.L., 163, 169
Foster, D.W., 625
Foster, H., 346
Foster, J.D., 743, 745
Foster, R.G., 410
Fowles, D.C., 472, 710
Fox, M.D., 280
Fox, N.A., 9, 11, 154, 270, 300, 302, 311, 319, 373, 377, 378, 381, 383, 502, 550, 555
Fox, S.E., 295, 381
Foxx, R.M., 642
Fraley, R.C., 251, 490
Francis, G., 90
Frank, D.A., 389–402
Frank, E., 493
Franke, B., 433
Frankenburg, F.R., 708
Franklin, J., 491
Franklin, M.E., 561, 572
Frazier, J., 669
Frazier, S.L., 131
Frazier, T.W., 431, 653, 654
Fredrickson, B.L., 134, 135
Freedman-Doan, P., 613
Freeman, L.N., 17
Freeman, M., 18
Freeman, R.D., 416
Freisthler, B., 96
Freitag, C.M., 636–638
French, D., 227, 228
French, N.H., 17
Frenn, K.A., 298, 331, 333, 374, 384

Freres, D.R., 135
Freshman, M., 563, 570
Freud, S., 18, 524
Freund, A.M., 132
Freyd, J.J., 762
Frick, P.J., 428, 478, 707
Fridell, S.R., 688
Friedel, S., 255
Friedman, H., 337
Friedman, J.N., 175
Friedman, R.J., 230
Friedrich, W.N., 762
Friemel, C.M., 627
Friis, S., 535
Friman, P.C., 644
Frith, C.D., 382
Frodl, T.S., 497–499
Frohlich, L., 163
Fromme, K., 608, 611
Frosch, C.A., 147, 150
Frosch, D.L., 230
Frost, L.A., 672
Frost, R.O., 563, 564, 567
Frustaci, K., 752
Frye, D., 567
Fu, R., 225–237
Fu, V.R., 228
Fudell, M., 209, 501
Fudge, H., 491
Fulker, D.W., 49, 51, 248, 534
Fuller-Rowell, T.E., 210
Fung, H., 236
Furey, W., 17
Furman, D.J., 273
Furman, W., 187
Furmark, T., 278
Furstenberg, F.F. Jr., 26, 33
Futh, A., 569

G
Gabard-Durnam, L., 657
Gaensbauer, T., 726
Gahagan, S., 395
Galambos, N.L., 601
Gale, C.R., 503
Galea, S., 114, 603
Galles, S., 502
Galvan, A., 609
Gamble, W., 150
Ganger, W., 762
Ganiban, J., 397, 398, 728
Gannon-Rowley, T., 95
Ganzel, B.L., 295
Ganzini, L., 522
Gar, N., 551
Garbe, P.L., 165
Garber, J., 165, 209, 215, 489–507
Garcia, A., 562, 567
García Coll, C.T., 130, 683

Garcia, E.E., 164
Garcia, R., 393
Garcia-Coll, C., 197, 300
Gardner, C.O., 50, 52, 56, 249, 506, 590, 593
Gardner, F., 454
Gardner, H., 5
Gardner, L.I., 396
Gardner, W., 7, 473
Gariépy, J.-L., 316
Garite, T.J., 390
Garmezy, N., 4, 6, 8, 17, 27, 28, 34, 125, 126,
    128, 129, 155
Garner, A.S., 174
Garofano, A., 164
Garon, N., 656
Garrard, W.M., 169
Garrison, C.Z., 743
Gartstein, M.A., 229, 231, 319
Garvin, M.C., 377, 378
Gass, K., 150
Gathercole, V.C.M., 659
Gatzke-Kopp, L.M., 297, 471, 522, 524, 531, 532, 537, 704
Gauvain, M., 205
Gazelle, H., 505
Ge, X., 49, 50, 334, 337–343, 346, 347, 503, 504
Gee, G., 215
Geen, T., 564
Geffken, G.R., 570
Geffner, M.E., 696
Geldhof, G., 190
Gelernter, J., 270
Geller, B., 491
Geller, D.A., 562, 564, 566
Gelman, S.A., 696
Gendall, K.A., 623
Gendreau, P.L., 471
Gentsch, J.K., 198
Georgiades, K., 88
Gerard, J.M., 147, 213
Gerber, A.J., 499
Gerdts, J., 654
Gerrard, M., 195, 608
Gershkovich, M., 536
Gershman, E.S., 186
Gershoff, E.T., 475
Gervai, J., 251
Geschwind, D.H., 272, 276
Gesell, A., 567
Gest, S.D., 234
Gettinger, M., 130
Geurts, H.M., 291
Ghahramani, N., 695
Ghashghaei, H.T., 266
Ghaziuddin, M., 653
Ghera, M.M., 300
Ghosh-Ippen, C., 769
Giancola, P.R., 532
Giannetta, J., 171
Gianotti, F., 414
Gibb, B.E., 168, 194, 501, 503–505

Gibbons, F.X., 195, 608
Gibbons, R.D., 114
Gibson, J.J., 5, 19
Gibson, S., 433
Gidlow, B., 768
Giedd, J.N., 268, 269, 296
Gil, A.G., 605
Giletta, M., 196
Gill, M., 433
Gillberg, C., 505
Gillespie, N., 110
Gillham, J.E., 135
Gillihan, S.J., 547
Gilliom, M., 452
Gilman, S.E., 503
Gilman, S.R., 276
Gil-Rivas, V., 208
Gingrich, J.A., 273
Ginsburg, G.S., 546, 554
Ginzburg, S., 75
Gipson, P.Y., 205
Girgus, J.S., 165, 206, 504
Gittelman-Klein, R., 553
Gjerde, P.F., 500
Gladstone, T.R.G., 127
Glass, J.D., 410
Glass, S., 704
Gleason, M.M., 299, 362–364, 379, 395
Glendinning, A., 707
Glenn, A.L., 710
Glover, G., 609
Glover, V., 255, 295, 434
Glovinsky, P.B., 415
Glowinski, A.L., 494, 495
Glucksman, E., 744, 748
Gmel, G., 96
Gnehm, H.E., 746
Goeke-Morey, M., 150
Goffinet, S., 762, 765
Gogtay, N., 268
Gold, A.L., 735
Goldberg, D.P., 229
Goldberg, S., 4, 206
Goldberger, E., 567
Golden, E., 127
Golding, J., 434
Goldin-Meadow, S., 659
Goldman, D., 589, 590
Goldman, S.J., 531, 534
Goldsmith, H.H., 312, 315, 430, 493, 535
Goldstein, D.B., 253
Goldstein, L.H., 288
Goldwin, M.A., 549, 689
Goldwyn, R., 37
Gollan, J.K., 500
Golombok, S.E., 695
Gomez, A., 771
Goncalves, S., 622
Goncy, E., 114
Gone, J.P., 528

Gonzales, N.A., 213
Gonzalez, L.M., 209
Gonzalez-Tejera, G., 493
Good, B., 746
Goodman, A., 73, 74, 230
Goodman, E., 215, 610
Goodman, G.S., 730
Goodman, M., 191, 709
Goodman, R., 73, 74, 97, 100, 132, 230
Goodman, S.H., 493, 504
Goodman, W.K., 562, 564
Goodnight, J.A., 311, 312, 315, 318, 323, 324
Goodwin, G.M., 278, 414
Goodwin, R.D., 499
Goodyer, I.M., 491, 495–497, 499, 501–503
Gootman, J.A., 167, 172
Gooze, R.A., 393
Gordis, E.B., 472, 473
Gordon, K.H., 526
Gordon, L.U., 206
Gordon, M., 169
Gordon, R., 96
Gorka, A., 614
Gorman, A., 190
Gorman-Smith, D., 130
Gosch, A., 74
Gotlib, I.H., 273, 495, 498, 501, 502, 506
Gotlib, I.J., 338
Gottesman, I., 7
Gottfredson, D.C., 172
Gottleib, G., 114
Gottlieb, G., 265, 272
Gottman, J.M., 453
Gould, G.G., 270, 271, 273
Gould, M.S., 528
Gould, S.J., 18, 38
Govindan, R.M., 382
Goy, E.R., 522
Goy, R.W., 695
Gozal, D., 418
Graae, F., 536
Graber, J.A., 209, 211, 332–336, 338–343, 345–348, 375, 623
Grace, S.L., 393
Graczyk, P.A., 504
Gradisar, M., 415
Grafodatskaya, D., 277
Graham, J., 171
Graham, S., 168, 191, 192, 196, 197
Gralen, S.J., 624
Granat, A., 394
Granger, D.A., 192, 291, 297, 472
Granic, I., 155, 314, 475, 591
Granot, D., 153
Grant, B.F., 228, 584, 589, 602
Grant, K.E., 205–218, 502
Grantham-McGregor, S., 168
Grapentine, W.L., 536
Grason, H., 97
Gray, J.A., 314, 499

Gray, M., 145
Gray, P.H., 395
Graziano, P.A., 430
Green, B.L., 744
Green, J.G., 94, 288, 394
Green, R., 688, 690, 692, 696
Green, T.M., 337
Greenberg, G.S., 592
Greenberg, M.T., 163, 168, 173, 178, 189, 450, 471, 476, 480
Greenberger, E., 230, 233, 234
Greene, R., 468
Greenfeld, T.K., 94
Greenfield, P.M., 226
Greenland, S., 88
Greenspan, R.J., 46
Greenwood, K.M., 413
Gregory, A.M., 548, 549, 552
Gregory, S.G., 277
Gresham, F.M., 667
Gress-Smith, J.L., 411
Grether, J.K., 103
Grey, I.K., 126
Grice, S.J., 267
Griesler, P.C., 189
Griessmair, M., 54
Griggs, C., 331, 333, 384
Griggs, J., 209
Grigorenko, E.L., 130
Grillon, C., 268, 550
Grills, A.E., 192
Grills-Taquechel, A.E., 556
Grilo, C.M., 704, 708, 709
Grimbos, T., 695
Grimm, K., 333
Grimminck, E., 768
Grisham, J.R., 562, 568
Groark, C.J., 357, 366
Grobin, A.C., 590
Groh, A.M., 552
Grolnick, W.S., 707
Gromoske, A.N., 129
Groom, M.J., 436
Gross, J.N., 476
Gross, R., 47
Grossman, H.J., 667
Grossman, J., 17
Grossman, K.E., 154
Grossmann, K.E., 357, 359
Grote, V., 397
Grotpeter, J.K., 190
Grover, R.L., 554
Groza, V.K., 357
Gruber, C.P., 689
Gruber, R., 409
Gruenewald, P.J., 96
Gruenewald, T., 288, 295
Grumbach, M.M., 332
Grunes, M.S., 572
Grusec, J.E., 149, 316

Grych, J.H., 145, 147, 150, 746
Guastella, A.J., 279
Guedeney, N., 491
Guendelman, M., 296
Guerra, N.G., 234
Guerry, J.D., 187
Guevremont, D.C, 440
Guimond, F.A., 155
Guiney, J., 549
Gulanick, M., 211
Gulley, B.L., 339
Gulsrud, A., 655
Gump, P., 177
Gundapuneedi, T., 498
Gunderson, B.H., 505
Gunderson, J.G., 706, 709, 710
Gunnar, M., 154, 165, 554
Gunnar, M.G., 334
Gunnar, M.R., 49, 173, 289–291, 298, 300, 302, 312,
        317, 331, 333, 334, 340, 348, 349, 371–385, 734
Gunnell, D.J., 521, 526
Gunter, T.D., 274
Gunzerath, L., 602
Guo, G., 252
Guo, J., 607, 612
Guo, M., 233
Guo, S., 392
Guralnick, M.J., 392
Guralnik, O., 767
Gureje, O., 229
Guroff, J.J., 761
Gurvits, I.G., 709
Gustafsson, P.A., 212
Gustafsson, P.E., 212
Guth, A., 414
Guth, S., 110
Guthrie, D., 750
Guthrie, W., 660
Gutman, L.M., 34
Guyer, A.E., 189, 268, 279, 689
Guzder, J., 710
Gwinn, A.M., 133

H
Ha, T., 450
Haas, E., 194
Hackett, L., 232
Hackett, R.J., 232
Hackman, D.A., 292
Hadders-Algra, M., 637
Hadwin, J.A., 551, 554
Haeffel, G., 501
Hagan, J., 346
Haggerty, K.P., 164
Haglund, N.G., 395
Hagtvet, K., 118
Hairston, I.S., 394
Haley, G., 17
Halim, M.L., 697

Halit, H., 267
Hall, J., 752
Hall, M., 693
Hallett, D., 38
Hallin, A.L., 395
Hallmayer, J., 495, 654
Hallquist, M., 110
Halperin, J.F., 427–442
Halperin, J.M., 427, 430, 432, 434, 473
Halpern, C.T., 114, 255
Halpert, J.A., 207
Hamaguchi, Y., 236
Hamer, D., 254
Hames, J.L., 133
Hamill, S.K., 635
Hamilton, D., 416
Hamilton, J.P., 273
Hammen, C., 110, 193, 207, 209, 211, 213, 215, 331
Hammen, C.C., 210
Hammen, C.L., 30, 211, 212, 491, 493, 495–497, 501,
        503–506
Hammock, E.A.D., 295
Hammond, M., 538
Hamon, M., 533
Hamre, B.K., 175, 176
Hamrick, N., 214
Han, G., 734
Hancock, G., 119
Hanish, L.D., 198, 475
Hankin, B.L., 90, 194, 209, 212, 213, 320, 490, 493, 495,
        496, 499–501, 503–505, 555
Hanna, C., 752
Hans, S.L., 476
Hansel, T.C., 743
Hansenne, M., 533
Hanson, J.L., 377
Happonen, M., 494
Har, A.F., 641
Harden, A., 676
Harden, K.P., 196, 250, 336, 338, 342, 343, 345, 347,
        625, 626
Hare, R.D., 468
Hare, T.A., 268, 609
Hariri, A.R., 46, 52, 53, 56, 265, 272, 273, 293, 296, 614
Harkness, K.L., 150, 151, 301, 491, 501, 503
Harkness, S., 226
Harley, M., 57
Harlow, H.F., 12
Harlow, M.K., 12
Harmer, C.J., 278
Harmon, R.J., 398
Harnish, J.D., 478
Harold, G.T., 150, 494
Harrington, H., 94
Harrington, R., 491, 494
Harris, A.R., 173
Harris, H.B., 392
Harris, J.C., 665, 666, 668, 669, 671
Harris, L., 525
Harris, P.L., 749

Harris, T., 528
Harrison, J., 527
Harrison, P.J., 56
Harry, J., 694
Hart, E.L., 428
Hart, H., 734
Hart, K.J., 638
Hart, S., 319
Harter, K., 148
Harter, S., 187
Hartup, W.W., 185, 187, 470
Harty, S.C., 432
Harvey, A.G., 409–420, 496, 499
Haselager, G.J.T., 146
Hasin, D.S., 97, 584, 585, 589, 603
Haskett, M.E., 735
Haslam, N., 110
Hasler, G., 498
Hastings, P.D., 229, 232, 291, 321, 341
Hatri, A., 268, 269
Hattie, J., 168
Hatzenbuehler, M.L., 92, 97, 192, 210, 707
Hauser, S.T., 127, 132
Havel, M., 414
Haw, C., 523
Hawes, D.J., 478
Hawi, Z., 433
Hawker, D.S.J., 554
Hawkins, D., 231
Hawkins, J.D., 115, 163, 164, 174, 176, 589,
        591, 592, 607
Hawkins, S.S., 97
Hawley, P.H., 190, 478
Haworth, C.M., 256
Hawton, K., 523, 525–528
Hawtrey, C.E., 643
Hay, D.F., 186
Hay, I., 707
Hayden, E.P., 500
Hayes, A.F., 211
Hayes, D.S., 186
Hayes, L.J., 451
Hayes, S.C., 451
Haynie, D.L., 334, 336, 337, 343, 612
Hayward, C., 331, 333, 336–338, 341, 493, 622
Hazel, N.A., 209, 210, 495
Hazen, N., 148
Hazen, R.A., 323
Hazlett, H., 659
He, J.P., 638
He, Y., 228, 235, 236
Healey, D.M., 427, 430, 434
Healy, L., 571
Healy-Farrell, L., 573
Heard, H.L., 522
Heath, A.C., 246, 249, 251, 494, 497, 593
Heath, N., 535
Hebebrand, J., 255
Heber, R., 668
Hébert, M., 762

Hechtman, L., 432
Heckman, J.J., 164, 169, 170
Hedeker, D., 114
Hedges, D.W., 752
Heekeren, H.R., 268, 269
Heiervang, E., 230
Heilbron, N., 190, 191
Heim, C., 301, 734
Heinrichs, M., 277
Heinrichs, N., 233
Heinz, A., 53, 273
Heitzeg, M.M., 588, 595
Helder, E., 382
Helenius, H., 535
Helmerhorst, F.M., 289
Helmers, K., 765
Helms, S.W., 188
Helstelä, L., 535
Helzer, J.E., 70, 110
Hemenway, D., 527
Hemmings, S.M., 566, 574
Hen, R., 273
Henderson, C., 97
Henderson, H.A., 271, 555
Henderson, K., 336, 337
Hendrie, N.W., 374
Henggeler, S.W., 461, 480, 481
Heninger, G.R., 564
Henly, S., 114
Hennessey, J.G., 436
Henquet, C., 56, 57
Henry, D.B., 131
Henry, J., 553
Henry, R., 211, 503
Henshaw, D., 567
Herbert, J., 495–497
Herman, R.A., 695
Hermans, H.J.M., 67
Hermelin, B., 652
Hernandez Jozefowicz, D.M., 331
Hernández-Guzmán, L., 336, 338
Heron, J., 56, 434, 636, 637
Herrenkohl, E.C., 726
Herrenkohl, R.C., 130, 726
Herrenkohl, T.I., 130
Herrera, C., 730
Herreros, F., 362
Hersen, M., 674
Hertzman, C., 287–289
Herzog, M., 475
Heslenfeld, D.J., 436
Hess, L.E., 440
Hesse, E., 360, 727, 728, 770
Hessel, E.T., 119, 193
Hetherington, E.M., 205, 247, 249, 251, 256
Hettema, J.M., 413, 548
Hevey, C., 707
Heylens, G., 695
Hiatt, S., 726
Hibell, B., 604

Hicks, B.M., 583–596, 709
Higuchi, S., 591
Hildebrandt, T., 625, 627
Hilgetag, C.C., 266
Hill, A.L., 431
Hill, B.K., 677
Hill, C.L., 564
Hill, D., 497
Hill, E., 93
Hill, J.E., 111, 196, 491
Hill, J.P., 337
Hill, K.G., 115, 607
Hill, N.E., 177
Hill, S.Y., 453
Hillman, J.B., 342
Hilt, L.M., 192, 210, 493
Hinde, R.A., 449
Hindmarsh, P.C., 696
Hines, M., 693–696
Hingson, R., 602
Hinney, A., 255
Hinshaw, S.P., 166, 192, 193, 429, 431, 432, 530, 531,
    533, 610
Hinton, D.E., 229
Hiripi, E., 621
Hironaka, L.K., 389–402
Hirsch, R., 397
Hirschfeld-Becker, D.R., 550
Hirsh-Pasek, K., 113
Hiruma, N., 230
Hitchens, K., 148
Hjern, A., 395
Ho, A.Y., 196
Ho, M., 209
Hoagwood, K., 171
Hoban, T.F., 410, 419
Hockley, C., 391
Hodapp, R.M., 27
Hodges, E.E., 192, 193
Hodges, J., 373, 376, 380
Hodgson, R., 563, 564, 567
Hoebeke, P., 639
Hoeft, F., 268
Hoek, H.W., 622
Hoeve, M., 145
Hoff, E., 115, 659
Hoffeld, W., 54
Hoffman, D.M., 173
Hoffman, K.B., 501
Hoffman, M.L., 707
Hoffmann, R., 496
Hofstadter, K.L., 644
Hofstra, M.B., 490
Holaday, M., 749
Hole, W., 674, 676
Holford, T.R., 94
Holguin, S.R., 594
Holland, E., 110
Holland, P., 637
Hollenstein, T., 155

Holliday, J., 196
Hollinsworth, T., 257
Hollon, S.D., 494
Holmbeck, G.N., 209, 210, 337, 610
Holmes, A., 52
Holmes, B.M., 709, 762
Holmes, T., 205–207
Holsboer, F., 47
Holshausen, K., 498
Holston, M.A., 173
Holt, M.K., 236
Holt, R., 186
Holton, A., 153, 453
Holton, J., 725
Honorado, E., 476
Hooe, E.S., 499
Hooman, N., 641
Hooper, S.R., 665, 746
Hope, V., 767
Hopmeyer, A., 189
Hoppe-Graff, S., 230
Hops, H., 452, 494, 504, 611
Hopwood, C.J., 256
Horn, J.L., 114
Hornstein, N.L., 762
Hornung, K., 726
Horowitz, K., 743
Horwood, L.J., 54, 56, 92, 146, 235, 258, 495, 499
Houlihan, A.E., 608
Houshyar, S., 197
Houston, I., 275
Houston, K., 523
Houts, A.C., 642, 643
Houts, R., 175, 333
Howe, A.C., 643
Howe, M.L., 730, 731
Howe, R., 411
Howe, T.R., 730
Howell, A.J., 413
Howell, C.T., 69
Howes, C., 150
Hoza, B., 505
Hsiao, C., 197
Hsu, H.C., 393
Hu, X.Z., 270, 495
Hua, J., 382
Huang, C.H., 271
Huang, H., 498, 499
Hubbard, J.A., 473
Hubbard, S., 610
Hublin, C., 640
Huddleston, E., 769
Huddleston, J., 334, 337, 338
Hudson, J.I., 621, 710
Hudson, J.L., 231, 543, 551
Hudziak, J.J., 72, 494, 695
Huebner, D., 92, 536
Huemer, J., 750, 751
Hueng, K., 654, 657
Huerta, M., 653

Huesmann, L.R., 152, 234
Huey, S.J. Jr., 228
Hughes, C.W., 146, 434, 476
Hughes, H.M., 746
Hughes, J.L., 491
Huisjes, H.J., 637
Huisman, M., 196
Huizinga, D., 31, 54, 131
Huizink, A.C., 251
Hulette, A.C., 762
Hulvershorn, L.A., 498
Hume, C.S., 696
Hummer, D.L., 414
Humpartzoomian, R.A., 299
Humphrey, N., 212
Hung, R.J., 57
Hunt, H.D., 178
Hunt, K.L., 744
Hunt, R.D., 436
Hupp, S.C., 668
Huppert, J.D., 571
Huq, N., 209
Hurd, Y.L., 625
Hurley, K.M., 397
Hurrelmann, K., 601, 605
Hurt, H., 171
Hus, V., 653
Hussey, P., 434
Hussong, A.M., 119, 589, 601
Huston, A.C., 145
Huston, L., 359
Huth-bocks, A., 749
Huzinec, C., 440
Hwang, C.P., 711
Hyde, J.S., 331, 493, 500
Hyde, L.W., 46, 53, 152, 265, 272, 274, 280, 614
Hyed, J., 493
Hyman, C., 185
Hymel, S., 166, 188
Hynan, M.T., 392
Hynes, M.E., 428

I

Iacono, W.G., 110, 249–251, 586, 588–592, 624, 625,
        709
Ialongo, N.S., 554, 610
Ianni, F., 604
Iannotti, R.J., 191, 745
Ichikawa, H., 414
Iervolino, A.C., 695
Ihle, L., 229
Ilg, F., 567
Illfeld, F.W., 528
Inderbitzen, H.M., 707
Indredavik, M.S., 395
Inge, A.P., 271
Inglis, D., 707
Ingoldsby, E.M., 452, 536
Ingram, R.E., 501, 506

Inoubli, A., 688
Insel, T.R., 254, 490
Ioannidis, J.P., 57
Iobst, E., 565
Ireland, M., 504
Irons, D.E., 591
Irons, M., 669
Irwin, M., 96
Israel, A., 111
Israel, S., 297
Ito, S., 292
Iughetti, L., 627
Ivanenko, A., 496
Ivanov, I., 432
Ivanova, M.Y., 69, 73, 74, 78
Ivarsson, T., 505
Ivy, A., 373
Izard, C.E., 147

J

Jaccard, J., 338
Jackowski, A., 752
Jackson, D.N., 167, 713
Jackson, E.C., 639
Jackson, J., 215
Jackson, K.M., 114, 607, 612
Jacobi, C., 622
Jacobs, J., 178
Jacobs, L., 146
Jacobs, R.H., 500
Jacobsen, R.H., 17
Jacobsen, T., 762
Jacobson, C.M., 709
Jacobson, K., 51
Jacobvitz, D.B., 148, 360
Jaffee, S.R., 90, 93, 503, 746, 747
Jager, J., 614
Jagiellowicz, J., 312
Jain, S., 126, 127, 130, 131
Jamieson, P., 608
Jan, J.E., 416
Jang, K.L., 711, 765
Janicki-Deverts, D., 287
Jankowski, M.K., 392
Jans, T., 564
Janssen, M.M., 228
Jardine, R., 593
Jaselskis, C., 677
Jaser, S.S., 499
Jayadev, S., 57
Jaycox, L.H., 171
Jechura, T.J., 414
Jedema, H.P., 53
Jeng, S.F., 393
Jenkins, C., 765
Jenkins, J.M., 146, 150, 252
Jenness, J.L., 209, 495
Jennings, P.A., 173
Jensen, B., 164

Jensen, P.S., 17, 111, 493
Jeon, H., 378, 382
Jeong, S.H., 765
Jessor, R., 592, 607, 609
Jessor, S.L., 592
Jesus Mari, J., 752
Ji, J., 343
Jimenez, A.M., 292
Jin, X., 362
Johansen, E.B., 532
John, O.P., 167
Johnson, A.E., 173, 375, 384
Johnson, C.M., 412
Johnson, D.E., 291, 374, 375
Johnson, J.G., 704, 708, 712, 713
Johnson, K., 496
Johnson, L.L., 686
Johnson, M., 112
Johnson, M.H., 267
Johnson, M.K., 33, 177
Johnson, R.J., 133, 608
Johnson, S.L., 395, 419, 502
Johnson, T.C., 770
Johnson, V.K., 148, 149
Johnson-Reid, M., 734
Johnston, J., 153
Johnston, L.D., 602–605, 610, 611, 613, 614
Johnstone, S.J., 377
Joiner, T.E. Jr., 133, 165, 500, 504, 521–523, 526, 528
Joinson, C., 636, 637, 639, 641, 643
Joireman, J., 472
Jollant, F., 533
Jones, D.J., 505, 589
Jones, G.V., 555
Jones, J., 669
Jones, K.M., 644
Jones, M.C., 336, 641
Jones, R.M., 268
Jones, S.M., 173, 478
Jones, W., 268, 658
Jonson-Reid, M., 724
Joormann, J., 273, 495, 501, 502
Jørgensen, T., 401
Jorm, A.F., 54
Jose, P.E., 198
Joseph, R.M., 269
Jouriles, E.N., 145–147, 746
Joy, M.E., 319
Joyce, P.R., 533, 706
Joyner, K., 92
Judd, C.M., 210, 320
Juffer, F., 48, 297, 357, 361, 363, 371, 372, 374, 381
Juraska, J.M., 627
Jutte, D., 11, 293
Juvonen, J., 191, 192, 336, 343

K
Kabat-Zinn, J., 173
Kadlec, M.B., 658
Kagan, J., 114, 132, 229, 234, 319, 605, 606

Kaijser, V.G., 685
Kalaydjian, A., 638
Kalick, S., 228
Kalin, N.H., 291, 503
Kalivas, P.W., 594
Källberg, H., 57
Källén, K.B., 395
Kallman, F.J., 7
Kalra, S.K., 565
Kaltiala-Heino, R., 338, 339, 345–347, 505, 623
Kaminer, D., 750
Kaminer, Y., 674
Kamphaus, R.W., 72
Kamphuis, J.H., 191
Kandel, D.B., 611, 612
Kandulu, R., 572
Kane, P., 500
Kang, N.J., 169
Kania, J., 169, 170
Kanner, L., 651
Kaplan, K.A., 409, 413, 420
Kaplan, N., 3
Kaplow, J.B., 548, 589, 731
Kapoor, A., 503
Kappeler, L., 253
Kaprio, J., 341, 593, 640
Karchemskiy, A., 752
Karere, G.M., 55
Karg, K., 49, 52, 58, 258, 533
Karippot, A., 418
Karl, A., 752
Karlamangla, A., 288
Karmiloff-Smith, A., 267
Karraker, K.H., 393
Karterud, S., 535
Karyl, J., 747
Kasari, C., 655, 659
Kasen, S., 713
Kashani, J.H., 492
Kashdan, T.B., 132, 135
Kashy, D.A., 626
Kastrom, T., 677
Katainen, S., 504
Kataoka, S.H., 171
Katikaneni, L.D., 394
Kato Klebanov, P., 92
Katz, B.N., 210
Katz, E.C., 608
Katz, L.F., 147
Katz, M., 208
Kaufman, J., 256, 495–497, 499, 503, 732, 752
Kaufman, N., 461
Kavanagh, K., 451, 461
Kawabata, Y., 236
Kawachi, I., 397, 503
Kawycz, N.J., 553
Kaysen, D., 747
Kazdin, A.E., 17, 18, 412, 456
Keane, S.P., 193, 430, 431
Kearney, C.A., 544
Keating, D.P., 287, 608

Keehn, B., 269
Keel, P.K., 625
Keeler, G., 88, 91, 492, 610, 743, 745, 746, 753
Keenan, K., 111, 476
Keenan-Miller, D., 209, 495
Kegel, C.A.T., 48
Keiley, M.K., 215, 313, 319
Keith, R.A., 693
Kelder, S.H., 228
Kellam, S.G., 455, 589
Keller, E., 625
Keller, M., 571
Keller, M.B., 31
Keller, M.C., 57
Keller, P.S., 297, 472
Keller, S.M., 743–754
Kelley, E., 660
Kelley, M.L., 525
Kelling, G.L., 177
Kellogg, C.K., 627
Kelly, A.B., 611
Kelly, M., 17
Kelly, S., 130, 527
Keltikangas-Jarvinen, L., 504
Kemeny, M.E., 173
Kempen, H.J.G., 67
Kenardy, J., 769
Kendall, P.C., 211, 610
Kendall-Tackett, K.A., 744
Kendler, K.S., 46, 50, 51, 246, 249–251, 494, 506, 548,
        589, 590, 593, 625
Kenkel, D., 602
Kenna, G.A., 585
Kennard, B.D., 491
Kennedy, C.E., 397
Kennedy, D., 659
Kennedy, J.L., 568
Kennedy, M.A., 54, 258, 495
Kennedy, P., 537
Kenny, D., 209
Kentgen, L.M., 497
Kerbeshian, J., 669
Kercher, A.J., 213
Kerig, P.K., 148, 149
Kerkhof, G.A., 175
Kern, L., 431
Kerns, K.A., 504, 551, 552
Kerr, A., 382
Kerr, D.C.R., 431, 452
Kerr, M., 196, 234, 235, 341, 611
Kerr, W.C., 94
Kersting, A., 392
Kerstjens, J.M., 395
Keshavan, M.S., 752
Keskivaara, P., 504
Kesler, R., 289
Kessen, W., 40
Kessler, R.C., 88, 90, 91, 93, 95, 103, 163, 169, 206,
        246, 249, 251, 489, 492, 493, 496, 547, 562,
        610, 621, 743
Keundig, H., 96

KewalRamani, A., 163
Key, A., 657
Keyes, C.L.M., 133
Keyes, K.M., 94–96, 603, 731
Khamis, V., 745, 746
Kheirandish, L., 418
Khoo, S.T., 611
Kiecolt-Glaser, J.K., 118
Kiel, E.J., 320, 323
Kiesner, J., 233, 611, 612
Kiff, C.J., 290, 311, 321
Kilgore, K., 153, 453
Kill, K.G., 174
Killen, J.D., 493, 623
Killgore, W.D.S., 268
Kilmer, R.P., 208
Kilpatrick, D.G., 270, 743
Kim, H.K., 257, 380, 505, 762
Kim, J.E., 129, 210, 729, 731, 735
Kim, K.J., 554, 762
Kim, P., 291, 295
Kim, S., 129, 321
Kim-Cohen, J., 54, 94, 130, 732, 735
Kimmel, E., 642
Kimmel, H.D., 77, 642
Kimmerly, N.L., 9
Kincaid, S.B., 592
King, B.H., 677
King, C., 522, 528, 529
King, D.W., 748
King, J.A., 291, 473
King, K.M., 211
King, L.A., 135
King, M., 166
King, N.J., 543, 546, 547, 553
King, R.A., 496, 567
King, S., 290
Kinnally, E.L., 53, 274, 275
Kinniburgh, K.M., 770
Kint, M.J.W., 554
Kirby, D.B., 178
Kirchner, H.L., 434
Kirkby, J., 413
Kirley, A., 433
Kirmizigul, P., 751
Kirsch, P., 277
Kirsh, S.J., 153
Kishiyama, M.M., 292
Kisiel, C., 762, 768
Kistin, C.J., 396
Kistler, D.J., 726, 727
Kistner, J.A., 228, 505
Klackenberg, G., 417
Klareskog, L., 57
Klassen, P., 694
Klebanov, P.K., 392
Kleber, H.D., 596
Klein, B.R., 762
Klein, D., 112
Klein, D.F., 553
Klein, D.J., 610

Klein, D.L., 311
Klein, D.N., 340, 490, 492, 499, 500, 522, 524, 703–714
Klein, M.H., 291
Klein, M.W., 461, 462
Klein, R.G., 428
Klein, W.M.P., 608
Kleinerman, R., 396
Kleinhans, N.M., 268
Kleinman, A., 226, 229, 746
Kleinman, J., 226, 229
Kleinman, M., 528
Kliemann, D., 268, 269
Kliewer, W., 211
Klimes-Dougan, B., 291, 341, 343, 348
Klin, A., 268, 658, 689
Klingberg, T., 434
Klinger, L.G., 497
Klinnert, M.D., 312
Kljakovic, M., 198
Klonsky, E.D., 531
Klorman, R., 312, 727
Kluft, R.P., 761, 764
Klump, K.L., 621–627
Knafo, A., 297, 695
Knapp, L., 674
Knapp, P., 111
Knauper, B., 103
Knibbe, R.A., 339
Knight, E., 492
Knight, K., 215
Knight, R.T., 292
Knol, D.L., 291
Knoll, J., 675
Knudson, G., 685
Knutelska, M., 767
Kobak, R.R., 150
Kobor, A., 118–119
Kobor, M.S., 293
Koch, M., 57
Kochanek, K.D., 521, 525
Kochanska, G., 236, 250, 255, 256, 319, 321, 322, 361, 472, 476
Kochenderfer, B.J., 190
Kochenderfer-Ladd, B., 192, 193
Koenen, K.C., 93, 131, 171, 275
Koenig, J.I., 503
Koenigs, M., 266
Koenigsberg, H.W., 709
Koga, S., 359
Kogan, N., 147
Kogos, J., 147
Kohl, P.L., 724
Kohlberg, L., 314
Koivisto, A.M., 339, 623
Kolevzon, A., 47
Kolko, D.J., 748
Kolpacoff, M., 257
Kondo, D.G., 498
Kong, A., 47, 253
Koopmans, J.R., 593

Koot, H.M., 235, 676
Kopp, C.B., 316
Korbin, J.E, 96
Korenman, S., 92, 399
Korja, R., 393, 394
Korman, E., 415
Korosi, A., 373
Kose, S., 295
Koskenvuo, M., 593, 640
Kostaki, A., 503
Kosterman, R., 174
Kosunen, E., 338, 339, 345, 346
Kotagal, S., 419
Kotchick, B.A., 93
Kotov, R., 311, 499
Kouros, C.D., 297
Kovacs, E.A., 315
Kovacs, M., 490–493, 502
Koverola, C., 752
Kowalik, J., 750
Krabbendam, L., 57
Kracke, B., 336, 338, 345
Kraemer, G.W., 503
Kraemer, H.C., 110, 393, 622
Krafchuk, E., 37
Kramer, L., 401
Kramer, M., 169, 170
Krantz, J.Z., 675
Kraper, C.K., 561–575
Krebs, N.F., 398
Kreppner, J.M., 371, 372, 376, 380, 381, 384, 385
Kreppner, R., 357
Kretchmar, M.D., 148
Kretsch, N., 625
Kreukels, B.P.C., 685, 693
Kreutzer, T., 90
Krieger, N, 88
Kring, A.M., 706
Kringlon, E., 7
Krishnakumar, A., 147, 402
Kroenenberg, M., 743
Kroenke, C.H., 294
Krohn, M.D., 612
Kronenberg, H.M., 625
Kroonenberg, P.M., 359
Krueger, R.F., 110, 249, 251, 586, 589, 590, 622, 703–705, 710, 712
Krueger, R.R., 590
Krug, E.G., 527
Krukowski, R.A., 69
Kruse, S., 640
Kuban, K.C., 395
Kubarych, T., 110
Kubena, A.A., 765
Kubu, C., 653
Kuehnle, K., 153
Kuehnle, T., 414
Kuhl, E., 110
Kuhl, P., 655
Kuhn, B.R., 411, 644

Kuhn, D., 707
Kujawa, A.J., 311, 493
Kumsta, R., 48, 55
Kung, H., 521
Kuntsche, E., 96
Kuo, D., 734
Kuo, W.-L., 119
Kuperminc, G.P., 743, 745
Kupersmidt, J.B., 187, 456, 707–708, 730
Kupfer, D.J., 110, 530
Kuppens, P., 110
Kurlakowsky, K.D., 500–501
Kurowski, C.O., 707
Kurtz, J.L., 133, 134
Kusche, C.A., 480
Kusel, S.J., 191
Kusumakar, V., 496
Kutcher, S.P., 496
Kuterovac, G., 747
Kwok, O., 119
Kwon, S., 655

L

La Greca, A.M., 186, 188, 194, 554, 743, 745
Laakso, A., 532
Laakso, M., 115
Lack, C.W., 571
Lacourse, E., 457, 469
LaCrosse, J., 314
Ladd, C.O., 301, 380
Ladd, G.W., 145, 190, 193
Ladouceur, C.D., 266, 333, 334
LaFavor, T.L., 384
LaFreniere, P.J., 231
LaGrange, B., 501
Lahey, B.B., 17, 251, 331, 428, 431, 432, 467–469, 473, 490, 493, 532, 710
Lai, K.Y.C., 74
Laird, N., 114
Laird, R.D., 156
Laitinen-Krispijn, S., 338, 339
Lakdawalla, Z., 501
Lalonde, C.E., 38
Lamarre, M., 683
Lamb, M.E., 7, 11, 711, 749
Lambert, L.E., 213
Lambert, N.M., 133–135
Lambert, S.F., 228, 342
Lambert, W.W., 235
Lamborn, S.D., 145
Lamm, C.I., 418
Lamminmäki, A., 694
Lamont, M.A., 669
Lamping, D.L., 74
Land, K.C, 95
Landa, R., 656
Landis, T.Y., 747
Landoll, R.R., 554
Landolt, M.A., 746

Landsverk, J.L., 762
Lane, S., 291, 312
Lane, T.L., 502
Laney, T., 209
Langer, D.A., 291
Langley, A.K., 171
Lanham, J.S., 396
Lanier, P., 734
Lansford, J.E., 156, 169, 187–189, 312, 318, 323, 324, 452, 478
Lanza, S., 111
Laporta, L.D., 762
Lapsly, A.-M., 357
Larroque, B., 395
Larsen, P.R., 625
Larson, D.W., 491
Larson, J., 611, 612
Larson, R.W., 172, 610
Larsson, H., 710
Larsson, I., 212
LaRusso, M.D., 173
LaSalle, J.M., 277
Laser, J.A., 762
Lash, T.L, 88
Last, C.G., 90
Latendresse, S.J., 590, 591
Latva, R., 393
Lau, J.Y.F., 273, 494, 501, 549, 550, 555
Lau, S., 166
Laub, J., 231
Laub, J.H., 113, 114, 127, 132, 457, 458, 462
Laucht, M., 271, 435
Laudon, M., 416
Lauer, P.A., 172
Lauritsen, J., 231
Laursen, B., 115, 194, 610
Laviola, G., 298
Law, P., 654
Lawlor, M.S., 173
Lawrence, A.A., 692
Lawrence, F., 119
Lawson, J.S., 730
Lazarus, R.S., 206
Le Bihan, C., 533
Le, T., 231
Leader, L.R., 503
LeBlanc, J., 496
Lechcier-Kimel, R., 228
Leckman, J.F., 562, 564, 567
LeCouteur, A., 652
LeDoux, J.E., 549
Lee, E.A., 707
Lee, J.M., 335, 613
Lee, K., 167
Lee, S.S., 55, 212, 428, 431, 432
Lee, T.M., 414, 480
Lee, V.E., 177
Leenaars, A.A., 523, 524, 529, 530
Leen-Feldner, E.W., 341
Lefkowitz, M.M., 17

Leggio, L., 585
Legrand, L.N., 110, 589
Lehmkuhl, H.D., 570
Lehr, T., 57
Lei, M.K., 48
Leibenluft, E., 689
Leiberman, A., 367
Leibowitz, G.S., 762
Leinonen, J.A., 505
Leis, J., 128
Leistico, A.-M.R., 707
LeMare, L., 188
Lemery, K.S., 312, 315
Lemery-Chalfant, K., 411
Lemeshow, S., 393
Lemogne, C., 274
Lemons, J.A., 398
Lenane, M.C., 564, 566
Leng, L., 225–237
Lengua, L.J., 290, 311, 312, 315, 320, 321, 476, 500,
      502, 745, 746
Lenox, K., 185
Lensing, S., 399
Lenzenweger, M., 112
Leonard, A.C., 394
Leonard, H., 564, 567
Leonard, S., 475
Lepine, J., 543
Leppanen, J.M., 498
Lerner, R.M., 4, 6, 14, 605, 606, 612, 614
Lesch, K.P., 270, 495
Lester, J., 233
Lester, K.J., 257, 554
Leukefeld, C., 605
Leung, P., 230
Levendosky, A., 749
Leventhal, B.L., 677
Leventhal, T., 96, 127
Levine, M.D., 645
Levine, M.P., 624
Levine, S., 289
Levitan, G.W., 666
Levitt, M.J., 146
Levitt, P., 295, 381, 654
Levy, J.C., 396
Levy, K.L., 709
Lewin, D.S., 411
Lewinsohn, P.M., 338, 490, 491, 493, 494, 500, 503, 506,
      528, 623
Lewis, A.V., 638
Lewis, C., 231
Lewis, D.A., 273
Lewis, D.C., 596
Lewis, D.O., 768
Lewis, G., 56, 258
Lewis, J., 726
Lewis, M., 3–20, 90, 209, 269, 358, 360, 361, 364, 605,
      606, 658, 659, 683, 748, 763, 764
Lewis, M.D., 312, 315, 565, 726
Lewis, M.H., 672, 674, 675

Lewis, T.L., 379
Li, B., 228, 232, 235
Li, D., 228, 235, 236, 420
Li, F., 188, 194, 451
Li, G., 94, 95
Li, Y., 115, 612
Li, Z., 232
Liang, J., 115
Liben, L.S., 683
Libero, D., 765
Lichtenstein, P., 625
Liddle, E.B., 436, 437
Lieberman, A.F., 672, 745, 769
Liebert, R.M., 636, 642
Liebowitz, M.R., 571
Liew, J., 232
Liggin, R., 171
Lilienfeld, S., 111
Limperopoulos, C., 395
Lin, C.C., 228
Lin, E., 229
Lin, M.-H., 476
Lin, S., 92
Lin, Y.H., 744
Linares, T.J., 434
Lind, P.A., 495
Lindblad, F., 395
Linden, M., 132
Lindquist, M., 119
Lindsey, E.W., 155
Lindström, K., 395
Lindström, M., 533
Linehan, M.M., 522, 525, 526, 534, 535, 709
Link, B.G., 97
Lionel, A.C., 434
Liotti, G., 764
Lippman, J., 750
Lipsey, M.W., 169
Lipsey, T.L., 747
Lipton, R., 357, 367
Lira, A., 273
Lissek, S., 268, 550
Litman, R., 524
Litt, I.F., 338
Little, B.R., 134, 136
Little, T.D., 192, 478, 536
Littner, M., 419
Liu, C., 208
Liu, D., 301
Liu, J., 230
Liu, K.A., 288
Liu, X., 97, 165
Livelsey, W.J., 765
Livesley, W.J., 711, 713
Lizardi, H., 704
Lizotte, A.J., 612
Llewellyn, N., 337, 343, 347, 502
Lloyd-Richardson, E.E., 525, 526, 610
Lo Coco, A., 233
Lobato, D.J., 675

LoBue, V., 555
Lochman, J.E., 185, 188, 456, 478, 480
Locke, J., 655
Locke, V., 205
Lockhat, R., 750
Loeber, R., 31, 96, 111, 313, 428, 453, 454, 457,
    468–471, 473, 710
Loehlin, J.C., 48, 249
Loening-Baucke, V., 635, 641
Lofthouse, N., 313
Lohr, S.L, 89
Loibl, L.M., 528
Loman, M.L., 384
Loman, M.M., 49, 290, 374
London, B.E., 168, 169
Loney, J., 428
Long, A.C., 745
Long, J.D., 331, 333, 384
Lonigan, C.J., 319, 323, 499, 550, 555, 746
Lonsdorf, T.B., 549
Lopez, A.D., 570, 669
Lopez, C., 192
Lopez, M.H., 164
Lopez, N.L., 431, 452
Lopez, S.J., 133, 134
Lopez-Duran, N., 490
Lorber, M.F., 472, 479
Lorberbaum, J.P., 295
Lord, C.E., 269, 652, 653, 658, 660
Lord, S.E., 331
Lorenz, F.O., 503, 554
Losada, M.F., 135
Lott, R.S., 677
Lou, X.Y., 532
Louis, T.A., 114
Love, R.A., 171
Lovejoy, M.C., 504
Low, H., 339
Low, S.M., 147, 611
Lowe, K., 669
Lowe, S.R., 131
Lowry, C.B., 688
Lozoff, B., 398, 410
Luan, J.A., 252
Lubetsky, M.J., 674
Lubke, G., 110
Luby, J.L., 492, 503
Ludolph, P.S., 709
Luecken, L.J., 411
Luijk, M.P., 251, 728
Luisi, S., 627
Luk, J.W., 191
Luke, D., 209
Lumley, M.N., 501, 503
Lund, L.K., 395
Lundberg, I., 56
Lunsing, R.J., 637
Luo, Q., 611
Lupien, S.J., 290, 300
Luskin, F.M., 173

Luthar, S.S., 34, 125–136, 155, 167, 213, 214, 296, 735
Luther, J.S., 767
Luthra, R., 743
Lutter, C.K., 396
Luyckx, K., 145
Luykx, J.J., 498
Luyster, R.J., 395, 657–660
Luyten, P., 549
Lykken, D.T., 248
Lyman, E.L., 125–136, 296
Lynam, D.R., 235, 315, 341, 428, 470, 605, 710
Lynch, K.G., 432
Lynch, M.E., 90, 337, 725
Lyneham, H.J., 543
Lynne, S.D., 339, 341
Lynne-Landsman, S.D., 342
Lynskey, M.T., 93, 494
Lyons, D.M., 208, 300
Lyons, J.S., 762, 768
Lyons, K.E., 173
Lyons-Ruth, K., 360, 365, 476, 531, 535, 709, 762, 764
Lythcott, M., 197
Lytton, H., 248, 696
Lyubchik, A., 762
Lyytinen, H., 115

M
Maas, I., 132
Maas, Y.G.H., 410
MacCallum, R.C., 110, 118
Maccoby, E.E., 144, 145
Macfie, J., 728, 729, 762
Machado, B.C., 622
Machado, P.P., 622
Macias, M.M., 394
Maciejewski, P.K., 734
MacIntosh, R., 215
Mackay, C.E., 278
MacKenzie, M.J., 331, 397
Mackinnon, A., 54
MacLean, W.E. Jr., 672
MacLennan, D., 130
MacMillan, H.L., 129
MacMillan, S., 498
MacQueen, G.M., 497, 498
Macri, S., 298
Madan, A., 323
Madden, P.A., 494
Madigan, S., 359, 360
Madras, B.K., 436
Maes, H.H., 710
Maggi, S., 130
Maggs, J., 601, 605, 609
Maggs, J.L., 585, 601–614
Maggs, J.M., 602
Magnabosco, J.L., 165
Magnusson, D., 31, 110, 114, 185, 333, 335, 336,
    338–341, 343, 345, 347
Mahabee-Gittens, E.M., 394

Maheu, F.S., 381, 382
Mahoney, J.L., 172
Mahoney, M.M., 414
Main, A., 320
Main, M., 3, 37, 359, 360, 727, 728, 770
Maing, D.M., 688
Makinodan, M., 292
Makki, M.I., 382
Malanchuk, O., 167
Malarkey, W.B., 118
Malecki, C., 209
Malhi, G., 565
Maliken, A., 567
Malloy, P., 428
Malmud, E., 171
Malone, M.J., 193
Malone, P.S., 187, 189, 450, 471
Malone, S.M., 588, 589
Malpaux, B., 416
Manassis, K., 319
Mancebo, M.C., 565
Mandelkron, R., 401
Mandell, D., 660
Mangelsdorf, S.C., 147, 150, 317, 393, 554
Manly, J.T., 129, 724, 736
Mann, B.J., 762
Mann, J.J., 532, 533
Mannarino, A.P., 744, 750, 751, 769
Manning, L.G., 146, 154
Mannuzza, S., 428, 431, 432
Manuck, S.B., 614
Marceau, K., 333
March, C.L., 431
March, J.S., 573, 574, 750
Marchant, P., 402
Marchessault, K., 710
Marcia, J., 609
Marcus, B.A., 644
Marcus, C.L., 418
Marcus, J., 322
Margolin, G., 152, 745, 747
Maris, R.W., 525–529
Markey, C., 337
Markham, J.A., 503
Markon, K.E., 70, 110, 589, 622
Markowitsch, H.J., 266
Marks, A.K., 130, 146
Marks, D.J., 430
Marks, I.M., 543, 565
Marks, R.P., 770
Marlin, D., 401
Marlow, L., 337
Marmorstein, N.R., 731
Marques, S., 365
Marriage, K., 17
Marriott, M., 498
Marsh, G.R., 414
Marsh, P., 188, 537, 606
Marshall, P.J., 377, 383
Marshall, R., 743

Martens, A., 704
Martens, P.M., 744
Martin, A., 129, 496
Martin, C., 198
Martin, C.L., 475, 683, 697
Martin, C.S., 734
Martin, J.A., 144, 145, 389
Martin, J.L., 573, 623
Martin, J.M., 490, 501
Martin, M., 555
Martin, M.J., 149, 151
Martin, N.C., 215, 501
Martin, N.G., 593
Martin-Glenn, M.L., 172
Martini, T.S., 229
Martins, C., 365
Martsolf, J.T., 669
Marttunen, M., 339, 623
Martyn, C.N., 503
Martyn-Nemeth, P., 211
Marvin, R.S., 148, 150, 380
Masaryk, T., 523
Maslowksy, J., 278
Maslowsky, J., 601–614
Masse, L.C., 589
Masten, A.S., 6, 34, 40, 126–129, 131–135, 195, 234,
    296, 342, 450, 499, 601, 606, 613, 711, 747
Masterpasqua, F., 16
Matas, L., 504
Mathew, S.J., 497
Mathieson, L.C., 735
Matijasevich, A., 397
Matson, J.L., 666, 669, 675–677
Matthews, D.B., 590
Matthews, K.A., 287, 291
Matthews, S.G., 503
Matthys, W., 468, 472, 532
Mattis, S.G., 546
Mattson, M.E., 601
Mattson, S.N., 434
Mattsson, A., 339
Maughan, A., 723, 728, 729, 736
Maughan, B., 113, 132, 174, 177
Maumary-Gremaud, A., 475
Maurer, D., 379
Maxfield, J., 194
Maxfield, M.G., 731
Maxwell, K.L., 450
Maxwell, L.E., 32
Maxwell, S.E., 210, 320
Mayberg, H.S., 498
Mayes, L.C., 9, 549
Mayes, T.L., 491
Mayeux, L., 190
Maynard, A.E., 226
Mayou, R.A., 748
Mays, V.M, 92
Mayseless, O., 153
Mazure, C.M., 564, 734
McAdams, D.P., 714

McBrair, M.C., 695
McBurnett, K., 468, 473
McCaffery, J.M., 610
McCall, R.B., 357, 362, 364, 366
McCandless, M.A., 193
McCann, J.B., 397
McCarthy, M.M., 627
McCartney, K., 255, 568, 593
McCartney, L., 568
McCarty, C.A., 501
McCaul, K.D., 608
McCauley, E., 501
McClarty, B., 752
McCleery, J., 401
McClelland, G.H., 210, 320
McClelland, S., 373, 374
McClure, E.B., 268, 278
McCluskey, C.P., 612
McConaughy, S.H., 17, 18, 69, 81
McCord, J., 131, 452, 536
McCormick, M.C., 392
McCoy, K., 146
McCracken, J., 571
McCrae, R.R., 134, 712
McCrory, E.J.P., 479
McDermid, S.A., 688
McDermott, J.M., 555
McDonald, R., 746
McDonough, S.C., 38
McDowell, E.E., 526–530
McEachern, A.D., 152, 454
McElhaney, K.B., 188, 606
McElwain, N.L., 149
McEwen, B.S., 154, 206, 215, 216, 288–290, 292, 295, 375, 497
McFadyen-Ketchum, S., 297
McFarland, F.C., 188, 606
McFarlane, A.C., 748
McGee, R., 91, 589
McGinn, L.K., 505
McGlashan, T.H., 531, 704
McGlinchey, E.L., 409–420
McGoron, L., 365
McGowan, P.O., 272
McGrath, J.J., 291
McGrath, M.L., 549, 642–644
McGraw, K., 153, 453
McGreenery, C.E., 761
McGue, M., 248–251, 586, 588–592, 611, 624, 625, 709
McGuffin, P., 52, 271
McGuigan, K.A., 610
McGuire, J.K., 693
McGuire, S., 251
McHale, J., 146
McHale, J.L., 147, 150
McHale, J.P., 147, 148
McHale, S.M., 146
McKay, D., 572
McKay, K.E., 473
McKay, M., 743

McKenzie, M.J., 38
McKeown, S.P., 528
McKinley, M.J., 186
McKinney, K.L., 336
McKinney, W.T., 506
McKinnon, M.C., 498
McKnew, D.H., 11, 31
McLaren, J., 668
McLaughlin, K.A., 11, 87–104, 192, 210, 213, 300, 377, 381, 383, 385, 707
McLaughlin, M.W., 167, 171
McLellan, A.T., 596
McLeod, B.D., 145, 551
Mclewin, L.A., 768
McLoyd, V.C., 287
McMahon, P.P., 761
McMahon, R.J., 480
McMahon, S.D., 205–218
McMakin, D.L., 414
McManus, B.M., 393
McMaster, L.E., 336, 337
McMillan, D.L., 667
McNally, R., 229, 269
McNamara, J.O., 767
McPartland, J., 653
McPherson, A.V., 735
Mead, H.K., 154, 471
Mead, J., 762
Mead, M., 226
Meaney, M.J., 6, 38, 47, 246, 252, 253, 255, 265, 272, 275, 289, 290, 293, 299, 301, 374, 494, 495
Medina, A., 152
Medina-Mora, M.E., 212
Medland, S.E., 549
Mednick, S.A., 710
Meece, D.W., 250
Meece, J.L., 168
Meehl, P.E., 110, 318, 490
Meesters, C., 323
Mehlum, L., 535
Mehta, M.A., 381, 382
Mehta, P.D., 110, 119
Meier, M.H., 57, 536
Meijer, A.M., 175
Meiklejohn, J., 173
Meininger, J.C., 228
Meiser-Stedman, R., 744, 748, 749
Mell, L.K., 565
Mellon, M.W., 642
Mellon, S.H., 294
Meltzer, L.J., 411
Meltzoff, A.N., 9, 745, 746
Melville, C.A., 678
Mendelsohn, J., 165
Mendelson, T., 173
Méndez, E., 212
Mendle, J., 332, 334, 336–339, 342–348, 608, 625
Mennin, D.S., 707
Mennuti, R.B., 163
Menolascino, F.J., 669

Menon, V., 268
Merali, Z., 289
Mercer, S.H., 236
Mercier, L., 496
Mercken, L., 196, 611
Mercy, J.A., 725
Meredith, W., 111
Merian, J., 521
Merikangas, K.R., 73, 165, 166, 492, 493, 638
Merlo, L.J., 570, 572
Mermelstein, R., 493, 501
Mersky, J.P., 129
Mertins, V., 54
Mervielde, I., 311, 319, 499, 712
Merz, A.B., 689
Merz, E.C., 364
Mesman, J., 48, 297, 321, 361
Messersmith, J., 613
Messing, M., 173
Messner, M., 727
Metalsky, G.I., 500
Metin, B., 437
Metz, S., 173
Meyer, A., 118
Meyer, H.A., 177
Meyer, I.H., 91, 92
Meyer, J.S., 54, 289
Meyer-Bahlburg, H.F.L., 686, 687
Meyer-Lindenberg, A., 46, 55, 56, 277, 279, 474, 711
Meyers, J., 590
Meyerson, D.A., 208, 210
Mezulis, A.H., 209, 331, 493, 500, 501
Micali, N., 569
Mick, E., 431
Miguel-Hidalgo, J.J., 498
Mihalic, S.F., 481
Mikolajewski, A., 319
Mikolajová, V., 765
Mikulincer, M., 552
Milevsky, A., 146
Milham, M.P., 437
Milich, R., 428, 429
Miller, A.L., 54, 258, 495, 709
Miller, B., 115
Miller, C.J., 70, 110, 430, 431
Miller, D.B., 215
Miller, D.P., 734
Miller, E.K., 594
Miller, G.E., 216, 289–291, 375
Miller, G.M., 436
Miller, J., 92
Miller, J.D., 410
Miller, J.E., 399
Miller, J.Y., 589
Miller, L.C., 70, 374, 376
Miller, M., 527
Miller, N., 501
Miller, P., 767
Miller, R.J., 175
Miller, S.M., 3, 209, 683

Miller, T.Q., 607
Miller, W.R., 413
Miller-Johnson, S., 475, 476
Mills, C.L., 128
Mills, R.S.L., 231
Mills-Koonce, R., 316
Milne, B.J., 94
Min, M.O., 434
Mindell, J.A., 410–412, 416, 418
Mineka, S., 209, 550, 554
Miniño, A.M., 521
Minkovitz, C.S., 97
Minor, K.L., 495, 501
Minuchin, P., 146
Minuchin, S., 148
Miranda, J., 506
Mirmiran, M., 410
Mirza, N.R., 273
Mischel, W., 8, 10, 18
Mishne, J.M., 642
Miskovic, V., 395
Mistlberger, R.E., 410
Mitchell, A.M., 497
Mitchell, R.E., 611
Mittelmark, M.B, 212
Mizuta, I., 230
Mletzko, T., 734
Mochida, G.H., 669
Moessinger, A., 393
Moffatt, M.E., 636
Moffit, T.E., 93, 468, 470
Moffitt, T.E., 49, 52, 90, 94, 115, 131, 167, 272, 334, 335, 338–342, 479, 499, 589, 606, 613, 710, 746
Moghaddam, B., 608
Mohay, H., 391
Mohr, N., 745
Moilanen, I., 110
Moilanen, K.L., 152, 450
Mokros, H.B., 17
Mokrova, I., 431
Molina, B.S., 431, 432
Molnar, B.E., 126, 743
Monahan, J., 457
Monahan, K.C., 612, 613
Mondloch, C.J., 379
Moneta, G., 610
Monk, C.S., 265–280, 608
Monk, T.H., 414, 415
Monroe, S.M., 150, 151, 208, 214, 216, 301, 491, 503, 505, 506
Monteiro, C., 399
Montgomery, D.F., 644
Montplaisir, J., 419
Moore, C.F., 503
Moore, D.R., 451
Moore, H., 553
Moore, J.H., 532
Moore, L., 196
Moorman, J.E., 165
Moos, B.M., 574

Moos, R.H., 574
Morabia, A., 88
Morales, J., 234
Moran, M., 490
Moraru, A., 373
More, D., 198
Morehouse, R.L., 496
Morenoff, J.D., 95
Moretti, M.M., 17
Morey, L.C., 706
Morey, R.A., 257
Morgan, C., 252
Morgan, R.T., 642
Morgenthaler, T.I., 418
Moriarty, A.E., 125
Morin, A.J.S., 500
Morin, C.M., 413
Morison, S.J., 380
Moritz, A.M., 636, 638, 641
Moritz, G., 752
Morris, A.S., 143, 152, 707
Morris, J.B. Jr., 639
Morris, M.C., 209, 501
Morris, N.M., 338
Morris, P.A., 225, 295
Morrison, F.J., 37, 175
Morrow, A.L., 590
Mors, O., 493
Mortensen, P.B., 104
Mortimer, J.T., 613
Moser, D.K., 392
Moser, J., 18
Moss, H.B., 601
Mostofsky, S.H., 436
Moulson, M.C., 378
Mounts, K.O., 393
Mounts, N.S., 145
Mowrer, O.H., 642
Mowrer, W.M., 642
Moylan, C.A., 130
Mrazek, D.A., 312, 397
Mrug, S., 323, 505
Muddasani, S., 497
Muehlenkamp, J.J., 709
Mueller, A., 688
Mueller, B.R., 47
Mueller, E., 186
Mulder, R.T., 392, 706
Mullaney, J., 583
Mullen, P.E., 623
Muller, R.T., 768
Muller-Nix, C., 393, 394
Mullins-Nelson, J.L., 707
Munafò, M.R., 56, 258, 270, 273
Munck, A.U., 289
Mundy, P.C., 271, 767
Murane, R., 163–165, 172
Muris, P., 323, 543, 547, 549, 550, 553–556
Murnen, S.K., 624
Murphy, A., 366

Murphy, C.C., 668
Murphy, J., 492
Murphy, K., 429
Murphy, L.B., 125, 642
Murphy, R.F., 178
Murphy, S., 635
Murphy, S.E., 278
Murphy, S.L., 521
Murray, C.J.L., 570
Murray, J., 710
Murray, K., 472
Murray, K.E., 436
Murray, K.T., 236
Murray, L.M., 550, 551
Murray, R.M., 57, 174
Murray-Close, D., 189, 706, 734
Murry, V.M.B., 49, 129, 132, 257, 339
Murtagh, D.R., 413
Musselman, D.L., 734
Mussen, P.H., 336
Mustillo, S., 88, 91, 492, 610
Muthén, B.O., 74, 75, 110, 112–115, 119
Muthén, L., 114
Muzet, A., 413, 415
Muzik, O., 382
Myers, J.M., 51, 589
Myers, L., 744
Myers, M.W., 189, 461, 476
Myers, S.S., 143, 707
Myers-Schulz, B., 266
Myrick, A.C., 771

N
Na, S., 393
Nachmias, M., 317, 554
Nadeem, E., 171
Nagin, D.S., 113, 115, 116, 118, 452, 457
Nahmias, C., 498
Naigles, L., 660
Najaka, S.S., 172
Najman, J.J., 210
Najman, J.M., 209, 212, 495
Nakamoto, J., 190
Nakamura, J., 135
Nakatani, E., 565
Nakonezny, P.A., 434
Nandi, A., 114
Nansel, T.R., 166, 191
Nasir, N.S., 164
Natale, V., 414
Nathanson, M., 745
Natsuaki, M.N., 338, 340–343, 345–348, 503, 732
Navarro, F., 644
Nazarov, A., 498
Neal, C., 295
Neal, J.W., 131
Neal, S., 473
Neal, Z.P., 131
Neale, B.M., 433

Neale, M.C., 50, 110, 246, 249, 251, 494, 548, 589
Nears, K., 735
Neary, E.M., 505, 563
Nebert, D.W., 257
Neckerman, H.J., 166
Nederhof, E., 257
Needell, B., 96
Negriff, S., 332, 334, 335, 337, 338, 341–343, 608
Negron, R., 536
Neiderhiser, J.M., 49, 249, 256, 347
Neild, R.C., 178
Neiman, S., 166
Nelson, C.A., 11, 295, 299, 300, 373, 376–378,
    381, 383, 657, 659
Nelson, D., 767
Nelson, E.C., 744
Nelson, E.E., 53
Nelson, M.M., 479
Nelson, N., 212
Nelson, S.E., 195, 456, 457, 461
Nelson-Gardell, D., 129
Nemeroff, C.B., 301, 734
Neppl, T.K., 130
Ness, A., 396
Nesse, R.M., 543
Neuhaus, E., 297, 532, 537
Neuman, G., 504
Neumann, D.L., 269, 553
Nevéus, T., 634, 635, 640
New, A., 709
Newcomb, A.F., 193
Newcorn, J.H., 432
Newhouse, P.A., 71
Newman, B., 93
Newman, D.L., 499, 589
Newman, J.P., 315, 319, 322, 323
Newman, S.C., 531
Newman, T.K., 55
Newschaffer, C., 654
Neziroglu, F., 572
Ng, T., 171
Ngun, T.C., 695
Ngwe, J.E., 115
Niaura, R., 610
Nicholls, D.E., 623
Nichols, K.E., 476
Nichols, P., 28
Nichols, T.R., 332, 339, 375
Nickerson, A.B., 171
Nickman, S.L., 383
Nicole, A., 393
Nielsen, E.O., 273
Nigg, J.T., 427, 430, 431, 433, 499, 588, 595
Nijenhuis, E.R.S., 763
Nijmeijer, J.S., 271
Nikulina, V., 54, 751
Nilsson, D., 765
Nishina, A., 192
Nissen, J.B., 493
Nissenson, K.J., 571

Nitschke, J.B., 278, 497
Nobile, M., 495
Nock, M.K., 478, 526, 528, 536
Noens, I.L., 689
Noftle, E.E., 133
Nolan, C.L., 497
Nolan, S.A., 504, 505
Nolen-Hoeksema, S., 90, 165, 169, 206, 209, 213, 214,
    228, 493, 501, 504, 707
Noll, J.G., 733, 762
Noll, R.B., 592
Nolte, T., 549, 552, 555
Nomura, Y., 435
Norasakkunkit, V., 228
Norcross, M.A., 268, 550
Nordentoft, M., 104
Nordquist, N., 270, 273
Norman, S., 393
Norris, A.W., 391
Northoff, G., 498
Norwood, W.D., 746
Notter, O., 198
Novak, M.A., 289
Nunez, J.L., 627
Nunnally, J.C., 73
Nurmi, J.E., 166, 194

O
Oades, R.D., 433, 436
Obeidallah, D., 341
Obel, C., 54, 230
Oberlander, T.F., 252, 294
Obermeyer, W.H., 165
O'Bleness, J.J., 361
Obradović, J., 126, 209, 290, 292, 295–298, 300, 302, 468
O'Brien, C.P., 596
O'Brien, L., 119, 609, 612
O'Brien, M., 431, 693
Obrosky, D.S., 492
O'Callaghan, M.J., 395
O'Carroll, P.W., 522
O'Connor, E.E., 127
O'Connor, J., 748
O'Connor, M.E., 623
O'Connor, M.J., 147
O'Connor, N., 652
O'Connor, S.M., 397
O'Connor, T.G., 49, 50, 245–258, 325, 362, 371, 376,
    380, 434, 534
Odgers, C., 113
O'Donnell, K., 255
O'Donnell, M.L., 748
O'Donovan, A., 294, 392
O'Donovan, M., 434, 654
Odouli, R., 103
Oesterle, S., 164
Oetting, W.S., 591
Offord, D.R., 31, 467, 493
Ogawa, J.R., 762, 764

Ogburn, E., 584
Ogliari, A.K., 549
Oh, S., 231
O'Hare, E., 504
Oishi, S., 133–135
Okawa, M., 414
Olafsen, K.S., 395
Oldehinkel, A.J., 210, 257, 500
Olds, R.S., 612
Olfson, M., 493
Olino, T.M., 499
Oliveira, P.S., 365
Oliver, P., 152
Oliveri, M.E., 206
Ollendick, T.H., 192, 543–556
Olley, A., 565
Olrick, J.T., 380
Olsen, B, 9
Olsen, E.M., 396, 401
Olsen, J.E., 145
Olson, D.R., 707
Olson, L.S., 172
Olson, S.L., 431, 452
Olthof, T., 706
Oltmanns, T.F., 703
Olvera, R.L., 498
Olweus, D., 191, 339, 462
O'Malley, P.M., 602, 603, 605, 610, 611, 613, 614
O'Neal, K.K., 475
O'Neil, K.A., 234, 610
O'Neill, M., 762
O'Nions, E.J.P., 273
Ontai, L.L., 130
Oomen, C.A., 300
Oort, F.J., 175
Oosterlaan, J., 291, 436
Oosterman, M., 291, 366
Opitz, J.M., 677
Oppenheimer, C.W., 212
Orav, E.J., 496
Oreland, L., 270, 273
O'Riley, A.A., 529
O'Riordan, M., 268
Ormel, J., 110, 210, 257, 500
Orn, H., 531
O'Roak, B.J., 253
Oroszi, G., 589
Orth, U., 707
Ortiz, L.R., 497
Oscar-Berman, M., 594
Osgood, D.W., 610, 612
O'Shea, T.M., 390
Oshri, A., 256, 731–733
Osofksy, H.J., 743, 745
Osofksy, J.D., 743
Ostendorf, F., 167
Oster-Granite, M.L., 676
Osterling, J., 656
Osterman, M.J., 389
Ostlund, H., 625, 627

Ostrowski, S.A., 746, 748
Ottet, M., 208
O'Tuathaigh, C.M.P., 57
Overbeek, G., 48, 49
Overton, W.F., 4, 5, 18
Owen, A., 685
Owen Blakemore, J.E., 683, 694
Owen, L.D., 189
Owen, M.J., 56, 434
Owens, D., 565
Owens, E.B., 431, 432, 476
Owens, J.A., 416
Owens-Stively, J., 410
Ozaki, S., 414
Ozer, E.J., 747, 748
Ozonoff, S., 653, 654, 656, 657

P
Paap, M.C., 686
Padawar, R., 692
Padawer, W., 642
Padilla-Walker, L.M., 197
Padyukov, L., 57
Page, B., 535
Pai, D., 382
Paikoff, R.L., 334, 337, 342, 343, 345
Pajer, K., 473
Palermo, S.D., 571
Paley, B., 144, 146–148, 504
Pals, J.L., 714
Panagiotides, H., 497
Pang, K.L., 429, 531
Pantell, M.S., 287
Papageorgiou, A., 393
Papandonatos, G.D., 610
Papežová, H., 765
Paradise, J., 745
Pardini, D.A., 456, 468
Pargament, K.I., 131
Pariente, C., 394
Paris, J., 531, 709, 710, 765
Park, C.L., 132
Park, I.J.K., 236, 504
Park, N., 132
Park, R.J., 497, 501
Parke, R.D., 153, 205, 730
Parker, J.G., 707, 730
Parker, K.C.H., 393
Parker, K.J., 208, 300, 375
Parker, S.W., 291, 312, 378
Parkhurst, J.T., 189, 190
Parritz, R.H., 317, 554
Partin, J.C., 635
Partin, J.S., 635
Partinen, M., 640
Parzer, P., 762
Pasch, L., 215
Pasterski, V., 687, 696
Pastor, D., 115

Pat-Horenczyk, R., 761
Patianna, V., 627
Patrick, C., 110
Patrick, J.C., 392
Patrick, M.E., 601–614
Patterson, C.J., 729, 730
Patterson, G.R., 37, 111, 152, 153, 156, 189, 313,
        314, 449–457, 460, 475, 477, 480, 534, 535,
        591, 612, 710
Patton, G.C., 331
Patton, R.G., 396
Paul, G., 504
Paul, J., 660
Paul, R., 658
Pauli-Pott, U., 255
Pauls, D.L., 433, 562, 564–566, 568
Paulus, M.P., 277, 278
Pawl, J.H., 672
Payne, A.V.L., 501
Paysnick, A.A., 129
Pearl, R., 233
Pearlin, L.I., 206
Pears, K.C., 380
Pease, T.E., 761
Pechtel, P., 752
Peck, S.C., 131, 164, 167
Peebles, C.D., 749
Peebles-Kleiger, M.J., 392
Peeke, L.G., 494, 501
Peeples, F., 96
Peets, K., 191
Pelayo-Terán, J.M., 56
Peleg, Y., 231
Pelham, W.E., 428, 431
Pellegrini, A.D.L., 458
Penckofer, S., 211
Penev, P., 413
Peng, B., 57
Pennan, A., 762
Pennebaker, J.W., 229
Pennington, B.F., 429, 431
Peper, J.S., 627
Pepler, D., 336, 337
Perel, J.M., 473, 751
Perez-Edgar, K., 555
Perez-Olivas, G., 551, 555
Pergamin-Hight, L., 270
Peris, T.S., 569, 570, 573, 574
Perkins, P., 625
Perrin, E.C., 376, 394
Perrin, S., 546, 548, 749
Perrine, N., 525
Perry, B.D., 752, 766, 767, 770
Perry, D.G., 191–193
Perry, L.C., 191
Perry, L.M., 292
Person, E.S., 690
Pervanidou, P., 751
Pesenti-Gritti, P., 549
Petersen, A.C., 333, 335, 338

Petersen, I.T., 109, 119, 311–325
Petersen, J., 401
Peterson, B.S., 499, 565
Peterson, C., 132, 135
Peterson, G., 762
Peterson, J.B., 532
Petit, G.S., 156
Petraitis, J., 607
Petras, H., 455
Pettit, G.S., 187, 188, 250, 297, 311–313, 315, 318,
        321–324, 478, 729, 730
Petukhova, M., 93
Pezawas, L., 273
Pfaff, D.W., 625
Phares, V., 69
Philibert, R.A., 48, 49, 255–257, 274, 275, 322
Philip, R.C., 267
Phillips, B.M., 323, 499, 550
Phillips, D.A., 129
Phillips, K.A., 566
Phillips, M.L., 266, 343
Phillips, N.K., 212
Phillips, W., 654
Piacentini, J.C., 536, 571, 573, 744
Piaget, J., 6, 15, 566
Pianta, R.C., 135, 175, 176
Piatti, V.C., 295
Picchietti, D.L., 419
Pickett, L., 678
Pickles, A., 51, 52, 110, 111, 132, 360, 376, 428, 491,
        657, 660
Pidada, S., 232
Piehler, T.F., 234, 476
Pierce, E.W., 431
Pierce, S., 291
Pierrehumbert, B., 393, 394
Pierson, R.K., 377
Pietrefesa, A., 565, 567
Pihl, R.O., 532
Pihlakoski, L., 491
Pijlman, F.T.A., 48, 297, 361
Pilgrim, C.C., 611, 612
Pilkington, L., 762
Pilkonis, P., 110
Pillai, A.G., 73, 382
Pina, A.A., 232, 573
Pine, D.S., 111, 267, 268, 549, 550, 555, 565, 689, 747
Pinto, A.O., 270
Pinto-Martin, J.A., 395
Piquero, A.R., 336, 337, 467
Pisecco, S., 440
Pisterman, S., 440
Pistis, M., 57
Pitchot, W., 533
Pitiot, A., 436
Pitman, R.K., 752
Pitner, S.L., 644
Pitts, S.C., 589
Piven, J., 269
Pivik, R.T., 496

Pizzagalli, D.A., 497, 752
Pjetri, E., 627
Plessen, K.J., 436
Pletnikov, M.V., 57
Pliszka, S.R., 436
Plomin, R., 48, 49, 51, 247–251, 253, 255, 256, 534, 669, 695, 710
Plotsky, P.M., 301, 380
Ploubidis, G.B., 74
Pluess, M., 55, 155, 296, 321
Plummer, N., 398
Poehlmann, J., 392–395
Poelmans, G., 433
Poikkeus, A., 115
Poindexter, B.B., 398
Polanczyk, G., 733
Poland, R.E., 496, 497
Polcari, A., 761
Pollack, M., 229
Pollak, S.D., 151, 300, 301, 312, 332, 333, 345, 374, 377, 378, 726, 727, 734
Pollard, C., 537
Pollard, R., 767
Pollock, J.I., 410
Pollock, R.A., 566
Polo, A., 214
Polo-Tomás, M., 93, 746
Pomerantz, E.M., 501
Ponirakis, A., 338
Poole, D.A., 749
Pope, H.G., 621
Popkin, B.M., 399
Porcelli, S., 252, 257
Porges, S.W., 154
Porter, C., 730
Porter, M.R., 188, 606
Portillo, N., 131
Posner, M.I., 452, 501
Possel, P., 497
Post, R.M., 491, 506, 761
Potapova, N., 532
Poteat, V.P., 166
Potijk, M.R., 395
Poulin, F., 131, 233, 452, 505, 536, 611
Poulter, M.O., 252
Poulton, R., 56, 94
Poustka, F., 192
Powell, N.P., 456
Power, C., 235
Power, T.J., 440
Powers, B., 490
Powers, C.J., 475, 480
Powers, J.L., 536
Powers, M.B., 547
Poznanski, E., 17
Prakash, K., 234
Pramstaller, P.P., 414
Prantzalou C., 554
Prater, K.E., 268
Preacher, K.J., 110, 211

Predieri, B., 627
Prescott, C.A., 258, 506, 589–591
Presnell, K., 338, 623
Presson, C.C., 609
Price, A.W., 743, 745
Price, J.L., 498
Price, J.M., 189
Price, L.H., 564
Price, R.K., 231, 468
Price-Evans, K., 553
Prichard, Z., 54
Primus, R.J., 627
Prinstein, M.J., 185–198, 234, 505, 526, 536, 611, 743
Prinzie, P., 191
Prom, E.C., 48
Propper, C., 255, 256, 316
Provencal, N., 293, 301
Provence, S., 357, 367, 396
Przybeck, T.R., 706
Puech, A.J., 533
Puess, M., 366
Puig-Antich, J.A., 417
Pukrop, R., 637
Punamaki, R.L., 505
Purcell, S., 131
Purdie, N., 168
Purdon, C., 563
Purington, A., 536
Purkis, H.M., 553
Purselle, D., 734
Puterman, E., 294
Putnam, F.W., 733, 744, 761, 762, 764, 765
Putnam, K.M., 497, 706
Putnam, S.P., 319
Puts, D.A., 695
Puttler, L.I., 591
Pyhala, R., 394
Pynoos, R.S., 744, 750

Q
Qin, J., 730
Quane, J.M., 611
Quay, H.C., 70, 532
Quevedo, K.M., 165, 334, 384
Quigley, K.S., 291
Quigley, M.A., 390, 391
Quihuis, G., 165
Quillian, R.E., 414
Quine, L., 675
Quinnell, F.A., 392

R
Rabban, M., 693
Raby, K.L., 317
Rachman, S., 562–564, 567
Racine, Y.A., 467
Radke-Yarrow, N., 11
Radtke, R.A., 414

Raes, A., 640
Rafferty, J., 215
Raghunath, N., 639
Rahe, T., 205
Rahman, Q., 695
Raichle, M.E., 280, 497
Raikkonen, K., 504
Raine, A., 459, 470, 472, 531, 710, 734
Rajkowska, G., 498
Ram, N., 333
Ramey, C.T., 165, 170
Ramey, S.L., 144, 165, 170
Ramirez, J.M., 299
Ramirez, J.S.B., 299
Ramirez, R., 211
Rammstedt, B., 167
Ramsay, D., 658
Ramsey, B., 563
Ramsey, E., 534
Ramstetter, C.L., 174
Rancourt, D., 187, 188, 190, 194
Rankin, B.H., 611
Rantanen, P., 339, 505, 623
Rao, U., 489–507
Rapee, R.M., 213, 231, 233, 543, 551–552
Raphaelson, Y.E., 291
Rapoport, J.L., 268, 269, 563, 564, 567
Rasbash, J., 252
Rasmussen, J.L., 147
Rasmussen, S.A., 562, 564
Rasumussen, S.A., 568
Rathouz, P.J., 251, 473
Rauch, S.L., 565, 752
Raudenbush, S.W., 96, 113, 114
Raval, P., 229
Raval, V., 229
Ravens-Sieberer, U., 74
Raver, C.C., 35
Raviv, A., 409
Raviv, T., 209
Ray, R.D., 266, 749
Raynor, P., 402, 491
Razza, R.P., 167
Read, J.P., 611
Ready, D.D., 177
Reardon, S.F., 605
Reavis, R.D., 193
Reboussin, B.A., 610
Redcay, E., 659
Reddy, Y.C., 565
Ree, M.J., 414, 416
Reed, A., 726
Reef, J., 72
Reese, H.W., 18
Reeves, M.A., 171
Regestein, Q.R., 414, 415
Regier, D.A., 95, 110, 120
Regnerus, M., 338
Rehm, J., 94
Rehm, L., 563

Reich, D.B., 708
Reich, S.M., 198
Reich, T.R., 583
Reichenberg, A., 47, 253
Reichow, B., 653
Reid, C.B., 278
Reid, J.B., 313, 451, 455, 480
Reid, J.C., 492
Reid, M.J., 454, 480
Reifman, A.S., 611
Reijneveld, S.A., 395
Reijntjes, A., 191, 192
Reilly, N., 503
Reimers, T.M., 644
Reinecke, J., 113
Reinecke, M.A., 500
Reinke, J., 133
Reis, H.T., 135
Reising, M.M., 210
Reiss, A.L., 749, 752
Reiss, D., 206, 247, 249, 251, 252, 256, 347
Reiss, S., 666, 676, 678
Remington, B., 431
Renk, K., 69
Repacholi, B.M., 9, 476
Repetti, R.L., 143, 154, 192
Repetti, R.S., 143, 150, 151, 154, 157
Reppert, S.M., 410
Resch, F., 762
Rescorla, L.A., 71–75, 77–80, 216, 228, 688
Resick, P., 747
Resnick, H.S., 743
Resnick, M.D., 504
Restifo, K., 152
Rettew, D., 564, 569
Reus, V.I., 294
Reuter, M., 156
Rey-Casserly, C., 392
Reyna, V.F., 608, 609
Reynolds, A.J., 129, 735, 736
Reynolds, B.M., 336, 343
Reynolds, B.R., 143
Reynolds, C.R., 72
Reynolds, K.D., 211
Rezai, A., 653
Reznick, J., 567
Rhead, M.J., 669
Rheingold, H.L., 4
Rhemtulla, M., 250
Rhodes, J.E., 131
Ribi, K., 746
Rice, F., 494, 495
Rice, J.P., 583
Richards, M.H., 338, 610
Richardson, G.S., 414
Richardson, M.E., 436
Rich-Edwards, J.W., 734
Richert, K.A., 752
Richey, J., 490
Richter, M.A., 568

Richter-Appelt, H., 687
Richters, J.E., 17, 18, 157
Richters, M., 362
Ricken, J., 414
Rickert, V.I, 412
Ricks, D., 314
Ridder, E.M., 235
Riddle, M., 546
Ridge, B., 322
Riegel, K.F., 5, 6
Riemann, R., 167
Rifkin, A., 770
Rigo, J., 398
Riis, J., 97
Rijsdijk, F., 710
Riley, A.W., 128
Riley, C., 365
Riley, E.R., 434
Riley, R.L., 762
Rimland, B., 652
Rimpela, A., 505
Rimpela, M., 338, 339, 346, 505, 623
Rintelmann, J., 496
Rios, R., 131
Rippey Massat, C., 171
Risch, N., 52, 252, 258
Risi, S., 505, 653
Risk, N., 231
Riso, L.P., 704
Rissanen, A., 623
Ritchie, M.D., 57
Ritter, G.W., 171
Ritter, K., 706
Ritterband, L.M., 643
Rivet, K., 608
Rivier, C.L., 154
Rizley, R., 725
Rizvi, S.L., 535
Rizzo, C.J., 505
Ro, E., 714
Robb, A.S., 751
Robers, S., 166
Roberson-Nay, R., 498
Robert, J.J., 496
Roberts, A., 171
Roberts, B.W., 708, 711, 712
Roberts, C.R., 226
Roberts, J.M., 711
Roberts, M.C., 133
Roberts, N., 17
Roberts, R.E., 226, 228, 494
Roberts, W., 130
Robins, L.N., 31, 58, 453, 468, 531
Robins, R.W., 133, 167, 706, 707
Robinson, L.R., 143, 707
Robinson, N.S., 187, 501, 505
Robinson, T.E., 532, 594
Robinson, W., 94
Robles, T.F., 143
Rock, P.F., 197

Rockhill, B., 93
Rockoff, J.E., 175
Rodgers, B., 235
Rodkin, P.C., 233
Rodriguez, M.L., 612
Rodriguez-Tomé, H., 337
Roelofs, J., 169
Roenneberg, T., 414
Roennebert, T., 410
Roesch, L., 493
Roeser, R.W., 131, 163–179, 331, 612
Roeyers, H., 437, 639
Roff, M.M., 185
Rogal, S., 751
Rogers, J.W., 434, 635
Rogers, S., 655, 656, 659
Rogosch, F.A., 49, 119, 128, 129, 210, 256, 258, 290,
    377–378, 537, 606, 726, 728–736
Rohde, P.M., 493, 500, 503, 528
Rohling, D., 637
Rohrmann, S., 192
Roiser, J.P., 273
Roisman, G.I., 251, 337, 357, 552
Rollnick, S, 413
Romans, S.E., 623
Romens, S., 113
Romeo, R.D., 384
Romer, D., 608
Romero, L.M., 206, 289
Romero-Canyas, R., 169
Romney, D.M., 696
Ronchi, P., 566
Rone, L., 481
Rones, M., 171
Rood, L., 169
Rosa, A., 57
Rose, A.J., 194
Rose, G., 87, 89
Rose, L., 745
Rose, R.J., 341, 593
Rose, S.A., 499
Roseby, V., 153
Rosen, C.L., 416
Rosén, I., 533
Rosen, K.M., 292
Rosen, L.H., 198
Rosen, P.M., 536
Rosenberg, M.S., 746
Rosenberg, T.K., 492
Rosenblat-Stein, S., 174
Rosenblum, K.L., 131
Rosenblum, L., 5
Rosenthal, D.R., 188
Rosenthal, S., 4, 358
Rosin, H., 692
Ross, C.A., 57, 761
Ross, L.E., 392
Ross, S., 535
Rossman, B.B.R., 746
Rosso, I.M., 498

Roth, J.H., 550
Roth, J.L., 172
Rothbart, M.K., 35, 155, 227, 311, 312, 314, 317–319,
    322, 323, 430, 452, 499, 501, 502, 567, 745
Rothenberger, A., 433
Rothman, K.J., 88
Rothschild, L., 704
Routh, D.K., 18
Rovet, J.F., 669
Rovine, M., 358
Rowan, B., 175
Rowden, L., 188
Rowe, D.C., 339
Rowe, J.W., 295
Rowe, M.L., 659
Rowlett, R., 677
Roy, A.K., 453
Roy, P., 360, 376, 380
Rozenman, M., 554
Rozin, P., 136
Rubia, K., 268, 377, 734
Rubin, B.R., 589
Rubin, K.H., 188, 228, 229, 231, 232, 234,
    235, 321, 707
Rubin, R.T., 473
Rubio-Stipec, M., 110, 492
Ruble, D.N., 683
Rucker, D.D., 110, 211
Rudolf, M.C.J., 402, 491
Rudolph, K.D., 119, 192, 193, 196, 207, 210, 212, 213,
    215, 297, 302, 331–349, 493, 494, 500–501–506,
    607, 608
Rueda, M.R., 452
Rueger, S., 209, 210
Rueter, M.A., 503, 504, 611
Ruiz-Pelaez, J.G., 391
Rumberger, R.W., 178
Ruscio, A.M., 562
Ruscio, J., 490
Russell, D.W., 195
Russell, S.T., 92, 166
Russell, V.A., 532
Russoniello, C.V., 746
Rust, J., 695
Ruths, S., 765
Rutter, M., 3, 4, 6, 8, 16, 17, 27, 32–34, 41, 45–60, 70,
    111, 119, 125–134, 174, 177, 248, 296, 313, 315,
    357, 360, 362, 363, 371, 372, 375, 376, 380, 383,
    384, 434, 490, 491, 493, 534, 605, 607, 614,
    652–654, 668, 669, 710, 725
Ruuska, J., 623
Ryan, C.E., 92
Ryan, C.N., 533, 536
Ryan, N.D., 343, 417, 492, 497, 752
Ryan, R.M., 129
Ryan, S.M., 551–552
Ryder, A.G., 229
Ryding, E., 533
Ryff, C.D., 133
Rynn, M.A., 278

S
Sable, J., 164
Sachdev, P., 565
Sachek, J., 430
Sachs, H.T., 665–679
Sack, C., 551
Sack, R.L., 415
Sadeh, A., 174, 409–411
Sadovnick, A.D., 668
Saeger, K., 692
Saffery, R., 294
Sagi-Schwartz, A., 359
Sagvolden, T., 532
Sahin, E., 294
Sahl, R., 676
Saigal, S., 395
Sakai, J., 231
Salekin, R.T., 707
Sallee, F.R., 746
Salmelin, R.K., 393
Salmivalli, C., 191
Salmon, K., 479, 746
Saltzman, H., 501
Salvator, A., 392
Salzberg, A.D., 17
Samek, D.R., 611
Sameroff, A.J., 5, 6, 13, 14, 17, 25–41, 131, 156, 165,
    166, 185, 209, 265, 314, 331, 397, 431, 452, 605,
    614, 683
Sami, N., 432
Sampson, R.J., 95, 96, 113, 114, 127, 132, 457, 458, 462
Samson, J.A., 761
Samuel, D.B., 110, 705, 712
Sanborn, K., 333, 337, 341
Sánchez, F.J., 695
Sanchez, J., 92, 536
Sanchez, M.M., 301, 380
Sandberg, D.E., 393, 687
Sanddal, N.D., 522
Sanders, S., 762
Sanderson, W.C., 505
Sandin, S., 47
Sandler, I.N., 211, 500, 502
Sandman, C.A., 677
Sandstrom, M.J., 190, 505
Sanikhani, M., 685
Sanislow, C.A., 704, 708
Santengelo, S.L., 271
Santiago, C., 209
Santiago, R., 692
Santonastaso, P., 621
Santos, I.S., 397, 399
Sapolsky, R.M., 154, 289, 295, 497
Saporta, A.S.D., 382
Sar, V., 765
Sari, F., 339
Sarin, S., 501
Sarsour, K., 11, 293
Sarter, M., 266
Sasser, T.R., 467–482

Sattora, A., 119
Sauder, C., 532
Saudino, K.J., 7, 319
Saunders, B.E., 743
Saunders, W.B., 163, 169
Savage, T.A., 171
Savas, H.A., 765
Savoie, L., 374
Savonlahti, E., 394
Sawa, A., 57
Sawyer, A.M., 481
Saxena, S., 565
Saylor, C.F., 17, 394
Saywitz, K.J., 744
Scahill, L., 564
Scaramella, L.V., 130, 503
Scarna, A., 414
Scarpa, A., 473
Scarr, S., 255, 593
Scerif, G., 436
Schaeffer, C., 461
Schaeffer, S., 12
Schaer, M., 208
Schafer, J., 119
Schafer, W.D., 9
Schafer-Kalkhoff, T., 215
Schagen, S.E., 696
Schalling, D., 339
Schalock, R.L., 665
Schaps, E., 176
Schatzberg, A.F., 268, 300
Scheepers, F.E., 468
Scheeringa, M.S., 744, 749, 750, 753
Scheib, E., 198
Schelleman-Offermans, K., 339
Schendel, D., 668
Schermerhorn, A.C., 150, 156, 311–325
Scheungel, C., 366
Schiefele, U., 168
Schlomer, G.L., 450
Schlotz, W., 48, 375, 384
Schlup, B., 572
Schmaling, K.B., 454
Schmeidler, J., 767
Schmidt, D.A., 414
Schmidt, J.D., 119, 193
Schmidt, L.A., 395
Schmidt, M.H., 289, 435
Schmidt, N.B., 554
Schmitt, J., 110
Schmitt-Rodermund, E., 335
Schnack, H.G., 627
Schneider, B.H., 228, 230, 233
Schneider, K., 770
Schneider, M.L., 57, 503, 627
Schneider-Rosen, K., 11, 492, 728
Schneiger, A., 461
Schniering, C.A., 213, 543, 551
Schnitker, S.A., 133
Schnurr, P.P., 392

Schoff, K., 147
Schofield, C.A., 168
Schofield, E., 551
Schonert-Reichl, K.A., 173
Schoppe-Sullivan, S.J., 147
Schore, A.N., 316
Schork, N., 270
Schorr, C., 744
Schote, A.B., 54
Schotsmans, P., 522
Schouten, E., 169
Schraedley, P.K., 338
Schramm, S., 178
Schrepferman, L.M., 152, 505, 534
Schroeder, C.S., 676
Schroeder, M.L., 713
Schroeder, S.R., 676
Schuder, M.R., 764
Schuengel, C., 291
Schuld, V., 762
Schulenberg, J.E., 585, 601–614
Schultz, R.T., 268
Schulz, K.M., 627
Schulz, P.M., 531
Schulz, U., 205
Schumann, C.M., 269
Schumann, G., 280, 591
Schwab-Stone, M., 493, 743, 745
Schwartz, C.E., 234
Schwartz, D., 190–192, 729, 730
Schwartz, S.M., 88, 413
Schwartzapfel, B., 692
Schwartz-Mette, R.A., 194
Schwarz, E.D., 752
Schwarz, N., 103
Schwarzer, R., 205
Schwarzwald, J., 748
Schweinberger, M., 196
Schwichtenberg, M.A.J., 392
Sciuto, G., 566
Scolton, K.L., 153
Scott, K.M., 731
Scott, S., 257, 325
Scourfield, J., 494
Seaton, E., 215, 747–748
Sebanc, A.M., 291, 312
Sebat, J., 654
Sedlak, A.J., 725, 746
Seedat, S., 745, 750, 751
Seeley, J.K., 503
Seeley, J.R., 338, 490, 493, 494, 503, 506, 528, 623
Seeman, T.E., 143, 192, 206, 288, 290, 295
Segal, N.L., 248
Segal, Z.V., 506
Segawa, E., 115
Seibt, J., 417
Seidel, W.F., 413
Seidman, E., 213
Seidman, L.J., 436
Seif, H., 166

Seifen, S., 637
Seifer, B., 17
Seifer, R., 28, 33, 34, 37, 165, 311, 312, 414
Seligman, M.E.P., 132, 165, 206
Seltzer, M.M., 660
Selye, H., 289
Semel, M., 749
Semer, N.L., 638
Semler, C.N., 414
Sen, S., 49, 258, 533
Sennhauser, F.H., 746
Sergeant, J.A., 291
Sergi Papiol, L.F., 57
Serketich, W.J., 231
Serocynski, A.D., 501
Seroczynski, A.D., 501
Serpell, L., 744
Serretti, A., 252
Sesack, S.R., 270
Sesma, A., 234
Sestan, N., 652, 654
Seth, S., 427, 429
Sethi, S., 637
Settle, C., 771
Seward, N., 416
Shackman, A.J., 151, 727
Shackman, J.E., 151, 727
Shad, M.U., 497, 498
Shaffer, D., 73, 91, 493, 536, 547
Shagle, S.C., 145
Shah, M.D., 401
Shah, P.E., 394
Shahar, G., 174
Shalev, I., 294
Shanahan, L., 491
Shanahan, M.J., 115, 605, 607
Shankman, S.A., 503, 706
Shannis, D., 295
Shannon, K.E., 154, 297, 532
Shannon, M.P., 746
Shapiro, D., 749
Sharkey, P., 96
Sharma, A., 249, 611
Sharpley, A.L., 414
Shaver, P.R., 552
Shaw, B., 115
Shaw, D.S., 127, 152, 450, 452–454, 476, 479, 502, 536
Shaw, H., 610
Shaw, J.A., 744, 747
Shaw, P., 434, 436
Shaw, R.J., 392
Shear, M.K., 493
Shedden, K., 49, 113, 258, 533
Shedler, J., 704
Sheeber, L., 504
Sheffield Morris, A., 478
Sheldon, K.M., 132–135
Shelton, T.L., 431, 440
Shen, Y., 654
Shenk, C.E., 733, 746

Shepard, S.A., 129
Sher, K.J., 114, 564
Sher, L., 532
Sherbourne, C., 115
Sheridan, J., 734
Sheridan, M.A., 11, 293, 300, 302, 377, 381, 383
Sherman, B.J., 131
Sherman, L., 452
Sherman, S.J., 609
Sherrill, J., 492
Sherrod, K.B., 397
Shibui, K., 414
Shields, A., 377–378, 729, 730
Shields, J., 7
Shih, J.H., 493, 503, 504
Shildrick, S., 551, 555
Shimamura, A.P., 752
Shin, J.U., 765
Shin, L.M., 752
Shin, N., 315, 317
Shin, S.H., 734
Shiner, R.L., 132, 311, 499, 708, 711, 712, 714
Shinn, L.K., 693
Shipra, M.P., 637
Shirar, L., 762
Shirk, S.R., 414
Shirm, S., 171
Shirtcliff, E.A., 208, 291, 295, 297, 332, 333, 341, 345, 349, 734
Shiyko, M.P., 346
Shneidman, E.S., 521–526
Shonkoff, J.P., 129
Short, E.J., 434
Shortt, A., 571
Shortt, J.W., 611
Showers, J., 401
Shreeram, S., 638, 639
Shrestha, S., 230
Shrout, P.E., 110
Shulha, H.P., 277
Sibille, E., 273
Sibug, R.M., 289
Siddaway, A.P., 744
Sidney, S., 288
Sieck, W.R., 674
Siegel, J.M., 338, 345, 346
Siegel, L., 749
Siegle, G.J., 414
Siever, L., 709
Sigman, M., 659
Silbereisen, R.K., 335, 336, 338, 345
Silberg, J., 341, 493, 494, 549
Silberg, J.L., 48, 51, 710, 761–771
Silberg, J.S., 763
Silberg, S.L., 770
Silberman, E.K., 761
Silbersweig, D., 709
Silk, J.S., 143, 145, 334, 343, 502, 707
Silk, K.R., 706
Sillaber, I., 47

Sillen, U., 640
Siller, M., 659
Silva, J.R., 365
Silva, P.A., 341, 499, 589
Silverman, M.M., 522, 525
Silverman, W.K., 232, 338, 543, 544, 554, 555, 743, 745, 750
Silvern, L., 747, 748
Silverthorn, N., 131
Sim, L., 766
Simakajornboon, N., 419
Simeon, D., 767
Simien, C., 497
Simmons, R.G., 334, 336
Simon, G.E., 229
Simon, M.B., 589
Simon, N.M., 294
Simon, T., 69
Simon, V.A., 189, 505
Simonds, L.M., 569
Simonoff, E., 468, 470, 669
Simons, A.D., 506
Simons, J., 609
Simons, R.L., 54, 55, 339, 341, 503, 504
Simonsen, E., 705, 713
Simpson, H.B., 571
Sinai, D., 411
Sinclair, L., 653
Sinclair, P., 196
Singer, B.H., 295
Singer, J., 112
Singer, L.T., 392, 434
Singh, A.L., 251
Singh, D., 686, 687, 689, 691, 693
Singh, N.N., 678
Singleton, R.A., 215
Sinha, P., 726, 727
Siperstein, G.N., 667
Sirof, B., 767
Sisk, C.L., 625–627
Sjaastad, J., 92
Skardhamar, T., 114
Skinner, E., 173
Skinner, K., 192
Skinner, M.L., 189, 456
Skitch, S.A., 209–211, 505
Skodol, A.E., 704–706
Skoog, T., 341
Skovgaard, A.M., 401
Skranes, J., 395
Slade, E., 171
Slavin, R.E., 164
Sleeper, L., 745
Sloan, D.M., 706
Slobodskaya, H.R., 231
Sloutsky, V.M., 378
Slutske, W.S., 536, 590, 593
Smallish, L., 428, 431, 432
Smeeth, L., 103
Smeraldi, E., 566

Smider, N.A., 291
Smiler, A.P., 696
Smith, B., 676
Smith, C., 747
Smith, D.P., 228
Smith, D.R., 731
Smith, E., 748
Smith, J.D., 453
Smith, J.R., 92
Smith, K.A., 745, 746
Smith, L.B., 314
Smith, M.T., 413
Smith, P., 744, 748, 749
Smith, R.S., 125, 126, 745
Smith, S.M., 280
Smith, S.R., 765
Smith Stover, C., 747
Smith, Y.L.S., 698
Smokowski, P.R., 211
Smolak, L., 624
Smolen, A., 209, 495
Smyke, A.T., 359, 365, 379, 380
Sneed, J.R., 704
Sneed, T.J., 642
Snidman, N., 132, 234
Snijders, T.A.B., 196
Snoek, H., 472, 532
Snow, D., 172
Snow, M.S., 762
Snow, R.E., 167, 174
Snowberg, K.E., 173
Snyder, C.R., 134
Snyder, J., 152, 153, 156, 452, 453, 455, 461, 475, 476, 505, 534, 611
Soares, I., 365
Sobol, B., 770
Sodhi, J., 627
Soenens, B., 552
Söhmen, T., 751
Sokol, B.W., 38
Sokolowski, M., 55
Solantaus, T.S., 505
Solomon, A., 490
Solomon, J., 359
Solomon, Z., 748
Sondik, E.J., 165
Sontag, L.M., 209, 211, 341, 343
Sonuga-Barke, E.J.S., 48, 55, 357, 363, 372, 375–377, 381, 384, 427–442
Soong, W.T., 213
Sopko, A.M., 393
Sorensen, M.J., 493
Soto, T.W., 561–575
Soukup, J., 765
Sourander, A., 535
Sousa, C., 130
South, S.C., 592
Southam-Gerow, M.A., 501
Sovner, R., 677
Spagnola, M., 736

Spanagel, R., 627
Spangler, G., 154, 359
Spatola, C.A.M., 549
Spear, L.P., 595, 601, 608, 627
Spector, T., 695
Spence, S.H., 544
Spezio, M.L., 269
Spiegel, K., 413
Spieker, S., 497
Spielman, A.J., 415
Spiker, D., 393
Spilsbury, J.C., 96
Spinelli, S., 53
Spinrad, T.L., 457, 501–502, 706
Spirito, A., 536, 638
Spitz, R., 357, 358, 366, 396
Spitznagel, E., 503
Spivack, G., 322
Splittgerber, F., 178
Sporn, J., 751
Spracklen, K.M., 188, 194, 451, 612
Springer, K.W., 734
Springer, T., 745
Srinath, S., 73
Sroufe, A.L., 358
Sroufe, L.A., 3, 7–9, 11, 13, 16, 18, 27, 32, 37, 41, 45,
    90, 150, 151, 154, 313, 315, 359, 490, 504, 592,
    709, 725, 727–729, 762
Stacey, J., 551
Stadler, C., 192
Staff, J., 613
Staff, R.T., 293
Stafford, L., 228
Stahlschmidt, M.J., 734
Stallard, P., 748, 750
Stamperdahl, J., 209, 292, 296
Stang, P.E., 163, 169
Stanger, C., 17, 18
Stansbury, K., 291
Stansbury, R., 228
Stansfeld, S., 235
Stanton, C., 610
Stark, L.J., 638, 643
Staron, V., 751
Starr, M.D., 9
Starr, R.H., 402
State, M., 652, 654
Stattin, H., 31, 166, 185, 196, 336, 341, 343, 347, 611
Staudinger, U.M., 132
Stavrakaki, C., 17
Steele, H., 9, 357–367
Steele, J., 413
Steele, K., 763
Steele, M., 9, 357–367
Steensma, T.D., 685, 686, 688, 693, 695, 698
Steer, R.A., 750, 769
Steere, J.C., 436
Steger, M.F., 132, 135
Stegge, H., 706
Steglich, C.E.G., 196

Steimke, R., 268, 269
Stein, A., 397
Stein, B.D., 171
Stein, D.J., 504, 562, 745, 750
Stein, G.L., 209, 210, 589
Stein, M.A., 165
Stein, M.B., 270, 277, 278, 752
Stein, S.M., 636
Steinberg, A.M., 744
Steinberg, L., 129, 143, 145, 268, 334, 337, 347, 450,
    456, 490, 707
Steinberg, L.D., 608, 609, 612, 613
Steiner, H., 750, 762
Steingard, R.J., 497
Steinhausen, H.C., 493
Steinmetz, J.L., 491
Steketee, G., 563, 568
Stellar, E., 295
Stellern, S.A., 361
Stengler-Wenzke, K., 571, 574
Stepanski, E.J., 413
Stephens, D., 132
Steptoe, A., 258
Sterba, S.K., 13, 14, 109–120
Sterling, L., 655
Sterling, P., 295
Stern, E., 709
Stern, H.P., 639
Stern, M., 393
Stevens, S., 55
Stevens, S.E., 376
Stevens, S.J., 413
Stevenson, J., 211, 410, 494, 551
Steward, D.S., 748
Steward, M.S., 748
Stewart, A., 115
Stewart, D.E., 393
Stewart, J., 287
Stewart, R.B., 148, 150
Stewart, R.C., 397
Stewart, S.E., 564, 565
Stice, E., 194, 209, 338, 339, 343, 493, 501, 610, 623
Stieben, J., 473
Stillion, J.M., 526–530
Stinson, F.S., 584
Stinson, K., 414
Stjernqvist, K., 395
Stocker, C.M., 146, 187
Stoiber, K.C., 130
Stolbach, B.C., 762, 765
Stoll, B.J., 389
Stolow, D., 209
Stone, D., 171
Stone, L.B., 194, 213
Stone, W., 657
Stoneman, Z., 675
Stoolmiller, M., 153, 247, 300, 505
Stoolmiller, M.M., 189
Stoolmiller, M.S., 453, 456, 457
Storch, E.A., 566, 570, 571, 573

Stormshak, E.A., 129, 146, 191, 454
Storvall, E.E., 339
Stouthamer-Loeber, M., 34, 167, 454, 471, 710
Stovall, K.C., 251, 366
St.Peter, C., 534
Straits, B.C., 215
Strakowski, S., 278
Strang-Karlsson, S., 395
Strathearn, L., 295
Strathman, A., 472
Strauman, T.J., 493
Straus, M.A., 747
Strauss, C.C., 17, 90
Strawn, J.R., 278
Strickland, J, 112
Strobel, K.R., 165
Strobino, D., 97
Stropes, J., 505
Stroud, L.R., 334
Stryker, L., 118
Stuhlmacher, A.F., 207
Stuhlman, M.W., 176
Sturge-Apple, M.L., 143–157, 732, 736
Sturm, R., 165
Sturman, D.A., 608
Stuvland, R., 747
Styne, D.M., 332
Su, M.S., 640
Suarez, M., 152
Subrahmanyam, K., 198
Subramanian, S.V., 126, 397
Subramanyam, M.A., 397, 399
Sucoff, C.A., 95
Sugden, K., 58
Sugimura, N., 192, 500
Suisman, J.L., 626
Sullivan, P., 654
Sullivan, P.B., 399
Sullivan, P.F., 494, 706
Sullivan, T., 118
Sumner, M.M., 291
Sun, Y.E., 293
Sung, M., 339
Suomi, S.J., 289
Super, C.M., 226
Supplee, L., 454
Sureshkumar, P., 641
Surguladze, S.A., 273
Surkan, P.J., 397
Susman, E.J., 151, 154, 331–345, 348, 472, 608, 733
Susser, E.S., 47, 87, 88, 92
Susser, M., 88
Sutera, S., 660
Sutphen, J.L., 639
Sutton, P.D., 389
Suvak, M.K., 566
Suwanlert, S., 225
Suway, J.G., 555
Svedin, C.G., 765
Svrakic, D.M., 706

Swaab, H., 688–689
Swain, J.E., 295
Swain-Campbell, N.R., 56
Swank, P.R., 746
Swanson, J.M., 440
Swartz, J.R., 265–280
Swearer, S.M., 166
Swedo, S.E., 564, 565, 567
Swift, M., 322
Swift, R.M., 585
Synder, C.R., 134
Szalacha, L.A., 177
Szasz, T.S., 10
Szatmari, P., 277, 654, 655
Szeinberg, A., 416
Szekely, E., 627
Szeto, K., 399
Szkrybalo, J., 683
Szumowski, E.K., 431
Szyf, M., 252, 374
Szymanski, L.S., 676
Szyszko, J., 666

T
Tabone, J.K., 129
Tackett, J.L., 252, 499, 703, 705, 708, 711, 714
Taga, K., 337
Tager–Flusberg, H., 651–661
Taillefer, S., 548, 549
Tajima, E.A., 130
Takacs, A., 118–119
Talbot, L.S., 409, 502
Talbott, M.R., 659
Talge, N.M., 295
Talwar, C., 136
Tamang, B.L., 230
Tamm, L., 434
Tamplin, A., 497
Tan, J., 209
Tanaka, C., 231
Tang, W., 391
Tankersley, L., 155
Tanner, J.L., 457
Tannock, R., 433
Tarter, R.E., 594
Tarullo, A.R., 290, 375–378, 380, 383, 384
Tasali, E., 413
Taska, L., 748, 764
Tassi, P., 413, 415
Tate, B.A., 414
Taub, B., 338
Tauras, J.A., 603
Taylor, A.Z., 54, 93, 131, 196, 197, 746
Taylor, B., 335
Taylor, C.B., 493
Taylor, C.M., 746
Taylor, E., 434
Taylor, J., 319
Taylor, L., 163, 165, 170, 171, 501

Taylor, M., 768
Taylor, R.D., 172, 747–748, 753
Taylor, S.E., 143, 169, 192
Taylor, Z.E., 290
Taywaditep, K.J., 694
Tazuma, L., 229
Teasdale, J.D., 491, 501
Teicher, M.H., 295, 761, 762
Teisl, M., 729, 730
Telch, M.J., 191
Tellegen, A., 6, 127, 128, 234, 248
Tenconi, E., 621
Terry, R., 185
Tesher, H.B., 295
Tessier, R., 391
Testiny, E.P., 17
Teunissen, H.A., 493
Thabet, A.A., 743–747
Thapar, A., 46, 52, 54, 434, 494
Tharner, A., 394
Thatcher, D.L., 734
Thatcher, J.E., 312, 727
Theall, K.P., 294, 295
Thede, L.L., 695
Thelen, E., 314
Thibodeau, E.L., 732
Thiébot, M.H., 533
Thienemann, M., 573
Thiéry, J.C., 416
Thirlwall, K., 551
Thomaes, S., 706
Thomas, A., 6, 14, 311, 499
Thomas, C., 481
Thomas, J.J., 622
Thomas, K.M., 268
Thomas, Y.F., 584
Thomason, M.E., 273
Thombs, D.L., 612
Thome-Granz, S., 636
Thompson, H., 573
Thompson, M., 427, 654, 657
Thompson, R.A., 7, 11, 129, 150, 157, 535, 726
Thompson, T., 171, 668, 676
Thomsen, A.H., 501
Thomsen, P.H., 493, 562
Thomson, R.A., 501
Thorlindsson, T., 233
Thornberry, T.P., 456, 457
Thornton, L.M., 625
Thorp, J.A., 390
Thorpy, M.J., 415
Thurm, A.E., 205, 207, 208
Tieman, W., 384
Tienari, P., 250
Tierney, A., 657
Tiet, Q.Q., 131
Tietjen, A.M., 226
Tikotzky, L., 411
Timbremont, B., 491
Timmermans, M., 235

Timmons-Mitchell, J., 481
Ting, A.H., 295
Tipsord, J.M., 449, 452
Tirella, L., 376
Tisak, J., 111
Tizard, B., 373, 376
Tizard, J., 668
Tobin, D.D., 697
Tobin-Richards, M.H., 335, 336
Todd, B.J., 627
Todd, M., 589
Todd, R.D., 497
Todd, R.M., 312, 315
Todorov, A.A., 274
Tolan, P.H., 130
Tolin, D.F., 563, 745
Tolley-Schell, S.A., 727
Tomany-Korman, S.C., 165
Tomarken, A.J., 497
Tomiyama, A.J., 294
Tomkins, S.S., 764
Tompson, M., 504
Tonetti, L., 414
Tonge, B.J., 676
Topitzes, J.W., 735
Torchia, M.G., 752
Tordjman, S., 271
Torgersen, S., 709, 711
Toro, R., 436
Torppa, M., 115
Torrance, N., 707
Tost, H., 498
Toth, S.L., 49, 90, 377–378, 492, 537, 723, 728–731, 734, 736, 762
Tottenham, N., 300, 381, 382, 385
Tout, K., 291
Touwen, B.C., 637
Towbin, K.A., 689
Townsend, E., 523
Tracy, K., 710
Trainor, C.D., 341
Tram, J., 501
Trancik, A., 288, 320
Träskman-Bendz, L., 533
Traue, H., 229
Treadwell, K.R., 750
Tremblay, R.E., 113, 114, 454, 457, 470, 473, 475, 589
Trentacosta, C.J., 479
Treuba, H.T., 176
Treutlein, J., 591
Tricamo, M., 625
Trickett, P.K., 343, 472, 608, 733, 734, 762, 765
Trickey, D., 744–746, 748, 753
Troelsen, K.B., 273
Troop-Gordon, W., 119, 192, 193, 297, 333, 340–342, 502, 607, 608
Trosbach, J., 571
Trost, K., 115
Trowell, J., 750
True, W.R., 590

Trueman, M., 190
Truglio, R., 490, 494
Trujillo, K., 768
Trull, T.J., 110, 703–705
Truman, J., 166
Truong, N.L., 166
Trzaskowski, M., 256
Trzesniewski, K.H., 168, 706, 707
Tsai, L., 677
Tschann, J., 215
Tseng, H.M., 744
Tu, S., 101, 104
Tubman, J.G., 605
Tucker, J.S., 610
Tucker-Drob, E.M., 250
Tueller, S., 110
Turgeon, L., 505
Turkewitz, R., 130
Turkheimer, E., 196, 250, 332
Turnbull, A.V., 154
Turner, H.A., 210–211
Tutkun, H., 765
Tuvblad, C., 531
Tuzun, U., 765
Twenge, J.M., 90, 228, 493
Tylenda, B., 665–679
Tyson, D.F., 177
Tyson, S., 762
Tzavidis, N., 210

U
Uchiyama, M., 414
Udry, J.R., 338
Uher, R., 46, 48, 52, 53, 256, 271
Uhrlass, D.J., 168, 503
Underwood, K., 190
Underwood, L., 289
Underwood, M.K., 198
Unis, A.S., 17
Urban, R., 118–119
Urberg, K.A., 611
Ursini, G., 276
Usher, B.A., 154, 291
Ustun, T.B., 229
Utz, R.L., 94

V
Vaglum, P., 535
Vaidya, C.J., 437
Vaillancourt, T., 166
Vaillant, G.E., 127, 132
Valavi, E., 641
Valdez, C.R., 128
Valentine, J.C., 131
Valentine, J.D., 747
Valentiner, D., 505
Valentino, K., 729, 731, 747
Valera, E.M., 436

Valois, R., 118
van Acker, R., 233
van Aken, M.A.G., 146, 167, 234
van Baal, G.C.M., 593, 627
van Beijsterveldt, C.E.M., 494, 695
van Beijsterveldt, T.C.E.M., 72
van Berckelaer-Onnes, I.A., 689
Van Berkel, C., 289
van Bokhoven, I., 473
Van Cauter, E., 413
Van de Water, J., 103
van den Berg, M.P., 251
van den Brink, W., 110
Van den Dries, L., 363
Van den Norortgate, W., 713
van den Oord, E.J.C.G., 72, 110
van der Ende, J., 72, 251, 338, 384, 490
Van der hart, O., 763
van der Kolk, B.A., 752, 753
van der Meere, J., 437
van der Valk, J.C., 72
Van der Vorst, H., 196
van Dulmen, M.H.M., 114, 291, 381, 592, 731
Van eerdewegh, P., 583
van Engeland, H., 472, 532
Van Erdeghem, S., 639
van Ewijk, H., 436
van Goozen, S.H.M., 472, 473, 532, 698
van Hasselt, V., 674
Van Hoeck, K., 637, 639
Van Hoecke, E., 639
van Hooff, A.J.L., 521, 522
Van Horn, P., 769
van Hulle, C.A., 251, 493
van IJzendoorn, H.W., 187
van IJzendoorn, M.H., 38, 48, 54, 155, 248, 252, 255,
      257, 270–272, 275, 296, 322, 357–359, 361, 363,
      366, 371, 374, 381, 552, 727
Van, I.M.H., 297
van Leeuwen, K.G., 499, 551, 712, 713
van Lier, P.A., 196, 235
van Lieshout, C.F.M., 146, 187
van Meurs, I., 72
Van Noppen, B., 568
van Os, J., 56
van Rossum, I., 472
Van Ryzin, M.J., 131, 298, 378, 459, 461
Van Vlierberghe, L., 551
Van Zalk, M.H.W., 234
Van Zalk, N., 234
Vande Walle, J., 639
Vandell, D.L., 186
Vander Stoep, A., 501
Vanderbilt, D.L., 389–402
Vanderbilt-Adriance, E., 127, 129, 134
Vanderburg, D.G., 751
Vanderburgh, R., 692
VanderLaan, D.P., 689, 696, 697
Vanderwert, R.E., 383
Vanmeenen, K., 728

Vannucci, R.C., 669
Vargo, B., 17
Varlinskaya, E.I., 608
Vartanian, L.R., 622
Vasey, M.W., 268, 323, 543–556
Vassilopoulos, S.P., 554
Vaughn, B.E., 315, 317
Vaurio, L., 434
Vazquez, D.M., 49, 154, 289–291
Veenstra, R., 500
Veenstra-VanderWeele, J., 271
Velazquez, L., 770
Velsor-Friedrich, B., 211
Venables, P.H., 710
Venter, J., 750
Verdeli, H., 131
Verhulst, F.C., 72, 210, 251, 338, 384, 490, 500
Vermeiren, R., 192
Vernberg, E.M., 191, 743, 744, 746, 747
Vernes, S., 654
Vernon-Smiley, M., 171
Véronneau, M.-H., 131, 189, 450, 461
Verrico, T., 419
Vest, A., 114
Vickerman, A., 745, 747
Victora, C.G., 397
Viding, E., 479, 707, 710
Viechtbauer, W., 708
Vietze, P.M., 397
Vigilante, D., 767
Vigod, S.N., 392
Vik, T., 395
Viken, R.J., 593
Vilain, E., 695
Villegas, L., 392
Viner, R.M., 623
Visscher, P.M., 26
Vitaro, F., 114, 192, 457, 472, 473, 478, 500, 505
Vivian, D., 636
Vogel, J., 747
Vogel-Farley, V., 657
Vogt, D.S., 748
Vohr, B.R., 391, 394
Vohs, K.D., 135
Volkmar, F.R., 268, 362, 653, 689
Volkow, N.D., 532, 594
Vollebergh, W.A., 251
Vollrath, M., 746
von Eye, A., 110, 114
von Gontard, A., 634, 636–639, 641
von Soest, T., 118
von Stauffenberg, C, 431
Vondra, J.I., 476, 729
Voracek, M., 528
Vorria, P., 255
Voss, H., 609
Vostanis, P., 743
Vreeman, R.C., 176
Vrieze, S.I., 590
Vyas, A., 382
Vygotsky, L.S., 225, 226

W
Wachs, T.D., 311, 315
Wade, T.M., 624
Wadsworth, K.N., 610
Wadsworth, M.E., 209, 501
Wager, T.D., 268
Wagner, A., 522
Wagner, C., 215
Wagner, E.F., 605
Wagner, J.B., 657
Wagner, K.D., 165, 493
Wahler, R.G., 452
Wakefield, A.J., 654
Wakefield, J., 57
Wakschlag, L.S., 476
Walberg, H.J., 163
Waldam, I.D., 532
Waldman, I.D., 110, 111, 251, 467, 490, 710
Walker, A., 492
Walker, C.E., 643
Walker, E.F., 154
Walker, J.L., 745
Wall, M., 603
Wall, S., 150, 315, 358
Wallace, J.F., 315, 319, 322
Wallace, J.M. Jr., 605
Wallace, L.E., 503
Wallen, K., 695
Wallenstein, S., 528
Waller, E.M., 194
Waller, N.G., 110, 490
Wallien, M.S.C., 685, 688–689, 691, 695, 697
Wallin, L., 392
Wallis, K.E., 631–346
Walls, T., 119
Walsemann, K., 215
Walsh, B.T., 622
Walsh, B.W., 536
Walsh, C.A., 669
Walsh, D.I., 135
Walsh, F., 130
Walsh, K., 677
Walter, H.J., 171
Walters, A.S., 419, 669, 674
Walters, E.E., 492
Walton, G.M., 176
Walton, K.E., 110, 708
Wan, M.W., 394
Wang, C., 725
Wang, J., 191, 252
Wang, L., 232, 235
Wang, M.C., 163
Wang, T., 393
Wang, Y., 320, 399
Wang, Z., 235
Wångby, M., 188
Wanner, B., 500
Ward, C.S., 735
Wardrop, J.L., 193
Ware, J., 114
Wareham, N.J., 252

Wargo, J.B., 188
Warren, K., 602
Warren, M.P., 209, 332, 333, 336, 338, 341
Warren, S., 359
Warzak, W.J., 639
Wasserman, D., 55
Wasserman, J., 55
Wasserstein, S.B., 194, 745
Watanabe, H.K., 17
Waterhouse, L., 173
Waters, A.M., 553, 563
Waters, E., 150, 315, 357, 358
Waters, F.S., 763, 769, 770
Waters, F.W., 771
Waters, T.L., 569, 573, 574
Watson, D.C., 499, 550, 706
Wayland, K.K., 188
Waysman, M., 748
Weaver, D.R., 410
Weaver, I.C.G., 252, 272, 549
Webb, C.A., 209
Weber, J., 399
Webster, S.E., 215
Webster-Stratton, C., 257, 454, 480, 538
Weeland, J., 48, 49
Weems, C.F., 554, 555, 749, 750
Weenink, D., 231
Weersing V.R., 554
Wehry, A.M., 278
Weichold, K., 335–337, 343
Weigel, C., 745
Weil, M.H., 391
Weile, B., 401
Weinberg, C., 93
Weinberger, D.R., 46, 53, 56, 265, 272
Weinfield, N.S., 762
Weinraub, M., 552
Weinstock, M., 503
Weir, J.M., 498, 499
Weisenberg, M., 748
Weisner, T.S., 38
Weiss, B., 225, 492
Weiss, G., 432
Weissberg, R.P., 163, 172
Weissman, L., 643, 644, 646
Weissman, M.M., 491, 493
Weist, M., 171
Weisz, J.R., 145, 225, 230, 501, 551
Weitzman, E.D., 415
Weksberg, R., 277
Welch, S.L., 623
Welch, S.S., 535
Weller, J., 750
Welles-Nystrom, B., 230
Wellman, H.M., 431, 452
Wells, A.M., 172
Wells, K.C., 480
Wells, T., 194
Welsh, J.D., 154
Weng, S.J., 268, 269, 277
Werner, E.E., 125, 126, 128, 129, 296, 745

Werner, H., 605
Werry, J.S., 678
Wertlieb, D., 745
Wessels, H., 711
West, P.D., 394
West, S.G., 114, 119, 500, 502
Westen, D., 704, 706, 712
Westenberg, P.M., 554
Wethington, E., 147, 295
Wethington, H.R., 751
Wetter, E.K., 212, 320, 499
Wewerka, S.S., 298, 331, 333, 384
Wexler, L.M., 528
Weyant, L.L., 432, 433
Whang, S.-M., 230
Wheelwright, S., 268, 689
Whitaker, A.H., 395, 563
Whitaker, J.S., 163
Whitaker, R.C., 393
White, B.A., 228
White, C.N., 710
White, H.R., 115, 471, 607, 731
White, J., 762
White, L.K., 555
Whitehand, C., 190
Whitehead, C., 706
Whiteside, S.P., 546, 548, 556, 572
Whiting, B.B., 228
Whiting, J.W.M., 631, 632
Whitlock, J.L., 536
Whitmore, K., 668
Whittle, S., 297
Wichers, M.C., 246
Wichstrom, L., 336, 338, 339, 345, 535, 562
Widaman, K.F., 707
Widiger, T.A., 110, 703–705, 711–713
Widom, C.S., 54, 709, 731
Widom, D.S., 732
Widow, R.K., 529
Wieland, S., 763, 770, 771
Wiens, M, 288
Wiers, C.E., 272, 276
Wiers, R.W., 594
Wiersema, R., 437
Wigal, T., 440
Wigfield, A., 168
Wigg, K., 496
Wiggins, J.L., 269, 273
Wiik, K.L., 255, 374, 381
Wilbur, M.B., 397
Wild, J., 688
Wilkerson, S.B., 172
Wilkinson-Ryan, T., 706
Willcutt, E.G., 427–429, 431
Wille, N., 74
Willems, P., 611
Willert, A., 132
Willett, J., 112
Williams, D.T., 770
Williams, J.M., 129, 336, 339, 340, 346
Williams, L.M., 274, 744

Williams, M., 491
Williams, S.M., 91, 532
Williamson, D.E., 492, 497, 498
Willis, K., 419
Willoughby, M., 112, 115, 255
Wilson, A.C., 320, 746
Wilson, B.J., 382
Wilson, D.B., 172
Wilson, J.D., 625
Wilson, J.G., 677
Wilson, J.K., 610
Wilson, J.Q., 177
Wilson, K.S., 186
Wilson, M.N., 453, 454, 669
Wilson, S.B., 550
Wimbarti, S., 230
Windischberger, C., 279
Windle, M., 151, 155, 323, 596, 601, 608
Windsor, J., 373
Wing, L., 652
Winner, E., 707
Winslow, E.B., 476
Winsper, C., 709
Winter, C.E., 195
Winter, M.A., 38, 148, 150
Winters, A., 469
Winzelberg, A.J., 173
Wirth, R.J., 112, 119
Wise, D., 747
Wise, M., 419
Wismer Fries, A.B., 378
Witkiewitz, K., 110
Wittchen, H.-U., 545, 547
Wohlgemuth, W.K., 414
Woitaszewski, S.A., 171
Wojslawowicz, J.C., 707
Wolchik, S.A., 500, 502
Wolf, A.W., 410
Wolff, P.H., 764
Wolfgang, B.J., 748
Wolfson, A.R., 175
Wolke, D., 709
Wolkowitz, O.M., 294
Wolosin, S.M., 436
Wolraich, M., 440
Wong, C., 655
Wong, M.C., 229
Wong, M.Y., 252
Wong, P.T.P., 133
Wong, W.I., 696
Woo, S., 504
Wood, H., 685, 688, 689, 696
Wood, J.J., 145, 551
Wood, M.D., 611
Woods, C.M., 563
Woods, K., 706
Woodward, L.J., 491
Woolf, J., 656
Woolly, D.P., 746
Woon, F.L., 752

Worthman, C.M., 40, 333, 337, 339, 493
Wotjak, C.T., 47
Wright, C.M., 396, 397, 399, 400
Wright, P., 194
Wu, J., 119
Wu, P., 726
Wu, Y.C., 744
Wugalter, S., 111
Wyatt, J.K., 413, 416
Wynne, L.C., 249

X
Xia, M., 504
Xu, J.Q., 521
Xue, Y., 96

Y
Yagmurlu, B., 378
Yang, B., 543
Yang, H.J., 213
Yang, R., 751
Yang, Y., 95
Yao, J., 391
Yao, S., 209
Yasui, M., 456, 461
Yates, T.M., 126–128, 133–135, 731, 769
Yau, W.Y., 595
Ye, Y., 94
Yeager, C.A., 768
Yeargin-Allsopp, M., 668
Yeung, W.J., 92
Yezigi, L., 638
Yildiz-Yesiloglu, A., 498
Yoerger, K., 152, 612
Yorbik, O., 492–494, 751
Yoshida, C.K., 103
Young, B.N., 231
Young, E., 493
Young, G.C., 642
Young, J.F., 495
Young, J.K., 627
Young, R., 392
Young, S.E., 695
Youngstrom, E.A., 147, 431, 653
Young-Wolff, K.C., 258
Yu, C.Y., 74, 75
Yuan, J., 57
Yucel, K., 498
Yule, W., 744, 748, 749
Yurgelon-Todd, D., 268

Z
Zachar, P., 110
Zaglul, H., 749
Zaharia, M.D., 289
Zahn-Waxler, C., 11, 154, 230, 291, 341, 745
Zak, R.S., 418

Zakama, A., 498
Zakhari, S., 602
Zald, D.H., 266
Zalecki, C.A., 437
Zalewski, M., 290, 311, 320, 321, 532
Zalsman, G., 497
Zammit, S., 56
Zanarini, M.C., 708–710
Zappulla, C., 233, 236
Zarrett, N.R., 131, 167, 605–607, 614
Zautra, A.J., 131, 135
Zavos, H.M., 256
Zax, M., 28, 33
Zeanah, C.H., 11, 300, 359, 360, 362–366, 373, 377–379,
    381, 383, 393, 744, 749, 753
Zehr, J.L., 627
Zeisel, S.H., 397
Zeiss, A., 490
Zelazo, P.D., 173, 382, 476, 567
Zelkowitz, P., 393, 710
Zelli, A., 152
Zentner, M., 311
Zera, M., 469
Zettergren, P., 188
Zeumer, D., 57
Zhang, C., 610
Zhang, G., 236, 257
Zhang, H., 564
Zhang, J., 166
Zhang, Q., 111
Zhang, S., 110

Zhang, T.-Y., 6, 253
Zhang, Y., 654
Zhao, S., 547
Zheng, M., 531
Zhou, E.S., 216, 289
Zhou, H., 232
Zhou, M., 273
Zhou, Q., 320
Zhu, X., 209
Zigler, E., 27, 34, 126, 136, 669
Zimerman, B., 491
Zimmer-Gembeck, M.J., 563
Zimmerman, M.A., 131, 704
Zink, C.F., 56
Zink, S., 638
Zins, J.E., 163, 172
Zirbel, C.S., 169
Zito, J.M., 430
Zohar, A., 567, 573
Zoratto, F., 298
Zoroglu, S.S., 765
Zubieta, J.K., 595
Zucker, K.J., 683–698
Zucker, R.A., 583–596, 601, 606, 608, 610
Zuckerman, B., 410
Zuckerman, M., 472, 609
Zungu-Dirwayi, N., 750
Zvolensky, M.J., 543, 544, 556, 609
Zwaigenbaum, L., 656, 658
Zweig-Frank, H., 765
Zwiers, M.P., 436

Subject Index

A

AAIDD. *See* American Association on Intellectual and Developmental Disabilities (AAIDD)

A-DES. *See* Adolescent Dissociative Experiences Scale (A-DES)

ADHD. *See* Attention-deficit/hyperactivity disorder (ADHD)

Adjustment disorders, 678

Adolescence. *See also* Depression; Dissociative disorders, children and adolescents
- ADHD, 429, 431, 439
- adulthood, 703
- and adults, 660
- aggression and violence, 451, 454
- ambulatory heart rate, 291
- amygdala, 269
- antisocial behavior, 457
- attachment disruption, 709
- Australian, 212
- Axis I disorders, 704
- BMI, 734
- BN, 623
- brain development, 659
- childhood, 733
- children's peer acceptance/rejection, 189
- Chinese, 209–210, 232
- conduct disorder, 710
- cross-cultural researchers, 228
- delinquency, 156
- developmental models, 475, 476, 530
- early maturation, 337
- emotion regulation, 706
- Euro–American, 234
- fear circuitry, 550
- feminine behaviors, 691
- friendships and progressions, 460
- health-risk behaviors, 188
- 5-HTTLPR, 273, 732
- inflexibility and hostility, 156
- Latino children, 228
- longitudinal study, middle childhood and preadolescent youth, 192

- Mexican, 212
- neighborhood-level poverty and segregation, 210
- neurobiological sensitivity to stress, 334
- PD and AG, 547
- peer
  - clustering, 458
  - deviant affiliation, 189
  - electronic interactions, 197–198
  - feedback, 187
  - -perceived popularity, 190
  - socialization processes, 194, 195
- polycystic ovary syndrome, 688
- posttraumatic growth, 208
- predict psychological problems, 208
- psychopathology, 207
- PTSD (*see* Posttraumatic stress disorder (PTSD))
- puberty, 338, 346, 624
- risk and opportunity, 383–384
- self-injure, BPD, 531, 535, 536
- social augmentation hypothesis, 189
- social behaviors, 187
- sociocultural context, 683
- Southeast Asian and North American, 230
- stress, 205–207
- stress exposure, 301
- substance (*see* Substance use)
- suicide rates, 527
- treatment approach, 698
- UCLA child, 215
- USA with Latino, 209
- US school population (*see* School mental health)
- Western groups, 233
- and young adulthood suicide, 527–528

Adolescent Dissociative Experiences Scale (A-DES), 765

Adrenocorticotropic hormone (ACTH), 53

Adulthood
- behavioral issues, 675
- con artists and "scams," 675
- description, 674
- self-motivation and time management, 675

M. Lewis and K.D. Rudolph (eds.), *Handbook of Developmental Psychopathology*,
DOI 10.1007/978-1-4614-9608-3, © Springer Science+Business Media New York 2014

Affect theory, 764. *See also* Dissociative disorders,
    children and adolescents
AG. *See* Agoraphobia (AG)
Aggression. *See also* Growth, psychological construct
    animal defensive, 471–472
    antisocial behaviors, 230
    antisocial personality disorder, 710
    appetitive motivational system, 472
    behavioral issues, 675
    children's behavioral competencies, 189
    Chinese, 197, 230
    cyber-victimization, 191
    delinquency, 205, 208, 236
    destructive behaviors, 677
    DHEAS, 339, 343
    English parents, 232
    maltreatment, 729
    MAOA-L, 474
    North America, 236
    peer victimization, 190, 192
    personality disorder, 731–732
    physical, example, 115
    physiological systems, 471
    predicted trajectories, 117
    preschool children, 230
    psychiatry, 668
    RCGM *vs.* LCGM aggression trajectories, 113
    self-control and adjustment, 235–236
    sexual abuse, 729
    social and relational, 187
    socialization experiences
        family and peers, 475
        interpersonal modeling and reinforcement, 475
        language and self-regulatory control skills, 476
        peer disliking, 476
        siblings and peers, 475
        social expectations and reasoning, 476–477
    sociometric and peer-perceived popularity, 190
    stress response system, 473–474
    threat/perceived harm, 472–473
    and violence (*see* Violence)
Agoraphobia (AG), 545, 547
Alcoholism
    abuse, 583
    AUD, 583
    beginning, mid-20s, 587
    behavioral disinhibition, 588–589, 595
    biopsychosocial matrix, 584
    causal structure, 584
    classification, 585
    consumption, 583
    dependence, defined, 583
    early onset, 589
    epidemiology, 584–585
    ethanol, 584
    gene–environment correlations, 593–594
    genetic influences, 589–591
    heavy drinking, 585–586
    internalizing symptoms, childhood and AUD,
        584, 589

    late adolescence and young adulthood, 586–587
    later-onset, 586
    legal status, 587
    liability, 595
    measures, binge drinking, 587
    middle adolescence, 587–588
    motivation, 596
    NESARC, 584–586
    neurocognitive deficits, 594–595
    prevalence rates, substance use disorders,
        586f, 587f
    psychiatric disorders, 584
    psychoactive effects, nicotine, 587
Alcohol use disorder (AUD). *See* Alcoholism
American Association on Intellectual and Developmental
        Disabilities (AAIDD)
    assumptions, 666
    and MR, 665
AN. *See* Anorexia nervosa (AN)
Angelman syndrome, 46
Anorexia nervosa (AN)
    and BED, 626
    and BN, 621
    and EDNOS, 622, 623
Antisocial behavior
    childhood
        coercion theory, 454
        community-level dynamics, 454
        peer contagion, 455
        violence and aggression, adolescence, 454
    violence
        adolescence and young adulthood, 457
        coercive joining, 459, 460
        early-adolescence peer behaviors, 458
        friendship dynamics, 458–459
        gangs, involvement, 461
        puberty, 456
        randomized interventions studies, 457
        self-organization, 456, 458
        threat–submission coercion dynamic, 460
Antisocial personality disorder (ASPD)
    ADHD, 531
    aggression and criminality, 710
    and BPD, 531, 711
    conduct disorder, 710
    developmental trajectory, 710
    genetic and environmental influences, 710
    genetic polymorphism, 710–711
    social and contextual variables, 710
    temperament styles, 710
Anxiety disorders
    and ASD, 265, 266
    clinical manifestations, 556
    cognitive factors, 554–555
    depression, 173, 317–318
    depression and somatic complaints, 228–230
    description, 543
    developmental issues, 546–547
    diagnostic categories, 544
    DSM-5, 544

epidemiology, 547–548
GAD, 546
genes and gene–environment interactions, 270–271
genetics, 548–549
imaging gene–environment interactions and
        epigenetics, 274–276
imaging genetics, 273–274
individual social, 233
integrative development, 555
internalizing problems, 165, 166
learning influences, 552–553
maltreatment and psychopathology, 731
mediated effects, 318
and mood disorders, 313, 678
neurobiology, 549–550
non-fearful children, 323
panic disorder, 545
parental influences
        children's fears, 550
        direct parental influences, 551–552
        indirect parental effects, 552
prefrontal-amygdala function, 267–268
SAD, 544–545
shyness-inhibition and adjustment, 234–235
SoP, 545
SPs, 545
stress, 553–554
temperament, 550
treatment studies, 278–279
ASD. See Autism spectrum disorders (ASD)
ASPD. See Antisocial personality disorder (ASPD)
Assessment, 468–469, 708, 713, 728, 730
        Achenbach System of Empirically Based, 216
        agreed-upon protocols, 763
        amygdala, 752
        assessment tools, 765
        biomedical tests, 687–688
        cognitive and adaptive behavior, 670
        communication, sensory, motor and behavioral
                factors, 666
        and contextual factors, 291
        fMRI, 275
        genetic influences, 256
        intra/inter individual change, 208
        minor stressors, 218
        multicultural assessment, psychopathology
                Analyses of variance (ANOVAs), 75
                ASEBA instruments, 74
                ASEBA multicultural norm, soceities, 74
                case of Kristin, age 5, 78–81
                case of Robert, age 11, 81–82
                CBCL/6-18 Total Problems scores, 75–76
                CIDI, 73
                Comparative Fit Index (CFI), 75
                confirmatory factor analyses (CFAs), 74
                constructing, 76–77
                DAWBA vs. DISC, 73
                multicultural norms, 75–77
                practical applications, 77–82

root mean square error of approximation
        (RMSEA), 74
standardized diagnostic interview (SDI), 73
standardized multicultural assessment, 73–75
Strengths and Difficulties Questionnaire
        (SDQ), 74
neurobiological, 302
psychological testing, 688
psychotherapy, 750
pubertal status and timing effects, 623
systems-level stressors, 215
Attachment, 552, 658, 672
        child insecurity, 149–150
        child–parent, 251
        crux treatment, 771
        disorganized-disoriented attachments,
                359–360, 764
        gene–environment studies, 251
        genetic influence, 251
        genotype–environment interactions, 255
        5-HTTLPR gene, 255
        insecure, 14 (see also Growth, psychological
                construct)
        parent–child relationship, 707
        parent–child security, 155
        prematurity
                maternal postnatal depression, 394
                parent–child relationships, 393
                preterm infants, 393
        psychopathology, 360–361
        relationships
                bizarre behaviors, 727
                frightened and frightening (FR), 728
                genetic variation, 728
                parent–child relationship, 727
                stage-salient developmental task, 728
        self-control and emotion regulation skills, 709
        social and affective sequelae, 379
        theory and psychoanalysis (see Psychopathology)
        Tomkins' affect theory, 764
Attention-deficit/hyperactivity disorder (ADHD),
        68, 271, 653, 677–678
        cognitive and motivational deficits, 441
        description, 427
        development
                children, 430
                cognitive and language, 431
                follow-up studies, 431–432
                preschool period, 431
                psychopathology perspective, 430
                school age, 431
        diagnostic issues
                clinical presentation, 430
                DSM-IV, 428, 429
                follow-up, children, 429
                inattention and hyperactivity impulsivity
                        symptoms, 428
        early deprivation, 376, 377
        endophenotypes, 657

Attention-deficit/hyperactivity disorder (ADHD) (*cont.*)
   epidemiology, 432–433
   etiological considerations, 427
   etiological models
      developmental psychopathology, 437–439
      environmental influences and gene–environment,
         433–435
      neurobiological mediators (*see* Neurobiological
         mediators, ADHD)
   externalizing behavior disorders, 531
   hyperactive and impulsive behaviors, 468
   multimodal treatment, 533
   normative peers, children, 193
   ODD, CD and ASPD, 532
   treatment
      behavioral interventions, 439
      developmental psychopathology, 441
      evidence-based psychosocial interventions, 440
      FDA, 439
      limitations, 440–441
      medication, 439–440
Autism spectrum disorders (ASD),
      313, 670, 672, 689, 690
   anxiety disorders (*see* Anxiety disorders)
   behavioral interventions, 661
   characterization, 265
   cognition and observable behavioral symptoms, 652
   complex disorder, 652
   Dawson's developmental model, 660
   disturbances in social behavior (Kanner and
      Asperger), 651–652
   DSM 5, 653
   DSM IV criteria, 652–653
   emotional regulation, 660
   environmental interactions, 271
   epigenetics, 277
   excitatory and inhibitory, 652
   genes and gene–environment interactions,
      271–272
   genetic studies (*see* Genetic(s))
   high-risk infants, 660
   5-HTTLPR, 271
   identification and treatment, 655
   imaging genetics, 276–277
   infants
      Dawson's model, 655, 657
      diffusion tensor imaging, 656
      endophenotypes, 656–657
      ERP, 656
      protective factors, 657
      risk, 656
      temperamental characteristics, 656
      vocalization and nonverbal communication, 656
   neurodevelopmental disorder, 651
   nongenetic factors, 654–655
   Parent–child interactions, 661
   PDD-NOS, 651
   prefrontal-amygdala function, 268–269
   psychoanalytic explanations, 652

   risk process and protective factors, 661
      (*see also* Risk)
   toddler years, infants
      adulthood, 660
      behavioral developmental trajectory, 657
      brain structure and function, 659
      canonical babbling, 658
      caregivers, children, 659
      comorbid intellectual disability, 658
      deficits, 657
      empathy and emotions, 658
      full-blown onset disorder, 659
      gestural communication, 658–659
      interpret and predict behavior, mental states, 658
      neurodevelopmental disorders, 658
      parental behavior, 659
      parent-based interventions, 659
      predictor, motor skills and social deficits, 660
      "regression," 657
      social communication symptoms, 659
      social impairments, 657
   treatment studies, 279
Avon Longitudinal Study of Parents and Children
      (ALSPAC), 56

B
BASC. *See* Behavior Assessment System for Children
      (BASC)
BED. *See* Binge eating disorder (BED)
Behavioral disinhibition, 588–589, 595
Behavioral genetics, 194, 196, 654
   applications, psychopathology and treatment,
      256–257
   description, 245
   genetic influence and hypotheses
      academic and social competence, young children,
         251–252
      ACE tripartite analytic model, 248
      developmental phenotypes, 251
      ENCODE project, 253
      epigenetic research, 252
      gene expression, 252
      genotype–environment correlations, 249
      heritability, 247
      monozygotic (MZ) and dizygotic (DZ), 246
      multilevel modeling, 252
      mutations, 253
      natural experiments, 246
      nature-nurture debate, 253
      nongenetic sources, 251
      parental divorce, 250
      parent-child relationships, 249
      pleiotropy, 251
      7-repeat DRD4 allele, 252
      shared and non-shared environment, 248
      sizable gene-gene interactions, 246
      sources, 247
      substantial change, 250

individual's genetic makeup, 258
and molecular genetic approaches, 245
OCD, 565
and psychopathology, 253–255
serotonergic neurons project, 533
serotonin transporter gene, 258
timing and programming, 255–256
trait impulsivity, 531, 532
Behavior Assessment System for Children (BASC), 71
BEIP. *See* Bucharest Early Intervention Project (BEIP)
Binge eating, 626
Binge eating disorder (BED), 626
Biobehavioral characteristics, 35. *See also*
        Regulation model
Biological factors
    BPD and BPD-related behaviors, 709
    CD development, 471
    nongenetic biological factors, 695
    puberty, 625
    stress, 209
Biological sensitivity
    allostatic load processes, 295
    amygdala-vmPFC resting-state connectivity, 301
    ANS and HPA axis dysregulation, 301
    autonomic nervous system regulation, 291–292
    behavioral and emotional pathologies, 301
    brain circuitry and function, 292–293
    BSCT, 296
    chronic HPA axis regulation, 298
    contextual factors, 302
    contextual stress, 296–297
    cortisol arousal/reactivity, 302
    early life experience, 287–289
    epigenetic modification, 293–294
    etiologic complexities, 287
    genetic polymorphisms, 296
    HPA axis regulation, 289–291
    5HTTLPR and BDNF genotype, 297
    individual's "stress reactivity," 296
    longitudinal studies, 298
    organismic factors, 296
    physiological assessment, 298
    positive and negative aspects, environments,
        297, 299–300
    rat and nonhuman primate studies, 300–301
    sensitive and critical periods, 295–296
    spontaneous dysregulation, 301
    subserve neurobiological sensitivity, 296
    telomeres, 294–295
    U-shaped association, 297
    white and ethnic minority children, 298
BMI. *See* Body mass index (BMI)
BN. *See* Bulimia nervosa (BN)
Body mass index (BMI), 734
Borderline personality disorder (BPD), 530, 534
    adults, 709
    and ASPD, 711
    biological factors, 709
    caregiver behaviors, 709

clinical features and comorbidity, adults, 708–709
    dysregulation, 708
    harsh treatment, 709
    impulse control disorders, 709–710
    self-control and emotion regulation skills, 709
    self-regulation and social interaction, 709
BPD. *See* Borderline personality disorder (BPD)
Brain structure and function,
        333, 381, 383, 627, 656, 659
    adulthood, 295
    alcoholism, 594–595
    amygdala and hippocampus, 752
    anxiety disorders (*see* Anxiety disorders)
    ASD (*see* Autism spectrum disorders (ASD))
    and biological development, 295
    and circuitry, 292–293
    cognitive and emotional capabilities, 300
    developmental psychopathology research, 265
    fMRI findings, 319
Bucharest Early Intervention Project (BEIP),
        373, 383
Bulimia nervosa (BN)
    and AN, 621
    and EDNOS, 622, 623
    influence, 622
    pubertal timing, 623
Bullying
    depression, 166
    homophobic forms, 166
    and peer victimization, 729–730

C
Caregiver–child relationships, 128
CBCL. *See* Child Behavior Checklist (CBCL)
CBT. *See* Cognitive-behavioral therapy (CBT)
CBT-I. *See* Cognitive behavioral treatments for insomnia
        (CBT-I)
CD. *See* Conduct disorder (CD)
CFAs. *See* Confirmatory factor analyses (CFAs)
CFA tests, 71
Chicago Parenting Center (CPC), 735–736
Child Behavior Checklist (CBCL), 71
Child, environment models
    epigenetic model
        gene expression, 16
        HPA axis, 16
    goodness-of-fit model
        mismatch., 14
        non-transformational feature, 15
        positive environmental experiences, 16
        sex-role behavior, 15
    interactional model
        interactive in nature, 13
        maladaptive behavior, 13
    transformational model
        colinearity and high correlations, 14
        insecure attachment, 14
        transactional models, 14

Childhood
  ADHD, 431, 436, 439
  adolescence, 706
  adulthood, 710–711
  adult mental health, 287
  and adult SES, 294
  aggression and violence, 452–454
  aggressive behavior, 478
  antisocial behavior, 454–455
  anxiety disorders, 548, 556
  ASD symptoms, 269
  attachment, 358
  behavioral characteristic, 229
  CD, 468
  child maltreatment, 725
  cortisol elevations, 301
  depression (*see* Depression)
  developmental sequence model, 478–479
  early deprivation (*see* Early childhood)
  education classroom, 673
  enuresis and encopresis (*see* Elimination disorders)
  externalizing problems, 166
  extracurricular and community activities, 673
  fraternal birth order effect, 696
  frustration and confusion, 673–674
  5HTR2A gene, 533
  internalizing and externalizing problems, 535
  longitudinal study, 192
  maternal care, 298
  normative school transitions, 178
  peer-assessed shy-withdrawn behavior, 234
  peers earlier, 185
  psychache, 524
  rejection, 188
  school functioning and peer difficulties, 165
  self-regulation and control, 231
  sex-typed behavior, 692
  sexual and physical abuse, 761
  slow learner, 673
  social subordination, 287–288
  stress-sensitive periods, 296
  suicidal behaviors, 526
  telomere length, 294
  trauma exposure, 753
  young children, 527
Child maltreatment
  and allostatic load
    cortisol regulation, 733
    hospital-based treatment, 734
    hyper-and hypocortisolism, 733
    hypotheses, 734
    multi-domain assessment, 734
    multiple interactive physiological systems, 733
  analysis, personality clusters, 732
  attachment relationships, 727–728
  attention and arousal
    atypical emotional environment, 726
    ERP, 727
    facial expression, 727
    learning, perceptual and memory systems, 727

    negative emotions, 726
    stage-salient developmental task, 726
  cascading effects, 731
  CRHR1, 733
  definitional and epidemiological issues, 723–725
  description, 723
  ecological-transactional model, 725
  equifinality and multifinality, 726
  5-HTTLPR, 732–733
  MAOA, 732
  memory
    autobiographical memory, 731
    defensive processing, 731
    hypothesized adverse effects, 730
    PTSD and dissociation, 730
    recall task, 731
  peer relations (*see* Peer(s))
  personality disorders, 731–732
  potentiating and compensatory factors, 725
  prevention and intervention
    burden, mental illness, 736
    CPC and NFP, 735–736
    CPP, 736
    effects, 735
  psychiatric symptoms and diagnoses, 731
  resilience, 734–735 (*see also* Resilience)
  self-system process
    defensive processing, 729
    early caregiving experiences, 728
    grandiose self-representations, 729
    neutral/negative emotions, 728
    physical and sexual abuse, 729
    preschool period, 728
    school-age maltreated children, 729
  stage-salient developmental tasks, 725–726
Child–Parent Psychotherapy (CPP), 736, 769–770
Child Protective Services (CPS), 724–725
CIDI. *See* Composite International Diagnostic
      Interview (CIDI)
Classification
  AAIDD, 666
  alcoholism, 585
  ASD (*see* Autism spectrum disorders (ASD))
  bisexual/homosexual, 691
  maltreated infants, 727–728
  MCS, 725
  PDS (*see* Personality disorders (PDs))
  prematurity, 390
  social transitioners, 693
CNVs. *See* Copy number variants (CNVs)
Cognitive-behavioral therapy (CBT), 572, 573
Cognitive behavioral treatments for insomnia
      (CBT-I), 413
Cognitive sequelae
  attention problems and hyperactivity,
      376–377
  emotion perception, 378
  executive functions, 377
  general intelligence, 376
  theory of mind (ToM), 377–378

Comorbid psychopathology, ID
    abnormal movements, 677
    adjustment disorders, 678
    aggressive/destructive behaviors, 677
    anxiety and mood disorders, 678
    attention and motivational deficits, 677–678
    description, 676
    efficacy, DSM diagnoses, 676
    SIB, 676–677
Comparative Fit Index (CFI), 75
Composite International Diagnostic Interview
        (CIDI), 73
Compulsions
    definitions, 562
    disorder (see Obsessive-compulsive disorder (OCD))
    pathology and non-pathology, 563–564
Conduct disorder (CD), 51, 169, 171
    aggressive responding, 471–474
    alcohol, 588
    categorical vs. dimensional approaches, 468–469
    characteristics, 467
    developmental course, 470–471
    developmentally linked disorders, 468
    prevention and intervention
        aggression and antisocial activity, 479
        approaches, 479
        cognitive-behavioral and social-emotional skill
            training, 480
        family programs, antisocial adolescents, 480–481
        multicomponent prevention programs, 481
        parent management training, 479–480
    socialization experiences, aggression, 474–477
    transactional models
        dual-pathway models, 478
        early-onset pathway, 478
        heterogeneity, 477–478
        parallel developmental processes, 477
        psychophysiological and social risk factors, 479
        sequential developmental processes, 477–479
    vs. depression, 313
Confirmatory factor analyses (CFAs), 71, 74
Conners Rating Scales (CRS), 71
Consciousness
    attention deficit disorders, 766
    depersonalization experience, 767
    marijuana, 767
    naltrexone, 766–767
    seizure disorders, 767
    self-hypnosis, component, 767
Contextual model. See also Unified theory of
        development
    multiple environmental risks, 33
    promotive factors, 34
    social contacts, 32
    social ecologies, analysis, 32
Control disorders, 709–710
    alcohol, 584
    effortful, 319, 320
    parental behavioral, 144
Copy number variants (CNVs), 654

Corticotropin-releasing hormone receptor 1 gene
        (CRHR1), 733
CPC. See Chicago Parenting Center (CPC)
CPP. See Child–parent psychotherapy (CPP)
CPS. See Child Protective Services (CPS)
CRHR1. See Corticotropin-releasing hormone receptor 1
        gene (CRHR1)
CRS. See Conners Rating Scales (CRS)
Culture, 666, 725, 746–748, 753
    deny/isolate distressing feelings, 359
    safe school, 176
    self and group-oriented, 197
    students, school environments, 174
Culture, social, behavioral and psychological problems
    cross-cultural researchers, 237
    description, 225
    internalizing and externalizing behaviors
        adolescents, 234
        aggression, self-control and adjustment, 235–236
        aggressive and antisocial behaviors, 230–231
        cross-cultural researchers, 228
        depression, anxiety and somatic complaints,
            228–230
        shyness-inhibition, social anxiety and adjustment,
            234–235
        socially active groups, 234
    maladaptive development
        anthropological perspective, 225
        contextual-developmental perspective, 227
        traditional perspectives, 225–227
    parent-child interaction, 237
    peer interaction, 237
    social attitudes and children's behaviors
        parental attitudes and socialization practices,
            231–232
        peer evaluations and responses, 232–234
    social evaluation and response, 236

D
Daytime sleepiness, 415–417
Delayed sleep phase syndrome (DSPS), 414–415
Delinquency, 205, 208
Depersonalization/derealization disorder, 767
Depression, 30, 95, 191, 194, 684, 696, 708, 713, 770
    ADHD, 677–678
    adolescence, 384
    adolescent, 301
    "anaclitic depression," 396
    ANS and HPA axis dysregulation, 301
    anxiety, 205, 208, 211, 212
    anxiety and somatic complaints across cultures,
        228–230
    Asian group-oriented societies, 236
    AUD, 588, 589, 592
    BPD, 531
    bullying, 166
    child/adolescent, 677
    childhood sexual abuse, 744
    chronic /stressors, 506

Depression (*cont.*)
    classic MZ-DZ twin design, 248
    continuity
        childhood to adulthood, 490–491
        symptoms, syndrome and disorder, 490
    cortisol dysregulation, 734
    CRHR1, 733
    description, 489
    diathesis-stress models, 506
    early life stress, 380
    epidemiology
        comorbidity, 493–494
        MDD, 492
        The National Comorbidity Survey-Adolescent
            Supplement, 492
        sex differences, 493
    Euro–Americans, 236
    genes and neural pathways, 506–507
    genetic factors
        behavioral genetic studies, 494–495
        molecular genetics, 495–496
    42-h meditation/emotion regulation training, 173
    and hormonal changes, 338
    5-HTTLPR, 732
    inflammatory processes, 375
    internalizing problems, 165
    interpersonal relationships
        family, 504–505
        peers, 505
    maternal, 290, 393, 397
    maturation, 340, 341, 346
    modern lifespan approach, 522–523
    mood disorders, 677
    negative cognitions, 500–501
    neurobiology
        maturational changes, 499
        neuroendocrine studies, 497
        neuroimaging studies, 497–498
        pediatric depressive disorders, 498
        sleep architecture and electrophysiological
            studies, 496–497
    old-age suicide, 529
    parental, 297
    phenomenology, 491–492
    prenatal, 392
    PTSD and maternal, 393
    pubertal processes, 626
    self-regulation and coping, 501–502
    social withdrawal and isolation, 673
    stressful life events and trauma, 502–504
    temperament, 499–500
    TF-CBT, 750
    tryptophan 5-monooxygenase (TPH1) gene, 533
    vs. conduct disorder, 313
    youth in academically oriented groups, 234
Developmental cascade models, 195–196
Developmental epidemiology
    advances in the surveillance, 88
    age–period–Cohort effects
        age effects, 94
        changes in risk and protective factors, 94
        depression, 95
    antisocial behavior, developmental taxonomy, 90
    definition, 87
    disease prevention, 88–89
    disparities, health outcomes, 88
    distribution of diseases, 88
    Durham Family Initiative (DFI), 89
    epidemiological data
        publicly available datasets, advantages, 97–100
        sampling datasets, characteristics, 99–100
        service utilization, 98
        using epidemiological data, 98–104
    geographic, social, and contextual influences
        collective efficacy, 96
        Moving to Opportunity (MTO) Study, 96
        neighborhoods, 96
    infectious disease epidemiology, 88
    multilevel and mechanistic perspectives, 88
    policy-level influences
        National tracking data, 97
        NHIS, 96
        SED, 98
        Strengths and Diffculties Questionnaire, 97
        YRBSS, 96
    population-level inferences
        exposure–outcome relationships, 93
        NCS-A, 93
        PARP, 93–94
        PTSD, 93
    populations, influence on, 89–90
    psychopathology
        lesbian, gay, or bisexual (LGB), 91
        MECA, 91
        mental disorders, prevalence, 91
        NCS-A, 91
        SED, 91
        sexual orientation and psychopathology, 91
    risk and protective factors
        childhood poverty and educational attainment, 92
        duration of exposure, 92
        high IQ and positive temperament, 93
        magnitude of exposure, 93
        pre-natal maternal malnutrition, 92
        timing of exposure, 92
    study, selection
        attrition, 102
        case–control studies, 103–104
        cross-sectional studies, 102–103
        cross-sequential cohorts, 101, 102
        depressive symptoms, 102
        exposure–outcome relationships, 101
Developmental pluralism, 153
Developmental psychopathology (DP). *See also* Stressors
    attachment theory and psychoanalysis, 3
    child by environment models, 13–16
    conceptual models, 209
    construction of reality, 19–20

environment
    development and psychopathology, 41
    unified theory of development, 29–38
    unifying theory of development, 39–41
environmental model, 9–12
friendship, friendship behaviors and friend influence,
        193–195
individuals and development
    molecular genetics, 28
    schizophrenia, psychiatric diagnoses, 29
maladaptive, definition, 16–18
modeling strategies (see DP research, modeling
        strategies)
models
    abnormal development, 4
    affordance, 5
    human nature, views, 4
    operant conditioning, 5
    passive child-active/passive environment model, 5
    relational developmental systems perspective, 4
    sex-role behavior, 4, 5
pathology, definition, 27–28
peer
    status, 187–190
    victimization, 190–193
prediction and the notion of sudden change, 18–19
prior experience
    environmental influences, 12
    long-term observation, 13
putative mechanisms, 186
roots
    mental disorders and health, 26
    nature-nurture dichotomy, 27
temperament, effects, 3–4
theoretical models, etiology, 206
trait or status model, 6–9
Developmental trajectories, 185–186, 189, 198
    bisexual/homosexual sexual orientation, 691–692
    clinical interview and sexual orientation, 690
    description, 690
    feminine behaviors, 691
    gender identity and sexual orientation, 691
"Deviancy training," 131
DFI. See Dissociation-focused interventions (DFI)
Diagnosis
    ADHD
        clinical presentation, 430
        DSM-IV, 428, 429
        follow-up, children, 429
        inattention and hyperactivity impulsivity
                symptoms, 428
    avoidance/numbing symptom cluster, 749
    behavioral developmental trajectory, 657
    CD, 467, 468
    clusters, experience symptoms, 749
    dissociative amnesia, 769
    DSM, 748
    EDNOS, 622, 626
    elimination disorders, childhood, 633
    enuresis/thumb-sucking, 749

feeding disorders, young children, 400
fMRI, 272
full-blown symptoms, 656
GD
    adolescent/adult criteria, 687
    developmental trajectories, 687
    DSD, 686
    DSM-5 diagnostic criteria, 685, 686
    gender-variant behavior, 687
    GID, 686–687
    physical inter-sex condition, 687
ID
    AAIDD, assumptions, 666
    cognitive function, 667
    cultural and familial factors, 669
    definition, 667
    description, 666
    developed fetuses, 669
    developmental speech and motor milestones, 667
    education services, 667
    genetic counseling and prenatal testing, 668
    genetics and environmental factors, 668–669
    infancy/early childhood, 667–668
    IQ scores falling, 667
    neurobiological factors, 669
    neurological impairments, 668
    "organic ID" and "cultural/familiar ID," 669
    population prevalence, 668
impairment/emotional distress, 749
lack, intervention, 749
language development, 749
MDD, 495
mood and anxiety disorders, 731
OCD, 561–562
PD
    adolescence, 708
    ASPD (see Antisocial personality disorder
            (ASPD))
    BPD (see Borderline personality disorder (BPD))
    depression and suicide, 708
    dynamic processes, 708
PDD-NOS, 652–653
researchers and clinicians, 749
social affective communication, 651
Diagnostic and Statistical Manual (DSM), 68
Diagnostic and Statistical Manual of Mental Disorders,
        5th edition (DSM-5), 703
FFM, 705
hybrid dimensional-categorical system, 705
PD-TS, 705
Dialectic integration of development, psychopathology
    "bottom-up" approach, 69
    developmental framework
        ADHD, 68
        DSM and ICD, 68
    multicultural assessment, 75–81
    psychometric advances, 71–72
    quantitative assessment
        actualizing assessment, 70–71
        BASC, 71

Dialectic integration of development, psychopathology
    (*cont.*)
    confirmatory factor analytic (CFA) tests, 71
    CRS, 71
    "dimensional" diagnostic criteria, 70
    EFA methods, 71
    multi-informant assessment, 71
    psychometric advances, 70–71
    quantitative multicultural approach, 67–68
    standardized assessment, behavioral, emotional, and
        social problems, 69
    traditional cross-cultural research, 67
Diffusion tensor imaging (DTI) technique, 498
Dimensional personality symptom item pool (DIPSI),
        713
DIPSI. *See* Dimensional personality symptom item pool
        (DIPSI)
Discrete behavioral states model, 764
Disinhibited social engagement disorder, 362
Disorder of sex development (DSD)
    physical inter-sex condition, 687
    polycystic ovary syndrome, 688
Disruptive behavior disorder, 50–51, 58, 154, 156, 233,
        236, 313, 566, 668, 670, 677. *See also*
        Gene–environment interactions (GxE)
Dissociation-focused interventions (DFI), 770
Dissociative amnesia, 769
Dissociative disorders, children and adolescents
    abnormal somatic experiences, 769
    A-DES, 765
    affective awareness, 764–765
    agreed-upon protocols, 763
    arousal, affects, 764
    assessment tools, 765
    brain's adaptive system, 763
    child clinicians familiar, 763
    childhood trauma, 761
    consciousness, 766–767
    depersonalization/derealization disorder, 765
    detoxification, 765
    diagnoses, 762–763
    discrete behavioral states model, 764
    disorganized attachment, 764
    fantasy-proneness hypnotizability/interpersonal
        sensitivity, 765
    fluctuations, 768
    hallucinatory experiences
        hearing voices, 767–768
        malevolent influence, child's behavior, 768
    incipient multiple personality disorder, 761
    measurable symptom, 762
    memory lapses, 768–769
    Multidimensional Inventory of Dissociation, 765
    natural disasters, 761
    posttraumatic stress disorder, 765–766
    risk-taking behaviors, 762
    screening measures, 766
    secondary and tertiary dissociation, 763
    self-conception, 763–764

    sexual and physical abuse, 761–762
    shame-based conceptions, 764
    symptoms, 766
    Tomkins' affect theory, 764
    treatment
        ARC and effective approaches, 770
        child–parent psychotherapy, 769–770
        cognitive interventions, 770
        creative interventions, 770
        crux, 771
        DFI, 770
        diencephalon, limbic system and cortex, 770
        disabling symptoms, 769
        hyperarousal, 771
        trauma-based disorders, 769, 771
    treatment model, 763
    war trauma, 762
DP research, modeling strategies
    growth (*see* Growth, psychological construct)
    longitudinal modeling, psychopathology
        complex probability samples, 119
        design and data considerations, 119
        distal outcome, 119
        equifinality, 119
        gene–environment interactions, 119
    modeling across developmental time
        change trajectory, superordinate latent
            construct, 119
        distal outcome, 119
        equifinality, 119
        multiple-informant data, 118
    psychiatric syndromes, categorical or continuous
        Bayesian methods, 112
        DSM-IV Axis I psychiatric syndromes, 110
        measurement invariance, 111
        noninvariance, 111
        statistical power, 110
        successive comorbidity, 111
        symptom-level data, 110
DSD. *See* Disorder of sex development (DSD)
DSM-5. See Diagnostic and Statistical Manual of Mental
        Disorders, 5th edition (DSM-5)
DSM-5 and DSM-IV
    clinical and epidemiological research,
        703–704
    comorbidity, 704
    definition, 703
    multiaxial and hybrid dimensional categorical
        classification, 703
    polythetic criteria, 703
    self- and informant-reports, 704
    stable traits and acute symptoms, 703
    transient developmental disturbances and mental
        disorders, 704
DSM IV criteria
    classification systems, 653
    core symptom domains, 652
    deficits, classic autism, 652–653
    phenotypic heterogeneity, 653

DSPS. *See* Delayed sleep phase syndrome (DSPS)
DTI technique. *See* Diffusion tensor imaging (DTI) technique
Durham Family Initiative (DFI), 89

E
Early childhood
  aggression and violence
    children's noncompliance, 453
    coercion dynamics, 453
    depression, 452
    Family Check-Up (FCU), 454
    Family Process Code, 453
    Markov models, 453
    parent–child interactions, 452
  caregiver's ability, 673
  deprivation
    BEIP, 373
    cognitive sequelae, 376–378
    description, 372
    experience-dependent neural development, 373
    experience-expectant neural systems, 373
    Greenough's argument, 373
    models, 373
    neurobiological correlates, 381–383
    physical health and growth, 374–376
    psychopathology, 371–372
    social and affective sequelae, 378–381
  language development, 672
  personal mastery, 672
  self-care skills, 673
Early onset
  alcoholism, 589
  OCD, 565
Eating disorders, 165, 521, 529
  BED, 626
  binge eating, 626
  biological/genetic risk, 626–627
  definitions, 621–622
  description, 621
  environmental/psychosocial influences, 626
  genes and neurobiological systems, 627
  puberty (*see* Puberty)
  symptoms, 622
  twin studies, estrogen, 626
Eating disorders not otherwise specified (EDNOS), 622, 623, 626
EDNOS. *See* Eating disorders not otherwise specified (EDNOS)
Educational resilience, 167
Elimination, 667, 668, 690, 704
  deficits, pragmatic language skills, 660
  early pubertal timing and dieting, 625, 626
Elimination disorders
  careful medical review, 642
  concomitant problems
    anxiety, 639

    attention, 638–639
    biophysical characteristics, 639–641
    breast-feeding, 640
    demographic variables, 641
    depression, 639
    genetic factors, 640
    hypercalciuria, 640–641
    school-related, disruptive and oppositional, 639
    self-esteem, attachment and prosocial skills, 638
    sleep apnea/disturbances, 640
  defecation, 632
  developmental considerations
    atypicalities, 633
    readiness, 632–633
    transient regression, 633
  diagnosis, 633, 641
  dichotomies, 634
  etiological frameworks, 631
  familial nature, 636
  fecal incontinence
    constipation, 635
    liquid stool, 635
    literature, 635
    nomenclature, 633, 634
    paradoxical constriction, sphincter, 635
    physical examination, 635
    retentive, 635
    soiling, 635
    vicious cycle, 635
  immaturity, 637
  improper diet, 637
  learning/skills deficit model, 636–637
  literature, 631, 633
  nocturnal enuresis, 637
  prevalence, 636
  psychodynamic formulation, 636
  risk factors, 638
  toilet training, 631
  treatment
    behavioral methods, 642–643
    constipation, 643–644
    cruel and barbarous methods, 642
    daytime and secondary incontinence, 643
    guidance, 645
    identification, readiness, 646
    record keeping, 644
    scheduled toilet sitting, 644–645
    secondary disorders, 645
    self-help skill, 645
    soft stool passage, 644
    soiling behavior and warm bath, 645
    systematic reinforcement, 645
    training modifications, 645
  urination (*see* Urination)
Emotional/behavioral problems
  educational resilience, 167
  psychological self-system processes, 167
  students with long-term academic, 178

Emotional disorders, 676
Emotion regulation, 210, 217, 531, 535, 536, 706
    adolescence and early adulthood, 706
    automatic and voluntary, 266
    coercive and conflictual relationships, 711
    cross-cultural difference, 229
    EEG asymmetry, 735
    internalizing problems, 227
    maltreated children, 726
    potential child-related protective processes, 660
    serotonin transporter and insecure attachment, 255
Enuresis and encopresis. See Elimination disorders
Environmental model
    abused children, 11–12
    active organism model, 10
    change as function, 11
    developmental process, 10
    environmental forces., types, 10
    environments, definition, 9
    maladaptive behavior development, 11
    peer relationships, 12
    positive and negative environment, 11
Environmental Risk (E-Risk), 93
Environmental Risk (E-Risk) Longitudinal Twin
        Study, 93
Environmental stressors, 496, 537
    AUD, 591–593
    5-HTTLPR, 274
    Val/Val alleles, 276
Epidemiology. See also Developmental epidemiology;
        Gender dysphoria (GD)
    ADHD, 432–433
    alcoholism, 584–585
    anxiety disorders
        comorbidity, 548
        continuity across age, 548
        GAD, 547
        PD and AG, 547
        SAD, 547
        SoP, 547
        SP, 547
    childhood sexual abuse, 743
    child maltreatment
        CPS, 724–725
        MCS, 724
        medical diagnosis, 723–724
        neglect and emotional, 724
        physical and sexual abuse, 724
        Prevent Child Abuse America, 725
    demographic factors, 654–655
    depression
        comorbidity, 493–494
        MDD, 492
        The National Comorbidity Survey—Adolescent
            Supplement, 492
        sex differences, 493
    genders and age, 744
    ID, 668
    natural disasters, 743
    prematurity, 389–390

    substance use, 601
    trauma exposure, 743, 744
Epigenetics
    ASD, 277
    behavioral genetics, 252
    child, environment models
        gene expression, 16
        HPA axis, 16
    effects, gene–environment interdependence, 58
    and gene expression, 253
    and HPA effects, 49
    imaging gene–environment interactions, 274–276
    imaging genetics, imaging gene–environment
        interactions, 272
    methylation, 312
    modifications, 288, 293–294
ERP. See Event-related brain potentials (ERP); Exposure
        and response prevention (ERP)
Event-related brain potentials (ERP), 656, 657, 727
Evolutionary model. See also Unified theory of
        development
    gene–environment interactions, 38
    punctuated equilibrium, 38
Exploratory factor analytic (EFA) methods, 71
Exposure and response prevention (ERP), 572
Externalizing disorders, 360–361

F
Failure to thrive (FTT)
    child characteristics, 398–399
    child's clinical presentation and growth
        parameters, 396
    description, 395–396
    feeding characteristics, 400–401
    interventions, 401–402
    mechanism, 396
    "organic" vs. "nonorganic," 397
    parent characteristics/risk factors, 397–398
    social context, 399–400
    2010 United Nations' surveys, 396
Family(ies), 185, 189, 194, 208, 212, 214
    Achenbach System of Empirically Based Assessment
        (ASEBA), 688
    adolescents and adults, 692
    African American community, 747
    alcoholism
        common life situations, 593
        history, AUD, 588, 591, 592
        money, 592
        obligations, 583
        prevalence, 586
    attachment insecurity, 150
    boundaries, 148–149
    cascade mechanisms, 153–154
    child/children
        adaptation, 156
        affiliative styles, 152–153
        attachment insecurity, 149–150
        defensive reactivity, 150–152

difficult temperament, 155
  mental health outcomes, 143, 154
coercion theory, 454
coercive and conflictual relationships, 711
coercive interaction patterns, 459
cultural contexts, 130
definition, 143–144
developmental pluralism, 153
development of psychopathology, 143
disadvantages, 170
downstream peripheral biology in adults, 289
Durham Family Initiative (DFI), 89
early pubertal timing and dieting, 626
ecological risk factors, 165
ecological-transactional model, 725
economic hardship, 170
emotional/behavioral problems, 170
environment models, 154
Family Check-Up (FCU), 454
family risk factors, 143–144
family systems theory, 144
G × E interactions, 130
grandmother involvement, 129–130
high-risk infants, 656
holism, 147–148
homosexual sexual orientation, 693
"indicated pharmacotherapies," 130
interdependency, 146–147
interparental relationship characteristics, 145–146
interpersonal processes, 709
maladaptive outcomes, 296
mechanisms, 149
mediational pathways, 147
mental illness, 736
OCD
  accommodation, 569–570
  cognitive development, 566–567
  diagnosis, 568–569
  environment, 568
  impact, 561
  parent and child behaviors, 568
  relationship and quality of life,
      568, 570–572
  symptom development, 568
organizational framework, graphical depiction,
    143, 144
parent–child subsystem, 144–145
positive behavior support, 457
positive parenting, 129
protective processes, 129
regulating conditions, 154–155
relationships with family members, 129
school connections, 177–178
sexual abuse, 724
sibling relationship quality, 146
social-emotional development, students,
    164, 170, 179
substance use, 610–611
summer vacation, wealthier, 172
systemic organizing parameters, 146
transactional models, 155–156

Family Check-Up (FCU), 454
Family Process Code, 453
Family stress, ID
  children and adolescents, 675–676
  siblings, 675
FFM. See Five-factor model (FFM)
Five-factor model (FFM), 705, 711, 712
FMRI. See Functional magnetic resonance imaging
    (fMRI)
Frightened and frightening (FR), 728
FTT. See Failure to thrive (FTT)
Functional magnetic resonance imaging (fMRI)
  anxiety disorders and ASD (see Autism spectrum
      disorders (ASD))
  brain
    anxiety disorders, treatment, 278–279
    ASD, treatment, 279
    pharmacological agent, 277
  developmental psychopathology
    cognitive processes, 279
    large-scale fMRI studies, 280
    longitudinal designs, 279–280
    social contexts and relationships
        characteristic, 279
  genes code, 265
  imaging genetic studies, 280
  neural activation, 267
  neuroimaging research, 267
  prefrontal amygdala cortex circuitry, 280
  studies, 498
  transactional model, 265

G
GAD. See Generalized anxiety disorder (GAD)
GD. See Gender dysphoria (GD)
Gender dysphoria (GD)
  assessment (see Assessment)
  behavior problems
    ASD, 689
    children and adolescents, 688
    clinical populations, 689
    gender-variant behavior, 690
    generic risk factors, 690
    hypothesized pathways, 690
    siblings, 689
    SRS, 689
    treatment, 690
  causal mechanisms
    male and female fetus, 694
    psychosexual differentiation, 694
    sex-dimorphic behavior, 694
    sibships, 694
  children and adolescents, 683
  clinical management
    adolescents, 697
    birth sex vs. gender identity, 698
    contra-sex hormonal therapy, 697–698
    treatment approach, 698
    well-designed comparative treatment
        approaches, 698

Gender dysphoria (GD) (*cont.*)
  cognitive-developmental factors, 697
  description, 683
  developmental trajectories, 690–692
  diagnosis (*see* Diagnosis)
  Diane's male behavior, 684
  Frank's female behavior, 684
  fraternal birth order effect, 695–696
  genetics, 695
  GID, 683
  maternal prenatal sex preference, 696
  predictors, gender identity (*see* Gender identity,
      predictors)
  prenatal sex hormones, 695
  psychosocial influences, 696
  referral rates, 684–685
  sex-dimorphic characteristics, 688
  sex-typed behavior, 688
  social reinforcement
    infancy and toddlerhood, 696
    parental reinforcement efforts, 696–697
    parent generation, 696
Gender identity disorder (GID)
  gender-variant behavior, 687
  physical inter-sex condition, 687
  sexual anatomy, 686
Gender identity, predictors
  childhood assessment, 693
  childhood, clinical evaluation and treatment, 692
  developmental malleability and plasticity, 692
  gender transition movement/subculture, 692
  gender-variant/cross-gender behavior, 692, 693
  homosexual, 694
  SES, 693
  sex difference, 693
  TAU, 692–693
Gene–environment correlations (rGE)
  active and evocative rGE, 49
  adaptive or maladaptive environment, 51
  adoption studies, 50
  heritability, 50
  parent-child relationship, 50
  passive/active/evocative rGE, 49
  peer deviance (PD) and conduct disorder (CD), 51
Gene–environment interactions (GxE)
  additive and multiplicative synergistic
      interactions, 52
  disruptive behavior, 51–52
  5-HTTLPR and forms of stress, 52
  intermediate phenotype, 53
  methodological issues, 51–52
  positive reasons, 51
  serotonin metabolites, 53
Gene–environment interdependence
  anomalies, reasons, 58
  chromosome anomalies, 58
  COMT and MAOA effects, 60
  congenital anomalies, 58
  copy-number variations (CNVs), 58
  epigenetic effects, 58

  GxE, 58–59
  5-HTTLPR GxE, 59
  MAOA gene, 59
  prenatal/postnatal effects, 59
  rGE, 58
Generalized anxiety disorder (GAD), 546, 547
Genetic(s), 206, 695
  adolescence, girls, 624
  antisocial behavior, 710
  anxiety, 548–549
  anxiety disorders, 273–274
  ASD, 276–277
  behavioral-genetics research, 196, 494–495
  biological factors, 709
  "broader autism phenotype," 654
  children's peer experiences, 196
  child's development, 669
  CNVs, 654
  disorganized attachment, 728
  environmental effects, 247–250
  environmental influences, 711
  epigenetics (*see* Epigenetics)
  estrogen, 625
  fantasy-proneness, hypnotizability/interpersonal
      sensitivity, 765
  human molecular, 302
  hypotheses, 246–247, 624
  impulsivity, 532
  influences on behavioral phenotypes, 250–253
  maltreatment and depression, 732
  molecular genetics, 495–496
  monozygotic and dizygotic twins, 653–654
  neurotransmitters/neurotrophins, 625
  OCD, 565
  ovarian hormones and sex-differention behaviors, 624
  polymorphisms, 296, 532
  prenatal testing, 668
  serotonin hypothesis, 533
  twin studies, 624–625
Genetic influences
  catechol-O-methyltransferase (COMT) effect, 46
  environments, 47
  genomic imprinting, 46
  GxE, 46
GID. *See* Gender identity disorder (GID)
Growth, psychological construct
  3 class-specific mean trajectories, 115
  complex interactions, 114
  individual trajectories, 112, 119–120
  interaction, 114
  LCGMs, 115, 116
  person-oriented research paradigm, 114
  physical aggression, example, 115
  predicted aggression trajectories, 117–118
  predicting, 114–118
  random coefficient growth modeling (RCGM), 112
  RCGM *vs.* LCGM aggression trajectories, 113–114
GxE, MAOA genotype and antisocial behavior
  animal models, 55
  hostile environment, 55

low-activity genotype animals, 55
low-MAOA-activity males, 54–55
overt antisocial behavior (ASB), 55
variable nucleotide repeat (VNTR), 54

H
Hallucinatory experiences
    hearing voices, 767–768
    malevolent influence, child's behavior, 768
Handbook of Developmental Psychopathology, 3
Hierarchical personality inventory for children (HiPIC), 712, 713
HiPIC. *See* Hierarchical personality inventory for children (HiPIC)
Holism, 147–148
HOME Scale, 9
Hyperarousal, 771
Hypercalciuria, 640–641

I
ID. *See* Intellectual disability (ID)
ID, diagnosis
    AAIDD, assumptions, 666
    clinical profile
        cognitive function, 667
        definition, 667
        developmental speech and motor milestones, 667
        education services, 667
        infancy/early childhood, 667–668
        IQ scores falling, 667
        neurological impairments, 668
    cultural and familial factors, 669
    description, 666
    developed fetuses, 669
    genetic counseling and prenatal testing, 668
    genetics and environmental factors, 668–669
    neurobiological factors, 669
    "organic ID" and "cultural/familiar ID," 669
    population prevalence, 668
Infancy, 672
Infant–parent patterns
    caregiving, 359
    cultural influences, 359
    disorganization, 359–360
    early childhood, 358
    and infant temperament, 358–360
    prevalence rates, 359
    strange situation, 358
Insomnia
    bedtime worry, rumination and vigilance, 414
    CBT-I, 413
    daytime coping, 414
    functional analysis, 413
    motivational enhancement (ME), 413
    relapse prevention, 414
    sleep and circadian education, 413
    sleep–wake window, 413
    wake up, 414
    wind down, 413–414

Intellectual disability (ID)
    AAIDD, 665
    children, handicaps, 670
    comorbid psychopathology (*see* Comorbid psychopathology, ID)
    development
        adolescence, 674
        adulthood, 674–675
        childhood, 672–673
        developmental disability, 671
        early childhood, 672–673
        infancy, 672
        skills, 672
        trajectories, 671–672
    developmental psychopathology, 666
    diagnosis (*see* Diagnosis)
    diagnostic overshadowing, 666
    evaluation
        cognitive and adaptive behavior, 670–671
        genetic disorder, 671
        neuroimaging and cytogenetic techniques, 671
        verbal and non-verbal intelligence tests, 671
    family stress (*see* Family stress, ID)
    MR, 665
    physical disabilities
        blindness and hearing impairment, 669
        comorbid psychopathology, 669
        dual diagnosis, 669
        internal and external triggers, 669–670
International Classification of Diseases (ICD), WHO, 68
International Society for the Study of Trauma and Dissociation (ISST-D), 762, 771
ISST-D. *See* International Society for the Study of Trauma and Dissociation (ISST-D)

L
Lesbian, gay and bisexual (LGB), 91
Life stress, 128, 207, 215, 527, 535, 714. *See also* Resilience
    alcohol (*see* Alcoholism)
    anxiety and depression, 380
    depression, 341
    description, 293
    HPA axis regulation, 298
    5-HTTLPR genotype, 274
    model human experiences, 301
    neural processing, 382
    telomere shortening, 294

M
Major depressive disorder (MDD), 490, 492, 493, 496
Maladaptive
    construction of reality
        father–child relationship, 19
        stimulus, 19
    discrete *versus* continuous behavior
        CBCL, 17
        DSM-like classification system, 16
        yes-no classification system, 17

Maladaptive (*cont.*)
  people's perceptions, 17
  prediction and sudden change
    ability of prediction, 18
    continuity, 18
    gradualism, 18
Maltreatment, 270, 535. *See also* Child maltreatment
  children, 210
  early childhood, 449
  homicide, 746
  RAD, 364
  sexual abuse, 762
Maltreatment classification system (MCS), 724
MAOA. *See* Monoamine oxidase A (MAOA)
MCS. *See* Maltreatment classification system (MCS)
MDD. *See* Major depressive disorder (MDD)
MECA. *See* Methods for the Epidemiology of Child and
    Adolescent Mental Disorders (MECA)
Memory
  autobiographical memory, 731
  defensive processing, 731
  hypothesized adverse effects, 730
  PTSD and dissociation, 730
  recall task, 731
Mental disorders, 704. *See also* Intellectual disability
    (ID)
Mental retardation (MR), 665, 667. *See also* Intellectual
    disability (ID)
Methodological matters
  publication bias, 57
  rule-based algorithms, 57
  serotonin transporter gene, 58
Methodology, 210, 216, 218, 724
  androphilia, 691
  behavioral interventions, 657
  genetic and nongenetic factors, 654
Methods for the Epidemiology of Child and Adolescent
    Mental Disorders (MECA), 91
Monoamine oxidase A (MAOA), 54, 732
Motivation
  adolescent substance use, 609–610
  alcoholism, 596
  appetitive motivational system, 472
  attention and motivational deficits, 677–678
  cognitive and motivational deficits, 441
  motivational enhancement (ME), 413
  self-motivation and time management, 675
Motivational enhancement (ME), 413
Moving to Opportunity (MTO), 96
MR. *See* Mental retardation (MR)
Multidimensional Inventory of Dissociation, 765
Multi-informant assessment, 71

N
Narcolepsy, 419–420
National Child Traumatic Stress Network (NCTSN), 769
National Comorbidity Survey Replication (NCS-R), 93
National Epidemiologic Survey on Alcohol and Related
    Conditions (NESARC), 584–586

National Health Interview Survey (NHIS), 96
Nature, 185, 197, 198, 211, 215, 675, 677, 696, 714, 745,
    746, 770
  ASD, 268
  human abilities, 169–170
  nature-nurture debate, 253
  puberty's effects, 331–333, 621
  siblings, 146
  subsystem relationships, 144
  tissue-specific, 252
Nature-nurture integration
  DP perspective, 45
  gene–environment correlations (rGE), 49–51
  gene–environment interactions (GxE), 51–53
  gene–environment interdependence, 58–60
  genetic influences, 46–47
  GxE, MAOA genotype and antisocial behavior,
    54–55
  methodological matters, 57–58
    publication bias, 57
    rule-based algorithms, 57
    serotonin transporter gene, 58
  nongenetic influences, 47–49
  rodent studies
    5-HTT gene, functional variation, 53
    plasticity genes, 54
  schizophrenia and other outcomes, 56–57
NCS-A. *See* US National Comorbidity Survey
    Replication Adolescent Supplement (NCS-A)
NCTSN. *See* National Child Traumatic Stress Network
    (NCTSN)
NESARC. *See* National Epidemiologic Survey on
    Alcohol and Related Conditions (NESARC)
Neurobiological mediators, ADHD
  brain chemistry, 436
  brain function, 436–437
  brain structure, 436
  mediational model, 435
Neurobiology
  of addiction, 594–595
  anxiety, 549–550
  depression, children and adolescents, 496–499
  genetics and, 566–567
  pediatric depression, 499
Neuroendocrine studies, 497
Neuroimaging studies
  amygdala, 498
  DTI technique, 498
  fMRI studies, 498
  hippocampus, 497–498
  sMRI studies, 497
Neuroscience
  burgeoning, 302
  developmental psychopathology, 265
  human molecular genetics, 302
  substance use, 608–609
Nongenetic influences
  active and evocative gene–environment, 48
  environmental influences, 48
  environment, objective and effective, 48

epigenetics and HPA effects, 49
experience, 48
longitudinal twin and parent design (LTAP), 48
maternal and paternal age effects, 47
prenatal/postnatal influences, 47
psychosocial influences, 48
Non-rapid eye movement (NREM), 409, 410
NREM. *See* Non-rapid eye movement (NREM)
Nurse Family Partnership (NFP), 735–736

O
"Objectively threatening," 218
Obsessive-compulsive disorder (OCD), 677, 678
    childhood and adolescence, 561
    cognitive developmental, 566–567
    comorbidity, 566
    data, 562
    definition, 561–562
    description, 561
    developmental model, 566–567
    early-onset, 565
    familial (*see* Family(ies))
    genetics, 565
    neuropsychological deficits, 565–566
    pathology and non-pathology, 563–564
    phenomenology, 564
    prevalence, 562
    symptoms and behaviors, 561, 562
    and temperament, 567–568
    treatment
        CBT, 572, 573
        ERP, 572
        family interventions, 572–573
        modalities, 573
        pharmacological, 572
        pre-and posttreatment measures, 573
        psychotherapies, 572
        symptom severity, 573
OCD. *See* Obsessive-compulsive disorder (OCD)
ODD. *See* Oppositional defiant disorder (ODD)
Oppositional defiant disorder (ODD), 468

P
Panic disorder (PD), 545, 547
Parasomnias, 417–418
Parenting, 189, 195, 210, 212, 217
    alcohol, 588, 591–593
    authoritarian styles, 145
    behavioral inhibition X challenging *vs.* harsh, 321
    behaviors and child psychopathology, 144–145
    BPD, 710
    broader autism phenotype, 654
    child adjustment, 707
    and child interactions, 726
    and child maladjustment, 156
    children's developing capacities, 144
    cross-gender identification, 692
    dance and martial arts classes, 673

direct parental influences, 551–552
early childhood, 452
education services, 667
emotional reaction, 451
environmental influences, 272, 569
frightened and frightening (FR), 728
indirect parental effects, 552
infant–parent patterns (*see* Infant–parent patterns)
maltreatment, early childhood, 449
management training, 479–480
NCTSN, 769
nonalcoholic, 588
parent–child interaction, 452, 453
positive, 129 (*see also* Family(ies))
power-assertive and directive, 231
prematurity, 392–393
risk/resiliency, 747
sex variation, 694
skills and frustration, 672
SRS, 689
temperament and adjustment, 316
trauma-related symptoms, 751
PARP. *See* Population attributable risk proportion (PARP)
PD. *See* Panic disorder (PD)
PDD-NOS. *See* Pervasive developmental disorder not otherwise specified (PDD-NOS)
PDDs. *See* Pervasive developmental disorders (PDDs)
PD-trait specified (PD-TS), 705
PD-TS. *See* PD-trait specified (PD-TS)
Peer(s), 208, 210, 211, 666, 673, 674. *See also* Peer relationships
    ADHD, 400, 431
    affiliations and contagion effects, 536–537
    aggressive behavior, 475
    antisocial behavior, 455
    assessed shy-withdrawn behavior, 234
    autobiographical memory, 769
    bullying and peer victimization, 729–730
    canonical babbling, 658
    cognitive and emotional processes, 730
    community-level dynamics, 454
    contagion dynamic, 451
    CRE programs, 169
    developmental pathways, 729
    deviant groups, 458
    disadvantage, 335
    disliking, 476
    evaluations and responses, 232–234
    exposure, 343
    infant rhesus monkeys, 289
    media and communication, 461
    middle childhood, 707
    networks, 475
    non-bully peers, 166
    on-time-/ late-maturing, 338, 339
    opposite-sex relationships, 336
    poor emotion regulation, 730
    poorer school functioning, 165
    pubertal development, 622

Peer(s) (*cont.*)
  relationships, 481
  self-esteem, 707
  self-organization, 456
  SES, 292
  sexual abuse, 729
  social difficulties, 163
  social ostracism, 690
  substance use, 611–612
  transgressions, 153
  victimization and aggression, 297
  victimization and coercion, 729
  youths' maturation, 333
Peer-assisted learning, 131
Peer deviance (PD), 51, 323
Peer relationships
  adaptive and maladaptive trajectories, 198
  adolescent's longitudinal, 198
  biological mechanisms and moderators, 196
  cascade models, 195–196
  cross-cultural considerations, 197
  delinquent/criminal activity, 185
  depression, 194
  developmental psychopathology (*See* Psychopathology)
  developmental trajectories, 185–186
  electronic peer interactions, 197–198
  elucidate mechanisms, 198
  environmental systems, 185
  externalizing symptoms, 188–189
  maladjustment, 191
  moderator, 194
  normative peer experiences, 186–187
  peer processes and children's symptoms, 195
  peer-rejected youth, 187, 188
  peer socialization, 194
  poor, 12
  psychopathology (*See* Developmental psychopathology (DP))
  race and ethnicity, 196–197
  social network analysis, 196
  substantial attention, 186
Periodic limb movement disorder (PLMD), 418–419
Personality disorders (PDs)
  child and adolescent personality traits
    adaptive and maladaptive personality, 712
    bottom-up approach, 712–713
    and DIPSI, 713
    emotional reactivity and regulation, 711
    and FFM, 711, 712
    and HiPIC, 712
    rank-order stability, 711–712
    temperament, 711
  child temperament and adult personality, 714
  core impairments
    Axes I and II disorders, 706
    bidirectional influences, 707
    child adjustment, 707
    children's self-esteem, 706
    emotion regulation, 706–708

    empathy and intimacy, 706
    "interpersonal" domain, 706
    interpersonal relationships, empathy, 707
    preschool period, 707
    "self" domain, 705–706
    social communication, 707
  description, 703
  developmental contexts and life stress, 714
  diagnosis of PD (*see* Diagnosis)
  DSM-IV and DSM-5, 703–705
  prevention and intervention efforts, 714
Personality pathology, 731. *See also* Personality disorders (PDs)
Personal model. *See also* Unified theory of development
  comorbidity, 31
  conduct disorder, 31–32
  depression, 30
Pervasive developmental disorder not otherwise specified (PDD-NOS), 651–653
Pervasive developmental disorders (PDDs), 651, 653, 670, 689
PFC. *See* Prefrontal cortex (PFC)
PLMD. *See* Periodic limb movement disorder (PLMD)
Population attributable risk proportion (PARP), 93
Positive psychology and resilience
  childhood, resilience
    autonomy or belief in oneself, 125
    stress, 126
    vulnerability and coping patterns, 125
  differences
    adversity, 132
    developmental issues, 132
    developmental psychopathology, 132, 133
    healthy or optimal development, 133
    positive outcomes, 133
    social acceptance, 133
  optimal outcomes, 136
  research (*see* Resilience)
  similarities
    competence, 134
    "doing well," definition, 134
    evidence and self-scrutiny, 135
    mutually beneficial salutary constructs., 134
Posttraumatic stress disorder (PTSD), 93, 212, 228, 730
  broad age range, 753
  Child Behavior Checklist, 765–766
  child's intrinsic and extrinsic, 744
  diagnosis and phenomenology (*see* Diagnosis)
  efficacy, pharmacotherapy, 754
  epidemiology, 743–744
  5-HTTLPR, 270
  neurobiological correlates
    amygdala, 752
    brain structures, 752
    child's development, 752
    hippocampus, 752
    influences, 752
    neural systems, 752
    prefrontal cortex, 752
    trauma exposure, 752–753

posttrauma factors
    African American community, 747–748
    emotional distress, 748
    influential/primary source, 747
    motor vehicle accidents, 748
    parental distress, 748
poverty exacerbates, 392
pretrauma/demographic variables, 753
pretrauma factors
    characteristics, 745
    cognitive resources, 744
    definition, 744
    emotional or cognitive maturity, 745
    female gender, 745
    gender and trauma type, 745
    homicide and maltreatment, 746
    natural disaster, 745
    sexual abuse, 745
    temperament, 745–746
    trauma-related and post-event variables, 744
sleep and eating problems, 393
sleep dysregulation, 393–394
trauma-related factors
    chronic trauma exposure, 747
    hurricane, 747
    interpersonal traumas, 746
    meta-analysis, 746
    "secondary stressors," 747
    type, violence, 746–747
treatment (see Treatment, PTSD)
Prader–Willi syndrome, 46
Prefrontal cortex (PFC), 533
Prematurity
    child outcomes, 394
    classification, 390
    epidemiology, 389–390
    influence on attachment, 393–394
    medical complications, 390
    neonatal intensive care, 390–392
    parental
        functioning, 392
        response, child, 392–393
    and social-emotional development, 394–395
    vulnerable child syndrome, 394
Psychopathology, 371–372, 437–439, 441. See also
        Child maltreatment; Developmental
        psychopathology (DP); Dissociative disorders,
        children and adolescents; Gender dysphoria
        (GD); Personality disorders (PDs);
        Psychopathology
    ADHD, 411, 437–439
    adolescents and young adults, 527
    anxiety (see Anxiety disorders)
    AUD, 583–585, 587, 594, 595
    BPD, 531
    early childhood deprivation, 371–372
    externalizing disorders, 339–340, 360–361
    internalization, 337–339
    PTSD (see Posttraumatic stress disorder (PTSD))
    puberty (see Puberty)
    and social changes, 334

PTSD. See Posttraumatic stress disorder (PTSD)
Puberty, 706–707, 710
    biological changes, 333–334
    breast development, 684
    contextual-amplification effects, 341–342
    description, 331
    direct and indirect effects, 333
    early deprivation, 375
    eating disorders
        boys, 623
        genetic and biological theories (see Genetic(s))
        girls, 623
        psychosocial theories, 624
        pubertal status and timing effects, 622–623
        pubertal timing, 622
        risk factors, 622
    effects
        biological, psychological and social, 337
        psychological, 336
        social, 336–337
    empirical research, 337
    hypothalamic-pituitary-adrenocortical (HPA)
        axis, 384
    indexes, 344–346
    individual differences, 340
    integrative models, 340
    interactive effects, 333
    interpersonal risk pathways, 343
    linkages, 340, 342
    nature and course
        adrenal steroid and gonadal hormones, 332
        developmental psychopathology, 331–332
        physical changes, 333
        "social stimulus value," 332
    personal-accentuation effects, 340–341
    personal risk pathways, 342–343
    predictors vs. consequences, 347–348
    process models, 342
    psychological and social changes, 334
    psychopathology (see Psychopathology)
    resilience, 348–349
    short vs. long-term pathways, 346–347
    sleep, 174
    status, 334–336
    tempo, 336
    timing, 335

R
RAD. See Reactive attachment disorder (RAD)
Rapid eye movement (REM), 409, 410
Reactive attachment disorder (RAD)
    abandoned/orphaned children, 365–366
    description, 362
    diagnostic nosology, 362–363
    disinhibited social engagement disorder, 362
    DSM IV-R, 362
    international adoptions, 363–364
    multiple models, attachment, 365
    and post-traumatic stress disorder, 363
    psychiatric classifications, 363

Regulation model. *See also* Unified theory
      of development
  bio-logical regulators, 35
  ice-cream-cone-in-a-can model, 35
  reactivity and self-regulatory, temperament, 35
  self-and other-regulation, relations, 36
  "self"-regulation, 35
  transactions, 36–37
REM. *See* Rapid eye movement (REM)
Representational model. *See also* Unified theory
      of development
  individual well-being, 38
  meaning systems, 38
  representations, definition, 37
Research design, 655
  behavioral genetics, 245–246
  child maltreatment (*see* Child maltreatment)
  genetic influence, 246
  natural experiments, 246
Resilience, 248, 253, 255, 361. *See also* Positive
      psychology and resilience
  adversity, 126
  commonalities, 127
  community processes
    "deviancy training," 131
    mentoring effects, 131
    peer-assisted learning, 131
    positive support strategies, 130
    risk modifiers, 130
    social organization processes, neighborhood, 131
  competence, 127
  crisis intervention, 171
  description, 734–735
  educational, 166, 167
  EEG asymmetry and emotion regulation, 735
  ego resiliency, 127
  emotional/behavioral risk, 168
  family processes
    cultural contexts, 130
    G × E interactions, 130
    grandmother involvement, 129–130
    indicated pharmacotherapies, 130
    positive parenting, 129
    protective processes, 129
    relationships with family members, 129
  individual attributes
    "constitutional" factors, 132
    IQ, low and high, 131
    positive personality traits, 132
    problem-solving skills, 131
  molecular genetics, 735
  multilevel investigation, 735
  personality characteristics and self-processes, 735
  personal trait, 1278
  positive adaptation, 127
  pretrauma, trauma-related and posttrauma
      factors, 744
  puberty, 348–349
  resilient adaptation, 128
  risk modifiers

    most influential, 129
    relatively modifiable, 129
  vulnerability
    attention to process, 128
    caregiver–child relationships, 128
    multivariate regressions, 128
    person-based analyses, 128
    promotive or protective factors, 128
    and protective process, 128
    protective processes, mechanisms
      or processes, 128
    variable-and person-based analyses, 128
"Resilient adaptation," 128
Restless leg syndrome (RLS), 418–419
Risk, 206, 216
  ADHD, 430, 431, 435, 441
  adolescence, 383–384, 674
  anxiety disorders, 550, 554
  ASPD, 710
  and attachment experiences, 360–361
  BN, 623
  BPD, 709
  CD, 468, 479, 481
  child maltreatment, 725
  Dawson's model, 655
  depression and suicide, 708
  early deprivation, 376
  endophenotypes, 657
  E-Risk Longitudinal Twin Study, 96
  estrogen activation, 626
  gene–environment interaction studies, 271
  hormone's effects, 625
  5-HTT gene, 275
  5-HTTLPR, 270, 273
  hypothesized pathways, 690
  infants, 655–656
  mental disorder, 666
  modifiers
    most inufluential, 129
    relatively modifiable, 129
  movement disorders, 677
  multifinality asserts, 726
  multiple environmental, 33
  natural disasters, 743
  NIS, 724
  parent characteristics, 397–398
  parent–child dyads, 249
  pretrauma child characteristics, 745
  and protective factors
    changes, 94
    childhood poverty and educational
      attainment, 92
    duration of exposure, 92
    high IQ and positive temperament, 93
    magnitude of exposure, 93
    pre-natal maternal malnutrition, 92
    timing of exposure, 92
  psychiatric disorders, 666
  psychological adjustment and psychosocial, 249
  psychopathology (*see* Psychopathology)

psychosis, 56
PTSD, 730
puberty, 621
secondary stressors, 747
sex-specific processes, 624
siblings, 654
social context, 399
stress, 377
stressful life events, 553
stress reactivity, 473
substance use, 608–613
suicide (*see* Suicide)
YRBSS, 96
RLS. *See* Restless leg syndrome (RLS)
Rochester Longitudinal Study (RLS), 28
Rodent studies
    5-HTT gene, functional variation, 53
    plasticity genes, 54
Root mean square error of approximation
        (RMSEA), 74

S
SAD. *See* Separation anxiety disorder (SAD)
Schizophrenia
    cannabis use in adolescence, 57
    dopamine system, COMT effects, 56
    "externalizing behavior," 55
    5-HTTLPR in amygdala activation, 56
    psychosis risk, 56
    Val158Met polymorphism GxE effect, 57
    Val/Val, Val/Met, Met/Met genotype, 56
Schooling
    academic and emotional/behavioral, 168
    academic and social-emotional development,
        178–179
    adolescents' mental health, 175
    child and adolescent development, 163
    crisis intervention, 170–171
    depression, 166
    follow-up studies, 167
    governments, 170
    homophobic forms, bullying, 166
    human capital investment model, 169–170
    long-term educational costs, 169
    psychological processes
        characteristic, 167
        self-regulation, 167–168
        self-representation, 168–169
        social cognition, 169
    school-linked services, 171–172
    school-wide reform
        climate, 176–177
        community-based service learning, 178
        family–school connections, 177–178
        opportunities, 177
        physical environment, 177
        scheduling, 174–175
        teacher quality, 175

teacher–student relationships, 175–176
    transitions, 178
    social-emotional learning, 172–173 (*see also*
        Social-emotional development)
    US school population
        co-occurring patterns, 166–167
        demographic characteristics, 164
        educational characteristics, 164–165
        mental health (*see* School mental health)
        physical health problems, 165
        poverty and achievement gaps, 165
School mental health
    administrators and teachers, 170
    developmental social policy, 170
    developmental systems framework, 163
    family and emotional/behavioral problems, 170
    long-term educational costs, 169
    psychological targets, 164
    social cognitive processes, 169
    substance use, adolescence, 612–613
    US school population
        bullying, 166
        daily functioning in and out, 165
        internalizing problems, 165–166
        LGBT, 166
        violence, 166
SCN. *See* Suprachiasmatic nuclei (SCN)
SED. *See* Serious emotional disturbance (SED)
Selective serotonin reuptake inhibitors (SSRIs),
        750, 751, 754
Self-inflicted injury (SII)
    definitional considerations, 525–526
    developmental challenges, 537
    deviant peer group affiliations, 536–537
    emotion dysregulation, 534–536
    empirical foundations, 523–525
    impulsivity, 531–534
Self-injurious behavior (SIB), 676–677
Self-injury and suicide risk. *See* Suicide
Separation anxiety disorder (SAD), 544–545, 547
Serious emotional disturbance (SED), 91, 98
Serotonin transporter polymorphism (5-HTTLPR),
        732–733
SES. *See* Socioeconomic (SES)
SIB. *See* Self-injurious behavior (SIB)
SIENA. *See* Simulation Investigation for Empirical
        Network Analyses (SIENA)
SII and suicide risk, definition, 525–526. *See also*
        Suicide
Simulation Investigation for Empirical Network
        Analyses (SIENA), 196
Sleep, 640, 653, 675, 677, 734, 764, 765, 767
    behavioral interventions, 420
    circadian sleep process, 410
    disorders
        breathing, 418
        daytime sleepiness, 415–417
        narcolepsy, 419–420
        older children and adolescents, 413–415

Sleep (*cont.*)
  parasomnias, 417–418
  RLS and PLMD, 418–419
  young children, 411–412
  disturbance
    children, 410–411
    knowledge and clinical skills, 409
  fatigue, 175
  homeostatic sleep process, 410
  NREM, 409, 410
  puberty causes, 174
  REM, 409, 410
  SCN, 410
Sleep apnea/disturbances, 640
Sleep architecture and electrophysiological studies, 496–497
SMRI. *See* Structural magnetic resonance imaging (sMRI)
Social and affective sequelae
  anxiety, 380–381
  attachment, 379
  cognitive functions, 378
  indiscriminate friendliness, 379–380
  socioemotional problems, 379
Social-emotional development
  learning programs, 172–173
  noncognitive, 170
  parent involvement, 177
  school-based mental health, 164
  self-regulation (SR), 167
Social phobia (SoP), 545, 547
Social policy, 170
Social responsiveness scale (SRS), 689
Socioeconomic (SES), 693
SoP. *See* Social phobia (SoP)
SP. *See* Specific phobia (SP)
Specific phobia (SP), 545, 547
SRS. *See* Social responsiveness scale (SRS)
SSRIs. *See* Selective serotonin reuptake inhibitors (SSRIs)
Standardized diagnostic interview (SDI), 73
Statistical modeling, 119, 120, 195–196, 301
Strengths and Difficulties Questionnaire (SDQ), 74, 97
Stressors
  child and adolescent research, stress, 205–207
  conceptual model, 207
  extant findings and promote incremental research, 207–208
  gender influences, 217
  mediation findings, 210–211
  mental health, 205
  moderate stress, 217
  moderation findings, 209–210
  "objectively threatening," 218
  prospective findings, 208–209
  reciprocal and dynamic findings, 213–214
  reciprocal and dynamic relations, 218
  specificity findings, 211–213
  stressful life experiences, 218
  stress research

  checklists, 214–215
  inadequate and inconsistent measurement, 214
  interviews, 215
  measurement, 214
  mimic minor stressors, 216
  "objectively threatening," 214
  physiologically focused laboratory measurement, 215–216
  reliability and validity, 216
  taxonomic organizations based on conceptual hypotheses, 217
Structural magnetic resonance imaging (sMRI), 497–498
Substance abuse, 171, 172, 211, 677
Substance use
  alcohol and drugs, 601
  biological and physical changes, 608
  cascading flow, 613
  celebrity deaths, 603
  cognitive and neurological changes, 608–609
  continuity and discontinuity, 605–606
  developmental
    framework, 605
    transitions, 606–607
  developmental framework, 605
  difficulties, 613
  epidemiology and etiology, 601
  European, 604
  exceptions, 603
  externalizing behaviors, 610
  family, 610–611
  grade levels, 603–604
  health and social effects, 602
  high school level, 614
  identity and motivations, 609–610
  individual, 607
  initiation and escalation, 613
  integration, 614
  interactions, 605
  late 1990s, 603
  literature, 601, 607
  marijuana and alcohol, 603
  and mechanisms, 608
  monitoring, 602, 613
  multiple transitions, 614
  onset and escalation, 601, 614
  opportunities, 605
  peers, 611–612
  physiological, 607
  prevalence, 602
  2011 rates, 603
  school and work, 612–613
  sensation seeking, 609
  sociodemographic variation, 602, 604–605
  sociological theories, 608
  symptoms, 610
  United States, 604
Suicide, 191, 708
  adolescence, rates, 527
  depression, 708
  lifespan

adolescent and young adulthood, 527–528
   childhood, 527
   midlife, 528–529
   old-age, 529
  models, 529–530
  mortality rates, 521, 522
  risk factors, 529
  self-inflicted injury (SII)
    definitional considerations, 525–526
    developmental challenges, 537
    deviant peer group affiliations, 536–537
    emotion dysregulation, 534–536
    empirical foundations, 523–525
    impulsivity, 531–534
  Shneidman's assertion, 529
  statistical snapshot, 526–527
  vulnerabilities/risk factors, 530
  young adulthood, 527–528
Suprachiasmatic nuclei (SCN), 410

T

TAU. *See* Treatment-as-usual (TAU)
Temperament, 192, 251, 270, 656
  adult personality, 714
  anxiety disorders, 550
  Big 3 and Big 5 models, 312
  biological processes, 324
  characteristics, 155
  child biological functioning, 312
  depression, 499–500
  description, 311
  developmental psychopathology, 311, 313
  differential linkage model, 318–320
  direct effects, 318
  effects, 3–4
  effortful control X environment, 323
  emotional and behavioral style, 745
  emotional reactivity and regulation, 711
  externalizing and internalizing problems, 313
  high IQ and, 93
  and infant–parent attachment, 358–359
  interactions, 323–324
  measurement, 317–318
  mediated effects, 318
  mediated mechanisms, 318
  mediator models, 320
  moderated effects, 318
  negative emotionality X environment, 321–322
  nonlinear processes, 318, 320–321
  and OCD
    ideation, high school, 567–568
    normative and pathological forms, 568
    styles, parenting environments, 568
  patterns, 325
  positive emotionality X environment, 322
  prosocial and autonomous skills, 324
  reactivity and self-regulatory, 35
  risk/resiliency, 744

self-regulation abilities, 324
social process model, 314–317
transactional processes, 325
TF-CBT. *See* Trauma-focused cognitive behavioral
    therapy (TF-CBT)
Theory of mind (ToM), 377–378
Timing and programming, 255–256
Trait or status model
  attachement construct, 7
  environments, role of, 9
  invulnerability/resilience model, 7
  mother–child relationship, 7
  problems, 8–9
  schizophrenic children, 7
  stress impact, 8
Transactional models, CD
  dual-pathway models, 478
  early-onset pathway, 478
  heterogeneity, 477–478
  parallel developmental processes, 477
  psychophysiological and social risk factors, 479
  sequential developmental processes, 477–479
Trauma-based disorders, 769
Trauma-focused cognitive behavioral therapy (TF-CBT),
    750, 751, 754
Treatment-as-usual (TAU), 692–693
Treatment, PTSD
  pharmacotherapy
    randomized controlled trials, 751
    SSRI, 751
    trauma-related symptoms, 751
  psychotherapy
    randomized controlled trial, 750
    TF-CBT, 750
    trauma-focused cognitive behavioral therapy, 750

U

Unified theory of development
  biopsychological self-system, 39
  biopsychosocial ecological system, 39
  contextual model
    multiple environmental risks, 33
    promotive factors, 34
    social contacts, 32
    social ecologies, analysis, 32
  evolutionary model
    gene–environment interactions, 38
    punctuated equilibrium, 38
  personal change, context, and regulation models, 40
  personal model
    comorbidity, 31
    conduct disorder, 31–32
    depression, 30
  puberty, 40
  regulation model
    bio-logical regulators, 35
    ice-cream-cone-in-a-can model, 35
    reactivity and self-regulatory, temperament, 35

Unified theory of development (*cont.*)
    self- and other- regulation, relations, 36
    "self"-regulation, 35
    transactions, 36–37
    representational model
        individual well-being, 38
        meaning systems, 38
        representations , definition, 37
    social institutions, 40
Urination
    incontinence
        classification, 634
        continuous *vs.* intermittent, 634
        DSM-5, 634
        monosymptomatic *vs.* nonmonosymptomatic
            enuresis, 635
        nocturnal *vs.* daytime, 634–635
        nomenclature, 633, 634*f*
    physiology, 631–632
US National Comorbidity Survey Replication Adolescent
        Supplement (NCS-A), 91

V
Violence
    antisocial behavior
        adolescence and young adulthood, 457
        coercive joining, 459, 460
        early-adolescence peer behaviors, 458
        friendship dynamics, 458–459

    gangs, involvement, 461
    puberty, 456
    randomized interventions studies, 457
    self-organization, 456, 458
    threat–submission coercion dynamic, 460
    aversive social behaviors and threats, 449
    coercion and contagion dynamics, 451–452
    collateral effects, 455–456
    "developmental cascade," 450
    developmental psychopathology, 462
    early childhood
        children's noncompliance, 453
        coercion dynamics, 453
        depression, 452
        Family Check-Up (FCU), 454
        Family Process Code, 453
        Markov models, 453
        parent–child interactions, 452
    interventions, 449
    microsocial and macrosocial dynamics, 450
    predictable and preventable, 449
    social networks, 449
    technological advancements, 461

Y
Youth Risk Behavior Surveillance System (YRBSS), 96
YRBSS. *See* Youth Risk Behavior Surveillance System
        (YRBSS)